BLACK'S
MEDICAL
DICTIONARY

BLACK'S MEDICAL DICTIONARY

Edited by Gordon Macpherson, MB, BS

Thirty-eighth edition

A & C BLACK · LONDON

38th edition published by
A & C Black (Publishers) Limited
35 Bedford Row, London WC1R 4JH

ISBN 0-7136-4019-7

A CIP catalogue record for this book
is available from the British Library

In its earlier editions *Black's Medical Dictionary* was edited by:
J. D. Comrie, MD — first to seventeenth editions, 1906–42
H. A. Clegg, FRCP — eighteenth edition, 1944
W. A. R. Thomson, MD — nineteenth to thirty-fourth editions, 1948–84
C. W. H. Havard, FRCP — thirty-fifth and thirty-sixth editions, 1987 and 1990
G. Macpherson, MB, BS – thirty-seventh edition, 1992

Typeset by Ace Filmsetting Ltd, Frome
Printed and bound in Great Britain by Mackays of Chatham, Kent

CONTENTS

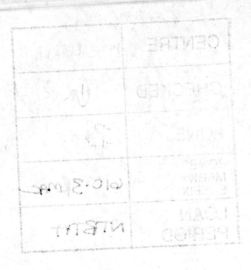

CENTRE	
CHECKED	N
PRICED	
COVER IMAGE SCREEN	6.10.3 pm
LOAN PERIOD	NIGHT

PREFACE

Black's Medical Dictionary was first published in 1906. In this, the 38th edition, over 30 specialists have contributed to updating existing and preparing new entries. The dictionary defines and explains over 5,000 terms relevant to medicine. Where appropriate, the texts provide a guide to treatments but medicine is evolving rapidly and the treatments described are based on current practice when this edition was prepared.

New drugs appear regularly and in general I have covered various groups of drugs rather than providing comprehensive lists of available drugs which is the province of formularies and pharmacopoeias. Where specific drugs are mentioned I use the generic or official name as given in the *British Pharmacopoeia*.

As well as five new appendices, many illustrations have been revised and several new ones added. I am grateful to Mrs Joanna Cameron for doing this important task so skilfully.

I am much indebted to the following experts who have helped to update the 38th edition: Dr J. I. Alexander, FRCA; Dr M. Anderson, FRCP; Mr N. Bates, BSc.; Dr M. M. Brown, MRCP; Mr C. Bulstrode, FRCS; Mr A. Campbell, BSc.; Mr K. K. Chan, FRCS; Dr G. Dalton, MRCP; Dr A. M. Denman, FRCP; Mr A. J. Dickinson, FRCS; Dr A. J. Dyson, FRCP; Dr G. Evans, MRCP; Dr M. Farrell, MRCPsych; Mr N. A. Frost, FRCS; Dr P. E. Gower, FRCP; Dr J. McGregor, MB; Dr I. McKinlay, FRCP; Dr J. M. S. Pearce, FRCP; Dr J. S. Price, FRCPsych.; Dr J. M. Shneerson, FRCP; Dr M. L. Snaith, FRCP; Dr R. Stanhope, FRCP; Mr J. H. Vickers, FRCS; Dr M. Weisz, FRCA; Mr S. J. Wood, FRCS; and Dr K. G. Wormsley, FRCP.

I owe special thanks to Dr Laurence Baker, Miss Linda Beecham, Ms Sharon Davies, Dr Stella Lowry, and Dr Alison Tonks, who have all in different ways contributed to ensuring the topicality of the 38th edition, and to Dr G. C. Cook, FRCP, who extensively revised many of the tropical medicine entries. Finally, my grateful thanks to Miss Margaret Baker, whose subeditorial skills have greatly improved the text.

GORDON MACPHERSON

A

ABDOMEN is the lower part of the trunk. Above, and separated from it by the diaphragm, lies the thorax or chest, and below lies the pelvis, generally described as a separate cavity though continuous with that of the abdomen. Behind are the spinal column and lower ribs, which come within a few inches of the iliac bones. At the sides the contained organs are protected by the iliac bones and down-sloping ribs but in front the whole extent is protected only by soft tissues. The latter consist of the skin, a varying amount of fat, three layers of broad, flat muscle, another layer of fat, and finally the smooth, thin peritoneum which lines the whole cavity. These soft tissues allow the necessary distension when food is taken into the stomach, and the various important movements of the organs associated with digestion. The shape of the abdomen varies; in children it may protrude considerably, though if this is too marked it may indicate disease. In healthy young adults it should be either slightly prominent or slightly indrawn, and should show the outline of the muscular layer, especially of the pair of muscles running vertically (recti), which are divided into four or five sections by transverse lines. In older people fat is usually deposited on and inside the abdomen.

Contents The principal contents of the abdominal cavity are the digestive organs, i.e. the stomach and intestines, and the associated glands, the liver and pancreas. The position of the stomach is above and to the left when the individual is recumbent, but may be much lower in the erect position. The liver lies above and to the right, largely under cover of the ribs, and occupying the hollow of the diaphragm.

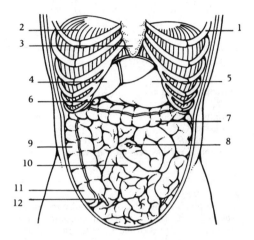

1 6th costal cartilage	7 transverse colon
2 diaphragm	8 position of umbilicus
3 xiphoid process	9 right flexure of colon
4 liver	10 small intestine
5 stomach	11 caecum
6 gall-bladder	12 appendix

Contents of abdomen in position.

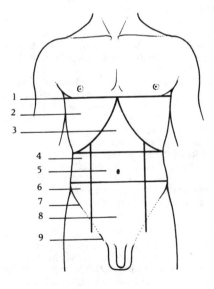

1 xiphisternal plane
2 hypochondriac region
3 epigastrium
4 right lumbar region
5 umbilical region
6 right iliac region
7 right anterior superior iliac spine
8 hypogastric region
9 inguinal region

Regions of the abdomen.

Against the back wall on either side lie the kidneys, protected by the last two ribs. From the kidneys run the ureters, or urinary ducts, down along the back wall to the bladder in the pelvis. The pancreas lies across the spine between the kidneys, and on the upper end of each kidney is a suprarenal gland. The spleen is positioned high up on the left and partly behind the stomach. The great blood vessels and nerves lie on the back wall, and the remainder of the space is taken up by the intestines or bowels (see INTESTINE). The large intestine lies in the flanks on either side in front of the kidneys, crossing below the stomach from right to left, while the small intestine hangs from the back wall in coils which fill up the spaces between the other organs. Hanging down from the stomach in front of the bowels is the omentum, or apron, containing much fat, and helping to protect the bowels. In pregnancy the uterus, or womb, as it increases in size, rises up from the pelvis into the abdomen, lifting the coils of the small intestine above it.

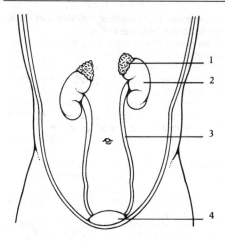

1 right adrenal gland
2 right kidney
3 right ureter
4 bladder

Position of renal system on rear wall of abdomen.

The *pelvis* is the part of the abdomen within the bony pelvis (see BONE), and contains the rectum or end part of the intestine, the bladder, and, in the male the prostate, in the female the uterus, ovaries, and Fallopian tubes.

ABDOMEN, DISEASES OF
(See under STOMACH, DISEASES OF; INTESTINE, DISEASES OF; DIARRHOEA; LIVER DISEASES; PANCREAS, DISEASES OF; GALL BLADDER, DISEASES OF; KIDNEYS, DISEASES OF; URINARY BLADDER, DISEASES OF; HERNIA; PERITONITIS; APPENDICITIS; TUMOUR.)
The abdomen contains the liver and gall bladder, stomach, appendix, small and large intestine, pancreas, kidneys and bladder, any of which may become diseased. There is a variety of different disease processes that can occur, including inflammation, ulceration, infection or tumour (see STOMACH, DISEASES OF). Abdominal disease may be of rapid onset, described as acute, or more long term when it is termed chronic. General symptoms of abdominal disease include:
PAIN This is usually ill defined but can be very unpleasant and is termed visceral pain. Pain is initially felt near the mid line of the abdomen. Generally, abdominal pain felt high up in the mid line originates from the stomach and duodenum. Pain that is felt around the umbilicus arises from the small intestine, appendix and first part of the large bowel, and low midline pain comes from the rest of the large bowel. If the diseased organ secondarily inflames or infects the lining of the abdominal wall – the peritoneum (q.v.) – peritonitis (q.v.) occurs and the pain becomes more defined and quite severe, with local tenderness over the site of the diseased organ itself. Hence the pain of appendicitis (q.v.) begins as a vague mid-line pain, and only later moves over to the right iliac fossa, when the inflamed appendix has caused localized peritonitis. Perforation (q.v.) of one of the hollow organs in the abdomen – for example, a ruptured appendix or a gastric or duodenal ulcer (see STOMACH, DISEASES OF) eroding the wall of the gut – usually causes peritonitis with resulting severe pain.
The character of the pain is also important. It may be constant, as occurs in inflammatory diseases and infections, or colicky (intermittent) as in intestinal obstruction.
SWELLING The commonest cause of abdominal swelling in women is pregnancy. In disease, swelling may be due to the accumulation of trapped intestinal contents within the bowel, the presence of free fluid (ascites) within the abdomen, or enlargement of one or more of the abdominal organs due to benign causes or tumour.
CONSTIPATION may be partial (only flatus can be passed), or complete (no faeces or flatus can be passed). It is often associated with abdominal swelling. In intestinal obstruction, the onset of symptoms is usually rapid with complete constipation and severe, colicky pain. In chronic constipation, the symptoms occur more gradually.
NAUSEA AND VOMITING may be due to irritation of the stomach, or intestinal obstruction, when it may be particularly foul and persistent. There are also important non-abdominal causes, such as in response to severe pain or motion sickness.
DIARRHOEA may indicate serious disease, especially if it is persistent or contains blood.
JAUNDICE is a yellow discoloration of the skin and eyes, and may be due to disease in the liver or bile ducts.
Diagnosis and treatment Abdominal diseases are often difficult to diagnose because of the multiplicity of the organs contained within the abdomen, their inconstant position and the vagueness of some of the symptoms. Correct diagnosis usually requires experience, often supplemented by specialized investigations. For this reason, it is wise to consult an experienced practitioner at an early stage, particularly if the symptoms are severe, persistent, recurrent, or resistant to simple remedies.

ABDUCENT NERVE is the sixth nerve rising from the brain and controls the external rectus muscle of the eye, which turns the eye outwards. It is particularly liable to be paralysed in diseases of the nervous system, thus leading to an inward squint.

ABDUCT means to move a part of the body – for example, a limb – away from the mid line.

ABLATION means the removal of any part of the body by a surgical operation.

ABORTIFACIENT is a drug which causes artificial abortion.

ABORTION is defined as the expulsion of a fetus showing no signs of life before the 28th week of pregnancy.

SPONTANEOUS ABORTION, often called miscarriage, may occur at any time before 28 weeks, although it is commonest in the first 12 weeks of pregnancy. Of all diagnosed pregnancies 15–20 per cent end in spontaneous abortion.

The upper limit in the United Kingdom definition has recently been reduced to 24 weeks' gestation to take account of the fact that viability of a fetus is possible from 24 weeks' gestation onwards.

Spontaneous abortions occurring in early pregnancy (q.v.) are thought to be particularly associated with fetal defects such as chromosomal abnormalities. They have also been attributed to a lack of progesterone secretion during the developing pregnancy, abnormalities of the shape of the uterine cavity, and maternal disorders such as diabetes mellitus, thyroid disease and problems with the immune system. An incomplete response of the maternal immune system to pregnancy seems of particular importance in women who suffer recurrent miscarriages, defined as three or more spontaneous abortions.

Factors such as increased maternal age, a high number of previous pregnancies and smoking predispose to spontaneous abortion.

Ultrasound scans (q.v.) have altered the management of abortions. These make it possible to distinguish between threatened miscarriages, where the women have experienced some vaginal bleeding, but the fetus is alive; inevitable abortion, where the neck of the womb has started to open up; incomplete abortion, where part of the fetus or placenta is retained; and complete abortions. Whereas bed rest may be useful in treating threatened abortions, an inevitable or incomplete abortion will normally require the evacuation of the uterus and a complete miscarriage should require no treatment at all.

Evacuation of the uterus involves administering a general anaesthetic, gentle dilatation of the neck of the womb (cervix), and removal of the remaining products of the pregnancy.

Maternal factors are thought to account more often for late abortions. These include an inappropriately early opening of the neck of the womb (cervical incompetence), structural abnormalities and infections of the uterus.

Ultrasound scan is important to assess the condition of the intrauterine fetus. If the fetus appears normal uterine contractions may be suppressed with drugs.

In cases of cervical incompetence, it may be possible to close the cervical canal with a suture, which is removed at 38 weeks' gestation.

THERAPEUTIC ABORTION Before this can take place, two doctors must agree that the continuation of the pregnancy would involve risk, greater than if the pregnancy were terminated, of injury to the physical or mental health of the mother or any existing child(ren). The legislation introduced in 1990 states that at the time of abortion the pregnancy should not have exceeded the 24th week.

There is no time limit on therapeutic abortion where the termination is done to save the mother's life, there is substantial risk of serious fetal handicap, or of grave permanent injury to the health of the mother.

About 175,000 terminations are performed a year on residents in England and Wales, fewer than 500 at over 20 weeks' gestation.

The mortality from therapeutic abortion is less than 1 per 100,000 women and, provided it is performed skilfully before 12 weeks of pregnancy, it is not associated with any reduction in fertility, increased rates of spontaneous abortion or preterm birth in subsequent pregnancies.

Methods of abortion Up to about 12 weeks into the pregnancy therapeutic abortion is performed by removing the contents of the uterus by suction under general anaesthetic after dilatation of the cervix.

In the future surgery may be avoided by using the drug mefepristone (RU 486), which causes abortion in about 85 per cent of cases.

Termination after 14 weeks usually requires induction of labourlike pains with PROSTAGLANDINS (q.v.).

ABO SYSTEM (see BLOOD GROUPS).

ABRASION means the rubbing off of the surface of the skin or of a mucous membrane due to some mechanical injury. Such injuries, though slight in themselves, are apt to allow entrance of dirt containing organisms and so to lead to an abscess or some severer form of inflammation.

Treatment The most effective form of treatment consists in the thorough and immediate cleansing of the wound with soap and water. An antiseptic such as 1 per cent cetrimide can then be applied, and a sterile dry dressing.

DENTAL ABRASION is a form of trauma in which the teeth are worn away. This may be by bruxism or excessive use of the toothbrush, particularly if an abrasive toothpaste is used. It usually occurs at the junction of the crown and root of the tooth and is worst on the upper left teeth in a right-handed person.

ABREACTION An emotional release caused by the recall of past unpleasant experiences. This is normally the result of psychoanalytical treatment in which psychotherapy, certain drugs, or hypnosis are used to effect the abreaction. The technique is used in the treatment of anxiety, hysteria, or other neurotic states.

ABRUPTIO PLACENTA Placental bleeding after the 24th week of pregnancy which may result in complete or partial detachment of the placenta from the wall of the womb. The woman may go into shock. The condition is sometimes associated with raised blood pressure and pre-eclampsia (q.v.).

ABSCESS is a localized collection of pus. A minute abscess is known as a pustule (see PUSTULE), a diffused production of pus is known as cellulitis or erysipelas (see ERYSIPELAS). An abscess may be acute or chronic. An acute abscess is one which develops rapidly within the course of a few days or hours. It is characterized by a definite set of symptoms.

Causes The direct cause is various bacteria. In a few cases the presence of foreign bodies, such as bullets or splinters, or contact with poisonous plants, such as poison ivy, may produce abscesses, but these foreign bodies may remain for life buried in the tissues without causing any trouble provided they are not contaminated with bacteria or other micro-organisms.

The micro-organisms most frequently found are *staphylococci*, and next to these *streptococci*, though the latter cause more virulent abscesses. Other abscess-forming organisms are *Pseudomonas pyocyanea* and *Escherichia coli*, which lives always in the bowels, and under certain conditions wanders into the surrounding tissues and produces abscesses.

The presence of micro-organisms is not sufficient to produce suppuration (see IMMUNITY; and INFECTION); *streptococci* can often be found on the skin and in the skin glands of perfectly healthy individuals. Given the proper micro-organisms in the tissues, whether they will produce abscesses or not depends upon the virulence of the organism and the individual's natural resistance.

When bacteria have gained access, for example, to a wound, they rapidly multiply, produce toxins, cause local dilatation of the blood-vessels, slowing of the blood-stream, and exudation of blood corpuscles and fluid. The leucocytes, or white corpuscles of the blood, collect around the invaded area, and destroy the latter either by actually devouring and digesting them (see PHAGOCYTOSIS), or by forming a toxin that kills them. If the body's local defence mechanisms fail to do this, the abscess will spread and may in severe cases cause generalized infection or septicaemia.

Symptoms The classic symptoms of inflammation are redness, warmth, swelling, pain and fever. When the cavity containing fluid has been formed, a sign, known as fluctuation, can be made out. The lymphatic glands in the neighbourhood may be swollen and tender in an attempt to stop the bacteria spreading to other parts of the body. Immediately the abscess is opened, or bursts, the pain disappears, the temperature falls rapidly to normal, the elasticity of the tissues around the cavity diminishes its bulk, and the healing of the small space left proceeds rapidly. If, however, the abscess discharges into an internal cavity, such as the bowel or bladder, it may heal very slowly, and the reabsorption of its poisonous products may cause general ill-health. When an abscess is deep-seated, an important sign for diagnosis is provided by examination of the blood. (See LEUCOCYTOSIS.)

Treatment Most local infections of the skin respond to antibiotics. If pus forms the abscess should be surgically opened and drained.

Abscesses can occur in any tissue in the body – for example, bones, brain, kidneys, lungs and appendix – but the principles of treatment are broadly the same: use of an antibiotic and, where appropriate, surgery.

A chronic abscess is one which takes weeks or months for its development. In some cases it is tuberculous, being caused by *Mycobacterium tuberculosis*, but other organisms such as the fungus actinomycosis or the staphyllococcus bacteria may be the cause.

ABSORPTION Uptake by the body tissues of fluids or other substances. For example, food is absorbed from the digestive tract into the blood and lymph systems. Food is absorbed mainly in the small intestine (jejunum and ileum), which is lined by multiple VILLI that increase its surface area.

ABSTRACT This is a dry powder produced by extracting the active principles from a crude drug with strong alcohol, mixing with sugar of milk, and drying. Abstracts are standardized so as to be twice the strength of the crude drug.

ACANTHOSIS NIGRICANS, is a darkly pigmented verrucous skin change, usually around the neck and axilla. It may be inherited but is most commonly acquired and is associated with adenocarcinoma, usually of the stomach (see CANCER), and certain hormonal disorders such as the polycystic ovary (q.v.), Addison's disease (q.v.) and Cushing's syndrome (q.v.).

ACARUS The group of animal parasites which includes *Sarcoptes scabiei*, the cause of the skin disease known as Itch, or Scabies. This parasite used to be known as *Acarus scabiei*. (See SCABIES.)

ACCIDENT PREVENTION IN THE HOME Every year 5,500 people are killed in accidents in British homes, a further 2.2 million need hospital treatment and 900,000 consult their GPs. Domestic accidents in England and Wales cost the health service over £300 million a year. Many of these accidents happen to children or old people, and many of them are preventable.

Children's accidents can often be predicted by their stage of development. Small babies are most at risk of being dropped or having hot drinks spilled on them. As they learn to roll, crawl, and walk they are at risk of falls. As they become more inquisitive they are prone to poisoning from medicines and household chemicals. Older children are at risk from road traffic accidents. Boys are twice as likely to have accidents as girls, and children from deprived backgrounds are at particular risk. Sensible precautions will prevent many accidents. Small babies should not be left unattended on raised surfaces, and manufacturers' instructions should be followed when using all nursery equipment.

Hot drinks should not be consumed anywhere near a baby or where a small child is running about. Heavy and dangerous objects should be moved out of children's reach, and parents should remember that children are quite capable of using toys as 'mounting blocks' to reach high shelves. All medicines and chemicals should be locked up. Bath water should be run from the cold tap first to ensure that a child does not get into a scalding running bath, and no child should be left unattended in a bath. Windows, especially on upper floors, should be fitted with locks that restrict the amount by which they can be opened, and stairgates can prevent many falls. By law all children's nightwear must be flameproof, but this does not remove the need for fireguards and care with naked flames and matches. Further information about preventing children's accidents can be obtained from the Child Accident Prevention Trust (see AP-PENDIX 2: ADDRESSES).

Old people may be frail and have impaired eyesight, hearing, and mobility that increase their risk of an accident. Special precautions, similar to those for children, may be needed for people suffering from dementia, but more general rules include ensuring adequate lighting (especially on stairwells), removing unnecessary furniture and other obstacles from main thoroughfares in the home, removing loose mats from hard floors, and wearing well-fitting shoes. Specific help like walking aids, grab rails, and bath aids may help some people.

Many aspects of home safety apply to people of all ages. Domestic fires account for three-quarters of the deaths and injuries in fires in Britain. Wiring should be checked every five years, and electrical equipment should be installed and maintained according to the manufacturers' instructions. Architectural glass is a major health hazard. Toughened glass is best as it breaks into cuboid pieces. Such safety glass should be used for domestic glazing (at least at low levels). Further information about accidents at home can be obtained from the Royal Society for the Prevention of Accidents (see APPENDIX 2: ADDRESSES).

Although many, if not all, accidents are potentially preventable, they continue to occur. Information on basic first aid can be found in APPENDIX 1: BASIC FIRST AID.

ACCOMMODATION   The process by which the refractive power of the lens of the eye is increased by constriction of the ciliary muscle, producing an increased thickness and curvature of the lens. Rays of light from an object further than 6 metres away are parallel on reaching the eye. These rays are brought to a focus on the retina mainly by the cornea. If the eye is now directed at an object closer than 6 metres away, the rays of light from this near object will be diverging by the time they reach the eye. In order to focus these diverging beams of light, the refracting power of the lens must increase. In other words the lens must accommodate.

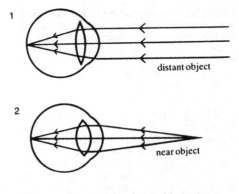

Diagram of eye in relaxed state (1) viewing a distant object and in an accommodated state; (2) with increased convexity of the lens for viewing a near object.

With age the lens loses its elasticity and thus becomes less spherical when tension in the zonule relaxes. This results in an increased long sightedness with age (*presbyopia*) requiring reading glasses for correction. (See AGEING.)

ACEBUTOLOL (see ADRENERGIC RECEPTORS).

ACE INHIBITORS (see ANGIOTENSIN-CONVERT-ING ENZYME INHIBITORS).

ACETABULUM is the cup-shaped socket on the pelvis in which rests the head of the femur or thigh-bone, the two forming the hip joint. (See HIP JOINT.)

ACETAZOLAMIDE is a drug which acts by inhibiting the enzyme carbonic anhydrase. This enzyme is of great importance in the production of acid and alkaline secretions in the body. Acetazolamide has proved of value in the treatment of glaucoma. There is some evidence that it is of value in the prevention of altitude sickness (q.v.).

ACETIC ACID is the active principle in vinegar. Three types are used in medicine: standard acetic acid used for testing urine; a glacial version used as a caustic for treating warts; dilute acid sometimes used in preparing cough medicines.

ACETOACETIC ACID is an organic acid produced by the liver when it is rapidly oxidizing fatty acids, a metabolic process which occurs, for example, during starvation. The acid produced is then converted to *acetone*, which is excreted.

ACETONE is a volatile, colourless organic compound of the *ketone* group produced by the partial oxidation of fatty acids. In some abnormal conditions, such as starvation, uncontrolled diabetes or prolonged vomiting, acetone and other ketones can accumulate in the blood (see KETONE). Acetone along with beta-hydroxybutyric and aceotacic acids may then appear in the urine, presaging developing coma.

ACETYLCHOLINE, an acetic acid ester of the organic base *choline*, is one of the substances which mediates the transmission of nerve impulses from one nerve to another, or from a nerve to the organ it acts on such as muscles. Its predominant role as a *neutotransmitter* is in the parasympathetic nervous system (q.v.), but it also plays an important part in the transmission of nerve impulses in the brain. Acetylcholine is rapidly destroyed by cholinesterase, an enzyme present in the blood. *Atropine* and *curare* stop acetylcholine acting at the muscle membranes, thus causing paralysis. *Anticholinergic* drugs such as physostigmine prolong the action of acetylcholine.

ACETYLCYSTEINE is a drug that is used in the treatment of fibrocystic disease of the pancreas (q.v.) and paracetamol poisoning (q.v.).

ACETYLSALICYLIC ACID (see ASPIRIN).

ACHALASIA is another term for spasm, but indicates not so much an active spasm of muscle as a failure to relax.

ACHALASIA OF THE CARDIA is a condition in which there is a failure to relax of the muscle fibres round the opening of the gullet, or oesophagus, into the stomach. (See OESOPHAGUS, DISEASES OF.)

ACHILLES TENDON A thick tendon that joins the calf muscles to the heel bone (calcaneus) and pulls up that bone. Named after the mythical Greek hero Achilles, who was reputedly vulnerable to his enemies only in his heel, the tendon is prone to rupture in middle-aged people playing vigorous sports such as squash or tennis.

ACHLORHYDRIA means an absence of hydrochloric acid from the stomach juice. If the condition persists after the administration of histamine, the person probably has atrophy of the stomach lining. Achlorhydria occurs in about 4 per cent of healthy people and in several conditions, including *pernicious anaemia*, carcinoma of the stomach and *gastritis*.

ACHONDROPLASIA is a form of growth retardation in which the arms and legs are abnormally short. It is a dominant hereditary condition, and the commonest form of retarded growth. It affects both sexes and, whilst many are stillborn or die soon after birth, those who survive have normal intelligence and a normal expectation of life and good health.

ACID BASE BALANCE The balance between the acid and alkaline elements present in the blood and body fluids. The normal hydrogen ion concentration of the plasma is a constant pH 7·4, and the lungs and kidneys have a crucial function in maintaining this figure. Changes in pH value will cause acidosis or alkalosis.

ACIDOSIS is a condition in which there is either (i) a production in the body of two abnormal acids – beta-hydroxybutyric and acetoacetic acids, or (ii) a diminution in the alkali reserve of the blood.
Causes The condition is usually due to faulty metabolism of fat which results in the production of beta-hydroxybutyric and acetoacetic acids. It occurs in diabetes mellitus (q.v.) when this is either untreated or inadequately treated, starvation, persistent vomiting, and delayed anaesthetic vomiting. It also occurs in the terminal stages of glomerulonephritis (see KIDNEYS, DISEASES OF) when it is due to failure of the kidneys. A milder form of it may occur in severe fevers, particularly in children. (See also ACETONE.)
Symptoms General lassitude, vomiting, thirst, restlessness, and the presence of acetone in the urine form the earliest manifestations of the condition. In diabetes a state of coma may ensue and the disease end fatally.
Treatment The underlying condition must always be treated: e.g. if the acidosis is due to diabetes mellitus (q.v.) insulin must be given. For the acidosis, alkalis should be given; e.g. bicarbonate of soda, either by mouth, or by injection if there is persistent vomiting or if the patient is unconscious. Glucose should also be given, and adequate fluids.

ACINUS is the name applied to each of the minute sacs of which secreting glands are composed, and which usually cluster round the branches of the gland-duct like grapes on their stem. (See GLANDS.)

ACNE A skin complaint common in adolescence. It arises from sebaceous glands associated with hair follicles, especially on the face, chest, and neck. There is increased sebum production, with the development of blackheads. Proliferation of bacteria in the ducts of the sebaceous glands leads to inflammation. Adolescent acne usually clears with time. Topical treatment with benzoyl peroxide (q.v.) or salicylic acid may help. Vitamin A creams and ultraviolet light are sometimes useful, and severe cases may benefit from oral antibiotics such as oxytetracycline. Very severe acne may respond to a three-month course of 13-cis-retinoic acid, but this is teratogenic and can cause liver problems. It can only be prescribed in hospital.

ACNE ROSACEA (see ROSACEA).

ACOUSTIC NEUROMA A slowly growing benign tumour in the auditory canal arising from the *Schwann* cells of the acoustic cranial nerve. The neuroma, which accounts for about 7 per cent of all tumours inside the *cranium*, may cause facial numbness, hearing loss, unsteady balance, headache, and tinnitus. It can usually be removed surgically, sometimes with microsurgical techniques that preserve the facial nerve.

ACRIFLAVINE, an aniline derivative, is an orange-red crystalline powder, readily soluble in water, with strong antiseptic powers.

ACROCYANOSIS is a condition, occurring especially in young women, in which there is persistent blueness of hands, feet, nose and ears as a result of slow circulation of blood through the small vessels of the skin.

ACRODYNIA (see ERYTHROEDEMA).

ACROMEGALY is a disorder caused by the increased secretion of growth hormone by an adenoma of the anterior pituitary gland. It results in excessive body growth of both the skeletal and the soft tissues. If it occurs in adolescence before the bony epiphyses have fused the result is gigantism. If it occurs in adult life the skeletal overgrowth is confined to the hands, feet, cranial sinuses and jaw. Most of the features are due to overgrowth of the cartilage of the nose and ear and the soft tissues which increase the thickness of the skin and lips. Viscera such as the thyroid and liver are also affected. The overgrowth of the soft tissues occurs so gradually that the patient and spouse are often unaware of the change. It is only relatives who have not seen the patient for many months or years who are aware of the striking change in physical appearance.

The local effects of the tumour commonly cause headache and, less frequently, impairment of vision, particularly of the temporal field of vision, as a result of pressure on the nerves to the eye. The tumour may damage the other pituitary cells giving rise to gonadal, thyroid or adrenocortical insufficiency. The diagnosis is confirmed by measuring the level of growth hormone in the serum and by an X-ray of the skull which usually shows enlargement of the pituitary fossa. The treatment consists of removal or irradiation of the pituitary adenoma. This may have to be done via a craniotomy if the tumour is large but can often be done by an approach through the nose and sphenoid sinus. Deep X-ray therapy to the pituitary fossa is also effective treatment but it may take several years for irradiation to achieve its maximum effect. Drugs, such as bromocriptine, which are dopamine agonists, lower growth hormone levels in acromegaly and are particularly useful as an adjunct to radiotherapy.

ACROMION is the part of the scapula, or shoulder blade, forming the tip of the shoulder and giving its squareness to the latter. It projects forward from the scapula, and, with the clavicle or collar-bone in front, forms a protecting arch of bone over the shoulder joint.

ACROPARAESTHESIA is a disorder occurring predominantly in middle-aged women in which there is numbness and tingling of the fingers.

ACTH (ADRENOCORTICOTROPIC HORMONE) is the commonly used abbreviation for corticotrophin (q.v.).

ACTINOMYCIN D is an antibiotic isolated from *Streptomyces antibioticus* and *Streptomyces chrysomallus*; it has an inhibitory action on neoplastic cells (see CYTOTOXIC).

ACTINOMYCOSIS is a chronic infectious condition caused by an anaerobic micro-organism *Actinomyces israelii* that often occurs as a *commensal* on the gums, teeth, and tonsils. Commonest in adult men, the sites most affected are the jaw, lungs, and intestine, though the disease can occur anywhere. Suppurating granulomatous tumours develop which discharge an oily, thick pus containing yellowish ('sulphur') granules. A slowly progressive condition, actinomycosis usually responds to antibiotic drugs but improvement may be slow and surgery is sometimes needed to drain infected sites. Early diagnosis is important. Treatment is with antibiotics such as penicillin and tetracyclines. The disease occurs in cattle in which it is called woody tongue.

ACUPUNCTURE is a traditional Chinese method of healing by inserting thin needles into certain areas beneath the skin and rotating them. Its rationale is that disease is a manifestation of a disturbance of Yin and Yang energy in the body, and that acupuncture brings this energy back into balance by what is described as 'the judicious stimulation or depression of the flow of energy in the various meridians'. What is still unclear to western doctors is why needling, which is the essence of acupuncture, should have the effect it is claimed to have. One theory is that the technique stimulates deep sensory nerves, promoting the production of pain-relieving endorphins (q.v.). Of its efficacy in skilled Chinese hands, however, there can be no question, and in China the technique is an alternative to anaesthesia for some operations. The technique is increasingly used in the West, by medically qualified doctors as well as other complementary medicine practitioners.

ACUTE An adjective to describe a disease of short duration that starts quickly and has severe symptons. It may also refer to a symptom, for example, severe pain. An ACUTE

ABDOMEN is a serious disorder of the abdomen requiring urgent treatment, usually surgery. ACUTE HEART FAILURE is the sudden stopping or defect in the action of the heart. ACUTE LEUKAEMIA is a rapid growth in the numbers of white blood cells which is fatal if untreated. The contrasting adjective is chronic.

ACYCLOVIR is an antiviral drug that is particularly useful in infections by herpes virus.

ADACTYLY   Absence of the digits.

ADDICTION   Ideas about dependence and addiction have changed over the past two centuries. It was not until the mid 18th century that excessive drinking, or 'inebriety' as it was then known, came to be regarded as some sort of disease. Definitions of dependence have been produced using criteria which help experimental research. The emphasis has been on the observable behaviour of the user of the addictive substance and how the addiction is learned, modified and reinforced. Some sociologists argue that consumption may be defined as abnormal (or deviant) if it exceeds the established norm of the community. The twenty-eighth report of the World Health Organization Expert Committee on Drug Dependence in 1993 defined drug dependence as 'a cluster of physiological, behavioural and cognitive phenomena of variable intensity, in which the use of a psychoactive drug (or drugs) takes on a high priority. The necessary descriptive characteristics are preoccupation with a desire to obtain and take the drug and persistent drug seeking behaviour. Determinants and the problematic consequences of drug dependence may be biological, psychological or social and usually interact.'

Drug dependence can have serious consequences for individuals, families, communities and even nations, with some countries' economies influenced by the production, export and consumption of addictive substances.

Different drugs cause different rates of dependence: tobacco is the commonest drug of addiction, heroin and cocaine cause high rates of addiction, whereas alcohol is much lower, with cannabis lower again. Smoking in the Western world reached a peak after the Second World War with almost 80 per cent of the male population smoking. The reports on the link between smoking and cancer in the early 1960s resulted in a decline that has continued to today when 26 per cent of the US population (28·1 per cent of men and 23·5 per cent of women) and in Britain 35 per cent of men and 29 per cent of women smoke cigarettes. Globally, tobacco consumption continues to grow, particularly in the developing world with multinational tobacco companies marketing their products aggressively.

Approximately 4 per cent of the population are dependent on alcohol and 2 per cent on other drugs, both legal and illegal, at any one time in Western countries. The way drugs are taken may vary from oral, nasal, inhalation or injection, and the route of use may influence the extent of reported dependence.

HIV and AIDS (q.v.) have added another dimension to the effects of dependence. Major national variations occur in the prevalence of HIV among injecting drug users. In Northern Europe around 15 per cent of injectors are seropositive to HIV – namely, they are infected. More recent data on hepatitis C (q.v.), a virus that is transmitted by similar means to HIV, show that 50–70 per cent of injectors in most countries are infected.

Over 40 distinct theories or models of drug misuse have been put forward. One is that the individual consumes drugs to cope with personal problems or difficulties in relations with others. The other main model emphasizes environmental influences such as drug availability, environmental pressures to consume drugs and sociocultural influences such as peer pressure. These complex multifactorial models are descriptive and clinical and are generally based on minimal experimental data.

By contrast to these models of why people misuse drugs, models of compulsive drug use, where individuals have a compulsive addiction, have been amenable to testing in the laboratory. Studies at cellular and nerve-receptor levels are atempting to identify mechanisms of tolerance and dependence for several substances. Classical behaviour theory is a key model for understanding drug dependence. This and current laboratory studies are being used to explain the reinforcing nature of dependent substances and are helping to provide an explanatory framework for dependence. Drug consumption is a learned form of behaviour. Numerous investigators have used conditioning theories to study why people misuse drugs. Laboratory studies are now locating the 'reward pathways' in the brain for opiates and stimulants where positive reinforcing mechanisms involve particular sectors of the brain. There is a consensus among experts in addiction that addictive behaviour is amenable to effective treatment and that the extent to which an addict complies with treatment makes it possible to predict a positive outcome. But there is a long way to go before the mechanisms of drug addiction are properly understood or ways of treating it generally agreed. Scientists, doctors, sociologists, law-enforcement agencies and governments will have to co-operate closely if solutions are to be found. (See also DRUG ADDICTION.)

ADDISON'S DISEASE   The cause of Addison's disease is a deficiency of the adrenocortical hormones cortisol, aldosterone and androgens due to destruction of the adrenal cortex. It occurs in about 1:25,000 of the population. Although the destruction of the adrenal cortex in Addison's original description was due to tuberculosis, a much more common cause today is auto-immune damage.

Rare causes of Addison's disease include metastases from carcinoma, usually of the bronchus, granulomata and haemochromatosis. **Symptoms** The clinical symptoms depend on the severity of the underlying disease process. The patient usually complains of anorexia, nausea and loss of weight. The skin becomes pigmentated due to the increased production of ACTH (q.v.). Faintness, especially on standing, is due to postural hypotension secondary to aldosterone deficiency. Women lose their axillary hair and both sexes are liable to develop mental symptoms such as depression. **Diagnosis** depends on demonstrating impaired serum levels of cortisol and inability of these levels to rise after an injection of ACTH. **Treatment** consists in replacement of the deficient hormones and this enable patients to lead a completely normal life and to enjoy a normal life expectancy.

ADENINE ARABINOSIDE is a nitrogen-containing base compound that is a constituent of the nucleic acids deoxyribonucleic acid (DNA) (q.v.) and ribonucleic acid (RNA) (q.v.).

ADENITIS means inflammation of a gland. (See LYMPHATICS.)

ADENO- is a prefix denoting relation to a gland or glands.

ADENOCARCINOMA A malignant growth of glandular tissue. This tissue is widespread throughout the body's organs and the tumours may occur, for example, in the stomach, ovaries, and uterus. Adenocarcinomas may be subdivided into those that arise from mucous or serous secreting glandular tissue.

ADENOIDS (see NOSE, DISEASES OF).

ADENOMA means a benign tumour composed of glandular tissue. It may arise in any part of the body in which glandular tissue occurs: e.g. the thyroid gland. It must be differentiated from an adenocarcinoma, which is a malignant tumour composed of glandular tissue. (See TUMOUR.)

ADENOVIRUSES are viruses containing double-stranded DNA which cause around 5 per cent of clinically recognized respiratory illnesses. Of the 40 or so known types only a few have been properly studied to establish how they produce disease. Adenoviruses cause fever and inflammation of the respiratory tract and mucous membranes of the eyes, symptoms resembling those of the common cold. Infections are generally benign and self limiting and treatment is symptomatic and supportive, although the elderly and people with chronic chest conditions may develop secondary infections which require antibiotic treatment.

ADHESION The abnormal union of two normally separate tissues. It may occur after inflammation or surgery. The result is often a fibrous band between the adjacent tissues. Examples are adhesions between joint surfaces – which reduce mobility of a joint – or, after operation, between loops of intestine, where the fibrous band may cause obstruction. Movement of the heart may be restricted by adhesions between the organ and its membranous cover, the pericardial sac.

ADIPOSE TISSUE or FAT is a loose variety of fibrous tissue, in the meshes of which lie cells, each of which is distended by several small drops, or one large drop, of fat. This tissue replaces fibrous tissue when the amount of food taken is in excess of the bodily requirements. (See DIET; OBESITY.)

ADIPOSIS DOLOROSA, also known as Dercum's disease, is a condition in which painful masses of fat develop under the skin. It is commoner in women than in men.

ADOPTION (see CHILD ADOPTION).

ADRENAL GLANDS, also known as SUPRARENAL GLANDS, are two organs situated one upon the upper end of each kidney. Each measure about 5 cm (2 inches) in length from above downwards, rather less than that from side to side; and each is about 6 mm (¼ inch) thick. The two together weigh about 7 grams. **Structure** Each suprarenal gland has an enveloping layer of fibrous tissue. Within this the gland shows two distinct parts: an outer, firm, deep-yellow, *cortical* layer, and a central, soft, dark-brown, *medullary* portion. The cortical part consists of columns of cells running from the surface inwards, whilst in the medullary portion the cells are arranged irregularly and separated from one another by large capillary blood-vessels. Both the blood vessels and the nerves of the suprarenal glands are large and numerous, considering the small size of the organ. **Functions** It has long been known that removal of the suprarenal glands in animals is speedily followed by great muscular prostration and death in a few days. In human beings, disease of the suprarenal glands is apt to bring on Addison's disease, in which the chief symptoms are increasing weakness and bronzing of the skin. The medulla of the glands produces a substance – adrenaline – the effects of which closely resemble those brought about by activity of the sympathetic nervous system: dilated pupils, hair standing on end, quickening and strengthening of the heart-beat, immobilization of the gut, increased output of sugar from the liver into the blood-stream. From the cortex of the gland are produced a series of hormones which play a vital, though as yet incompletely elucidated, rôle in the metabolism of the body. Some (such as aldosterone) control the electrolyte balance of the body, others are concerned in carbohydrate metabolism, whilst others again are concerned with sex physiology. Cortisone is the most important hormone of the adrenal cortex and is essential for life. (See ADRENALINE; ADDISON'S DISEASE; CORTISONE.)

ADRENALINE is the secretion of the adrenal medulla (see ADRENAL GLANDS). Its effect is similar to stimulation of the *sympathetic nervous system* as occurs when a person is excited, shocked or frightened. In the *United States Pharmocopoeia* it is known as epinephrine. It is also prepared synthetically. Among its important effects are raising of the blood pressure, increasing the amount of glucose in the blood, and constricting the smaller blood-vessels.

It is applied directly to wounds on gauze or lint to check haemorrhage. Injected along with some local anaesthetic it permits painless, bloodless operations to be performed on the eye, nose, etc. It is injected hypodermically to relieve asthma, and to stimulate the heart in collapsed conditions.

ADRENERGIC RECEPTORS are the sites in the body on which adrenaline (q.v.) and comparable stimulants of the sympathetic nervous system (q.v.) act. Drugs which have an adrenaline-like action are described as being adrenergic. There are four different types of adrenergic receptors, known as alpha$_1$, alpha$_2$, beta$_1$, and beta$_2$, respectively. Stimulation of alpha receptors leads to constriction of the bronchi, constriction of the blood vessels with consequent rise in blood-pressure, and dilatation of the pupils of the eyes. Stimulation of beta$_1$ receptors quickens the rate and output of the heart, whilst stimulation of beta$_2$ receptors dilates the bronchi.

For long it had been realized that in certain cases of asthma adrenaline had not the usual beneficial effect of dilating the bronchi during an attack; rather it made the asthma worse. This was due to its acting on both the alpha and beta adrenergic receptors. A derivative, isoprenaline, was therefore produced which acted only on the beta receptors. This had an excellent effect in dilating the bronchi, but unfortunately also affected the heart, speeding it up and increasing its output – an undesirable effect which meant that isoprenaline had to be used with great care. In due course drugs were produced, such as salbutamol, which act predominantly on the beta$_2$ adrenergic receptors in the bronchi and have relatively little effect on the heart.

The converse of this story was the search for what became known as beta-adrenoceptor-blocking drugs, or beta-adrenergic-blocking drugs. The theoretical argument was that if such drugs could be synthesized, they could be of value in taking the strain off the heart – for example: stress → stimulation of the output of adrenaline → stimulation of the heart → increased work for the heart. A drug that could prevent this train of events would be of value,

for example, in the treatment of angina pectoris (q.v.). Now there is a series of beta-adrenoceptor-blocking drugs of use not only in angina pectoris, but also in various other heart conditions such as disorders of rhythm, as well as high blood-pressure. They are also proving of value in the treatment of anxiety states by preventing disturbing features such as palpitations. Some are useful in the treatment of migraine. (see BETA-ADRENOCEPTOR-BLOCKING DRUGS).

ADRENOCORTICOTROPHIC HORMONE (ACTH) A hormone which is released into the body during stress. Made and stored in the anterior pituitary gland, ACTH regulates the production of Corticosteroid hormones from the Adrenal Gland. ACTH is vital for the growth and maintenance of the adrenal cortical cells. Its production is in part controlled by the amount of hydrocortisone in the blood and also by the hypothalmus. The hormone is used to test adrenal function and treat conditions such as asthma.

ADRENOGENITAL SYNDROME or CONGENITAL ADRENAL HYPERPLASIA An inherited condition, the adrenogenital syndrome or congenital adrenal hyperplasia is an uncommon disorder affecting about one baby in 7,500. The condition is present from birth and the victim suffers from various enzyme defects as well as a block on the production of hydrocortisone and aldosterone by the adrenal gland. In girls the syndrome produces virilization of the genital tract, which may become enlarged. The metabolism of salt and water is disturbed causing dehydration, low blood pressure, and loss of weight. Enlargement of the adrenal glands occurs and the affected individual may also develop excessive pigmentation in the skin. Treatment requires replacement of the missing hormones and, if started early, may lead to normal sexual development.

ADULT RESPIRATORY DISTRESS SYNDROME (ARDS) A form of acute respiratory failure in which a variety of different disorders give rise to pulmonary injury by what is thought to be a common pathway. It has a high mortality (about 70 per cent).

The exact aetiology is unknown, but it is thought that, whatever the stimulus, activation of neutrophils (which may then be sequestered in the lungs) releases cytotoxic substances – substances that damage or kill cells – such as oxygen-free radicals and proteases which damage the alveolar capillary membranes. Once these are damaged protein-rich oedema fluid leaks into the alveoli and interstitial spaces. Surfactant (q.v.) is also lost. This impairs gas exchange and gives rise to the clinical and pathological picture of acute respiratory failure.

The typical patient with ARDS has rapidly worsening hypoxaemia (lack of oxygen in the blood), often requiring mechanical ventilation, which contrasts with the relative lack of physical signs. There are all the signs of respiratory failure (see TACHYPNOEA, TACHYCARDIA, CYANOSIS, etc.), though the chest may be clear apart from a few crackles. Radiographs show bilateral, patchy, peripheral shadowing sparing the cardio and costophrenic angles. Blood gases will show a low PaO$_2$ (concentration of oxygen in pulmonary arterial blood) and usually a high PaCO$_2$ (concentration of carbon dioxide in pulmonary arterial blood). The lungs are 'stiff' – they are less effective because of the loss of surfactant and the non-cardiogenic pulmonary oedema. The causes of ARDS may be broadly divided into the following:

MICROBIOLOGICAL – pulmonary, distant, or generalized infection by bacteria, fungi, or viruses.

ACTIVATION OF HOST DEFENCE – massive transfusion, transfusion reaction, cardiopulmonary bypass, etc., may cause activation of neutrophils (q.v.) via complement pathways.

CHEMICAL – this includes drugs, inhaled toxic gases and smoke, and metabolic disorders like uraemia (q.v.) and pancreatitis (see pancreas, diseases of).

PHYSICAL – trauma to the lung, gastric aspiration, aspiration of water, etc. The principles of management are supportive, with treatment of the underlying condition if that is possible. Oxygenation is improved by increasing inspired oxygen concentration and mechanical ventilation of the lungs. Attempts are made to reduce the formation of pulmonary oedema by careful management of fluid balance. Secondary infections are treated if they arise, as are the possible complications of prolonged ventilation with low lung compliance (e.g., pneumothorax (q.v.)). There is some evidence that giving surfactant through a nebulizer or aerosol may help to improve lung effectiveness and reduce oedema. There is little evidence that steroids are of use. Some experimental evidence supports the use of free radical scavengers and antioxidants, but these are not commonly used. In severe cases extracorporeal gas exchange has been advocated as a supportive measure until the lungs have healed enough for adequate gas exchange. (See also RESPIRATORY DISTRESS SYNDROME AND HYALINE MEMBRANE DISEASE.)

ADVERSE REACTIONS TO DRUGS Any drug may produce unexpected or unwanted adverse reactions including *anaphylaxis*. Although new drugs are subjected to extensive laboratory testing and are tried on selected patients in controlled clinical studies, adverse reactions may come to light when they are widely prescribed for patients. It is essential, therefore, that doctors report such reactions to the authorities, in the case of the United Kingdom to the Committee on Safety of Medicines (CSM). A special 'yellow card' reporting mechanism exists for this purpose which can be used for established as well as new drugs. Patients who think that a drug they are taking is producing side-effects should tell their doctor.

Examples of adverse reactions include skin eruptions, nausea, bleeding, jaundice, sleepiness, headaches, and tremors. To prevent adverse reactions doctors should prescribe a drug only if it is essential, check if the patient suffers from an allergy and, if he or she is taking other drugs, prescribe only the amount of medicine required and give clear instructions on use and known side-effects.

AEDES AEGYPTI is the scientific name of the mosquito which conveys to man (by biting) the viruses of yellow fever and of dengue or 'breakbone fever'. (See DENGUE; and YELLOW FEVER.)

AEGOPHONY is the bleating or punchinello tone given to the voice as heard by *auscultation* (q.v.) with a stethoscope, when there is a small amount of fluid in the pleural cavity.

AEROPHAGY means air-swallowing, and is the name applied to a habit which some persons, especially when suffering from dyspepsia, contract of swallowing mouthfuls of air.

AEROSOL (see INHALANTS).

AETIOLOGY is the part of medical science dealing with the causes of disease.

AFFERENT An adjective to describe nerves, blood vessels, or lymphatic vessels that conduct their electrical charge or contents inwards to the brain, spinal cord or relevant organ.

AFIBRINOGENAEMIA is a condition in which the blood will not clot because fibrin (q.v.) is absent. It is characterized by haemorrhage. There are two forms: (*a*) a congenital form, and (*b*) an acquired form. The latter may be associated with advanced liver disease, or may occur as a complication of labour. Treatment consists of the intravenous injection of fibrinogen and blood transfusion.

AFTERBIRTH (see PLACENTA).

AFTERPAINS are pains similar to but feebler than those of labour, occurring in the two or three days following childbirth.
Causes are generally the presence of a blood-clot or retained piece of placenta which the womb is attempting to expel.

AGAMMAGLOBULINAEMIA is a condition found in children, in which there is no gamma-globulin (q.v.) in the blood. These children are particularly susceptible to infections as they are unable to form antibodies to any infecting micro-organism.

breathing owing to spasm of the bronchioles (q.v.), swollen joints, nausea and headaches. Severe allergic reactions may cause a person to go into shock (q.v.). Prevention is the best treatment with the sensitive individual avoiding the food or other factor such as pollen known to cause an allergic reaction. This may require extensive testing to establish the allergen. Sometimes an allergy may be cured by desensitizing the individual with small doses of the allergen (see IMMUNOTHERAPY). Severe allergic symptoms may require treatment with sympathomimetic drugs (q.v.) such as adrenaline, with antihistamines (q.v.) or with steroids. Expert medical attention is needed for patients with severe reactions.

ALLOCHEIRIA is the name for a disorder of sensation in which sensations are referred to the wrong part of the body.

ALLOGRAFT is a piece of tissue or an organ, such as the kidney, transplanted from one to another of the same species: e.g. from man to man. It is also known as a homograft.

ALLOPATHY is a term applied sometimes by homoeopathists to the methods used by regular practitioners of medicine and surgery. The term literally means curing by inducing a different kind of action in the body, and is an erroneous designation.

ALLOPURINOL is a drug of value in the treatment of gout. It acts by suppressing the formation of uric acid. It is also being used in treatment of uric acid stone in the kidney.

ALOPECIA is another name for baldness. (See BALDNESS.)

ALOPECIA AREATA is the term given to the disorder in which the hair comes out in patches, resulting in shiny, smooth, bald areas. (See BALDNESS.)

ALPHA FETOPROTEIN A protein produced in the gut and liver of the fetus. Abnormality in the fetus, such as neural tube defect, may result in raised levels of alpha fetoprotein in the maternal blood. In Down's syndrome levels may be abnormally low. In either case screening of the pregnancy should be done, including amniocentesis to check the amount of alpha fetoprotein in the amniotic fluid. The protein may also be produced in some abnormal tissues in the adult, for example, in patients with liver cancer.

ALTERNATIVE MEDICINE (see COMPLEMENTARY MEDICINE).

ALTITUDE SICKNESS This condition, also known as mountain sickness, occurs in mountain climbers or hikers who have climbed too quickly to heights above 3000 m, thus failing to allow their bodies to acclimatize to altitude. The lower atmospheric pressure and shortage of oxygen result in hyperventilation – deep, quick breathing – and this reduces the amount of carbon dioxide in the blood. Nausea, anxiety, and exhaustion are presenting symptoms and seriously affected individuals may be acutely breathless because of pulmonary oedema (excess fluid in the lungs). Gradual climbing over two or three days should prevent mountain sickness. In serious cases the individual must be brought down to hospital as a matter of urgency. Most attacks, however, are mild.

ALVEOLITIS means inflammation of the alveoli (see ALVEOLUS) of the lungs caused by an allergic reaction. When the inflammation is caused by infection it is called pneumonia and when by a chemical or physical agent it is called pneumonitis. It may be associated with systemic sclerosis or rheumatoid arthritis.
EXTRINSIC ALLERGIC ALVEOLITIS is the condition induced by the lungs becoming allergic (see ALLERGY) to various factors or substances. It includes bagassosis (q.v.), farmer's lung (q.v.), mushroom-worker's lung (q.v.) and budgerigar-fancier's lung (q.v.). It is characterized by the onset of shortness of breath, tightness of the chest, cough and fever. The onset may be sudden or gradual. Treatment consists of removal of the affected individual from the offending material to which he has become allergic. Corticosteroids (q.v.) give temporary relief.

ALVEOLUS is a term applied to the sockets of the teeth in the jaw-bone. The term is also applied to the minute divisions of glands and the air sacs of the lungs.

ALZHEIMER'S DISEASE is a degenerative disorder of the cerebral cortex that produces a dementia (q.v.) in middle to late life. The commonest cause of dementia, the disease's onset is insidious and the first manifestation is usually failing memory. The cause is unknown, although various theories have been proposed, one being that the condition results from the deposition of aluminium in the brain cells. Heredity may play a part. There is no cure. Relatives can obtain help and advice from the Alzheimer's Disease Society (see APPENDIX 2: ADDRESSES).

AMANTADINE is a drug which is being used in the treatment of certain virus infections, and is proving of value in the prevention of certain forms of influenza. It is also used in the treatment of Parkinsonism (q.v.).

AMAUROSIS is the term applied to blindness in which there is no obvious lesion of the eye, the blindness being caused by disease of the optic nerve, retina or brain, or being due to hysteria.

AMAUROSIS FUGAX is the term given to sudden transitory impairment, or loss of, vision. It usually affects only one eye, and is commonly due to circulatory failure. In its simplest form it occurs in normal people on rising suddenly from the sitting or recumbent position, when it is due to the effects of gravity. It also occurs in migraine. A not uncommon cause, particularly in elderly people, is transient ocular ischaemia (see ISCHAEMIA), resulting from blockage of the circulation to the retina (see EYE) by emboli (see EMBOLISM) from the common carotid artery or the heart. Treatment in this last group of cases consists of control of the blood pressure if this is raised, as it often is in such cases; the administration of drugs that reduce the stickiness of blood platelets such as aspirin. In some instances removal of the part of the carotid artery from which the emboli are coming may be indicated.

AMBIVALENCE is the term applied to the psychological state in which a person concurrently hates and loves the same object or person.

AMBLYOPIA means defective vision for which no recognizable cause exists in any part of the eye. It may be due to such causes as defective development or excessive use of tobacco or alcohol. The most important form is that associated with squinting (q.v.), or gross difference in refraction between the two eyes. It has been estimated that in Britain around 5 per cent of young adults have amblyopia due to this cause.

AMELIA   This is absence of the limbs, usually a congenital defect.

AMENORRHOEA is the absence of the menstrual flow during the time of life at which it should occur. (See MENSTRUATION.) If menstruation has never occurred the amenorrhoea is termed primary. If it ceases after having once become established it is known as secondary amenorrhoea. The only value of these terms is that some patients with either chromosome abnormalities or malformations of the genital tract fall into the primary category. Otherwise the age of onset of symptoms is more important.

The causes of amenorrhoea are numerous and treatment requires dealing with the primary cause. The commonest cause of amenorrhoea is pregnancy. Hypothalamic disorders such as psychological stress or anorexia nervosa also cause amenorrhoea. Poor nutrition or loss of weight by dieting may cause it and any serious underlying disease such as tuberculosis or malaria may also result in the cessation of periods. The excess secretion of prolactin, whether this is the result of a micro-adenoma

(see ADENOMA) of the pituitary gland or whether it is drug induced will cause amenorrhoea and possibly galactorrhoea (q.v.) as well. Malfunction of the pituitary gland will result in a failure to produce the gonadotrophic hormones with consequent amenorrhea. Excessive production of cortisol, as in Cushing's syndrome, or of androgens, as in the adreno-genital syndrome or the polycystic ovary syndrome, will result in amenorrhoea. Amenorrhoea occasionally follows the use of the oral contraceptive pill and may be associated with both hypothyroidism and obesity. It is thus important to take a careful history with emphasis on psychological factors, weight fluctuations and the use of drugs that may stimulate the release of prolactin, and it is also important to look for evidence of virilization.

A gynaecological examination is necessary in primary amenorrhoea to exclude malformations of the genital tract. Estimations of the gonadotrophic hormone levels will reveal whether the amenorrhoea is primary ovarian failure or secondary to pituitary disease. In view of the frequent psychosomatic origins of amenorrhoea, reassurance of the patient is of great importance, in particular with reference to marriage and the ability to conceive. When weight loss is the cause of amenorrhoea restoration of body weight alone can result in spontaneous menstruation. Patients with raised concentrations of serum gonadotrophin hormones have primary ovarian failure. It is not amendable to treatment. Cyclical oestrogen/progestogen therapy will usually establish withdrawal bleeding. If the amenorrhoea is due to mild pituitary failure menstruation may return after treatment with clomiphene. Clomiphene is a non-steroidal agent which competes for oestrogen receptors in the hypothalamus. The patients who are most likely to respond to clomiphene are those who have some evidence of endogenous oestrogen and gonadotrophin production.

AMENTIA is the failure of the intellectual faculties to develop normally.

AMETHOCAINE is a powerful local anaesthetic which is used in selected circumstances when a prolonged effect is required.

AMETROPIA (see REFRACTION).

AMIKACIN is a semi-synthetic derivative of kanamycin (q.v.) which is used to treat infections caused by micro-organisms resistant to gentamicin (q.v.) and tobramycin (q.v.).

AMILORIDE is a diuretic that acts without causing excessive loss of potassium (see DIURETICS).

AMINES are substances derived from ammonia or amino-acids (q.v.) which play an important part in the working of the body, including the brain and the circulatory system. They include adrenaline (q.v.), noradrenaline (q.v.) and histamine (q.v.). (See also MONOAMINE OXIDASE INHIBITORS.)

AMINO-ACID is the name given to the ultimate products of digestion of protein foods and from which the protein materials of the body are again built up. They are organic acids in which one or more hydrogen atoms have been replaced by the chemical group NH_2. (See PROTEIN.)

AMINOCAPROIC ACID is a drug used to treat hereditary angioedema, a serious anaphylactic reaction of the skin and respiratory tract resulting from a deficiency in the body's immunological defence mechanisms.

AMINOGLUTETHIMIDE is a drug that inhibits the synthesis of adrenal corticorteroids. It is proving of value in the treatment of cancer of the breast in post-menopausal women.

AMINOGLYCOSIDES These are a group of antibiotics that are usually kept for use in severe infections. They are effective against a wide range of bacteria but can cause side-effects that include damage to the kidneys and inner ear. Amikacin (q.v.), gentamycin, kanamycin, neomycin and streptomycin are important examples of this group of drugs.

AMINOPHYLLINE is the name given to a combination of theophylline and ethylenediamine. It is used in the treatment of bronchial asthma.

AMITRIPTYLINE (see ANTIDEPRESSANTS).

AMMONIA is a compound of hydrogen and nitrogen that occurs naturally. The solution is colourless with a pungent smell; it is used in urine testing. In humans certain inherited defects in the metabolism of ammonia can cause neurological symptoms including mental retardation.

AMNESIA means loss of memory.

AMNIOCENTESIS is the piercing of the amniotic sac in the pregnant uterus through the abdominal wall to withdraw a sample of amniotic fluid for prenatal testing.

AMNION is the tough fibrous membrane which lines the cavity of the womb during pregnancy, and contains from 0·5 to 1 litre (one to two pints) of fluid in which the embryo floats. It is formed from the ovum along with the embryo, and in labour the part of it at the mouth of the womb forms the 'bag of waters'. (See LABOUR.) When a child is 'born with a caul', the caul is a piece of amnion. (See CAUL.)

AMNIOSCOPY is the insertion of a viewing instrument (amnioscope) through the abdominal wall into the pregnant uterus to examine the inside of the amniotic sac. The growing fetus can be viewed directly and its condition and sex assessed without disturbing the pregnancy. The amniotic sac may also be viewed late in pregnancy through the cervix or neck of the womb using an instrument called the fetoscope.

AMNIOTIC FLUID The clear fluid contained within the amnion that surrounds the fetus in the womb and protects it from external pressure. The fluid, mainly water, is produced by the amnion and is regularly circulated, being swallowed by the fetus and excreted through the kidneys back into the amniotic sac. By the 35th week of pregnancy there is about one litre of fluid but this falls to half a litre at term. The amniotic sac normally ruptures in early labour releasing the fluid or 'waters'.

AMOEBA is a minute protozoan organism consisting of a single cell, in which a nucleus is surrounded by protoplasm that changes its shape as the protozoon progresses or absorbs nourishment. Several varieties are found under different conditions within the human body. One variety, *Entamoeba coli*, is found in the large intestine of man without any associated disease; another, *Entamoeba gingivalis*, is found in the sockets of the teeth associated with pyorrhoea; another, *Entamoeba histolytica*, is the causative organism of amoebic dysentery (see DYSENTERY). Two, *Acanthamoeba* and *Naegleria fowleri*, cause the infection of the brain known as meningoencephalitis (q.v.). *Entamoeba histolytica* may also cause meningoencephalitis. Other forms are found in the genital organs.

AMOEBIASIS (see DYSENTERY).

AMOXYCILLIN (see PENICILLIN, ANTIBIOTIC).

AMPHETAMINES are a group of drugs closely related to adrenaline and act by stimulating the sympathetic nervous system. When taken by mouth they have a profound stimulating effect on the brain, producing a sense of well-being and confidence and seemingly increasing the capacity for mental work. They are, however, drugs of dependence and their medical use is now strictly limited, for example, to the treatment of narcolepsy.

Because they inhibit appetite, they rapidly achieved a reputation for slimming purposes, but they should not be used for this purpose. The dangers of amphetamines far outweigh their advantages.

AMPHORIC is an adjective denoting the kind of breathing heard over a cavity in the lung. The sound is like that made by blowing over the mouth of a narrow-necked vase.

AMPHOTERICIN is a mixture of antifungal substances derived from *Streptomyces nodosus*, which is proving of value in the treatment of certain of the diseases classified under the heading of mycosis (q.v.). It is, however, a very toxic substance and is therefore only used in those infections in which the outlook is otherwise hopeless. It is also proving of value in the treatment of certain cases of amoebic meningoencephalitis. (See MENINGOENCEPHALITIS.)

AMPICILLIN (see PENICILLIN, ANTIBIOTIC).

AMPOULE is a small glass container having one end drawn out into a point capable of being sealed so as to preserve its contents sterile. It is used for containing solutions for hypodermic injection.

AMPUTATION is the severing of a limb, or part of a limb from the rest of the body. The leg is the most common site of amputation. It is usually performed as a controlled operation and may be required for a variety of reasons. In the young, severe injury is the most common cause, when damage to the limb is so extensive as to make it non-viable or functionally useless.

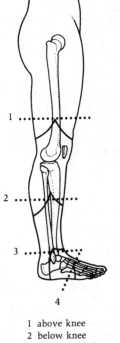

1 above knee
2 below knee
3 Syme's heel flap
4 midtarsal

Amputation sites of lower limb.

In the elderly, amputation is more often the result of vascular insufficiency, resulting in gangrene or intractable pain.

The aim is to restore the patient to full mobility with a prosthetic (artificial) limb, which requires both a well-fitting prosthesis (q.v.) and a well-healed surgical wound. If this is not possible, the aim is to leave the patient with a limb stump that is still useful for balancing, sitting and transferring. Common types of lower-limb amputation are shown in the illustration. The Symes amputation can be walked upon without requiring a prosthesis. The below-knee amputation preserves normal flexion of the knee, and virtually normal walking can be achieved with a well-fitting artificial limb. Learning to walk is more difficult following an above-knee amputation, but some well-motivated patients can manage well. After any amputation it is not unusual for the patient to experience the sensation that the limb is still present. This is called a phantom limb and the sensation may persist for a long time. (See PROSTHESES, PHANTOM LIMB.)

AMSACRINE (see CYTOTOXIC).

AMYLASE is an enzyme (q.v.) in pancreatic juice which facilitates the conversion of starch to maltose. (See PANCREAS.)

AMYL NITRITE is a volatile, oily liquid prepared by the action of nitric and nitrous acids upon amyl alcohol. It resembles other nitrites in its power of relieving spasms and dilating blood-vessels, and it acts with great rapidity when inhaled, producing its effects in a few seconds.

AMYLOIDOSIS, or WAXY DISEASE, is the condition in which deposits of complex protein, known as amyloid, are found in various parts of the body. It is a degenerative condition resulting from various causes such as chronic infection, including tuberculosis and rheumatoid arthritis.

AMYLOSE is the name applied to any carbohydrate of the starch group.

ANABOLIC STEROIDS The nitrogen-retaining effect of androgen is responsible for the larger muscle mass of the male. This is called an anabolic effect. Attempts have been made to separate the anabolic effects of hormones from their virilizing effects. This is only partially successful. Thus anabolic steroids have the property of protein building so that when taken they lead to an increase in muscle bulk and strength. All the anabolic steroids have some androgenic activity but they cause less virilization than androgens in women. Androgenic side-effects may result from any of these anabolic compounds, especially if they are given for prolonged periods. All these compounds should therefore be used with caution in women, and are contra-indicted in men with prostatic carcinoma. Jaundice due to stasis of bile in the intrahepatic canaliculi is a hazard, and the depression of pituitary gonadotrophin production is a possible complication.

Anabolic steroids have been used to stimulate protein anabolism in debilitating illness and to promote growth in children with pituitary dwarfism and other disorders associated with interference of growth. Stimulation of protein anabolism may also be of value in acute renal failure, and the retention of nitrogen and calcium is of probable benefit to patients with osteoporosis (q.v.) and to patients receiving corticosteroid therapy. Anabolic steroids may stimulate bone marrow function in hypoplastic anaemia.

Anabolic steroids have been widely abused by athletes aiming to improve their strength, stamina and speed. They should not be used for this purpose and athletes using them face bans from official competitions.

The anabolic steroids in therapeutic use include nandrolone and stanozolol.

ANAEMIA is the condition characterized by inadequate red blood cells and/or haemoglobin in the blood. It is considered to exist if haemoglobin levels are below 13 grams per 100 ml in males and below 12 grams per 100 ml in adult non-pregnant women. No simple classification of anaemia can be wholly accurate, but the most useful method is to divide anaemias into: (a) microcytic hypochromic anaemia, (b) megaloblastic hyperchromic anaemia, (c) aplastic anaemia, (d) haemolytic anaemia. In Britain, anaemia is much more common among women than in men. Thus, around 10 per cent of girls have anaemia at the age of 15, whilst in adult life the incidence is over 30 per cent between the ages of 30 and 40, around 20 per cent at 50, and around 30 per cent at 70. Among men the incidence is under 5 per cent until the age of 50, and it then rises to 20 per cent at the age of 70. Ninety per cent of all cases of anaemia in Britain are microcytic, 7 per cent are macrocytic, and 3 per cent are haemolytic or aplastic. (See also SICKLE-CELL ANAEMIA; and THALASSAEMIA.)

MICROCYTIC HYPOCHROMIC ANAEMIA This corresponds to a large extent with what used to be known as 'secondary anaemia'. It takes its name from the characteristic changes in the blood.

Causes (1) *Loss of blood* (a) As a result of trauma. This is perhaps the simplest example of all, when, as a result of an accident involving a large artery, there is severe haemorrhage. (b) Menstruation. The regular monthly loss of blood which women sustain as a result of menstruation always puts a strain on the blood-forming organs. If this loss is excessive, then over a period of time it may lead to quite severe anaemia. (c) Child-birth. A considerable amount of blood is always lost at child-birth, and if this

is severe, or if the woman was anaemic during pregnancy, a severe degree of anaemia may develop. (d) Bleeding from the gastro-intestinal tract. The best example here is anaemia due to 'bleeding piles' (see PILES). Such bleeding, even though slight, if maintained over a long period of time, is a common cause of anaemia in both men and women. The haemorrhage may be more acute and occur from a duodenal or gastric ulcer, when it is known as haematemesis (q.v.). (e) Certain blood diseases, such as purpura (q.v.) and haemophilia (q.v.), which are characterized by bleeding.

(2) *Defective blood formation* (a) This is the main cause of anaemia in infections. The microorganism responsible for the infection has a deleterious effect upon the blood-forming organs, just as it does upon other parts of the body. (b) Toxins. In conditions such as chronic glomerulonephritis and uraemia there is a severe anaemia due to the effect of the disease upon blood formation. (c) Drugs. Certain drugs, such as aspirin and the non- steroidal anti-inflammatory drugs, may cause occult gastro-intestinal **bleeding**.

(3) *Inadequate intake of iron* The daily requirement of iron for an adult is 12 mg, and 15 to 20 mg during pregnancy. This is well covered by an ordinary diet, so that by itself it is not a common cause. But if there is a steady loss of blood, as a result of heavy menstrual loss or 'bleeding piles', the intake of iron in the diet may not be sufficient to maintain adequate formation of haemoglobin.

(4) *Inadequate absorption of iron* This may occur in diseases of intestinal malabsorption.

In many cases the anaemia is found to be due to a combination of two or more of these causes. A severe form of this anaemia in women, known as chlorosis, used to be common, but it is seldom seen nowadays.

Symptoms These depend upon whether the anaemia is sudden in onset, as in severe haemorrhage, or gradual. In all cases, however, the striking sign is pallor, the depth of which depends upon the severity of the anaemia. The colour of the skin may be misleading, except in cases due to severe haemorrhage, as the skin of many people is normally pale. The best guide is the colour of the internal lining of the eyelid. When the onset of the anaemia is sudden the patient complains of weakness and giddiness, and he loses consciousness if he tries to stand or sit up. The breathing is rapid and distressed, the pulse is rapid, and the blood-pressure is low. In chronic cases the tongue is often sore (glossitis), and the nails of the fingers may be brittle and concave instead of convex (koilonychia). In some cases, particularly in women, the Plummer-Vinson syndrome is present. This consists of difficulty in swallowing and may be accompanied by huskiness; in these cases glossitis is also present. There may be slight enlargement of the spleen, and there is usually some diminution in gastric acidity.

Changes in the blood The characteristic change is a diminution in both the haemoglobin and the red cell content of the blood. There is a relatively greater fall in the haemoglobin than in the red cell count. If the blood is examined under a microscope the red cells are seen to be paler and smaller than normal. These small red cells are known as microcytes.

Treatment consists primarily of giving sufficient iron by mouth to restore, and then maintain, a normal blood picture. The main iron preparation now used is ferrous sulphate, 200 mg, thrice daily after meals. When the blood picture has become normal, the dosage is gradually reduced. A preparation of iron is available which can be given intravenously, but this is only used in cases which do not respond to iron given by mouth, or in cases in which it is essential to obtain a quick response.

If, of course, there is haemorrhage, this must be arrested, and if the loss of blood has been severe it may be necessary to give a blood transfusion. Care must be taken to ensure that the patient is having an adequate diet. If there is any underlying metabolic, oncological, toxic or infective condition, this, of course, must be adequately treated after appropriate investigations.

MEGALOBLASTIC HYPERCHROMIC ANAEMIA There are various forms of anaemia of this type, such as those due to nutritional but the most important is that known as PERNICIOUS ANAEMIA.

PERNICIOUS ANAEMIA Up until about seventy years ago its cause was unknown and it was an invariably fatal disease. In 1926, two Americans, G. R. Minot and W. P. Murphy, reported that pernicious anaemia responded to treatment with liver. This discovery ranks in importance with that of insulin in the treatment of diabetes mellitus. This form of treatment is based upon the now well-proved fact that pernicious anaemia is due to lack of what is known as the *intrinsic factor*. For the formation of normal red blood corpuscles a substance known as the extrinsic factor is necessary. The efficient absorption of this factor into the body is dependent on the presence of intrinsic factor which is produced normally by the mucosa lining the distal part of the stomach. It is the inability of the patient to produce the intrinsic factor that leads to the onset of pernicious anaemia. In a normal person with adequate amounts of intrinsic factor, approximately 70 per cent of the extrinsic factor (which is vitamin B_{12} and is present in meat and other foods) in the daily diet is absorbed into the body. In patients with pernicious anaemia, however, less than 2 per cent is absorbed.

Symptoms Pernicious anaemia is a disease of middle age, being rare under the age of 40 years. It affects both men and women. The onset is usually insidious, so that the anaemia is usually well developed before medical advice is sought. In addition to the general symptoms and signs already described in the section on microcytic anaemia, the important features of pernicious anaemia are as follows. The patient, who is often prematurely grey-haired, has a characteristic lemon-yellow complexion. The tongue is often sore and appears thinner, smoother, and redder than usual. There is often soreness and excoriation of the corners of the mouth – a condition known as cheilosis. There may be slight enlargement of the spleen. There is a complete absence of free hydrochloric acid in the stomach, even after the injection of histamine.

One of the most serious complications of pernicious anaemia is a disease with the cumbersome title of SUBACUTE COMBINED DEGENERATION OF THE CORD. This, as the name indicates, is a degenerative condition of the spinal cord, and the importance of recognizing its onset is that it can be cured by adequate treatment of the anaemia. Its early manifestations are a sensation of tingling or 'pins and needles' in the legs, accompanied by stiffness. Later, if untreated, the stiffness becomes progressively worse, finally leading to paralysis.

Changes in the blood The red cells are larger than normal, i.e. macrocytes and they appear to be redder than normal. They also vary in shape (poikilocytosis) and in size (anisocytosis). Occasionally a few primitive red cells (normoblasts) may be found. The total white cell count is diminished: i.e. there is leucopenia. The final diagnosis depends upon an examination of the bone marrow, which is found to contain megaloblasts.

Treatment consists of the administration of vitamin B_{12} in the form of hydroxocobalamin. It is given by injection. It must always be remembered that a patient with pernicious anaemia requires to take vitamin B_{12} for the rest of his or her life.

APLASTIC ANAEMIA is a disease in which the red blood corpuscles are very greatly reduced and in which no attempt appears to be made in the bone marrow towards their regeneration. It is more accurately called hypoplastic anaemia as the degree of impairment of bone marrow function is rarely complete. The cause in many cases is not known, but in rather less than half the cases the condition is due to some toxic substance, such as benzol or certain drugs, or ionizing radiations. The patient becomes very pale, with a tendency to haemorrhages under the skin and mucous membranes, and the temperature may at times be raised. The red blood corpuscles diminish steadily in numbers. Treatment consists primarily of regular blood transfusions. Although the disease is often fatal, the outlook has improved in recent years. About 25 per cent of patients recover when adequately treated, and others survive for several years. In severe cases promising results are being reported from the use of bone marrow transplantation.

HAEMOLYTIC ANAEMIA results from the excessive destruction, or haemolysis (q.v.), of the red blood cells. This haemolysis may be due to undue fragility of the red blood cells, when the condition is known as congenital haemolytic anaemia, or acholuric jaundice.

ANAEROBE is the term applied to bacteria having the power to live without air. Such organisms are found growing freely, deep in the soil, as, for example, the tetanus bacillus.

ANAESTHESIA The loss of sensation or feeling. It may be caused by a disease process, but its common usage describes a reversible process for abolishing sensation to allow painful procedures such as surgery to occur without pain or distress to the patient.

Anaesthesia is provided by a trained specialist who, in most countries, is a qualified medical practitioner. The anaesthetist will assess the patient's fitness for anaesthesia, choose and perform the appropriate type of anaesthetic, whilst monitoring and caring for the well-being of the patient, and, following reversal of the anaesthetic, supervise the recovery and post-operative analgesia for the patient. Anaesthesia can be broadly divided into general and local.

GENERAL ANAESTHESIA Under general anaesthesia patients are given a combination of drugs to render them reversibly unconscious during a painful procedure. A so called 'balanced' anaesthetic provides unconsciousness, analgesia, and a greater or lesser degree of muscle relaxation. By using a combination of drugs the side-effects of any individual drug are minimized, while achieving the optimum anaesthetic effect.

A general anaesthetic may be divided into induction, maintenance, and recovery (or reversal). Historically anaesthesia has been divided into four stages (see below) but these are only seen clearly with a purely inhalational induction and maintenance.
Stage 1: onset of induction to unconsciousness.
Stage 2: stage of excitement.
Stage 3: plane 1 – deep regular breathing
plane 2 – cessation of eye movement
plane 3 – surgical anaesthesia
plane 4 – diaphragmatic paralysis.
Stage 4: overdosage.

Induction merely means putting the patient to sleep. Most often this is performed by means of an intravenous injection, though an inhalation technique can be used instead. The most widely used agents are short-acting barbiturates, thiopentone, and methohexitone, whilst two newer agents etomidate and propofol are also used.

The maintenance of anaesthesia is usually by administration of oxygen and nitrous oxide containing a volatile anaesthetic agent. Anaesthetic machines and vaporizers provide a constant percentage of each constituent set by the anaesthetist. They are administered to the patient via a breathing circuit either through a mask or an endotracheal tube. For some operations the patient may be paralysed with a muscle relaxant, in which case their lungs will be artificially ventilated by a machine (see ARTIFICIAL VENTILATION OF THE LUNGS). Often opioids are given to supplement analgesia, as may a local anaesthetic block.

The most commonly used volatile agents in the UK are halothane (a halogenated hydrocarbon), isoflurane and enflurane (isomers of a halogenated ether). On a world-wide basis ether and chloroform are still often used. The mode of action of these agents is not fully understood, though there are several theories, but by whatever action they reversibly depress conduction of impulses in central nervous tissue and thereby produce unconsciousness.

Reversal of anaesthesia will occur when the patient is allowed to breathe oxygen or oxygen-enriched air and excrete via the lungs the volatile anaesthetic agent previously absorbed. Muscle relaxants and occasionally the effects of opioids are pharmacologically reversed.

Ketamine is an unusual anaesthetic sometimes used for general anaesthesia but more often for painful procedures such as burns dressings. It produces a dissociative anaesthesia under which patients may open their eyes and move but are unaware of what is happening. Though it is an excellent analgesic and depresses ventilation less than most other anaesthetics, it produces hallucinations and nightmares.

LOCAL ANAESTHETICS are drugs which reversibly block the conduction of impulses in nerves. They therefore abolish the motor and sensory function in the areas served by that particular nerve. Many drugs have local anaesthetic actions but all the ones used to produce local anaesthesia clinically are amide or ester derivatives of aromatic acids. If absorbed systemically in toxic amounts, they produce central-nervous-system and cardiovascular side-effects. Local anaesthesia may be used to supplement general anaesthesia, as the sole method if coexisting medical conditions make general anaesthesia unsuitable, or for the relief of chronic or acute pain. Several techniques are used as listed below:

Local infiltration – small quantities of local anaesthetic are infiltrated subcutaneously to produce a small area of anaesthetized skin. Similarly, deeper tissues may be infiltrated and anaesthetized. This technique is useful for removing small superficial lesions and suturing skin.

Nerve blocks – local anaesthetic is injected in the proximity of nerve plexuses or individual nerves. Once it has diffused into the nerve, surgical anaesthesia in the area subserved by the nerve is achieved. More than one nerve may need to be blocked.

Spinal – small volumes (2–4 ml) of local anaesthetic are injected into the cerebrospinal fluid (CSF) (q.v.) by means of a spinal needle inserted through the tissues of the back and the dura mater (q.v.). A dense symmetrical motor and sensory block is produced in the lower body. The height of the block is dependent on the volume of local anaesthetic injected, the position of the patient, and individual variation. If the block is too high, the respiratory muscles are paralysed and respiratory arrest occurs. Because the sympathetic nerves are also blocked, hypotension may occur as the blood vessels in the blocked area vasodilate. A spinal headache may occasionally complicate a spinal anaesthetic, possibly because of continuing leakage of CSF through the dural puncture.

Epidural – as with a spinal, anaesthesia is produced in the lower body. The spinal nerves are blocked in the epidural space by injection of local anaesthetic through a fine-bore plastic catheter inserted through a special needle (Tuohy needle). Because of the catheter the block can be augmented if necessary as it begins to wear off. This makes it ideal for the relief of labour pains as well as for operations below the waist. Potential complications are hypotension and headache (due to accidental dural puncture with the Tuohy needle – a rare occurrence). There is a risk of spinal-cord compression by clot or abscess because of the confined space within which it lies. For this reason both spinal and epidural anaesthesia are contraindicated in patients who are receiving anticoagulant drugs or who have generalized or local sepsis.

ANALEPTIC means a restorative medicine, or one which acts as a stimulant of the central nervous system: for example caffeine.

ANALGESIA means loss of the power to feel pain without loss of consciousness. The condition may occur as the result of disease in or damage to nerves. Analgesia can be produced intentionally by the use of pain-killing drugs called *analgesics*. (See also AUDIOANALGESIA; CRYOANALGESIA.)

ANALGESICS are drugs that relieve pain. Unlike local anaesthetics they do not abolish other modalities of sensation. There are many drugs with different modes of action available, and the choice of analgesic will depend on the type and severity of the pain. Mild or moderate pain is usually treated with simple analgesics such as paracetamol, aspirin, or one of the wide range of drugs known collectively as non-steroidal anti-inflammatory drugs (q.v.) (NSAIDS).
Paracetamol acts within the central nervous system by inhibiting prostaglandin (q.v.) biosynthesis. It causes hepatic damage in overdosage.
The NSAIDS (including aspirin) have both central and peripheral action. They inhibit prostaglandin synthetase (cyclo-oxygenase) – an enzyme necessary for the production of certain prostaglandins implicated in the development of inflammation. A central, antipyretic, action also occurs. Side-effects include gastrointestinal bleeding from gastric erosions, inhibition of platelet (q.v.) aggregation, fluid retention, and a variable propensity for renal papillary damage.
Severe pain is often treated using opioid drugs. These mimic the action of naturally occurring analgesics (endorphins and enkephalins (qq.v.) at opioid receptors in the brain and spinal cord. They also produce euphoria, which helps in coping with pain. Respiratory depression, vomiting, constipation, and itching are possible side-effects. The older drugs are naturally occurring purified plant alkaloids (q.v.) (e.g. morphine and papaveretum). Semi-synthetic drugs such as diamorphine (heroin) are also useful and there is now a plethora of synthetic opioids which have various strengths and durations of action (e.g., pethidine, fentanyl, alfentanyl, and sufentanyl).

ANALYSIS means a separation into component parts by determination of the chemical constituents of a substance. The process of analysis is carried out by various means: e.g chromatographic analysis by means of the adsorption column; colorimetric analysis by means of various colour tests; densimetric analysis by estimation of the specific gravity; gasometric analysis by estimating the different gases given off in some process; polariscope analysis by means of the polariscope; volumetric analysis by measuring volumes of liquids. Analysis is also sometimes used as an abbreviation for psycho-analysis (q.v.).

ANAPHYLAXIS is an abnormal response of the body to a foreign substance (antigen); the affected tissues release histamine which causes local or systemic attack. An example is the pain, swelling, eruption, fever and sometimes collapse that may occur after the injection of tetanus antitoxin or immunization against diseases such as diphtheria or measles. The serum used in such injections is the trigger. Some people may suffer from anaphylaxis as a result of allergy to a particular food or substance such as animal hair or plant leaves. On rare occasions a person may be so sensitive that anaphylaxis may lead to profound shock and collapse which, unless the affected person receives urgent medical attention, may cause death.

ANAPLASIA means the state in which a body cell loses its distinctive characters and takes on a more primitive form; it occurs, for example, in cancer, when cells proliferate rapidly.

ANASTOMOSIS is the direct intercommunication of the branches of two or more *veins* or *arteries* without any intervening network of *capillary* vessels. The term also describes the surgical joining of two hollow vessels, nerves or organs to form an intercommunication

ANATOMY is the science which deals with the structure of the bodies of men and animals. Brief descriptions of the anatomy of each important organ are given under the headings of the various organs. It is studied by dissection of bodies bequeathed for the purpose or of the bodies of those who die in hospitals and similar institutions, unclaimed by relatives.

ANCROD is an enzyme (q.v.) present in the venom of the Malayan pit viper which destroys the fibrinogen in blood and thereby prevents the blood clotting. In other words it is an anticoagulant (q.v.).

ANCYLOSTOMIASIS is a parasitic infection caused by the nematodes *Ancylostoma duodenale* and *Necator americanus* which results in hookworm disease. These infections are exceedingly common in tropical and developing countries – millions of people being affected. Classically, *A. duodenale* occurred in the Far East, Mediterranean littoral, and Middle East, and *N. americanus* in tropical Africa, Central and South America, and the Far East; however, in recent years, geographical separation of the two human species is less distinct. In areas where standards of hygiene and sanitation are unsatisfactory, larvae (embryos) enter via intact skin, usually the feet. 'Ground itch' occasionally occurs as larvae enter the body. They then undergo a complex life-cycle, migrating through the lungs, trachea, and pharynx. Adult worms are 5–13 (mean 12) mm in length; their normal habitat is the small intestine – especially jejunum – where they adhere to the mucosa by hooks, thus causing seepage of blood into the lumen. A worm-pair produces large numbers of eggs, which are excreted in faeces; when deposited on moist soil they remain viable for many weeks or months. Clinical manifestations include microcytic hypochromic anaemia, hypoalbuminaemia (low serum protein) and, in a severe case, oedema. A chronic infection in childhood can give rise to physical, mental, and sexual retardation. Treatment is with one of the benzimidazole compounds, usually mebendazole or albendazole; however, in developing countries, cheaper preparations are used, including tetrachloroethylene, bephenium hydroxynaphthoate, and pyrantel embonate. Anaemia usually responds to iron supplements; blood transfusion is rarely indicated.

ANCYLOSTOMA BRAZILIENSIS A nematode infection of dogs, which in humans causes local disease (larva migrans) only, usually on the soles of the feet. It is usually acquired by walking on beaches contaminated with dog faeces in places such as the Caribbean.

ANDROGEN is the general term for any one of a group of hormones which govern the development of the sexual organs and the secondary sexual characteristics of the male. Testosterone, the androgenic hormone formed in the interstitial cells of the testis, controls the development and maintenance of the male sex organs and secondary sex characteristics. In small doses it increases the number of spermatozoa produced, but in large doses it inhibits the gonadotrophic activity of the anterior pituitary gland and suppresses the formation of the spermatozoa. It is both androgenic and anabolic in action. The anabolic effect includes the ability to stimulate protein synthesis and to diminish the catabolism of amino acids, and this is associated with retention of nitrogen, potassium, phosphorus and calcium. Doses in excess of 10 mg daily to the female may produce virilism.

Unconjugated testosterone is rarely used clinically because its derivatives have a more powerful and prolonged effect, and testosterone itself requires implantation into the subcutaneous fat, using a trocar and cannula for maximum therapeutic benefit. Testosterone propionate is prepared in an oily solution, as it is insoluble in water. It is effective for three days and is therefore administered intramuscularly twice weekly. Testosterone phenylpropionate is a long-acting micro-crystalline preparation, which, when given by intramuscular or subcutaneous injection, is effective for two weeks. Methyl-testosterone is only weakly active by mouth though it is absorbed sublingually. It does however produce a cholestatic jaundice in a significant proportion of patients and is therefore better avoided. Mesterolone is an effective oral androgen and is less hepatoxic. It does not inhibit pituitary gonadotrophic production and hence spermatogenesis is unimpaired. Testosterone undecanoate has recently been introduced and may well prove to be the oral androgen of choice.

The androgens in therapeutic use which can be given by mouth include: mesterolone, methyltestosterone, testosterone, testosterone undecanoate. Those that can be given by injection include: testosterone propionate, testosterone phenylpropionate, testosterone enanthate, testosterone esters and drostanolone.

ANENCEPHALY is the term given to the condition in which a child is born with a defect of the skull and absence of the brain. Anencephaly is the most common major malformation of the central nervous system. It has an incidence of 0·65 per 1,000 live births. There is complete absence of the cerebral hemispheres and overlying skull and the brain stem and cerebellum are atrophic. If the pregnancy goes to term the infants rapidly die but in 50 per cent of pregnancies associated with anencephaly spontaneous abortion occurs. It is possible to detect the presence of anencephaly in the fetus by measuring the level of alpha foeto protein in the mother's serum or in the amniotic fluid. (See SPINA BIFIDA.)

ANEUPLOIDY is the state in which there is an abnormal number of chromosomes (q.v.): e.g. Down's syndrome (q.v.) and Turner's syndrome (q.v.).

ANEURINE is an alternative name for vitamin B₁. (See THIAMINE.)

ANEURYSM An aneurysm is a localized swelling or dilatation of an artery due to weakening of its wall. The commonest sites are the aorta, the arteries of the legs, the carotids and the subclavian arteries. Aneurysms may also form in the arteries at the base of the brain (the circle of Willis (q.v.)), usually due to an inherited defect of the arterial wall. Aneurysms usually arise in the elderly, with men affected more commonly than women. The commonest cause is degenerative atheromatous disease, but other rarer causes include trauma, inherited conditions such as Marfan's syndrome, or acquired conditions such as syphilis (q.v.) or polyarteritis nodosa (q.v.). Once formed, the pressure of the circulating blood within the aneurysm causes it to increase in size. At first, there may be no symptoms or signs, but as the aneurysm enlarges it becomes detectable as a swelling which pulsates with each heartbeat. It may also cause pain due to pressure on local nerves or bones. Rupture of the aneurysm may occur at any time, but is much more likely when the aneurysm is large. Rupture is usually a surgical emergency, because the bleeding is arterial and therefore considerable amounts of blood may be lost very rapidly, leading to collapse, shock and even death. Rupture of an aneurysm in the circle of Willis causes subarachnoid haemorrhage.

Treatment Treatment is usually surgical. Once an aneurysm has formed the tendency is for it to enlarge progressively regardlessof any medical therapy. The surgery is often demanding and is therefore usually undertaken only when the aneurysm is large and the risk of rupture is therefore increased. The patient's general fitness for surgery is also an important consideration. The surgery usually involves either bypassing or replacing the affected part of the artery using a conduit made of either vein or a manmade fibre which has been woven or knitted into a tube.

ANGINA is a feeling of constriction or suffocation often accompanied by pain (see ANGINA PECTORIS).

ANGINA PECTORIS is pain in the centre of the chest. Usually exercise – sometimes acute anxiety – brings it on and pain may be severe and felt also in the arms and the jaw. The condition, which is aggravated by cold weather, is the result of the heart's demand for blood being greater than the coronary arteries can provide. This failure is usually due to narrowing of the coronary arteries by *atheroma*; rarely, it may be caused by congenital defects in the arteries rendering them incapable of carrying sufficient blood to meet increased demands from the body. Angina may be relieved or prevented by such drugs as *glyceryl trinitrate* and *propanolol*. If drug treatment does not work, surgery on the coronary arteries such as *angioplasty* or *bypass grafts* may be necessary. People who suffer from angina pectoris need advice on their lifestyle, in particular about diet, exercise and avoidance of smoking or excessive alcohol consumption. They may have high blood pressure, which will also require medical treatment.

ANGIOCARDIOGRAPHY means X-raying of the heart after injection into it of a radio-opaque substance.

ANGIOGRAPHY means rendering the blood-vessels visible on an X-ray film by injecting into them a radio-opaque substance. In the case of arteries this is know as *arteriography*; the corresponding term for veins being *venography* or *phlebography*. This procedure demonstrates whether there is any narrowing of the lumen of the vessel.

ANGIOMA is a tumour composed of blood-vessels. (See TUMOUR and NAEVUS.)

ANGIONEUROTIC OEDEMA is a painless swelling in the sub-cutaneous tissues or the sub-mucosa, usually occurring around the face and especially affecting the eyes, lips and tongue. It is similar in many ways to nettle rash (see URTICARIA). It is caused primarily by food allergy. There is also an hereditary form which is transmitted as an autosomal dominant trait and is due to an enzyme deficiency that inactivates one of the mediators of inflammation called Complement. (See AMINOCAPROIC ACID.)

ANGIOPLASTY A method of treating blockage or narrowing of a blood vessel or heart valve by inserting a balloon into the constriction to reopen it. The technique is used to treat a narrowed artery in the heart or a limb. About 65 per cent of patients treated benefit, but when symptoms persist or recur the procedure may be repeated. There is a small risk of damage to the vessel or valve.

ANGIOTENSIN is a peptide that occurs in two forms I and II. The former results from the action of the enzyme *renin* on alpha globulin (a protein) produced by the liver and passed into the blood. During passage of the blood through the lungs angiotensin I is converted into an active form, angiotensin II, by an enzyme. This active form constricts the blood vessels and stimulates the release of two hormones *vasopressin* and *aldosterone* which raise the blood pressure. (See ANGIOTENSIN-CONVERTING ENZYME (ACE) INHIBITORS).

ANGIOTENSIN-CONVERTING ENZYME INHIBITORS The enzyme that converts angiotensin I to angiotensin II is called angiotensin-converting enzyme. Angiotensin II controls the blood pressure and is the most potent endogenous pressor substance produced in the body; angiotensin I has no such pressor activity. Inhibition of the enzyme that converts angiotensin I to angiotensin II will thus have marked effects on lowering the blood pressure and ACE inhibitors have a valuable role in treating heart failure. Captopril was the first ACE inhibitor to be synthesized. It lowers peripheral resistance by causing arteriolar dilatation and thus lowers blood pressure. Other drugs such as enalapril and lisinopril have since been developed. Some kidney disorders increase the production of angiotensin II and so cause hypertension.

ANGITIS, or ANGIITIS, means inflammation of a vessel such as a blood-vessel, lymph-vessel, or bile-duct.

ÅNGSTRÖM UNIT (called after the Swedish physicist) is a measurement of length and equals 1/10000 micrometre, or one-hundred-millionth of a centimetre. It is represented by the symbol Å and is used to give the length of electro-magnetic waves.

ANHIDROSIS is an abnormal diminution in the secretion of sweat. This may be caused by diseases or a congenital defect.

ANISOCYTOSIS This refers to a variation in the size of red blood cells.

ANKLE is the joint between the leg bones (tibia and fibula) above, and the talus (the Roman dice-bone) below. It is a very strong joint with powerful ligaments binding the bones together at either side, many sinews running over it, and bony projections from the leg bones, which form large bosses on either side, called the outer and inner malleoli, extending about 12 mm (half an inch) below the actual joint. Two common injuries near the ankle are a sprain, on the inner side, consisting of tearing of the internal ligament; and fracture of the fibula (Pott's fracture) on the outer side. (See also JOINTS, DISEASES OF.)

ANKYLOSING SPONDYLITIS (see SPINE AND SPINAL CORD, DISEASES AND INJURIES OF).

ANKYLOSIS is a term meaning the condition of a joint in which the movements are restricted by fibrous bands, or by malformation, or by actual union of the bones. (See JOINTS, DISEASES OF.)

ANKYLOSTOMA (see ANCYLOSTOMIASIS).

ANODYNES are curative measures which soothe pain. They act by removing the cause of pain, by soothing the irritated nerves of the painful part, or by paralysing the part of the brain by which the painful impression is received. Substances which destroy the power of feeling altogether are called anaesthetics (q.v.), those which destroy only the power of feeling pain are analgesics (q.v.).
Varieties Alkaline applications are anodynes to bee-stings. Prolonged application of either cold or heat is an anodyne in inflammation. Chloroform, camphor and menthol are local anodynes, while internally various synthetic products like aspirin soothe pain in distant parts.
Uses Opium is the oldest and most powerful anodyne, but can only be used in cases of excessive pain, because of its tendency to habit-formation. Barbiturates dull pain, but with it the mental faculties, so that they also interfere with the performance of everyday duties. Aspirin and paracetamol seem to have the power of dulling only that part of the brain which perceives the pain, and so are most suitable in slighter pains which do not incapacitate though they interfere with ordinary duties. (For further details, see NEURALGIA; HEADACHE; INFLAMMATION; and the various drugs named.)

ANOPHELES is the generic name of a widely distributed group of mosquitoes, certain species of which transmit to man the parasitic protozoa *Plasmodium*, the agent that causes malaria. *Anopheles maculipennis* and *A. bifurcatus* are both found in England and can both transmit the malaria parasite.

ANOREXIA means loss of appetite. (See APPETITE.)

ANOREXIA NERVOSA (see EATING DISORDERS).

ANOSMIA means loss of sense of smell. (See NOSE, DISEASES OF.)

ANOVULAR Absence of ovulation. Anovular menstruation occurs when a woman takes the contraceptive pill.

ANOXAEMIA means reduction of the oxygen content of the blood below normal limits.

ANOXIA is the term applied to that state in which the body tissues have an inadequate supply of oxygen. This may be because the blood in the lungs does not receive enough oxygen, or because there is not enough blood to receive the oxygen, or because the blood stagnates in the body. (See OXYGEN.)

ANTABUSE (see DISULFIRAM).

ANTACIDS have long been used to treat gastrointestinal disorders, including peptic ulcer, and are still widely used. They neutralize the hydrochloric acid secreted in the stomach's digestive juices and relieve pain and the discomfort of indigestion. A large number of proprietary preparations are on sale to the public and most contain compounds of aluminium or magnesium or a mixture of the two. Other agents include activated dimethicome – an antifoaming agent aimed at relieving flatulence, alginates, which protect against reflux oesophagitis and surface anaesthetics. Antacids commonly prescribed by doctors include aluminium hydroxide, magnesium carbonate and magnesium trisilicate. Sodium bicarbonate and calcium and bismuth compounds are also used, though the latter is best avoided as it may cause neurological side-effects.

ANTAGONIST (*a*) The action of one drug in opposing the action of another. (*b*) A muscle the contraction of which opposes that of another muscle called the *agonist* (q.v.). When the agonist contracts the antagonist relaxes.

ANTE- is a prefix meaning before or forwards.

ANTEFLEXION means the abnormal forward curvature of an organ in which the upper part is sharply bent forward. The term is especially applied to forward displacement of the uterus.

ANTENATAL is a term applied to conditions occurring before birth. It is used with reference both to mother and child. (For Antenatal Clinics, see MATERNITY AND CHILD WELFARE.)

ANTEPARTUM An adjective describing an event before labour starts in pregnancy.

ANTERIOR An adjective that describes or relates to the front part of the body, limbs, or organs.

ANTERIOR TIBIAL SYNDROME (see MUSCLE).

ANTEVERSION is the term applied to the forward tilting of an organ, especially of the uterus.

ANTHELMINTICS are substances which cause the death or expulsion of parasitic worms.

ANTHRACOSIS is the change which takes place in the lungs and bronchial glands of coal miners, and others, who inhale coal dust constantly. The lungs are amazingly efficient in coping with this problem. During a working lifetime a coalminer may inhale around 5000 grams of dust, but at post-mortem examination it is rare to find more than about 40 grams in his lungs. The affected tissues change in colour from greyish pink to jet black, owing to loading with minute carbon particles. (See PNEUMOCONIOSIS.)

ANTHRAX is a very serious disease occurring in sheep and cattle, and in those who tend them or handle the bones, skins and fleeces, even long after removal of the latter from the animals. It is sometimes referred to as malignant pustule, wool-sorters' disease, splenic fever of animals or murrain. It is now a rare condition in the United Kingdom. The cause is a bacillus (*B. anthracis*) which grows in long chains and produces spores of great vitality. These spores retain their life for years, in dried skins and fleeces; they are not destroyed by boiling, freezing, 5 per cent carbolic lotion, or, like many bacilli, by the gastric juice. The disease is communicated from a diseased animal to a crack in the skin, e.g. of a shepherd or butcher, or from contact with contaminated skins or fleeces. Nowadays skins are handled wet, but if

they are allowed to dry so that dust laden with spores is inhaled by the workers an internal form of the disease results. Instances have occurred of the disease being conveyed on shaving brushes made from bristles of diseased animals.

Symptoms (*a*) EXTERNAL FORM This is the 'malignant pustule'. After inoculation of some small wound, a few hours or days elapse, and then a red, inflamed swelling appears, which grows larger till it covers half the face or the breadth of the arm, as the case may be. Upon its summit appears a bleb of pus, which bursts and leaves a black scab, perhaps 12 mm (half an inch) wide. At the same time there is great prostration and fever. The inflammation may last ten days or so, when it slowly subsides and the patient recovers, if surviving the fever and prostration.

(*b*) INTERNAL FORM This takes the form of pneumonia with haemorrhages, when the spores have been drawn into the lungs, or of ulcers of the stomach and intestines, with gangrene of the spleen, when they have been swallowed. It is usually fatal in two or three days.

Prevention is most important by disinfecting all hides, wool and hair coming from areas of the world. An efficient vaccine is now available. Treatment consists of the administration of large doses of penicillin or of one of the tetracyclines.

ANTI- is a prefix meaning against.

ANTIBIOTIC is the term used to describe any antibacterial agent derived from micro-organisms. Such agents destroy or inhibit the growth of other micro-organisms. Examples are penicillin, cephalosporin, aminoglycosides, streptomycin, and tetracycline.

Penicillin was the first antibiotic to be discovered and used in the 1940s. The discovery and isolation in 1958 of the penicillin nucleus, 6-amino penicillanic acid (6-PNA) allowed many new penicillins to be synthesized. These are now the largest single group of antibiotics used in clinical medicine. Most *staphylococci* have now developed resistance to benzylpenicillin, the early form of the drug, because they produce penicillinases, enzymes which break down the drug. Other types of penicillin such as cloxacillin and flucoxacillin are not affected and are used against penicillin-resistant staphylococci..

The cephalosporins are derived from the compound cephalosporin C which is obtained by fermentation of the mould cephalosporium. The cephalosporin nucleus 7 Amino cephalosporanic (7-ICA) acid has been the basis for the production of the semi-synthetic compounds of the cephalosporin nucleus. The first semi-synthetic cephalosporin, cephalothin, appeared in 1962; it was followed by cephaloridine in 1964. The original cephalosporins had to be given by injection but more recent preparations can be given by mouth. The newer preparations are less readily destroyed by beta lactamases and so they have a much broader spectrum of anti-

ANTIBODIES 30

bacterial activity. The newer cephalosporins include cephalexin, cefazolin, cephacetrile, cephapirin, cefamandole, cefuroxine, cephrodine, cefodroxil and cefotaxine. Inactivation of beta lactamase is the basis of bacterial resistance to both the penicillins and the cephalosporins so that attempts to prepare these antibiotics with resistance to beta lactamase is of great importance. A synthetic inhibitor of beta lactamase called clavulanic acid has recently been synthesized. This is used in combination with the penicillins and cephalosporins to prevent resistance. The cephamycins are a new addition to the beta lactam antibiotics. They are similar in structure to the cephalosporins but are produced, not by fungi, but by actinomycetes.

ANTIBODIES are substances in the blood which destroy or neutralize various toxins or 'bodies' (e.g. bacteria), known generally as antigens. The antibodies are formed, usually, as a result of the introduction into the body of the antigens to which they are antagonistic, as in all infectious diseases.

ANTICHOLINERGIC An action or drug that inhibits the activity of acetylcholine (q.v.).

ANTICOAGULANTS are drugs which prevent coagulation of the blood. The main ones now in use are heparin (q.v.), phenindione (q.v.) and warfarin (q.v.). Heparin is a natural anticoagulant which directly affects the blood-clotting process and acts quickly. The other two are synthetic agents and take longer to act; they affect blood coagulation factors. Anticoagulants destroy blood clots in embolism and thrombosis. Patients who are on anticoagulants require to be carefully monitored under medical supervision, and should carry an Anticoagulant Card with instructions about the use of whatever anticoagulant drug they may be taking.

ANTICONVULSANT A drug that reduces or prevents the severity of an epileptic convulsion or seizure. The nature of the fit and the patient's reaction influences the type of anticonvulsant used. Anticonvulsants inhibit the high level of electrical activity in the brain that causes the fit. Among regularly used anticonvulsants are carbamazepine, clonazopam, diazepam, phenobarbitone, phenytoin, primidone, and sodium valporate (SEE EPILEPSY).

ANTIDEPRESSANTS are drugs which relieve depressive illness, characterized by depressed or absent effect, poor concentration, loss of interest, low self-esteem and changes in sleep and appetite (SEE MENTAL ILLNESS). Although some may cause sedation, they are quite different from the minor tranquillizers such as the benzodiazepines. Tolerance and habituation do not occur so they are not addictive.

Unlike the sedative effect, which lasts about eight hours, the antidepressant effect takes two to four weeks to develop, and the reason for this delay is not known. The antidepressant should be continued for at least six months after recovery in order to prevent relapse.

The tricyclic antidepressants were introduced in the late 1950s. They affect a number of brain transmitters and peripheral nerve receptors. Their antihistaminic action is thought to cause sedation, and their anticholinergic action causes dry mouth, constipation, tremor, blurring of vision and occasionally retention of urine and, for men, difficulties with erection and ejaculation.

Many tetracyclic and other compounds have been introduced with the same pharmacological profile as the tricyclics; some of them have been withdrawn because of serious side-effects.

The latest wave of antidepressants are called selective serotonin re-uptake inhibitors (SSRIs) because they share the tricyclic action on serotonin but lack the tricyclic action on other transmitters such as noradrenaline (q.v.). They are thought to be as effective as the tricyclics and to be safer in overdosage. Because their patents have not yet run out, they are very much more expensive.

The other major group of antidepressants is the monoamine oxidase inhibitors (MAOIs), such as phenelzine, which are thought to be more helpful in the 'atypical depressions' characterized by an excess, rather than a deficiency, of appetite and sleep. They can cause episodes of hypertension after the ingestion of foods containing tyramine, such as cheese, broad beans and meat extracts. Recently a new group of MAOIs has been introduced, such as moclobemide, in which the inhibition of the enzyme is reversible, and these are thought to be safer.

ANTIDIURETIC HORMONE (ADH) (see VASOPRESSIN).

ANTIDOTES are remedies which neutralize the effects of poisons. Thus acids have alkalis as antidote and vice versa.

ANTIEMETIC A drug that counteracts nausea and sickness. Some antihistamines and anticholinergics have an antiemetic effect. They are used to combat motion sickness or nausea and vomiting brought on by other drugs.

ANTIGEN is the term applied to a substance which causes the formation of antibodies: it is usually a protein that is foreign to the body.

ANTIHISTAMINE DRUGS are drugs which antagonize the action of histamine (q.v.) and are therefore of value in the treatment of certain allergic conditions. They are also of some value in the treatment of vasomotor rhinitis. They reduce rhinorrhoea and sneezing but are usually less effective in relieving nasal congestion.

All antihistamines are also useful in the treatment of urticaria and certain allergic skin rashes, insect bites and stings. They are also used in the treatment of drug allergies. Chlorpheniramine or promethazine injections are useful in the emergency treatment of angioneurotic oedema and anaphylaxis.

There is little evidence that any one antihistamine is superior to another and patients vary considerably in their response to them. The antihistamines differ in their duration of action and in the incidence of side-effects such as drowsiness. Most are short-acting, but some (such as promethazine) work for up to twelve hours. They all cause sedation but promethazine, trimeprazine and dimenhydrinate tend to be more sedating while chlorpheniramine and cyclizine are less so, as are astemizole, oxatomide and terfenadine. Patients should be warned that their ability to drive or operate machinery may be impaired and that the effects of alcohol may be increased.

ANTIHYPERTENSIVE DRUGS A group of drugs which are used to treat high blood pressure (hypertension). Untreated hypertension leads to strokes, heart attacks and heart failure. The high incidence of hypertension in western countries has led to intensive research to discover antihypertensive drugs and many have been marketed. The drugs may work by reducing the power of the heart beat, by dilating the blood vessels or by increasing the excretion of salts and water in the urine (diuresis). Antihypertensive treatment has greatly improved the prognosis of patients with high blood pressure by cutting the frequency of heart and renal failure (q.v.), stroke (q.v.), and coronary thrombosis (q.v.). Among the groups of drugs now in use are diuretics (q.v.), beta-adrenoceptor-blocking agents (q.v.), calcium-channel blockers (q.v.), ACE inhibitors (q.v.), vasodilators and centrally acting agents such as methyldopa.(See HYPERTENSION; MALIGNANT HYPERTENSION.)

ANTIMETABOLITES are a group of drugs which have been introduced for the treatment of certain forms of malignant disease. Chemically, they closely resemble substances (or metabolites) which are essential for the life and growth of cells. When introduced into the body they are 'mistaken', so to speak, by the cell for the corresponding metabolite, thereby preventing the cell from making use of the metabolite, or substance, which is essential for its growth. By this means the life of the cell is affected and it ultimately dies.

ANTIMONY is the name applied to a metal and also to its sulphide, a black powder found in nature. The tartrate of potassium and antimony is commonly known as tartar emetic in reference to its chief property. The preparations of antimony, some of which are used in the treatment of tropical diseases such as kala-azar, are all irritants; hence in large doses they are poisons.

ANTIMUSCARINE is a pharmacological effect that inhibits the action of acetylcholine (q.v.), a chemical neurotransmitter released at the junctions (synapses) of parasympathetic nerves (q.v.) and at the junctions between nerves and muscles.

ANTIPERISTALSIS is a movement in the bowels and stomach by which the food and other contents are passed upwards, instead of in the proper direction. (See PERISTALSIS.)

ANTI-PSYCHOTIC DRUGS (see NEUROLEPTICS).

ANTIPYRETICS are measures used to reduce temperature in fever.
Varieties Cold-sponging, wet-pack, baths and diaphoretic drugs such as quinine, salicylates and aspirin.
Uses (see under above headings).

ANTISEPTICS prevent the growth of disease-causing micro-organisms without damaging living tissues.

Among chemicals used are boric acid, carbolic acid, hydrogen peroxide and products based on coal tar, such as cresol. Chlorhexidines, iodine, formaldehyde, flavines, alcohol and hexachlorophane are also used. Antiseptics are applied to prevent infection – for example, in preparing the skin before operation. They are also used to treat infected wounds.

ANTISPASMODICS (see SPASMOLYTICS).

ANTITOXINS, ANTITOXIC SERUM (see IMMUNOLOGY: serum therapy).

ANTIVENINE, or ANTIVENOM, is the name given to SNAKE VENOM ANTISERUM, which is produced by the injection of venom from poisonous animals such as snakes, spiders or scorpions into animals in small but increasing doses. The animal becomes immune to the particular venom injected. Native tradition in countries in Africa and Asia has it that a comparable method provides protection against snake bites in the treatment given by traditional snake doctors who specialize in the treatment of snake bites. The antiserum prepared from the serum of such immunized animals is effective in neutralizing venom injected by the bite of a snake of the same species. No antiserum effective against all venoms is available. The custom is for each country to prepare antisera able to neutralize the venoms of indigenous snakes. The antivenom active against the venom of the adder is known as Zagreb antivenom. To be of any use, it must be administered as soon as possible after the snake bite. (See BITES AND STINGS.)

ANTROSTOMY is the operation in which an opening is made through the nose into the maxillary antrum. (See ANTRUM.)

ANTRUM means a natural hollow or cavity. The *maxillary antrum* is now known as the maxillary sinus (see SINUS). The *mastoid antrum* is situated in the mastoid process, the mass of bone felt behind the ear. It may become the seat of an abscess in cases of suppuration of the middle ear (see EAR, DISEASES OF). The *pyloric antrum* is the part of the stomach immediately preceding the pylorus (q.v.).

ANURIA is a condition in which no urine is voided. (See KIDNEYS, DISEASES OF: glomerulonephritis; URINE.)

ANUS is the opening at the lower end of the bowel. It is kept closed by two muscles, the external and internal sphincters. The latter is a muscular ring which extends about 25 mm (1 inch) up the bowel, is nearly 6 mm (¼ inch) thick, and is kept constantly contracted by the action of a nerve centre in the spinal cord. In disease of the spinal cord the muscle may be paralysed, and inability to retain the motions results.

ANUS, DISEASES OF (see RECTUM, DISEASES OF).

ANXIETY STATE (see NEUROSIS).

ANXIOLYTICS are drugs for the relief of anxiety. They will induce sleep when given in large doses at night and so are hypnotics as well. Conversely most hypnotics will sedate when given in divided doses during the day. Prescription of these drugs is widespread but physical and psychological dependence occurs as well as tolerance to their effects. This is particularly true of the barbiturates which are now limited in their use, but also applies to the benzodiazepines. Withdrawal syndromes may occur if drug treatment is stopped too abruptly. Hypnotic sedatives and anxiolytics should therefore not be prescribed indiscriminately, but reserved for short courses. Among the anxiolytics are the widely used benzodiazepines (q.v.), the rarely used barbiturates, and the occasionally prescribed drugs such as buspirone (q.v.) and beta-blockers like propanolol (q.v.) and oxprenolol (q.v.).

AORTA is the large vessel which opens out of the left ventricle of the heart and carries blood to all the body. It is about 45 cm (1½ feet) long and 2·5 cm (1 inch) wide. Like other arteries it possesses three coats, of which the middle one is much the thickest. This consists partly of muscle fibre, but is mainly composed of an elastic substance, called elastin. The aorta passes first to the right, and lies nearest the surface behind the end of the second right rib-cartilage; then it curves backwards and to the left, passes down behind the left lung close to the backbone, and through an opening in the diaphragm into the abdomen, where it divides, at the level of the navel, into the two common iliac arteries, which carry blood to the lower limbs. Its branches, in order, are: two coronary arteries to the heart wall; the brachiocephalic, left common carotid, and left subclavian arteries to the head, neck and upper limbs; several small branches to the oesophagus, bronchi, and other organs of the chest; nine pairs of intercostal arteries which run round the body between the ribs; one pair of subcostal arteries which is in series with the intercostal arteries; four (or five) lumbar arteries to the muscles of the loins; coeliac trunk to the stomach, liver and pancreas; two mesenteric arteries to the bowels; and suprarenal, renal and testicular arteries to the suprarenal body, kidney, and testicle on each side. From the termination of the aorta rises a small branch, the median sacral artery, which runs down into the pelvis. In the female the ovarian arteries replace the testicular.

The chief diseases of the aorta are atheroma and aneurysm. (See ARTERIES, DISEASES OF; ANEURYSM; and COARCTATION OF THE AORTA.)

AORTIC REGURGITATION The back flow of blood through the aortic valve of the heart into the left ventricle caused by an incompetent valve. The failure to close may be caused by a congenital defect or by damage from disease. The defect may be cured by surgical replacement of the damaged valve with an artificial valve. (See HEART DISEASES.)

AORTIC STENOSIS Narrowing of the aortic valve which obstructs the flow of blood through it with serious effects on the heart and the circulation. The muscle in the left ventricle works harder to compensate for the obstruction and thickens as a result. Stenosis is usually caused by the deposition of calcium on the valve and is commonly associated with atheroma. Untreated, the condition leads to heart failure, but nowadays the stenosis can be treated surgically.

AORTIC VALVE The valve that controls the flow of blood from the aorta to the left ventricle of the heart. (See HEART.)

AORTITIS means a degenerative condition of the lining of the aorta. It is usually produced by syphilis.

AORTOGRAPHY is the technique of rendering the aorta visible in an X-ray film by injecting a radio-opaque substance into it. (See also ANGIOGRAPHY.)

APERIENTS are medicines which produce a natural movement of the bowels. (See CONSTIPATION; PURGATIVES.)

APEX is the pointed portion of any organ which has a conical shape. The apex of each lung reaches about 3·5 to 5 cm (1½ or 2 inches) above the collar-bone into the neck. In health the apex of the heart can be felt below the fifth rib immediately inside the nipple.

APEX BEAT   This is the beat of the apex of the heart, which can be felt through the skin to the left of the breastbone between the fifth and sixth ribs.

APGAR SCORE is a method of assessing a baby's condition at birth, in which a value of 0, 1 or 2 is given to each of five signs: colour, heart-rate, muscle tone, respiratory (or breathing) effort, and the response to stimulation. A total score of 10 indicates that the newborn child is in excellent condition.

APHAKIA is a term which means absence of the lens of the eye.

APHASIA means a loss of the power of speech, due to injury to the centres which govern this act in the brain. The higher of these centres, which have to do with forming the ideas of speech, putting words together in sentences, and governing the movements of mouth, tongue and larynx, lie on the surface of the cerebral hemispheres, especially of the left; while the lower centres, which directly bring the muscles of the voice organs into action, under superintendence of the higher ones, are in the medulla or hind brain.
Causes   The cause is destruction of a portion of the brain, including one of these higher centres, owing to rupture of a blood-vessel, and haemorrhage into the brain tissue; or owing to blocking of a blood-vessel by an embolus (see EMBOLISM), or by clotting of the blood on the diseased wall of a vessel (see THROMBOSIS), any one of which cuts off the supply of blood to the part concerned. The causes are thus the same as in a stroke, and aphasia may be one of the symptoms of a stroke especially when the right side of the body is paralysed, or may occur by itself, according to the extent of brain involved. Other diseases, such as tumours, may also be the cause, the important factor being interference with the functions of certain definite areas of the brain.
Varieties   It was first pointed out by Broca that the inferior frontal gyrus on the left side of the brain in right-handed persons, and vice versa in left-handed persons, is, after death, found to be diseased in those who have, in life, suffered from inability to speak, although the intelligence and powers of silent reading and of writing may have remained. Such a condition is known as *motor aphasia*. But the state is generally more complicated. In addition to Broca's speech area, which governs the movements of the tongue, mouth and larynx that frame words to express ideas, there is a centre in the middle frontal gyrus of the left side, which regulates the power of writing intelligibly, and disease of this region produces loss of power to write rationally, even though the hand remains quite able to hold a pen, this condition being known as *agraphia*. These two forms involve loss of power of *production* of speech and writing, but there are corresponding losses of power of *perception* known as *word blindness* and *word deafness*, the two conditions being grouped together as *sensory aphasia*. In the former of these the afflicted person is unable to read correctly, though his vision is perfect, and he may be able to spell and even to write, though not to read what he writes. This condition is due to disease in the angular gyrus. In word deafness the disability consists in failure to understand what is said, and, though the sufferer hears perfectly, the sounds are to him like those of a foreign tongue which he does not understand; in this case the disease lies in the superior temporal gyrus. There are still more complicated forms in which the disease affects, not the surface of the brain, but the strands of nerve fibres, which run from one centre to another and reduce the working of the whole arrangement to a system.

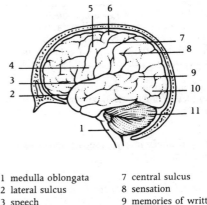

1 medulla oblongata	7 central sulcus
2 lateral sulcus	8 sensation
3 speech	9 memories of written
4 movements of tongue	words
5 movements of trunk	10 sight
6 movements of leg	11 cerebellum

Areas on the left surface of cerebrum associated with definite functions.

Symptoms   The disorder generally follows a stroke and exists along with some paralysis on the right side of the body. *Aphasia* may come on suddenly and last only a few hours or days, being due then to a temporary circulatory disturbance in the brain. Generally it is permanent, and, naturally, a person with aphasia has always some mental impairment. Sometimes he is absolutely without the power of speech. When the condition is one of *sensory aphasia*, names of persons, of places, even of the commonest household articles.

Treatment This is as in stroke, of which the condition often forms a part (see STROKE). The condition is seldom much improved if it has lasted more than a week without improvement. But in some patients improvement is achieved by teaching the afflicted person to read and speak just as one would teach a child, a new part of the brain apparently being educated.

APHONIA means loss of voice. It is caused by some disorder in the throat or in the nerves proceeding to the throat muscles, or by hysteria. (See VOICE AND SPEECH.)

APHTHOUS ULCER A small painful ulcer in the lining (mucosa) of the mouth. It is usually self limiting.

APICECTOMY is the minor operation carried out to try to save a tooth which has an abscess on it or which does not respond to root treatment. In this the abscess and the apex of the tooth are removed.

APLASIA The complete or partial failure of tissue or an organ to develop.

APNOEA A general term meaning the cessation of breathing. Apnoea is a medical emergency. Death soon follows if breathing is not quickly restored. Apnoea may be caused by an obstruction to the airway, for example by the tongue during general anaesthesia, or by a disturbance of the mechanisms that control breathing. Rapid heavy breathing reduces the blood levels of carbon dioxide and can lead to a brief period of apnoea.

APO- is a prefix implying separation or derivation from.

APODIA Absence of the foot.

APOMORPHINE is a crystalline alkaloid closely related to morphine and having a powerful emetic action. Apomorphine hydrochloride is given hypodermically in doses of 2 to 8 mg in cases of poisoning by non-corrosive agents in which the patient is unable to swallow or a very rapid emetic action is desired. It is also used to control motor fluctuations in Parkinson's disease that cannot be controlled by levodopa.

APONEUROSIS is the term applied to the white fibrous membrane which serves as an investment for the muscles and which covers the skull beneath the scalp.

APOPLEXY (see STROKE).

APPENDICECTOMY, or appendectomy, is the operation for the removal of the appendix vermiformis.

APPENDICITIS This is an inflammatory condition of the appendix, and is a common surgical emergency, affecting mainly adolescents and young adults. It is usually due to a combination of obstruction and infection of the appendix, and has a variable clinical course ranging from episodes of mild self-limiting abdominal pain to life-threatening illness. Abdominal pain beginning in the centre of the abdomen but which later shifts position to the right iliac fossa is the classical symptom. The patient usually has accompanying fever and sometimes nausea, vomiting, loss of appetite, diarrhoea, or even constipation. The precise symptoms vary with the exact location of the appendix within the abdomen. In some individuals the appendix may 'grumble' with repeated mild attacks which resolve spontaneously. In an acute attack, the inflammatory process begins first in the wall of the appendix but, if the disease progresses, the appendix can become secondarily infected and pus may form within it. The blood supply may become compromised and its wall may become gangrenous. Eventually the appendix may rupture, giving rise to a localized abscess in the abdomen or, more rarely, free pus within the abdomen which causes generalized peritonitis (q.v.). Rupture of the appendix is a serious complication and the patient may be severely unwell.

Treatment The best treatment is prompt surgical removal of the diseased appendix, usually with antibiotic cover. If performed early, before rupture occurs, the procedure is normally straightforward and recovery swift. If the appendix has already ruptured and there is abscess formation or free intra-abdominal pus, surgery is still the best treatment but postoperative complications are more likely, and full recovery may be slower. (See PERITONITIS.)

APPENDIX is a term applied to appendages of several hollow organs. The epiploic appendices are a number of tags of fat hanging from the outer surface of the large intestine. The appendices of the larynx are two pouches, one on either side between the false and true vocal cords. The term appendix is most commonly applied to the vermiform appendix of the large intestine. It is a tubular prolongation of the large intestine with an average length of 9 or 10 cm and a width of 6 mm. It lies in the right lower corner of the abdomen and has peritoneal, muscular and mucous coats similar to those of the rest of the intestine.

APPETITE is the craving for the food necessary to maintain the body and to supply it with sufficient energy to carry on its functions. The ultimate cause of appetite is a question of supply and demand in the muscles and various organs, but the proximate cause is doubtful.

Unlike hunger, it is probably an acquired, rather than an inborn, sensation. Whatever other factors may be concerned, the tone of the stomach is of importance. Important factors in stimulating appetite are anticipation and the sight and smell of well-cooked food. Individuals who eat unsuitable substances such as faeces are described as suffering from *pica*, which occurs sometimes during pregnancy, in children, in hysteria, and often in mental disorders. The two chief disorders, however, are excessive increase of appetite and diminution or loss of appetite.

Excessive appetite may be simply a bad habit, due to habitual over-indulgence in good food, and resulting in gout, obesity, etc., according to the other habits and constitution of the person. It may also be a sign of diabetes mellitus or thyrotoxicosis. (See EATING DISORDERS.)

Diminished appetite is a sign common to almost all diseases causing general weakness, because the activity of the stomach and the secretion of gastric juice fail early when vital power is low. It is the most common sign of dyspepsia due to gastritis (see DYSPEPSIA) and of cancer of the stomach. In some cases it is a manifestation of stress or strain such as domestic worry or difficulties at work. Indeed, appetite seems to be particularly susceptible to emotional disturbances, as is evidenced by the linked conditions of bulimia (pathological overeating) and anorexia nervosa (pathological dieting). These are dealt with under their respective headings.

APPROVED NAMES is the term used for names devised or selected by the British Pharmacopoeia Commission for new drugs. The intention is that if any of the drugs to which these Approved Names are applied should eventually be included in the *British Pharmacopoeia* the Approved Name should be its official title. The issue of an Approved Name, however, does not imply that the substance will necessarily be included in the *British Pharmacopoeia* or that the Commission is prepared to recommend the use of the substance.

APRAXIA means loss of power to carry out regulated movements. Although there is no muscle weakness or incoordination, there is difficulty in formulating movement patterns.

APYREXIA means absence of fever.

ARACHNODACTYLY, or MARFAN'S SYNDROME, is a congenital condition characterized by extreme length and slenderness of the fingers and toes and, to a lesser extent, of the limbs and trunk, laxity of the ligaments, and dislocation of the lens of the eye. The antero-posterior diameter of the skull is abnormally long, and the jaw is prominent. There may also be abnormalities of the heart.

ARACHNOID MEMBRANE is one of the membranes covering the brain and spinal cord (see BRAIN). Arachnoiditis is the name applied to inflammation of this membrane.

ARBOVIRUSES are a group of around 200 viruses, which are transmitted to man by arthropods (q.v.). They include the viruses of dengue (q.v.) and yellow fever (q.v.) which are transmitted by mosquitoes.

ARC EYE   Damage to the corneal surface of the eye caused by ultraviolet light (q.v.) from arc welding. A painful condition, it usually heals if the eyes are covered with pads for a day or two. It can be prevented by the proper use of protective goggles. A similar condition occurs in snow blindness or when someone fails to protect the eyes when using sun-tan lamps.

ARCUS SENILIS (see EYE DISEASES).

ARENAVIRUSES are a group of viruses, so called because under the electron microscope they have a sand-sprinkled (Latin, *arenosus*) appearance. Among the diseases in man for which they are responsible are lassa fever (q.v.) in West Africa, Argentinian haemorrhagic fever (mortality rate 3 to 15 per cent), a similar disease in Bolivia (mortality rate 18 per cent), and lymphocytic choriomeningitis, in which deaths are uncommon.

AREOLA literally means a small space, and is the term applied to the red or dusky ring round the nipple, or round an inflamed part. Increase in the duskiness of the areola on the breast is an important early sign of pregnancy.

ARGYLL ROBERTSON PUPIL is a condition (described originally by Dr Argyll Robertson) in which the pupils contract when the eyes converge on a near object, but fail to contract when a bright light falls on the eye. It is found in several diseases, especially in locomotor ataxia and neurosyphilis, an advanced manifestation of syphilis (q.v.).

ARGYRIA, or ARGYRIOSIS means the effect produced by taking silver salts over a long period, and consists of a deep duskiness of the skin, especially of the exposed parts.

ARM is the part of the upper limb between the shoulder and elbow, but is generally taken to include also the forearm and shoulder regions. The upper limb is attached to the body by the strong pectoral muscles in front and by several powerful muscles springing from the spine and ribs behind. The great mobility of the shoulder is largely due to the fact that the only contact with the bones of the trunk takes place between the collar-bone and the upper end of the sternum or breast-bone, the shoulder- blade sliding freely between the muscles of the back as the arm is raised and lowered. The bones of the arm are the clavicle or collar-bone and the scapula or shoulder-blade lying at the upper part of the chest, the humerus, a single bone in the upper arm, and the radius and ulna lying side by side in the forearm. Eight small bones compose the wrist (or carpus) and connect the hand with the lower end of the radius.

The shoulder-joint is of the ball-and-socket variety, the head of the humerus resting against the glenoid cavity of the shoulder-blade. The elbow is a hinged joint formed at the lower end of the humerus above, while the ulna forms the chief part of the joint below, the radius resting lightly against the humerus. When the hand is rotated so as to lie palm up or back up, the radius in the first case lies alongside the ulna and in the latter crosses over it. The chief muscle which bends the elbow is the biceps in front of the upper arm, while the triceps lying behind straightens the limb. A group of muscles attached at the inner side of the elbow act to bend the wrist and fingers; another group of muscles attached to the outer side of the elbow have the general action of straightening and bending backwards the wrist and fingers.

One large artery (brachial artery) runs down the inner side of the upper arm corresponding to the seam of the coat sleeve in position. At the elbow this divides into two branches, the radial and ulnar arteries. The radial artery can be felt pulsating near the wrist and is generally known as the pulse. The ulnar artery lies to the inner side of the forearm, deeply imbedded in muscles. A large group of nerves lies at the inner side of the armpit, and these nerves run downwards to supply the muscles and skin of the arm. The ulnar nerve can readily be felt behind the inner side of the elbow, where it is exposed to bruising and is popularly known as the 'funny bone'. The large radial nerve runs down the back of the upper arm and the outer side of the forearm. At the back of the upper arm it is often damaged, leading then to the condition known as drop-wrist (q.v.), in which the hand hangs helpless and cannot be raised.

The collar-bone, by reason of its exposed position, is liable to fracture from falls on the shoulder, and the radius is often broken by falls on the palm of the hand. The shoulder-joint, on account of its great mobility, is prone to be dislocated in twists of the upper arm, but the elbow-joint is seldom injured. A small bursa or cavity lies between the skin and the end of the ulna at the point of the elbow, and this is often inflamed as the result of injury, and in the same way as the bursa in front of the knee is affected in the condition known as housemaid's knee. (See BURSITIS.)

ARMPIT, or AXILLA, is the pyramidal hollow between the upper arm and chest, bounded in front by the pectoral or breast muscles, behind by the shoulder-blade and its muscles, and running up to a point beneath the collar-bone. It contains the axillary vessels and nerves which run to the arm, also much fatty tissue, many sweat glands and lymphatic glands. The latter

are important, because in poisoned wounds of the arm they may become inflamed, resulting in abscess; and still more, because in cancer of the breast they may become infected with cancer, and have to be removed with the breast. Wounds in the armpit are dangerous on the outer, front, and back walls, because large blood vessels run there.

ARRHYTHMIA means any variation from the normal regular rhythm of the heart-beat. The condition is produced by some affection interfering with the mechanism which controls the beating of the heart, and includes the following disorders: sinus arrhythmia, atrial fibrillation, atrial flutter, heart block, extrasystole, pulsus alternans, and paroxysmal atrial tachycardia, ventricular tachycardia and ventricular fibrillation. (See HEART DISEASES.)

ARROWROOT is a West Indian plant (*Maranta arundinacea*). As sold, it is a white powder, consisting of almost pure starch, derived from the root of the plant. It is used as an invalid food, because it is easy to digest, but it must, of course, be combined with other forms of nourishment.

ARSENIC is a metal, but is better known by its oxide, white arsenic, by two arsenites of copper, Scheele's green and emerald green, and by two sulphides of arsenic, orpiment or king's yellow, and realgar. It has been traditionally used in many industrial and commercial products but use is now greatly restricted. If taken – or given – over long periods, larger and larger doses can be tolerated, till at last a quantity many times the poisonous dose has no apparent ill-effect.

Most poisoning occurs through accidental ingestion, though arsenic has been used to murder people. Industrial poisoning, once common, is now rare. Poisoning may be acute or chronic, the former causing inflammation of the stomach lining, resulting in nausea, vomiting, diarrhoea, and sweating. Chronic poisoning manifests as tiredness, weakness, loss of hair and dry and pigmented skin. Treatment includes the administration of dimercaprol. (See POISONS and APPENDIX 2: ADDRESSES.)

ARTEFACT (See artifact).

ARTERIES are vessels which convey oxygenated blood away from the heart to the tissues of the body, limbs, and internal organs. In the case of most arteries, the blood has been purified by passing through the lungs, and is consequently bright red in colour, but in the pulmonary arteries which convey it to the lungs it is unoxygenated, dark, and like the blood in veins.

The arterial system begins at the left ventricle of the heart with the aorta (see AORTA), which gives off branches that subdivide into smaller and smaller vessels, the final divisions, called

1 external carotid
2 superior and inferior thyroid
3 brachiocephalic (innominate)
4 internal thoracic
5 lateral thoracic
6 brachial
7 superior mesenteric
8 inferior mesenteric
9 radial
10 ulnar
11 obturator
12 inferior gluteal
13 femoral
14 deep femoral
15 perforating
16 deep palmar arch
17 superficial palmar arch

18 digital
19 anterior tibial
20 peroneal (fibular)
21 arcuate
22 medial malleolar
23 plantar arch
24 superficial temporal
25 occipital
26 internal carotid
27 vertebral
28 common carotid
29 left subclavian
30 aortic arch
31 outline of heart
32 axillary
33 intercostal aortic
34 aorta
35 coeliac
36 left renal
37 spermatic
38 common iliac
39 internal iliac
40 external iliac
41 internal pudendal
42 descending genicular
43 popliteal
44 posterior tibial
45 dorsalis pedis

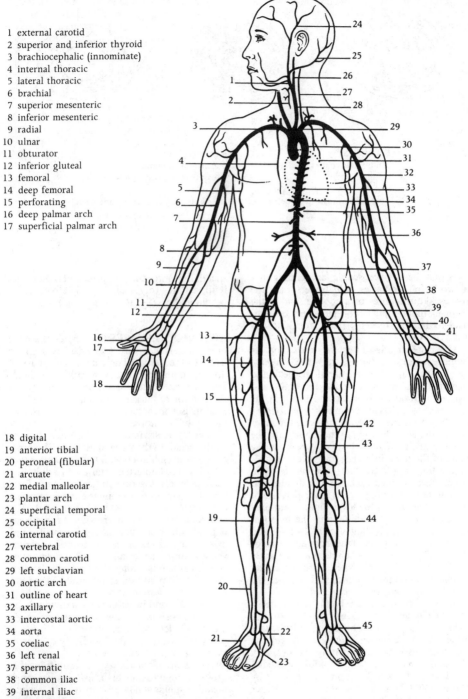

Diagram of body's arterial system.

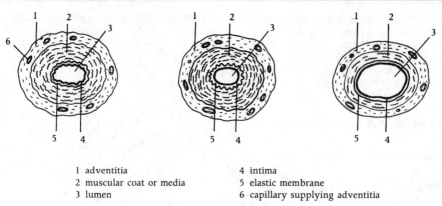

1 adventitia
2 muscular coat or media
3 lumen

4 intima
5 elastic membrane
6 capillary supplying adventitia

Cross-sections showing structures of (left to right) artery, arteriole and vein.

arterioles, being microscopic, and ending in a network of capillaries, which perforate the tissues like the pores of a sponge, and bathe them in blood that is collected and brought back to the heart by veins. (See CIRCULATION OF THE BLOOD.)

The chief arteries after the *aorta* and its branches (see AORTA) are: (1) the *common carotid*, running up each side of the neck and dividing into *internal carotid* to the brain, and *external carotid* to the neck and face; (2) the *subclavian* to each arm, continued by the *axillary* in the armpit, and the *brachial* along the inner side of the arm, dividing at the elbow into the *radial* and the *ulnar*, which unite across the palm of the hand in arches that give branches to the fingers; (3) the two *common iliacs*, in which the aorta ends, each of which divides into the *internal iliac* to the organs in the pelvis, and the *external iliac* to the lower limb, continued by the *femoral* in the thigh, and the *popliteal* behind the knee, dividing into the *anterior* and *posterior tibial* arteries to the front and back of the leg. The latter passes behind the inner ankle to the sole of the foot, where it forms arches similar to those in the hand, and supplies the foot and toes by *plantar branches*.

Structure: The arteries are highly elastic, dilating at each heart-beat as blood is driven into them, and forcing it on by their resiliency (see PULSE). Every artery has *three coats*: (*a*) the outer or adventitia, consisting of ordinary strong fibrous tissue; (*b*) the middle or media, consisting of muscular fibres supported by elastic fibres, which in some of the larger arteries form distinct membranes; and (*c*) the inner or intima, consisting of a layer of yellow elastic tissue on whose inner surface rests a layer of smooth plate-like endothelial cells, over which flows the blood. In the larger arteries the muscle of the middle coat is largely replaced by elastic fibres, which render the artery still more expansile and elastic. When an artery is cut across, the muscular coat instantly shrinks, drawing the cut end within the fibrous

sheath that surrounds the artery, and bunching it up, so that a very small hole is left to be closed by blood-clot. (See HAEMORRHAGE.)

ARTERIES, DISEASES OF   Arteries are the blood vessels that convey blood away from the heart to the tissues. The commonest cause of arterial disease is a degenerative condition known as atherosclerosis. Less commonly, inflammation of the arteries occurs. This inflammation is known as arteritis and occurs in a variety of conditions.

ATHEROSCLEROSIS is due to the deposition of cholesterol into the walls of arteries. The process starts in childhood with the development of fatty streaks lining the arteries. In adulthood these progress, scarring and calcifying to form irregular narrowings within the arteries eventually leading to blockage of the vessel. The consequence of the narrowing or blockage depends on which vessels are involved – diseased cerebral vessels cause strokes, coronary vessels cause angina and heart attacks, renal vessels cause renal failure and peripheral arteries cause limb ischaemia (localized bloodlessness).

Risk factors predisposing individuals to atherosclerosis include age, male gender, raised plasma cholesterol concentration, high blood pressure, smoking, a family history of atherosclerosis, diabetes and obesity.

ARTERITIS occurs in a variety of conditions that produce inflammation in the arteries. Examples include syphilis – now rare in Britain – which produces inflammation of the aorta with subsequent dilatation (aneurysm formation) and risk of rupture; giant cell arteritis (temporal arteritis), a condition usually affecting the elderly, which involves the cranial arteries and leads to headache, tenderness over the temporal arteries and the risk of sudden blindness; Takayasau's syndrome, predominantly affecting young females, involves the aortic arch and its major branches, leading to the absence of pulses in affected vessels; polyarteritis nodosa is a condition causing multiple small nodules to form on the smaller arteries. General symptoms such as fever, malaise, weakness, anorexia and weight loss are accompanied by local manifestations of ischaemia (bloodlessness) in different parts of the body.

ARTERIOGRAPHY (see ANGIOGRAPHY).

ARTERIOLE is a small artery.

ARTERIO-VENOUS ANEURYSM is an abnormal communication between an artery and a vein. It is usually the result of an injury, such as a stab or a gunshot wound, which involves both a neighbouring artery and vein.

ARTERITIS means inflammation of an artery. (SEE ARTERIES, DISEASES OF.)

ARTHRALGIA   Pain in a joint in which there is no swelling or other indications of arthritis.

ARTHRITIS refers to any condition of joints of the limbs or spine associated with inflammatory or structural change. It is distinguished from arthralgia which simply implies joint pain with or without any inflammatory or structural change. The two main categories of arthritis are osteoarthritis, in which the primary change is thought of as mechanical failure of articular cartilage, and rheumatoid arthritis, in which the primary problem is a chronic inflammation of the synovial lining, of joints, tendon sheaths and bursae. Other less common forms of inflammatory arthritis include psoriatic arthritis, Reiter's syndrome, colitic arthritis and Behçet's syndrome. Spondarthritis refers to an inflammatory arthritis with involvement of the spine and is often associated with the HLA B27 tissue type. (See OSTEOARTHRITIS; RHEUMATOID ARTHRITIS; RHEUMATIC FEVER.)

ARTHRODESIS is the operation for fixing a joint in a given position, from which it cannot be moved. It results in a pain-free, stable, strong joint in certain cases of joint disease such as osteoarthrosis of the knee.

ARTHROPATHY is a term applied to any form of joint disease.

ARTHROPLASTY is the term applied to the operation for the making of a new joint as, for example, in advanced cases of osteoarthrosis of the hip, or the loosening of a fixed or stiff joint.

ARTHROPODS are segmented invertebrates with jointed legs. They include a wide range of organisms, such as scorpions, mites, ticks, spiders and centipedes (see ARBOVIRUSES).

ARTHROSCOPE: An instrument that enables the operator to see inside a joint cavity and, if necessary, take a biopsy or carry out an operation.

ARTICULAR means anything connected with a joint: e.g. articular rheumatism.

ARTICULATION is a term employed in two senses in medicine, either meaning the enunciation of words and sentences or meaning the type of contact between the surfaces of joints – these surfaces are called articular surfaces.

ARTIFACT (ARTEFACT) A foreign body found in living tissue viewed under a microscope. It is usually caused by faulty preparation of a specimen with the result that disease or abnormality seems to be present.

ARTIFICIAL INSEMINATION In this method of fertilization semen is collected either by the husband (AIH) or by a donor (AID) through masturbation and introduced into the upper vagina around the time of ovulation.

AIH is thought to be particularly useful for men with retrograde ejaculation or erectile impotence.

AID may be considered when the partner's sperm count is either very low or zero. Insemination can be made with fresh or frozen semen. Donors should be tested for sexually transmitted diseases and their identity remain unknown to the infertile couple. The pregnancy rate over six months is 50–60 per cent.

ARTIFICIAL INTELLIGENCE is the so far unsuccessful target of research workers to develop a computer that thinks like a human.

ARTIFICIAL KIDNEY (see KIDNEY, ARTIFICIAL).

ARTIFICIAL LIMBS AND OTHER PARTS   (see PROSTHESES).

ARTIFICIAL RESPIRATION (see APPENDIX 1: BASIC FIRST AID).

ARTIFICIAL VENTILATION OF THE LUNGS   Normally, on inspiration, air is drawn into the lungs by a subatmospheric pressure within the pleural space. This is achieved by expanding the lungs using the intercostal muscles and the diaphragm. Expiration is achieved by reversing the process and, when breathing heavily, contracting the abdominal muscles. To produce ventilation artificially this cycle of air flowing in and out of the lungs must be reproduced (see LUNGS). This may be achieved using intermittent positive or negative pressure as described below.

INTERMITTENT POSITIVE PRESSURE (ITP) – The simplest form of intermittent positive-pressure ventilation is mouth-to-mouth resuscitation (see APPENDIX 1: BASIC FIRST AID) where an individual blows his or her own expired gases into the lungs of an apnoeic person via the mouth or nose. Similarly gas may be blown into the lungs via a face mask (or down an endotracheal tube) and a self-inflating bag or an anaesthetic circuit containing a bag which is inflated by the flow of fresh gas from an anaesthetic machine, gas cylinder, or piped supply. In all these examples expiration is passive.

For more prolonged artificial ventilation it is usual to use a specially designed machine or ventilator to perform the task. The ventilators used in operating theatres when patients are anaesthetized and paralysed are relatively simple devices. Generally they consist of bellows which fill with fresh gas and which are then mechanically emptied (by means of a weight, piston, or compressed gas) via a circuit or tubes attached to an endotracheal tube into the patient's lungs. Adjustments can be made to the volume of fresh gas given with each breath and to the length of inspiration and expiration. Expiration is usually passive back to the atmosphere.

On the intensive-care unit, where patients are not usually paralysed, the ventilators are more complex. They have electronic controls which allow the user to programme a variety of pressure waveforms for inspiration and expiration. There are also programmes that allow the patient to breathe between ventilated breaths or to trigger ventilated breaths, or inhibit ventilation when the patient is breathing.

Indications for artificial ventilation are when the patient is unable to breathe adequately on his own. This may be due to injury or disease of the central nervous, cardiovascular, or respiratory systems or drug overdose. Artificial ventilation is performed to allow time for healing and recovery. Sometimes the patient is able to breathe but it is considered advisable to control ventilation – e.g. in severe head injury. Some operations require the patient to be paralysed for better or safer surgical access and this may require ventilation. With lung operations or very unwell patients ventilation is also indicated.

Artificial ventilation usually bypasses the physiological mechanisms for humidification of inspired air, so care must be taken to humidify inspired gases. It is important to monitor the efficacy of ventilation – e.g. by using blood gas measurement, pulse oximetry, and tidal carbon dioxide, and airways pressures.

Artificial ventilation is not without its hazards. The use of *positive pressure* raises the mean intrathoracic pressure. This can decrease venous return to the heart and cause a fall in cardiac output (q.v.) and blood pressure. Positive-pressure ventilation may also cause pneumothorax (q.v.), but this is rare. While patients are ventilated, they are unable to

breath and so accidental disconnection from the ventilator may cause hypoxia and death. NEGATIVE-PRESSURE VENTILATION is seldom used nowadays. The chest or whole body, apart from the head, is placed inside an airtight box. A vacuum lowers the pressure within the box causing the chest to expand. Air is drawn into the lungs through the mouth and nose. At the end of inspiration the vacuum is stopped, the pressure in the box returns to atmospheric, and the patient exhales passively. This is the principle of the 'iron lung' which saved many lives during the polio epidemics of the 1950s. These machines are cumbersome and make access to the patient difficult. In addition, complex manipulation of ventilation is impossible.

Jet ventilation is a relatively modern form of ventilation which utilizes very small tidal volumes (see LUNGS) from a high-pressure source at high frequencies (20–100/min). First developed by physiologists to produce low stable intrathoracic pressures whilst studying carotid-body reflexes (q.v.), it is sometimes now used in intensive therapy units for patients who do not achieve adequate gas exchanges with conventional ventilation. Its advantages are lower intrathoracic pressures (and therefore less risk of pneumothorax and impaired venous return) and better gas mixing within the lungs.

ARYTENOID is the name applied to two cartilages in the larynx.

ASBESTOSIS is a form of pneumoconiosis (q.v.), in which widespread fine scarring occurs in the lungs, leading to severe breathing disability. The main hazard, however, is the risk of cancer (mesothelioma) of the lung or pleura, or sometimes of the ovary. It is caused by the inhalation of mainly blue or brown asbestos dust, either during mining or quarrying, or in one of the many industries in which it is used: e.g. as an insulating material, in the making of paper, cardboard and brake linings. A person suffering from asbestosis is entitled to compensation as the disease is legally prescribed. About 900 people a year in the UK claim compensation, and 400 of these are for mesothelioma.

ASCARIASIS is the disease produced by infestation with the roundworm, *Ascaris lumbricoides*, also known as the maw-worm. Superficially it resembles a large earthworm. The male measures about 17 cm (7 inches) and the female 23 cm (9 inches) in length. It is a dirt disease, most prevalent where sanitation and cleanliness are lacking, particularly in the tropics and subtropics. Consumption of food contaminated by the ova (eggs), especially salad vegetables, is the commonest cause of infection. In children, infection is commonly acquired by crawling or playing on contaminated earth, and then sucking their fingers. After a complicated life-cycle in the body the adult worms end up in the intestines, whence they may be passed in the stools. A light infection may cause no symptoms. A heavy infection may lead to colic, or even obstruction of the gut. Occasionally a worm may wander into the stomach and be vomited up.

Treatment consists of the administration of levamisole, a piperazine derivative, pyrantel embonate, or mebendazole.

ASCITES is an accumulation of fluid in the abdomen. The causes include heart failure, cancer, cirrhosis of the liver and infections.

ASCORBIC ACID (VITAMIN) is a substance present in various natural sources such as fruits and vegetables, or synthetically prepared. (See VITAMIN.)

ASEPSIS is a term, used in distinction from 'antisepsis', to mean that principle in surgery by which, instead of strong germicides like corrosive sublimate or carbolic acid being applied to wounds, all the dressings, swabs, and instruments used are sterilized by steaming, boiling, or dry heat. Thin, sterilized, india-rubber gloves are worn by surgeons and prevent risk of infection from the hands. Aseptic surgery has the advantage that the germ-destroying activity of the tissues and their healing power after wounds are not lessened by antiseptics which decrease the vitality of the tissues. Healing is therefore surer and more rapid after an aseptic operation. (See also ANTISEPTICS.)

ASH stands for ACTION ON SMOKING AND HEALTH. It is a charity founded by the Royal College of Physicians in 1971 and supported by the DOH. Its aim is to alert and inform the public to the dangers of smoking and to try to prevent the disability and death which it causes. It gathers a wide range of information about smoking and disseminates it to the public to increase knowledge about the dangers of smoking and how to give up the habit. It commissions surveys on public attitudes to smoking and brings together working groups on such subjects as giving up smoking and how to prevent children from starting to smoke. It is largely due to the efforts of ASH that the majority of adults in the United Kingdom (more than six out of ten) are now non-smokers. ASH works on their behalf by pressing proprietors of public space to provide more smoke-free areas and advising them how to create and operate them. Hundreds of smokers who would like to give up smoking contact ASH for information every month. ASH has a small headquarters staff in London with other national and regional branches in Scotland, Wales, and Northern Ireland. More branches are opening every year. Further information can be obtained from ASH (see APPENDIX 2: ADDRESSES).

ASPARAGINASE is an enzyme that breaks down the amino-acid, asparagine. This is of no significance to most cells in the body as they can make asparagine from simpler constituents.

Certain tumours, however, are unable to do this and therefore, if they cannot receive ready-made supplies of the amino-acid, they die. It is on this basis that asparaginase is proving of promise in the treatment of tumours which, by the administration of asparaginase, are deprived of an essential metabolite – and perish.

ASPARTANE is an artificial sweetener 200 times as sweet as sugar but without the bitter after-taste of saccharine.

ASPERGILLOSIS is a disease caused by invasion of the lung by the fungus, *Aspergillus fumigatus*. The infection is acquired by inhalation of air-borne spores of the fungus which settle and grow in damaged parts of the lung such as healed tuberculous cavities, abscesses, or the dilated bronchi of bronchiectasis (q.v.).

ASPERGILLUS is the name applied to a group of fungi including the common moulds. Several of these are capable of infecting the lungs and producing a disease resembling pulmonary tuberculosis.

ASPHYXIA means literally absence of pulse, but is the name given to the whole series of symptoms which follow stoppage of breathing and of the heart's action. Drowning is one cause but obstruction *of the air passages* may occur as the result of a foreign body or in some diseases, such as croup, diphtheria, swelling of the throat due to wounds or inflammation, asthma (to a partial extent), tumours in the chest (causing slow asphyxia), and the external conditions of suffocation and strangling. Placing the head in a plastic bag results in asphyxia and poisonous gases also cause asphyxia, for example, carbon monoxide gas, which may be given off by a stove or charcoal brazier in a badly ventilated room can kill people during sleep. (See CARBON MONOXIDE.) Several gases, such as sulphurous acid (from burning sulphur), ammonia, and chlorine (from bleaching-powder), cause involuntary closure of the entrance to the larynx, and thus prevent breathing. Other gases, such as nitrous oxide (or laughing-gas), chloroform, and ether, in poisonous quantity, stop the breathing by paralysing the respiration centre in the brain.

Symptoms In most cases death from asphyxia is due to insufficiency of oxygen supplied to the blood. The first signs are rapid pulse and gasping for breath. Next comes a rise in the blood pressure, causing throbbing in the head, with lividity or blueness of the skin, due to failure of aeration of the blood, followed by still greater struggles for breath and by general convulsions. The heart becomes over-distended and gradually weaker, a paralytic stage sets in, and all struggling and breathing slowly cease. When asphyxia is due to charcoal fumes, coal-gas, and other narcotic influences, there is no convulsive stage, and death ensues gently and may occur in the course of sleep.

Treatment So long as the heart continues to beat, recovery may be looked for with prompt treatment. The one essential of treatment is to get the impure blood aerated by artificial respiration. Besides this, the feeble circulation can be helped by various methods. (See APPENDIX 1: BASIC FIRST AID, choking, cardiac/respiratory arrest.)

ASPIRATION means the withdrawal of fluid or gases from the natural cavities of the body or from cavities produced by disease. It may be performed either for curative purposes, or, very often, a small amount is drawn off for diagnosis of the nature or origin of the fluid. An instrument called an aspirator is used to remove blood and fluid from a surgical operation site – for example, the abdomen or the mouth (in dentistry).

Pleurisy with effusion is a condition requiring aspiration, and a litre or more of fluid may be drawn off by an aspirator or a large syringe and needle. *Chronic abscesses* and *tuberculous joints* may call for its use, the operation being done with a small syringe and hollow needle. *Pericarditis with effusion* is another condition in which aspiration is sometimes performed. The spinal canal is aspirated by the operation of lumbar puncture. (See LUMBAR PUNCTURE.) In children the ventricles of the brain are sometimes similarly relieved from excess of fluid by piercing the fontanelle (soft spot) on the infant's head. (See HYDROCEPHALUS.)

ASPIRIN, or ACETYLSALICYLIC ACID, is a white crystalline powder which is used like sodium salicylate as a remedy for reducing inflammation and fever. It has some action in relieving pain and producing sleep and is therefore often used for headache and slighter degrees of insomnia. Daily doses are now used in the prevention of coronary thrombosis. The dose is 75 to 300 mg. Aspirin should be used with caution in children and in people with dyspepsia or gastric ulcers. (See ANALGESICS.)

ASPIRIN POISONING may not be common in relation to the vast amounts that are consumed every year, but nevertheless it is a worrying problem.

In ordinary doses it may induce bleeding from the stomach. This is usually quite mild, but it can be severe. In small doses it can produce a severe allergic reaction in individuals who are sensitive to it. This takes the form of asthma and angioneurotic oedema.

When an overdose is taken, there is marked over-breathing, sweating and vomiting. Later the individual becomes restless and irritable, and there may be convulsions before consciousness is finally lost.

Treatment The stomach should be washed out, preferably with an alkaline solution, and a litre of 5-per-cent sodium bicarbonate should be left in the stomach. If there has been much loss of fluid by sweating and vomiting, fluids may need to be given intravenously. In severe cases oxygen may need to be administered.

ASSISTED CONCEPTION There are two types of assisted conception: in vitro fertilization (IVF) and gamete intrafallopian transfer (GIFT).

IN VITRO FERTILIZATION In this technique the female partner receives drugs to enhance ovulation. Just before ovulation several ripe eggs are collected under ultrasound guidance or through a laparoscope. The eggs are incubated with the prepared sperm. About 40 hours later, once the eggs have been fertilized, up to three embryos are transferred into the mother's uterus via the cervix. Pregnancy should then proceed normally. About one in five IFV pregnancies results in the birth of a child. The success rate falls rapidly if the female partner is aged 40 and over.

Indications In women with severely damaged fallopian tubes IVF offers the only chance of pregnancy. The method is also used in couples with unexplained infertility, male-factor infertility where the sperm count is only slightly abnormal, and in women who have suffered an early or surgical menopause. In these cases donor eggs are used.

Almost one quarter of pregnancies are multiple. Twin or triplet pregnancies are associated with many more problems such as premature labour. As the likelihood of multiple pregnancy increases with the number of eggs replaced into the uterus, recent legislation in the United Kingdom has recommended that no more than three eggs are transferred in each IVF cycle.

It is also important to monitor the preovulation phase in the woman by ultrasound scan so that not too many eggs develop, as this may lead to hyperstimulation of the ovaries which can cause the development of ovarian cysts.

GAMETE INTRAFALLOPIAN TRANSFER This method of fertilization may be used provided at least one fallopian tube is healthy and patent. As with IVF, ovulation is usually stimulated in the female partner. The woman then undergoes a laparoscopy just before ovulation during which the ripe eggs are picked up from the ovaries and injected into the fallopian tube together with prepared sperm from the husband. Fertilization then takes place as it does in natural conception.

GIFT is indicated in couples with unexplained infertility, minor male- or cervical-factor infertility. Associated problems are similar to IVF and are mainly related to an increased rate of multiple pregnancies.

The success rate for GIFT is about 17 per cent.

ASTEREOGNOSIS means the loss of the capacity to recognize the nature of an object by feeling it, and indicates a lesion (e.g. tumour) of the brain.

ASTHENIA means want of strength.

ASTHENOPIA means a sense of weakness in the eyes, coming on when they are used. As a rule it is due to long-sightedness, slight inflammation, or weakness of the muscles that move the eyes. (See VISION.)

ASTHMA is a disorder of breathing characterized by narrowing of airways within the lung. The main symptom is breathlessness. A major feature of asthma is the variability in the degree of airway narrowing. This reversibility of the obstruction may occur spontaneously or as a result of treatment.

Cause Recent research has emphasized the importance of inflammation in the wall of the airways in asthma. This produces swelling in the airway wall which narrows the lumen and there is also contraction of the smooth muscle in the wall of the airway. The narrowing of the airways in the lung is responsible for the great difficulty in breathing which is the characteristic feature of asthma. The inflamed airway is irritable and further narrowing occurs in response to non-specific irritants and specific triggers. There is a large number of substances to which the asthmatic subject may be hypersensitive and contact with these may be responsible for an attack. These include pollens, skin scales of certain animals such as cats, dogs and horses, the house dust mite (*Dermatophagoides* species), certain industrial agents such as platinum salts (see OCCUPATIONAL DISEASES). In some asthmatic patients substances in the diet may be important, either colourings and additives or specific foodstuffs.

Asthmatic subjects have a genetic predisposition to form antibodies of the IgE class against allergens which they meet, particularly if these are inhaled. Skin tests may demonstrate this production of antibodies but there are often positive responses to many allergens and further investigation is usually necessary to accept that the particular allergen is important in the patient's asthma.

Asthma is often at its worst in the early hours of the morning causing disturbance of sleep. In some cases this may be related to specific allergens such as feathers in pillows, but usually it is just part of the pattern of daily variation in asthma. Non-specific factors such as dust, cold air, emotional disturbance and stress may exacerbate asthma and increase the sensitivity to other precipitants of asthma.

Asthma often runs in families and the genetic basis is under investigation. Asthmatic subjects often suffer from other allergic conditions such as hay fever and eczema as do other members of their family. Asthma most often begins in early childhood, by the age of 7. Asthma affects around 10 per cent of children, usually in a mild form. In this age group boys are affected twice as often as girls. Mildly affected children may grow out of their asthma and in adults the prevalence is nearer 5 per cent and males and females are equally affected. Asthma may come on at any age and, when it develops for the first time in adults, it is often more persistent with fewer identifiable precipitating factors. The death rate for asthma in the United Kingdom is around 1,000 per year and is steady or increasing slightly.

The prevalence of asthma varies around the world. In most developed countries rates are similar to the UK, although it is commoner in Australia and New Zealand. Asthma in children in developed countries has been rising during the past decade. Whether this is due to pollution is unclear but it may be a factor. In less developed countries rates are lower but rise with increasing urbanization.

The term asthma is sometimes used in cardiac asthma. This describes the breathlessness associated with pulmonary oedema (q.v.) and left-sided heart failure. The term is used less than it was and should be abandoned.

Symptoms The major symptoms of asthma are breathlessness and cough. Occasionally coughing may be the only symptom of asthma and this is more common in children when night-time coughing attacks may be mistaken for bronchitis and treated inappropriately with antibiotics.

The amount of airway narrowing can be measured as the peak expiratory-flow rate by a simple meter. The hallmark of asthma is variability of airway narrowing; this may be intermittent mild breathlessness often precipitated by an obvious cause such as exercise or severe life-threatening attacks. Some asthma attacks have a sudden onset but routine recordings of peak expiratory-flow rate show that there is often a period of gradual decline for some days before the acute attack. A change in treatment during this decline will often prevent the severe attack and hospital admission.

The breathlessness of an acute attack of asthma produces distress in breathing out through the narrowed airways but the associated overinflation of the lungs results in difficulties in inspiration. The noise of turbulent air in narrowed airways produces wheezing noises, particularly on expiration. In a severe attack the breathing rate and the pulse rate increase and the patient may find it easier to breathe sitting up with the shoulders raised. In very severe attacks the patient may be too breathless to speak and reduced oxygen in the blood may result in the blueish colour of cyanosis. These features, together with lack of response to the usual inhaled treatment, indicate that the attack is very severe and urgent hospital treatment is necessary.

When asthma is poorly controlled for a long time in childhood, the chest may be left overexpanded. Chronic severe asthma may eventually result in airway narrowing which is no longer reversible in response to treatment but has become fixed.

Treatment The first important consideration in the management of asthma is avoidance of precipitating factors. Sometimes this is possible where a specific animal, occupational exposure or foodstuff is involved. More often the problem is a widespread allergen such as pollen or house dust mite which is difficult or impossible to avoid. Exposure to specific allergens may produce prolonged reaction in the airways which remain more susceptible to other precipitants for days afterwards. Exercise should be considered differently. Although it may provoke asthma, it does not increase problems encountered with other substances and it is beneficial for asthmatics to stay fit. Exercise should continue with appropriate medication such as beta-agonist beforehand.

In some countries desensitization is commonly practised. This is done by taking an allergen to which the patient is sensitive and trying to produce tolerance by giving small injections of the substance and gradually increasing the dose. Antibodies which block the asthmatic response may develop. Severe reactions occur occasionally. There is a dispute about the effectiveness and desensitization is rarely used in the UK now.

There are two main forms of drug treatment. Bronchodilator drugs are used to dilate the airways and relieve breathlessness. They may also prevent problems when taken before exposure. The most useful group of bronchodilators are the beta adrenergic agonists. There are a range of these and the commonest-used drugs are salbutamol and terbutaline. These drugs should be used usually to control symptoms and not as regular therapy on their own. Other bronchodilators are anticholinergics such as ipratropium bromide and the theophylline group.

The second group of drugs are the suppressors or anti-inflammatory drugs. These are inhaled corticosteroids, sodium cromoglycate and nedocromil. When bronchodilators are used more than once a day regularly, then an anti-inflammatory agent should be considered. Sodium cromoglycate is often useful in children, inhaled corticosteroids are usually needed in adults. These prophylactic drugs must be taken regularly to be effective. This requires careful patient preparation and explanation.

All the drugs mentioned, apart from theophyllines, are best taken by inhalation into the respiratory tract. This means that only a small dose is necessary, little of the drug gets in to the rest of the body and few side-effects occur. Careful instruction is necessary to make sure the patient can use the inhalation device effectively. There are enough types of inhaler device currently available to suit almost anybody. Large doses of corticosteroids by inhalation can produce some systemic effects but are much less of a problem than steroid tablets. They can also produce local effects in the mouth such as candidiasis (thrush).

Newer drugs are being developed to deal with various aspects of the inflammatory process in asthma. At present inhaled corticosteroids are the most effective and are relatively free of adverse effects. They should be considered when a drug such as salbutamol (Ventolin) is being used more than once every day.

Asthmatic patients should stay fit using a warm-up period and a drug such as salbutamol or terbutaline prior to exercise.

Specific breathing exercises are of little use. Every asthmatic should have a treatment plan to deal with exacerbations and a peak-flow meter available to measure the severity of the problem. Alternative therapies such as hypnosis have been used with some effect in selected patients.

Advice and support for research into asthma is provided by the National Asthma Campaign (see APPENDIX 2: ADDRESSES).

ASTIGMATISM is an error of refraction in the eye due to the cornea (the clear membrane in front of the eye) being unequally curved in different directions, so that rays of light in different meridians cannot be brought to a focus together on the retina. The curvature, instead of being globular, is egg-shaped, longer in one axis than the other. The condition causes objects to seem distorted and out of place, a ball for instance looking like an egg, a circle like an ellipse. The condition is remedied by suitable spectacles of which one surface forms part of a cylinder. (See SPECTACLES.)

ASTROVIRUSES are small round viruses with no distinctive features, which have been isolated from the stools of infants with gastroenteritis (see DIARRHOEA).

ASYMPTOMATIC The lack of any symptoms of disease whether or not a disease is present.

ASYNERGIA means the absence of harmonious and co-ordinated movements between muscles having opposite actions – e.g. the flexors and extensors of a joint – and is a sign of disease of the nervous system.

ASYSTOLE means arrest of the action of the heart.

ATAVISM means the principle of inheritance of disease or bodily characters from grandparents or remoter ancestors, the parents not having been affected by these.

ATAXIA means loss of co-ordination, though the power necessary to make the movements is still present. Thus an ataxic person may have a good grip in each hand but be unable to do any fine movements with the fingers, or, if the ataxia be in the legs, he throws these about a great deal in walking, though he can lift the legs and take steps quite well. This is due to a sensory defect or to disease of the cerebellum. (See FRIEDREICH'S ATAXIA; LOCOMOTOR ATAXIA.)

ATELECTASIS means collapse of a part of the lung, or failure of the lung to expand at birth.

ATENOLOL is a drug that antagonizes beta adrenergic receptors (q.v.) and is of value in the treatment of high blood-pressure, angina and arrythmias. One of its practical advantages is that only one dose a day need be taken. Atenolol, being a beta-blocking drug, may precipitate asthma, an effect that may be dangerous. Among the side-effects are fatigue and disturbed sleep. (See ADRENERGIC RECEPTORS.)

ATHEROMA is a degenerative change in the inner and middle coats of arteries. (See ARTERIES, DISEASES OF.)

ATHEROSCLEROSIS is a form of arteriosclerosis, in which there is fatty degeneration of the middle coat of the arterial wall. (See ARTERIES, DISEASES OF: arteriosclerosis.)

ATHETOSIS is the name for slow, involuntary, writhing, and repeated movements of the face, tongue, hands and feet, caused by disease of the brain. It is usually a manifestation of cerebral palsy (q.v.). Drugs used to treat Parkinson's disease can also cause athetosis.

ATHLETE'S FOOT is a somewhat loose term applied to a skin eruption on the foot, usually between the toes. It is commonly due to ringworm (q.v.), but may be due to other infections, or merely excessive sweating of the feet. It usually responds to careful foot hygiene and the use of antifungal powder.

ATLAS is the name applied to the first cervical vertebra. (See SPINAL COLUMN.)

ATONY means want of tone or vigour in muscles and other organs.

ATOPY, meaning out of place, is a form of hypersensitivity characterized, amongst other features, by a familial tendency. It is due to the propensity of the affected individual to produce large amounts of reagin antibodies which stick to mast cells in the mucosa so that when the antigen is inhaled histamine is released from the mast cell. It is the condition responsible for asthma and hay fever. (See also ALLERGY.) It is estimated that 10 per cent of the human race are subject to atopy. (See also DERMATITIS.)

ATRESIA means the absence of a natural opening, or closure of it by a membrane. Thus atresia may be found in new-born infants preventing the bowels from moving, and, in young girls after puberty, absence of the menstrual flow may be due to such a malformation.

ATRIAL NATRIURETIC PEPTIDE The atria of the heart contain peptides with potent diuretic and vaso-dilating properties. It has been known since 1980 that extracts of human atria have potent diurectic and natriuretic effects in animals (see DIURETICS). In 1984 three polypeptide species were isolated from human atria and were called alpha, beta and gamma human atrial natriuretic peptides. Plasma concentration of immuno-reactive atrial natriuretic peptide can now be measured. The levels are low in healthy subjects and are increased in patients with congestive heart failure. Infusion of the peptides into human volunteers causes a natriuresis and diuresis. Atrial natriuretic peptide is thus the most recently isolated hormone.

ATRIAL SEPTAL DEFECT (see HEART DISEASES, Congenital heart disease).

ATRIUM is the name now given to the two upper cavities of the heart. These used to be known as the auricles of the heart. The term is also applied to the part of the ear immediately internal to the drum of the ear. (Plural: ATRIA.)

ATROPHY occurs when normal tissue or an organ wastes because the constituent cells die. Undernourishment, disease, injury, lack of use or ageing may cause atrophy. Muscular atrophy occurs in certain neurological diseases such as poliomyelitis or muscular dystrophy. The ovary atrophies at the menopause. (See MUSCLES, DISEASES OF).

ATROPINE is the active principle of belladonna, the juice of the deadly nightshade. Because of its action in dilating the pupils it was at one time used as a cosmetic to give the eyes a full, lustrous appearance. It acts by antagonizing the action of the parasympathetic nervous system (q.v.). It temporarily impairs vision by paralysing accommodative power. (See ACCOMMODATION.) It inhibits the action of some of the nerves in the autonomic nervous system (q.v.). The drug relaxes smooth muscle. It has the effect of checking the activity of almost all the glands of the body, including the sweat glands of the skin and the salivary glands in the mouth. It relieves spasm by paralysing nerves in the muscle of the intestine, bile-ducts, bladder, stomach, etc. It has the power, in moderate doses, of markedly increasing the rate of the heart-beats, though by very large doses the heart, along with all other muscles, is paralysed and stopped.

Uses In eye troubles, atropine drops are used to dilate the pupil for more thorough examination of the interior of the eye, or to draw the iris away from wounds and ulcers on the centre of the eye; they also soothe the pain due to light falling on an inflamed eye, and are further used to paralyse the ciliary muscle and so prevent accommodative changes in the eye while the eye is being examined with the ophthalmoscope (q.v.). Atropine is used before general anaesthesia to reduce secretions in the bronchial tree. It is given by injection. The drug can also be used to accelerate the heart rate in bradycardia (q.v.) as a result of coronary thrombosis.

ATROPINE or BELLADONNA POISONING
This may occur from children's eating the berries or leaves of the deadly nightshade. The appearance of a patient with atropine poisoning has been described as: 'hot as a hare, red as a beet, blind as a bat, dry as a bone, and mad as a wet hen'. The warning symptoms are: (1) great dryness of the mouth and throat, (2) wide dilatation of the pupils, (3) increased rate of the heart's action. The person becomes restless and may go into coma with respiratory failure and convulsions.
Treatment The swallowed material should be got rid of by washing out the stomach followed by charcoal. If breathing becomes feeble, artificial respiration must be performed. The patient should be given plenty to drink but as atropine affects bladder control catheterization may be needed. A sedative, such as diazepam, is given to control the excitement, and in severe cases neostigmine, which is a specific antidote, can be given. (See POISONS and APPENDIX 2: ADDRESSES.)

AUDIOANALGESIA is a method of relieving the pains of childbirth. It is produced by the patient listening through headphones to a combination of white sound and music. The intensity of the sound is controlled by the woman herself according to the intensity of her pain. Experience suggests that the method is successful in women who are well adapted, like music and have some understanding of labour and delivery.

AUDIOMETRY is the testing of hearing.

AUDITORY NERVE (see VESTIBULOCOCHLEAR NERVE).

AURA is a peculiar feeling which persons, subject to epileptic seizures, have just before the onset of an attack. It may be a sensation of a cold breeze, a peculiar smell, a vision of some animal or person, an undefinable sense of disgust, or the like, but it is very important for persons who experience it, because it gives warning that a fit is coming and may enable a place of safety or seclusion to be reached.

AURAL Relating to the ear.

AURICLE is a term applied both to the pinna or flap of the ear and also to the ear-shaped tip of the atrium of the heart.

AURISCOPE is an instrument for examining the ear. The source of illumination may be incorporated in the instrument, as in the electric auriscope, or it may be an independent light which is reflected into the ear by means of a forehead mirror.

AUSCULTATION is a term in medicine applied to the method employed by physicians for determining, by listening, the condition of certain internal organs. The ancient physicians appear to have practised a kind of auscultation, by which they were able to detect the presence of air or fluids in the cavities of the chest and abdomen.

In 1819, the French physician, Laennec, introduced the method of auscultation by means of the stethoscope. Initially a wooden cylinder, the stethoscope has evolved into a binaural instrument consisting of a small expanded chest-piece and two flexible tubes, the ends of which fit into the ears of the observer. Various modifications of the binaural stethoscope have been introduced.

The numerous conditions affecting the lungs can be recognized by means of auscultation and the stethoscope. The same is true for the heart, whose varied and often complex forms of disease can, by auscultation, be identified with striking accuracy. But auscultation is also helpful in the investigation of aneurysms and certain diseases of the oesophagus and stomach. The stethoscope is also a valuable aid in the detection of some forms of uterine tumours, especially in the diagnosis of pregnancy.

AUSTRALIAN ANTIGEN An antigen associated with the hepatitis B virus (see HEPATITIS). The infection occurs in around 0·1 per cent of the population in Britain and the blood of people with it must not be used for transfusion. The name originated because the antigen was first discovered in an Australian aborigine.

AUTISM The term autism was introduced by Kanner in 1943 to describe a disharmony of development in which children are unable to mature socially despite excellent motor skill. Thus, despite their manual dexterity they are unable to form emotional bonds, even with their parents. Because of their disregard of other people they are refractory to discipline. Although they may acquire some language, they communicate little.

Advice and information on autism may be obtained from the National Autistic Society (see APPENDIX 2: ADDRESSES).

AUTO- is a prefix meaning self.

AUTOANTIBODY An antibody produced by a person's immune system that acts against the body's own tissues resulting in autoimmunity (q.v.).

AUTOCLAVE This is one of the most effective ways of ensuring that material, e.g. surgical dressings, is completely sterilized and that even the most resistant bacteria with which it may be contaminated, are destroyed. Its use is based upon the fact that water boils when its vapour pressure is equal to the pressure of the surrounding atmosphere. This means that if the pressure inside a closed vessel be increased, the temperature at which water inside the vessel boils, will rise above 100 °C. By adjusting the pressure, almost any temperature for the boiling of the water will be obtained. This is now one of the most widely used methods of sterilization in hospitals and laboratories.

AUTOGENOUS means self-generated and is the term applied to products which arise within the body. It is applied to bacterial vaccines manufactured from the organisms found in discharges from the body and used for the treatment of the person from whom the bacteria were derived.

AUTOIMMUNITY is a reaction to an individual's own tissues (self-antigens) to which tolerance has been lost (see IMMUNITY). Autoantibodies are not necessarily harmful and are commonly encountered in healthy persons. Autoimmune disease ensues when the immune system attacks the target cells of the autoimmune reaction. Examples are destruction of circulating red blood cells by autoantibodies in some forms of haemolytic anaemia and thyroiditis in which the thyroid gland is infiltrated by auto-reactive T and B lymphocytes. Systemic lupus erythematosus (see LUPUS) is another autoimmune disease. These diseases include diabetes mellitus (q.v.) and rheumatoid arthritis (q.v.) (see IMMUNOLOGY).

AUTO-INTOXICATION means literally self-poisoning, and is any condition of poisoning brought about by substances formed in or by the body.

AUTOLYSIS means the disintegration and softening of dead cells brought about by enzymes in the cells themselves.

AUTOMATISM means the performance of acts without conscious will, as, for example, after an attack of epilepsy or concussion of the brain. In such conditions the person may perform acts of which he is neither conscious at the time nor has any memory afterwards. It is especially liable to occur when persons suffering from epilepsy, mental subnormality, or concussion consume alcoholic liquors. It may also occur following the taking of barbiturates or psychedelic drugs (q.v.). There are, however, other cases in which there are no such precipitatory factors. Thus it may occur following hypnosis, mental stress or strain, or conditions such as fugues (q.v.) or somnambulism (see SLEEP). The condition is of considerable importance from a legal point of view, because acts done in this state, and for which the person committing them is not responsible, may be of a criminal nature. According to English law, however, it entails complete loss of consciousness, and only then is it a defence to an action for negligence. A lesser impairment of consciousness is no defence.

AUTONOMIC NERVOUS SYSTEM is part of the nervous system which regulates the bodily functions that are not under conscious control. These include regulating the heart beat, intestinal movements, salivation, sweating, etc. It consists of two main divisions – the SYMPATHETIC and the PARASYMPATHETIC SYSTEMS (qq.v.). The smooth muscles, heart and most glands are connected to nerve fibres from both systems and their proper functioning depends on the balance between these two. (See NERVES.)

AUTOPSY means a post-mortem examination, or the examination of the internal organs of a dead body. (See NECROPSY.)

AUTO-SUGGESTION is a peculiar mental state, which sometimes occurs after accidents, in which the will and judgement are partially perverted, so that slight or temporary injuries are greatly exaggerated in the imagination, and the person believes himself to be affected by some serious disability. Examples of this are found in paralysed and insensitive limbs following some minor bruise, for example in a railway accident, and the blindness, deafness, or inability to speak, which sometimes followed concussion in soldiers, especially when the injury was received in the dark. This state is also called 'traumatic suggestion'. The condition often approaches very near to, or is mingled with, the condition of malingering, in which the person consciously suggests to himself or produces some disability from an ulterior motive, as, for example, in some of the prolonged cases of disability following a trifling injury for which a person is in receipt of compensation. The term is also applied to the reverse process, by which, either as a result of suggestion by another person, or suggestion applied by the will-power of the person affected, a cure of such a condition is accomplished.

AVASCULAR Without a blood supply. Avascular necrosis is the death of a tissue because the blood supply has been cut off.

AVERSION THERAPY is a form of psychological treatment in which such an unpleasant response is induced to his psychological aberration that the patient decides to give it up. Thus the victim of alcoholism is given a drug that makes the subsequent drinking of alcoholic liquors so unpleasant by inducing nausea and vomiting that he decides to give up drinking. (See ALCOHOL; and DISULFIRAM.) Another commonly used method of inducing aversion is an electric shock. Aversion therapy may help in the treatment of alcoholism, drug addiction, sexual deviations, such as transvestism, and compulsive gambling.

AVITAMINOSIS is the condition of a human being or an animal deprived of one or more vitamins.

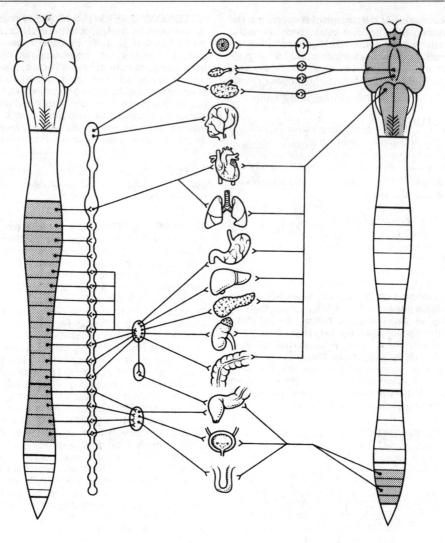

Schematic diagram of autonomic nervous system. (Left) Sympathetic nerves leaving middle section of spinal cord to connect via the vertebral ganglion (sympathetic trunk) to organs. (Right) Parasympathetic nerves leaving the brain and lower spinal cords to connect to organs.

AVULSION Forcible tearing away of one tissue from another. For example, a tendon may be avulsed from the bone to which it is attached or a nerve may be injured and torn away from the tissue in which it runs.

AXILLA is the anatomical name for the armpit. (See ARMPIT.)

AXIS is the name applied to the second cervical vertebra. (See SPINAL COLUMN.)

AXON Nerve fibre: an elongated projection of a nerve cell or neurone that carries an electrical impulse to the tissue at the end of the axon. Large axons are covered by a sheath of insulating myelin which is interrupted at intervals by nodes of Lanvier, where other axons branch out. An axon may be more than a metre long. It ends by branching into several filaments called telodendria and these are in contact with muscle or gland membranes and other nerves.

AZATHIOPRINE is a cytotoxic and an immunosuppressive drug. In the first of these capacities it is proving of value in the treatment of acute leukaemia. As an immunosuppressive agent, by reducing the antibody response of the body it is proving of value in facilitating the success of transplant operations by reducing the chances of the transplanted organ, e.g. the kidney, being rejected by the body. It is also proving of value in the treatment of auto-immune diseases. (See CYTOTOXIC.)

AZOOSPERMIA is the condition character-ized by lack of spermatozoa in the semen.

AZOTAEMIA means the presence of urea and other nitrogenous bodies in greater concentra-tion than normal in the blood. The condition is generally associated with advanced types of kidney disease.

B

BABINSKI REFLEX is an abnormal response of the plantar reflex. When a sharp body is drawn along the sole of the foot, instead of the toes bending down towards the sole as usual, the great toe is turned upwards and the other toes tend to spread apart. This response may be obtained in normal infants, but after the age of about two years its presence indicates some severe disturbance in the upper part of the central nervous system.

BACAMPICILLIN (see ANTIBIOTIC).

BACILLUS This is a big group (genus) of Gram-positive rodlike bacteria. Found widely in the air and soil – commonly as spores – they feed on dead organic matter. As well as infect-ing and spoiling food, some are pathogenic to humans, causing, for example, anthrax, con-junctivitis and dysentery. They are also the source of some antibiotics (See under MICROBI-OLOGY.)

BACITRACIN is a polypeptide antibiotic de-rived from *Bacillus licheniformis*. It is active against the same range of bacteria as penicillin.

BACK The back consists mainly of the spinal column and hinder parts of the ribs, and the wide-spreading iliac or haunch bones with the sacrum below. The bones are covered by thick and powerful muscles, which above support and move the head and which below pass round the flanks and downwards into the lower limbs. The skin covering the back is not very sensitive and is not greatly subject to painful conditions. The powerful muscles, of which the chief is the erector spinae, are vulnerable to minor injuries, the result of twists and strains, and also to rheumatic affections (see LUMBAGO). Diseases and injuries of the spinal column and spinal cord are of a very serious nature (see SPINAL COLUMN; SPINAL CORD).

BACKACHE is a symptom of many diseases. In addition to being the result of local causes, pain may be referred to the back from diseases in deep-seated organs. Medical causes which include inflammatory conditions, neoplasms and metabolic disorders are generally readily recognized but in total they are involved in only 1 or 2 per cent of all cases of chronic persistent backache. Similarly, sensations of pain experi-enced in the back but originating elsewhere in the body are usually identified by clinical history and laboratory investigations. A large majority of episodes of back pain stem from mechanical or structural disorders. Within this category diagnosis of a prolapsed intervertebral disc as the cause of suffering is relatively straightforward. In many other instances, how-ever, the mechanical abnormalities giving rise to pain remain the subject of speculation. Among the many known causes of back pain are:
(1) Mechanical and traumatic causes.
(*a*) Musculo tenderness and ligament strain.
(*b*) Fractures of the spine.
(*c*) Prolapsed intravertebral disc.
(*d*) Spondylosis.
(*e*) Congenital anomalies.
(2) Inflammatory causes.
(*a*) Osteomyelitis.
(*b*) Tuberculosis.
(*c*) Brucellosis.
(*d*) Paravertebral abcess.
(*e*) Spondyloarthropathy.
(*f*) Ankylosing spondylitis.
(*g*) Reiter's syndrome.
(*h*) Psoriatic arthropathy.
(3) Neoplastic causes.
(*a*) Primary benign tumours.
(*b*) Primary malignant tumours.
(*c*) Metastatic disease.
(4) Metabolic bone disease.
(*a*) Osteoporosis.
(*b*) Osteomalacia.
(*c*) Paget's disease.
(5) Referred pain.
(*a*) Posterior duodenal ulcer.
(*b*) Carcinoma of the pancreas.
(*c*) Pelvic disease[d]prolapse of the womb. Ovarian inflammation and tumours.
(6) Psychogenic causes.
(*a*) Anxiety.
(*b*) Depression.
  People with backache can obtain advice from the National Back Pain Association, (see AP-PENDIX 2: ADDRESSES).

BACLOFEN is a powerful muscle relaxant acting at the spinal level. It is used chiefly to relieve chronic severe muscle spasm and is also useful in treating some cases of multiple sclero-sis (q.v.). The major side-effects are sedation and hypotonia (loss of muscle tone).

BACTERAEMIA is the condition in which bacteria are present in the bloodstream.

BACTERIA are micro-organisms of a simple primitive form, though somewhat larger and more complex than viruses (see MICROBIOLOGY). Although responsible for a large number of human infections (q.v.), many of these may be successfully treated with antibiotics (q.v.), though resistant strains of bacteria do develop – increasingly so with the extensive use of antibiotics.

BACTERICIDE strictly means anything which kills bacteria, but is usually applied to drugs and antiseptics which do this. Hence *bactericidal*.

BACTERIOLOGY (See MICROBIOLOGY).

BACTERIOPHAGE is the term given to a virus (q.v.) which has a bacterium (q.v.) as its host. Containing either single-stranded or double-stranded DNA or RNA (qq.v.), a particular phage generally may infect one or a limited number of bacterial strains or species. After infection, once phage nucleic acid has entered the host cell, a lytic or a lysogenic cycle may result, depending on the phage and host types. Some (virulent) phages always induce a lytic cycle, whereby the bacterial synthetic machinery is programmed to produce viral components, which are assembled into virus particles and released on bacterial lysis (disintegration). Other (temperate) phages induce a non-lytic, or lysogenic, state, in which phage nucleic acid integrates stably into and replicates with the bacterial chromosome. The relationship can revert to a lytic cycle and production of new phages. In the process the phage may carry small amounts of donor bacterial DNA which may be expressed in a new host individual during lysogeny: the production of diphtheria toxin by *Corynebacterium diphtheriae* and of erythrogenic toxin by *Streptococcus pyogenes* are well-known examples of the effects of lysogeny.

BACTERIOSTATIC Preventing bacterial growth and cell division.

BACTERIURIA means the presence of bacteria in the urine, usually a sign of infection in the kidneys, bladder, or urethra.

BACUP stands for the British Association of Cancer United Patients and their families and friends. It was founded by Dr Vicky Clement-Jones after she was treated for ovarian cancer and it became fully operational on 31 October 1985. The aim of the association is to provide an information service to cancer patients who want to know more about their illness or who need practical advice on how to cope with it. It does not seek to replace the traditional relationship between the doctor and patient, nor does it recommend specific treatment for particular patients; but its aim is to help patients to understand more about their illness so that they can communicate more effectively and freely with their medical advisors and their families and friends.

For full details of information and counselling services see APPENDIX 2: ADDRESSES.

BAGASSOSIS is an industrial lung disease occurring in those who work with bagasse, which is the name given to the broken sugar cane after sugar has been extracted from it. Bagasse, which contains 6 per cent silica, is used in board-making. The inhalation of dust causes an acute lung affection, and subsequently in some cases a chronic lung disease. (See ALVEOLITIS.)

BAL is the abbreviation for *British Anti-Lewisite*. (See DIMERCAPROL.)

BALANITIS is inflammation of the glans penis (q.v.). Acute balanitis is associated with allergic dermatitis (q.v.) and herpes genitalis (q.v.). Diabetics are at increased risk of non-specific secondary infections; if recurrent balanitis occurs, circumcision is usually indicated.

BALANTIDIASIS is a form of dysentery caused by a protozoon known as *Balantidium coli*, a common parasite in pigs, which are usually the source of infection. It responds to metronidazole.

BALDNESS, or alopecia, is the loss of hair from the body – chiefly from the scalp, though it may also occur at other sites. It may be patchy or diffuse, sudden in onset or slowly progressive, reversible or irreversible, depending on the cause.
Causes MALE PATTERN BALDNESS (androgen-dependent) increases with age, ethnic variation, genetic influence on age of onset/severity; ALOPECIA AREATA (q.v.), generalized or localized sudden hair loss, common, genetic predisposition; TELOGEN EFFLUVIUM is the self-limiting thinning of hair often seen in women four to nine months after having a baby; CHRONIC DISCOID LUPUS ERYTHEMATOSUS, patchy hair loss; SYSTEMIC LUPUS ERYTHEMATOSUS, diffuse hair loss, reversible with treatment; ENDOCRINE (chiefly hypothyroidism and hypopituitarism), diffuse hair loss, not always reversible with treatment; NUTRITIONAL (chronic iron deficiency and generalized malnutrition), diffuse hair loss, reversible; DRUG-INDUCED: mainly cytotoxic drugs, androgens (in women), excess vitamin A and synthetic retinoids; fungal infections, localized hair loss, reversible; LICHEN PLANUS, localized hair loss, permanent.
Treatment Irreversible hair loss is best treated with a well-made wig, which will greatly improve the patient's morale. Grafting hair-bearing skin to the scalp has had limited success. Many 'cures' are offered, few succeed.
ALOPECIA AREATA, or patchy baldness, is common on the scalp, but may affect the hair all

over the body. It occurs principally in adolescents and young adults. The cause is not known. It is doubtful whether treatment makes any difference. The hair regrows spontaneously in a majority of cases, though sometimes lighter in colour, or even white. Ultra-violet light is beneficial in some cases. The more extensive the areas of baldness, and the more often it recurs, the worse the outlook for regrowth of the hair.

BALLOTTEMENT The technique of examining a fluid-filled part of the body for the presence of a floating object. For example, a fetus can be pushed away by a finger inside the mother's vagina. The fetus floats away from the examining finger and then bounces back on to it.

BALSAMS are substances which contain resins and benzoic acid. Balsam of Peru, balsam of tolu, and Friars' balsam (compound tincture of benzoin) are the chief. They are traditional remedies given internally for colds, and aid expectoration, while locally they are used to cover abrasions and stimulate ulcers.

BANDAGES are pieces of material used to support injured parts or to retain dressings in position.
Types *Triangular bandages* are made by taking a piece of calico 1 metre square and cutting it across cornerwise to form two triangles. The cut side of each is called the 'base', and the opposite right-hand corner is called the 'point'. *Crepe bandages*, which have a one-way stretch, consist of characteristic fabric of plain weave in which the warp threads are of cotton and wool and the weft threads are of cotton. They are used in the treatment of mild sprains and strains, and as compression bandages over paste bandages in the treatment of varicose ulcers. Much of the elasticity is lost during use, but can be restored by washing in soapy water. *Domette bandages* consist of union fabric of plain weave, in which the warp threads are of cotton or viscose, or of a combined cotton and viscose yarn, and the weft threads are of wool. It is used mainly for orthopaedic purposes, especially where a high degree of warmth, protection and support is needed. *Elastic bandages* provide firm support as in the treatment of varicose veins. *Plaster of Paris bandages* are impregnated with calcium sulphate and used as a form of splint. (See PLASTER OF PARIS.) *Netelast* is an elasticated tubular net of cellular cotton and elastic. It can be applied easily and quickly, can be washed and sterilized, and is available in different sizes. *Tubegauz* consists of seamless, circular cotton tubular material, which can be applied easily and quickly to any part of the body. *Tubifast* is a tubular bandage made from rayon with fine interwoven threads. It has a one way stretch which provides light pressure and so ensures that it holds itself in position.
    For more detailed instruction in bandaging the reader is referred to *First Aid Manual*, the authorized manual of the St John's Ambulance Association, St Andrew's Ambulance Association and British Red Cross Society (6th edition, 1992, London: Dorling Kindersley).

BARAGNOSIS means the inability on the part of a patient to recognize that an object placed in the hand has weight, a condition due to disease of the brain.

BARANY'S TEST is a test for gauging the efficiency of the balancing mechanism (the vestibular apparatus) by applying hot or cold air or water to the external ear.

BARBER'S ITCH (see SYCOSIS).

BARBITURATES are a group of drugs which are based on the structure of barbituric acid. Substitutions or alterations within the basic structure produce drugs which reversibly depress the central nervous system by inhibiting the transmission of impulses between certain neurones. Thus they cause drowsiness or unconsciousness (depending on dose), reduce the cerebral metabolic rate for oxygen and depress respiration but may accentuate pain in small doses. Their use as sedatives and hypnotics has largely been superseded by more modern drugs with more suitable pharmacological properties. Some members of this group of drugs, for instance, phenobarbitone, have selective anticonvulsant properties and are used in the treatment of grand mal (q.v.) convulsions and status epilepticus (see EPILEPSY). The short-acting drugs thiopentone and methohexitone are widely used to induce general anaesthesia. Barbiturates are metabolized by the cytochrome P450 enzyme system in the liver. They are potent hepatic enzyme inducers and may therefore increase the metabolism of other drugs. This characteristic is used therapeutically in hyperbilirubinaenia (raised concentration of bile salts in the blood) and kernicterus (q.v.). Their use is contraindicated in porphyria (q.v.) (See also DRUG ADDICTION.)

BARIUM SULPHATE is a radio-opaque white powder used in X-ray studies of the stomach and gastro-intestinal tract.

BARORECEPTOR Specialized nerve ending which acts as a stretch receptor in the carotid sinus, aortic arch, atria, pulmonary veins, and left ventricle. Increased pressure in these structures increases the rate of discharge of the baroreceptors. This information is relayed to the medulla and is important in the control of blood pressure.

BARRIER CREAMS are substances applied to the skin before work to prevent damage by irritants. They are also used in medicine: e.g. for the prevention of bedsores and napkin rashes.

There are three main types of barrier creams: a *dust barrier* to protect the skin against sensitizing dusts and against substances which, if absorbed, will produce systemic poisoning; a *water-repellent barrier* for those whose hands are constantly exposed to water, alkalis, and water-soluble oils; an *oil-repellent* or *water-miscible barrier*, which is a protective against oils, greases and solvents, and which facilitates their removal without the use of abrasives or oil solvents.

Silicones (q.v.), which are water repellent, are being used increasingly as barrier creams.

The hands should be clean and dry before applying a barrier cream. The cream should be applied sparingly to the whole of the hands. To get the full value from silicone creams, they should be applied twice daily for ten days before exposing the hands to irritants; after this a once-daily application should be sufficient.

The use of barrier creams must not be allowed to lead to any slackening in the attention paid to other more important protective measures, such as standards of cleanliness in workshops and the wearing of protective clothing.

BARRIER NURSING is the nursing of a patient suffering from an infectious disease in such a way that the risk of his passing on the disease to others is effectively reduced. Thus, precautions are taken to ensure that all infective matter, such as stools, urine, sputum, discharge from wounds, and anything that may be contaminated by such infective matter, such as nurses' uniforms, bedding and towels are so treated that they will not convey the infection. (See NURSING.)

BARTHOLIN'S GLANDS Two small glands opening either side of the external vaginal orifice. Their secretions help to lubricate the vulva.

BASAL CELL CARCINOMA Commonly called 'rodent ulcer' this tumour presents on the skin of the face as a shallow ulcer with a raised, rolled edge. The condition can be successfully treated with curettage and cautery (See CAUSTICS AND CAUTERIES), cryotherapy (q.v.), surgical removal or radiotherapy (q.v.). If untreated it erodes slowly into the underlying structures of the face and head.

BASAL GANGLION Grey matter near the base of the cerebral hemispheres, consisting of the corpus striatum (caudate nucleus and lenticular nucleus (globus pallidus and putamen)), claustrum, and amygdaloid nucleus. The basal ganglia are involved in the subconscious regulation of voluntary movement, and disorders in this region cause dyskinesias.

BASAL METABOLISM (see METABOLISM).

BASILIC VEIN is the prominent vein which runs from near the bend of the elbow upwards along the inner side of the upper arm. It is generally the vein opened in venesection for blood-letting.

BASOPHIL A type of white cell or leucocyte which has coarse granules in its cytoplasm (q.v.) that stain purple-black with certain chemicals. Basophils contain histamine (q.v.) and heparin (q.v.) and have the ability to ingest foreign particles.

BASOPHILIA is a term applied to the blueish appearance under the microscope of immature red blood corpuscles when stained by certain dyes. This appearance, with the blue areas collected in points, is seen in lead poisoning and the condition is called punctate basophilia. The term basophilia may also mean an increase in the numbers of basophil cells in the blood.

BAT EARS is the term commonly applied to prominent ears. The condition may be familial, but this is by no means the rule. Strapping the ears firmly back has no effect and is merely a waste of time and an embarrassment to the child. In cases in which the condition is proving a definite embarrassment to the child, it can be rectified by plastic surgery.

BATHER'S ITCH, also called SWIMMER'S ITCH, WATER ITCH, and SCHISTOSOME DERMATITIS, is the term given to a blotchy rash on the skin occurring in those bathing in water which is infested with the larvae of certain trematode worms known as *Schistosomes* (see SCHISTOSOMIASIS). The worm is parasitic in snails. The skin rash is caused by penetration of the skin by the free-swimming larval cercaria. Bather's itch is common in many parts of the world, including USA, Canada, Central and South America, Australasia, Malaysia and Japan. It has also been found in Wales, France, and Germany.

BCG VACCINE BCG (*Bacillus Calmette-Guérin*) vaccine, which was introduced in France in 1908, is the only vaccine that has produced significant immunity against the tubercle bacillus and at the same time has proved safe enough for use in human subjects. The original work of Calmette and Guérin has now been amply confirmed by investigators in many parts of the world. BCG vaccination is usually considered for five main groups of people. (1) Schoolchildren: the routine programme in schools usually covers children aged between 10 and 14. (2) Students, including those in teacher training colleges. (3) Children and new-born infants of Asian origin because of the high incidence of tuberculosis in this ethnic group. (4) Health workers, such as nurses, and others likely to be exposed to infection in their work. (5) Household contacts of people known to have active tuberculosis and new-born infants in households where there is a history of tuberculosis. A pre-vaccination tuberculin test is necessary in all age-groups except new-born infants, and only those with negative tuberculin reactions are vaccinated. Complications are few and far between. A local reaction at the site of vaccination usually occurs between two and six weeks after vaccination, beginning as a small papule that slowly increases in size. It may produce a small ulcer. This heals after around two months, leaving a small scar. (See IMMUNITY; TUBERCULIN.)

BEÇHET'S SYNDROME This is a syndrome of unknown aetiology. It is characterized by oral and genital ulceration, iridocyclitis and arthropathy. Thrombophlebitis is a common complication and involvement of the central nervous system may occur.

BECLOMETHASONE DIPROPIONATE is a corticosteroid that is proving of value as a cream or ointment in the treatment of certain skin diseases. It is also of value by inhalation in the treatment of asthma and hay fever, and by insertion into the nose in the treatment of perennial rhinitis. (See NOSE, DISEASES OF.)

BED BUG, or *Cimex lectularius,* is a wingless, blood-sucking insect, parasitic on man. It is a flat, rusty brown insect, 5 mm long and 3 mm wide, with an offensive, never forgotten smell, which cannot fly. The average life is 3 to 6 months, but it can live for a year without food. The bed bug remains hidden during the day in cracks in walls and floors, and in beds. It does not transmit any known disease. Eggs hatch out into larvae in 6 to 10 days, which become adult within about 12 weeks. A temperature of 44 °C kills the adult in an hour. Various agents have been used to disinfect premises, such as sulphur dioxide, ethylene oxide mixed with carbon dioxide, hydrogen cyanide and heavy naphtha, but insecticide is the most effective disinfecting agent.

BED SORES, or PRESSURE SORES, are areas of inflamed skin, tending to ulcerate and become infected, which appear on the body or limbs of people confined to bed or a wheelchair for long periods.
Causes Sores are particularly likely to occur in people who are thin, elderly, or debilitated. People with neurological diseases are particularly at risk. The direct cause is pressure on area of skin that restricts local circulation.
Symptoms The patient often feels no pain. Sores commonly form where the bones show through the skin in the lower part of the back, on the heels, on the haunch, on the ankles, on the elbows, or on the shoulder blades. Redness of the skin over a prominence quickly turns blue and dusky. Then a black slough forms and comes away, leaving a raw surface which widens if not carefully treated.
Treatment The best treatment is preventive,

by keeping the patient's back, buttocks and heels scrupulously clean and dry; by examining night and morning for any sign of redness; and especially by changing the patient's position so as to relieve the various prominences from constant pressure. The twice-daily smearing of the skin with barrier creams (q.v.) containing silicone, such as dimethicone cream may help.

BED WETTING Known medically as enuresis, bed wetting is the involuntary passage of urine at night. It can occur at all ages but is a particular problem with children and the elderly. Enuresis in children usually stops as they grow older but, when it persists, the child (and parents) need advice. Treatment is by positive reinforcement of bladder control, alarm systems such as the 'pad and bell', or occasionally by drugs.
Constipation is a common cause of urinary incontinence – and hence bedwetting – in the elderly and should be treated. Enuresis in the elderly may also be due to organic disease or to mental deterioration and confusion. Appropriate investigation, treatment and nursing should be arranged.

BEER (see ALCOHOL).

BEE STINGS (see BITES AND STINGS).

BEHAVIOUR THERAPY A form of psychiatric treatment based on learning theory. Symptoms are considered to be conditioned responses, and treatment is aimed at removing them, regardless of the underlying diagnosis. Desensitization, operant conditioning, and aversion therapy are examples of behaviour therapy.

BELCHING (see ERUCTATION).

BELLADONNA (see ATROPINE).

BELL'S PALSY refers to the isolated paralysis of the facial muscles on one or both sides, of unclear cause, though damage to the seventh cranial, or facial nerve (q.v.), possibly of viral origin, is thought likely. Occurring in both sexes at any age, it presents with a facial pain on the affected side, followed by an inability to close the eye or smile. The mouth appears to be drawn over to the opposite side, and fluids may escape from the angle of the mouth. Examination reveals flattening of the lines of expression, with inability to wrinkle the brow or whistle.
Treatment Oral steroids, if started early, increase the rate of recovery, which occurs in over 90 per cent of patients, usually starting after two or three weeks and complete within three months. Permanent loss of function with facial contractures occurs in about 5 per cent of patients. Recurrence of Bell's palsy is unusual.

B ENDORPHIN A naturally occurring painkiller which is produced by the pituitary as part of a prohormone (pre-pro-opianomelanocortin). It is an agonist at opioid receptors, and its release is stimulated by pain and stress.

BENDS (see COMPRESSED AIR ILLNESS).

BENIGN Not harmful. Used especially to describe tumours that are not malignant.

BENNETT'S FRACTURE, so-called after an Irish surgeon, Edward Hallaran Bennett (1837–1907), is a longitudinal fracture of the first metacarpal bone, which also involves the carpometacarpal joint.

BENZEDRINE is a proprietary name for amphetamine sulphate (see AMPHETAMINES).

BENZHEXOL is one of the antimuscarinic class of drugs used to treat Parkinsonism (q.v.). It has a moderate effect on tremor and rigidity, but tardive dyskinesia – involuntary movements – is not improved, and indeed may be made worse. Taken alone it is useful in mild cases of Parkinsonism, or to supplement the action of levodopa (q.v.) in more severe cases. Psychiatric disturbance may result in susceptible patients, necessitating discontinuation of treatment.

BENZOCAINE is a white powder with soothing properties used as a sedative for inflamed and painful surfaces.

BENZODIAZEPINES A large family of drugs used as hypnotics, anxiolytics, tranquillizers, anticonvulsants, premedicants, and for intravenous sedation. They differ in their duration of action, metabolites, and lipid solubility. Short-acting ones are used as hypnotics (q.v.), longer acting ones as hypnotics and tranquillizers (q.v.), and those with high lipid solubility act rapidly if given intravenously. They act at a specific central- nervous-system receptor or by potentiating the action of inhibitory neurotransmitters. They have advantages over other sedatives by having some selectivity for anxiety rather than general sedation. They do not induce hepatic enzymes and are safer in overdose. Unfortunately they may cause aggression, amnesia, excessive sedation, or confusion in the elderly. Those with long half lives or with metabolites having long half lives may produce a hangover effect, and dependence on these is now well recognized.

BENZOTHIADIAZINES, or THIAZIDES, are a group of diuretics (q.v.) which are effective when taken by mouth. They act by inhibiting the reabsorption of sodium and chloride in the renal tubules. They also have a blood-pressure-lowering effect. Chlorothiazide was the first member of this group to be introduced. Their main use is to relieve oedema in heart failure.

All thiazides are active by mouth with an onset of action within one to two hours, and a duration of twelve to twenty-four hours. Chlorthalidone is a thiazide-related compound that has a longer duration of action and only requires to be given on alternate days. The other thiazide drugs available include bendrofluazide, cyclopenthiazide, hydrochlorothiazide, hydroflumethiazide, indapamide, mefruside, methyclothiazide, metolazone and polythiazide. The loop diuretics are more potent than the thiazides. They are so called because they inhibit re-absorption from the ascending loop of Henle in the renal tubules. Frusemide, bumetanide, and ethacrynic acid are the three most important loop diuretics.

BENZYL BENZOATE is widely used as a lotion in the treatment of scabies (q.v.).

BENZYLPENICILLIN (see PENICILLIN).

BEREAVEMENT There is significantly increased psychiatric and physical morbidity following bereavement. Psychosomatic disorders, common neuroses, affective disorders, alcoholism and suicide may occur. The bereaved who are most at risk are those whose lives are complicated by crises other than bereavement and those who see their families as unsupportive. In the case of those who have been widowed, those whose marriage was ambivalent are particularly at risk and this is sometimes associated with an unrealistic idealization of the dead partner. Treatment should be directed towards encouragement of the expression of sorrow, anger, guilt, anxiety and helplessness and reassurance about the normality of the physiological accompaniments of grief.

BERIBERI (Singhalese: *beri* = extreme weakness.) Formerly a major health problem in many Asian countries, beriberi is a nutritional deficiency disease, resulting from prolonged deficiency of the water-soluble vitamin thiamine (vitamin B_1). It is often associated with deficiencies of other members of the the vitamin B complex. A major public health problem in countries where highly polished rice constitutes the staple diet, beriberi also occurs sporadically in alcoholics (Wernicke's encephalopathy) and in people suffering from chronic malabsorptive states. Clinical symptoms include weakness, paralysis – involving especially the hands and feet (associated with sensory loss, particularly in the legs) – and 'burning sensations' in the feet (dry beriberi). Alternatively, it is accompanied by oedema, palpitations, dilated heart, and cardiac involvement (wet beriberi). Death usually results from cardiac failure. Thiamine deficiency can be confirmed by estimating erythrocyte transketolase concentration; blood and urine thiamine levels can be measured by high-pressure liquid chromatography. Treatment consists of large doses of vitamin B_1 (thiamine) (q.v.) – orally or intramuscularly –

a diet containing other vitamins of the B group, and rest.

INFANTILE BERIBERI   This is the result of maternal thiamine deficiency; although the mother is not necessarily affected, the breast-fed baby may develop typical signs (see above). Optic and third cranial, and recurrent laryngeal nerves may be affected; encephalopathy can result in convulsions, coma, and death.

BERYLLIOSIS is a disease of the lungs caused by the inhalation of particles of beryllium oxide.

BETA-ADRENOCEPTOR-BLOCKING DRUGS   antagonize the beta effects of the sympathetic nervous system, particularly affecting the heart, bronchi, pancreas, liver and peripheral vasculature. Various drugs are available (including atenolol, metoprolol, and propranolol), differing in their cardiac selectivity. Used mainly to control hypertension, angina, tachydysrhythmias, and myocardial reinfarction, they slow the heart and have a hypotensive action, with a risk of inducing cardiac failure. Beta blockers cause bronchoconstriction and they should be avoided in patients with a history of asthma or obstructive airways disease, in whom brochospasm may be induced. They should be used cautiously in diabetics, as they may interfere with the metabolic and autonomic responses to hypoglycaemia.

BETAMETHASONE is a corticosteroid (q.v.) which has an action comparable to that of prednisolone, but in much lower dosage. In the form of betamethasone valerate it is used as an application to the skin as an ointment or cream.

BETATRON (see RADIOTHERAPY).

BEZAFIBRATE is a drug that lowers the level of lipids in the blood (see HYPERLIPIDAEMIA).

BEZOAR   A mass of ingested foreign material found in the stomach, usually in children or people with psychiatric illnesses. It may cause gastric obstruction and require surgical removal. The commonest type consists of hair and is known as a trichobezoar.

BICARBONATE OF SODA, or BAKING SODA, is an alkali, sometimes used as a home remedy for indigestion or soothing insect bites.

BICEPS   A term used for a muscle that has two heads. The *biceps femoris* flexes the knee and extends the hip and the *biceps brachii* supinates the forearm and flexes the elbow and shoulder.

BICUSPID   Having two cusps. The premolars

are bicuspid teeth, and the mitral valve is a bicuspid valve.

BIFID   Split into two parts.

BIFOCAL LENS   A spectacle lens in which the upper part is shaped to assist distant vision and the lower part is for close work such as reading.

BIFURCATION   The point at which a structure (for example, a blood vessel) divides into two branches.

BIGUANIDES are a group of oral hypoglycaemic drugs, of which metformin (q.v.) is the only one available for treatment, used to treat non-insulin-dependent diabetics, when strict dieting and treatment with sulphonylureas (q.v.) have failed. It acts mainly by reducing gluconeogenesis (q.v.) and by increasing peripheral utilization of glucose. Hypoglycaemia is unusual, unless taken in overdose. Gastrointestinal side-effects such as anorexia, nausea, vomiting, and transient diarrhoea are common initially, and may persist, particularly if large doses are taken. Metformin should not be given to patients with renal failure, in whom there is a danger of inducing lactic acidosis.

BILATERAL   Occurring on both sides of the body.

BILE is a thick, bitter, greenish-brown fluid, secreted by the liver and stored in the gallbladder (see LIVER: gall bladder). Consisting of water, mucus, bile pigments, and various salts, it is discharged through the bile ducts into the intestine a few centimetres below the stomach. This discharge is increased shortly after eating, and again a few hours later. It helps in the digestion and absorption of food, particularly fats, and is itself reabsorbed, passing back through the blood of the liver. In jaundice (q.v.), obstruction of the bile ducts prevents discharge, leading to a build-up of bile in the blood and deposition in the tissues. The skin becomes greenish-yellow, while the stools become grey or white and the urine dark. Vomiting of bile is a sign of intestinal obstruction, but may occur in any case of persistent retching or vomiting, and should be fully investigated.

BILHARZIASIS is another name for schistosomiasis (q.v.).

BILIRUBIN is the chief pigment in human bile. It is derived from haemoglobin (q.v.) which is the red pigment of the red blood corpuscles. The site of manufacture of bilirubin is the reticulo-endothelial system (q.v.). When bile is passed into the intestine from the gall-bladder, part of the bilirubin is converted into stercobilin and excreted in the faeces. The remainder is reabsorbed into the blood-stream, and of this portion the bulk goes back to the liver to be re-excreted into the bile, whilst a small proportion is excreted in the urine as urobilinogen.

BILIVERDIN is the chief pigment of bile in herbivora and birds. It is a precursor of bilirubin in the production of the latter from haemoglobin, and there is a small amount in human bile.

BINAURAL Relating to both ears.

BINOCULAR Relating to both eyes. Binocular vision involves focusing on an object with both eyes simultaneously and is important in judging distance.

BINOVULAR TWINS are twins who result from the fertilization of two separate ova. (See MULTIPLE BIRTHS.)

BIO-AVAILABILITY refers to the proportion of a drug reaching the systemic circulation after a particular route of administration. The most important factor is first-pass metabolism – that is, pre-systemic metabolism in either the intestine or the liver. Many lipid soluble drugs such as beta blockers, some tricyclic anti-depressants, and various opiate analgesics (qq.v.) are severely affected. Food may affect bioavailability by modifying gastric emptying, thus slowing drug absorption. Ingested calcium may chelate with drugs such as tetracyclines, further reducing their absorption.

BIOFEEDBACK is a technique whereby an auditory or visual stimulus follows on from a physiological response. Thus, a subject's electrocardiogram (q.v.) may be monitored, and a signal passed back to the subject indicating his heart rate: e.g. a red light if the rate is between fifty and sixty beats a minute; a green light if it is between sixty and seventy a minute. Once the subject has learned to discriminate between these two rates he can then learn to control his heart rate. How this is learned is not clear, but it is claimed that by this biofeedback it is possible to control the heart rate and blood-pressure, relax spastic muscles, and even bring migraine under control.

BIOPSY means the removal and examination of tissue from the living body for diagnostic purposes. For example, a piece of a tumour may be cut out and examined to determine whether it is cancerous.

BIOTIN is one of the dozen or so vitamins included in the vitamin B complex. It is found in liver, eggs, and meat, and it is also synthesized by bacteria in the gut. Absorption from the gut is prevented by avidin, a constituent of egg-white. The daily requirement is small: a fraction of a milligram daily. Gross deficiency results in disturbances of the skin, a smooth tongue and lassitude.

BIRD FANCIER'S LUNG, or PIGEON BREEDER'S LUNG as it is sometimes known, is a form of extrinsic allergic alveolitis resulting from sensitization to birds. In bird fanciers skin tests have revealed sensitization to birds' droppings, eggs, protein and serum, even through there has been no evidence of any illness. (See ALVEOLITIS).

BIRTH-MARKS are of various kinds. The most common are port-wine marks (see NAEVUS). Pigment spots are found, very often raised above the surface and more or less hairy, being then called moles (see MOLE).

BIRTH RATE Using the number of birth registrations as a guide, it was estimated that 640,000 live births took place in England in 1993, a 2-per-cent drop on 1992. Of these, 31 per cent occurred outside marriage. The fertility rate for women in their early 30s has been fairly constant over the past three years, while the rate for older women has been steadily rising.

BISACODYL is a laxative which acts by stimulation of the nerve endings in the colon by direct contact with the mucous lining.

BISEXUAL Having the qualities of both sexes. The term is used to describe people who are sexually attracted to both men and women.

BISMUTH salts are used to treat various bowel irritations. The salicylate and subnitrate are often given internally to check irritative diarrhoea; the stools are turned black. Subgallate is given in the form of suppositories to treat haemorrhoids. Various bismuth-containing antacids are on sale; they should generally be avoided, as they have a potentially neurotoxic effect.

BITES AND STINGS Animals' bites are best treated as puncture wounds which should simply be washed and dressed. Antibiotics may be given to minimize the risk of infection, and tetanus toxoid given if appropriate. Should rabies (q.v.) be a possibility, then further treatment must be considered. Bites and stings of venomous reptiles, amphibians, scorpions, snakes, spiders, insects and fish may result in clinical effects characteristic of that particular poisoning. In some cases specific antivenoms may be given to reduce the severity of illness or save the victim's life.

Many snakes are non-venomous (e.g. pythons, garter snakes, king snakes, boa constrictors) but may still inflict painful bites and cause local swelling. Most venomous snakes belong to the viper and cobra families and are common in Asia, Africa, Australia, and South America. Victims of bites may experience various effects including swelling, paralysis of bitten area, blood-clotting defects, palpitations, respiratory difficulty, convulsions and other toxic effects on the nervous and cardiovascular systems. Victims should be treated as for shock – namely kept at rest, warm, and given oxygen if required, but they should take nothing by mouth. The site of the bite should be immobilized but a tourniquet must not be used. All victims should be promptly transferred to a medical facility. When appropriate and available, antivenoms, which are available at certain hospitals or medical centres, should be administered as soon as possible.

Similar management is appropriate for bites and stings by spiders, scorpions, sea-snakes, venomous fish and other marine animals and insects.

BITES AND STINGS IN THE UK   The adder (*Vipera berus*) is the only venomous snake native to Britain and is a timid animal that only bites when provoked. People rarely die from adder bites. Only 14 deaths have been recorded in the UK since 1876, the last of these in 1975. Adder bites may result in marked swelling, weakness, collapse, shock, and in severe cases hypotension, non-specific changes in the heart's electrical conduction cycle, and peripheral leucocytosis (rise in numbers of white cells in the blood). Victims of adder bites should be transferred to hospital quickly but passively, even if they have no obvious symptoms, with the affected limb being immobilized and the site of the bite left alone. Local incisions, suction, use of tourniquets, ice packs or permanganate must not be attempted. Hospital management may include use of a specific antivenom, Zagreb®.

The weever fish is found in the coastal waters of the British Isles, Europe, the eastern Atlantic, and the Mediterranean Sea. It possesses venomous spines in its dorsal fin. Stings and envenomation commonly occur when an individual treads on the fish. The victim may experience a localized but increasing pain over two hours. As the venom breaks down when heated (heat-labile), immersion of the affected area in water at approximately 40 °C or as hot as can be tolerated for 30 minutes should ease the pain. Cold applications will worsen the discomfort. Simple analgesics and antihistamines may be given.

Bees, wasps and hornets are insects of the Order Hymenoptera in which the females possess stinging apparatus at the end of the abdomen. Stings may cause local pain and swelling but rarely cause severe toxicity. Generalized (systemic) anaphylactic reactions (q.v.) can occur in sensitive individuals which may be fatal so they should try and avoid situations where they might get stung. If they are stung, emergency medical treatment is required with the victim receiving adrenaline to reverse the state of severe shock. Deaths caused by upper-airway blockage due to stings in the mouth or neck regions are reported. In victims of stings the stinger should be removed by flicking or scraping but not squeezing or pulling as more venom may enter the wound. The site should be cleaned. Antihistamines and cold applications may bring relief. For anaphylactic reactions adrenaline, by intramuscular injection, may be required.

BLACK DEATH is an old name for plague. (See PLAGUE.)

BLACKHEADS (see ACNE).

BLACKWATER FEVER Acute intravascular haemolysis and renal failure, associated with severe *Plasmodium falciparum* infection. The complication is frequently fatal. It is associated with haemoglobinuria, jaundice, fever, vomiting, and severe anaemia. in an extreme case the patient's urine appears black. Tender enlarged liver and spleen are usually present. The precise aetiology remains obscure, but the disease is clearly triggered by quinine usage at subtherapeutic dosage in the presence of *P. falciparum* infection, especially in the nonimmune individual. Now that quinine is rarely used for chemoprophylaxis of this infection (it is reserved for treatment), blackwater fever has become very unusual. Treatment is as for severe complicated *P. falciparum* infection with renal impairment; dialysis and blood transfusion are usually indicated. When inadequately treated, the mortality rate may be over 40 per cent but, with satisfactory intensive therapy, this should be reduced substanially.

BLADDER, DISEASES OF See URINARY BLADDER, DISEASES OF. For diseases of the gall-bladder see GALL-BLADDER, DISEASES OF. (See also URINE.)

BLADDERS are sacs formed of muscular and fibrous tissue and lined by a mucous membrane, which is united loosely to the muscular coat, so as freely to allow increase and decrease in the contained cavity. Bladders are designed to contain some secretion or excretion, and communicate with the exterior by a narrow opening through which their contents can be discharged. In man there are two, the *gall-bladder* and the *urinary bladder*.

GALL-BLADDER   This is situated under the liver in the upper part of the abdomen, and its function is to store the bile, which it discharges into the intestine by the bile duct. For further details, see LIVER.

URINARY BLADDER   This is situated in the pelvis, in front of the last part of the bowel. The bladder, in the full state, rises up into the abdomen and holds about 570 ml (a pint) of urine. Two fine tubes, called the ureters, lead into the bladder, one from each kidney; and the urethra, a tube as wide as a lead pencil when distended, leads from it to the exterior, a distance of 4 cm (1½ inches) in the female and 20 cm (8 inches) in the male.

Structure The wall of the bladder is similar in structure to that of the bowels, and consists of four coats. The inner surface is lined by a soft mucous membrane covered by epithelial cells of irregular shape. This is attached to the muscular coat by a loose, fibrous, sub-mucous coat, in which run numerous blood-vessels. In the muscular coat the muscle fibres are arranged in several layers, and run in various directions, thereby adding greatly to the strength of the wall. On its upper and back part, the bladder possesses a covering of serous membrane, formed by part of the general peritoneal lining of the abdominal cavity, but this outermost coat does not extend down to the base of the bladder, where the latter lies in close contact with the other pelvic organs. The bladder is suspended in position by numerous ligaments, four of which are fibrous bands, while the remaining five are formed by thickened portions of the peritoneum. The base of the bladder is directed downwards and backwards, and in this part are the three openings of the ureters and urethra. The exit from the bladder is kept closed by a muscular ring, which is relaxed every time water is passed.

BLEEDER is a term applied to persons in whom it is difficult to stop bleeding when some small wound has been sustained. (See HAEMO-PHILIA.)

BLEEDING (see HAEMORRHAGE; and VENESECTION).

BLENORRHOEA means an excessive discharge of mucus or slimy material from a surface, such as that of the eye, nose, bowel, etc. The word catarrh is used with the same meaning, but also includes the idea of inflammation as the cause of such discharge.

BLEOMYCIN is an antibiotic, obtained from *Streptomyces verticillus*, that is being used with a certain amount of success in the treatment of cancer of the upper part of the gut, the genital tract and lymphomas. (See CYTOTOXIC.)

BLEPHARITIS means inflammation of the eyelids. (See EYE DISEASES.)

BLEPHAROSPASM (see EYE DISEASES.)

BLIGHTED OVUM, or BLIGHTED FETUS, is the term used to describe a condition in which apparently normal development of the embryo and its surrounding membranes continues for a short time and then the embryo dies, leaving the membranes alive for a little longer. The causes are not clear but are assumed to be either defects (possibly hereditary) in the ovum or fertilizing sperm, or some fault in the mother's womb. (See ABORTION; FETUS.)

BLINDNESS The statutory definition for the purposes of registration as a blind person under the National Assistance Act, 1948, is that the person is 'so blind as to be unable to perform any work for which eyesight is essential'. Generally this is vision worse than 6/60 in the better eye, or with better acuity than this but where 'the field of vision is markedly contracted in the greater part of its extent'. Partial sight has no statutory definition but there are Department of Health guidelines for registering a person partially sighted. Generally these are vision of 6/24 or worse with some contraction of the peripheral field, or better with gross field defects. The World Health Organization has estimated that there are over 40 million binocularly blind people in the world. The causes of blindness vary with age and degree of development of the country. In Western society the commonest causes are 'other retinal disease, glaucoma, diabetic retinopathy and senile cataract'. (See also VISION.)

Any blind person, or his or her relatives, can obtain help and advice from the Royal National Institute for the Blind (see APPENDIX 2: ADDRESSES).

NIGHT BLINDNESS (NYCTALOPIA) An inability to see in the dark. It can be associated with retinitis pigmentosa or Vitamin A deficiency.

BLIND SPOT (see VISION, FIELD OF).

BLISTERS AND COUNTER-IRRITANTS, formerly used to treat inflammatory skin conditions, are rarely employed nowadays, having been largely superseded by topical steroids.

BLOOD consists of cellular components suspended in plasma. It circulates through the blood vessels carrying oxygen and nutrients to the organs and removing carbon dioxide and other waste products for excretion. In addition, it is the vehicle by which hormones and other humoral transmitters reach their sites of action.
Composition The cellular components are red cells or corpuscles (erthrocytes, q.v.), white cells (leucocytes and lymphocytes, qq.v.), and platelets.

The cells are biconcave discs with a diameter of 7.5μm. They contain haemoglobin, which is an iron containing porphyrin compound, which takes up oxygen in the lungs and releasesit to the tissue.

The white cells are of various types - nomenclature depending on their morphology. They can leave the circulation to wander through the tissues. They are involved in combating infection, wound healing, and rejection of foreign bodied. Pus consists of the bodies of dead white cells.

Platelets are the smallest cellular components and play an important role in blood coagulation.

Erythrocytes are produced by the bone marrow in adults and have a life span of about 120

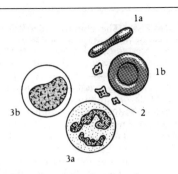

1 red blood cell (erythrocyte): (a) side view
  (b) plan view
2 platelets
3 white blood cells (leucocytes): (a) neutrophil
  or granular leucocyte; (b) lymphocyte

Red and white blood cells and platelets.

days. White cells are produced by the bone marrow and lymphoid tissue. Plasma consists of water, electrolytes (q.v.), and plasma proteins. It comprises 48-58 per cent of blood volume. Plasma proteins are produced mainly by the liver and certain types of white cells. Blood volume and electrolyte composition are closely regulated by complex mechanisms involving the kidneys, adrenal glands, and hypothalamus (qq.v.).

Haemoglobin		
concentration:	men	14–18 g/dl
	women	12–16 g/dl
Erythrocyte count:	men	4·5–6·0 × 10^{12}/l
	women	3·5–5·0 × 10^{12}/l
Mean corpuscular volume		76–96 fl.
Mean corpuscular haemoglobin concentration		31–35 g/dl
Mean corpuscular haemoglobin		27–32 pg
White cell count:		4–10 × 10^9/l
Neutrophils		40–75%
Eosinophils		1–6%
Basophils		0–1%
Monocytes		2–10%
Lymphocytes		20–50%
Platelet count:		150–400 × 10^9/l
Packed cell volume:	men	42–52%
	women	37–47%

Range of normal blood count.

BLOOD BANK A department in which blood products are prepared, stored, and tested prior to transfusion into patients.

BLOOD BRAIN BARRIER A functional semi-permeable membrane separating the brain and cerebrospinal fluid from the blood. It allows small and lipid soluble molecules to pass freely but is impermeable to large or ionized molecules and cells.

BLOOD CLOT A blood clot arises when blood comes into contact with a foreign surface, for example, damaged blood vessels, or when tissue factors are released from damaged tissue. An initial platelet plug is converted to a definitive clot by the deposition of fibrin, which is formed by the clotting cascade and erythrocytes.

BLOOD CORPUSCLE (see ERYTHROCYTE and LEUCOCYTE).

BLOOD COUNT The number of each of the cellular components per litre of blood. It may be calculated using a microscope or by an automated process.

BLOOD, DISEASES OF (see ANAEMIA; LEUKAEMIA).

BLOOD DONOR An individual who donates his or her own blood for use in patients of compatible blood group who require transfusion.

BLOOD GASES Specifically this describes the measurement of the tensions of oxygen and carbon dioxide in blood. However, it is usually used to describe the analysis of a sample of heparinized arterial blood not only for gases but for acid base assessment. This includes measurement of oxygen, carbon dioxide, oxygen saturation, pH, bicarbonate, and base excess (the amount of acid required to return a unit volume of the blood to normal pH).

BLOOD GROUPS People are divided into four main groups in respect of a certain reaction of the blood. This depends upon the capacity of the serum of one person's blood to agglutinate the red blood corpuscles of another's in certain circumstances. The reaction depends on antigens, known as agglutinogens, in the red corpuscles and antibodies, known as agglutinins, in the serum. There are two of each, the agglutinogens being known as A and B. Anyone's blood corpuscles may have (1) no agglutinogens, (2) agglutinogen A, (3) agglutinogen B, (4) agglutinogens A and B: these are the four groups.

In blood transfusion, the person giving and the person receiving the blood must belong to the same blood group, or a dangerous reaction will take place from the agglutination that occurs when blood of a different group is present.

Group	Agglutinogens in the corpuscles	Agglutinins in the plasma	Frequency in Great Britain
AB	A and B	None	2 per cent
A	A	Anti-B	46 per cent
B	B	Anti-A	8 per cent
O	Neither A nor B	Anti-A and Anti-B	44 per cent

The four main blood groups

Rhesus factor In addition to these A and B agglutinogens (or antigens) there is another one known as the Rhesus (or Rh) factor, so named because there is a similar antigen in the red blood corpuscles of the Rhesus monkey. About 84 per cent of the population have this Rh factor in their blood and are therefore known as 'Rh-positive'. The remaining 16 per cent who do not possess the factor are known as 'Rh-negative'.

The practical importance of the Rh factor is that, unlike the A and B agglutinogens, there are no naturally occurring Rh antibodies, but such antibodies may develop in an Rh-negative person if the Rh antigen is introduced into his or her circulation. This can occur (a) if an Rh-negative person is given a transfusion of Rh-positive blood, (b) if an Rh-negative mother married to an Rh-positive husband becomes pregnant and the fetus is Rh-positive. If this happens, the mother develops Rh antibodies which can pass into the fetal circulation, where they react with the baby's Rh antigen and cause haemolytic disease of the fetus and newborn. This means that the child may be stillborn or become jaundiced shortly after birth (see HAEMOLYTIC DISEASE OF THE NEW-BORN).

As about one in six expectant mothers is Rh-negative a blood-group examination is now considered an essential part of the antenatal examination of a pregnant woman. All such Rh-negative expectant mothers are now given a 'Rhesus card' showing that they belong to the rhesus-negative blood group. This card they should always carry with them. Rh-positive blood should never be transfused to an Rh-negative girl or woman.

BLOOD-LETTING (see VENESECTION).

BLOOD-POISONING (see SEPTICAEMIA)

BLOOD-PRESSURE is that pressure which must be applied to an artery in order to stop the pulse beyond the point of pressure. It may be roughly estimated by feeling the pulse at the wrist, or more accurately measured using a sphygmomanometer (q.v.). It is dependent on the pumping force of the heart, together with the volume of blood, and on the elasticity of the blood vessels. The blood pressure is biphasic, being greatest (systolic pressure) at each heartbeat and falling (diastolic pressure) between beats. The average systolic pressure is around 100 mm Hg (q.v.) in children, 120 mm Hg in young adults, and generally rises with age as the arteries get thicker and harder. Diastolic pressure in a healthy young adult is about 80 mm Hg, and a rise in diastolic pressure is often a more sure indicator of hypertension than a rise in systolic pressure. The latter is more labile and sensitive to changes of body position and emotional mood. Hypertension (q.v.) has various causes, most important of which are kidney disease (q.v.), essential hypertension (q.v.), and mental stress. Systolic pressure may well be over 200 mm Hg. Abnormal hypertension is often accompanied by arterial disease (q.v.), with an increased risk of strokes, heart attacks, and heart failure (qq.v.). Various anti-hypertensive drugs (q.v.) are available; they should be carefully evaluated, considering the patient's full clinical history, before use.

Hypotension (q.v.) may result from superficial vasodilation (for example, after a bath, or in fevers) and in weakening diseases or heart failure. The blood pressure generally falls on standing, leading to temporary postural hypotension – a particular danger in elderly people.

BLOOD TEST Removal of venous, capillary, or arterial blood for haematological, microbiological, or biochemical laboratory investigations.

BLOOD TRANSFUSION (see TRANSFUSION OF BLOOD).

BLOOD VESSEL Tubes through which blood is conducted from or to the heart. Blood from the heart is conducted via arteries and arterioles through capillaries and back to the heart via venules and then veins. (See ARTERIES and VEINS).

'BLOWING' OF CANS means the presence of gas in cans of food, the gas resulting from putrefaction or fermentation of the food, or from the action of fruit on the metal of the container, producing hydrogen. The ends of the can or tin bulge and give a tympanitic note on percussion. The food in such cans should not be eaten.

BODY MASS INDEX (BMI) provides objective criteria of size to enable an estimation to be made of an individual's level or risk of morbidity (q.v.) and mortality. The BMI, which is derived from the extensive data held by life insurance companies, is calculated by dividing a person's weight by the square of his or her height (kilograms/metres^2). Acceptable BMIs range from 20–25 and any figure above 30 characterizes obesity. The index may be used (with some modification) to assess children and adolescents. (See OBESITY.)

BOILS, or FURUNCLES, are small tender areas of inflamed skin containing pus. They often start in the roots of hairs and are usually caused by *Staphylococcus aureus* infection. A large number of boils close together is called a carbuncle. Boils usually heal quickly when the pus is released, but antibiotics are sometimes required. Anyone liable to recurrence of boils should be investigated to exclude diabetes mellitus.

BOLUS A lump of food prepared for swallowing by chewing and mixing with saliva. The term is also used to describe the rapid intravenous injection of fluid or a drug, as opposed to a slower infusion.

BONDING The formation of a close selective attachment, as in the relationship between a mother and her baby.

BONE forms the framework upon which the rest of the body is built up. The bones are generally called the skeleton, though this term also includes the cartilages which join the ribs to the breast- bone, protect the larynx, etc.

Structure of bone Bone is composed partly of fibrous tissue, partly of bone matrix comprising phosphate and carbonate of lime, intimately mixed together. As the bones of a child are composed to the extent of about two-thirds of fibrous tissue, whilst those of the aged contain one-third, the toughness of the former and the brittleness of the latter are evident. The shafts of the limb bones are composed of *dense bone*, the bone being a hard tube surrounded by a membrane, the periosteum, and enclosing a fatty substance, the marrow; and of *cancellous bone*, which forms the short bones and the ends of long bones, in which a fine lace-work of bone fills up the whole interior, enclosing marrow in its meshes. The marrow (see BONE MARROW) of the smaller bones is of great importance. It is red in colour, and in it red blood corpuscles are formed. Even the densest bone is tunnelled by fine canals (Haversian canals) in which run small blood-vessels, nerves and lymphatics, for the maintenance and repair of the bone. Round these Haversian canals the bone is arranged in circular plates called lamellae, the lamellae being separated from one another by clefts, known as lacunae, in which single bone-cells are contained. Even the lamellae are pierced by fine tubes known as canaliculi lodging processes of these cells. Each lamella is composed of very fine interlacing fibres.

GROWTH OF BONES Bones grow in thickness from the fibrous tissue and lime salts laid down by cells in their substance; while the long bones grow in length from a plate of cartilage (epiphyseal cartilage) which runs across the bone about 1·5 cm or more from its ends, and which on one surface is also constantly forming bone till the bone ceases to lengthen about the age of sixteen or eighteen. The existence of this cartilage is important to bear in mind, because in children an injury to it may lead to diminished growth of the limb.

REPAIR OF BONE is effected by cells of microscopic size some called osteoblasts, elaborating the materials brought by the blood, and laying down strands of fibrous tissue, between which bone earth is later deposited; while other cells, known as osteoclasts, dissolve and break up dead or damaged bone. When a fracture has occurred, and the broken ends have been brought into contact, these are surrounded by a mass of blood at first; this is partly absorbed and partly organized by these cells, first into fibrous tissue and later into bone. The mass surrounding the fractured ends is called the callus, and for some months it forms a distinct thickening, which is gradually smoothed away, leaving the bone as before the fracture. If the ends have not been brought accurately in contact a permanent thickening results.

VARIETIES OF BONES Apart from the structural varieties, bones fall into four classes: (*a*) long bones like those of the limbs; (*b*) short bones composed of cancellous tissue like those of the wrist and the ankle; (*c*) flat bones like those of the skull; (*d*) irregular bones like those of the face or the vertebrae of the spinal column (or backbone).

THE SKELETON consists of over 200 bones. It is divided into an AXIAL part, consisting of the skull, the vertebral column, the ribs with their cartilages, and the breast-bone; and an APPENDICULAR portion consisting of the four limbs. The hyoid bone in the neck, together with the cartilages protecting the larynx and windpipe, may be described as the VISCERAL skeleton.

AXIAL SKELETON The *skull* consists of the cranium, which has eight bones, viz. occipital, two parietal, two temporal, one frontal, ethmoid, and sphenoid; and of the face, which has fourteen bones, viz. two maxillae or upper jawbones, one mandible or lower jaw-bone, two malar or cheek bones, two nasal, two lacrimal, two turbinal, two palate bones, and one vomer bone. (For further details, see SKULL.) The *vertebral column* consists of seven vertebrae in the cervical or neck region, twelve dorsal vertebrae, five vertebrae in the lumbar or loin region, the sacrum or sacral bone (a mass formed of five vertebrae fused together and forming the back part of the *pelvis*, which is closed at the sides by the haunch-bones), and finally the coccyx (four small vertebrae representing the tail of lower animals). The vertebral column has four curves: the first forwards in the neck, the second backwards in the dorsal region, the third forward in the loins, and the lowest, involving the sacrum and coccyx, backwards. These are associated with the erect attitude, develop after a child learns to walk, and have the effect of diminishing jars and shocks before these reach internal organs. This is still further aided by discs of cartilage placed between each pair of vertebrae. Each vertebra has a solid part, the body in front, and behind this a ring of bone, the series of rings one above another forming a bony canal, up which runs the spinal cord to pass through an opening in the skull at the upper end of the canal and there join the brain. (For further details, see *spinal column*.) The *ribs*, twelve in number, on each side, are attached behind to the twelve dorsal vertebrae, while in front they end a few inches away from the breast-bone, but are continued forwards by cartilages. Of these the upper seven reach the breast-bone, these ribs being called true ribs, the next three are joined each to the cartilage above it, while the last two have their ends free and are called floating ribs. The *breast-bone*, or sternum, is shaped something like a short sword, about 15 cm (6 inches) long, and rather over 2·5 cm (1 inch) wide.

APPENDICULAR SKELETON   The *upper limb* consists of the shoulder region and three segments – the upper arm, the forearm, and the wrist with the hand, separated from each other by joints. In the shoulder lie the clavicle or collar-bone (which is immediately beneath the skin, and forms a prominent object on the front of the neck), and the scapula or shoulder-blade behind the chest. In the upper arm is a single bone, the humerus. In the forearm are two bones, the radius and ulna; the radius, in the movements of alternately turning the hand palm up and back up (called, respectively, supination and pronation), rotating round the ulna, which remains fixed. In the carpus or wrist are eight small bones – the scaphoid, lunate, triquetral, pisiform, trapezium, trapezoid, capitate, and hamate. In the hand proper are five bones called metacarpals, upon which are set the four fingers, each containing the three bones known as phalanges, and the thumb with two phalanges.

The *lower limb* consists similarly of the region of the haunch and three segments – the thigh, the leg, and the foot. The haunch-bone is a large flat bone made up of three – the ilium, the ischium, and the pubis, fused together, and forms the side of the pelvis or basin which encloses some of the abdominal organs. The thigh contains the femur, and the leg contains two bones – the tibia and fibula. In the tarsus are seven bones: the talus (which forms part of the ankle joint), the calcaneus or heel-bone, the navicular, the lateral, intermediate, and medial cuneiforms, and the cuboid. These bones are so shaped as to form a distinct arch in the foot both from before back and from side to side. Finally, as in the hand, there are five metatarsals and fourteen phalanges, of which the great toe has two, the other toes three each.

Besides these named bones there are others sometimes found in sinews, called sesamoid bones, while the numbers of the regular bones may be increased by extra ribs or diminished by the fusion together of two or more bones.

BONE, DISEASES OF   Bone is not an inert scaffolding for the human body. It is a living, dynamic organ, being continuously remodelled in response to external mechanical and chemical influences and acting as a large reservoir for calcium and phosphate. It is as susceptible to disease as any other organ but responds in a way rather different from the rest of the body.

In economic terms the most important disease of bone is OSTEOPOROSIS in the elderly, a gradual loss of bone mass with age. Its cause is not known but it is more common in women, especially after the menopause. It may be responsible in a large part for the epidemic of fractured neck of femur currently occurring in the developed world. Its course may be slowed by calcium supplements, exercise, and hormone-replacement therapy, but there is no known cure.

OSTEOMALACIA or rickets is the loss of minerali-zation of the bone rather than simple loss of bone mass. It is caused by vitamin D deficiency and is probably the most important bone disease in the Third World. In sunlight the skin can synthesize vitamin D, but normally rickets is caused by a poor diet, or a failure to absorb food normally (malabsorbtion). In rare cases vitamin D cannot be converted to its active state due to the congenital lack of the specific enzymes and the rickets will fail to respond to treatment with vitamin D. Malfunction of the parathyroid gland or of the kidneys can disturb the dynamic equilibrium of calcium and phosphate in the body and severely deplete the bone of its stores of both calcium and phosphate.

Congenital diseases of bone are rare but may produce certain types of dwarfism or a susceptibility to fractures (osteogenesis imperfecta). Primary bone tumours are also rare, but secondaries from carcinoma of the breast, prostate and kidneys are relatively common. They may form cavities in a bone, weakening it until it breaks under normal load (a pathological fracture). The bone eroded away by the tumour may also cause problems by causing high levels of calcium in the plasma.

Infection of bone (osteomyelitis) occurs most commonly after an open fracture, or in newborn babies. Once established it is very difficult to eradicate. The bacteria appear capable of lying dormant in the bone for the life of the patient and are not easily destroyed with antibiotics. At any time the infection can break out again causing further damage.

Paget's disease (q.v.) is a common disease of bone in the elderly, caused by overactivity of the osteoclasts (cells concerned with removal of old bone, before new bone is laid down by osteoblasts). The bone affected thickens and bows and may become painful. Treatment with calcitonin and diphosphonates may slow down the osteoclasts, and so hinder the course of the disease, but there is no cure.

If bone loses its blood supply (avascular necrosis) it eventually fractures or collapses. If the blood supply does not return, bone's normal capacity for healing is severely impaired.

For the following diseases see separate articles RICKETS; ACROMEGALY; OSTEOMALACIA; OSTEOPOROSIS; OSTEOGENESIS IMPERFECTA.

Tumours of bone can be benign (non-cancerous) or malignant (cancerous). Most malignant tumours found in bone have spread there from another organ, such as the breast, lung or gut. OSTEOID OSTEOMA is a harmless small growth which can occur in any bone. Its pain is typically removed by aspirin.

EWING'S TUMOUR is a malignant growth affecting long bones, particularly the tibia (calf bone). The presenting symptoms are a throbbing pain in the limb and a high temperature. Treatment is combined surgery, radiotherapy and chemotherapy.

OSTEOSARCOMA is a malignant tumour of bone with a peak incidence between the ages of 10 and 20. It typically involves the knees, causing a warm tender swelling. Removal of the growth with bone conservation techniques can often replace amputation as the definitive treatment. Chemotherapy can improve long-term survival.

MYELOMA is a generalized malignant disease of blood cells which produces tumours in bones which have red bone marrow such as the skull and trunk bones. These tumours can cause pathological fractures.

BONE MARROW is the soft substance occupying the interior of bones. There are two kinds: yellow marrow, which contains a large amount of fat, is found within the shaft of long limb bones; while red marrow, which has a highly cellular structure, occupies the space within the ribs, sternum, vertebral bodies, and the ends of the long bones. Bone marrow is the site of formation of the erythrocytes (q.v.), granular leucocytes (q.v.), and platelets (q.v.).

BONE TRANSPLANT The insertion of a piece of bone from another site or from another person to fill a defect, provide supporting tissue, or encourage the growth of new bone.

BORAX, or BIBORATE OF SODA, acts in much the same ways as boric acid, but without its acid reaction.
Uses Its chief use is in the form of a lotion (about 1 part to 30 of water) in all forms of itching and chapping of the skin. In thrush (q.v.) and other forms of irritation about the mouth in children the honey of borax, smeared on several times a day, is very soothing. To clean the mouth as well as soothe it, borax in honey wiped over the gums and tongue is very efficient. As in the case of boric acid, it should not be used in infants and young children.

BORBORYGMUS means flatulence in the bowels.

BORNHOLM DISEASE, also known as devil's grip, and epidemic myalgia, is an acute infective disease due to Coxsackie viruses (q.v.), and characterized by the abrupt onset of pain around the lower margin of the ribs, headache, and fever. It occurs in epidemics, usually during warm weather, and it is more common in young people than the old. The illness usually lasts seven to ten days. It is practically never fatal. The disease is named after the island of Bornholm in the Baltic, where several epidemics have been described.

BOTULINUM TOXIN The toxin of the anaerobic bacterium *Clostridium botulinum* (q.v.) is now routinely used to treat focal dystonias (q.v.) in adults. These include blepharospasm (see EYE DISEASES), spasmodic torticollis (q.v.), muscular spasms of the face, squint and some types of tremor. Injected close to where the nerve enters the affected muscles, the toxin blocks nerve transmissions for up to four months, so relieving symptoms. The toxin is also being tried out in cerebral palsies, and research is continuing.

BOTULISM A rare type of food poisoning with a mortality greater than 50 per cent, caused by the presence of the exotoxin of the anaerobic bacterium *Clostridium botulinum*, usually in contaminated tinned or bottled food. Symptoms develop a few hours after ingestion.

The toxin has two components, one having haemaglutinin activity and the other neurotoxic activity which produces most of the symptoms. It has a lethal dose of as little as 1 mg/kg and is highly selective for cholinergic nerves. Thus the symptoms are those of autonomic parasympathetic blockade (dry mouth, constipation, urinary retention, mydriasis, blurred vision) and progress to blockade of somatic cholinergic transmission (muscle weakness). Death results from respiratory muscle paralysis. Treatment consists of supportive measures and 4 aminopyridine and 3, 4 di-aminopyridine, which may antagonize the effect of the toxin.

BOUGIES are solid instruments for introduction into natural passages in the body either in order to apply medicaments which they contain or with which they are coated, or, more usually, in order to dilate a narrow part or stricture of the passage. Thus we have, for example, urethral bougies, oesophageal bougies, rectal bougies, made usually of flexible rubber or, in the case of the urethra, of steel.

BOVINE SPONGIFORM ENCEPHALOPATHY A fatal disease of cattle, equivalent to scrapie in sheep and similar to human Creutzfeldt-Jakob disease or kuru. It has recently reached epidemic proportions, generating public concern that it may be transmissible to humans. The disease is probably transmitted by ingestion of infected animal products and has a long incubation period – up to five years. The causative agent has not yet been identified but may be a slow-acting virus.

BOWELS (see INTESTINE).

BOWEN'S DISEASE This is a form of carcinoma *in situ* in the skin. It presents as an isolated scaling plaque. Round papules appear on the chest and back. It is due to abnormal keratin in the hair follicles and is a genetically determined disease.

BOW LEGS, or GENU VARUM: A deformity of the legs which comprises outward curvature between knee and ankle. It may be normal in infancy and occurs in osteoarthrosis, rickets, and other metabolic bone disease. In early childhood it may correct with growth, but in other cases surgical correction by *osteotomy* or ephiphyseal stapling is possible.

BOXING INJURIES rank eighth in frequency among sports injuries. According to the 'Report on the Medical Aspects of Boxing' issued by the Committee on Boxing of the Royal College of Physicians of London in October 1969, of 224 ex-professional boxers examined, 37 showed evidence of brain damage which was disabling in thirteen.

The subject remained a contentious one and in 1984 a report of a working party of the British Medical Association was published. It concluded that there are two main ways in which boxing may lead to structural damage to the brain. The first type of damage occurs as an acute episode in which one or more severe blows leads to loss of consciousness and occasionally to death. Death in the acute phase is usually due to intracranial haemorrhage and this carries a mortality of 45 per cent even with the sophisticated surgical techniques currently available. The second type of damage develops over a much longer period and is cumulative, leading to the atrophy of the cerebral cortex and brain stem. The repair processes of the brain are very limited and even after mild concussion it may suffer a small amount of permanent structural damage. Brain scanning techniques now enable brain damage to be detected during life. Brain damage of the type previously associated with the punch-drunk syndrome is now being detected before obvious clinical signs have developed. Evidence of cerebral atrophy has been found in relatively young boxers including amateurs and those whose careers have been considered successful. The tragedy is that brain damage can only be detected after it has occurred. Many doctors are opposed to boxing, even with the present medical precautions taken by those responsible for running the sport.

BRACHIAL means 'belonging to the upper arm'. There are, for example, a brachial artery, and a brachial plexus of nerves through which run all the nerves to the arm. The brachial plexus lies along the outer side of the armpit, and is liable to be damaged in dislocation at the shoulder.

BRACHYCEPHALIC means short-headed and is a term applied to skulls the breadth of which is at least four-fifths of the length. Brachycephaly is a characteristic of the Alpine race.

BRACHYDACTYLY is a term applied to the conditions in which the fingers or toes are abnormally short.

BRADYCARDIA means slowness of the beating of the heart with corresponding slowness of the pulse (below 60 per minute). (See HEART DISEASES.)

BRADYKINESIA refers to the slow, writhing movements of the body and limbs that may occur in various brain disorders (see ATHETOSIS).

BRADYKININ is a substance derived from plasma proteins, which plays an important role in many of the reactions of the body, including inflammation (q.v.). Its prime action is in producing dilatation of arteries and veins. It has also been described as 'the most powerful pain-producing agent known'.

BRAILLE   A system of printing or writing for the blind using tangible dots or points to represent the characters.

BRAIN   The brain and spinal cord together form the central nervous sytem, the twelve nerves passing on each side from the brain, and the thirty-one from the cord being called the peripheral nervous system, while the complex chains of nerves and ganglia lying within the chest and abdomen, and acting to a large extent independently of the other two systems, though closely connected with them, make up the autonomic system, and govern the activity of the viscera.

Divisions   The brain in its simplest form in lowly vertebrate animals is a thickened part at the front end of the spinal cord, developed in order to govern the organs of special sense, viz. smell, sight, hearing, and taste, lodged near at hand. Higher in the scale, in fishes for example, there are marked bulgings of nervous matter forming the fore-brain, the mid-brain, and the hind-brain, and that part connected with the nerves of the eyes appears to be the highest

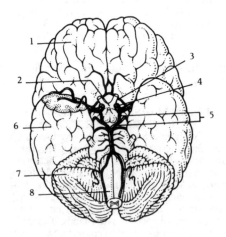

1 frontal lobe of cerebrum
2 optic chiasma
3 anterior cerebral artery
4 internal carotid artery
5 circle of Willis
6 temporal lobe of cerebrum
7 cerebellum
8 medulla oblongata (leading to spinal cord)

Brain viewed from below showing arterial network (circle of Willis),

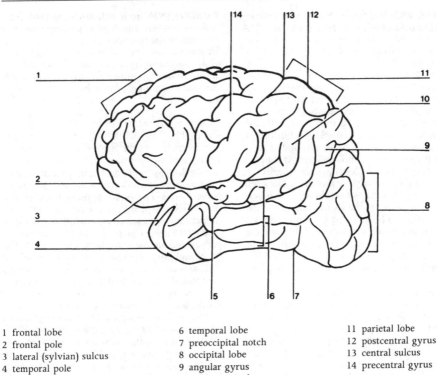

1 frontal lobe
2 frontal pole
3 lateral (sylvian) sulcus
4 temporal pole
5 superior temporal sulcus

6 temporal lobe
7 preoccipital notch
8 occipital lobe
9 angular gyrus
10 supramarginal gyrus

11 parietal lobe
12 postcentral gyrus
13 central sulcus
14 precentral gyrus

Side view of the brain.

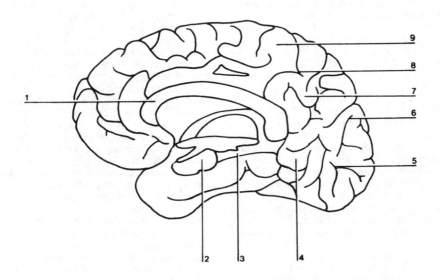

1 sulcus of corpus callosum
2 uncus
3 hippocampal sulcus

4 lingual gyrus
5 calcarine sulcus
6 cuneus

7 precuneus
8 subparietal sulcus
9 paracentral lobule

Vertical section through the middle of the brain.

governing part. In man, however, the part in front of this is specially developed, and not only forms the great bulk of the entire brain, but governs the activities of the rest. This part is called the cerebrum.

The CEREBRUM forms the great bulk of the brain in amount and consists of two cerebral hemispheres which occupy the entire vault of the cranium and are incompletely separated from one another by a deep median cleft, the longitudinal cerebral fissure. At the bottom of this cleft the two hemispheres are united by a thick band of some 200 million transverse nerve fibres: the corpus callosum. Other clefts or fissures, or sulci as they are known, make deep impressions, dividing the cerebrum into lobes. Of these the chief are the lateral sulcus and the central sulcus. The lobes of the cerebrum are the frontal lobe in the forehead region, the parietal lobe on the side and upper part of the brain, the occipital lobe to the back, and the temporal lobe lying just above the region of the ear.

Numbers of shallower infoldings of the surface called furrows or sulci separate raised areas called convolutions or gyri. The outer 3 mm or thereabouts of the cerebral hemispheres consists of grey matter largely made up of ganglion cells, while in the deeper part the white matter consists of medullated nerve fibres connecting different parts of the surface and passing down to the lower parts of the brain. Among the white matter lie several rounded masses of grey matter, the lentiform and caudate nuclei. In the centre of each cerebral hemisphere is an irregular cavity, the lateral ventricle, each of which communicates with that on the other side and behind with the 3rd ventricle through a small opening, the interventricular foramen, or foramen of Monro.

The BASAL NUCLEI consist of two large masses of grey matter imbedded in the base of the cerebral hemispheres in man, but forming the chief part of the brain in many animals. Between these masses lies the 3rd ventricle, from which the infundibulum, a funnel-shaped process, projects downwards into the pituitary body, and above lies the pineal gland. This region includes the important *hypothalamus*.

The MID-BRAIN, or *mesencephalon*, is a stalk about 20 mm long connecting the cerebrum with the hind-brain. Down its centre lies a tube, the cerebral aqueduct, or aqueduct of Sylvius, connecting the 3rd and 4th ventricles. Above this aqueduct lie the corpora quadrigemina, and beneath it are the crura cerebri, strong bands of white matter in which important nerve fibres pass downwards from the cerebrum.

The PONS is a mass of nerve fibres, some of which run crosswise and others are the continuation of the crura cerebri downwards.

The CEREBELLUM lies towards the back, underneath the occipital lobes of the cerebrum.

The MEDULLA OBLONGATA is the lowest part of the brain, in structure resembling the spinal cord, with white matter on the surface and grey matter in its interior. This is continuous through the large opening in the skull, the foramen magnum, with the spinal cord. Between the medulla, pons, and cerebellum lies the 4th ventricle of the brain.

Structure The brain is made up of grey and white matter. In the cerebrum and cerebellum the grey matter is arranged mainly in a layer on the surface, though both have certain grey masses imbedded in the white matter. In the other parts the grey matter is found in definite masses called nuclei, from which the nerves spring. The grey matter consists mainly of cells in which all the activities of the brain begin. These cells vary considerably in size and shape in different parts of the brain, though all give off a number of processes, some of which form nerve fibres. The cells on the surface of the cerebral hemispheres, for example, are very numerous, being set in layers five or six deep. In shape these cells are pyramidal, giving off processes from the apex, from the centre of the base, and from various projections elsewhere on the cell. The grey matter is everywhere penetrated by a rich supply of blood-vessels, and the nerve cells and blood-vessels are supported in a fine network of fibres, known as neuroglia. The white matter consists of nerve fibres, each of which is attached, at one end, to a cell in the grey matter, while, at the other end, it splits up into a tree-like structure round another cell in another part of the grey matter in the brain or spinal cord. The fibres have insulating sheaths of a fatty material, which, in the mass, gives the white matter its colour, and they convey messages from one part of the brain to the other (association fibres), or, grouped into bundles, leave the brain as nerves, or pass down into the spinal cord, where they end near, and exert a control upon, cells from which in turn spring the nerves to the body. Both grey and white matter are bound together by a felt-work called neuroglia. The general arrangement of fibres can be best understood by describing the course of a motor nerve fibre. Arising in a cell on the surface in front of the central sulcus, such a fibre passes inwards towards the centre of the cerebral hemisphere, the collected mass of fibres as they lie between the lentiform nucleus and optic thalamus being known as the internal capsule. Hence the fibre passes down through the crus cerebri, giving off various small connecting fibres as it passes downwards. After passing through the pons it reaches the medulla, and at this point crosses to the opposite side (decussation of the pyramids). Entering the spinal cord, it passes downwards to end finally in a series of branches (arborization) which meet and touch (synapse) similar branches from one or more of the cells in the grey matter of the cord (see SPINAL CORD).

Size The weight of the average male brain is 1·4 kg, ranging from 1·24 to 1·68 kg, of the female brain 1·25 kg, ranging from 1·13 to 1·51 kg, but brains have been found as heavy as 1·8 kg, or, in exceptional cases, even more. The maximum mass of brain tissue is reached at the age of 20, and then decreases steadily.

Functions The cerebrum is associated with the intellectual faculties in man, and also exerts a guiding influence over the rest of the nervous system. It is not, however, necessary to actual life. If the cerebrum of a frog is destroyed it still breathes and its heart beats, it can hop if pinched, and swim if put in water, but when left alone it sits still till it perishes. If the same happens to a pigeon it can fly when thrown in the air, and can alight, but it does not fly away when threatened, nor will it take food, having lost even the instinct to preserve life. If, on the other hand, the cerebellum of a pigeon is destroyed, the bird cannot maintain its balance, the cerebellum being concerned in the regulation of muscular movements and in preserving the equilibrium of the body.

Plato recognized three mental faculties, which he placed, respectively, in the liver, heart, and brain, these organs being supposed to secrete the 'animal spirits' appropriate to each faculty; and this view was accepted by the medical writers of antiquity. In the Middle Ages the Arabian physicians, however, following Galen's opinion, placed the different mental faculties in the several ventricles of the brain, this theory being adopted by Duns Scotus, Thomas of Aquino, and referred to by Burton in his *Anatomy of Melancholy*.

Descartes (1596–1650) had the fanciful idea that the pineal body was the seat of the mind. After his time it was thought that the whole brain must act together in every process, from the fact that, in cases of severe injury to the head, much substance can be lost from some parts of the brain without impairment of any one definite function or memory.

But it is now known that definite areas of the surface are associated with definite functions. The earliest systematic attempt to localize the functions of the brain to certain areas was made by Gall and Spurzheim, who founded the system of phrenology in the first quarter of the nineteenth century. Although this system was proved to be wrong both as regards the functions of the brain and the philosophic analysis of mental processes, the criticism it called forth gave a great impetus to the attempt to localize the functions of the brain in definite spots. Between 1820 and 1840 it became established that, in people who have lost the power of speech during life, the brain shows some disease in the left frontal lobe after death, and in 1861 Broca made the first definite discovery in cerebral localization by proving that the faculty of speech is governed by a centre in the region of the inferior frontal gyrus, named (after him) Broca's convolution. His discovery was followed later by the important observation of Hughlings Jackson that certain forms of epilepsy, associated with movements beginning in a definite limb, are caused by disease affecting the part of the brain that borders on the central sulcus, and this discovery was confirmed and extended by many experimenters and physicians. Fritsch, Hitzig, Ferrier, Sherrington, Grünbaum and others have shown that definite areas near the central sulcus are associated with the movement of definite parts. Further, the occipital lobes are associated with the sense of sight, the temporal lobe with hearing, and the inner surface of the same lobe with taste and smell. The purely intellectual faculties are probably associated with the frontal lobes, which seem to govern nothing else. The cerebellum has to do with the powers of balancing and of regulating movements. The medulla and pons have important functions, governing many of the processes most essential to life, e.g. those of respiration, rate of the heart, swallowing, vomiting, and giving off all the nerves which arise from the brain, except the first four.

MEMBRANES The brain is separated from the skull by three membranes: the dura mater, a thick fibrous membrane; the arachnoid mater, a more delicate structure; and the pia mater, adhering to the surface of the brain, and containing the blood-vessels which nourish it. Between each pair is a space containing fluid on which the brain floats as on a water-bed. The fluid beneath the arachnoid membrane mixes with that inside the ventricles through a small opening in the 4th ventricle, called the median aperture, or foramen of Magendie.

These fluid arrangements have a great influence in preserving the brain from injury.

NERVES: Twelve nerves come off the brain:

I.	Olfactory, to the nose (smell).	
II.	Optic, to the eye (sight).	
III.	Oculomotor	
IV.	Trochlear	to eye-muscles.
V.	Abducent	
VI.	Trigeminal, to skin of face.	
VII.	Facial, to muscles of face.	
VIII.	Vestibulocochlear, to hear (hearing and balancing).	
IX.	Glossopharyngeal, to tongue (taste).	
X.	Vagus, to heart, larynx, lungs, and stomach.	
XI.	Spinal accessory, to muscles in neck.	
XII.	Hypoglossal, to muscles of tongue.	

BLOOD-VESSELS Four vessels carry blood to the brain: two internal carotid arteries in front, and two vertebral arteries behind. These communicate to form a circle (circle of Willis) inside the skull, so that if one is blocked the others, by dilating, take its place. The chief branch of the internal carotid artery on each side is the middle cerebral, and this gives off a small but very important branch which pierces the base of the brain and supplies the region of the internal capsule with blood. The chief importance of this vessel lies in the fact that the blood in it is under specially high pressure, owing to its close connection with the carotid artery, so that haemorrhage from it is liable to occur and thus give rise to apoplexy. Two veins, the internal cerebral veins, bring the blood away from the interior of the brain, but most of the small veins come to the surface and open into large venous sinuses, which run in grooves in the skull, and finally pour their blood into the internal jugular vein that accompanies the carotid artery on each side of the neck.

BRAIN, DISEASES OF The human brain is a highly complex network of nerve cells and their interconnecting 'wires' or axons. Its diseases consist of either expanding masses (lumps or tumours); or of areas of shrinkage (atrophy) due to degeneration, or to loss of blood supply, usually from blockage of an artery.

TUMOURS All masses cause varying combinations of headache and vomiting – symptoms of raised pressure within the inexpansible bony box formed by the skull; general or localized epileptic fits; weakness of limbs or disordered speech; and varied mental changes. Tumours may be primary, arising in the brain, or secondary deposits from tumours arising in the lung, breast or other organs. Some brain tumours are benign and curable by surgery; examples include MENINGIOMAS and PITUITARY TUMOURS. The symptoms depend on the size and situation of the mass. Abscesses, or blood clots (HAEMATOMAS) on the surface or within the brain may resemble tumours. Some are removable. GLIOMAS are primary malignant tumours, which despite surgery and radiotherapy usually have a bad prognosis.

Clinical examination and brain scanning (CT, or computerized tomography (q.v.); magnetic resonance imaging (MRI) (q.v.)) are safe, accurate methods of demonstrating the tumour, its size, position and treatability.

STROKES When a blood vessel, usually an artery, is blocked by a clot, thrombus or embolism, the local area of the brain fed by that artery is damaged (see STROKE). The resulting infarct (softening) causes a stroke. The cells die and a patch of brain tissue shrinks. The obstruction in the blood vessel may be in a small artery in the brain, or a larger artery in the neck. Aspirin, anti-clotting, and other drugs reduce recurrent attacks, and a small number of people benefit if a narrowed neck artery is cleaned out by an operation, endarterectomy. Similar symptoms develop abruptly if a blood vessel bursts, causing a cerebral haemorrhage. The symptoms of a stroke are sudden weakness or paralysis of the arm and leg of the opposite side to the damaged area of brain (HEMIPARESIS); and sometimes loss of half of the field of vision to one side (HEMIANOPIA). The speech area is in the left side of the brain controlling language in right-handed people. In 60 per cent of left handers, the speech area is on the left side and in 40 per cent on the right side. If the speech area is damaged, difficulties in both understanding words, and in saying them, develops (see DYSPHASIA).

DEGENERATIONS (ATROPHY) For reasons often unknown, various groups of nerve cells degenerate prematurely. The illness resulting is determined by which groups of nerve cells are affected. If those in the deep basal ganglia are affected, a movement disorder occurs, such as Parkinson's disease, hereditary Huntington's chorea, or, in children with birth defects of the brain, athetosis and dystonias. Modern drugs, such as dopamine drugs (q.v.) in Parkinson's disease (q.v.), and other treatments can improve the symptoms and reduce the disabilities of some of these diseases.

DRUGS AND INJURY Alcohol in excess, the abuse of many sedative drugs and artificial brain stimulants – such as cocaine, LSD and heroin (see DRUG ADDICTION) can damage the brain; the effects can be reversible in early cases. Severe head injury can cause localized or diffuse brain damage (see HEAD INJURY).

CEREBRAL PALSY Damage to the brain in children can occur in the uterus during pregnancy or can result from rare hereditary and genetic diseases. Stiff spastic limbs, movement disorders and speech defects are common. Some of these children are mentally backward. Physical and rehabilitation therapies may be beneficial.

DEMENTIAS In older people, a diffuse loss of cells, mainly at the front of the brain, causes Alzheimer's disease, the main feature being loss of memory, attention and reasoned judgement (dementia). It affects about 5 per cent of the over-80s, but is not simply due to ageing processes. Most patients require routine tests and brain scanning to indicate other treatable causes of dementia. Response to current treatments is poor. Like Parkinson's disease it progresses slowly over many years. It is uncommon for these diseases to run in families. Rarely, multiple strokes can cause dementia.

INFECTIONS in the brain are uncommon. Viruses such as measles, mumps, herpes, AIDS, and, rarely, immunization cause encephalitis: a diffuse inflammation (see AIDS; and ENCEPHALITIS). Bacteria may infect the membrane covering the brain causing meningitis. Antibiotics have allowed a cure or good control of symptoms in most cases of meningitis, but early diagnosis is essential. Severe headaches, fever, vomiting and increasing sleepiness are the principal symptoms which demand urgent advice from the doctor, and usually admission to hospital. If infection spreads from an unusually serious sinusitis or from a chronically infected middle ear, or from a penetrating injury of the skull, an abscess may slowly develop. Brain abscesses cause insidious drowsiness, headaches and at a late stage weakness of the limbs or loss of speech; a high temperature is *seldom* present. Early diagnosis, confirmed by brain scanning, is followed by antibiotics and surgery in hospital, but the outcome is good in only half the patients.

BRAIN INJURIES Most blows to the head cause no loss of consciousness and no brain injury. If someone is knocked out for a minute or two, there has been a brief commotion of the brain cells (CONCUSSION), but no after-effects. Most leave hospital within 1 to 3 days, have no organic signs, recover and return quickly to work without further complaints.

SEVERE HEAD INJURIES cause unconsciousness for hours or many days, followed by loss of memory before and after that period of unconsciousness. The skull may be fractured, there may be fits in the first week, and there may develop a blood clot in the brain (intracerebral haematoma), or within the membranes covering the brain (extradural, and subdural haematomata). These clots compress the brain and the pressure inside the skull rises with urgent life-threatening consequences. They are identified by neurologists and neurosurgeons, confirmed by brain scans (computed tomography, magnetic resonance imaging (qq.v.)), and require urgent surgical removal. Recovery may be complete, or in very severe cases can be marred by physical disabilities, epilepsy, and by changes in intelligence, rational judgement, and behaviour. Symptoms generally improve in the first two years.

A minority of those with MINOR HEAD INJURIES have complaints and disabilities which seem disproportionate to the injury sustained. Referred to as the Post-traumatic Syndrome, this is not a diagnostic entity. The complaints are headaches, forgetfulness, irritability, slowness, poor concentration, fatigue, dizziness (usually not vertigo), intolerance of alcohol, light and noise, loss of interests and initiative, depression, anxiety, and impaired libido. Reassurance and return to light work help these symptoms to disappear, in most cases within three months. Psychological illness and unresolved compensation claims feature in many with implacable complaints.

People who have had brain injuries, and their relatives, can obtain help and advice from Headway National Head Injuries Association (see APPENDIX 2: ADDRESSES).

BRAIN-STEM DEATH When brain damage results in the irreversible loss of brain function, including brain-stem function, the individual is incapable of life without the aid of a ventilator. Criteria have been developed to recognize that 'death' has occurred and allow cessation of ventilation. The British criteria require that the patient is deeply unconscious and unable to breathe spontaneously.

All reversible pharmacological, metabolic, endocrine, and physiological causes must be excluded, and there should be no doubt that irreversible brain damage has occurred. Diagnostic tests are performed by two senior doctors which confirm that brain-stem reflexes are absent. These tests must be repeated after a suitable interval before death can be declared. The tests for brain death are:

(1) Fixed, dilated pupils
(2) Absent corneal reflex
(3) Absent vestibulo-ocular reflex
(4) No cranial motor response to somatic stimulation
(5) Absent gag and cough reflexes
(6) No respiratory effort in response to apnoea and adequate arterial CO_2.

BRAN is the meal derived from the outer covering of a cereal grain. It contains little or no carbohydrate, and is mainly used to provide roughage (q.v.) in the control of bowel function and the prevention of constipation.

BRANCHIAL CYST A cyst arising in the neck from remnants of the embryological branchial clefts. They are usually fluid filled and will therefore transilluminate.

BREASTS, or MAMMARY GLANDS, occur only in mammals and provide milk for feeding the young. These paired organs are usually fully developed only in adult females, but are present in rudimentary form in juveniles and males. In women, the two breasts overlie the second to sixth ribs on the front of the chest. On the surface of each breast is a central pink disc called the areola, which surrounds the nipple. Inside, the breast consists of fat, supporting tissue and glandular tissue, which is the part that produces milk following childbirth. Each breast consists of twelve to twenty compartments arranged radially around the nipple. Each compartment opens on to the tip of the nipple via its own duct through which the milk flows. The breast enlargement that occurs in pregnancy is due to development of the glandular part in preparation for lactation. In women beyond childbearing age, the glandular part of the breasts reduces (called involution) and the breasts become less firm and contain relatively more fat.

BREASTS, DISEASES OF In normal life, the female breasts undergo hormone-controlled enlargement at puberty, and also in pregnancy. The glandular part of the breast undergoes shrinkage (involution) later in life, after the menopause. Besides these normal changes, the breast can be affected by many different diseases. Common symptoms include pain, nipple discharge or retraction, and the formation of a lump within the breast. Despite recent publicity given to breast cancer, benign disease is much commoner than cancer, especially in young women.

BENIGN DISEASES These include inflammation of the breast (mastitis), abscess formation, and benign breast lumps.

Inflammation/mastitis/abscess Women who are breast feeding are particularly prone to inflammation of their breasts (mastitis), because infection may enter the breast via the nipple. Prompt treatment with antibiotics may arrest the process, before a breast abscess forms. Overflow of the contents of abnormal or blocked ducts (duct ectasia) can cause a non-bacterial inflammation in the surrounding breast tissue. Anti-inflammatory drugs, not antibiotics, are the appropriate treatment. If an abscess does form, it should be surgically drained regardless of the exact cause.

Nipple complaints The commonest symptoms are nipple retraction, discharge, and skin change. Mammary duct ectasia (above) with or without local mastitis is the usual benign cause of all of these complaints.

Breast lumps Breast lumps are either solid or cystic. Simple examination may fail to distinguish between the two, but if a simple, benign cyst is aspirated, it usually disappears. If the fluid is bloodstained, or if a lump still remains, malignancy is a possibility. The commonest solid benign lump is a fibroadenoma. This occurs mainly in women of childbearing age, and is a painless, mobile lump. Small ones can usually be safely left alone.

MALIGNANT DISEASE Cancer of the breast occurs most commonly in post-menopausal women, and presents classically as a slowly growing, painless, firm lump. Rarer symptoms, such as a bloodstained nipple discharge, or eczematous skin change over the nipple may also suggest the presence of breast cancer. Any lump in the breast should be carefully assessed in order to exclude malignancy, although in younger women a benign cause is still more likely. The usual investigations are a combination of mammography (q.v.) and aspiration of a lump to obtain a tissue sample for laboratory examination. These two tests reliably diagnose most breast cancers.

The treatment of breast cancer remains controversial. In some cases, mastectomy (removal of the breast) is still necessary, but if the disease is still contained locally, local excision of the lump is now commonly performed. It is generally accepted that sampling of the glands in the armpit of the same side should also be performed to check for spread of the disease beyond the breast, as this helps decide whether additional treatments, such as chemo- or radiotherapy would be of benefit. Screening programmes, involving regular mammography are now established in the United Kingdom and in other countries. These aim to detect more tumours at an early and curable stage.

BREAST SCREENING A set of investigations aimed at the early detection of breast cancer. It includes self-screening by monthly examination of the breasts and formal programmes of screening by palpation and mammography in special clinics. In Britain the Forrest report* recommended triennial mammographic screening by invitation of all women aged 50–64 and screening of older women on demand, but whether this is the most cost-effective system is currently under debate.

BREATH, DISORDERS OF The manner in which breathing is affected is described under RESPIRATION. (See also BREATHLESSNESS; CHEST DISEASES; LUNGS, DISEASES OF.)

BAD BREATH, or halitosis, in an individual can be unpleasant for others, even though he or she may be unaware of it.

Causes Frequent causes are bad teeth, infections of the gums (e.g. Vincent's angina), chronic tonsillitis, and indigestion. Besides these, bronchiectasis (q.v.) may produce a very unpleasant odour. A 'mousey' odour of the breath is often detectable during menstruation or

premenstrually. In certain diseases there may be a characteristic odour of the breath: e.g. a sweet odour in cases of diabetes mellitus verging on coma; a musty odour (foetor hepaticum) in severe acute liver failure; a urine-like odour in uraemia (q.v.). Certain drugs, notably paraldehyde and disulfiram, also give a characteristic odour to the breath, as do certain foodstuffs, notably garlic.

Treatment Careful attention to the hygiene of the mouth is essential, or the dental treatment of any defective teeth or infection of the gums. Any other relevant disorders should be treated. The smell may be temporarily relieved by an appropriate mouth wash or lozenges, several varieties of which are available commercially.

BREATH-HOLDING Breath-holding attacks are not uncommon in infants and toddlers. They are characterized by the child's suddenly stopping breathing in the midst of a bout of crying evoked by pain, some emotional upset, or loss of temper. The breath may be held so long that the child goes blue in the face. The attack is never fatal and the condition disappears spontaneously after the age of 3 to 5 years, but once a child has acquired the habit it may recur quite often.

The attacks require no treatment as recovery is spontaneous and rapid. In no circumstances should the parents dramatize the situation by slapping, pinching, or drenching the child with water.

BREATHING (see RESPIRATION).

BREATHLESSNESS may be due to any condition which renders the blood impure or deficient in oxygen, and which therefore produces excessive involuntary efforts to gain more air. Exercise is a natural cause and acute anxiety may provoke breathlessness in otherwise healthy people. Deprivation of oxygen – for example, in a building fire – will also cause the victim to raise his breathing rate. Many diseased *conditions of the lungs* diminish the area available for breathing: e.g. pneumonia, tuberculosis, emphysema, bronchitis, collections of fluid in the pleural cavities, and pressure by a tumour or aneurysm.

Pleurisy causes short, rapid breathing to avoid the pain of deep inspiration.

Narrowing of the air passages may produce sudden and alarming attacks of difficult breathing, especially among children: e.g. in croup, asthma, and diphtheria (see these headings).

Almost all *affections of the heart* cause breathlessness, especially when the person undergoes any special exertion.

Anaemia is a frequent cause.

Obesity is often associated with shortness of breath.

Among the *general diseases* which may interfere with breathing, uraemia (q.v.) and the coma which may occur in diabetes mellitus must be noted.

(*Forrest P. *Breast Screening: Report to the Health Ministers of England, Wales, Scotland and Northern Ireland by a Working Group Chaired by P. Forrest.* London: HMSO, 1986.)

BREATH SOUNDS The transmitted sounds of breathing, heard when a stethoscope is applied to the chest. Normal breath sounds are described as *vesicular*. Abnormal sounds may be heard when there is increased fluid in the lungs or fibrosis (crepitation or crackles), when there is bronchospasm (rhonchi or wheezes), or when the lung is consolidated (bronchial breathing). Absent breath sounds occur with pleural effusion, pneumothorax, or after pneumonectomy.

BREECH PRESENTATION Buttock presentation. The baby lies within the uterus so that it would be delivered buttocks first. This mode of delivery carries an increased risk of damage to baby and mother but with modern obstetric techniques the outcome of labour, though often prolonged, is usually satisfactory. If fetal distress develops the infant can be delivered by Caesarean section.

BRIGHT'S DISEASE (see KIDNEYS, DISEASES OF: glomerulonephritis).

BRITISH NATIONAL FORMULARY is a pocket book for those concerned with the prescribing, dispensing and administration of medicines in Britain. It is produced jointly by the Royal Pharmaceutical Society and the British Medical Association and is revised twice yearly.

BRITTLE BONE DISEASE is another name for osteogenesis imperfecta (q.v.).

BROMIDES introduced in 1857 as the first effective treatment for epilepsy (q.v.), have been largely superseded by barbiturates and more recent anticonvulsants (q.v.). They are also obsolete in their use as general sedatives and hypnotics (q.v.). Bromide is notoriously cumulative in the body, replacing chloride, and low doses taken over long periods may cause poisoning, or bromism (q.v.).

BROMIDROSIS means the excretion of evil-smelling perspiration. (See PERSPIRATION.)

BROMISM refers to a group of symptoms consisting of acne, with increased mucus secretion, headache, foul breath, tremors and incoordination, indicating that too much bromide is being taken. The bromide should be stopped and sodium chloride (5–10 g) with water (4 l) given daily.

BROMOCRIPTINE is an ergot (q.v.) alkaloid which is being successfully used in the treatment of acromegaly (q.v.). It is also proving of value in the treatment of Parkinsonism (q.v.), the suppression of lactation, and the pain in the breast that sometimes precedes menstruation.

BROMPTON MIXTURE is a prescription of somewhat variable constituents, but consisting basically of morphine, cocaine and whisky (or rum) which was used as an effective pain-reliever, particularly in the terminal stages of painful diseases such as cancer.

BRONCHIAL TUBES (see AIR PASSAGES; BRONCHUS; LUNGS).

BRONCHIECTASIS is a condition characterized by dilatation of the bronchi. This is the result as a rule of infection of the bronchial tree leading to obstruction of the bronchi. As a result of the obstruction the affected individual cannot get rid of the secretions in the bronchi beyond the obstruction. This accumulates and becomes infected and gradually weakens the wall of the bronchi which dilate and become an increasingly large deposit of infected material. The initial infection may be due to bacterial or viral pneumonia or the infection of the lungs complicating measles or whooping-cough. Other causes are obstruction of the bronchi by tuberculosis, cancer of the lung or the inhalation into the lungs of a foreign body, such as a tooth during dental extraction. It usually starts in childhood but may not manifest itself until adult life. It manifests itself by the coughing up of large amounts of putrid, foul-tasting, foul-smelling expectoration, which may contain blood. The condition is not immediately dangerous to life, but as a rule it results in a gradual deterioration of health, with night sweats, clubbing of the fingers and toes (see CLUBBING), and an aggravated form of chronic bronchitis. **Treatment** consists of getting rid of the accumulated secretion in the dilated bronchi by means of what is known as postural drainage. This consists of the patient lying on the affected side over the edge of the bed with a pillow under him, and the head well down, so as to drain the affected area. This allows the infected secretion to drain to the trachea (or windpipe) whence it is coughed up. This should be carried out for a quarter of an hour night and morning. It helps to increase the amount of secretion got rid of if someone percusses, or firmly taps, on the chest over the affected area. At the same time the patient should take deep breaths and cough firmly to dislodge the secretion and get rid of it. Should there be a flare-up of the condition, as there often is, this postural drainage should be done four times a day. If the odour is particularly unpleasant, this may be kept in check by inhalations of creosote, or by vaporizing creosote and other aromatic substances in steam near the bed. If there should be a flare-up of the condition due to infection, this is controlled by antibiotics. If the condition is localized to one lobe of the lung, an operation (lobectomy) may be performed to remove the affected lung. Patients with bronchiectasis should be immunized against influenza every autumn, should not smoke, and should ensure that they have a well-balanced diet and as much fresh air as possible.

BRONCHIOLES is the term applied to the finest divisions of the bronchial tubes.

BRONCHIOLITIS is the name sometimes applied to bronchitis affecting the finest bronchial tubes, also known as capillary bronchitis.

BRONCHITIS is inflammation of the bronchial tubes. This may occur as an acute transient illness or as a chronic condition.

ACUTE BRONCHITIS is due to an acute infection, viral or bacterial, of the bronchi. This is distinguished from pneumonia by the anatomical site involved – bronchitis affects the bronchi whilst pneumonia affects the lung tissue. The infection causes a productive cough, and fever. Secretions within airways sometimes lead to wheezing. Sometimes the specific causative organism may be identified from the sputum. The illness is normally self limiting but, if treatments are required, bacterial infections respond to a course of antibiotics.

CHRONIC BRONCHITIS is a clinical diagnosis applied to patients with chronic cough and sputum production. For epidemiological studies it is defined as cough productive of sputum on most days during at least three consecutive months for not less than two consecutive years.

In the past industrial workers regularly exposed to heavily polluted air commonly developed bronchitis. The main aetiological factor is smoking. This leads to an increase in size and number of bronchial mucous glands. These are responsible for the excessive mucus production within the bronchial tree causing a persistent productive cough. The increased number of mucous glands along with the influx of inflammatory cells may lead to airway narrowing. When airway narrowing occurs, it slows the passage of air producing breathlessness. Other less important causative factors include exposure to pollutants and dusts. Infections do not cause the disease but frequently produce exacerbations with worsening of symptoms.

Treatments involve the use of antibiotics to treat the infections that produce exacerbations of symptoms. Bronchodilators (drugs that open up the airways) help to reverse the airway narrowing that causes the breathlessness. Cessation of smoking reduces the speed of progression.

BRONCHODILATOR This type of drug reduces the tone of smooth muscle in the bronchioles and therefore increases their diameter. Such drugs are used in the treatment of asthma and other causes of bronchoconstriction. As bronchiolar tone is a balance between sympathetic and parasympathetic activity, most bronchodilators are either B2 receptor agonists or cholinergic receptor antagonists, although theophyllines are also useful.

BRONCHOGRAPHY means rendering the outline of the bronchial tree visible on an X-ray film by means of the injection of a radio-opaque substance through the larynx. This is a simple procedure carried out under general anaesthesia and allows the accurate location of, for example, a lung abscess, bronchiectasis (q.v.), or a tumour in the lung.

BRONCHOPHONY means the resonance of the voice as heard by auscultation over the site of the large bronchial tubes, and, in diseased conditions, conveyed beyond these by cavities or solidification of parts of the lung.

BRONCHOPLEURAL FISTULA An abnormal communication between the tracheobronchial tree and the pleural cavity (see LUNGS). Most commonly occurring from breakdown of the bronchial stump following *pneumonectomy*, it may also be caused by trauma, neoplasia, or inflammation.

BRONCHO-PNEUMONIA (see PNEUMONIA).

BRONCHOSCOPE is an instrument constructed on the principle of the telescope, which on introduction into the mouth is passed down through the larynx and windpipe and enables the observer to see the interior of the larger bronchial tubes. The bronchoscope has largely been superseded by fibreoptic bronchoscopy. (See FIBREOPTIC ENDOSCOPY.)

BRONCHUS, or bronchial tube, is the name applied to tubes into which the windpipe divides, one going to either lung. The name is also applied to the divisions of these tubes distributed throughout the lungs, the smallest being called bronchioles.

BRUCELLOSIS, also known as UNDULANT FEVER, MALTA FEVER, MEDITERRANEAN FEVER.

Causes In Malta and the Mediterranean littoral the causative organism is the *Brucella melitensis* which is conveyed in goat's milk. In Great Britain, the USA, and South Africa, the causative organism is the *Brucella abortus*, which is conveyed in cow's milk. This is the organism which is responsible for contagious abortion in cattle. In Great Britain brucellosis is largely an occupational disease and is now prescribed as an industrial disease (see OCCUPATIONAL DISEASES), and insured persons who contract the disease at work can claim industrial injuries benefit. The incidence of brucellosis in the UK has fallen from over 300 cases a year in 1970 to single figures in the 1990s.

Symptoms The characteristic features of the disease are undulating fever, drenching sweats, pains in the joints and back, and headache. There are, however, many atypical cases, and the diagnosis may be difficult. The liver and spleen may be enlarged. The diagnosis is confirmed by the finding of *Br. abortus*, or antibodies to it, in the blood. Recovery and convalescence tend to be slow.

Treatment Treatment is directed towards re-

lieving the symptoms. The condition responds well to one of the tetracycline antibiotics, and also to gentamicin and co-trimoxazole, but relapse is all too common. In chronic cases a combination of streptomycin and one of the tetracyclines is often more effective.
Prevention It can be prevented by boiling or pasteurizing all milk used for human consumption. In Scandinavia, the Netherlands, Switzerland and Canada the disease has disappeared following its eradication in animals. Brucellosis has been eradicated from farm animals in the United Kingdom.

BRUISES, or CONTUSIONS, result from injuries to the deeper layers of the skin or underlying tissues, with variable bleeding, but without open wounds. Bruises range from a slight bluish discoloration, due to minimal trauma and haemorrhage, to a large black swelling in more severe cases. Diseases such as haemophilia (q.v.) and scurvy (q.v.), which reduce coagulation (q.v.), should be suspected when extensive bruises are produced by minor injuries. Bruises change colour from blue-black to brown to yellow, gradually fading as the blood pigment is broken down and absorbed. Minor bruises may be prevented by applying pressure and cold compresses after the injury; but once bruising has occurred, the time taken to disappear is roughly proportional to the amount of bleeding. Bruising in the abdomen or in the back in the area of the kidneys should prompt the examining doctor to assess whether there has been any damage to internal tissues or organs.

BRUIT and **MURMUR** are words used to describe abnormal sounds heard in connection with the heart, arteries, and veins on auscultation.

BRUXISM or TOOTH GRINDING is the habit of grinding the teeth, usually while asleep and without being aware of it. The teeth may feel uncomfortable on wakening. It is very common in children and is of no significance, although more severe forms, even during the waking period, may occur in the mentally retarded. In adults it may be associated with stress or a malpositioned tooth or an overfilled tooth. It is also found in some patients taking drugs, such as fenfluramine and levodopa, which cause minor tremors and reduced muscle control. If the bruxism persists, then excessive wear may result in the loss of enamel and cause pain. Treatment is not very successful unless a cause can be found and removed. A plastic splint fitted over the teeth may help.

BUBO means a swelling of a lymphatic gland in the groin in venereal disease or in plague. (See PLAGUE.)

BUCCAL   Relating to the mouth or inside of the cheek.

BUDGERIGAR-FANCIER'S LUNG is a form of extrinsic allergic alveolitis, resulting from sensitization to budgerigars, or parakeets as they are known in North America. Skin tests have revealed sensitization to the birds' droppings and/or serum. As it is estimated that budgerigars are kept in 5–6 million homes in Britain, current figures suggest that anything up to 900 per 100,000 of the population are exposed to the risk of developing this condition. (See ALVEOLITIS.)

BUERGER'S DISEASE (see THROMBOANGIITIS OBLITERANS).

BULBAR PARALYSIS (see PARALYSIS).

BULIMIA means insatiable appetite of psychological origin. This eating disorder symptom may be of psychological origin or be the result of neurological disease, for example, a lesion of the hypothalamus (q.v.), Bulimia nervosa is linked to anorexia nervosa and is sometimes called the binge and purge syndrome. Bulimia nervosa is characterized by overpowering urges to eat large amounts of food followed by induced vomiting or abuse of laxatives to avoid any gain in weight. Most of the cases are prone to being overweight and all have a morbid fear of obesity. They indulge in bouts of gross overeating, or 'binge rounds' as they describe them, to 'fill the empty space inside'. By their bizarre behaviour, most of them manage to maintain a normal weight. It is most common in women in their 20s. The condition is accompanied by irregular menstruation, often amounting to amenorrhoea. Although there are many similarities to anorexia nervosa, it differs in that there is no attempt at deceit, and it is freely admitted that there is an eating disorder and there is distress about the symptoms it produces. In spite of this, the response to treatment, which is as in anorexia nervosa, is far from satisfactory. (See EATING DISORDERS.)

BULLA is another word for blister.

BUMETANIDE is a diuretic (q.v.) which is active when taken by mouth. It acts quickly – within half-an-hour – and its action is over in a few hours. (See BENZOTHIADIAZINES, DIURETICS.)

BUNDLE BRANCH BLOCK   An abnormality of the conduction of electrical impulses through the ventricles of the heart, resulting in delayed depolarization of the ventricular muscle. The electrocardiograph (see ELECTROCARDIOGRAM) shows characteristic widening of the QRS complexes. Abnormalities of the right and left bundle branches cause delayed contraction of the right and left ventricles respectively.

BUNDLE OF HIS, or atrioventricular bundle, is a bundle of special muscle fibres which pass from the atria to the ventricles of the heart and which form the pathway for the impulse which makes the ventricles contract, the impulse originating in the part of the atria known as the sinuatrial node.

BUNIONS (see CORNS AND BUNIONS).

BUPIVACAINE is a local anaesthetic, about four times as potent as lignocaine (q.v.). It has a slow onset of action (up to 30 minutes for full effect), but its effect lasts up to eight hours, making it particularly suitable for continuous epidural analgesia in labour (q.v.). It is commonly used for spinal anaesthesia, particularly lumbar epidural blockade (see ANAESTHESIA). It is contra-indicated in intravenous regional anaesthesia, or Bier's block (q.v.).

BURKITT'S LYMPHOMA Malignant lymphoma in children previously infected with Epstein Barr virus (q.v.). It occurs mainly in the jaw and abdominal organs. It is common in parts of Africa where malaria is endemic.

BURNING FEET is a syndrome (q.v.) characterized by a burning sensation in the soles of the feet. It is rare in temperate climes but widespread in India and the Far East. The precise cause is not known, but it is associated with malnutrition, and lack of one or more components of the vitamin B complex is the likeliest cause.

BURNING MOUTH is a traditional description of pain in the mouth. It is most commonly associated with faulty dentures. (See TEETH, DISEASES OF.) Other causes include infections of the mouth. (See MOUTH, DISEASES OF.) It sometimes occurs during the menopause and diabetic subjects are liable to complain of it, especially if their diabetes is not under control. Vitamin deficiency, particularly of certain members of the vitamin B complex, may be responsible. Fungal infection following the administration of antibiotics can also cause soreness in the mouth.

BURNS AND SCALDS Burns are injuries caused by dry heat, scalds by moist heat, but the two are similar in symptoms and treatment. Severe burns are also caused by contact with electric wires, and by the action of acids and other chemicals. The burn caused by chemicals differs from a burn by fire only in the fact that the outcome is more favourable, because the chemical destroys the bacteria on the part, so that less suppuration follows.

Severe and extensive burns are most frequently produced by the clothes, for example, of a child, catching fire. This applies especially to cotton garments, which blaze up quickly. It should be remembered that such a flame can immediately be extinguished by making the individual lie on the floor so that the flames are uppermost, and wrapping him in a rug, mat, or blanket. As prevention is always better than cure, particular care should always be exercised with electric fires and kettles or pots of boiling water in houses where there are young children or old people. Equally important is it that children's night-clothes and frocks be made of non-inflammable material. Pyjamas are also much safer than nightdresses. Severe scalds are usually produced by escape of steam in boiler explosions.

Degrees of burns The French surgeon Dupuytren divided burns into six degrees, according to their depth. In practice, however, today burns are referred to as either *superficial* (or partial thickness) burns when there is sufficient skin tissue left to ensure regrowth of skin over the burned site; and *deep* (or full thickness) when the skin is totally destroyed and grafting will be necessary.

Symptoms Whilst many domestic burns are minor and insignificant, more severe burns and scalds can prove to be very dangerous to life. The main danger is due to shock (q.v.). This arises as a result of loss of fluid from the circulating blood at the site of the burn. This loss of fluid leads to a fall in the volume of the circulating blood. As the maintenance of an adequate blood volume is essential to life, the body attempts to compensate for this loss by withdrawing fluid from the uninjured areas of the body into the circulation. This, however, in turn, if carried too far begins to affect the viability of the body cells. As a sequel, essential body cells, such as those of the liver and kidneys, begin to suffer, and the liver and kidneys cease to function properly. This will show itself by the development of jaundice (q.v.) and the appearance of albumin in the urine. (See PROTEINURIA.) In addition, the circulation begins to fail with a resultant lack of oxygen (see ANOXIA) in the tissues, and the victim becomes cyanosed (see CYANOSIS), restless and collapsed and, in some cases, death ensues. In addition, there is a strong risk of infection occurring. Particularly is this the case with severe burns which leave a large raw surface exposed and very vulnerable to any micro-organisms. The combination of shock and infection can all too often be life-threatening unless expert treatment is immediately available.

The immediate outcome of a burn is largely determined by its extent. This is of more significance than the depth of the burn. To assess the extent of a burn in relation to the surface of the body, what is known as the Rule of Nine has been evolved. The head and each arm cover 9 per cent of the body surface, whilst the front of the body, the back of the body, and each leg each cover 18 per cent, with the perineum (or crutch) accounting for the remaining 1 per cent. The greater the extent of the burn, the more seriously ill will the victim become from loss of fluid from his circulation, and therefore the more prompt should be his removal to hospital for expert treatment. The depth of the burn, unless this is very great, is mainly of import when the question arises as to how much surgical treatment, including skin grafting, will be required.

Treatment This depends upon the severity of the burn. In the case of quite minor burns or scalds, all that may be necessary if they are seen immediately is to hold the part under cold running water until the pain is relieved. Cooling is one of the most effective ways of relieving the pain of a burn. If the burn involves the distal part of a limb, e.g. the hand and forearm, one of the most effective ways of relieving pain is to immerse the burned part in lukewarm water and add cold water until the pain disappears. As the water warms and pain returns more cold water is added. After some three to four hours, pain will not reappear on warming, and the burn may be dressed in the usual way. Thereafter a simple dressing – e.g. a piece of sterile gauze covered by cotton-wool, and on top of this a bandage or a piece of Elastoplast – should be applied. The part should be kept at rest and the dressing kept quite dry until healing takes place. Blisters should be pierced with a sterile needle, but the skin should not be cut away. No ointment or oil should be applied, and an antiseptic is not usually necessary.

In slightly more severe burns or scalds, it is probably advisable to use some antiseptic dressing. These are the cases which should be taken to a doctor – whether a general practitioner, a factory doctor, or a casualty officer in hospital. There is still no general consensus of expert opinion as to the best 'antiseptic' to use. Among those recommended are chlorhexidine, and antibiotics such as bacitracin, neomycin and polymixin. An alternative is to use a Tulle Gras dressing which has been impregnated with a suitable antibiotic.

In the case of severe burns and scalds, the only sound rule is immediate removal to hospital. Unless there is any need for immediate resuscitation, such as artificial respiration, or attention to other injuries there may be, such as fractures or haemorrhage, nothing should be done on the spot to the patient except to make sure that he is as comfortable as possible and to keep him warm, and to cover the burn with a sterile (or clean) cloth such as a sheet, pillowcases, or towels wrung out in cold water. If pain is severe, morphine should be given – usually intravenously. Once the victim is in hospital, the primary decision is as to the extent of the burn, and whether or not a transfusion is necessary. If the burn is more than 9 per cent of the body surface in extent, a transfusion is called for. The precise treatment of the burn varies, but the essential is to prevent infection if this has not already occurred, or, if it has, to bring it under control as quickly as possible. The treatment of severe burns has made great advances, with quick transport to specialized burns units, modern resuscitative measures, the use of skin grafting and other artificial covering techniques and active rehabilitation programmes, offering victims a good chance of returing to normal life.

Chemical Burns Phenol or lysol can be washed off promptly before they do much damage. Acid or alkali burns should be neutralized by washing them repeatedly with sodium bicarbonate or 1 per cent acetic acid, respectively. Alternatively, the following buffer solution may be used for either acid or alkali burns: monobasic potassium phosphate (70 grams), dibasic sodium phosphate (70 grams) in 850 millilitres of water. (See also PHOSPHORUS BURNS.)

BURSAE are natural hollows in the fibrous tissues, lined by smooth cells and containing a little fluid. They are situated at points where there is much pressure or friction, and their purpose is to allow free movement without stretching or straining the tissues: for example, on the knee-cap or the point of the elbow, and, generally speaking, where one muscle rubs against another or against a bone. They develop also beneath corns and bunions, or where a bone comes to press in an unwonted manner on the skin.

BURSITIS means inflammation within a bursa. Acute bursitis is usually the result of injury, injury especially on the knee or elbow, when the prominent part of the joint becomes swollen, hot, painful, and red.

Chronic bursitis is due to too much movement of, or pressure on, a bursa, with fluid building up in the bursa. Fluid may need to be drained and the affected area rested. Excision of a chronically inflamed bursa is sometimes necessary. For example, the condition of housemaid's knee is a chronic inflammation of the patellar bursa in front of the knee, due to too much kneeling.

Chronic bursitis about the sinews round the wrist and ankle is generally called a ganglion. (See GANGLION.)

BUSPIRONE is an anxiolytic drug to be used only for short periods. It acts as a tranquillizer to relieve anxiety and is taken by mouth. Side-effects include nausea, dizziness and headaches.

BUSULPHAN is a preparation allied to the nitrogen mustard group of compounds (q.v.), with an action on dividing cells similar to that of irradiation. It is proving of value in the treatment of chronic myeloid leukaemia. (See CYTOTOXIC.)

BUTYROPHENONES are a group of drugs, including haloperidol, which are proving to be effective in the treatment of psychotic illness.

BYSSINOSIS is a pneumoconiosis (q.v.), or chronic inflammatory thickening of the lung tissue, due to the inhalation of dust in textile factories. It is found chiefly among cotton and flax workers and, to a lesser extent, among workers in soft hemp. It is rare or absent in workers in jute and the hard fibres of hemp and sisal.

C

CACHET means an oval capsule, generally made of rice paper, for enclosing a dose of unpleasant medicine. Cachets are softened by moistening with water prior to swallowing.

CACHEXIA is the feeble state produced by serious disease, such as cancer.

CADMIUM POISONING is a recognized hazard in certain industrial processes, such as the manufacture of alloys, cadmium plating and glass blowing. Sewage sludge, which is used as fertilizer, may be contaminated by cadmium from industrial sources. Such cadmium could be taken up into vegetable crops. Cadmium levels in sewage are carefully monitored; surveys performed of people eating their own vegetables, grown in gardens fertilized with contaminated sludge, have shown no adverse health effects. Where an excess of cadmium is consumed it causes gastroenteritis, resulting in diarrhoea and vomiting. The most important source of cadmium is food, particularly some vegetables (cabbage, spinach, lettuce, kale, rhubarb and celery) when grown on soils fertilized with large amounts of contaminated sewage sludge. Smoking of cigarettes is the second major source of intake. The EEC Directive on the Quality of Water for Human Consumption lays down 5 milligrams per litre as the upper safe level.

CAECUM is the dilated commencement of the large intestine lying in the right lower corner of the abdomen. Into it the small intestine and the appendix vermiformis open, and it is continued upwards through the right flank as the ascending colon.

CAESAREAN SECTION is the operation used to deliver a baby through its mother's abdominal wall. It is performed when the risks to mother or child of vaginal delivery are thought to outweigh the problems associated with operative delivery. One of the commonest reasons for Caesarean section is 'disproportion' between the size of the fetal head and the maternal pelvis. The need for a Caesarean should be assessed anew in each pregnancy. It is no longer true that a woman who has had a Caesarean section in the past will automatically have one for subsequent deliveries. Caesarean section rates vary dramatically from hospital to hospital, and especially between countries, emphasizing that the criteria for operative delivery are not universally agreed.

The operation is usually performed through a low, horizontal 'bikini line' incision. A general anaesthetic in a heavily pregnant woman carries increased risks, and nowadays the operation is often performed under regional – epidural or spinal – anaesthesia. This also allows the mother to see her baby as soon as it is born, and the baby is not exposed to agents used for general anaesthesia. If a general anaesthetic is needed (usually in an emergency), exposure to these agents may make the baby drowsy for some time afterwards.

Another problem with delivery by Caesarean section is, of course, that the mother must recover from the operation whilst coping with the demands of a small baby.

CAESIUM-137 An artificially produced radioactive element that is used in radiotherapy treatment (q.v.).

CAFFEINE is a white crystalline substance obtained from coffee, of which it is the active principle. Its main actions are as a cerebral stimulant, a cardiac stimulant, and as a diuretic. It is also of value in some cases of asthma. It is a constituent of many tablets for the relief of headache, usually combined with aspirin and paracetamol. Granular effervescent citrate of caffeine forms a useful, non-intoxicating stimulant in headache due to tiredness.

CAISSON DISEASE (see COMPRESSED AIR ILLNESS).

CALAMINE, or CARBONATE OF ZINC, is a mild astringent used, as calamine lotion, to soothe and protect the skin in many conditions such as eczema and urticaria.

CALCANEUS is the heelbone or os calcis.

CALCICOSIS is the term applied to disease of the lung caused by the inhalation of marble dust by marble-cutters.

CALCIFEROL, or VITAMIN D$_2$, is a crystalline substance extracted from irradiated ergosterol, and has the same action as vitamin D. Man attains vitamin D in two ways: from food naturally containing or fortified with vitamin D, or from its production in the skin by the action of ultraviolet light on the precursor 7-dehydrocholesterol. The vitamin D produced in the skin and occurring naturally in food products is cholecalciferol or vitamin D$_3$ while the product used for food fortification or prescribed as calciferol is the synthetic compound ergocalciferol or vitamin D$_2$. The biological activity of both ergocalciferol and cholecalciferol is the same and both are metabolized in identical manner. Cholecalciferol itself has little, if any, biological activity and it is metabolized in the liver and subsequently in the kidney to produce the active metabolite one alpha 25-dihydroxy vitamin D and this is known as calcitriol. One alpha cholecalciferol (alfacalcidol) is a synthetic analogue which is rapidly converted to the active metabolite.

The action of vitamin D is to increase the

absorption of calcium from the gut and to increase the calcium release from bone. If there is a deficiency of vitamin D from the diet, or if vitamin D is not absorbed adequately, or if renal disease prevents the hydroxylation of cholecalciferol to dihydroxycholecalciferol, the bone disease of osteomalacia (q.v.) will result. This is a particularly common condition in the Asian immigrant population in Britain who tend to take a diet low in vitamin D and also tend to avoid sunlight on the skin so that the production of ergocalciferol is impaired.

The treatment of osteomalacia is to provide vitamin D. For low-dose treatment the most widely used preparation is calcium with vitamin D (BPC.). (See APPENDIX 5: VITAMINS.)

CALCIFICATION is the process of deposit of lime salts.

CALCITONIN is a hormone produced by the thyroid gland (q.v.) which lowers the concentration of calcium in the blood.

CALCIUM is the metallic element present in chalk and other forms of lime. The chief preparations used in medicine are calcium carbonate (chalk), calcium chloride, calcium gluconate, calcium hydroxide (slaked lime), liquor of calcium hydroxide (lime-water), calcium lactate, and calcium phosphate (see LIME). Although still commonly used in the treatment of chilblains, there is little evidence that calcium is of any real value in this condition. Calcium gluconate is freely soluble in water and is used in conditions in which calcium should be given by injection. Calcium chloride is sometimes used in the resuscitation of patients with cardiopulmonary collapse.

Calcium is a most important element in diet; the chief sources of it are milk and cheese. Calcium is especially needed by the growing child and the pregnant and nursing mother. The uptake of calcium by the baby is helped by vitamin D (see CALCIFEROL). A deficiency of calcium may cause tetany (q.v.) and an excess result in the development of calculi (stones) in the kidneys or gall-bladder.

The recommended daily intakes of calcium are: 500 mg for children, 700 mg for adolescents, 500–900 mg for adults and 1200 mg for pregnant or nursing mothers.

CALCIUM-CHANNEL BLOCKERS, OR CALCIUM ANTAGONISTS, inhibit the inward flow of calcium through the specialized slow channels of cardiac and arterial smooth-muscle cells. By thus relaxing the smooth muscle, they have important applications in the treatment of hypertension and angina. They should generally be avoided in heart failure, however, as further cardiac depression may cause clinical deterioration. Sudden withdrawal may exacerbate angina. Various types of calcium-channel blockers are available in the United Kingdom. These differ in their sites of action, leading to notable differences in their therapeutic effects. All the drugs are rapidly and completely absorbed, but extensive first-pass metabolism in the liver reduces bio-availability to around one fifth. Their hypotensive effect is additive with that of beta-blockers; they should, therefore, be used with great caution, if at all, together. They are particularly useful when beta-blockers are contra-indicated, for example, in asthmatics.

Verapamil, the longest available, is used to treat angina and hypertension. It is the only calcium-channel blocker effective against cardiac arrhythmias and it is the drug of choice in terminating supraventricular tachycardia. It may precipitate heart failure, and cause hypotension at high doses; it should never be used with beta-blockers. Nifedipine and diltiazem act more on the vessels and less on the myocardium than verapamil; they have no anti-arrhythmic activity. They are used in the prophylaxis and treatment of angina, and in hypertension. Nicardipine and similar drugs act mainly on the vessels, but are valuable in the treatment of hypertension and angina. They are useful as both adjuncts and alternatives to beta-blockers.

CALCULI is the general name given to concretions in, for example, the bladder, kidneys, gall-bladder.

CALIBRE is a talking book service which is available to all blind and handicapped people who can supply a doctor's certificate certifying that they are unable to read printed books in the normal way. Its catalogue contains over 370 books for adults and over 250 for children, and additions are being made at the rate of around three a week. Full details can be obtained from Calibre (see APPENDIX 2: ADDRESSES).

CALLIPER is a two-pronged instrument with pointed ends, for the measurement of diameters, such as that of the pelvis in obstetrics.

CALLIPER SPLINT is one that is applied to the broken leg in such a way that in walking the weight of the body is taken by the hip bone and not by the foot.

CALLOSITIES are thickenings of the outer skin or epidermis. (See CORNS AND BUNIONS.)

CALLUS is the new tissue formed round the ends of a broken bone. (See FRACTURES.)

CALORIE is the name applied to a unit of energy. Two units are called by this name. The small calorie, or gram calorie, is the amount of heat required to raise one gram of water one degree centigrade in temperature. The large Calorie or kilocalorie, which is used in the study of dietetics and physiological processes, is the amount of heat required to raise one kilogram of water one degree centigrade in temperature.

The number of Calories required to carry on the processes necessary for life and body warmth, such as the beating of the heart, the movements of the chest in breathing, and the chemical activities of the secreting glands, is, for an adult person of ordinary weight, somewhere in the neighbourhood of 1600 Calories. For ordinary sedentary occupations an individual requires about 2500 Calories, for light muscular work slightly over 3000 Calories, and for hard continuous labour about 4000 Calories daily.

Under the International System of Units (SI) (see APPENDIX 6: MEASUREMENTS IN MEDICINE) the kilocalorie has been replaced by the joule, the abbreviation for which is J (1 kilocalorie=4186·8 J). As the term calorie, however, is so well established in medical writing, it has been retained in this edition. Conversion from Calories (or kilocalories) is made by multiplying by 4·186, but a factor of 4·2 is simpler and accurate enough for all practical purposes.

CALVARIA is another name for the skull cap or vault of the head.

CALYX means a cup-shaped cavity, the term being especially applied to the recesses of the pelvis of the kidney.

CAMPHOR is a solid, crystalline, oily substance distilled from the wood of a species of laurel grown in Japan and Formosa, or made synthetically. Liniment of camphor and camphorated oil (28·5 g of camphor in 228 ml of olive oil) are useful as a mild counter-irritant to produce a warm glow when rubbed into the chest in bronchitis and similar conditions.

CAMPYLOBACTER is a species of microorganism found in farm and pet animals, and there is increasing evidence of its transmission from such sources to man. Outbreaks of infection with it have occurred following the drinking of unpasteurized milk from infected cows and eating undercooked meat and poultry. It causes diarrhoea, and it is considered that it may be responsible for 8 per cent of sporadic cases of infective diarrhoea as a result of the inflammation of the small intestine (enteritis) that it produces. During 1989 over 32,000 cases were reported in England, a reflection of the continuing increase in the diagnosis and reporting of the disease since its implication in gastrointestinal disease was recognized in the mid-1970s.

CANALICULUS means a small channel, and is applied to (*a*) the minute passage leading from the lacrimal pore on each eyelid to the lacrimal sac on the side of the nose; (*b*) any one of the minute canals in bone.

CANCELLOUS is a term applied to loose bony tissues as found in the ends of the long bones.

CANCER is the general term used to refer to a malignant tumour, irrespective of the tissue of origin. 'Malignancy' indicates that (i) the tumour is capable of progressive growth, unrestrained by the capsule of the parent organ and/or (ii) capable of distant spread via lymphatics or the blood stream resulting in development of secondary deposits of tumour known as 'metastases'. Microscopically, cancer cells appear different from the equivalent normal cells in the affected tissue. In particular they may show a lesser degree of differentiation (i.e. they are more 'primitive'), features indicative of a faster proliferative rate and disorganized alignment in relationship to other cells or blood vessels. The diagnosis of cancer usually depends upon the observation of these microscopic features in biopsies, i.e. tissue removed surgically for such examination.

Cancers are classified according to the type of cell from which they are derived as well as the organ of origin. Hence cancers arising within the bronchi, often collectively referred to as 'lung cancer', include both adenocarcinomas (derived from glandular epithelium) and squamous carcinomas (derived from squamous epithelium). Sarcomas are cancers of connective tissue, including bone and cartilage. The behaviour of cancers and their response to therapy vary widely depending on this classification as well as on numerous other factors such as growth rate, differentiation in cell and characteristics and size at the time of presentation. It is entirely wrong to see cancer as a single disease entity with a universally poor prognosis.

Incidence In most western countries cancer is the second most important cause of death after heart disease and accounts for 20–25 per cent of all deaths. There is wide international variation in the most frequently encountered types of cancer, reflecting the importance of environmental factors in the development of cancer. In the UK as well as the USA, carcinoma of the bronchus (q.v.) is the most common. Since it is usually inoperable at the time of diagnosis, it is even more strikingly the leading cause of cancer deaths. In women, breast cancer is most common, accounting for a quarter of all cancers; nevertheless, fewer than a half of women in whom breast cancer is discovered will die from the disease. Other common sites are as follows: males – colon and rectum, prostate and bladder; females – colon and rectum, uterus, ovary and pancreas.

In England and Wales in 1989 over 205,700 people were registered as suffering from cancers of all types. Over 36,800 of them had lung cancer, over 27,100 had large bowel cancer, nearly 28,000 breast cancer and more than 8,000 uterine cancer. The incidence of cancer varies with age, the older a person is the more likely is he or she to develop the disease: the over 85s have an incidence about nine times greater than those in the 25–44 age group.

Causes of cancer In most cases the causes of cancer remain unknown. Rapid advances have, however, been made in the past two decades in understanding the differences between cancer cells and normal cells at the genetic level. It is now widely accepted that cancer results from acquired changes in the genetic make-up of a particular cell or group of cells which ultimately lead to a failure of the normal mechanisms regulating their growth. It appears that in most cases a cascade of changes is required for cells to behave in a truly malignant fashion; the critical changes affect specific key genes (q.v.), known as oncogenes, which are involved in growth regulation.

Since small genetic errors occur within cells at all times, most but not all of which are repaired, it follows that some cancers may develop as a result of an accumulation of random changes which cannot be attributed to environmental or other causes. The environmental factors known to cause cancer such as radiation and chemicals (including tar from tobacco, asbestos, etc.) do so by increasing the overall rate of acquired genetic damage. Certain viral infections can induce specific cancers (e.g. Hepatitis B virus and hepatoma, Epstein Barr virus and lymphoma (qq.v.)) probably by inducing alterations in specific genes. Hormones may also be a factor in the development of certain cancers such as those of the prostate and breast. Where there is a particular family tendency to certain types of cancer, it now appears that one or more of the critical genetic abnormalities required for development of that cancer may have been inherited. Where environmental factors such as tobacco smoking or asbestos are known to cause cancer, then health education and preventive measures can reduce the incidence of the relevant cancer.

Treatment Many cancers can be cured by surgical removal if they are detected early, before there has been spread of significant numbers of tumour cells to distant sites. Important within this group are breast, colon and skin cancer (melanoma). The probability of early detection of certain cancers can be increased by screening programmes in which (ideally) all people at particular risk of development of such cancers are examined at regular intervals. Routine screening for cervical cancer and breast cancer is currently practised in the UK.

If complete surgical removal of the tumour is not possible because of its location or because spread from the primary site has occurred, an operation may nevertheless be helpful to relieve symptoms (e.g. pain) and to reduce the bulk of the tumour remaining to be dealt with by alternative means such as radiotherapy or chemotherapy. In some cases radiotherapy is preferable to surgery and may be curative, for example, in the management of tumours of the larynx or of the uterine cervix. Certain tumours are highly sensitive to chemotherapy and may be cured by the use of chemotherapeutic drugs alone. These include testicular tumours, leukaemias (q.v.), lymphomas (q.v.) and a variety of tumours occurring in childhood. These tend to be rapidly growing tumours composed of primitive cells which are much

more vulnerable to the toxic effects of the chemotherapeutic agents than the normal cells within the body.

Unfortunately neither radiotherapy nor currently available chemotherapy provides a curative option for the majority of common cancers if surgical excision is not feasible. New effective treatments in these conditions are urgently needed. Nevertheless the rapidly increasing knowledge of cancer biology will almost certainly lead to novel therapeutic approaches – including probably genetic techniques utilizing the recent discoveries of oncogenes (genes that can cause cancer) – at least by the early twenty-first century. Where cure is not possible, there often remains much that can be done for the cancer-sufferer in terms of control of unpleasant symptoms such as pain. Many of the most important recent advances in cancer care relate to such 'palliative' treatment, and include the establishment in the UK of palliative care hospices.

Families and patients can obtain valuable help and advice from Marie Curie Cancer Care, Cancer Relief Macmillan Fund, or the British Association of Cancer United Patients (see APPENDIX 2: ADDRESSES).

CANCRUM ORIS, also called WATER CANKER or NOMA, is a gangrenous ulcer about the mouth which affects weakly children, especially after some severe disease, such as measles. It is due to the growth of bacteria in the tissues.

CANDIDA CANDIDIASIS or MONILIASIS is an infection due to the fungus *Candida albicans*. It is the most common fungal infection. When it infects the mouth it is called thrush and appears as white patches on the throat and tongue. Although it can occur in any debilitated patient, it is particularly common in individuals on prolonged antibiotic treatment. It is cured by the anti-fungal agent Nystatin given as lozenges so that it is retained in the mouth. Candida infections are also common in skin folds and the vulva. Candida is also a common cause of vaginal infection which presents as a vaginal discharge and responds to Nystatin pessaries. Generalized fungal infection may occur in individuals in whom the immune system is compromised, as in patients with AIDS or patients on immunosuppressive drugs. Such more generalized infections require systemic treatment with the anti-fungal drug ketoconazole given by mouth or amphotericin by intravenous injection.

CANINE TEETH, or EYE-TEETH (see TEETH).

CANKER is the name applied to small ulcers which form about the mouth and lips as the result of some local irritation, e.g. a jagged tooth, or in a condition of dyspepsia and deteriorated general health. (See MOUTH, DISEASES OF.)

CANNABIS is one of the oldest euphoriants. Cannabis does not cause physical dependence but its abuse leads to passivity, apathy and inertia. Acute adverse effects of cannabis include transient panic reactions and toxic psychoses. The panic reactions are characterized by anxiety, helplessness and loss of control and may be accompanied by florid paranoid thoughts and hallucinations. The toxic psychoses are characterized by the sudden onset of confusion and visual hallucinations. Even at lower doses cannabis can precipitate functional psychoses in vulnerable individuals. The acute physical manifestations of short-term cannabis abuse are conjunctival suffusion and tachycardia.

CANNABIS INDICA consists of the flowering tops of *Cannabis sativa*.

CANNED FOOD has remained popular despite initial prejudices. Efficient modern methods of canning preserve both the purity and the nutritional value of food, much of which would otherwise be difficult or impossible for many people to obtain.

Canning involves two essential processes: (1) heat treatment of the food and (2) expulsion of all air, followed by hermetic sealing. Aseptic canning, in which sterilized food is then sealed in sterilized cans, may simplify this process, resulting in cans of nutritious and tasty food that may safely be kept for long periods.

Food poisoning from canned food is rare unless contamination occurs after the can is opened, although outbreaks of typhoid fever have resulted from cans cooled in contaminated water, and several outbreaks of staphylococcal poisoning have occurred, particularly from food canned faultily abroad. All canned food is carefully inspected at the factory, if made in this country, or at import. Any defects such as leaking, rusting, or bulging of the cans are grounds for rejection, and any signs of decomposition or dubious canning quality should provoke immediate suspicion.

CANNULA is a tube for insertion into the body, designed to fit tightly round a trocar, a sharp pointed instrument which is withdrawn from the cannula after insertion, so that fluid may run out through the latter.

CANTHARIDES, or SPANISH FLY, is a powder made of the body and wings of a dried beetle, *Cantharis vesicatoria*, which inhabits Spain, Italy, Sicily and Southern Russia.

Action It is an irritant, first, to the part with which it is brought in contact, and, secondly, to the genital and urinary organs by which it is discharged from the body.

Uses Its only use is for blistering (see BLISTERS AND COUNTER-IRRITANTS), and it may be applied as a plaster, in a paste, or painted on in ethereal solution called liquor epispasticus but it is seldom used now.

CANTHUS is the name applied to the angle at either end of the aperture between the eyelids.

CAPILLARIES are the minute vessels which join the ends of the arteries to the commencement of the veins. Their walls consist of a single layer of fine, flat transparent cells, bound together at the edges, and the vessels form a meshwork all through the tissues of the body, bathing the latter in blood with only the thin capillary wall interposed, through which gases and fluids readily pass. These vessels are less than 0·025 mm in width. (See CIRCULATION OF THE BLOOD.)

CAPSULE is a term used in several senses in medicine. The term is applied to a soluble case, usually of gelatine, for enclosing small doses of unpleasant medicine. *Enteric-coated capsules*, which have been largely superseded by enteric-coated tablets, are capsules treated in such a manner that the ingredients do not come in contact with the acid stomach contents but are only released when the capsule disintegrates in the alkaline contents of the intestine.

The term is also applied to the fibrous or membranous envelope of various organs, as of the spleen, liver or kidney. It is also applied to the ligamentous bag surrounding various joints and attached by its edge to the bones on either side.

CAPTOPRIL is a drug that has been introduced for the treatment of patients with severe hypertension (q.v.) resistant to other hypertensive agents. It acts by lowering the concentration in the blood of angiotensin II which is one of the factors responsible for high blood-pressure. (See ANGIOTENSIN; RENIN.)

CAPUT MEDUSAE is the term describing the abnormally dilated veins that form round the umbilicus in cirrhosis of the liver.

CAPUT SUCCEDANEUM is the temporary swelling which is sometimes found on the head of the new-born infant. It is due to oedema in and around the scalp, caused by pressure on the head as the child is born. It is of no significance and quickly disappears spontaneously.

CARBACHOL is a drug which stimulates the parasympathetic nervous system. It is given, for example, for paralysis of the gut, for glaucoma (q.v.) and for retention of urine due to atony.

CARBAMAZEPINE is a drug which is proving of value in the treatment of trigeminal neuralgia (see TRIGEMINAL NEURALGIA). It is also of value in the treatment of certain cases of epilepsy. Because of its occasional action in causing aplastic anaemia and jaundice it must only be used under careful medical supervision.

CARBARYL is a broad-spectrum insecticide effective against lice. It was introduced because lice began to show resistance to DDT and gamma benzene hexachloride (qq.v.). It is particularly effective against head lice. (See INSECTS IN RELATION TO DISEASE.)

CARBENOXOLONE is a derivative of glycyrrhizinic acid, the active principle of liquorice, which is sometimes used to treat ulceration of the oesophagus, but its side-effects necessitate careful monitoring.

CARBIMAZOLE is at present one of the most widely used drugs in the treatment of hyperthyroidism. It acts by interferring with the synthesis of thyroid hormone in the thyroid gland.

CARBOHYDRATE is the term applied to an organic substance in which the hydrogen and oxygen are usually in the proportion to form water. Carbohydrates are all, chemically considered, derivatives of simple forms of sugar and are classified as monosaccharides (e.g. glucose), disaccharides (e.g. cane sugar), polysaccharides (e.g. starch). Many of the cheaper and most important foods are included in this group, which comprises sugars, starches, celluloses and gums. When one of these foods is digested, it is converted into a simple kind of sugar and absorbed in this form. In the disease known as diabetes mellitus (q.v.), the most marked feature consists of an inability on the part of the tissues to assimilate and utilize the carbohydrate material. Each gram of carbohydrate is capable of furnishing slightly over 4 Calories of energy. (See DIET.)

CARBOLIC ACID, or PHENOL, was the precursor of all antiseptics (q.v.). It paralyses and then destroys most forms of life, particularly lowly organisms such as bacteria, while also softening tissues. It has been superseded by less penetrative and harmful antiseptics, though it is still used in calamine lotion for its anaesthetic effect.

CARBON DIOXIDE, or CARBONIC ACID, is formed by the body during metabolism and is exhaled by the lungs (see AIR, VENTILATION). Seen in sparkling waters and wines, it is also used in baths as a stimulant to the skin. Combined with oxygen in cylinders, it is used to control breathing in anaesthesia and in cases of carbon monoxide poisoning.

CARBON MONOXIDE is a colourless and odourless gas, the presence of which in a room is undetectable by the occupants. Hence its danger because it has 300 times the affinity for oxygen that haemoglobin (q.v.) has. It converts haemoglobin into carboxyhaemoglobin, and thereby deprives the tissues of the body of oxygen, as there is no haemoglobin left to pick up oxygen in the lungs and carry it throughout the body. As the gas is odourless, the occupants of the room – or garage – have no idea that they are breathing it. The result is that they become unconscious in the contaminated atmosphere and, all too often, by the time they are found, they are dead. Carbon monoxide has a special action on the ganglia at the base of the brain, and, if sufficient amounts are inhaled, permanent destructive changes occur in this vital part of the nervous system. What makes carbon monoxide poisoning all the more dangerous is its insidious onset. One of the commonest causes of carbon monoxide poisoning used to be coal gas but this risk has been brought under control in Britain since natural gas was introduced; this contains no carbon monoxide. Natural gas is not absolutely safe, however, because when burned in the absence of sufficient oxygen, or, whenever, for any reason, combustion is incomplete, carbon monoxide is formed. The risk is particularly high with water heaters in inadequately ventilated bathrooms. Care about maintaining adequate ventilation must be observed with all forms of heating derived from carbon-containing fuel. Perhaps the greatest risk in this respect today is from the use of oil heaters in rooms in which all sources of ventilation, such as windows and ventilators, have, in effect, been hermetically sealed. This is one of the major reasons why deaths in the home from carbon monoxide poisoning, other than piped gas, have increased. The exhaust gas

Degree of saturation of haemoglobin with carbon monoxide per cent	Signs and symptoms
0 to 10	No symptoms
10 to 20	Tightness across the forehead
	Possibly headache
	Flushed skin
	Yawning
20 to 30	Headache
	Dizziness
	Palpitations on exercise
30 to 40	Severe headache
	Weakness
	Dizziness
	Nausea
	Collapse (possibly)
40 to 50	As above, with increased respiratory rate and pulse rate, and more possibility of collapse
50 to 60	Syncope
	Coma
	Cheyne-Stokes' respiration
60 to 70	Coma
	Weakened action of the heart and breathing
	Death imminent or actually takes place
70 to 80	Respiratory failure
	Death
90	Immediate arrest of the heart

The manifestations of carbon monoxide poisoning, according to the amount of carbon monoxide in the blood. The limit of safety is 18 to 20 per cent

of petrol vehicles is also dangerous. This is why the engine of a car must *never* be switched on in a garage unless the garage doors are open. The main manifestations of carbon monoxide poisoning are shown in the table above. One of the most striking signs of carbon monoxide poisoning is the cherry-red appearance of the victim's face. This is due to the large amount of carboxyhaemoglobin in the blood.

Carbon monoxide, which has a deleterious effect on arteries, aggravating the arterial disease which occurs in high blood-pressure (see ESSENTIAL HYPERTENSION) and coronary thrombosis (q.v.), is present in cigarette smoke.

Treatment Urgent treatment is necessary with the victim moved into the fresh air, the airway cleared and 100-per-cent oxygen given as soon as possible. Artificial respiration may be required (see APPENDIX 1: BASIC FIRST AID) and admission to hospital is advisable since complications can occur. (See POISONS and APPENDIX 2: ADDRESSES.)

CARBOXYHAEMOGLOBINAEMIA is the term applied to the state of the blood in carbon monoxide poisoning, in which this gas combines with the haemoglobin, displacing oxygen from it. (See CARBON MONOXIDE.)

CARBUNCLE like a boil, is an infection of a hair follicle and sebaceous gland or of a sweat gland, but unlike a boil it does not remain localized but spreads more deeply. The infecting organism is usually a staphylococcus. (See BOILS; KIDNEYS, DISEASES OF.)

CARCINOGENESIS is the means or method whereby the changes responsible for the induction of cancer (q.v.) are brought about.

CARCINOMA is a type of cancer (q.v.).

CARCINOMATOSIS The spread of cancer cells from their original site of growth to other tissues in the body. Such a spread of cancer, which takes place mainly via blood and lymph vessels, is usually fatal.

CARDIA is a term applied to the upper opening of the stomach which lies immediately behind the heart.

CARDIAC ARREST occurs when the pumping action of the heart stops. This may be because the heart stops beating (see ASYSTOLE) or because the heart muscle starts contracting too fast to pump effectively (ventricular systole, the period when the heart contracts). Coronary thrombosis is the most frequent cause of arrest. Irreversible brain damage and death result without prompt treatment. Heart massage, defibrillation and artificial respiration, are customary treatment. Other causes of cardiac arrest are respiratory arrest, anaphylactic shock, and electrocution. (See APPENDIX 1: BASIC FIRST AID: cardiac/respiratory arrest.)

CARDIAC CATHETERIZATION A diagnostic procedure in which a tube is inserted into a blood vessel and threaded through to the chambers of the heart to monitor blood flow, blood pressure, blood chemistry, and the output of the heart, and to take a sample of heart tissue. It is only performed for life-threatening conditions.

CARDIAC CYCLE The various sequential movements of the heart that comprise the rhythmic relaxation and expansion of the heart muscles as first the atria contract and force the blood into the ventricles (diastole) which then contract (systole) to pump the blood round the body. (See ELECTROCARDIOGRAM.)

CARDIAC DISEASE (see HEART DISEASES).

CARDIAC MASSAGE is the procedure used to restart the action of the heart if it is suddenly arrested. For long the only recognized method of doing this was by opening the chest wall and massaging the heart directly by hand. This is perfectly feasible if the heart stops beating during an operation. Elsewhere, however, it is seldom a practicable proposition.

Recently it has been shown that in many cases the arrested heart can be made to start beating again by rhythmic compression of the chest wall.

This is done by placing the patient on a hard surface – a table or the floor – and then placing the heel of the hand over the lower part of the sternum and compressing the chest wall firmly, but not too forcibly, at the rate of 60 to 80 times a minute. At the same time artificial respiration must be started by the mouth-to-mouth method. (See APPENDIX 1: BASIC FIRST AID.)

CARDIAC MUSCLE The muscle, unique to the heart, which comprises the walls of the atria and ventricles. It consists of long broadening cells (fibres) with special physiological characteristics which enable them to keep contracting and expanding indefinitely.

CARDIAC OUTPUT The volume of blood pumped out by the ventricles during each cardiac cycle.

CARDIAC PACEMAKER The natural pacemaker is the sinuatrial node, found at the base of the heart (q.v.). The heart normally controls its rate and rhythm; heart block occurs when impulses cannot reach all parts of the heart. This may lead to arrhythmia (q.v.), or even cause the heart to stop (see HEART DISEASES). Artificial pacemakers may then be used; in the

United Kingdom these are required for around one person in every 2000 of the population. Usually powered by mercury or lithium batteries, lasting up to ten years, they are either fixed to the outside of the chest or implanted in the armpit, and connected by a wire passing through a vein in the neck to the heart. Normally adjusted to deliver 65 to 75 impulses a minute, they also ensure a regular cardiac rhythm. Patients with pacemakers may be given a driving licence provided that their vehicle is not likely to be a source of danger to the public, and that they are receiving adequate and regular medical supervision from a cardiologist.

Although there are numerous possible sources of electrical interference with pacemakers, the overall risks are slight. Potential sources include anti-theft devices, airport weapon detectors, surgical diathermy, ultrasound, and short-wave heat treatment. Nevertheless, many pacemaker patients lead active and fulfilling lives, achieving high standards in many sports.

CARDIAC TAMPONADE Compression of the heart due to abnormal accumulation of fluid within the fibrous covering of the heart (pericardium). The result is irregular rhythm and death if the fluid is not removed.

CARDIOANGIOGRAPHY means rendering the outline of the heart visible on an X-ray film by injecting a radio-opaque substance into it.

CARDIOLOGY is the term applied to that branch of medical science devoted to the study of the diseases of the heart.

CARDIOMYOPATHIES are diseases of heart muscle of unknown cause. There are three distinct varieties: (1) *Hypertrophic cardiomyopathy* is characterized by massive ventricular hypertrophy. This hypertrophied muscle is not efficient and cannot relax adequately so that the ventricles do not fill properly during diastole. (2) *Congestive cardiomyopathy* is characterized by dilatation of both ventricles causing severe impairment of contraction. (3) *Restrictive cardiomyopathy* – organic material collects around the endocardium and myocardium which restricts the inflow of blood to the ventricles.

The disorder usually presents with congestive cardiac failure for which there does not appear to be a known cause.

CARDIOPLEGIA A procedure whereby the heart is stopped by reducing its temperature (hypothermia), by injecting the muscle with a solution of salts or by electrostimulation. This enables surgeons to operate safely on the heart.

CARDIOPULMONARY BYPASS A procedure in which the body's circulation of blood is kept going when the heart is intentionally stopped to enable heart surgery to be carried out. A heart-lung machine substitutes for the heart's pumping action and the blood is oxygenated at the same time.

CARDIOSPASM means the spasmodic contraction of the muscle surrounding the opening of the oesophagus into the stomach: also termed *achalasia of the cardia*. (See OESOPHAGUS, DISEASES OF.)

CARDIOVASCULAR SYSTEM This refers to the whole circulatory system: the heart, the systemic circulation (the arteries and veins of the body) and the pulmonary circulation (the arteries and veins of the lungs). Blood circulates throughout the cardiovascular system bringing oxygen and nutrients to the tissues and removing carbon dioxide and other waste products.

CARDIOVERSION A way of reinstating the heart's normal rhythm in patients with an abnormally fast or irregular beat. A carefully timed direct-current shock is administered to the chest wall of a patient under general anaesthetic.

CARIES, dental decay, is the material remaining after the calcified structure of the tooth has been removed in dental disease. This is probably initiated by bacteria. As the decay is removed a hole develops and the tooth may collapse.

CARMINATIVES are preparations to relieve flatulence, and any resulting griping, by the bringing up of wind, or eructation (q.v.). Their essential constituent is an aromatic volatile oil, usually of vegetable extraction.

CARNEOUS MOLE is an ovum which has died in the early months of pregnancy. It usually requires no treatment and evacuates itself.

CAROTENE is a colouring matter of carrots, other plants, butter and yolk of egg, and is the precursor of vitamin A, which is formed from carotene in the liver. (See VITAMIN and APPENDIX 5: VITAMINS.)

CAROTID BODY is a small reddish-brown structure measuring 5 to 7 × 2·5 to 4 millimetres, situated one on each side of the neck, where the carotid artery divides into the internal and external carotid arteries. Its main function is in controlling breathing so that an adequate supply of oxygen is maintained to the tissues of the body. Oxygen levels are controlled by a reflex operating between the carotid body and the respiratory centre in the brain.

CARPAL TUNNEL SYNDROME is a condition characterized by attacks of pain and tingling in the first three or four fingers of one or both hands, which usually occur at night. It is caused by pressure on the median nerve as it passes under the strong ligament that lies across the front of the wrist. It often responds to rest induced by fixing the wrist in a plaster splint. If it does not respond to this treatment, the pressure is relieved by surgical division of the compressing ligament.

CARPUS is the Latin term for the wrist, composed of eight small bones firmly joined together with ligaments, but capable of a certain amount of sliding movement over one another. (See WRIST.)

CARRIERS OF DISEASE (see INFECTION).

CARTILAGE is a hard but pliant substance forming parts of the skeleton, e.g. the cartilages of the ribs, of the larynx and of the ears. Microscopically, cartilage is found to consist of cells arranged in twos or in rows, and embedded in a ground-glass-like material devoid of blood-vessels and nerves. The end of every long bone has a smooth layer of cartilage on it where it forms a joint with other bones (articular cartilage), and in young persons up to about the age of sixteen there is a plate of cartilage (epiphyseal cartilage) running right across the bone about 12 mm (half an inch) from each end. The latter, by constantly thickening and changing into bone, causes the increase in length of the bone. (See BONE.) In some situations there is found a combination of cartilage and fibrous tissue, as in the discs between the vertebrae of the spine. This fibro-cartilage, as it is known, combines the pliability of fibrous tissue with the elasticity of cartilage. (For cartilages of the knee, see KNEE.)

CARUNCLE is the name applied to any small fleshy eminence, whether normal or abnormal.

CASEATION is a process which takes place in the tissues in tuberculosis and some other chronic diseases. The central part of a diseased area, instead of changing into pus and so forming an abscess, changes to a firm cheese-like mass which may next be absorbed or may be converted into a calcareous deposit and fibrous tissue, and so healing results with the formation of a scar.

CASEIN is that part of milk which forms cheese or curds. It is produced by the union of a substance, caseinogen, dissolved in the milk, with lime salts also dissolved in the milk, the union being produced by the action of rennin, a ferment from the stomach of the calf. The same change occurs in the human stomach as the first step in the digestion of milk, and therefore when milk is vomited curdled it merely shows that digestion has begun.

CASTRATION is literally defined as deprivation of the power of generation. In practical terms this involves surgical removal of both ovaries (q.v.) or testicles (q.v.). Such an operation is most commonly associated with the treatment of malignant lesions. In women who have reached the menopause, bilateral oophorectomy is routinely performed during hysterectomy (q.v.), especially in cases of uterine carcinoma, and is usually performed when removing an ovarian tumour or malignant cyst. In men, orchidectomy is routine for testicular tumours, and is common when treating prostatic cancer. It is no longer performed on young boys as a means of preserving the alto voice, the 'castrato' role having been superseded by the countertenor.

CASTS of hollow organs are found in various diseases. Membranous casts of the air passages are found in diphtheria and in one form of bronchitis, and are sometimes coughed up entire. Casts of the interior of the bowels are passed in cases of mucous colitis associated with constipation, and casts of the microscopic tubules in the kidneys passed in the urine form one of the surest signs of glomerulonephritis.

CATALEPSY is a nervous affection in which part or all of the body becomes rigid. Often associated with schizophrenia, it is characterized by the adoption of strange – often statue-like – poses (catatonia (q.v.)), which may pass off within a few minutes, or may last for several hours or, rarely, days. Typically brought on by a sudden mental trauma, it may occur with prolonged depression or some other serious mental illness (q.v.), and occasionally with epilepsy (q.v.). Successful treatment must depend upon due recognition of all precipitating factors and circumstances.

CATAPLEXY is a condition in which the patient has a sudden attack of muscular weakness affecting the whole body. (See also NARCOLEPSY.)

CATARACT An opacity of the lens sufficient to cause visual impairment.
Causes Frequently there is no specific cause. Lens opacities become commoner with increasing age and probably 90 per cent of people over 75 have them. A smaller proportion of people suffer visual impairment, when the term cataract is usually applied. Apart from age, other risk factors for cataract development include diabetes (q.v.), high myopia (see REFRACTION), use of corticosteroids (q.v.), renal failure, eye trauma, eye surgery and uveitis (q.v.). There are also associations with dystrophia myotonica (q.v.), atopic dermatitis (q.v.), infrared radiation and X-rays and suspected relationships

with smoking, heavy alcohol consumption, diet and exposure to ultraviolet rays (q.v.). Cataracts are rarely found in infancy or childhood. In these age groups possible causes include hereditary factors, metabolic disorders and infections transmitted to the fetus in pregnancy.

Symptoms No symptoms are specific to cataract. Patients commonly complain of blurred or misty vision and sometimes excessive glare from car head-lamps or sunlight.

Diagnosis The diagnosis of cataract should be approached with caution because of the variable relationship of lens opacities to symptoms and the possibility of mistakenly attributing the cause of visual disturbance to cataract.

Treatment The subject's lens is surgically removed and usually replaced by a synthetic intra-ocular lens implant. This can be performed as a day case with the patient receiving a local anaesthetic. There is usually no need to perform surgery in adults unless they request it. Occasionally a cataract is removed for other reasons: to improve the view into the eye for the doctor (e.g. in diabetes), or when one of the very rare complications of cataract occurs (glaucoma (q.v.) or uveitis).

CATARRH is a state of irritation of the mucous membranes, particularly those of the air passages, associated with a copious secretion of mucus. This complaint, so prevalent in damp and cold weather, usually begins as a nasal catarrh or coryza, with a feeling of weight about the forehead and some difficulty in breathing through the nose, increased on lying down. Fits of sneezing, accompanied with a profuse watery discharge from the nostrils and eyes, soon follow, while the sense of smell and to some extent that of taste become considerably impaired. Sore throat, fever and bronchial irritation may occur, causing hoarseness and cough. Sometimes the vocal apparatus becomes so much inflamed (laryngeal catarrh) that temporary loss of voice results. After two or three days the symptoms begin to abate, though sometimes infection spreads to the lungs. (See BRONCHITIS; CHILLS AND COLDS.)

CATATONIA is a syptom in which an individual takes up odd postures often accompanied by muteness or semicoma. The arms and legs may be moved passively by someone else into positions that the sufferer then holds for many hours. Catatonia occurs in schizophrenia. It may also be associated with organic brain disease such as encephalitis lethargica (see ENCEPHALITIS), tumours and carbon monoxide intoxication.

CATECHOLAMINES are substances produced in the body from the dietary amino-acids (q.v.), phenylalanine and tyrosine. They include adrenaline (q.v.), noradrenaline (q.v.) and dopamine which have varying functions, usually as neurotransmitters, in the sympathetic and central nervous systems (qq.v.). Their chemical structure is based on a benzene ring with hydroxyl and amine side-chains.

CATGUT is used in surgery for tying cut arteries and stitching wounds. It is made from the fibrous coat of the intestines of animals, especially of the sheep, requires very careful purification, and in the tissues is gradually absorbed – in about five to ten days – as it is itself an animal substance. Hardened catgut is catgut which has been treated with a suitable hardening agent to prolong the time taken for it to be absorbed; catgut hardened by treatment with chromium compounds is known as chromicized catgut.

CATHARTICS are substances which produce an evacuation of the bowels. (See PURGATIVES.)

CATHETERS are hollow tubes used for passing into various organs of the body, either for investigational purposes or to give some form of treatment. They are used under strict sterile conditions.

Varieties *Cardiac catheters* are introduced through a vein in the arm and passed into the heart in order to diagnose some of the more obscure forms of congenital heart disease, and often as a preliminary to operating on the heart. *Endotracheal catheters* are used to pass down the trachea into the lungs, usually in the course of administering anaesthetics (q.v.). *Eustachian catheters* are small catheters that are passed along the floor of the nose into the Eustachian tube (q.v.) in order to inflate the ear. *Nasal catheters* are tubes passed through the nose into the stomach to feed a patient who cannot swallow: so-called nasal feeding. *Rectal catheters* are catheters passed into the rectum in order to give injections. *Suprapubic catheters* are catheters passed into the bladder through an incision in the lower abdominal wall just above the pubis, either to allow urine to drain away from the bladder, or to wash out an infected bladder. *Ureteric catheters* are small catheters that are passed up the ureter into the pelvis of the kidney, usually to determine the state of the kidney, either by obtaining a sample of urine direct from the kidney or to inject a radio-opaque substance preliminary to X-raying the kidney. (See PYELOGRAPHY.) *Urethral catheters* are catheters that are passed along the urethra into the bladder, either to draw off urine or to wash out the bladder. It is these last three types of catheters that are most extensively used.

'CAT SCANNER' (see CT SCANNER).

CAT-SCRATCH FEVER is a disease, probably due to a virus, which is characterized by enlargement of the glands. In spite of the name, there is a history of a cat scratch in only about half the cases; in others the infection is acquired through a puncture of the skin by a splinter or thorn. The glandular swelling is usually slight and of short duration, but in some cases may go on to abscess formation which requires aspiration. The infection is not controlled by penicillin.

CAUDA A tail or a tail-like structure. For example, the cauda equina is a collection of nerve roots from the lumbar sacral and coccygeal spinal nerves that runs down inside the spinal column until it leaves it through their respective openings.

CAUL is the piece of amnion which sometimes covers a child when he or she is born.

CAULIFLOWER EAR is the term applied to the distortion of the external ear produced by repeated injury in sport. Initially it is due to a

haematoma (q.v.) in the auricle (see EAR). To prevent deformity the blood should be drawn off from this haematoma as soon as possible, and a firm pressure bandage then applied. Subsequent protection can be given to the ear by covering it with a few layers of two-way stretch strapping wound round the head.

CAUSALGIA A severe burning pain in a limb in which the sympathetic and somatic nerves have been damaged.

CAUSTICS AND CAUTERIES are used to destroy tissues, the former by chemical action, the latter by their high temperature. (See ELECTROCAUTERY.)

CAVERNOUS BREATHING indicates a peculiar quality of the respiratory sounds heard on auscultation over a cavity in the lung.

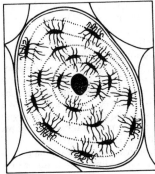

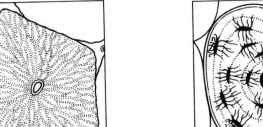

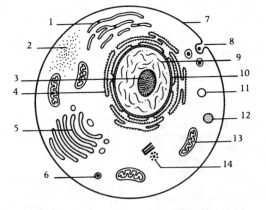

1 smooth endoplasmic reticulum
2 free ribosomes
3 nucleolus
4 rough endoplasmic reticulum
5 Golgi apparatus
6 microbody
7 cell membrane

8 exocytosis of secretory product
9 nuclear envelope
10 chromatin
11 glycogen granule
12 lysosome
13 mitochondrion
14 centrosomes (at right-angles to each other)

(Top left) Liver cell. (Top right) Bone cell. (Bottom) Diagrammatic representation of cell structure.

CAVERNOUS SINUS A channel for venous blood placed either side of the sphenoid bone at the base of the skull behind the eye sockets. Blood drains into it from the eye, the nose, the brain and part of the cheek and leaves via the internal jugular and facial veins.

CEFOXITIN is a semi-synthetic antibiotic, given by injection, which is used in the treatment of infections due to Gram-negative micro-organisms such as *Proteus* which are resistant to many other antibiotics.

CELLS are the microscopic particles which build up the tissues, of which they are the smallest structural divisions. There are around 10 billion in the human body.

Every cell consists essentially of a cell-body of soft albuminous material called cytoplasm, in which lies a kernel or nucleus which seems to direct all the activities of the cell. Within the nucleus may be seen a minute body, the nucleolus; and there may or may not be a cell-envelope around all. (See also MITOCHONDRIA.)

Cells vary much in size, ranging in the human body from 0·0025 mm to about 0·025 mm.

All animals and plants consist at first of a single cell (the egg-cell, or *ovum*), which begins to develop when fertilized by the sperm-cell derived from the opposite sex. Development begins by a division into two new cells, then into four, and so on till a large mass is formed. These cells then arrange themselves into layers, and form various tubes, rods, and masses which represent in the embryo the organs of the fully developed animal. (See FETUS.)

When the individual organs have been laid down on a scaffolding of cells, these gradually change in shape and in chemical composition. The cells in the nervous system send out long processes to form the nerves, those in the muscles become long and striped in appearance, and those which form fat become filled with fat droplets which distend the cells. Further, they begin to produce, between one another, the substances which give the various tissues their special character. Thus, in the future bones, some cells deposit lime salts, and others form cartilage; while, in tendons, they produce long white fibres of a gelatinous substance. In some organs the cells change little: thus the liver consists of columns of large cells packed together, while many cells, like the white blood corpuscles, retain their primitive characters almost entire.

Thus cells are the active agents in forming the body, and they have a similar function in repairing its wear and tear. Tumours (q.v.), and especially malignant tumours, have a highly cellular structure, the cells being of an embryonic type, or, at best, forming poor imitations of the tissues in which they grow.

CELLULITIS means an inflammation taking place in cellular tissue and usually refers to infection in the subcutaneous tissue. The word is erroneously used in the slimming business to refer to excess fatty tissue in the arms, buttocks and thighs. (See ABSCESS; ERYSIPELAS.)

CELLULOSE is a carbohydrate substance forming the skeleton of most plant structures. It is colourless, transparent, insoluble in water and is practically unaffected by digestion. In vegetable foods it therefore adds to the bulk, but it is of no value as a food-stuff. It is found in practically a pure state in cotton-wool.

CEMENT (see TEETH).

CEMENT BURNS arise as a result of prolonged contact of the skin with builders' cement. They are due to quicklime which constitutes 65 per cent of cement. As they are chemical, and not thermal, burns, the victim feels no immediate pain and therefore allows the contact to persist. The precautions that should be taken include adequate protection of the hands and feet, and avoidance of prolonged contact of the skin with cement. Cement, especially varieties containing chromium compounds, is a common cause of contact dermatitis (see DERMATITIS).

CENSOR is a term applied to the mental influence which prevents certain subconscious thoughts and wishes from coming into consciousness unless they are disguised so as to be unrecognizable.

CENTRAL NERVOUS SYSTEM This comprises the nervous tissue of the brain and spinal cord but does *not* include the cranial and spinal nerves and the autonomic nervous system. This latter group makes up the peripheral nervous system.

CENTRAL VENOUS PRESSURE The pressure of blood within the right atrium of the heart as measured by a catheter and manometer.

CENTRE is a term applied to a collection of nerve cells which give off nerve fibres and control some particular function: e.g. the speech centre and the vision centre in the brain.

CEPHALOSPORINS have been described as 'a valuable and versatile group of broad-spectrum, non-toxic antibiotics'. Most of them available at the moment are semi-synthetic derivatives of cephalosporin C, an antibiotic originally derived from a sewage outfall in Sardinia. They include cephaloridine, cephalothin, cephalexin, cephradine, and cephalozin. The term is sometimes used to include a group of semi-synthetic antibiotics with a comparable range of antibacterial action, but derived from a species of streptomyces. Strictly speaking this group, which includes cefoxitin, should be described as cephamycins. The indications for the use of individual members of the group vary. Some are active when given by mouth. Some have to be given by injection. One of their valuable features is that they are sometimes active against micro-organisms that have become resistant to penicillin, such as the gonococcus.

CERATE is a medicinal preparation, intended for external application, made with a basis consisting of wax in whole or in part which can be spread on the skin without melting: e.g. camphor cerate, compound menthol cerate.

CEREAL is the term applied to any plant of the nature of grass bearing an edible seed. The important cereals are wheat, oats, barley, maize, rice and millet. Along with these are usually included tapioca (derived from the cassava plant), sago (derived from the pith of the sago palm) and arrowroot (derived from the root of a West Indian plant), all of which consist almost entirely of starch. Semolina, farola and macaroni are preparations of wheat.

	per cent
Water	10 to 12
Protein	10 to 12
Carbohydrate	65 to 75
Fat	0·5 to 8
Mineral matter	2

Composition of cereals

Cereals consist predominantly of carbohydrate. They are therefore an excellent source of energy. On the other hand, their deficiency in protein and fat means that to provide a balanced diet, they must be supplemented by other foods rich in protein and fat, such as meat, milk and eggs.

	Water	Protein	Fat	Carbohydrate	Cellulose	Ash
Wheat	12·0	11·0	1·7	71·2	2·2	1·9
Oatmeal	7·2	14·2	7·3	65·9	3·5	1·9
Barley	12·3	10·1	1·9	69·5	3·8	2·4
Rye	11·0	10·2	2·3	72·3	2·1	2·1
Maize	12·5	9·7	5·4	68·9	2·0	1·5
Rice (polished)	12·4	6·9	0·4	79·4	0·4	0·5
Millet	12·3	10·4	3·9	68·3	2·9	2·2
Buckwheat	13·0	10·2	2·2	61·3	11·1	2·2

Composition of certain cereals.

CEREBELLUM AND CEREBRUM (see BRAIN).

CEREBRAL PALSY is the term used to describe a group of conditions characterized by varying degrees of paralysis and occurring in infancy or early childhood. In some 80 per cent of cases this takes the form of spastic paralysis: hence the lay description of them as 'spastics'.

The incidence is believed to be around 2 or 2·5 per 1000 of the childhood community. In the majority of cases the abnormality dates from before birth or occurs during birth. Among the pre-natal factors are some genetic malformation of the brain, a congenital defect of the brain, or some adverse effect on the fetal brain as by infection during pregnancy. Among the factors during birth that may be responsible are trauma to the child or prolonged lack of oxygen such as can occur during a difficult labour. This last factor is considered by some to be the most important single factor. In some 10 to 15 per cent of cases the condition is acquired after birth, when it may be due to kernicterus (q.v.), infection of the brain, cerebral thrombosis or embolism, or trauma. The congenital form is commoner in boys than girls, and a high proportion of the cases are first-born children.

The disease manifests itself in many ways. The victim may be spastic or flaccid, or the slow, writhing involuntary movements, known as athetosis, may be the predominant feature. These involuntary movements often disappear during sleep and may be controlled, or even abolished, in some cases by training the child to relax. The paralysis varies tremendously. It may involve the limbs on one side of the body (hemiplegia), both lower limbs (paraplegia), or all four limbs (tetraplegia). Mental subnormality is not uncommon.

The outlook for life is good, only the more severely affected cases dying in infancy. Although there is no cure, much can be done to help these disabled children, particularly if the condition is detected at an early stage. Little can be done to help those who have severe mental subnormality, but much can be done for those with normal intelligence by team work, giving attention to education, physiotherapy, occupational therapy and speech training. In this way many of these handicapped children are now reaching adult life as useful members of the community. Much help in dealing with these children can be obtained from SCOPE (formerly the Spastics Society), and the Scottish Council for Spastics (see APPENDIX 2: ADDRESSES).

CEREBROSPINAL FLUID is the fluid within the ventricles of the brain and bathing its surface and that of the spinal cord. Normally a clear, colourless fluid, its pressure when an individual is lying on one side is 50 to 150 mm water. A lumbar puncture (q.v.) should not be done if the intracranial pressure is raised (see HYDROCEPHALUS).

The cerebrospinal fluid provides useful information in various conditions and is invaluable in the diagnosis of acute and chronic inflammatory diseases of the nervous system. Bacterial meningitis results in a large increase in the number of polymorphonuclear leucocytes, while a marked lymphocytosis is seen in viral meningitis and encephalitis, tuberculous meningitis and neurosyphilis. The total protein content is raised in many neurological diseases, being particularly high with neurofibromas and Guillan-Barré syndrome, while the immunoglobulin G fraction is raised in multiple sclerosis, neurosyphilis, and connective-tissue disorders. The glucose content is raised in diabetes, but may be very low in bacterial meningitis, when appropriately stained smears or cultures often define the infecting organism.

CEREBROVASCULAR ACCIDENT (see STROKE.)

CERUMEN is the name for the wax-like secretion found in the external ear.

CERVICAL means anything pertaining to the neck, or to the neck of the womb.

CERVICAL CANCER Cancer of the cervix, the neck of the womb, is one of the most common cancers affecting women throughout the world. In some areas its incidence is increasing. This cancer has clearly identifiable precancerous stages with abnormal changes occurring in the cells on the surface of the cervix. These changes can be detected by a cervical smear test. Early cancer can be cured by diathermy, laser treatment, electrocoagulation or cryosurgery. If the disease has spread into the body of the cervix or beyond, more extensive surgery and possibly radiotherapy may be needed. The cure rate is 95 per cent if treated in the early stages but may fall as low as 10 per cent in some severe cases. About 4500 patients are diagnosed as having cervical cancer every year in the United Kingdom and about 2500 die from it. The sexual behaviour of a woman and her male partners influences the chances of getting this cancer. The earlier a woman has sexual intercourse and the more partners she has, the greater is the risk of developing the disease.

CERVICAL SMEAR This test detects abnormal changes in the cells of the cervix and this enables an affected woman to have early treatment. The National Health Service has arrangements to check women regularly. A woman's first test should be within six months of her first experience of intercourse and thereafter at three-yearly intervals for the rest of her life. The test is simple, with some cells being scraped off the cervix with a spatula and the tissue then being examined microscopically.

CERVICAL VERTEBRAE The seven bones of the top end of the backbone that form the neck. The first cervical vertebra is the atlas and this articulates with the base of the skull. The axis is the second vertebra, which contains a shaft of bone that allows the atlas to rotate on it, thus permitting the head to turn. (See SPINAL COLUMN.)

CERVICITIS means inflammation of the cervix uteri or neck of the womb.

CERVIX UTERI is the neck of the womb or uterus and is placed partly above and partly within the vagina. (See UTERUS.)

CETRIMIDE (also known as CETAVLON) is the official name for a mixture of alkyl ammonium bromides. It is a potent antiseptic, and as a 1-per-cent solution is used for cleaning and disinfecting wounds, and in the first-aid treatment of burns. As it is also a detergent, it is particularly useful for cleaning the skin, and also for cleansing and disinfecting greasy and infected bowls and baths.

CHAFING OF THE SKIN, commonly seen in infants and elderly people, is caused by the constant rubbing of two moist surfaces, typically at the natural folds such as the groins, armpits, and elbows. Clothes and ill-fitting shoes may also cause friction and pressure. It is best prevented by keeping the skin clean and dry.

CHAGAS' DISEASE, or American trypanosomiasis, is a disease widespread in Central and South America, and caused by the *Trypanosoma cruzi*. The disease is transmitted by the biting bugs, *Panstrongylus megistus* and *Triatoma infestans*. It occurs in an acute and a chronic form. The former, which is most common in children, practically always affects the heart, and the prognosis is poor. The chronic form is commonest in adolescents and young adults and the outcome depends upon the extent to which the heart is involved. There is no effective drug treatment. It has been suggested that Charles Darwin acquired the disease during his historic voyage on *The Beagle* and that it was the chronic form that turned him into an invalid for 40 years of his life after his return home and ultimately was responsible for his death in 1882. (See also SLEEPING SICKNESS.)

CHALAZION (see EYE DISEASES).

CHALICOSIS is a disorder of the lungs found among stonecutters, and due to the inhalation of fine particles of stone.

CHALK is calcium carbonate.

CHALK-STONES (see GOUT).

CHALYBEATE tonics or waters are those containing salts of iron. (See IRON.)

CHAMOMILE TEA is a bitter made by infusing chamomile flowers in boiling water for fifteen minutes and then straining. It is used cold in wineglassful doses.

CHANCRE means the primary lesion of syphilis.

CHANCROID means a soft or non-syphilitic venereal sore. It is caused by a micro-organism known as *Haemophilus ducreyi*. It is usually acquired by sexual contact, and responds well to treatment with sulphadimidine (q.v.). Fewer than 100 cases are diagnosed in Britain annually.

CHANGE OF LIFE (see CLIMACTERIC; MENSTRUATION).

CHAPPED HANDS occur in cold weather, when reduced sweat and sebaceous activity leads to decreased natural protection of the skin. Prolonged immersion in soapy water, followed by exposure to cold air, results in cracking of the skin.
   Prevention consists of minimizing exposure to detergents and soapy water, and wearing rubber gloves for all routine household duties. The hands should be kept dry and warm, and an oily barrier cream (q.v.) may be applied. Chapped hands should have an aqueous or oily cream applied regularly at bedtime, after which they should be covered by thin cotton gloves. Cracked fingertips are best treated with a tincture of benzoin and collodion.

CHAPPED LIPS (see LIPS).

CHARCOAL as used in medicine is a black powder prepared from vegetable matter by carbonization and activation. Available as granules, tablets, or biscuits, its value results from its ability to adsorb both gases and chemicals. Its two main uses are in the treatment of flatulence, supposedly by absorbing intestinal gas, and in treating overdoses of many drugs such as aspirin, paracetamol, antidepressants, barbiturates, and morphine. The dosage required is much larger for poisoning, and it is most useful if given within an hour of ingestion of the poison. It can adsorb ipecacuanha, therefore it should not be given until the emetic has taken effect. Methionine (an antidote to paracetamol) is also adsorbed, and the two should not be given together. It is occasionally applied as deodorant to foul skin ulcers.

CHARCOT-LEYDEN CRYSTALS are sharp crystals found in the sputum of those suffering from asthma, and of those affected by some blood diseases.

CHARCOT'S JOINTS is the name applied to a painless swelling and disorganization of the joints which is the result of damage to the pain fibres that occurs in diabetic neuropathy and tabes dorsalis. (See TABES.)

CHEILOSIS is an eczematous condition of the lips, especially at the angles of the mouth, and believed to be due to deficiency in the diet of one of the vitamins in the vitamin B complex – riboflavin. ANGULAR STOMATITIS and PERLÈCHE are other terms used to describe the condition, which may be associated with a red, sore tongue; fine desquamation at the junction of nose and lip, just inside the nose, and in the ears; eczema of the scrotum and perineum.

CHEIROPOMPHOLYX is the term applied to a disease of the skin in which little blisters filled with clear fluid suddenly appear on the hands and fingers. (See also POMPHOLYX.)

CHELATING AGENTS are compounds that will render an ion (usually a metal) biologically inactive by incorporating it into an inner ring structure in the molecule. (Hence the name from the Greek *chele*=claw.) When the complex formed in this way is harmless to the body and is excreted in the urine, such an agent is an effective way of ridding the body of toxic metals such as mercury. The main chelating agents are dimercaprol (q.v.), penicillamine (q.v.) and sodium calciumedetate.

CHEMOSIS Swelling of the conjunctiva (see EYE) of the eye, usually caused by inflammation from injury or infection.

CHEMOTAXIS means the property possessed by certain cells of attracting or repelling other cells.

CHEMOTHERAPY is the treatment of disease by chemical substances. In the modern sense it dates from the discovery by Paul Ehrlich, in 1910, of the action of Salvarsan ('606') in destroying the spirochaete of syphilis. This organic arsenical preparation revolutionized the treatment of syphilis. The next great advance in chemotherapy was the introduction of the sulphonamides in 1935. Just as Salvarsan had revolutionized the treatment of syphilis so did the sulphonamides revolutionize the treatment of infections with the streptococcus, pneumococcus, gonococcus and similar organisms. They remained supreme in the treatment of such infections as septicaemia, pneumonia, and certain forms of meningitis, until the introduction of penicillin during the 1939–45 War. Subsequently a series of new antibiotics (q.v.) have been discovered, including streptomycin, chloramphenicol, the tetracyclines and the cephalosporins. Over-use of chemotherapeutic drugs has stimulated widespread resistance among pathogenic micro-organisms previously susceptible to them. This is a worrying development.

Chemotherapy has also played an important rôle in tropical medicine: e.g. mepacrine and proguanil for the treatment of malaria; the amidines in the treatment of sleeping sickness in man, and the sulphones in the treatment of leprosy.

In recent years it has played an increasing and effective part in the treatment of cancer (q.v.), the drugs used being described as cytotoxic. As these drugs also damage normal tissue great care has to be exercised in their use. (see CYTOTOXIC).

CHENODEOXYCHOLIC ACID is one of the bile acids (see BILE), which is used in the treatment of cholesterol gall-stones (see GALL-BLADDER, DISEASES OF).

CHEST, or THORAX, is the upper part of the trunk. It is enclosed by the breast-bone(sternum) and the twelve ribs which join the sternum by way of cartilages and are attached to the spine behind. At the top of the thorax the opening in between the first ribs admits the windpipe (trachea), the gullet (oesophagus (q.v.)) and the large blood vessels. The bottom of the thorax is separated from the abdomen below by the muscular diaphragm (q.v.) which is the main muscle of breathing. Other muscles of respiration, the intercostal muscles, lie in between the ribs. Overlying the ribs are layers of muscle and soft tissue including the breast tissue.

Contents The trachea divides into right and left main bronchi which go to the two lungs (q.v.). The left lung is slightly smaller than the right. The right has three lobes (upper, middle and lower) and the left lung has two lobes (upper and lower). Each lung is covered by two thin membranes lubricated by a thin layer of fluid. These are the pleura and similar structures cover the heart (pericardium). The heart lies in the middle, displaced slightly to the left. The oesophagus passes right through the chest to enter the stomach just below the diaphragm. Various nerves, blood vessels and lymph channels run through the thorax. The thoracic duct is the main lymphatic drainage channel emptying into a vein on the left side of the root of the neck.

CHEST, DEFORMITIES OF The healthy chest is gently rounded all over, its contour being more rounded in women by the breast tissue. In cross section it is oval shaped with a longer dimension from side to side than back to front.
BARREL CHEST is found in long-standing asthma or chronic bronchitis and emphysema when the lungs are chronically enlarged. The anterio-posterior dimension of the chest is increased and the ribs are near horizontal. In this position they can produce little further expansion of the chest and breathing often relies on accessory muscles in the neck lifting up the whole thoracic cage on inspiration.
PIGEON CHEST is one in which the cross-section

of the chest becomes triangular with the sternum forming a sort of keel in front. It may be related to breathing problems in early life.
RICKETY CHEST is uncommon now and is caused by rickets in early life (see RICKETS). There is a hollow down each side caused by the pull of muscles on the softer ribs in childhood. The line of knobs produced on each side where the ribs join their costal cartilages is known as the rickety rosary.
PECTUS EXCAVATUM is quite a common abnormality where the central tendon of the diaphragm seems to be too short so that the lower part of the sternum is displaced inwards and the lower ribs are prominent. When severe it may displace the heart further to the left side.
LOCAL ABNORMALITIES in the shape of the chest occur when there is a deformity in the spine such as scoliosis which alters the angles of the ribs. The chest wall may be locally flattened when the underlying lung is reduced in size locally over a prolonged period. (See SPINE AND SPINAL CORD, DISEASES AND INJURIES OF.) This may be seen over a scarred area of lung such as that seen in pulmonary tuberculosis (q.v.).

CHEST DEVELOPMENT is affected by underlying disorders in the lungs. Local disease in the lungs may reduce the volume of all or part of one lung and lead to a local deformity in the overlying ribs. Long-standing narrowing of the airways such as that seen in asthma (q.v.) or emphysema (q.v.) may lead to a general expansion of the chest wall.

The muscles of respiration can be developed to some extent by training, either general fitness training or specific respiratory muscle work such as playing an instrument which involves blowing against a high resistance.

CHEST DISEASES The lungs and the heart are within the chest but the term chest disease usually refers to abnormalities of the lungs. However, lung problems are often intimately associated with heart disorders. The lungs are the site of gas exchange in the body where oxygen is brought into the blood and the waste product, carbon dioxide, removed. Smoking is a very important cause of lung disease and is responsible for most cases of lung cancer, chronic bronchitis and emphysema.
Symptoms *Breathlessness* is a common complaint in lung disease. Abnormalities in other systems such as the heart and the blood may cause breathlessness but lung problems are the most common cause. Shortness of breath limits exercise in many lung conditions. These are particularly diseases such as asthma, chronic bronchitis and emphysema which narrow the airways into the lungs (obstructive lung disorders) and those conditions which limit the expansion of the lungs (restrictive disorders) such as lung fibrosis, pneumonia, lung collapse or fluid around the lung (pleural effusion). Breathlessness also occurs when the muscles of the chest wall and diaphragm are weak or the chest wall is deformed. *Cough* is another com-

mon sympton and is caused by irritation at some site in the lungs or the airways to the lungs. Cough may be dry or produce sputum or phlegm. The colour of the sputum is yellow or green when infection is present. *Haemoptysis* is the production of sputum containing blood and is a symptom which should always be taken seriously and investigated. The lungs themselves do not produce painful sensations but inflammation of the lining around the lung (the pleura) leads to a pain which is worse on breathing, coughing and sometimes on movement (pleuritic pain).

Signs of lung disease may be seen outside the chest, for example, the blue coloration of the lips and skin (cyanosis) which occurs when the lungs are unable to bring enough oxygen into the blood.

Treatment Oxygen is useful in many lung diseases. In some patients with chronic lung disease the amount of oxygen needs to be carefully controlled. Antibiotics (q.v.) are used for pneumonia and other chest infections, with special antibiotics used over many months for tuberculosis. In asthma drugs can be used by inhalation directly into the airways. They can widen the airways and relieve breathlessness and also reduce the inflammation in the walls of the airways in the lungs. In cancer of the lung surgery may cure the disease but often it is not possible to remove the tumour and alternative treatments such as radiotherapy and chemotherapy may be used.

CHEYNE-STOKES BREATHING is a type of breathing seen in some serious nervous affections, such as brain tumours and stroke, and also in the case of persons with advanced disease of the heart or kidneys. When well marked it is a sign that death is impending, though milder degrees of it do not carry such a serious implication in elderly patients. The breathing gets very faint for a short time, then gradually deepens till full expirations are taken for a few seconds, and then gradually dies away to another quiet period, again increasing in depth after a few seconds and so on in cycles.

CHIASMA This is an X-shaped crossing. The optic chiasma is where the nerve fibres from the nasal half of each retina cross over the mid line to join the optic tract from the other side.

CHICKENPOX, or VARICELLA, is an acute contagious disease predominantly of children, though it may occur at any age, characterized by feverishness and an eruption on the skin. The name, chickenpox, is said to be derived from the resemblance of the eruption to boiled chick-peas.

Causes The disease occurs in epidemics affecting especially children under the age of ten years. It has no connection with smallpox, to which it bears a superficial resemblance. It is due to the varicella zoster virus, and the condition is an extremely infectious one from child to child. Although an attack confers life-long immunity, the virus may lie dormant and manifest itself in adult life as *herpes zoster* or shingles (see HERPES ZOSTER).

Symptoms There is an incubation period of fourteen to twenty-one days after infection, and then the child becomes feverish or has a slight shivering, or may feel more severely ill with vomiting and pains in the back and legs. Almost at the same time, an eruption consisting of red pimples which quickly change into vesicles filled with clear fluid appears on the back and chest, sometimes about the forehead, and less frequently on the limbs. These vesicles appear over several days and during the second day may show a change of their contents to turbid, purulent fluid and within a day or two they burst, or, at all events, shrivel up and become covered with brownish crusts. The small crusts have all dried up and fallen off in little more than a week and recovery is almost always complete.

Treatment The child must be isolated from susceptible children for a week from the appearance of the rash or until all the vesicles are dry, but there is no need to wait until the scabs have separated. Calamine lotion or a simple dusting powder relieves the itchiness. No other treatment beyond isolation is required.

CHIGGER is another name for *Trombicula autumnalis*, popularly known as the harvest mite (see BITES AND STINGS).

CHILBLAIN, or ERYTHEMA PERNIO, is an inflamed condition of the hands or feet, or occasionally of the ears, and should not be confused with cracked or chapped hands (q.v.). Most commonly found in childhood, it is associated with generally poor health, though there may also be a genetic predisposition. Precipitating factors include under-feeding, poor clothing, and a defective circulation; and diabetics, or those with ill-fitting footwear, are at particular risk. Prevention with good food and warm clothing, and regular exercise to maintain the circulation, is the best treatment.

CHILD ABUSE The physical or emotional mistreatment of a child. Neglect, physical injury, and sexual abuse are all forms of child abuse and they may be caused by parents, relatives, or carers. Greater awareness of the problem has led to an increase of reported incidents, but whether the incidence of abuse is actually rising is uncertain. Physical abuse or non-accidental injury is the most easily recognized form. Victims of sexual abuse may not reveal their experiences until adulthood and often not at all. Where child abuse is suspected, full investigation of the circumstances is necessary, and this may mean admitting a child to hospital or to local authority care. Abuse may be the result of impulsive action by adults or it may be premeditated, for example, the continued sexual exploitation of a child over several years. Premeditated physical assault is rare but is liable to cause serious injury to a child and requires urgent action when identified. Adults will go to some lengths to cover up persistent abuse. The child's interests are paramount but the parents may well be under severe stress and also require sympathetic handling.

CHILD ADOPTION Adoption was relatively uncommon until the Second World War with only 6,000 adoption orders annually. This peaked at nearly 25,000 in 1968 as adoption became more socially acceptable and the numbers of babies born to lone mothers rose in a climate hostile to single parenthood.

Adoption declined as the availability of babies fell with the introduction of the Abortion Act, 1968, improving contraceptive services and increasing acceptability of single parenthood.

However, with 10 per cent of couples suffering infertility, the demand continued, leading to the adoption of those previously perceived as difficult to place, i.e. physically, intellectually and/or emotionally disabled children and adolescents, those with terminal illness and children of ethnic-minority groups.

Recent controversies regarding homosexual couples as adoptive parents, adoption of children with or at high risk of HIV/AIDS, transcultural adoption and the increasing use of intercountry adoption to fulfil the needs of childless couples have provoked urgent consideration of the ethical dilemmas of adoption and its consequences for the children, their adoptive and birth families and society generally.

Detailed statistics have been unavailable since 1984 but in general there has been a downward trend with relatively more older children being placed. In 1989 7,044 adoption orders were granted (with an approximately equal ratio of boys to girls); 16 per cent were under 1 year, 26 per cent 1–4 years, 32 per cent 5–9 years, 19 per cent 10–14 years and 7 per cent 15–17 years old. Detailed reasons for adoption (i.e. interfamily, step-parent, intercountry, etc.) are not available but approximately one-third were adopted from local-authority care.

In the UK *all* adoptions (including interfamily and step-parent adoption) *must* take place through a registered adoption agency which may be local-authority based or provided by a registered voluntary agency. All local authorities must act as agencies, the voluntary agencies often providing specialist services to promote and support the adoption of more difficult-to-place children. Occasionally an adoption allowance will be awarded.

Adoption orders cannot be granted until a child has resided with its proposed adopters for 13 weeks. In the case of new-born infants the mother cannot give formal consent to placement until the baby is 6 weeks old, although informal arrangements can be made before this time.

In the UK the concept of responsibility of birth parents to their children and their rights to continued involvement after adoption are acknowledged by the Children Act, 1989. However, in all discussions the child's interests remain paramount. The Act also recognizes adopted children's need to have information regarding their origins.

BAAF – British Agencies for Adoption and Fostering – is the national organization of adoptive agencies, both local authority and voluntary sector. The organization promotes and provides training service, development and research, has several specialist professional subgroups (i.e. medical, legal, etc.) and produces a quarterly journal.

PPIAS – Parent to Parent Information Service on Adoptive Services – is an effective national support network of adoptive parents who offer free information, a 'listening ear' and, to members, a quarterly newsletter.

National Organization for Counselling Adoptees and their parents (NORCAP), is concerned with adopted children and birth parents who wish to make contact.

The Registrar General operates an Adoption Contact Register for adopted persons and anyone related to that person by blood, half blood or marriage. Information can be obtained from the Office of Population Censuses and Surveys. For the addresses of these organizations see APPENDIX 2: ADDRESSES.

CHILD DEVELOPMENT Children develop new skills in predictable patterns which can be observed as series of milestones along the road to maturity. Up to the age of 3 years milestones are traditionally charted in four areas: (1) *motor* – a reflection of physical strength; (2) *social interaction* with parents and strangers; (3) *language* – including hearing – and (4) *fine co-ordination* – including vision. Health-care professionals use these milestones to assess overall developmental progress and as an aid to pinpoint specific problems. Whilst the sequence is generally similar, the age at which a child reaches a given milestone is variable, even within one family, and reflects the child's physical health, environment and personality. If a child has a limited disability, one area of development may lag behind the others. A deaf child will have delayed language but will smile, walk and build towers at the expected time. A mild delay in all areas may reflect personality, chronic hospitalization or poor environmental stimulation, but a severe generalized delay suggests major brain dysfunction.

A child should at 6 months (1) roll over from front to back, (2) reach for and shake a rattle, (3) look round to see where noises are coming from and (4) transfer a cube from one hand to the other; at 1 year (1) walk holding on to furniture, (2) hold and drink from a cup, (3) use four words with meaning and (4) pick up a small object between thumb and forefinger; at 18 months (1) climb on to furniture, (2) pull socks off, (3) attempt to join in rhymes and (4) build a tower of three bricks; at 2 years (1) kick a ball, (2) tell about experiences, (3) name five toys and (4) copy vertical and horizontal lines; at 3 years (1) hop on one foot, (2) wash hands, (3) know first name and (4) copy a circle.

After the age of 3 the discovery of major developmental problems is unlikely. However, deafness and learning disabilities may go unappreciated until the child is much older.

CHILLS AND COLDS, though generally trivial, may serve as a prelude to serious disease. The 'common cold' is caused by a virus, transmitted by sneezing or coughing between members of families, schools, or people working together. It may be precipitated by breathing in damp and chilly air, though some people – particularly the elderly – are at greater risk.
Symptoms Nasal catarrh with a frontal headache is common, while inflammation of the sinuses (q.v.), sometimes spreading to the middle ear with mild fever, may occur. Rarely lasting more than a few days, it may be followed by tonsillitis (q.v.) or laryngitis (q.v.), while secondary respiratory infections such as bronchitis (q.v.), or even pneumonia (q.v.), may occur in predisposed individuals. Although mild, a cold often causes a short period of immuno-depression, which may lead to more serious diseases such as measles, whooping cough, influenza and tuberculosis.
Treatment A couple of days' bedrest provides relief for the sufferer, while also reducing the exposure of others to his infection. Vaccines seem to be ineffectual in the prevention of colds. Prompt medical advice should be sought in cases of prolonged or severe secondary infections.

CHIMERA is an organism, whether plant, animal or human being, in which there are at least two kinds of tissue differing in their genetic constitution.

CHIROPODY is that part of medical science which is concerned with the health of the feet. The modern chiropodist is a specialist capable of providing a fully comprehensive foot-health service. This includes the palliation of established deformities and dysfunction both as short-term treatment for immediate relief of painful symptoms and long-term management to secure optimum results. This requires the backing of effective appliances and footwear services. It also involves curative footcare, including the use of various therapeutic techniques, including minor surgery and the prescription and provision of specialized and individual appliances. Chiropody also has a preventative role which includes inspection of children's feet and the detection of foot conditions requiring treatment and advice and also foot-health education. The chiropodist is trained to recognize medical conditions which manifest themselves in the feet, such as circulatory disorders, diabetes mellitus and diseases causing ulceration.

The scope of practice of chiropodists is defined by the Society of Chiropodists as comprising the maintenance of the feet in healthy condition and the treatment of their disabilities by methods covered by the syllabus of training hitherto approved by the Department of Health. A chiropodist should confine his practice to this field of work and to such forms of advice and treatment as his training and experience qualify him to give. The only course of training in the United Kingdom recognized for the purpose of state registration by the Chiropodists Board of the Council for Professions Supplementary to Medicine is the Society of Chiropodists 3-year full-time course. The course includes instruction and examination in the relevant aspects of anatomy and physiology, local analgesia, medicine and surgery, as well as in podology and therapeutics. For the registered address of the Society of Chiropodists see APPENDIX 2: ADDRESSES.

CHIROPRACTOR is a term applied to a person who practises chiropractic. It is mainly a system of physical manipulations of minor displacements of the spinal column. These minor displacements, or subluxations (q.v.) of the spine are believed to affect the associated or neighbouring nerves. By manipulating the affected part of the spinal column the patient's complaint, whatever it may be – for example, backache – is relieved. Information can be obtained from the Chiropractic Advancement Association (see APPENDIX 2: ADDRESSES).

CHLAMYDIA is a genus of micro-organisms which include those responsible for non-specific urethritis (q.v.), ornithosis (q.v.), psittacosis (q.v.), and trachoma (q.v.). They are also widespread in birds and animals. Chlamydia can be sexually transmitted and 36,000 cases were reported in England in 1988.

CHLOASMA This is an increase in the melanin pigment of the skin as a result of hormonal stimulation. It is commonly seen in pregnancy and sometimes in women on the contraceptive pill. It mainly affects the face.

CHLORAL HYDRATE is a drug used for the short-term treatment of insomnia. When taken in moderate doses it produces a near natural sleep, with no change in the REM/NON-REM ratio (see REM SLEEP, SLEEP). Particularly useful for older people, it starts to act within 30 minutes, and is effective for about eight hours. It is dangerous in large doses, however, and frequent use may lead to habituation. Alcohol should be avoided, and patients should be warned that their ability to drive or operate machinery may be affected by drowsiness.

CHLORAMBUCIL is a derivative of nitrogen mustard (q.v.), which is proving of value in the treatment of chronic lymphatic leukaemia (see

LEUKAEMIA and Hodgkin's disease (q.v.)). It is given by mouth. (See CYTOTOXIC.)

CHLORAMPHENICOL is an antibiotic derived from a soil organism, *Streptomyces venezuelae*. It is also prepared synthetically. It is active against a wide range of organisms, but its most striking feature is its activity against certain rickettsias (q.v.). It has proved effective in the treatment of typhus, scrub typhus, Rocky Mountain spotted fever, typhoid and paratyphoid fevers. Its activity against certain organisms not susceptible to the sulphonamides and penicillin is proving of value. Particularly is this true of its use in the treatment of meningitis due to *H. influenzae*. It is given by mouth.

It is an antibiotic, however, that must be administered with discrimination because in certain individuals it may cause aplastic anaemia (see ANAEMIA), particularly if given for too long a period or in repeated courses.

CHLORDANE is an insecticide which has been used sucessfully against flies and mosquitoes resistant to DDT, and for the control of ticks and mites. It requires special handling as it is toxic to man when applied to the skin.

CHLORDIAZEPOXIDE is a widely used anti-anxiety drug. (See TRANQUILLIZERS, BENZODIAZEPINES.)

CHLORHEXIDINE, also known as HIBITANE, is an antiseptic which has a bacteriostatic action against many bacteria.

CHLORINATED LIME, also known as CHLORIDE OF LIME, is a white powder made by passing chlorine gas over slaked lime. It is a powerful bleaching agent and disinfectant, useful for household tasks, and effective in the disinfection of swimming pools and drinking water. When mixed with acidulated water, it gives off chlorine, a greenish gas with a pungent, choking smell, and highly toxic to all forms of bacterial life. Because of the adverse effects of chlorine on the environment steps are being taken to reduce the use of products containing it.

CHLORINE (see CHLORINATED LIME, and SODIUM HYPOCHLORITE).

CHLORMETHIAZOLE is a useful hypnotic particularly for elderly patients because of its freedom from hang-over effect. It is particularly useful in the acute withdrawal symptoms of alcoholism. The drug's sedative effects are a useful adjunct to regional anaesthesia and may also be of help in eclampsia (q.v.). Dependence may occur occasionally and therefore the length of period for which the drug is used should be limited. Side-effects include sneezing, conjunctival irritation and occasional headache.

CHLOROFORM is a colourless, volatile liquid, half as heavy again as water, and, unlike ether, non-inflammable. It was discovered by Liebig in 1831, and is a compound of carbon, hydrogen, and chlorine ($CHCl_3$). It does not dissolve to a large amount in water, but mixes readily with alcohol or ether. It dissolves sulphur, phosphorus, fats, resins, and most substances which contain a large proportion of carbon; it is therefore very useful as a cleansing agent. It was introduced into medicine in 1847 by Sir J. Y. Simpson, who was then in search of a substance which could produce unconsciousness for operative purposes more conveniently than ether, introduced a short time previously by Morton in America. (See ANAESTHESIA.)

Uses Chloroform is used as a solvent of fats, resins, etc., in many chemical processes. It is now rarely used in medicine.

CHLOROMA, or GREEN CANCER, is the name of a disease in which greenish growths appear under the skin, and in which a change takes place in the blood resembling that in leukaemia.

CHLOROPHYLL is the name of the green colouring matter of plants. Its main use is as a colouring agent, principally for soaps, oils and fats. It is also being found of value as a deodorant dressing to remove, or diminish, the unpleasant odour of heavily infected sores and wounds.

CHLOROQUINE, which is a 4-aminoquinoline, was introduced during the 1939–45 War for the treatment of malaria. It has also been found of value in the treatment of the skin condition known as chronic discoid lupus erythematosus, and of rheumatoid arthritis.

CHLOROTHIAZIDE is a potent benzothiadiazine (q.v.) diuretic which is active when taken by mouth. It has also a blood-pressure-lowering effect when used in conjunction with other hypotensive drugs.

CHLOROXYLENOL is an antiseptic which is used for treating cuts, abrasions and wounds. It is also widely used in obstetric practice. It is only slightly soluble in water (1 in 3000).

CHLORPROMAZINE is chemically related to the antihistamine drug, promethazine. One of the first antipsychotic drugs to be marketed, it is used extensively in psychiatry on account of its action in calming psychotic activity without producing undue general depression or clouding of consciousness. The drug is used particularly in schizophrenia and mania.

CHLORPROPAMIDE is one of the oral hypoglycaemic agents. It is a sulphonamide derivative and acts by stimulating the release of insulin from the pancreas. As it has a prolonged action, it need only be given once a day. Those taking chlorpropamide should bear in mind that in around 10 per cent of people it causes undue sensitivity to alcohol, resulting in severe flushing of the face, headache and a feeling of intoxication. (See also DIABETES MELLITUS, SULPHONYLUREAS.)

CHLORTETRACYCLINE (See TETRA-CYCLINES.)

CHOKING is the process which results from an obstruction to breathing situated in the larynx (see AIR PASSAGES). It may occur as the result of disease causing swelling round the glottis (the entrance to the larynx), or of some nervous disorders that interfere with the regulation of the muscles which open and shut the larynx, but generally it is due to the irritation of a piece of food or other substance introduced by the mouth, which provokes coughing but only partly interferes with breathing. As the mucous membrane lining the upper part of the latter is specially sensitive, coughing results in order to expel the cause of irritation. At the same time, if the foreign body is of any size, lividity of the face appears, due to partial suffocation (see ASPHYXIA).

Treatment The choking person should take slow, deep inspirations, which do not force the particle further in (as sudden catchings of the breath between the coughs do), and which produce more powerful coughs. If the coughing is weak, one or two strong blows with the palm of the hand over either shoulder blade, timed to coincide with coughs aid the effect of the coughing. In the case of a child the patient may be held up by the legs, when the substance causing the obstruction is more readily dislodged.

If this fails to dislodge the foreign body, what is known as the Heimlich manoeuvre should be tried. If the victim is standing or sitting, stand behind him and wrap your arms round his waist. Grasp the closed fist of the bottom hand with the other hand, and place the thumb side of the first against the abdomen slightly above the navel and below the ribs. Then press your fist against the abdomen with a quick upward thrust. Repeat several times if necessary. If the victim is lying down, whether semi-conscious or unconscious, kneel astride his hips facing him. With one hand on top of the other, place the heel of the bottom hand on the abdomen slightly above the navel and below the ribs. Press into the abdomen with a quick upward thrust. Repeat several times if necessary. Should the victim vomit, turn him quickly on his side and wipe out his mouth to prevent him inhaling the vomited material. Another method in adults is to draw the thighs up towards the body with the knees bent. The thighs are then pressed suddenly and violently into the abdomen. If this fails, call the doctor.

CHOLAGOGUES are substances which increase the flow of bile by stimulating evacuation of the gall-bladder. The great majority of these act only by increasing the activity of the digestive organs, and so producing a flow of bile already stored up in the gall-bladder. Substances which stimulate the liver to secrete more bile are known as CHOLERETIC.

CHOLANGIOGRAPHY is the process whereby the bile ducts and the gall-bladder are rendered radio-opaque and therefore visible on an X-ray film. (See SODIUM DIATRIZOATE.)

CHOLANGITIS is the term applied to inflammation of the bile ducts.

CHOLECYSTECTOMY means the removal of the gall-bladder by operation.

CHOLECYSTITIS means inflammation of the gall-bladder (see GALL-BLADDER, DISEASES OF).

CHOLECYSTOGRAPHY is the term applied to the process whereby the gall-bladder is rendered radio-opaque and therefore visisble on an X-ray film. (See SODIUM DIATRIZOATE.)

CHOLECYSTOKIN is the hormone (q.v.) released from the lining membrane of the duodenum (q.v.) when food is taken, and which initiates emptying of the gall-bladder.

CHOLELITHIASIS means the presence of gall-stones in the bile- ducts and/or in the gall-bladder. (See GALL-BLADDER, DISEASES OF.)

CHOLELITHOTOMY is the removal of gall-stones from the gall-bladder or bile ducts, when cholecystectomy (q.v.) or lithotripsy (q.v.) are inappropriate or not possible. It involves a cholecystomy, an operation to open the gall-bladder.

CHOLERA is bacterial infection caused by *Vibrio cholerae* – which causes systemic disease by the production of a toxin which results in a net flux of water and electrolytes towards the small-intestinal lumen. This causes profuse watery diarrhoea, and resultant dehydration and electrolyte imbalance. The small intestine is not affected structurally. Formerly known as the Asiatic cholera, the disease has occurred in epidemics and pandemics for many centuries. In 1823, it broke out of Asia, and extended into Asia Minor and Russia. It traversed Europe, arriving at Sunderland, England, in October 1831; London was affected in January 1832. It subsequently spread through much of North and Central America. The second pandemic originated in 1841 in India and China and extended in a similar direction to that of the first. The third began, also in the east, in 1850 and entered Europe in 1853; it was a major problem in North and South America. During this epidemic, Dr John Snow, a London anaesthetist, carried out seminal epidemiological work in Soho, London, which established that the source of infection was contaminated drinking water derived from the Broad Street pump. Several smaller epidemics involved Europe in the latter years of the 19th century, but none has arisen in Britain or the United States for many years. In 1971, the *El Tor* biotype of *V. cholerae* emerged and replaced much of the classical infection in Asia and, to a much lesser extent, Europe; parts of Africa were seriously affected. Recently a non-01 strain has arisen and is causing much disease in Asia. Cholera remains a major health problem (this is technically the seventh pandemic) in many countries of Asia, Africa and South America. It is one of three quarantinable infections.

Incubation period varies from a few hours to 5 days. Watery diarrhoea may be torrential and the resultant dehydration and electrolyte imbalance complicated by cardiac failure commonly causes death. The victim's skin elasticity is lost, the eyes are sunken, and the radial pulse may be barely perceptible. Urine production may be completely suppressed. Diagnosis is by detection of *V. cholerae* in a faecal sample. Treatment consists of rapid rehydration. Whereas the intravenous route may be required in a severe case, in the vast majority of patients oral rehydration (using an appropriate solution containing sodium chloride, glucose, sodium bicarbonate, and potassium) gives satisfactory results. Proprietary rehydration fluids do not always contain adequate sodium for rehydration in a severe case. Antibiotics, e.g. tetracycline and doxycycline, reduce the period during which *V. cholerae* is excreted (in children and pregnant women, furazolidone is safer); in an epidemic, rapid resistance to these, and other antibiotics has been clearly demonstrated. Prevention consists of improving public health infrastructure – in particular, the quality of drinking water. When supplies of the latter are satisfactory, the infection fails to thrive. Although a vaccine was first produced by Haffkine in 1893, immunization techniques remain unsatisfactory; they should not be mandatory for entry to any country. Improved vaccines are currently undergoing development and clinical trial.

CHOLERETIC is the term applied to a drug that stimulates the flow of bile (q.v.).

CHOLESTASIS A reduction or stoppage in the flow of bile (q.v.) into the intestine caused either by a blockage such as a stone in the bile duct or by liver disease disturbing the production of bile. The first type is called extrahepatic biliary obstruction and the second intrahepatic cholestasis. The patient develops jaundice and itching and passes dark urine and pale faeces.

CHOLESTEROL is a sterol, which is one of a class of solid alcohols; these are waxy materials derived from animal and vegetable tissues. It is widely distributed throughout the body, being especially abundant in the brain, nervous tissue, adrenal glands and skin. It is also found in egg yolk and gall-stones. It plays an important role in the body, being essential for the production of the sex hormones, as well as the repair of membranes. It is also the source from which bile acids are manufactured. The total amount in the body of a man weighing 70 kilograms (10 stones) is around 140 grams, and the amount present in the blood is 3·6 to 7·8 m.mol per litre or 150 to 250 milligrams per 100 millilitres.

A high blood-cholesterol level – that is, one over 6 m.mol per litre or 238 mg per 100 ml – is undesirable as there appears to be a correlation between a high blood cholesterol and atheroma (q.v.), the form of arterial degenerative disease associated with coronary thrombosis and high blood-pressure. This is well exemplified in diabetes mellitus (q.v.) and myxoedema (q.v.), two diseases in which there is a high blood cholesterol, sometimes going as high as 20 m.mol per litre; patients with these diseases are known to be particularly prone to arterial disease. There is also a familial disease known as hypercholesterolaemia, in which members of affected families have a blood cholesterol of around 18 m.mol per litre, or more, and are particularly liable to premature degenerative disease of the arteries.

The rising incidence of arterial disease in western countries in recent years has drawn attention to this relationship between high levels of cholesterol in the blood and arterial disease. The available evidence indicates that there is a relationship between blood-cholesterol levels and the amount of fat consumed. Thus, in Cape Town it has been shown that in men aged 45 the mean blood-cholesterol level was 234 mg per 100 ml in the European community and 166 mg per 100 ml in the Bantu community, and this was correlated with the basic difference between the diets of the two communities: 40 per cent of the calories in the European's diet was fat, compared with 20 per cent or less in the Bantu's diet. The suggestion was therefore made that the rising incidence of coronary heart disease, and other manifestations of arterial disease, such as high blood-pressure and strokes, might be arrested by persuading those living in western communities, such as Western Europe and USA, to eat less fat. One of the troubles is that the blood-cholesterol level bears little relationship with the amount of cholesterol consumed, most of the cholesterol in the body being produced by the body itself.

On the other hand, diets high in saturated fatty acids, chiefly animal fats such as red meat, butter and dripping, tend to raise the blood-cholesterol level; while foods high in unsaturated fatty acids, chiefly vegetable products such as olive and sunflower oils, and oily fish such as mackeral and herring, tend to lower it. There is a tendency in western society to eat too much animal fat, and current health recommendations are for everyone to decrease saturated-fat intake, increase unsaturated-fat intake, increase daily exercise, and avoid obesity. This advice is particulary important for people with high blood-cholesterol level, with diabetes mellitus (q.v.), or a history of coronary thrombosis.

CHOLESTYRAMINE is a drug that is proving of value in the treatment of the pruritus, or itching (q.v.), which occurs in association with jaundice. This it does by 'binding' the bile salts in the gut and so preventing their being reabsorbed into the bloodstream, where their excess in jaundice is responsible for the itching. It is also proving useful in reducing the level of cholesterol and triglycerides in the blood and thereby, like clofibrate (q.v.), helping to reduce the incidence of coronary artery heart disease. (See CORONARY THROMBOSIS; HYPERLIPIDAEMIA.)

CHOLINE is one of the many constituents of the vitamin B complex. Lack of it in the experimental animal produces a fatty liver. It is found in egg-yolk, liver, and meat. The probable daily human requirement is 500 mg, an amount amply covered by the ordinary diet. Choline can be synthesized by the body (see APPENDIX 5: VITAMINS).

CHOLINERGIC A description of nerve fibres that release acetylcholine (q.v.) as a neurotransmitter (q.v.).

CHONDROMA is a tumour composed in part of cartilage. (See TUMOUR.)

CHORDA A nerve fibre, tendon or cord.

CHOREA, or ST VITUS'S DANCE, is the occurrence of short, purposeless involuntary movements of the face, head, hands and feet. Movements are sudden, but the affected person may hold the new posture for several seconds. Chorea is often accompanied by athetosis (q.v.) when it is termed choreoathetosis. Choreic symptoms are often due to disease of the basal ganglion in the brain. The withdrawal of phenothiazines may cause the symptoms, as can the drugs used to treat Parkinson's disease (q.v.). Types of chorea include Huntington's (q.v.), Sydenham's (q.v.), which affects children, and senile.

CHORIOCARCINOMA is a form of cancer affecting the chorion (q.v.), in the treatment of which particularly impressive results are being obtained from the use of methotrexate.

CHORION is the more external of the two fetal membranes. (See PLACENTA.)

CHORIONIC GONADOTROPHIC HORMONE A hormone produced by the placenta (q.v.) during pregnancy. It is similar to the pituitary gonadotrophins, which are blocked during pregnancy. Large amounts appear in a woman's urine when she is pregnant and are used as the basis for pregnancy tests. Human gonadotrophins are used to treat delayed puberty and premenstrual tension.

CHOROID (see EYE).

CHOROIDITIS (see UVEITIS).

CHOROID PLEXUS An extensive web of blood vessels occurring in the ventricles of the brain and producing the cerebrospinal fluid. (See BRAIN.)

CHRISTMAS DISEASE is a hereditary disorder of blood coagulation which can only be distinguished from haemophilia (q.v.) by laboratory tests. It is so called after the surname of the first case reported in this country. About one out of every ten patients clinically diagnosed as haemophiliac has in fact Christmas disease. It is due to lack in the blood of Factor IX.

CHROMAFFIN is a term applied to certain cells and organs in the body, such as part of the adrenal glands, which have a peculiar affinity for chrome salts. These cells and tissues generally are supposed to secrete substances which have an important action in maintaining the tone and elasticity of the blood-vessels and muscles.

CHROMIC ACID is used in several industries, particularly in chromium plating. Unless precautions are taken it may lead to dermatitis of the hands, arms, chest and face. It may also cause deep ulcers, especially of the nasal septum and knuckles.

CHROMOSOMES are the rod-shaped bodies to be found in the nucleus of every cell in the body. They contain the genes, or hereditary elements, which establish the characteristics of an individual. Composed of a long double coiled filament of DNA (q.v.), they occur in pairs – one from the maternal, the other from the paternal – and human beings possess forty-six, made up of twenty-three pairs. The number of chromosomes is specific for each species of animal. Each chromosone can duplicate an exact copy of itself between each cell division. (See GENETIC CODE; GENETICS; HEREDITY; MEIOSIS; SEX CHROMOSOMES.)

CHRONIC A persistent or recurring condition. The disease, which may or may not be severe, often starts gradually and changes will be slow. Opposite of ACUTE.

CHYLE is the milky fluid which is absorbed by the lymphatic vessels of the intestine. The absorbed portion consists of fats in very fine emulsion, like milk, so that these vessels receive the name of lacteals (L. *lac*, milk). This absorbed chyle mixes with the lymph and is discharged into the thoracic duct, a vessel as large as a quill, which passes up through the chest to open into the jugular vein on the left side of the neck, where the chyle mixes with the blood.

CHYLURIA means the passage of chyle (q.v.) in the urine. This results in the passing of a milky-looking urine. It is one of the manifestations of filariasis (q.v.), where it is due to obstruction of the lymphatics (q.v.) by the causative parasite.

CHYME is the name given to the partly digested food as it issues from the stomach into the intestine. It is very acid and grey in colour, containing salts and sugars in solution, and the animal food softened into a semi-liquid mass. It is next converted into chyle.

CHYMOPAPAIN is an enzyme (q.v.) obtained from the paw-paw, which is being used in the treatment of prolapsed intervertebral discs (q.v.). When injected into the disc it dissolves it.

CHYMOTRYPSIN is an enzyme (q.v.) produced by the pancreas (q.v.) which digests protein. It is used as an aid in operations for removal of a cataract (see ZONULOLYSIS), and also by inhalation to loosen and liquefy secretions in the windpipe and bronchi.

CICATRIX is another word for scar.

CILIA is a term applied to minute, lash-like processes which are seen with the aid of the microscope upon the cells covering certain mucous membranes: e.g. the trachea (or windpipe) and nose and which maintain movement in the fluid passing over these membranes. They are also found on certain bacteria which have the power of rapid movement.

CILIARY BODY That part of the eye that connects the iris and the choroid. The ciliary ring is next to the choroid, the ciliary processes comprise many ridges behind the iris, to which the lens's suspensory ligament is attached, and the ciliary muscle, which contracts to change the curvature of the lens and so adjust the accommodation of the eye. (See EYE.)

CIMETIDINE is a drug (known as an H_2 antagonist (q.v.)) that is widely used in the treatment of peptic ulcer (q.v.). It acts by reducing the hyperacidity of the gastric juice by antagonizing histamine receptors in the stomach.

CIMEX LECTULARIUS (see BED BUG).

CINCHONA is the general name for several trees in the bark of which quinine is found. This bark is also known as Jesuit's bark, having been brought first to notice by Spanish priests in South America and brought to Europe first by the Countess of Cinchon, wife of the Viceroy of Peru, in 1640. The red cinchona bark is that which contains most quinine, and from which it is usually prepared. (See QUININE.) Various extracts and tinctures are made direct from cinchona bark, and used in place of quinine.

CINNAMON is the bark of *Cinnamomum zeylanicum*, a species of laurel grown in Sri Lanka (Ceylon). It has a stimulating action upon the stomach, and assists digestion; hence its use as a condiment. It is also an antispasmodic.

CIRCLE OF WILLIS, or CIRCULUS ARTERIOSUS, is a circle of arteries at the base of the brain, which is formed by the junction of the basilar, posterior cerebral, internal carotid and anterior cerebral arteries. Congenital defects may occur in these arteries and lead to the formation of aneurysms (q.v.). (See diagram, BRAIN.)

CIRCULATION OF THE BLOOD This principle was demonstrated for the first time by William Harvey in 1628. Harvey proved, first of all, mainly by the examination of living animals, that the arteries contain only blood. Secondly, he showed by three main propositions that this blood must go round from arteries to veins in a continuous circuit. (1) The quantity of blood passing from the veins into the heart in the course of a whole day is so great that it is quite impossible it could all be manufactured from the food. (2) The blood in the arteries passes in a constant stream to all the members of the body, and does not return by the same route. (3) The blood in the veins flows incessantly to the heart, and does not ebb and flow, as is shown by the valves in veins and in the heart, and by the fact that veins when pressed on do not fill from above. Having proved these points, he assumed there must be 'pores in the flesh' through which the blood 'percolated' from the ends of the arteries to the commencements of the veins. The last link in the evidence was supplied some thirty years later by Malpighi, an Italian scientist, who with the help of the microscope showed these 'pores' to be the minute vessels now called capillaries.

The course of the circulation is as follows The veins pour their blood, coming from the head, trunk, limbs and abdominal organs, into the right atrium of the heart. This contracts and drives the blood into the right ventricle, which then forces the blood into the lungs by way of the pulmonary artery. Here it is contained in thin-walled capillaries, over which the air plays freely, and through which gases pass readily out and in. The blood gives off carbon dioxide

(CO$_2$) and takes up oxygen (see RESPIRATION), and passes on by the pulmonary veins to the left atrium of the heart. The left atrium expels it into the left ventricle, which forces it on into the aorta, by which it is distributed all over the body. Passing through capillaries in the various tissues, it enters the veins, which ultimately unite into two great veins, the superior and the inferior vena cava, these emptying into the right atrium. This complete circle is accomplished by any particular drop of blood in about half a minute.

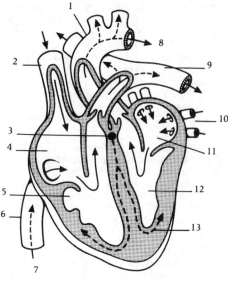

1 aorta	8 bloodflow to body
2 superior vena cava	9 left pulmonary artery
3 bundle of His	10 pulmonary veins
4 right atrium	11 left atrium
5 right ventricle	12 left ventricle
6 inferior vena cava	13 course of electroneural
7 bloodflow from body	impulses

Diagram of the heart and attendant blood vessels opened from the front to show the flow of blood.

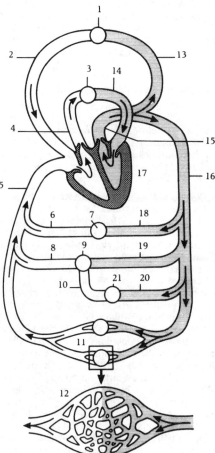

1 head and neck	12 capillary bed
2 superior vena cava	13 carotid artery
3 lungs	14 pulmonary vein
4 pulmonary artery	15 aorta
5 inferior vena cava	16 descending aorta
6 renal vein	17 heart
7 kidney	18 renal artery
8 hepatic vein	19 hepatic artery
9 liver	20 mesenteric and
10 hepatic portal vein	gastric artery
11 limbs	21 gut

Schematic plan of the body's circulation

In one part of the body there is a further complication. The veins coming from the bowels, charged with food material and other products, split up, and their blood undergoes a second capillary circulation through the liver. Here it is relieved of some food material and purified, and then passes into the inferior vena cava, and so to the right atrium. This is known as the portal circulation.

The circle is maintained always in one direction by four valves, situated one at the outlet from each cavity of the heart. (See HEART.)

The blood in the arteries going to the body generally is bright red, that in the veins dull red in colour, owing to the former being charged with oxygen, the latter with carbon dioxide (see RESPIRATION). For the same reason the blood in the pulmonary artery is dark, that in the pulmonary veins bright. There is no direct communication between the right and left sides of the heart, the blood passing from the right ventricle to the left atrium through the lungs.

In the embryo, before birth, the course of circulation is somewhat different, owing to the fact that no nourishment comes from the bowels nor air into the lungs. Accordingly, two large arteries pass out of the navel, and convey blood to be changed by contact with maternal blood (see PLACENTA), while a large vein brings

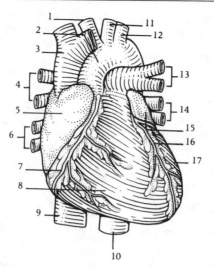

1 brachiocephalic trunk
2 aortic arch
3 superior vena cava
4 right pulmonary artery
5 right atrium
6 right superior and inferior pulmonary veins
7 right coronary artery
8 right ventricle
9 inferior vena cava

10 descending aorta
11 left common carotid artery
12 left subclavian artery
13 left pulmonary artery
14 left superior and inferior pulmonary veins
15 left atrium
16 branches of left coronary artery
17 left ventricle

Anterior view of heart showing main blood vessels including coronary arteries.

this blood back again. There are also communications between the right and left atria, and between pulmonary artery and aorta. The latter is known as the ductus arteriosus. At birth all these extra vessels and connections close and rapidly shrivel up.

CIRCUMCISION A surgical procedure to remove the prepuce of the penis in males and a part or all of the external genitalia in females. Circumcision is mainly done for religious or ethnic reasons. There is virtually no medical or surgical reason for circumcision in the male new-born infant. The prepuce is not normally retractable in infancy so this is not an indication for circumcision. By the age of one the prepuce is retractable in most boys. The Americans are more enthusiastic about circumcision, and the reason offered is that cancer of the penis occurs only when a foreskin is present. This is however a rare disease. In the uncircumcised adult there is an increased transmission of herpes and cytomegaloviruses during the reproductive years but this can be reduced by adequate cleansing. Phimosis is an indication for circumcision. Haemorrhage, infection and meatal stenosis are rare complications of circumcision. Circumcision in women is a damaging procedure, the results of which can cause psychological and sexual problems and complications in child-birth, and which has no known benefit to the woman's health, though cultural

pressures have resulted in its continuation in some Muslim and African countries.

CIRRHOSIS, or FIBROSIS, is a diseased condition, in which the proper tissue is replaced by fibrous tissue similar to scar tissue. The name cirrhosis was originally given by Laennec to the disease as occurring in the liver, because of its yellow colour. (See LIVER DISEASES.)

CIRSOID ANEURYSM is the term applied to the condition in which a group of arteries become abnormally dilated and tortuous.

CISPLATIN is a toxic drug with an alkylating action that gives it useful anti-tumour properties, especially against solid tumours such as ovarian and testicular cancers (see CYTOTOXIC).

CITRIC ACID is responsible for the sharp taste associated with citrus fruits, such as lemons and limes, and other fruits such as currants and raspberries. Although chemically different, it is similar in action and appearance to tartaric acid, obtained from grapes and other fruits, and similar to malic acid, found in apples and pears.
Uses   These acids stimulate the flow of saliva, and hence act to allay thirst and create a feeling of coolness, valuable in the treatment of fever.

They are changed on absorbtion into alkaline substances, which act to correct acidity, and hence are useful, when taken as effervescent drinks, in the treatment of irritable stomach.

CLAUDICATION A cramplike pain that occurs in the legs on walking. It may cause the sufferer to limp or, if severe, stop him or her from walking. The usual cause is narrowing or blockage of the arteries in the legs due to atherosclerosis. Intermittent claudication occurs when a person has to stop every so often to let the pain, caused by the build-up of waste products in the muscles, to subside. The condition may be improved by the patient's walking for an hour a day (resting when the pain starts). Oxpentifylline, a vasodilator, may help, as may calcium-channel-blocking drugs. Patients must avoid all tobacco products.

CLAUSTROPHOBIA means the fear of being in a confined space, or the fear experienced while in it.

CLAVICLE is the bone which runs from the upper end of the breast- bone towards the tip of the shoulder across the root of the neck. It supports the upper limb, keeps it out from the side, and gives breadth to the shoulders. The bone is shaped like an '*f*' with two curves, which give it increased strength. It is, however, liable to be broken by falls on the hand or on the shoulder, and is the most frequently fractured bone in the body. (See FRACTURES.)

CLAW-FOOT, or PES CAVUS, is a familial deformity of the foot characterized by an abnormally high arch of the foot accompanied by shortening of the foot, clawing of the toes and inversion, or turning inwards, of the foot and heel. Its main effect is to impair the resilience of the foot resulting in a stiff gait and aching pain. Milder cases are treated with special shoes fitted with a sponge rubber insole. More severe cases may require surgical treatment.

CLAW-HAND is a condition of bending and wasting of the hand and fingers, especially of the ring and little fingers. The condition is generally due to paralysis of the ulnar nerve. A somewhat similar condition is produced by contraction of the fibrous tissues in the palm of the hand, partly due to rheumatic changes and partly to injury caused by the constant pressure of a tool against the palm of the hand. (See DUPUYTREN'S CONTRACTURE.)

CLAW-TOES (see CLAW-FOOT).

CLEFT FOOT is a rare congenital abnormality characterized by the absence of one or more toes and a deep central cleft that divides the foot into two. It is sometimes known as lobster foot or lobster claw. It may be accompanied by other congenital defects, such as cleft hand, absent permanent teeth, cleft lip and palate, absence of the nails, and defects of the eye.

CLEFT HAND is a rare congenital abnormality characterized by the absence of one or more fingers and a deep central cleft that divides the hand into two. It is sometimes known as lobster hand. It may be accompanied by other congenital defects, such as cleft foot, absent permanent teeth, cleft lip and palate, absence of the nails and defects of the eye.

CLEFT PALATE is the term applied to a fissure in the roof of the mouth (palate) and/or the lip which is present at birth. It is found in varying degrees of severity in about 1 in 700 children. Modern plastic surgery can greatly improve the appearance of the baby and often further cosmetic surgery later will not be necessary. The parent of the child who has cleft lip and/or palate will be given detailed advice specific to his case. In general the team of specialists involved are the paediatrician, plastic surgeon, dentist or orthodontic specialist, and speech therapist. (See PALATE, MALFORMATIONS OF.)

CLICKING FINGER is a condition in middle-aged people in which the victim finds on wakening in the morning that he or she cannot straighten the ring or middle finger spontaneously, but only by a special effort, when it suddenly straightens with a painful click. Hence the name. In due course the finger remains bent at all times unless a special effort is made to straighten it with the other hand. The condition is due to a swelling developing in one of the tendons of the affected finger. If the tendon sheath is slit open surgically, the condition is relieved. Many cases recover spontaneously if the patient is prepared to wait.

CLICKING THUMB is a comparable condition sometimes found in the new-born baby, and occasionally in adults. In the baby, surgery should not be resorted to, as the condition practically always clears up spontaneously. In the adult it can be such a nuisance that it should probably be operated on at a fairly early stage.

CLIMACTERIC was a word originally applied to the end of certain epochs or stages in the life of an individual, at which some great change was supposed to take place. (See also MENOPAUSE.)

CLINDAMYCIN is an antibiotic which is used in the treatment of serious infections. This restriction is imposed because it is liable to cause severe colitis. It is active against a wide range of micro-organisms.

CLINICAL means literally 'belonging to a bed', but the word is used to denote anything associated with the practical study or observation of sick people as clinical medicine, clinical thermometers.

CLINICAL PSYCHOLOGY Psychology is the scientific study of behaviour. It may be applied in various settings including education, industry and health care. Clinical psychology is concerned with the practical application of research findings in the fields of physical and mental health. Training in clinical psychology involves a degree in Psychology followed by postgraduate training. Clinical psychologists are specifically skilled in applying theoretical models and objective methods of observation and measurement and in therapeutic interventions aimed at changing patient's dysfunctional behaviour, including thoughts and feelings as well as actions. Dysfunctional behaviour is explained in terms of normal processes and modified by applying principles of normal learning, adaption and social interaction.

Clinical psychologists are involved in health care in the following ways: (1) Assessment of thoughts, emotions and behaviour using standardized methods. (2) Treatment based on theoretical models and scientific evidence about behaviour change. Behaviour change is considered when it contributes to physical, psychological or social functioning. (3) Consultation with other health-care professionals about problems concerning emotions, thinking and behaviour. (4) Research on a wide variety of topics including the relationship between stress, psychological functioning and disease, the aetiology of problem behaviours, methods and theories of behaviour change. (5) Teaching other professionals about normal and dysfunctional behaviour, emotions and functioning.

Clinical psychologists may specialize in work in particular branches of patient care, including surgery, psychiatry, geriatrics, paediatrics, mental handicap, obstetrics and gynaecology, cardiology, neurology, general practice and physical rehabilitation. Whilst the focus of their work is frequently the patient, at times it may encompass the behaviour of the health-care professionals.

CLINICAL TRIALS Voltaire defined medical treatment as the act of pouring drugs, of which one knew nothing, into a patient, of whom one knew less. This derisive appraisal of the therapeutics of his time was nearly true as there were virtually no drugs of significant therapeutic value and any benefit the patient received was usually a placebo effect.

The development of effective medical treatment only dates back 50 years or so. When useful drugs did become available in the 1940s and the 1950s doctors realized the importance of evaluating their effectiveness. This lead to the introduction of the so-called clinical trials. Systematic measures were introduced to assess the efficacy initially of new medicines and, later, of surgical operations. This is now done by controlled, randomized clinical trials which compare the new treatment under evaluation either with a placebo or the previous standard treatment. If possible this is done on a double blind basis when neither the patient nor the doctor knows at the time whether the test treatment or the control is being administered: this enables bias to be removed. Such trials have to be done to recognized ethical standards with the procedure properly explained to the participating subjects.

CLINICS (see MATERNITY AND CHILD WELFARE).

CLITORIS A small sensitive organ comprising erectile tissue at the top of the female genitalia where the labial folds meet below the pubic bone. During sexual excitement the clitoris enlarges and hardens and may be the focus of orgasm.

CLOBAZAM is a benzodiazepine (q.v.) used to treat anxiety.

CLOFAZIMINE is a drug used in the treatment of leprosy.

CLOFIBRATE (see HYPERLIPIDAEMIA).

CLOMIPHENE is a drug that stimulates ovulation, or the production of ova, through the medium of the pituitary gland. It is thus being used in the treatment of female infertility. One of its hazards is that, if given in too big doses, it may produce multiple births.

CLOMIPRAMINE is an antidepressant drug. (See ANTIDEPRESSANTS.)

CLONAZEPAM is a drug that is proving of value in some cases of epilepsy, and in the restless-legs syndrome (q.v.). (See TRANQUILLIZER.)

CLONE A group of cells genetically identical to each other that have arisen from one cell by asexual reproduction (see CLONING).

CLONIC is a word applied to short spasmodic movements.

CLONIDINE is a drug originally introduced for the treatment of high blood-pressure. It is an alpha$_2$ adrenoreceptor agonist. It may also help in the prevention of attacks of migraine. If it is used in the treatment of high blood-pressure, its use must not be stopped abruptly as this may result in a sudden rise of blood-pressure within a matter of hours to a dangerously high level.

CLONING, from the Greek *klon* meaning a cutting such as is used to propagate plants, is essentially a form of asexual reproduction. The initial stages have been successfully achieved in rabbits. In essence the technique consists of destroying the nucleus of the egg and replacing it with the nucleus from a body cell of the same species – either a male or a female. This provides the egg with a full complement of chromosomes (q.v.) and it starts to divide and grow just at it would if it had retained its nucleus and been fertilized with a spermatozoon. The vital difference is that the embryo resulting from this cloning process owes nothing genetically to the female egg. It is identical in every respect with the animal from which the introduced nucleus was obtained.

CLONUS A succession of intermittent muscular relaxations and contractions usually resulting from a sustained stretching stimulus. An example is the clonus stimulated in the calf muscle by maintaining sustained upward pressure on the sole of the foot. The condition is often a sign of disease in the brain or spinal cord.

CLOSTRIDIUM is the genus, or variety, of micro-organisms that produce spores which enable them to survive under adverse conditions. They normally grow in soil, water and decomposing plant and animal matter, where they play an important part in the process of putrefaction (q.v.). Among the important members of the group, or genus, are *Clostridium welchii, Cl. septicum* and *Cl. oedematiens,* the causes of gas gangrene (see GANGRENE); *Cl. tetani,* the cause of tetanus (q.v.); and *Cl. botulinum,* the cause of botulism (q.v.).

CLOT is the term applied to any semi-solid mass of blood, lymph or other body fluid. Clotting in the blood is due to the formation of strings of fibrin produced by the action of a ferment. Milk clots in a similar manner in the stomach when exposed to the action of the ferment rennin. Clotting occurs naturally when blood is shed and comes in contact with tissues outside the blood-vessels. It occurs also at times in diseased vessels (*thrombosis*), producing serious effects upon the tissues supplied or drained by these vessels. Clots also form sometimes in the heart when the circulation is feeble and irregular. (See COAGULATION; EMBOLISM; THROMBOSIS.)

CLOTRIMAZOLE is a drug that is proving of value in the treatment of certain fungal or yeast infections, such as aspergillosis (q.v.) and cryptococcosis (q.v.).

CLOTTING TIME (see COAGULATION).

CLOVES are the unexpanded flower-buds of a species of myrtle, *Eugenia caryophyllus,* from the Indian Archipelago. Oil of cloves is an antiseptic, checks griping, and masks bad breath. It may be taken in doses of 2 or 3 drops on a lump of sugar, or one tablespoonful of infusion of cloves may be similarly used. Cotton-wool dipped in clove oil and put in a hollow tooth relieves toothache temporarily.

CLOXACILLIN is an antibiotic (q.v.) used to treat infections caused by penicillinase-producing staphylococci (q.v.). (See PENICILLIN, ANTIBIOTIC.)

CLUBBING is the term applied to the thickening and broadening of the finger tips and, less commonly, the tips of the toes, that occurs in certain chronic diseases of the lungs and heart. It is due to interstitial oedema especially at the nail bed leading to a loss of the acute angle between the nail and the skin of the finger. It is associated with lung cancer, empyema, bronchietasis and congenital cyanotic heart disease.

CLUB-FOOT, or TALIPES, is a deformity in which the foot is permanently twisted at the ankle-joint, so that the sole no longer rests on the ground in standing.
Classification The foot can be twisted in four directions. The heel may be pulled up so that the person walks on his toes (*talipes equinus*), or the toes may be bent up so that he walks on his heel only (*talipes calcaneus*), or the sole may look inwards so that he walks on the outer edge of the foot (*talipes varus*), or outwards so that he walks on the inside of the foot (*talipes valgus*). These are usually combined, the heel being drawn up and the sole turned inwards (*equino-varus*) or the heel resting on the ground and the sole looking outwards (*talipes calcaneo-valgus*). A more important division is into those cases in which the deformity exists at birth, which are generally at first fairly easily rectified; and into those cases which are acquired later in life as the result of some disease, which do not yield to such simple treatment.
Causes The cases found at birth are due to some arrest of development resulting in a structural deformity of both the forefoot and hindfoot (*talipes equino-varus*), or faulty positioning of the fetus in the womb (*talipes calcaneo-valgus*). The former occurs in 1–2 per 1000 live births in the UK. It is two to three times as common in boys as in girls, and is frequently bilateral. It tends to run in affected families, with an incidence 20–30 times that in the normal population. Despite numerous theories, its cause remains unknown; it is often associated with other abnormalities or forms part of a specific syndrome. Those cases acquired later may be caused by neurological conditions, with spasm of the muscles on the affected side (cerebral palsy), or paralysis of the muscles on the other side (poliomyelitis), or by rigidity due to the scar following a burn or inflammation.

Treatment should start as soon as possible after birth. Early treatment involves repeated gentle manipulations, maintaining the correction obtained with adhesive strapping, plaster of Paris or metal splints. The precise method used depends on the surgeon's preferences and the ability of the parents to bring the patient at frequent intervals for treatment. The response is often excellent, particularly with *talipes calcaneo-valgus*. A tendency to relapse when the child starts walking may be corrected by a wedge on the heel of the shoe. Surgery is usually indicated in more severe cases, and certainly if the initial conservative treatment has not resulted in full clinical and radiological correction after 12–14 weeks. In those cases resulting from disease or injury after birth, treatment involves splinting, strengthening the weakened muscles by massage and electrical stimulation. In severe cases, surgery involving tendon transplantation may be indicated.

CLUSTER HEADACHES   This is a distinct entity separate from migraine, although it is sometimes referred to as migrainous neuralgia. The name derives from the fact that the headaches cluster in periods of six to twelve weeks at certain times of the year. The headache is usually on one side and often around the eye. Lacrimation and running of the nose are frequently associated. A chronic form in which attacks persist for more than six months exists. Prophylactic treatment with Lithium carbonate is usually effective.

COAGULATION of the blood is the process whereby bleeding (or haemorrhage) is normally arrested in the body. It is part of the process of haemostasis (q.v.) which is the arrest of bleeding from an injured or diseased blood vessel. Haemostasis depends on the combined activities of vascular, platelet (q.v.) and plasma (q.v.) elements which are offset by processes to restrict the accumulation of platelets and fibrin (q.v.) to the damaged area. The three-stage process of cogulation is complex, involving many different substances. It is simply summarized in the following diagram:

prothrombin + calcium + thromboplastin
|
thrombin + fibrinogen
|
fibrin

Prothrombin and calcium are normally present in the blood. Thromboplastin is an enzyme which is normally found in the blood platelets and in tissue cells. When bleeding occurs from a blood-vessel there is always some damage to tissue cells and to the blood platelets. As a result of this damage, thromboplastin is released and comes in contact with the prothrombin and calcium in the blood. In the presence of thromboplastin and calcium prothrombin is converted into thrombin, which

in turn interacts with fibrinogen, a protein always present in the blood, to form fibrin. Fibrin consists of needle-shaped crystals, which, with the assistance of the blood platelets, form a fine network in which the blood corpuscles become enmeshed. This meshwork, or clot as it is known, gradually retracts until it forms a tight mass which prevents any further bleeding. It will thus be seen that clotting, or coagulation, does not occur in the healthy blood-vessel because there is no thromboplastin present. There is now evidence suggesting that there is an anti-thrombin substance present in the blood in small amounts, and that this substance antagonizes any small amounts of thrombin that may be formed as a result of small amounts of thromboplastin being released. The clotting or coagulation time is the time taken for blood to clot and can be measured under controlled conditions to ensure that it is normal (three to eight minutes). In certain diseases – haemophilia, for example – clotting time is greatly extended.

COAGULUM is the Latin term for a clot.

COARCTATION OF THE AORTA is a narrowing of the aorta in the vicinity of the insertion of the ductus arteriosus. It is a congenital abnormality. Satisfactory results are now obtained from surgical treatment.

COBALAMINS are a group of substances which have an enzyme action (SEE ENZYME) and are essential for normal growth and nutrition. (See also CYANOCOBALAMIN; HYDROXOCOBALAMIN.)

COBALT-60 is a radioactive isotope which is being used in the treatment of malignant disease. (See RADIOTHERAPY.)

COBALT EDETATE is an antidote for cyanide poisoning (q.v.).

COCAINE   Coca leaves are obtained from two South American plants, *Erythroxylum coca* and *Erythroxylum truxillense*, and contain an alkaloid, cocaine, which has marked effects as a stimulant, and, locally applied, as an anaesthetic by paralysing nerves of sensation. The dried leaves have been used from time immemorial by the South American Indians, who chew them mixed with a little lime. Their effect is to dull the mucous surfaces of mouth and stomach, with which the saliva, produced by chewing them, comes into contact, thus blunting, for long periods, all feeling of hunger. The cocaine, being absorbed, produces on the central nervous system a stimulating effect, so that all sense of fatigue and breathlessness vanishes for the time. It was by the use of coca that the Indian post-runners of South America were able to achieve their extraordinary feats of endurance. The continued use of the drug, however, results in emaciation, loss of memory, sleeplessness and general breakdown. Addiction to cocaine or a derivative, 'crack', is now a serious social problem in many countries. (See DRUG ADDICTION.)

Uses Before the serious effects that result from its habitual use were realized, the drug was sometimes used by hunters, travellers and others to relieve exhaustion and breathlessness in climbing mountains, to steady the nerves, and to dull hunger. The chief use in medicine is by local application to dull pain. Internally it is prescribed along with morphine or heroin for the relief of pain in advanced cancer. (See BROMPTON MIXTURE.) Here the risk of addiction is a secondary consideration. Otherwise it is practically only used in the treatment of diseases of the eye, and diseases of the ear, nose and throat. In the eye it is used as an anaesthetic in the form of eye-drops. It is also used in the form of lamellae to induce anaesthesia of the eye. A 5-per-cent spray solution is used to anaesthetize the throat and nose, whilst pastilles and lozenges containing 1·5 to 10 mg are used to reduce irritation of the throat and hoarseness. Artificial chemical compounds closely allied to cocaine are injected hypodermically in order to render painless small operations, such as amputation of the fingers, and by injection into the spinal canal to enable major operations to be done on the lower limbs without pain. (See PROCAINE.)

COCCUS is the name applied to a rounded form of bacterium. (See MICROBIOLOGY.)

COCCYDYNIA, or COCCYGODYNIA, means the sensation of severe pain in the coccyx.

COCCYX is the lower end of the spinal column, resembling a bird's beak and consisting of four nodules of bone, which represent vertebrae, and correspond to the tail in lower animals. They are deeply buried in the muscles in man, but in occasional cases they project backwards, and are surrounded by a fold of skin, so as to form an actual tail.

COCHLEA is the part of the inner ear concerned with hearing. (See EAR.)

CODEINE is one of the active principles of opium (q.v.). In the form of codeine phosphate it is widely prescribed for the relief of a useless, irritative cough, and also along with aspirin for the relief of headaches and rheumatic pains. It tends to be somewhat constipating.

COD-LIVER OIL is derived from the fresh liver of the cod (*Gadus callarius*). It is a rich source of vitamin D, used in the prevention and treatment of rickets, and vitamin A. Human milk contains more than enough vitamin D for the breast-fed baby, provided the mother has a balanced diet, with adequate exposure to

sunlight, or is taking vitamin supplements during pregnancy and lactation if considered necessary. All baby foods in the UK contain added vitamins, and therefore supplementation is unnecessary until weaning begins, and the baby starts taking cow's milk, which contains less vitamin D than human milk.

COELIAC DISEASE is a wasting disease of childhood in which there is inability to absorb fat from the intestines; there is therefore an excess of fat in the stools. It is the result of a constitutional intolerance of gluten (a constituent of wheat flour) which damages the lining membrane of the small intestine. This in turn interferes with the absorption of fat. Treatment is by means of a gluten-free diet. People with coeliac disease, or parents or guardians of coeliac children can obtain help and guidance from the Coeliac Society of the United Kingdom, (see APPENDIX 2: ADDRESSES). (See also GLUTEN; MALABSORPTION SYNDROME; SPRUE.)

COELIOSCOPY is a method of viewing the interior of the abdomen in patients in whom a tumour or some other condition requiring operation may be present but cannot with certainty be diagnosed. The examination is carried out by making a minute opening under local anaesthesia, and inserting an endoscope, a long flexible instrument bearing an electric lamp and telescopic lenses like that for examining the bladder (cystoscope), into the abdominal cavity. Certain of the abdominal organs can then be directly inspected in turn.

COGNITION The mental processes by which a person acquires knowledge. Among these are reasoning, creative actions and solving problems.

COITUS is sexual intercourse.
COITUS INTERRUPTUS (see CONTRACEPTION).

COLCHICUM, the bulb of *Colchicum autumnale*, or meadow-saffron, has long been used as a remedy for gout. How it acts is not quite certain.
Uses: Its main use is in gout, for which colchicine, the active principle of colchicum, in doses of 0·5 mg every one or two hours until the pain is relieved, followed by 0·5 mg thrice daily for about a week, is the form generally employed. Demecolcine, a derivative of colchicine, is sometimes of value in the treatment of chronic myelogenous leukaemia.

COLD, INJURIES FROM (see CHILBLAIN; FROSTBITE; HYPOTHERMIA; also CHILLS AND COLDS).

COLD SORES (see HERPES SIMPLEX).

COLD, USES OF The application of cold to the surface of the body is capable of influencing

the progress of disease in deep- seated parts to a considerable extent by acting on the blood at the surface, or through the nerves which end in the skin. Cold is applied for five chief purposes:
(a) *To subdue pain* In headache, a wet cloth to the forehead, or sponging with an evaporating mixture of vinegar and water, or eau-de-Cologne and water, is a well-known remedy. Sprains, if treated by holding the injured joint at once under running water, are much relieved. Later on, however, cold applications do harm, rather than good, by preventing the absorption of the effused blood. The pain of pleurisy may also be relieved by the application of an ice-bag to the side. Small operations may be done painlessly after freezing the skin of the part by spraying ethyl chloride over it.
(b) *To lessen inflammation* Ice-bags are used in inflammatory conditions to prevent the formation of an abscess.
(c) *To reduce high temperature* In any fever, sponging the arms and legs, one by one, with tepid water, is harmless and often very soothing.
(d) *To stop haemorrhage* In cases of increasing haemorrhage under the skin, for example, a bruised and blackening eye or a sprain, the amount of bleeding, and consequent discoloration, are lessened by applying compresses containing ice or some cooling lotion.
(See also HYPOTHERMIA; CRYOANALGESIA; CRYOSURGERY.)

COLD WEATHER ITCH is a common form of itchiness that occurs in cold weather. It is characterized by slight dryness of the skin, and is particularly troublesome in the legs of old people. The dryness may be accompanied by some mild inflammation of the skin. It may be exacerbated by excessive central heating. Over-washing with soap should be avoided. A non-alkaline substitute for soap such as Aqueous Cream BP is often beneficial. Relief is obtained from the use of emollients such as E45, applied regularly and always after a bath. Rough winter clothing should not be worn next to the skin.

COLDS (see CHILLS AND COLDS).

COLECTOMY is the operation for removing the colon.

COLESTIPOL (see HYPERLIPIDAEMIA).

COLIC This term is generally used for an attack of spasmodic pain in the abdomen. It is usually relieved by simple pressure, with no attendant fever – thus helping to distinguish it from inflammatory conditions.
SIMPLE COLIC often results from the build-up of indigestible material in the alimentary tract, leading to spasmodic contractions in the muscular lining. Other causes include habitual constipation, with accumulation of faecal material; and as an accompaniment of neurological disorders. Major risks include sudden

obstruction of the bowel from twisting, intussusception, or as a result of a tumour or similar condition. (See INTESTINE, DISEASES OF; INTUSSUSCEPTION.)
LEAD COLIC (*Syn.* painter's colic, *colica Pictonum*, Devonshire colic, dry belly-ache) is due to the absorption of lead into the system. This disease had been observed and described long before its cause was discovered. Its occurrence in an epidemic form among the inhabitants of Poitou was recorded by Francis Citois, in 1617, and the disease was thereafter termed *colica Pictonum*. It was supposed to be due to the acidity of the native wines, but it was afterwards found to depend on lead contained in them. (See LEAD POISONING.)
BILIARY COLIC and RENAL COLIC are the terms applied to that violent pain which is produced, in the one case where a biliary calculus or gall-stone passes down from the gall-bladder into the intestine, and in the other where a renal calculus descends from the kidney along the ureter into the bladder. (See GALL-BLADDER, DISEASES OF; and KIDNEYS, DISEASES OF.)
Treatment This consists of means to relieve the spasmodic pain, and removal where possible, of the underlying cause.
   Pressure on the abdomen, achieved by laying a baby across the nurse's arm, or with a hot-water bottle in older patients, often results in partial – if not complete – relief. Carminatives (q.v.) or anti-spasmodics (see SPASMOLYTICS) may also help.

COLIFORM Description of a gram negative bacterium found in the faeces. It covers the bacterial groups *Enterobacter, Escherichia,* and *Klebsiella.*

COLISTIN is an antibiotic isolated from the soil organism, *Bacillus polymyxa* var. *colistinus.* It is active against many Gram-negative organisms, and is proving of value in the treatment of gastro-intestinal and genito-urinary infections.

COLITIS means inflammation of the colon, the first part of the large intestine. *Mucous colitis,* once a fashionable disease, is now recognized not to be a form of colitis and has been named *mucomembranous colic,* or *spastic* or *irritable colon.* It is caused by painful spasms of the colon and may be due to anxiety. Treatment consists of dealing with the underlying nervous condition, the avoidance of all aperients, and a full diet without an excess of roughage. *Acute catarrhal colitis* occurs as part of an acute gastro-enteritis, usually due to food poisoning. The treatment is as for acute diarrhoea (q.v.).
ULCERATIVE COLITIS, the most important form, is an acute condition of unknown cause. Suggested causes include an abnormal immune response, possibly to bacteria or certain foods. Predominantly a disease of young adults, it is very liable to relapse. There is a strong familial tendency, with an association between

ulcerative colitis, ankylosing spondylitis and Crohn's disease.

Symptoms The onset may be sudden or insidious. In the acute form there is severe diarrhoea and the patient may pass up to twenty stools a day. The stools, which may be small in quantity, are fluid and contain blood, pus and mucus. There is always fever, which runs an irregular course. In other cases the patient first notices some irregularity of the movement of the bowels, with the passage of blood. This becomes gradually more marked. There is seldom actual pain except immediately prior to the passage of a stool, but there is always a varying amount of abdominal discomfort. The constant diarrhoea leads to emaciation and weakness, and there is always a well-marked anaemia. The acute form may be rapidly fatal, but as a rule the acute phase passes into a chronic stage. The chronic form is liable to run a prolonged course, and the majority of cases are subject to relapses for many years.

Treatment Non-specific, though complete bedrest is essential during the acute stage, with a high-protein, low-residue diet. Corticosteroids, given by mouth or enema, help to control the diarrhoea. The anaemia is treated with iron supplements, with blood infusions if necessary. Blood cultures should be taken, repeatedly if the fever persists. If septicaemia is suspected, broad-spectrum antibiotics should be given. Surgery to remove part of the affected colon may be necessary. After recovery, the patient should remain on a low-residue diet, and avoid unnecessary exposure to cold and damp. Sulphasalazine (q.v.) is helpful in the prevention of recurrences.

Patients and their relatives can obtain help and advice from the National Association for Colitis and Crohn's Disease (see APPENDIX 2: ADDRESSES).

COLLAGEN is the most abundant protein in the body. It is the major structural component of many parts of the body and occurs in many different forms. Thus it exists as thick fibres in skin and tendons. It is also an important constituent of the heart and blood vessels. With calcium salts it provides the rigid structure of bone. It also occurs as a delicate structure in the cornea of the eye, and in what is known as the basement membrane of many tissues including the glomeruli of the kidneys and the capsule of the lens of the eye. It plays a part in many diseases, hereditary and otherwise. Among the inherited abnormalities of collagen are those responsible for aneurysms of the circle of Willis (q.v.) and for osteogenesis imperfecta (q.v.). On boiling it is converted into gelatin.

COLLAGEN DISEASES is a general term for a group of diseases, including acute rheumatism and rheumatoid arthritis, characterized by changes in the tissue collagen. Although the precise cause is unknown, they are thought to be a sensitization reaction to an unknown toxin, and repond to corticosteroid treatment.

COLLAPSE is a condition of extreme weakness particularly involving the nervous system. It forms the final stage of many severe diseases, such as cholera, typhoid fever, and irritant poisoning. It is closely allied to the condition of surgical shock, but, whilst in collapse from the conditions mentioned the chief feature is feebleness of the heart's action, in shock there are numerous other prominent symptoms. (See SHOCK.)

Symptoms The face is pale and drawn, the forehead sometimes covered with cold sweat, the eyes sunken and glassy. The voice is weak, the breathing shallow, and the pulse rapid and feeble or imperceptible. The temperature is usually reduced to 35·6 or 36·1 °C (96 or 97 °F). Generally the patient lies on his back, paying no attention to what is proceeding around him.

Treatment The patient should be allowed to lie quietly on his back in a darkened room, well covered, and surrounded by hot bottles to maintain the body heat. Stimulants are also necessary.

COLLAR-BONE (see CLAVICLE).

COLLARGOL is a form of colloidal silver which mixes readily with water and any albuminous fluids, and has an antiseptic action. It is used especially for application to the eyes in inflammatory conditions.

COLLES'S FRACTURE is a fracture of the lower end of the radius close to the wrist, caused usually by a fall forwards on the palm of the hand, in which the lower fragment is displaced backwards. (See FRACTURES.)

COLLODIONS consist basically of a thick, colourless, syrupy liquid, made by dissolving gun-cotton (pyroxylin) in a mixture of ether and alcohol or with acetone. When painted on the skin the solvent evaporates, leaving a tough protective film behind that is useful for covering wounds. *Flexible collodion*, or collodion as it is often referred to, contains 1·6 per cent of pyroxylin, with colophony, castor oil and alcohol (90 per cent) in solvent ether. It should be kept in a well-sealed container. Being relatively elastic, it does not crack through the movements of the skin.

COLLOID is the name given to a type of cancer of internal organs, in which a glue-like substance collects in the interior of the tumour. The term is also applied to substances existing in a colloidal solution, and to the viscid iodine-containing material in the spaces of the thyroid gland.

COLLOIDAL SOLUTIONS are solutions in which a substance very finely divided into particles is suspended in another substance, as, for example, metals like silver and iron suspended in the form of minute particles in water or glycerin. The two constituents of the colloidal solution are called phases – the particles being known as the internal phase, and the medium in which they are suspended, the continuous or external phase. The term, suspensoid, is applied to colloids in which the particles consist of pure solid, and the term, emulsoid, is applied to those in which the particles absorb some of the liquid in which they are suspended.

COLOBOMA simply means a defect, but its use is usually restricted to congenital defects of the eye. These may involve, the lens, the iris, the retina or the eyelid.

COLON is the first part of the large intestine. (See INTESTINE.)

COLONIC IRRIGATION Washing out the large bowel with an enema of water or other medication.

COLONOSCOPE is an endoscope (q.v.) for viewing the interior of the colon. It is made of fibre glass which ensures flexibility, and incorporates a system of lenses for magnification and a lighting system.

COLOSTOMY is the operation for the establishment of an artificial opening into the colon. This acts as an artificial anus. The operation is carried out when there is an obstruction in the colon or rectum that cannot be overcome, or in cases, such as cancer of the rectum in which the rectum and part of the colon have to be removed. Such a colostomy opening can be trained to function in such a way that the patient can carry on a normal life, eating a more or less normal diet. Anyone wishing help or advice in the practical management of a colostomy should get in touch with the British Colostomy Association (See APPENDIX 2: ADDRESSES.) (See STOMA.)

COLOSTRUM is the first fluid secreted by the mammary glands for two or three days after childbirth. It contains less casein and more albumin than ordinary milk.

COLOUR BLINDNESS (see VISION, Defective colour vision).

COLPORRHAPHY is an operation designed to strengthen the pelvic floor in cases of prolapse of the uterus. The surgeon excises redundant tissue from the front vaginal wall (anterior colporrhaphy) or from the rear wall (posterior colporrhaphy), thus narrowing the vagina and tightening the muscles.

COLPOSCOPY is the method of examining the vagina and cervix by means of the binocular instrument known as the colposcope. It is proving of particular value in the early detection of cancer of the cervix.

COMA is a state of profound unconsciousness, in which the patient cannot be roused, and reflex movements are absent. Signs include long, deep, sighing respirations, a rapid, weak pulse, and low blood pressure. Usually the result of a stroke (q.v.), it may also be due to high fever, diabetes mellitus, glomerulonephritis, alcohol, epilepsy, cerebral tumour, meningitis, injury to the head, overdose of insulin, carbon monoxide poisoning, poisoning from opium and other narcotic drugs. Though usually of relatively short duration, and terminating in death, unless yielding to treatment, it may occasionally be long-lasting. The longest recorded case is that of the woman who died in the USA in 1978 at the age of 43, after having been in a coma for thirty-seven years following an operation for removal of her appendix. (See UNCONSCIOUSNESS.)

COMEDONES (see ACNE).

COMMENSAL is the term applied to microorganisms which live in or on the body (e.g. in the gut or respiratory tract, or on the skin) without doing any harm to the individual.

COMMINUTED FRACTURE A break in a bone in which the broken ends splinter into pieces. It is usually the result of a crushing force which also damages surrounding tissues such as nerves, blood vessels and muscles. Such a fracture is harder to set than a simple (clean) break. (See FRACTURES.)

COMMISSURE means a joining, and is a term applied to strands of nerve fibres which join one side of the brain to the other, to the band joining one optic nerve to the other, to the junctions of the lips at the corners of the mouth, etc.

COMMITTEE ON SAFETY OF MEDICINES (CSM) The Committee for Safety of Drugs was set up in 1963 in response to the thalidomide disaster. When the Medicines Act became law in 1971 this Committee was replaced by the Committee on Safety of Medicines. The CSM is an advisory committee which scrutinizes drugs at three stages: before clinical trials (clinical trial certificate stage), before a drug is advertised or marketed (product licence stage), or after marketing, the stage at which most doctors first have a direct interest in its work. Until 1981 the first stage in the assessment of new products required the granting to the company concerned of a clinical trial certificate, without which the product could not be tested in man. The issue of a trial certificate requires detailed animal evidence of toxicology and of teratogenic effects. A product licence is normally valid for five years, after which it has to be renewed. Before such a licence is granted efficacy must be shown for each of the proposed indications and appropriate warnings about side effects, contra-indications and interactions given.

COMMON COLD (see CHILLS AND COLDS).

COMMUNICABLE DISEASE This is an infectious or contagious disease, which can be passed from one person to another. Direct physical contact, the handling of an infected object or the transfer by droplets coughed or breathed out are all ways in which microorganisms can be transmitted. The government produces a list of notifiable diseases (q.v.), which includes all the dangerous communicable diseases.

COMMUNITY HEALTH COUNCIL A local group of people appointed to represent the views of the local community on services provided by Britain's National Health Service (q.v.). The councils are funded by the state, have no executive powers, but publish an annual report. Members have access to hospitals and the public can contact them about local services and ways of making complaints about hospital care. (see NATIONAL HEALTH SERVICE).

COMMUNITY PHYSICIAN A doctor who works in the specialty that encompasses preventive medicine (q.v.), epidemiology (q.v.) and public health (q.v.).

COMPATIBILITY The extent to which a person's defence systems will accept invading foreign substances, for example, an injection of a drug, a blood transfusion or an organ transplant. When incompatibility occurs there is usually a rapid antibody attack on the invading antigen with a severe local or system reaction in the individual receiving the antigenic substance.

COMPENSATION is a term applied to the counterbalancing of some defect of structure or function by some other special bodily development. The body possesses a remarkable power of adapting itself to even serious defects, so that disability due to these passes off after a time. The term is most often applied to the ability possessed by the heart to increase in size, and therefore in power, when the need for greater pumping action arises in consequence of a defective valve or some other abnormality in the circulation. A heart in this condition is, however, more liable to be prejudicially affected by strains and diseased processes, and the term 'failure of compensation' is applied to the symptoms that result when this power becomes temporarily insufficient.

COMPLEMENT is a normal constituent of blood serum which plays an important part in the antibody-antigen reaction which is the basis of many immunity processes. (See IMMUNITY.)

COMPLEMENTARY MEDICINE Also called alternative medicine, this type of medicine covers systems of care based on treatment methods or theories of disease that differ from those taught in Western-orientated medical schools. These systems include, for instance, chiropractic (q.v.), herbal remedies, holistic or 'whole person' medicine (q.v.), homoeopathy (q.v.), naturopathy – the use of natural substances to treat disease, reflexology – stimulation of nerves and blood vessels by foot massage, and faith healing. Acupuncture and osteopathy are alternative techniques increasingly used by medical practitioners, as is hypnosis. Registered osteopaths are now recognized in law and some other complementary-medicine techniques have training courses of varying standards.

The reason that the medical profession has been reluctant to recognize the often undoubted value of some complementary medical treatments is lack of any rigorous scientific testing of them. Even so, many patients turn to complementary medicine for treatment. The extent to which registered medical doctors use or ignore 'alternatives' varies greatly. In the United Kingdom the General Medical Council only permits 'shared care' of a patient if the registered practitioner retains overall responsibility, a requirement inimical to most alternative practitioners.

COMPLEMENT SYSTEM This is part of the body's defence mechanism that comprises a series of 20 serum peptides (q.v.) that are sequentially activated to produce three significant effects. These are the release of small peptides which provoke inflammation and attract phagocytes (q.v.); secondly, a substance (component C3b) is deposited on the membranes of invading bacteria or viruses and attracts phagocytes to destroy the microbes; thirdly, the activation of substances that damage cell membranes – called lytic components – which hasten the destruction of 'foreign' cells.

COMPLEX is the term applied to a combination of various actions or symptoms. The term is particularly applied to a set of symptoms occurring together in mental disease with such regularity as to receive a special name.

COMPLEXION (see ACNE; SKIN DISEASES; SUNBURN).

COMPLIANCE is the extent to which a patient follows the advice of a doctor or other health professional, especially in respect of drug or other treatments. This is generally increased if the patient understands the condition, and the basis for the proposed treatment.

COMPRESS is the name given to a pad of linen or flannel wrung out of water and bound to the body. It is generally wrung out of cold water, and may be covered with a piece of waterproof material. It is used to subdue pain or inflammation. (See COLD, USES OF.) A hot compress is generally called a fomentation. (See FOMENTATION.)

COMPRESSED AIR ILLNESS or CAISSON DISEASE affects workers in compressed air, such as underwater divers and workers in caissons. Its chief symptoms are pains in the joints and limbs (bends), pain in the stomach, headache and dizziness, and paralysis. Sudden death may occur. The condition is caused by the accumulation of bubbles of nitrogen in different parts of the body, usually because of too rapid decompression.

COMPRESSION SYNDROME (see MUSCLES, DISEASES OF).

COMPUTED TOMOGRAPHY or COMPU-TERIZED TOMOGRAPHY Tomography is an X-ray examination technique in which only structures in a particular plane produce clearly focused images. Whole-body computed tomography was introduced in 1977 and has already made a major impact in the investigation and management of medical and surgical disease. The technique is particularly valuable where a mass distorts the contour of an organ, e.g. a pancreatic tumour, or a lesion which has a density different from that of surrounding tissue, e.g. a metastasis in the liver. Computed tomography can distinguish soft tissues from cysts or fat, but in general soft tissue masses have similar appearances, so that distinguishing an inflammatory mass from a malignant process may be impossible. Computed tomography is particularly useful in patients with suspected malignancy. It can also define the extent of the cancer by detecting enlarged lymph nodes, indicating lymphatic spread. The main indications for computed tomography of the body are: mediastinal masses, suspected pulmonary metastases, adrenal disease, pancreatic masses, retroperitoneal lymph nodes, intra- abdominal abscesses, orbital tumours and the staging of cancer.

CONCEPTION signifies the complex set of changes which occur in the ovum and in the body of the mother at the beginning of pregnancy. The precise moment of conception is that at which the male element, or spermatozoon, and the female element, or ovum, fuse together. Only one-third of these conceptions survive to birth, whilst 15 per cent are cut short by spontaneous abortion or stillbirth. The remainder – over one half – are lost very early during pregnancy without trace. (See FETUS.)

CONCUSSION OF THE BRAIN (see BRAIN injuries).

CONDITIONED REFLEX The development of a specific response by an individual to a specific stimulus. The best-known conditioned reflex is the one described by Ivan Pavlov in which dogs that became accustomed to being fed when a bell was sounded salivated on hearing the bell even if no food was given. The conditioned reflex is an important part of behavioural theory.

CONDOM A thin rubber or plastic sheath placed over the erect penis before sexual intercourse. It is the most effective type of barrier contraception and is also valuable in preventing the transfer between sexual partners of pathogenic organisms such as gonococci, which cause gonorrhoea, and human immuno-deficiency virus, which may lead to AIDS.

CONDYLE is the name given to a rounded prominence at the end of a bone: for example, the prominences at the outer and inner sides of the knee on the thigh-bone (or femur). The projecting part of a condyle is sometimes known as an *epicondyle*, as in the case of the condyle at the lower end of the humerus (q.v.) where the epicondyles form the prominences on the outer and inner side of the elbow.

CONDYLOMA means a localized, rounded swelling of mucous membrane about the opening of the bowel, and the genital organs, sometimes known as 'genital warts' or 'ano-genital warts'. There are two main forms of them: *Condyloma latum*, which is syphilitic in origin, and *Condyloma acuminatum*, which often occurs in association with venereal disease, but is only indirectly due to it, being primarily a virus infection.

CONE (1) A light-sensitive cell in the retina of the eye that can also distinguish colours. The other type of light-sensitive cell is called a rod. There are around six million cones in the human retina and these are thought to comprise three types that are sensitive to the three primary colours of red, blue, and green. (2) A cone biopsy is a surgical technique in which a conical or cylindrical section of the lower part of the neck of the womb is excised.

CONGENITAL deformities, diseases, etc., are those which are either present at birth, or which, being transmitted direct from the parents, show themselves some time after birth.

CONGENITAL ADRENAL HYPERPLASIA (see ADRENOGENITAL SYNDROME and GENETIC DISORDERS).

CONGESTION means the accumulation of blood in a part due to over-filling of its blood-vessels. The condition may be due to some weakness of the circulation (see CIRCULATION,

DISORDERS OF), but as a rule is one of the early signs of inflammation (see ABSCESS; INFLAMMATION).

CONJUGATE DEVIATION is the term for describing the persistent and involuntary turning of both eyes in any one direction, and is a sign of a lesion in the brain.

CONJUNCTIVA (see EYE).

CONJUNCTIVITIS (see EYE DISEASES).

CONNECTIVE TISSUE This tissue holds together the different structures in the body. It comprises a matrix of substances called mucopolysaccharides in which are embedded a variety of specialist tissues and cells. These include elastic (yellow), collagenous (white) and reticular fibres as well as fibroblasts, macrophages and mast cells (q.v.). This variety is assembled in differing proportions to provide structures with varying functions: bone, cartilage, tendons and ligaments as well as fatty and elastic tissues.

CONSANGUINOUS A relationship by blood: siblings are closely consanguinous, cousins, and grandparents and grandchildren less so.

CONSERVATIVE TREATMENT Medical treatment which involves the minimum of active interference by the practitioner. For example, a disc lesion in the back might be treated by bed rest in contrast to surgical intervention to remove the damaged disc.

CONSOLIDATION is a term applied to solidification of an organ, especially of a lung. The consolidation may be of a permanent nature due to formation of fibrous tissue, or may be temporary, as in acute pneumonia.

CONSTIPATION is a condition in which the bowels are opened infrequently or incompletely, as a result of which the motions are dry and hard. Although one daily movement of the bowels is most common in health, the exact frequency may vary, though less than three times a week is generally regarded as constipation. It is a chronic condition, and must be distinguished from acute obstruction, a much more severe condition. (See INTESTINE, DISEASES OF.) The stools may vary considerably in colour, consistency, and amount, according to the nature and quantity of food and drink taken. **Causes** The most common causes are (1) habit, (2) 'a greedy colon', which absorbs water too quickly, (3) a spastic colon, in which the muscles remain in a state of spasm, (4) lack of tone in the muscle, sometimes due to a diet with inadequate vitamin B_1, (5) a low-roughage diet. Of these, poor habit is the most important. The

condition is usually aggravated by the use of aperients and purgatives. Uncommon causes, such as tumour, result in stricture of the bowel, leading to obstruction.
Symptoms and effects The stools are dark, hard, and passed with difficulty, and in small amount. In severe, persistent cases there may be swelling of the abdomen, from the retention of large masses of the remnants from digestion. Colic may occur in long-standing cases, in which the accumulation in the lower part of the bowel is beginning to affect the rest of the gut. Piles, which are a cause of increasing constipation, are often brought on by inattention to the bowels to begin with.
Treatment If there is no organic cause, such as tumour or other source of mechanical obstruction, attention to daily habit is the most important matter. Daily exercise should be encouraged, and a habit of regularly opening the bowels, at the same time each day, should be cultivated. A high-roughage diet is important, with plenty of fruit and vegetables. A cereal rich in bran is helpful, and wholemeal bread should be preferred.

CONSTITUTION, or DIATHESIS, means the general condition of the body, especially with reference to its liability to certain diseases.

CONSULTANT In Britain's health service a consultant is the senior career post for a fully qualified specialist. He or she normally sees patients referred by general practitioners – hence the historical term 'consultant' – or emergency cases admitted direct to hospital. NHS consultants are also allowed to do a certain amount of private practice. A consultant has to undergo several years of specialist training in hospital as a 'junior' doctor or dentist and pass higher examinations. There were over 21,000 consultants in the United Kingdom in 1993 and over 32,000 GPs for a population of more than 57 million.

CONSUMPTION (see TUBERCULOSIS).

CONTACT LENSES are lenses worn in contact with the eye, behind the eyelids and in front of the cornea. They may be worn for cosmetic, optical or therapeutic reasons. The commonest reason for wear is cosmetic, many short-sighted people preferring to wear contact lenses instead of glasses. Optical reasons for contact-lens wear include cataract surgery (usually unilateral extraction) and the considerable improvement in overall standard of vision experienced by very short-sighted people by wearing contact lenses instead of glasses. Therapeutic lenses are those used in the treatment of eye disease, 'bandage lenses' are used in certain corneal diseases: contact lenses can be soaked in a particular drug and then put on the eye so that the drug slowly leaks out on to the eye. Contact lenses may be hard, soft or gas permeable. Hard lenses are more optically accurate (because they are rigid), cheaper and more durable than soft. The main advantage of soft lenses is that they are more comfortable to wear. Gas-permeable lenses are so called because they are more permeable to oxygen than other lenses, thus allowing more oxygen to reach the cornea.

CONTAGION means the principle of spread of disease by direct contact with the body of an affected person.

CONTINUED FEVERS are typhus, typhoid and relapsing fevers, so called because of their continuing over a more or less definite space of time.

CONTINUOUS POSITIVE AIRWAYS PRESSURE A method for treating babies who suffer from alveolar collapse in the lung as a result of hyaline membrane disease (respiratory distress syndrome) (q.v.).

CONTRACEPTION A means of avoiding pregnancy despite sexual activity. There is no ideal contraceptive, and the choice of method depends on balancing considerations of safety, effectiveness, and acceptability. The best choice for any couple will depend on their ages and personal circumstances and may well vary with time. Contraceptive techniques can be classified in various ways, but one of the most useful is into 'barrier' and 'non-barrier' methods.
BARRIER METHODS These involve a physical barrier which prevents sperm from reaching the cervix. Barrier methods reduce the risk of spreading sexually transmitted diseases, and the sheath is the best protection against HIV infection (see AIDS/HIV) for sexually active people. The efficiency of barrier methods is improved if they are used in conjunction with a spermicidal foam or jelly, but care is needed to ensure that the preparation chosen does not damage the rubber barrier.
Condom (sheath) This is the most commonly used barrier contraceptive. It consists of a rubber sheath which is placed over the erect penis before intromission and removed after ejaculation. The failure rate, if properly used, is about 4 per cent.
Diaphragm or *cap* A rubber dome that is inserted into the vagina before intercourse and fits snugly over the cervix. It should be used with an appropriate spermicide and is removed six hours after intercourse. A woman must be measured to ensure that she is supplied with the correct size of diaphragm, and the fit should be checked annually or after more than about 7 lbs. change in weight. The failure rate, if properly used, is about 2 per cent.
NON-BARRIER METHODS These do not provide a physical barrier between sperm and cervix and so do not protect against sexually transmitted diseases, including HIV.
Coitus interruptus This involves the man's withdrawing his penis from the vagina before ejaculation. Because some sperm may leak

before full ejaculation, the method is not very reliable.
Safe period This involves avoiding intercourse around the time when the woman ovulates and is at risk of pregnancy. The safe times can be predicted using temperature charts to identify the rise in temperature before ovulation or by careful assessment of the quality of the cervical mucus. This method works best if the woman has regular menstrual cycles. If used carefully it can be very effective and is free from side-effects, but it requires a highly motivated couple to succeed. It is approved by the Catholic church.
Spermicidal gels, creams, pessaries, etc. These are supposed to prevent pregnancy by killing sperm before they reach the cervix, but they are unreliable and should be used only in conjunction with a barrier method.
Intrauterine contraceptive device (coil) This is a small metal or plastic shape placed inside the uterus that prevents pregnancy by disrupting implantation. Some people regard it as a form of abortion, so it is not acceptable to all religious groups. There is a significantly increased risk of pelvic infection and eventual infertility in women who have used coils, and in many countries their use has declined substantially. They must be inserted by a specially trained health worker, but once in place they permit intercourse at any time with no prior planning. Increased pain and bleeding may be caused during menstruation, but, if severe, these may indicate that the coil is incorrectly sited, and that its position should be checked.
Hormonal methods These include the combined oestrogen and progesterone and progesterone-only contraceptive pills, as well as longer-acting depot preparations. They modify the woman's hormonal environment and prevent pregnancy by disrupting various stages of the menstrual cycle, especially ovulation. The combined oestrogen and progesterone pills are very effective and are the most popular form of contraception. A wide range of preparations is available and the *British National Formulary* contains details of the commonly used varieties.
The main side-effects are an increased risk of cardiovascular disease. The lowest possible dose of oestrogen should be used, and many preparations use phasic preparations in which the dose of oestrogen varies with the time of the cycle. The progesterone- only or 'mini' pill does not contain any oestrogen and must be taken at the same time every day. It is not as effective as the combined pill, but failure rates of less than 1-per-100 woman years can be achieved. It has few serious side-effects, but may cause menstrual irregularities. It is suitable for use by mothers who are breast feeding. Depot preparations include intramuscular injections, subcutaneous implants, and intravaginal rings. They are useful in cases where the woman cannot be relied on to take a pill regularly but needs effective contraception. Their main side-effect is their prolonged action, which means that users cannot suddenly decide that they would like to become pregnant.

Sterilization Permanent contraception can be achieved by sterilizing either the male or female partner. The operation on men is easier and safer. Although sterilization can sometimes be reversed, this cannot be guaranteed and couples should be counselled in advance that the method is irreversible. There is a small but definite failure rate with sterilization, and this should also be made clear before the operation is performed.

Post-coital contraception This is, in effect, a high dose of the combined oral contraceptive given within 72 hours of unprotected intercourse. It can cause nausea and vomiting. It is useful in an emergency, e.g. if a sheath splits during intercourse or after rape, but, if a woman requests it repeatedly because she is forgetting to use her usual method of contraception, further counselling and a change of regular method is indicated.

CONTRACTURE means the permanent shortening of a muscle or of fibrous tissue. Contraction is the name given to the temporary shortening of a muscle.

CONTRAST MEDIUM A material that is used to increase the visibility of the body's tissues and organs during radiography. A common example is the use of barium which is given by mouth or as an enema to show up the alimentary tract.

CONTRE-COUP means an injury in which a bone, generally the skull, is fractured, not at the spot where the violence is applied, but at the exactly opposite point.

CONTROLLED DRUGS In the United Kingdom controlled drugs are those preparations referred to under the Misuse of Drugs Act, 1971. The act prohibits activities related to the manufacture, supply and possession of these drugs and they are classified into three groups which determine the penalties for offences involving their misuse. For example, class A includes cocaine, diamorphine, morphine, LSD and pethidine (qq.v.). Class B includes amphetamines, barbiturates, cannabis, codeine and pentazocine (qq.v.). Class C includes drugs related to amphetamines such as diethylpropion and chlorphentermine, meprobamate (q.v.) and most benzodiazepines (q.v.).

The Misuse of Drugs Regulations, 1985, define the classes of person authorized to supply and possess controlled drugs and lay down the conditions under which these activities may be carried out. In the Regulations drugs are divided into five schedules specifying the requirements for supply, possession, prescribing and record-keeping. Schedule 1 contains drugs, such as cannabis, which are not used as medicines. Schedules 2 and 3 contain drugs which are subject to the prescription requirements of the Act (see below). They are distinguished in the *British National Formulary* (BNF) (q.v.) by the symbol CD and they include morphine, diamorphine (heroin), other opioid analgesics, barbiturates, amphetamines, cocaine and diethylpropion. Schedules 4 and 5 contain drugs such as the benzodiazepines which are subject to minimal control. A full list of the drugs in each schedule can be found in the BNF.

Prescriptions for drugs in schedules 2 and 3 must be signed and dated by the prescriber, who must give his address. The prescription must be in the prescriber's own handwriting and provide the name and address of the patient and the total quantity of the preparation in both words and figures. The pharmacist is not allowed to dispense a controlled drug unless all the information required by law is given on the prescription.

The Misuse of Drugs (Notification and Supply of Addicts) Regulations, 1973, govern the notification of addicts. This is required in respect of the following commonly used drugs: cocaine, dextromoramide, diamorphine, dipipanone, hydrocodone, hydromorphone, levorphanol, methadone, morphine, opium, oxycodone, pethidine, phenazocine and piritramide.

Any doctor who suspects that his patient may be addicted to one of these drugs must notify the Chief Medical Officer at the Home Office in writing within seven days. Notification in writing must be confirmed annually if the patient is still being treated by the doctor. The Home Office maintains an Index of Addicts which is available to doctors on a confidential basis.

CONTUSION (see BRUISES).

CONVALESCENCE means the condition through which a person passes after having suffered from some acute disease, and before complete health and strength are regained.

CONVERGENCE (1) Inward turning of the eyes to focus on a near point with the result that a single image is registered by both retinas. (2) The coming together of various nerve fibres to form a nerve tract that provides a single pathway from different parts of the brain.

CONVOLUTIONS (see BRAIN).

CONVULSIONS are rapidly alternating contractions and relaxations of the muscles, causing irregular movements of the limbs or body generally, usually accompanied by unconsciousness. Generally a symptom of some other trouble, often of a minor nature in children, they are rarely a danger to life. Nevertheless a cause of alarm, they should always be taken seriously.

Causes The most common cause of convulsions in adults is epilepsy (q.v.), and it can also cause them in infants and children. The relative frequency of non-epileptic convulsions in infants and young children is probably due to an instability of the immature nervous system. An American investigation showed that in a large group of otherwise normal children, some 6 per cent had had one or more convulsions.

In young infants convulsions may be due to *birth injuries*, usually the result of a difficult labour. The convulsions in these cases are due to damage of the brain, either by bleeding from torn blood-vessels or concussion of the brain. In older infants convulsions may be due to the irritability of the brain often associated with *rickets*, a condition known as tetany. Other metabolic causes include hypoglycaemia and hypokalaemia. A sudden *rise of temperature*, such as may occur in any infection, may induce convulsions in an infant and young child.

Diseases of the brain, such as meningitis, encephalitis and tumours, or any disturbance of the brain due to bleeding, blockage of a blood-vessel, or irritation of the brain by a fracture of the skull, may also be responsible for convulsions.

Asphyxia, such as may occur in a young child during a paroxysm of whooping-cough, may also bring on convulsions.

Treatment Tepid sponging may help if there is fever, and a spoon or spatula should be put between the child's teeth if there is a possibility of his biting his tounge. Unless particularly severe, the movements seldom need be restrained. If the convulsions persist, it may be necessary to give parenteral benzodiazepines. As rule a sedative, or an injection of one of the barbiturates, controls the convulsions. Once these are under control, the cause of the convulsions must be sought and the necessary treatment given

COOLEY'S ANAEMIA (see THALASSAEMIA).

COOMB'S TEST A sensitive test that detects antibodies (q.v.) to the body's red cells (see ERYTHROCYTE). There are two methods: one, the direct, identifies those antibodies that are bound to the cells; the other, indirect, method identifies those circulating unattached in the serum.

CO-ORDINATION means the governing power exercised by the brain as a whole, or by certain centres in the nervous system, to make various muscles contract in harmony, and so produce definite actions, instead of meaningless movements. It is bound up intimately with the complex sense of localization, which enables a person with his eyes shut to tell, by sensations received from the bones, joints and muscles, the position of the various parts of his body. The power is impaired in various diseases, such as locomotor ataxia. It is tested by making the patient shut his eyes, moving his hand in various directions, and then telling him to bring the point of the forefinger steadily to the tip of the nose, or by other simple movements.

COPPER is an essential nutrient for man, and all tissues in the human body contain traces of it. The total amount in the adult body is 100 to 150 mg. Many essential enzyme systems are dependent on traces of copper. On the other hand, there is no evidence that dietary deficiency of copper ever occurs in man. Infants are born with an ample store, and the normal diet for an adult contains around 2 mg of copper a day. It is used in medicine as the two salts, sulphate of copper (blue stone) and nitrate of copper. The former is, in small doses, a powerful astringent, and in larger doses an irritant. Both are caustics when applied externally. Externally, either is used to rub on unhealthy ulcers and growths to stimulate the granulation tissue to more rapid healing.

COPROLALIA is the condition in which insane people give utterance to filthy and obscene words.

COPULATION The act of coitus or sexual intercourse when the man inserts his erect penis into the woman's vagina and after a succession of thrusting movements ejaculates his semen.

CORDOTOMY, or CHORDOTOMY, is the surgical operation of cutting the antero-lateral tracts of the spinal cord to relieve otherwise intractable pain. It is also sometimes known as tractotomy.

CORNEA (see EYE).

CORNEAL GRAFT (KERATOPLASTY) If the cornea becomes damaged or diseased and vision is impaired, it can be removed and replaced by a corneal graft. The graft is taken from the cornea of a human donor. Some of the indication for corneal grafting include keratoconus, corneal dystrophies, severe corneal scarring following herpes simplex, alkali burns or injury. Because the graft is a foreign protein, there is a danger that the recipient's immune system may set up a reaction causing rejection of the graft. Rejection results in oedema of the graft with subsequent poor vision. Once a corneal graft has been taken from a donor, it should be used as quickly as possible. Corneas can be stored for a short while in tissue-culture medium at low temperature.

The Department of Health has drawn up a list of suitable eye-banks to which people can apply to bequeath their eyes, and an official form is now available for the bequest of eyes. (See also DONORS; TRANSPLANTATION.)

CORNS AND BUNIONS A corn is a localized thickening of the cuticle or epidermis, of a conical shape, the point of the cone being directed inwards and being known as the 'eye' of the corn. A general thickening over a wider area is called a callosity. Bunion is a condition found over the joint at the base of the great toe, in which not only is there thickening of the skin, but the head of the metatarsal bone becomes prominent. Hammer-toe is a condition of the second toe, often caused by short boots, in which the toe becomes bent at its two joints in such a way as to resemble a hammer.

Corns and bunions are caused by badly fitting shoes, hence the importance of children and adults wearing properly fitted footwear. Corns can be pared after softening in warm water or painted with salicylic acid collodion or other proprietary preparations. Bad corns may need treatment by a chiropodist (q.v.). Bunions may require surgical treatment.

CORONARY is a term applied to several structures in the body encircling an organ in the manner of a crown. The coronary arteries are the arteries of supply to the heart which arise from the aorta, just beyond the aortic valve, and through which the blood is delivered to the muscle of the heart. Disease of the coronary arteries is a very serious condition producing various abnormal forms of heart action and the disease, angina pectoris.

CORONARY ANGIOPLASTY A technique of dilating atheromatous obstructions in coronary arteries by inserting a catheter with a balloon on the end into the affected artery. It is passed through the blockage (guided by X-ray fluoroscopy) and inflated.

CORONARY ARTERIES The right coronary artery arises from the right sinus of the valsalva and passes into the right atrio-ventricular groove to supply the right ventricle, part of the intraventricular septum and the inferior part of the left ventricle. The left coronary artery arises from the left sinus and divides into an anterior descending branch which supplies the septum and the anterior and apical parts of the heart, and the circumflex branch which passes into the left antrio-ventricular groove and supplies the lateral posterior surfaces of the heart. Small anastomoses exist between the coronary arteries and they have the potential of enlarging if the blood flow through a neighbouring coronary artery is compromised. (See CIRCULATION for diagram of heart and coronary arteries.) Coronary artery disease is damage to the heart caused by the narrowing or blockage of these arteries. It commonly presents as angina pectoris (q.v.) or acute myocardial infarction (see CORONARY THROMBOSIS).

CORONARY ARTERY VEIN BYPASS GRAFTING (CAVBG) When coronary arteries, narrowed by disease, cannot supply the heart muscle with sufficient blood the cardiac circulation may be improved by grafting a section of vein from the leg to bypass the obstruction. Around 10,000 people in the United Kingdom have this operation annually and the results are usually good. It is a major procedure that lasts several hours.

CORONARY THROMBOSIS is the acute, dramatic manifestation of ischaemic heart disease, one of the major killing diseases of western civilization. In 1992, ischaemic heart disease was responsible for about 134,000 deaths in England, compared with an annual average of over 109,000 in England and Wales in the period 1958 to 1960, but between 1980 and 1989 the figures fell by over 20 per cent. The alternative name for ischaemic heart disease is coronary artery disease. The underlying cause is disease of the coronary arteries, which carry the blood supply to the heart muscle (or myocardium). This results in narrowing of the arteries until finally they are unable to transport sufficient blood for the myocardium to function efficiently. One of three things may happen. If the narrowing of the coronary arteries occurs gradually, then either the individual concerned will develop angina pectoris (q.v.) or he will develop signs of a failing heart. (See HEART DISEASES.)

If the narrowing occurs suddenly or leads to complete blockage, or occlusion, of a major branch of one of the coronary arteries, then the victim collapses with acute pain and distress. This is the condition commonly referred to as a coronary thrombosis because it is usually due to the affected artery suddenly becoming completely blocked by thrombosis (q.v.). More correctly, it should be described as coronary occlusion, because the final occluding factor need not necessarily be thrombosis. Alternatively, it is sometimes referred to as myocardial infarction, this describing the destructive changes produced in the myocardium by lack of its blood supply. (See INFARCTION.)

Causes The precise cause is not known, but there is a wide range of factors which play a part in inducing coronary artery disease. Heredity is an important factor. It is commoner in men than in women. It is more common in those in sedentary occupations than in those who lead a more physically active life and the disease is more likely to occur in those with high blood-pressure than in those with normal blood-pressure. It is more common among smokers than non-smokers. The Royal College of Physicians in its report 'Smoking and Health' (1983) stated that 30 per cent of heart disease deaths are attributable to smoking. It is often associated with a high level of cholesterol (q.v.) in the blood. This in turn has been linked with an excessive consumption of animal, as opposed to vegetable, fats. In this connection the important factors seem to be the saturated fatty acids of animal fats which would appear to be more likely to lead to a high level of cholesterol in the blood than the unsaturated fatty acids of vegetable fats. As more research on the subject is carried out the arguments continue about the relative influence of the different factors.

Symptoms The presenting symptom is the sudden onset, often at rest, of acute, agonizing pain in the front of the chest. This rapidly radiates all over the front of the chest and often down over the abdomen. It is often accompanied by nausea and vomiting, so that suspicion may be aroused of some acute abdominal condition such as gall-stone colic or a perforated peptic ulcer. The victim soon becomes collapsed, with a pale, cold sweating skin, rapid pulse and difficulty in breathing. There is usually some rise in temperature.

Treatment is immediate relief of the pain by injections of morphine. Thrombolytic drugs should be given as soon as possible and continued. Subsequent treatment includes the continued administration of drugs to relieve the pain, the administration of drugs that may be necessary to deal with the heart failure that commonly develops and the irregular action of the heart that quite often develops, and the administration of oxygen. Patients are usually admitted to coronary care units, where they receive constant supervision. Such units maintain an emergency, skilled, round-the-clock staff of doctors and nurses, as well as all the necessary resuscitation facilities that may be required.

The outcome varies considerably. The first few days are critical ones and, if survived, the outlook is quite good with a first coronary thrombosis, provided the patient does not have a high blood-pressure and is not overweight. Following recovery, there should be a gradual return to work, care being taken to avoid any increase in weight, unnecessary stress and strain, and to observe moderation in all things. Smoking should be stopped. At one time, patients who had had a coronary thrombosis were kept in bed for prolonged periods. Today, however, in uncomplicated cases the aim is to get them up and about as soon as possible. Most patients are in hospital for a week to ten days and back at work in three months or sooner.

CORONAVIRUSES, so called because in electron micrographs the spikes projecting from the virus resemble a crown, are a group of viruses which have been isolated from people with common colds, and have also been shown to produce common colds under experimental conditions. Their precise significance in the causation of the common cold is still undetermined.

CORONER An independent legal officer of the Crown who is responsible for deciding whether to hold a postmortem and an inquest in cases of sudden or unexpected or unnatural death. He presides over an inquest, if held, sometimes with the help of a jury. Coroners are usually lawyers or doctors who have been qualified for at least five years. In Scotland the coroner is known as the procurator fiscal.

CORPORA QUADRIGEMINA form part of the mid-brain. (See BRAIN.)

CORPULENCE (see OBESITY).

COR PULMONALE is another name for pulmonary heart disease, which is characterized by hypertrophy and failure of the right ventricle of the heart as a result of disease of the lungs or disorder of the pulmonary circulation.

CORPUSCLE means a small body. (See BLOOD.)

CORPUS LUTEUM is the mass of cells formed in the ruptured Graafian follicle in the ovary from which the ovum is discharged about fifteen days before the onset of the next menstrual period. When the ovum escapes the follicle fills up with blood. This is soon replaced by cells which contain a yellow fatty material. The follicle and its luteal cells constitute the corpus luteum. The corpus luteum begins to disappear after ten days, unless the discharged ovum is fertilized and pregnancy ensues. In pregnancy the corpus luteum persists and grows and secretes the hormone, progesterone (q.v.).

CORRIGAN'S PULSE is the name applied to the collapsing pulse found with incompetence of the aortic valve. It is so called after Sir Dominic John Corrigan (1802–80), the famous Dublin physician, who first described it.

CORROSIVES are poisonous substances which corrode or eat away the mucous surfaces of mouth, gullet and stomach with which they come in contact. Examples are strong mineral acids like sulphuric, nitric and hydrochloric acids, caustic alkalis, and some salts like chlorides of mercury and zinc. (See POISONS.)

CORROSIVE SUBLIMATE, or PERCHLORIDE OF MERCURY, is a powerful antiseptic and an irritant poison. It is not to be confounded with subchloride of mercury or calomel. (See ANTISEPTICS; MERCURY.)

CORTEX The tissues that form the outer part of an organ and which are positioned just below the capsule or outer membrane. Examples are the cerebal cortex of the brain and the renal cortex of the kidney.

CORTICOSTEROIDS is the generic term for the group of hormones with a cortisone-like action. Many chemical modifications of the cortisone molecule have been prepared in an attempt to dissociate therapeutic action from side effects. Analogues are already available with no mineralo-corticoid effects and steroids with a gluco-corticoid activity and no inflammatory action have been synthesized. The main corticosteroid hormones currently available are cortisone, hydrocortisone, prednisone, prednisolone, methyl prednisolone, triamcinolone, dexamethasone, beta-methasone and paramethasone. They are used clinically in three quite distinct circumstances. First they constitute replacement therapy in states of adrenocortical insufficiency or hypopituitarism. In this situation the dose is physiological, namely the equivalent of the normal adrenal output under similar circumstances, and it is not associated with any side effects. Secondly, steroids are used to depress secretory activity of the adrenal cortex in conditions where this is abnormally high or where the adrenal cortex is producing abnormal hormones, as occurs in some hirsute women. The third application for corticosteroids is in suppressing the manifestations of disease in a wide variety of inflammatory and allergic conditions and in reducing antibody production in a number of auto-immune diseases. The inflammatory reaction is normally part of the body's defence mechanism and is to be encouraged rather than inhibited. However, in the case of those diseases in which the body's reaction is disproportionate to the offending agent, the steroid hormones can inhibit this undesirable response and although the underlying condition is not cured as a result it may resolve spontaneously. When such compounds are used for anti-inflammatory properties, the dose must be pharmacological; that is it must exceed the normal physiological requirement. Indeed, the necessary dose may exceed the normal maximum output of the healthy adrenal gland, which is about 250 to 300 mg cortisol per day. When doses of this order are used there are inevitable risks and side effects. A drug-induced Cushing's syndrome will result.

Corticosteroid treatment of short duration, as in angioneurotic oedema of the larynx or other allergic crises, may at the same time be life-saving and without significant risk. Prolonged therapy of such connective-tissue disorders, such as polyarteritis with its attendant hazards, is generally accepted because there are no other agents of therapeutic value. Similarly the absence of alternative medical treatment for such conditions as auto-immune haemolytic anaemia and auto-immune thrombocytopenia purpura establishes steroid therapy as the treatment of choice, which few would dispute. The place of steroids in such chronic conditions as rheumatoid athritis, asthma and eczema, is more debatable.

Although one must be aware of the side-effects, it is possible to become so obsessed with the risks of therapy as to underestimate the misery and danger of unrelieved chronic asthma or the incapacity, frustration and psychological trauma of rheumatoid arthritis. On the other hand, a form of treatment with the hazards of steroid therapy should never be undertaken lightly or until other established remedies have failed.

The incidence and severity of side-effects are related to the dose and duration of treatment. Prolonged daily treatment with 15 mg of prednisolone, or more, will cause hyper-cortisonism. Less than 10 mg prednisolone a day may be tolerated by most patients indefinitely. When used in pharmacological doses, steroid therapy is associated with certain side-effects which are so common as to be almost invariable but are not usually of serious consequence. These include gain in weight, fat distribution of the cushingoid type, acne and hirsutism, amenorrhoea, striae and increased bruising tendency. The more serious complications which fortunately occur much less frequently include infection, dyspepsia and peptic ulceration, gastrointestinal haemorrhage, adrenal suppression, osteoporosis, psychosis, diabetes mellitus, myopathy and potassium depletion.

CORTICOTROPHIN is the *British Pharmacopoeia* name for the adrenocorticotrophic hormone of the pituitary gland, also known as ACTH. It is so called because it stimulates the functions of the cortex of the suprarenal glands. This results, among other things, in an increased output of cortisone, Although first isolated from the pituitary gland in 1933, it was not until the discovery, in 1949, of the effect of cortisone and corticotrophin in rheumatoid arthritis that it came into general use. No means of synthesis has yet been discovered, and the only available sources are the pituitary glands of animals. It is only active when given by intravenous or intramuscular injection, but there are preparations available, which give a more prolonged action and which are given subcutaneously. As its action is predominantly the same as that of cortisone, the action of the two is discussed together in the section on cortisone (q.v.).

CORTISOL is another name for hydrocortisone (q.v.).

CORTISONE, originally known as Compound E, was isolated from beef adrenal glands in 1936 by workers at the Mayo Clinic. Its chemical name is 11-dehydro-17-hydroxycorticosterone. Mainly because of difficulties in obtaining adequate amounts, little interest was taken in it until, in 1949, Hench and Kendall and their colleagues demonstrated its dramatic, if transitory, effect in rheumatoid arthritis. The precise mode of action of cortisone is still not known. Among other things, it prevents (or delays) the proliferative changes in the tissues which are the normal response to infection and in allergic conditions. Among the conditions which have been shown to benefit from cortisone are rheumatoid arthritis, rheumatic fever, gout, certain eye conditions, certain skin conditions and Addison's disease.

Cortisone has two disadvantages which will always tend to restrict its use. One is that in chronic conditions such as rheumatoid arthritis the effect of cortisone is merely temporary, and tends to stop when administration is stopped. The other is that cortisone has certain toxic effects, and therefore it must only be used under medical supervision.

For all practical purposes corticotrophin (q.v.) and cortisone have the same action. (See also BETAMETHASONE; DEXAMETHASONE;

HYDROCORTISONE; PREDNISOLONE; PREDNISONE; AND TRIAMCINOLONE.)

CORYZA is the technical name of a 'cold in the head'.

COSTAL means anything pertaining to the ribs.

COSTALGIA means pain in the ribs.

COT DEATH (see SUDDEN INFANT DEATH SYNDROME).

CO-TRIMOXAZOLE is an antibacterial agent which is proving of value in a wide range of infections. It is a combination of two antibacterial agents: trimethoprim and sulphamethoxazole.

COTTON WOOL, or ABSORBENT COTTON as it is now technically named by the *British Pharmacopoeia*, is a downy material made from the hairs on cotton plant seeds (GOSSYPIUM HERBACEUM). It is used in medicine for a great variety of purposes.

COUGH is a sudden indrawing of air with the glottis (q.v.) wide open. This is followed by a blowing out of air against a closed glottis. The glottis then suddenly opens and the air in the lungs is expelled under high pressure – up to 300 millimetres of mercury and at a speed of 960 kilometres (600 miles) an hour. Its purpose is to rid the air passages and windpipe of what are colloquially known as foreign bodies, including the excessive mucus and other secretions produced in infections of the lungs and upper air passages, such as bronchitis and sore throat. As such secretions contain many micro-organisms, it is clear what an important part coughing plays in spreading the common cold and other infections of the nose, throat and lungs. It is a reflex action (q.v.) produced by stimulation of nerve endings in the air passages and may therefore be induced by irritation of these nerve endings by inflammation without any secretion. This results in the dry irritable cough which can be such a troublesome feature of the early and late stages of acute bronchitis, tracheitis (q.v.) and laryngitis (q.v.). Conversely the inability to cough in inflammatory conditions of the lungs, such as bronchitis and bronchopneumonia, especially in old folk, is an ominous sign, and every effort must be made to stimulate coughing so far as this is possible.

COUGH SYNCOPE is the loss of consciousness that may be induced by a severe spasm of coughing. This is the result of the high pressure that may be induced in the chest – over 200 millimetres of mercury – by such a spasm. This prevents the return of blood to the heart, the veins in the neck begin to bulge and the blood-pressure falls. This may so reduce the blood flow to the brain that the individual feels giddy and may then lose consciousness. (See FAINTING.)

COWPOX is a disease affecting the udders of cows, on which it produces vesicles. It is communicable to man, and there has for centuries been a tradition that persons who have caught this cowpox from cows do not suffer afterwards from smallpox. This formed the basis for Jenner's experiments on vaccination. (See VACCINATION.)

COXALGIA means pain in the hip-joint.

COXA VARA is a condition in which the neck of the thigh-bone is bent so that the lower limbs are turned outwards and lameness results.

COXSACKIE VIRUSES are a group of viruses so-called because they were first isolated from two patients with a disease resembling paralytic poliomyelitis, in the village of Coxsackie in New York State. Thirty distinct types have now been identified. They constitute one of the three groups of viruses included in the family of enteroviruses (q.v.). They are divided into two groups: A and B. Despite the large number of types of group A virus (24) in existence, evidence of their role in causing human disease is limited. Some, however, cause aseptic meningitis, and others cause a condition known as herpangina (q.v.). Hand, foot and mouth disease (q.v.) is another disease caused by the A group. All 6 types of group B virus have been associated with outbreaks of aseptic meningitis, and they are also the cause of Bornholm disease (q.v.). Epidemics of type B_2 infections tend to occur in alternate years.

CRAB-LOUSE is another name for *Pediculus pubis*, a louse that infests the pubic region. (See PEDICULOSIS.)

CRACKED-POT SOUND is a peculiar resonance heard sometimes on percussion of the chest over a cavity in the lung, resembling the jarring sound heard on striking a cracked pot or bell. It is also heard on percussion over the skull in patients with diseases of the brain such as haemorrhages and tumours, and in certain cases of fracture of the skull.

CRADLE is the name applied to the cage which is placed over the legs of a patient in bed, in order to take the weight of the bed-clothes off the legs.

CRADLE CAP, or CRUSTA LACTEA as it is technically known, is the form of seborrhoea of the scalp which is not uncommon in nursing infants. It usually responds to an ointment containing equal parts of Salicylic Acid Ointment of the *British National Formulary*, Sulphur Ointment BP, and White Soft Paraffin BP.

CRAMP is a painful spasmodic contraction of muscles, most commonly occurring in the limbs, but also apt to affect certain internal organs. NIGHT CRAMP is most common in the elderly, during pregnancy, in diabetics and in those with peripheral vascular disease. It comes on suddenly, often during sleep, the patient being aroused by an agonizing feeling of pain in the calf of the leg or back of the thigh. This painful disorder can be relieved by firmly grasping or briskly rubbing the affected part with the hand. SWIMMER'S CRAMP includes usually spasm of the arteries as well as of the muscles, due to cold and exertion. The limbs should be massaged and the victim kept warm.
HEAT CRAMPS are painful contractions of muscles occurring in men (e.g. stokers) working in high temperatures. The cramps are due to excessive loss of salt in the sweat, and can be cured, and prevented, by giving salt water to drink. (See also HEAT STROKE.)

CRANIAL NERVES are those arising from the brain. (See BRAIN.)

CRANIUM is the part of the skull enclosing the brain as distinguished from the face.

CREAM is the oily or fatty part of milk from which butter is prepared. Various medicinal preparations are known also as cream, e.g. *cold cream*, which is a simple ointment containing rose-water, beeswax, borax, and almond oil scented with oil of rose.

CREATINE is a nitrogenous substance, methyl-guanidine-acetic acid. In the adult human body there are about 120 grams of it, and 98 per cent of this is present in the muscles. Much of the creatine in muscle is combined with phosphoric acid as phosphocreatine, which plays an important part in the chemistry of muscular contraction.

CREATINE KINASE is an enzyme (q.v.) which is proving of value in the investigation and diagnosis of muscular dystrophy (see MYOPATHY), in which it is found in the blood in greatly increased amounts.

CREATININE is the anhydride of creatine and is derived from it. It is purely a waste product.

CREATININE CLEARANCE A method of assessing the function of the kidney by comparing the amount of creatinine – a product of body metabolism which is normally excreted by the kidneys – in the blood with the amount appearing in the urine.

CREEPING ERUPTION is a skin condition caused by the invasion of the skin by the larvae of various species of nematode worms. It owes its name to the fact that as the larva moves through and along the skin it leaves behind it a long creeping thin red line. (See STRONGYLOIDIASIS.)

CREMATION (see DEAD, DISPOSAL OF THE).

CREOSOTE is a clear, yellow liquid, of aromatic smell and burning taste, prepared by distillation from pine-wood or from beech-wood. It mixes readily with alcohol, ether, chloroform, glycerin, and oils.
It is a powerful antiseptic and disinfectant. Creosote is an ingredient of some disinfectant fluids.

CREPITATIONS is the name applied to certain sounds which occur along with the breath sounds, as heard by auscultation, in various diseases of the lungs. They are signs of the presence of moist exudations in the lungs or in the bronchial tubes, are classified as fine, medium, and coarse crepitations, and resemble the sound made by bursting bubbles of various sizes.

CREPITUS means a grating sound. It is found in cases of fractured bones when the ends rub together; also in cases of severe chronic arthritis by the rubbing together of the dried internal surfaces of the joints.

CRESOL is an oily liquid obtained from coal tar. It is a powerful antiseptic and disinfectant. **Uses**: It is used combined with soap to form a clear saponaceous fluid known as lysol, which can be mixed with water in any proportions. For the disinfection of drains it is used at a dilution of 1 in 20; for heavily infected linen 1 in 40; for floors and walls 1 in 100.

CRETINISM is a disease which is due to defective thyroid function in fetal life or early in infancy. The clinical recognition of hypothyroidism (q.v.) during the first week or months of life is difficult. The physical signs include growth retardation, a typical facies, a hoarse voice, coarse or thin hair and a large tongue, umbilical hernia and large anterior fontanelle. If the diagnosis is delayed numerous neurological abnormalities occur with abnormal gait, speech difficulties and poor co-ordination. If the disorder is not treated early mental retardation will be permanent. An early diagnosis, therefore, necessitates biochemical screening if the benefits of early treatment are to be utilized. Without early diagnosis one third of patients with cretinism will require special schooling and one quarter will have an I.Q. of less than 70.
Screening programmes for congenital hypothyroidism exist in North America, some

European countries and the United Kingdom. The incidence of primary hypothyroidism detected by such programmes is about 1:4400 live births. The screening programmes utilize cord blood serum, or capillary serum taken by a heel prick on day 5; the blood is used to assay the level of Serum Thyroxine and Serum TSH.

Treatment consists in giving thyroxine (q.v.) regularly.

CREUTZFELDT-JAKOB DISEASE is a rapidly progressive dementia occurring between the ages of forty and sixty-five. It is an uncommon disease in which dementia develops rapidly so that a normal healthy individual can be totally helpless within a year. The disease can be transmitted to animals by the innoculation of brain tissue from patients with the disease, after an incubation period of 11 to 71 months. The transmissible agent is thought to be a slow virus.

CRISIS is a word used with several distinct meanings. (1) The traditional meaning is that of a rapid loss of fever and return to comparative health in certain acute diseases. For example, pneumonia, if allowed to run its natural course, ends by a crisis, usually on the eighth day, the temperature falling in twenty-four hours to normal, the pulse and breathing becoming slow and regular, and the patient passing from a partly delirious state into natural sleep. The opposite mode of ending to crisis is by lysis: for example, in typhoid fever, where the patient slowly improves during a period of a week or more, without any sudden change. (2) A current use of the word crisis, and still more frequently of critical, is to signify a dangerous state of illness in which it is uncertain whether the sufferer will recover or not.

CROHN'S DISEASE is a chronic inflammatory disease that may occur in any part of the gut. The terminal ileum, colon and junction between the anus and rectum are particularly vulnerable. Ulcers (q.v.), fistulae (q.v.) and granulomatous tissue develop and the whole bowel may be affected. The cause is unknown, though the disorder may have an immunological origin. Steroids, given systematically and locally, may improve symptoms. Metrohidazole and azathioprine may help. The aim of treatment is to control the patient's symptoms. (See APPENDIX 2: ADDRESSES: Colitis and Crohn's Disease.)

CROUP is a household term for a group of diseases characterized by swelling and partial blockage of the entrance to the larynx, occurring in children and characterized by crowing inspiration. There are various causes including diphtheritic laryngitis (see DIPHTHERIA) and acute laryngitis. It is an account of this last condition which will be given here. (See also LARYNGO-TRACHEO-BRONCHITIS.)

Croup tends to occur in epidemics, particularly in autumn and early spring, and is almost exclusively viral in origin, commonly due to influenza or other respiratory viruses. It is always potentially dangerous, particularly in young children and infants, in whom the relatively small laryngeal airway may easily be blocked, leading to suffocation.

Symptoms Attacks generally come on at night, following a cold caught during the past couple of days. The breathing is hoarse and croaking (croup), with a barking cough and harsh respiratory noise. The natural tendency for the laryngeal airway to collapse is increased by the child's desperate attempts to overcome the obstruction. Parental anxiety, added to the child's, only exacerbates the situation. After struggling for up to several hours, the child finally falls asleep. The danger of recurrence, even fatal, must be borne in mind, however, and following one attack all children should be specially guarded against cold and damp until they have outgrown the tendency.

Treatment All cases of severe croup should be admitted to hospital for observation. Many improve on reaching the warm, confident atmosphere, but in the occasional child with progressive airways obstruction tracheostomy or intubation will be essential to prevent brain damage or even death. There is little evidence that putting the child in a cold mist tent or giving antibiotics or corticosteroids is of any value. Of greater importance is the reassurance of the child, and careful observation for signs of deterioration.

CRUCIATE LIGAMENTS are two strong ligaments in the interior of the knee-joint, which cross one another like the limbs of the letter X. They are so attached as to become taut when the lower limb is straightened, and they prevent over-extension or bending forwards at the knee. They are sometimes strained or torn as a result of sporting injuries or vehicle accidents. Surgery may be needed to repair the damage.

CRURAL means something connected with the leg.

CRUSH SYNDROME is the term given to a condition in which kidney failure occurs in patients who have been the victims of severe crushing accidents. The fundamental injury is damage to muscle. The limb swells. The blood volume falls. Blood urea rises; there is also a rise in the potassium content of the blood. Urgent treatment in an intensive therapy unit is required and renal dialysis may well be necessary. The patient may survive; or he dies with renal failure. Post-mortem examination shows degeneration of the tubules of the kidney, and the presence in them of pigment casts.

CRUTCH-PALSY (see DROP-WRIST).

CRYOANALGESIA is the induction of analgesia (q.v.) by the use of cold produced by means of a special probe. The use of cold for the relief of pain dates back to the early days of man. Two millennia ago, Hippocrates was recommending snow and ice packs as a preoperative analgesic. The modern probe allows a precise temperature to be induced in a prescribed area. Among its uses is in the relief of chronic pain which will not respond to any other form of treatment. This applies particularly to chronic facial pain.

CRYOPRECIPITATE When frozen plasma is allowed to thaw slowly at 4 °C, a proportion of the plasma protein remains undissolved in the cold thawed plasma and stays in this state until the plasma is warmed. It is this cold insoluble precipitate that is known as cryoprecipitate. It can be recovered quite easily by centrifuging. Its value is that it is a rich source of Factor VIII, which is used in the treatment of haemophilia (q.v.).

CRYOSCOPY means the method of finding the concentration of blood, urine, etc., by observing their freezing-point.

CRYOSURGERY is the use of cold in surgery. Its advantages include little associated pain, little or no bleeding, and excellent healing with little or no scar formation. Hence its relatively wide use in eye surgery. The coolants used include liquid nitrogen with which temperatures as low as -196 °C can be obtained, carbon dioxide (-78 °C) and nitrous oxide (-88 °C).

CRYOTHERAPY is the term applied to the treatment of disease by refrigeration. The two main forms in which it is now used are HYPO-THERMIA (q.v.) and refrigeration anaesthesia.

CRYPTOCOCCOSIS is a rare disease due to infection with a yeast known as *Cryptococcus neoformans*. Around 5 to 10 cases are diagnosed annually in the United Kingdom. It usually involves the lungs in the first instance, but may spread to the meninges and other parts of the body; including the skin. It responds well as a rule to treatment with amphotericin B, clotrimazole, and flucytosine.

CRYPTOCOCCUS is a genus of yeasts. *Cryptococcus neoformans* is widespread in nature and present in particularly large numbers in the faeces of pigeons. It occasionally infects man, as a result of the inhalation of dust contaminated by the faeces of pigeons, causing the disease known as cryptococcosis.

CRYPTORCHIDISM means an undescended testis. The testes normally descend into the scrotum during the seventh month of gestation. Until then the testis is an abdominal organ. If the testes do not descend before the first year of life they usually remain undescended until puberty and even then descent is not achieved in some instances. Fertility is impaired when one testis is affected and is usually absent in the bilateral cases. The incidence of undescended testis in full-term children at birth is 3·5 per cent, falling to less than 2 per cent at one month and 0·7 per cent at one year. Because of the high risk of infertility undescended testes should be brought down as early as possible and at the latest by the age of two. Sometimes medical treatment with human chorionic gonadotrophin is helpful but frequently surgical interference is necessary. This is the operation of orchidopexy.

CT SCANNER The machine which combines the use of a computer and X-rays to produce cross-sectional images of the body (see COMPUTED TOMOGRAPHY).

CULDOSCOPY is a method of examining the pelvic organs in women by means of an instrument comparable to a cystoscope (q.v.) inserted into the pelvic cavity through the vagina. The instrument used for this purpose is known as a culdoscope.

CUPPING is a traditional practice, now rarely used, for treating cases of deep-seated congestion by drawing blood to the surface. It causes sudden dilatation of the superficial blood-vessels, and so probably contracts those of underlying organs. But whatever the explanation, it gives relief in difficulty of breathing due to asthma, bronchitis and pleurisy and brings relief in lumbago and various forms of rheumatic pain.

CUPRUM is the Latin word for copper.

CURARE, known also as CURARA, WOORALI, WOURARI, URARI, and TICUNAS, is a dark-coloured extract from some trees of the *Strychnos* family. It is used by the South American Indians as an arrow poison, and is extremely potent, its action depending upon a crystalline alkaloid: *d*-tubocurarine chloride. This alkaloid paralyses the nerve endings in muscle. For many years it was considered to be much too dangerous for use in man, but research has shown that the pure alkaloid can be used with safety. Its main use is in anaesthesia, where the muscular relaxation it produces is of invaluable assistance to the surgeon. With the aid of tubocurarine adequate muscular relaxation can be obtained with a lesser degree of anaesthesia than would be required were the drug not being used. It is a drug, however, that should only be used by a skilled anaesthetist. Its action is antagonized by neostigmine. It has also been used in the treatment of spastic conditions.

CURDLED MILK (see CASEIN).

CURETTE is a spoon-shaped instrument used in surgery for scooping out the contents of any cavity of the body: e.g. the uterine cavity.

CUSHING'S SYNDROME was described in 1932 by Harvey Cushing, the American neurosurgeon. It is due to the excess production of cortisol. It can thus result from an adrenal tumour secreting cortisol or from a pituitary tumour secreting ACTH and stimulating both adrenal cortexes to hypertrophy and secrete excess cortisol. It is sometimes the result of ectopic production of ACTH from non-endocrine tumours in the lung and pancreas. The patient gains weight and the obesity tends to have a characteristic distribution over the face, neck and shoulder and pelvic girdles. Purple striae develop over the abdomen and there is often increased hairiness or hirsutism. The blood pressure is commonly raised and the bone softens as a result of osteoporosis. The best test to establish the diagnosis is to measure the amount of cortisol in a 24-hourly specimen of urine. Once the diagnosis has been established it is then necessary to undertake further tests to determine the cause.

CUTANEOUS means belonging to the skin. (See SKIN; SKIN DISEASES.)

CUTICLE (see SKIN).

CUTS (see WOUNDS).

CYANIDE POISONING Prussic, or hydrocyanic, acid is a very deadly poison with a sweet smell and pleasant taste, paralysing every part of the nervous system with which it comes in contact.

As a poison it acts with great rapidity, and, since potassium cyanide is used in some laboratory and industrial processes, and is almost as deadly in its effects as the acid, those using the cyanide should be acquainted with the treatment .

Symptoms After a large dose, the poison is very rapidly diffused through the body, and only a few minutes or seconds elapse before the symptoms appear. These are slowness of breathing, slowness and irregularity of the heart's action, and blueness of the face and lips. In a few minutes, insensibility with gradual stoppage of breathing and of the heart occurs, preceded in some cases by convulsions.

The suddenness and character of the symptoms and the sweet smell of prussic acid on the breath signal the cause.

Treatment Urgent hospital admission is required. Treatment is based on removal of the victim from the source, immediate emesis and stomach wash out and the administration of nitrites, which convert cyanide in the blood into the harmless cyanmethaemoglobin. Amyl nitrite is given by inhalation for 30 seconds every two minutes and also, if the victim can still swallow, 0·5 gram of sodium nitrite in 10 millilitres of water, by mouth. Oxygen is administered. Injections of sodium nitrite and sodium thiosulphate are then given, as well as analeptics. Cyanide emergency kits are available. The victim must be watched carefully for forty-eight hours. Another antidote is cobalt edetate.

CYANIDES are salts of hydrocyanic or prussic acid. They are highly poisonous, and are also powerful antiseptics. (See CYANIDE POISONING; WOUNDS.)

CYANOCOBALAMIN is the name given by the British Pharmacopoeia Commission to vitamin B_{12}. It is a red cobalt-containing substance, and it owes its name to the fact that it contains cyanide and cobalt. Vitamin B_{12} was first isolated in 1948 and was found to be an effective substitute for liver in the treatment of pernicious anaemia. (See ANAEMIA.) It has now been replaced by hydroxocobalamin (q.v.) as the standard treatment for this condition. (See COBALAMINS.)

CYANOSIS is a condition of blueness seen particularly about the face and extremities, accompanying states in which the blood is not properly oxygenated in the lungs. It appears earliest through the nails, on the lips, and the tips of the ears, and over the cheeks. It may be due to blockage of the air passages, or to disease in the lungs, or to a feeble circulation, as in heart disease. (See METHAEMOGLOBINAEMIA.)

CYBERNETICS is the science of communication and control in the animal and in the machine.

CYCLAMATES are artificial sweetening agents which are about 30 times as sweet as cane sugar. After being in use since 1965, they were banned by Government decree in 1969 because of adverse reports received from the USA.

CYCLICAL OEDEMA This is a syndrome in women characterized by irregular intermittent bouts of generalized swelling. Sometimes the fluid retention is more pronounced before the menstrual period. The eye lids are puffy and the face and fingers feel stiff and bloated. The breasts may feel swollen and the abdomen distended and ankles may swell. The diurnal weight gain may exceed 4 kg. The underlying disturbance is due to increased loss of fluid from the vascular compartment, probably from leakage of protein from the capillaries increasing the tissue osmotic pressure. Recent evidence suggests a decrease in the urinary excretion of dopamine may contribute as this catecholamine has a natriuretic action. This may explain why drugs that are dopamine antagonists, such as chlorpromazine, may precipitate or aggravate cyclical oedema. Conversely bromocriptine, a dopamine agonist, may improve the oedema.

CYCLIZINE HYDROCHLORIDE is an antihistamine drug (q.v.) which is mainly used for the prevention of sickness, including sea-sickness.

CYCLOPHOSPHAMIDE is a nitrogen mustard derivative (q.v.) which is proving of value in the treatment of various forms of malignant disease, including Hodgkin's disease and chronic lymphocytic leukaemia. (See CYTOTOXIC.)

CYCLOPLEGIA denotes paralysis of the ciliary muscle of the eye, which results in the loss of the power of accommodation in the eye. (See ACCOMMODATION.)

CYCLOPROPANE is one of the most potent of the anaesthetics given by inhalation. Its advantages are that it acts quickly, causes little irritation to the lungs, and its effects pass off quickly.

CYCLOSERINE is an antibiotic derived from an actinomycete, which is of value in the treatment of certain infections of the genitourinary tract, and of limited value in the treatment of tuberculosis.

CYCLOSPORIN A is a drug used to prevent the rejection of transplanted organs such as the heart and kidneys. (See TRANSPLANTATION.)

CYCLOTHYMIA is the state characterized by extreme swings of mood from elation to depression, and vice versa.

CYCLOTRON is a machine in which positively charged particles are so accelerated that they acquire energies equivalent to those produced by millions of volts. From the medical point of view its interest is that it is a source of neutrons. (See RADIOTHERAPY.)

CYESIS is another term for pregnancy.

CYPROHEPTADINE is an antihistamine drug (q.v.).

CYPROTERONE ACETATE is an anti-androgen. It inhibits the effects of androgens at receptor level and is therefore useful in the treatment of hirsutism in women and in the treatment of severe hypersexuality and sexual deviation in men. (See OESTROGEN.)

CYSTECTOMY The surgical excision of the bladder. When this is done, usually to treat cancer of the bladder, an alternative means of collecting urine from the kidneys must be arranged. The ureters of the kidney are usually transplanted into a loop of bowel which is brought to the surface of the abdomen to form a stoma (q.v.) that exits into an externally worn pouch.

CYSTIC DUCT The tube that runs from the gall bladder and joins up with the hepatic duct (formed from the bile ducts) to form the common bile duct. The bile produced by the liver cells is drained through this system and enters the small intestine to help in the digestion of food.

CYSTICERCOSIS rarely occurs except in Central Europe, Ethiopia, South Africa, and part of Asia. It results from ova being swallowed or regurgitated into the stomach from an adult pork tapeworm in the intestine. In the stomach the larvae escape from the eggs and are absorbed. They are carried in the blood to various parts of the body, most commonly the subcutaneous tissue and skeletal muscle, where they develop and form cysticerci. When superficial, they may be felt under the skin as small pea-like bodies. Although they cause no symptoms here, cysts may also develop in the brain. Five years later the larvae die, and the brain-tissue reaction may result in epileptic fits, obscure neurological disorders, and personality changes. The cysts calcify at this stage, though to a greater degree in the muscles than the brain, allowing them to be seen radiologically. Epilepsy starting in adult life, in anyone who has previously lived in an endemic area, should suggest the possibility of cysticercosis.
Treatment Most important is prevention of the initial tapeworm infection, by ensuring that pork is well cooked before eating it. Nurses and others attending to a patient harbouring an adult tapeworm must be careful to avoid ingesting ova from contaminated hands. The tapeworm itself can be destroyed with niclosamide (q.v.). Brain infections are treated with sedatives and anti-convulsants, surgery rarely being necessary. Most patients make a good recovery.

CYSTIC FIBROSIS is the commonest serious genetic disease in Caucasian children, with an incidence of about 1 per 2000 births. It is an artosomal recessive disorder of the mucus-secreting glands of the lungs, the pancreas, the mouth, and the gastro-intestinal tract, as well as the sweat glands of the skin. It is characterized by failure to gain weight in spite of a good appetite, by repeated attacks of bronchitis, and the passage of loose, foul-smelling and slimy stools. A simple, cheap, reliable test for detecting the disease by examination of the stools has now been evolved, which permits the early diagnosis of the disease. As yet there is no reliable method of detecting carriers of the disease or of detecting affected children before birth by antenatal tests. Treatment consists basically of regular physiotherapy and postural drainage, antibiotics and the taking of pancreatic enzyme tablets and vitamins. The earlier treatment is started, the better the results.

Whereas two decades ago, only 12 per cent of affected children survived beyond adolescence, today 75 per cent survive into adult life, and an increasing number are surviving into their 40's. Parents of children with cystic fibrosis, seeking help and advice, can obtain this from the Cystic Fibrosis Trust (see APPENDIX 2: ADDRESSES).

CYSTITIS means inflammation of the bladder. The presenting symptom is usually dysuria; that is, a feeling of discomfort when urine is passed and frequently a stinging or burning pain in the urethra. There is also a feeling of wanting to pass water much more often than usual and yet there is very little urine present when the act is performed. Cystitis may be associated with a dragging ache in the lower abdomen. The urine usually looks dark or stronger than normal. It is frequently associated with haematuria, which means blood in the urine and is the result of the inflammation. It is a common problem; over half the women in Britain suffer from it at some time in their life. The cause of the disease is a bacterial infection of the bladder, the germs having entered the urethra and ascended into the bladder. The most common organism responsible is called E. coli. This organism normally lives in the bowel where it causes no harm. It is therefore likely to be present on the skin around the anus so that there is always a potential for infection. The disease is much more common in women because the urethra, vagina and anus are very close together and the urethra is much shorter in the female than it is in the male. It also explains why women commonly suffer cystitis after sexual intercourse and honeymoon cystitis is a very common presentation of bladder inflammation. In most cases the inflammation is more of a nuisance than a danger but the infection can spread up to the kidneys and cause pyelitis (q.v.) which is a much more serious disorder.

In cases of cystitis the urine should be cultured to grow the responsible organism. The relevant antibiotic can then be prescribed. Fluids should be taken freely not only for an acute attack of cystitis but also to prevent further attacks, because if the urine is dilute the organism is less likely to grow. Bicarbonate of soda is also helpful as this reduces the acidity of the urine and helps to relieve the burning pain, and inhibits the growth of the bacteria. Careful hygiene, in order to keep clean down below, is also important. (See URINARY BLADDER, DISEASES OF.)

CYSTOCOELE is a prolapse of the base of the bladder in a woman. The pelvic floor muscles may be weakened after childbirth and, when the woman strains, the front wall of the vagina bulges. Stress incontinence often accompanies a cystocoele and surgical repair is then advisable (see COLPORRHAPHY).

CYSTOGRAM is an X-ray picture of the urinary bladder.

CYSTOMETER is an instrument for measuring the pressure in the urinary bladder.

CYSTOSCOPE is an instrument for viewing the interior of the bladder. It consists of a narrow tube carrying a small electric lamp at its end, a small mirror set obliquely opposite an opening near the end of the tube, and a telescope which is passed down the tube and by which the reflection of the brightly illuminated bladder wall in the mirror is examined. It is of great value in the diagnosis of conditions like ulcers and small tumours of the bladder.

Fine catheters can be passed along the cystoscope, and by the aid of vision can be inserted into each ureter and pushed up to the kidney, so that the urine from each kidney may be obtained and examined separately in order to diagnose which of these organs is diseased.

CYSTS are hollow tumours, containing fluid or soft material. They are almost always simple in nature.

Varieties RETENTION CYSTS: In these, in consequence of irritation or other cause, some cavity which ought naturally to contain a little fluid becomes distended or the natural outlet from the cavity becomes blocked. Wens are caused by the blockage of the outlet from sebaceous glands in the skin, so that an accumulation of fatty matter takes place. Ranula (q.v.) is a clear swelling under the tongue, due to a collection of saliva in consequence of an obstruction to a salivary duct. Cysts in the breasts are, in many cases, the result of blockage in milk ducts, due to inflammation. Cysts also form in the kidney as a result of obstruction to the free outflow of the urine.

DEVELOPMENTAL CYSTS: Of these, the most important are the huge cysts that originate in the ovaries. The cause is doubtful, but the cyst probably begins at a very early period of life, gradually enlarges, and buds off smaller cysts from its wall. The contents are usually a clear gelatinous fluid. Very often both ovaries are affected, and the cysts may slowly reach a great size, often, however, taking a lifetime to do so.

A similar condition sometimes occurs in the kidney, and the tumour may have reached a great size in an infant even before birth (congenital cystic kidney).

Dermoid cysts are small cavities, which also originate probably early in life, but do not reach any great size till fairly late in life. They appear about parts of the body where clefts occur in the embryo and close up before birth, such as the corner of the eyes, the side of the neck, the middle line of the body. They contain hair, fatty matter, fragments of bone, scraps of skin, even numerous teeth.

HYDATID CYSTS are produced in many organs, particularly in the liver, by a parasite which is the larval stage of a tapeworm found in dogs. They occur in people who keep dogs and allow them to contaminate their food. (See TAENIASIS.)

CYTARABINE is an antimetabolite substance that interferes with cellular division (see CYTOTOXIC).

CYTO- is a prefix meaning something connected with a cell or cells.

CYTOGENETICS is the study of the structure and functions of the cells of the body, with particular reference to the chromosomes (q.v.).

CYTOLOGY is the study of cells.

CYTOMEGALOVIRUSES are a group of viruses belonging to the herpesvirus group. They are so-called from the swollen appearance of infected cells (*cytomegalo* = large cell). Their importance is that they are responsible for the condition of cytomegalic disease of the newborn. The virus is transmitted from the mother either to her unborn baby while still in the uterus or to the baby during birth. In some cases the baby may show no evidence of infection, but in others it may cause a fatal disease characterized by jaundice and an enlarged liver and spleen. In those who recover from this severe form of the disease, there may be permanent mental retardation. In England and Wales, around 400 babies a year are born mentally retarded because the mother was infected with the virus in pregnancy.

CYTOMETER is an instrument for counting and measuring cells.

CYTOPLASM is the name given to the protoplasm (q.v.) of the cell body. (See CELLS.)

CYTOTOXIC means being destructive to cells. Many cytotoxic drugs are now available for the treatment of cancer and to suppress the immune system to prevent rejection of organ transplants. In some patients with cancer the treatment with cytotoxic drugs, or chemotherapy (q.v.), is given with the aim of curing the disease. Under these circumstances some degree of drug-related toxicity is acceptable. Patients with acute leukaemia and lymphomas as well as some carcinomas can be be cured with cytotoxic drugs. They are frequently used in combination because of the enhanced response achieved when given in this way.

The cytotoxic drugs include: (1) the alkylating agents which act by damaging DNA, thus interfering with cell reproduction. Cyclophosphamide, ifosfamide, chlorambucil, kelphalan, busulphan, thiotepa and mustine are examples of alkylating agents.

(2) There are a number of cytotoxic antibiotics used in the treatment of cancer – doxorubicin, bleomycin, actinomycin D, mithramycin and amsacrine are examples. They are used primarily in the treatment of acute leukaemia and lymphomas.

(3) Antimetabolites – these drugs combine irreversibly with vital enzymes systems of the cell and hence prevent normal cell division. Methotrexate, cytarabine, fluorouracil, mercaptopurine and azathioprine are examples.

(4) Another group of cytotoxic drugs are the vinca alkaloids such as vincristine and vinblastine.

(5) Some newer cytotoxic drugs have been introduced, such as cisplatin. This cytotoxic agent is particularly useful in the treatment of carcinoma of the ovary and teratomas of the testis.

D

DACRYOCYSTITIS (see EYE DISEASES).

DACTYLITIS means inflammation of a finger or toe.

DANAZOL inhibits pituitary gonadotrophin secretion and is used in the treatment of endometriosis, menorrhagia and gynaecomastia. The dose is usually of the order of 100 mg twice daily and side-effects may include nausea, dizziness, flushing and skeletal muscle pain. It is mildly androgenic.

D and C (DILATATION AND CURETTAGE): Scraping the lining of the uterus using a curette after opening up the cervix using a series of dilators. Incomplete abortions (q.v.) and uterine polyps (q.v.) may be treated by this procedure, but it is usually used to obtain tissue samples to assist in diagnosis.

DANDRUFF, or SCURF, is the white scales cast off from the scalp. (See SEBORRHOEA.)

DANGEROUS DRUGS (see CONTROLLED DRUGS).

DANTROLENE is a muscle-relaxing drug, indicated for chronic severe spasticity of voluntary muscle such as may occur after a stroke or in cerebral palsy and multiple sclerosis. Unlike most other relaxants, it acts directly on the muscle, thus producing fewer central-nervous-system side-effects. It is contraindicated if liver function is impaired and is not recommended for children or for acute muscle spasm. It may cause drowsiness, resulting in impaired performance at skilled tasks and driving.

DAPSONE is one of the most effective drugs in the treatment of leprosy. An antibacterial drug, its use may cause nausea, vomiting and, occasionally, it may harm nerves, the liver and red blood cells. During treatment blood tests are done to check on liver function and the number of red cells in the blood.

The drug is also used to treat dermatitis herpetiformis, a rare skin disorder.

DARTOS is the thin muscle just under the skin of the scrotum which enables the scrotum to alter its shape.

DAY BLINDNESS is a condition in which the patient sees better in a dim light or by night than in daylight. It is only found in conditions in which the light is very glaring, as in the desert and on snow, and is relieved by resting the retina, for example by wearing coloured glasses for a time.

DAYDREAMS occur when an individual during waking hours imagines enjoyable or exciting events or images. Most people daydream at some stage during their lives but it tends to occur when someone is stressed or unhappy. Children and teenagers in particular may sometimes daydream a lot. This should not usually worry their parents or teachers unless their work suffers or it affects the individual's personal relationships.

In those circumstances professional advice should be sought from a doctor or counsellor.

DDT is the generally used abbreviation for the compound which has been given the official name of dicophane. It was first synthesized in 1874, but it was not until 1940 that, as a result of research work in Switzerland, its remarkable toxic action on insects was discovered. This work was taken up and rapidly expanded in Great Britain and the USA, and one of its first practical applications was in controlling the spread of typhus. This disease is transmitted by the louse, one of the insects for which DDT is most toxic. Its toxic action against the mosquito has also been amply proved, and it thus rapidly became one of the most effective measures in controlling malaria. DDT is toxic to a large range of insects in addition to the louse and the mosquito; these include house-flies, bed-bugs, clothes-moths, fleas, cockroaches, and ants. It is also active against many agricultural and horticultural pests, including weevils, flour beetles, pine sawfly, and most varieties of scale insect.

DDT has thus had a wide use in medicine, public health, veterinary medicine, horticulture, and agriculture. Unfortunately, the indiscriminate use of DDT is potentially hazardous, and its use is now restricted or banned in several countries, including the United Kingdom.

The danger of DDT is that it enters the biological food chain with the result that animals at the end of the food chain such as birds or predators may build up lethal concentrations of the substance in their tissues.

In any case an increasing number of species of insects were becoming resistant to DDT. Fortunately, newer insecticides have been introduced which are toxic to DDT-resistant insects, but there are doubts whether this supply of new insecticides can be maintained as insects develop resistance to them.

DEAD, DISPOSAL OF THE Practically, only three methods have been used from the earliest times: burial; embalming; cremation.

BURIAL is perhaps the earliest and most primitive method. It was customary to bury the bodies of the dead in consecrated ground around the churches till the earlier half of the nineteenth century, when the utterly insanitary state of churchyards led to legislation for their better control, and now that cemeteries are supposed to be situated outside towns and in proper sites, the interment of the dead should seldom be a menace to the health of the living. Burials in Britain take place usually upon production of a certificate from a registrar of deaths, to whom notice of the death, accompanied by a medical certificate, must be given without delay by the nearest relatives.

EMBALMING is still used occasionally. The process consists in removing the internal organs by small openings and filling the body cavities with various aromatics of antiseptic power, the skin being swathed in bandages or otherwise protected from the action of the air. Bodies are also preserved by injecting the blood-vessels with strong antiseptics like perchloride of mercury. In certain circumstances bodies become naturally changed to a non-putrefying substance known as adipocere. (See PUTREFACTION.)

CREMATION provides a much speedier reduction of the body to its simple components than does burial, and one devoid of any harmful tendencies to the living. Not the least of its advantages is the amount of space that is saved. It is being used to an increasing extent.

In order to prevent any abuse, special certificates are required, and the necessary forms for these are obtained from the cremating authority. The law does not distinguish in England or the USA between cremation and burial, but special formalities are insisted upon by the crematorium authorities. The process of incineration takes between one and two hours. About 2·3 to 3·2 kg (5 to 7 pounds) of ash result from the combustion of the body, and there is no admixture with that from the fuel.

DEAD FINGERS (see RAYNAUD'S DISEASE).

DEADLY NIGHTSHADE is the popular name of *Atropa belladonna*, from which atropine is procured. Its poisonous black berries are sometimes eaten by children. (See ATROPINE.)

DEAD SPACE Gas exchange only occurs in the terminal parts of the pulmonary airways. That portion of each breath that is taken into the lungs but does not take part in gas exchange is known as dead space. Anatomical dead space describes air in the airways up to the terminal bronchioles. Physiological dead space also includes gas in alveoli which are unable to take part in gas exchange because of structural abnormalities or disease.

DEAFNESS is the term commonly used for hearing impairment. The Medical Research Council Institute of Hearing Research National Study of Hearing conducted between 1980 and 1982 showed that some 16 per cent of the adult British population have a mild hearing impairment (25 dB HL loss for the speech frequencies), while 4 per cent have a moderate loss (45 dB HL) and 1 per cent a severe loss (65 dB HL).

In most people, this is a sensorineural hearing impairment, commonly known as *nerve deafness*. This means that the abnormality is located in the inner ear (the cochlea), the auditory nerve or in the brain itself. The prevalence of this type of hearing impairment rises greatly in elderly people to the extent that over 50 per cent of the over-70s have a moderate hearing impairment. In most cases, no definite cause can be found, but excessive exposure to noise, either at work (e.g. shipyards and steelworks) or from gunfire and explosions, may contribute.

Conductive hearing impairment is the other main classification. Here there is an abnormality of the external or middle ear preventing the normal transmission of sound waves to the inner ear. This is most commonly due to chronic otitis media where there is inflammation of the middle ear, often with a perforation of the ear drum. It is thought that in the majority of cases this is a sequela of childhood middle-ear disease. Wax does not interfere with hearing unless it totally obstructs the ear canal or is impacted against the tympanic membrane, often due to injudicious use of cotton buds.

Conductive hearing impairment can, in many cases, be treated by an operation on the middle ear or by the use of a hearing aid. Sensorineural hearing impairments can be treated only with a hearing aid. In the UK hearing aids are available free on the NHS. Most NHS hearing aids are ear-level hearing aids, that is, they fit behind the ear with the sound transmitted to the ear via a mould in the external ear. The older body-worn hearing aids are now prescribed only for particular cases where an ear-level aid is unsuitable. Increasingly, however, smaller hearing aids are becoming available which fit within the ear itself and it is becoming much more common for people to wear hearing aids in both ears. The use of certain types of hearing aid may be augmented by fittings incorporated into the aid which pick up sound directly from television sets or from telephones, and from wire loop systems in halls, lecture theatres and classrooms. More recently bone-anchored hearing aids have been developed where the hearing aid is attached directly to the bones of the skull using a titanium screw. This type of hearing aid is particularly useful in children with abnormal or absent ear canals who cannot therefore wear conventional hearing aids. Even though it is estimated that over 10 per cent of the adult population in the UK might benefit from the use of a hearing aid, fewer than 4 per cent have ever tried one. Those people with a hearing impairment which is so profound ('stone deaf') that they cannot be helped by a hearing aid can sometimes now be fitted with an electrical implant in their inner ear (a cochlear implant).

Congenital hearing loss accounts for a very small proportion of the hearing-impaired population. It is important to detect at an early stage as, if undetected and unaided, it may lead to delayed or absent development of speech. The commonest cause of hearing difficulties in childhood is otitis media with effusion (glue ear). This usually resolves spontaneously, though if it persists, surgical intervention may be required usually involving insertion of a ventilation tube (see GROMMET) into the ear drum, often combined with removal of the adenoids (see NOSE, DISEASES OF).

Advice and information on deafness and hearing aids may be obtained from the Royal National Institute for Deaf People (see APPENDIX 2: ADDRESSES).

DEAMINATION is the process of removal of the amino group, NH_2, from amino-acids not required for building up body protein. This is carried out mainly in the liver by means of an enzyme, deaminase. The fatty acid residue is either burnt up to yield energy, or is converted into glucose.

DEATH, CAUSES OF Although the final cause of death is usually failure of the vital centres which govern the beating of the heart and the act of breathing, the practical question is the disease or injury which leads to this failure.

The principal causes of death in England in 1992 were ischaemic heart disease, which accounted for 30 per cent of all male deaths and 23 per cent of all female deaths, cerebral vascular disease, which accounted for 9 per cent of all male deaths and 15 per cent of all female deaths. Cancer of the respiratory organs accounted for 9 per cent of all male deaths and cancer of the digestive organs for 8 per cent of all male deaths, whereas cancer of the digestive organs accounted for 7 per cent of all female deaths.

DEATH CERTIFICATE A certificate required by law to be signed by a medical practitioner stating the main and any contributary causes of a person's death.

DEATH RATE In 1993, the death rate in England was 11·1 per thousand, a rise from the figure of 10·8 in 1992.

DEATH, SIGNS OF   There are some minor signs, such as relaxation of the facial muscles, which produces the staring eye and gaping mouth of the *Hippocratic countenance*, as well as a loss of the curves of the back, which becomes flat by contact with the bed or table; *discoloration of the skin*, which becomes of a wax-yellow hue, and loses its pink transparency at the finger-webs; *absence of blistering and redness* if the skin is burned (Christison's sign); and *failure of a ligature* tied round the finger to produce, after its removal, the usual change of a white ring, which, after a few seconds, becomes redder than the surrounding skin in a living person.

The only certain sign of death, however, is *stoppage of the heart*, and to ensure that this is permanent it is necessary to listen over the heart, that is, over the chest at the inner side of the nipple, for five minutes. This can be done by means of a stethoscope or by listening directly with the ear on the chest. *Stoppage of breathing* should also be noted, and this can be confirmed by observing that a mirror held before the mouth shows no haze, that a feather placed on the upper lip does not flutter, or that the reflection on the ceiling from a cup of water placed on the chest of the dead person shows no movement. An important sign is that if a cut is made in the skin or a vessel is opened no bleeding takes place after death.

In the vast majority of cases there is no difficulty in ensuring that death has occurred. The introduction of organ transplantation, however, and of more effective mechanical means of resuscitation, such as respirators, whereby an individual's heart can be kept beating almost indefinitely, has raised difficulties in a minority of cases. To solve the problem in these cases the concept of '*brain death*' has been introduced. In this context it has to be borne in mind that there is no legal definition of death. Death has traditionally been diagnosed by the irreversible cessation of respiration and heart-beat. In the Code of Practice drawn up in 1983 by a Working Party of the Health Departments of Great Britain and Northern Ireland, however, it is stated that 'death can also be diagnosed by the irreversible cessation of brain-stem function'. This is described as 'brain death'. The brain-stem consists of the mid-brain, pons and medulla oblongata which contain the centres controlling the vital processes of the body such as consciousness, breathing and the beating of the heart (see BRAIN). This new concept of death, which has been widely accepted in medical and legal circles throughout the world, means that it is now legitimate to equate brain death with death, that the essential component of brain death is death of the brain-stem, and that a dead brain-stem can be reliably diagnosed at the bedside.

Four points are important in determining the time that has elapsed since death. *Hypostasis*, or congestion, begins to appear as livid spots on the back, often mistaken for bruises, three hours or more after death. It is due to the blood running into the vessels in the lowest parts. *Loss of heat* begins at once after death, and the body has become as cold as the surrounding air after 12 hours, though this is delayed by hot weather, death from asphyxia, and some other causes. *Rigidity*, or rigor mortis, begins in six hours, takes another six to become fully established, remains for twelve hours and passes off during the succeeding twelve hours. It comes on quickly when extreme exertion has been indulged in immediately before death. Conversely it is slow in onset and slight in death from wasting diseases. It is slight or absent in children. It begins in the small muscles of the eyelid and jaw and then spreads over the body. *Putrefaction* is variable in time of onset, but usually begins in 2 or 3 days, as a greenish tint over the abdomen. (See PUTREFACTION.)

DEBILITY means a state of weakness.

DEBRIDEMENT   The surgical removal of foreign material and damaged tissue from a wound.

DECIBEL is the unit of hearing. One decibel is the least intensity of sound at which a given note can be heard. The usual abbreviation for decibel is dB.

DECIDUA is the name of the soft coat which lines the interior of the womb during pregnancy and which is cast off at birth.

DECOCTION is a preparation made by boiling various plants in water and straining the fluid.

DECOMPENSATION means a failing condition of the heart in a case of valvular disease.

DECONGESTANTS   Drugs which relieve nasal congestion and stuffiness. They may be given orally or by nasal spray, and most are sympathomimetics which cause vasoconstriction in the nasal mucosa.

DECUBITUS refers to the positions taken up in bed by patients suffering from various conditions such as pneumonia, peritonitis, or severe exhaustion. Such patients are liable to develop bed sores (q.v.), or decubitus ulcers.

DECUSSATION is a term applied to any point in the nervous system at which nerve fibres cross from one side to the other: e.g. the decussation of the pyramidal tracts in the medulla, where the motor fibres from one side of the brain cross to the other side of the spinal cord.

DEFAECATION means the act of opening the bowels. (See CONSTIPATION; DIARRHOEA.)

DEFIBRILLATION If a heart is fibrillating (see VENTRICULAR FIBRILLATION) the application of a large electric shock via paddles applied to the chest wall causes simultaneous electrical depolarization of all the cardiac cells and may allow the pacemaker to re-establish sinus rhythm. One paddle is placed below the right clavicle and the other over the cardiac apex. Care must be taken that no one is in contact with the patient or the bed when the shock is given, to avoid electrocution.

DEFICIENCY DISEASE is the term applied to any disease resulting from the absence from the diet of any substance essential to good health: e.g. one of the vitamins.

DEFORMITIES may be present at birth, or they may be the result of injuries, or disease, or simply produced by bad habits, like the curved spine occasionally found in children. (See BURNS; CHEST, DEFORMITIES OF; CLUB-FOOT; FINGERS; FLAT-FOOT; KNOCK-KNEE; LEPROSY; PALATE, MALFORMATIONS OF; PARALYSIS; RICKETS; SCAR; SKULL; SPINE AND SPINAL CORD, DISEASES AND INJURIES OF; JOINTS, DISEASES OF.)

DEGENERATION means a change in structure or in chemical composition of a tissue or organ by which its vitality is lowered or its function interfered with. Degeneration is of various kinds, the chief being fatty, fibroid (see CIRRHOSIS), calcareous, waxy, colloid, and mucoid.

Causes of degeneration are, in many cases, very obscure. In some cases heredity plays a part, particular organs, for example the kidneys, tending to show fibroid changes in successive generations. Fatty, fibroid, and calcareous degenerations are part of the natural change in old age. Defective nutrition may bring them on prematurely, as may excessive and long-continued strain upon an organ like the heart. Various poisons, like alcohol, play a special part in producing the changes, and so do the poisons produced by various diseases, particularly syphilis and tuberculosis.

DEGLUTITION means the act of swallowing. (See CHOKING.)

DEHYDRATION Removal of water. A reduction in the water content of the body. It may be caused by an inadequate intake or abnormal losses through sweating, vomiting, diarrhoea, or diuresis. The initial symptom is thirst which progresses to confusion and exhaustion. Rehydration may be produced by drinking, but in severe cases intravenous treatment may be necessary.

DELHI BOIL is a form of chronic sore occurring in Eastern countries, caused by a protozoan parasite, *Leishmania tropica*. (See LEISHMANIASIS.)

DELIRIUM is a condition of altered consciousness in which there is disorientation (as in a confusional state), incoherent talk and restlessness but with hallucination, illusions or delusions also present.

DELIRIUM (CONFUSION) The *milieu intérieur* of some old people is so fragile that acute confusion or acute brain syndrome is a common effect of physical illness. Elderly people are often referred to as being 'confused'; unfortunately this term is often inappropriately applied to a wide range of eccentricities of speech and behaviour as if it were a diagnosis. It can be applied to a patient with the early memory loss of dementia (q.v.), forgetful, disorientated and wandering; to the dejected old person with depression, often termed Pseudo-Dementia (Arie); to the patient whose consciousness is clouded in the delirium of acute illness; to the apranoid deluded sufferer of late-onset schizophrenia or even to the patient presenting with the acute dysphasia and incoherence of a stroke.

DELIRIUM TREMENS is the form of delirium most commonly due to withdrawal from alcohol, if dependent on it. There is restlessness, fear or even terror accompanied by vivid, usually visual, hallucinations or illusions. The level of consciousness is impaired and the patient may be disorientated for time, place and person.

Treatment is, as a rule, the treatment of causes. (See also ALCOHOL.) As the delirium in fevers is due partly to high temperature this should be lowered by tepid sponging (see COLD, USES OF). Careful nursing is one of the keystones of successful treatment, which includes ensuring that ample fluids are taken and nutrition is maintained.

DELIVERY means the final expulsion of the child in the act of birth. (See LABOUR.)

DELTA WAVES is the term given to abnormal electrical waves observed in the electro-encephalogram. (See ELECTRO-ENCEPHALOGRAPHY.) The frequency of the normal alpha waves is ten per second. That of the delta waves is seven or less per second. They occur in the region of tumours of the brain, and in the brains of epileptics.

DELTOID is the powerful triangular muscle attached above to the collar-bone and shoulder-blade, and below, by its point, to the humerus, nearly half-way down the outer side of the upper arm. Its action is to raise the arm from the side, and it covers and gives roundness to the shoulder.

DELUSIONS are errors in judgment, regarding simple facts, which interfere with the ordinary conduct of life. Thus a man may have the delusion that he has no stomach and refuse to take food. No amount of argument or demonstration will convince the subject of a delusion as to the error of his belief. The existence of a delusion, of such a nature as to influence conduct seriously is one of the most important signs in reaching a decision to arrange for the compulsory admission of the patient to hospital for observation. (See MENTAL ILLNESS.)

DEMENTIA   Severe dementia occurs in 5 per cent of individuals aged over 65; mild intellectual impairment is present in an additional 10–15 per cent (benign senile forgetfulness); the incidence of significant dementia rises to 20 per cent in those aged over 80. The predominant causes of dementia are Senile Dementia of the Alzheimer Type (SDAT) and Multi-Infarct Dementia (MID), occurring in a ratio of 70:30, and both types must be distinguished from the reversible Dementia Syndrome which develops over a few months. SDAT is characterized by defects in orientation, memory, intellectual function, judgement and activity; it is an acquired persistent loss of intellectual function with impairments in at least three of the following spheres of mental activity; language, memory, visio-spatial skills, personality and cognition (e.g. abstraction, judgement, mathematics). These defects in function tend to be preceded by memory loss, specifically, short term, occurring in the two to three years prior to presentation.

DEMOGRAPHY   The study of populations and factors affecting their health.

DE MORGAN SPOTS are small haemangiomas (q.v.) which occur in the skin of middle-aged people. No more than 3 mm in diameter, they are rarely widespread and are of no malignant significance.

DEMYELINATION   Destruction of the MYELIN SHEATH (see MYELIN) around NERVE FIBRES (see NERVES) which interferes with the nerve function. It can occur after injury to the nerve, but is particularly associated with multiple sclerosis.

DENDRITIC ULCER   A branching ulcer on the surface of the cornea caused by herpes simplex infection.

DENGUE   The term is Spanish, of African origin. The disease was first described by B. Rush in Philadelphia in 1780, and is also known as dengue fever, breakbone fever, and dandy fever, among others. Both endemic and epidemic in tropical and subtropical regions, it is also an acute arboviral infection caused by a flavivirus (family *togaviridae*) – of which there are four – transmitted by mosquitoes of the sub-genus Stegomyia, genus *Aëdes* – especially *Aëdes aegypti*. Four serotypes are distinct. Incubation period is 5–8 days, and is followed by abrupt onset of symptoms; fever, facial erythema – with intense itching (which spreads throughout the body), sore throat, running

eyes, and painful muscles and joints are common accompaniments. The symptoms subside within a few days and are frequently succeeded by a relapse similar to the first; this diphasic response is often accompanied by a typical 'saddle-back' temperature chart. Further relapses may occur, and joint pains continue for some months. In uncomplicated dengue the mortality rate is virtually zero. Diagnosis is by virus isolation or demonstration of a rising antibody-concentration in the acute phase of infection. There is no specific treatment, but mild analgesics can be used to relieve the pains, and calamine lotion the pruritus. Prevention can be achieved by reduction of the mosquito-vector population.

DENGUE HAEMORRHAGIC FEVER   This is a more severe form of the disease which usually occurs in young children; it is largely confined to the indigenous population(s) of south-east Asia. It is accompanied by significant complications and mortality. Immunological status of the host is considered important in pathogenesis.

DENERVATION   Interruption of the nerve supply to an organ or other structure.

DENTINE (see TEETH).

DENTIST is a person who diagnoses disease in the mouth, treats it and prevents its recurrence. There are a number of different groups. There is the *general dental practitioner* who is concerned with primary dental care. The *community dental practitioner* is part of the public-health team and is largely concerned with monitoring dental health and treating the young and the handicapped. In the *hospitals and dental schools* are those who are involved in only one of the specialities. The *restorative dentist* is concerned with the repair of teeth damaged by trauma and caries, and the replacement of missing teeth. The *orthodontist* is involved in the correction of jaws and teeth which are misaligned or irregular. This is done with appliances which may be removable or fixed to the teeth which are then moved with springs or elastics. *Oral and maxillofacial surgeons* are those who carry out surgery to the mouth and face. This not only includes removal of buried teeth but also treatment for fractured facial bones, removal of cancers and the repair of missing tissue and the cosmetic restoration of facial anomalies such as cleft palate or large or small jaws.

DENTITION (see TEETH).

DENTURE   A plate or frame bearing false teeth. It may be complete (replacing all the teeth in one jaw) or partial.

DEODORANTS are substances which remove or lessen objectionable odours. Some, which have a powerful odour, simply cover other smells, but the most effective act by giving off oxygen, so as to convert the objectionable substances into simple and harmless ones.

Varieties Volatile oils of plants, such as eucalyptus and turpentine, chlorine water and chlorinated lime, peroxide of hydrogen, charcoal, dry earth, sawdust, and potassium permanganate are among the most powerful.

Uses The main use is to purify sewage, bilgewater, and water- closets. Many powerful deodorants act, at the same time, as disinfectants. They are also used in sick-rooms to cover the smell of discharges, and the like. For the manner of use see under the individual deodorants. (See also PERSPIRATION.)

DEPILATION is the process of destroying hair; substances and processes used for this purpose being known as depilatories. The purpose may be effected in three ways: (1) by removing the hairs at the level of the skin surface; (2) by pulling the hairs out (epilation); (3) by destroying the roots and so preventing the growth of new hairs.

Shaving is the most effective way of removing superfluous hairs. Rubbing morning and night with a smooth pumice-stone is said to be helpful. The alkaline sulphides used as depilatories tend to erode the skin as well as the hairs. Electrolysis and diathermy have a limited use.

DEPOLARIZING NEUROMUSCULAR BLOCKADE (see NEUROMUSCULAR BLOCKADE).

DEPRESSION (see MENTAL ILLNESS).

DEPRESSOR is the name given to a nerve by whose stimulation motion, secretion, or some other function is restrained or prevented: e.g. the depressor nerve of the heart slows the beating of this organ.

DEQUALINIUM CHLORIDE is an antibacterial and antifungal compound which is of value in the treatment of infections of the mouth, gums, and throat, and in certain skin conditions.

DERBYSHIRE NECK is a colloquial name for goitre, which was fairly common in Derbyshire. (See GOITRE.)

DERMABRASION, or 'surgical planing', is a method of removing the superficial layers of the skin, which is sometimes useful in the removal of tattoos and superficial blemishes of the skin.

DERMATITIS is synonymous with eczema in all respects; although the lay term 'eczema' usually refers to atopic or endogenous eczema (see below), there are many other causes. Susceptibility to dermatitis is genetically determined in some cases, in others environmental irritants and allergens are implicated. Symptoms typically include itching, dryness or crack-

ing and, occasionally, soreness of the skin. Physical signs include redness (erythema), scaling and vesiculation (tiny blisters just beneath the surface of the skin).

ATOPIC DERMATITIS characteristically occurs in young patients 3 months–16 years old) with a personal or family history of hay fever, allergic rhinitis or asthma (atopy). There is a strong genetic component to this form of dermatitis which may be aggravated by various common allergens, including the house dust mite, cat and dog dander, and grass pollen. IRRITANT AND CONTACT ALLERGIC DERMATITIS results from direct toxic (irritant) or immunologically active (allergic) substances with the skin in susceptible individuals. Common irritants include bleaches, detergents and solvents; common allergens include nickel (in cheap jewellery, zip fasteners etc.), lanolin (in moisturizing creams and lotions) and colophony (in sticking plasters). Dermatitis which occurs as a result of exposure to irritants or allergens in the workplace is known as OCCUPATIONAL DERMATITIS. STASIS DERMATITIS (commonly known as varicose eczema) occurs predominantly in elderly patients with venous insufficiency, often in association with leg ulcers. Rarely, dermatitis may be caused by exposure to sunlight (PHOTODERMATITIS), to certain plant allergens (PHYTODERMATITIS) or by ingestion of drugs. ENDOGENOUS DERMATITIS, which tends to occur in middle-aged or elderly patients, is the term used when no obvious precipitating cause can be found.

Treatment of all types of dermatitis is similar: it involves identification of an underlying cause, if any, and taking appropriate avoidance or treatment measures. Application of emollients and steroids to affected skin is often sufficient to alleviate symptoms in most cases. Systemic immunosuppressive drugs may be required for control of severe disease which may, rarely, be life threatening..

Patient information can be obtained from the National Eczema Society (see APPENDIX 2: ADDRESSES).

DERMATOGLYPHICS is the study of the patterns made by the ridges and crevices of the hands and the soles of the feet. It has become an important study in medicine because of the help it provides in the diagnosis of certain diseases, such as mongolism. It is also proving of value in certain other congenital diseases. Thus, a recent study showed abnormal palmar findings in 64 per cent of patients with congenital heart disease (q.v.) compared with only 17 per cent of patients with acquired heart disease.

DERMATOME (1) Embryological tissue which has developed from the somites to become the dermis and subcutaneous tissue. The cutaneous area that is derived from each dermatome is supplied by a single dorsal spinal nerve root. (2) A surgical instrument for removing very thin slices of skin for grafting.

DERMATOMYOSITIS is an auto-immune disease, characterized by erythema of the skin and wasting of the muscles.

DERMATOPHYTES These are fungal infections. They are commonly seen as athlete's foot, scalp ringworm, tinea corporis and nail infection. They are due to fungi that normally inhabit the keratin tissue of the skin, hair and nails.

DERMOGRAPHIA, also known as DERMO-GRAPHISM and URTICARIA FACTITIA, is a condition in which tracings made on the skin leave a distinct swollen, reddish mark. It occurs in allergic individuals, in whom the stimulus of scratching the skin produces an excessive amount of histamine. (See ALLERGY.)

DERMOID CYST (see CYSTS).

DESFERRIOXAMINE is a chelating agent which is proving of value in the treatment of iron poisoning and thalassaemia.

DESQUAMATION means the scaling off of the superficial layer of the epidermis.

DETACHED RETINA Separation of the retina from the choroid in the eye. It may be due to trauma or be secondary to tumour or inflammation of the choroid and causes blindness in the affected part of the retina. It can be treated surgically using photocoagulation.

DETERGENTS are substances which clean the skin surface. This means that, strictly speaking, any soap, or soap-like substance used in washing, is a detergent. At the present day, however, the term is largely used for the synthetic detergents which are now used on such a large scale. These are prepared by the cracking and oxidation of high petroleum waxes with sulphuric acid. The commoner ones in commercial preparations are aryl alkyl sulphate or sulphonate and secondary alkyl sulphate.

In view of their widespread use they appear to cause relatively little trouble with the skin, but more trouble has been reported with the so-called 'biological' detergents that were introduced some years ago. They are so named because they contain an enzyme (q.v.) which destroys protein. As a result they are claimed to remove proteins – stains such as blood, chocolate, milk or gravy, which are relatively difficult for ordinary detergents to remove. Unfortunately these 'biological' detergents may cause dermatitis of the hands. In addition, they have been reported to cause asthma in those using them, and even more so in workers manufacturing them.

DETOXICATION means reduction or removal of the toxic properties of poisons or remedies. (See VACCINE.)

DEVIANCE Variation from normal. Often used to describe sexual behaviour.

DEVONSHIRE COLIC is caused by drinking cider which has been stored in contact with lead, so that colic comes on as a result of lead poisoning. (See COLIC; LEAD POISONING).

DEXAMETHASONE is a corticosteroid derivative. As an anti-inflammatory agent it is approximately 30 times as effective as cortisone and eight times as effective as prednisolone. On the other hand, it has practically none of the salt-retaining properties of cortisone.

DEXTRAN is the name given to a group of polysaccharides which was first discovered in sugar-beet preparations which had become infected with certain bacteria. A homogeneous preparation of it, with a consistent molecular weight and free from protein, is used as a substitute for plasma for transfusion purposes. Dextrans are slowly metabolized, which makes them valuable for the expansion and maintenance of blood volumes in shock arising from conditions such as burns and septicaemia. They are also useful in the prophylactic treatment of post-surgical thromboembolism (q.v.)

DEXTRIN is a soluble carbohydrate substance into which starch is converted by diastatic ferment or by heat. It is thus contained in toast, the crust of bread, biscuits, and breakfast foods. It is a white or yellowish powder which, dissolved in water, forms mucilage. Animal dextrin, also known as glycogen (q.v.), is a carbohydrate stored in the liver after meals, often in considerable amounts.

DEXTROCARDIA The heart is situated on the right of the chest in a mirror image of its usual position. This may be associated with similar inversion of the abdominal organs – situs inversus.

DEXTROMORAMIDE is a potent, habit-forming analgesic, or pain-reliever, which is active whether taken by mouth or given by injection.

DEXTROSE is another name for purified grape sugar or glucose.

DIA- is a prefix meaning through or thoroughly.

DIABETES INSIPIDUS is a disease characterized by excessive thirst and the passing of large volumes of urine which have a low specific gravity and contain no abnormal constituents. It is either due to a lack of the antidiuretic hormone normally produced by the hypothalamus and stored in the posterior pituitary gland, or to a defect in the renal tubules which prevents them responding to the antidiuretic hormone vasopressin. When the disorder is due to a vasopressin insufficiency, a primary or secondary tumour in the area of the pituitary stalk is responsible for one third of cases. In another one third of cases there is no apparent cause and such idiopathic cases are sometimes familial. A further one third of cases result from a variety of lesions including trauma, basal meningitis and granulomatous lesions in the pituitary stalk area. When the renal tubules fail to respond to vasopressin this is usually because of a genetic defect transmitted as a sex-linked recessive characteristic and the disease is called nephrogenic diabetes insipidus. Metabolic abnormalities such as hypercalcaemia and potassium depletion render the renal tubule less sensitive to vasopressin and certain drugs such as lithium and tetracycline may have a similar effect.

If the disease is due to a deficiency of vasopressin, treatment should be with the analogue of vasopressin called desmopressin which is more potent than the natural hormone and has less pressor activity. It also has the advantage in that it is absorbed from the nasal mucosa and so does not require to be injected.

Nephrogenic diabetes insipidus cannot be treated with desmopressin. The urine volume can, however, usually be reduced by half by a thiazide diuretic. Diabetes insipidus is a relatively rare condition and must be differentiated from diabetes mellitus (q.v.) which is an entirely different disease.

DIABETES MELLITUS is a condition characterized by a raised concentration of glucose in the blood because of a deficiency in the production and/or action of insulin (q.v.), a pancreatic hormone made in special cells called the islet cells of Langerhans.

Mering and Minkowski in 1889 found that diabetes followed removal of the pancreas from animals. In 1909 it was established that the defect was due to the failure of the pancreas to produce a hormone which was given the name insulin. However it was not until 1921 that two research workers, Banting and Best, first isolated insulin.

Symptoms Thirst, polyuria, weight loss despite eating, and recurrent infections, e.g. balanitis (q.v.) and vulval infections, are the main symptoms.

However, subjects with non-insulin-dependent diabetes may have the disease for several years without symptoms and diagnosis is often made incidentally or when presenting with a complication of the disease.

Classification INSULIN-DEPENDENT DIABETES MELLITUS (IDDM) (juvenile-onset diabetes, Type I diabetes) describes subjects with a severe deficiency or absence of insulin production. Insulin therapy is essential to prevent ketosis (q.v.) – a disturbance of the body's acid/base balance and an accumulation of ketones in the tissues. The onset is most commonly during childhood, but can occur at any age. Symptoms are acute and weight loss is common.

NON-INSULIN-DEPENDENT DIABETES MELLITUS (NIDDM) (maturity-onset diabetes, Type II diabetes): this may be further sub-divided into obese and non-obese groups. This type usually occurs after the age of 40 years with an insidious onset. Subjects are often overweight and weight loss is uncommon. Ketosis rarely develops. Insulin production is reduced but not absent.

DIABETES ASSOCIATED WITH OTHER CONDITIONS (a) Due to pancreatic disease, e.g. chronic pancreatitis; (b) secondary to drugs, e.g. glucocorticoids (q.v.); (c) excess hormone production, e.g. growth hormone (acromegaly, q.v.); (d) insulin receptor abnormalities; (e) genetic syndromes.

GESTATIONAL DIABETES   Diabetes occurring in pregnancy and resolving afterwards.

Aetiology Insulin-dependent diabetes occurs as a result of autoimmune destruction of beta cells within the pancreas. Genetic influences are important and individuals with certain HLA tissue types (HLA DR3 and HLA DR4) are more at risk. However, the risks associated with the HLA genes are small. If one parent has IDDM, the risk of a child's developing IDDM by the age of 25 years is 1·5–2·5 per cent and the risk of a sibling of an IDDM subject's developing diabetes is about 3 per cent.

Non-insulin-dependent diabetes has no HLA association, but the genetic influences are much stronger. The risks of developing diabetes vary with different races. Obesity, decreased exercise and ageing increase the risks of disease development. The risk of a sibling of a NIDDM subject's developing NIDDM up to the age of 80 years is 30–40 per cent.

Treatment of diabetes aims to prevent symptoms, restore carbohydrate metabolism to as near normal as possible and to minimize complications. Concentration of glucose, fructosamine and glycated haemoglobin in the blood are used to give an indication of blood-glucose control.

Insulin-dependent diabetes requires insulin for treatment. Non-insulin-dependent diabetes may be treated with diet, oral hypoglycaemic agents (q.v.) or insulin.

DIET   Many NIDDM diabetics may be treated with diet alone. For those subjects who are overweight, weight loss is important, although often unsuccessful. A diet high in complex carbohydrate, high in fibre, low in fat and aiming towards ideal body weight is prescribed. Subjects taking insulin need to eat at regular intervals in relation to their insulin regime and missing meals may result in hypoglycaemia, a lowering of the amount of glucose in the blood.

ORAL HYPOGLYCAEMICS are used in the treatment of non-insulin- dependent diabetes in addition to diet, when diet alone fails to control blood sugar levels. (a) Sulphonylureas act mainly by increasing the production of insulin. (b) Biguanides, of which only Metformin is available, may be used alone or in addition to sulphonylureas (q.v.). Its main actions are to

lower the production of glucose by the liver and improve its uptake in the peripheral tissues.
INSULIN   All insulin is injected – mainly by syringe but sometimes by insulin pump – because it is inactivated by gastrointestinal enzymes. There are three main types of insulin preparation: (a) short action (approximately 6 hours), with rapid onset; (b) intermediate action (approximately 12 hours); (c) long action, with slow onset and lasting for up to 36 hours. Human, porcine and bovine preparations are available. Much of the insulin now used is prepared by genetic engineering techniques from micro-organisms. There are many regimens of insulin treatment involving different combinations of insulin. Regimens vary depending on the requirements of the patients, most of whom administer the insulin themselves. Carbohydrate intake, energy expenditure and the presence of infection are important determinants of insulin requirements on a day-to-day basis.
Complications   The risks of complications increase with duration of disease.
DIABETIC EYE DISEASE   (a) retinopathy, (b) cataract. Regular examination of the fundus enables any abnormalities developing to be detected and treatment given when appropriate to preserve eyesight.
NEPHROPATHY   Subjects with diabetes may develop kidney damage which can result in renal failure.
INCREASED RISKS are present of (a) heart disease, (b) peripheral vascular disease and (c) cerebrovascular disease.
NEUROPATHY   (a) Symmetrical sensory polyneuropathy, damage to the sensory nerves that commonly presents with tingling, numbness of pain in the feet or hands. (b) Asymmetrical motor diabetic neuropathy presenting as progressive weakness and wasting of the proximal muscles of legs. (c) Mononeuropathy, individual motor or sensory nerves may be affected. (d) Autonomic neuropathy, which affects the autonomic nervous system, has many presentations, including impotence, diarrhoea or constipation and postural hypotension.
SKIN LESIONS   There are several skin disorders associated with diabetes including (a) Necrobiosis lipoidica diabeticorum usually occurring as an unsightly area on the shin. (b) Ulcers, which most commonly occur on the feet due to peripheral vascular disease, neuropathy and infection. Foot care is very important.
DIABETIC KETOACIDOSIS occurs when there is insufficient insulin present to prevent ketone (q.v.) production. This may occur before the diagnosis of IDDM or when insufficient insulin is being given. The presence of large amounts of ketones in the urine indicates excess ketone production and treatment should be sought immediately. Coma and death may result if the condition is left untreated.
DIABETIC HYPOGLYCAEMIA occurs when amounts of glucose in the blood become low. This may occur in subjects taking sulphonylureas or insulin. Symptoms usually develop when the glucose concentration falls below 2·5 mmol/l.

They may, however, occur at higher concentrations in subjects with persistent hyperglycaemia – an excess of glucose – and at lower levels in subjects with persistent hypoglycaemia. Symptoms include confusion, hunger and sweating. Refined sugar followed by complex carbohydrate will return the glucose concentration to normal. If the subject is unable to swallow, glucagon may be given intramuscularly or glucose intravenously, followed by oral carbohydrate, once the subject is able to swallow.

Although there are complications associated with diabetes, many subjects live to an old age. People with diabetes or their relatives can obtain advice from the British Diabetic Association (see APPENDIX 2: ADDRESSES).

DIAGNOSIS is the art of distinguishing one disease from another, and is essential to scientific and successful treatment. The name is also given to the opinion arrived at as to the nature of a disease. It is in diagnosis more than in treatment that the highest medical skill is required, and, for a diagnosis, the past and hereditary history of a case, the symptoms complained of, and the signs of disease found upon examination are all weighed. Many methods of laboratory examination are also used at the present day in aiding diagnosis.

DIALYSIS is the process whereby crystalloid and colloid substances are separated from a solution by interposing a semipermeable membrane, such as cellophane, between the solution and pure water. The crystalloid substances pass through the membrane into the water until a state of equilibrium, so far as the crystalloid substances are concerned, is established between the two sides of the membrane. The colloid substances do not pass through the membrane.

Dialysis is available as either *haemodialysis* or *peritoneal dialysis*. In the former blood is removed from the circulation either through an artificial arterio-venous fistula (junction) or a temporary or permanent internal catheter in the jugular vein. It then passes through an artificial kidney ('dialyser') to remove toxins (e.g. potassium and urea) by diffusion and excess salt and water by ultrafiltration from the blood into dialysis fluid prepared in a 'proportionator' (often referred to as a 'kidney machine'). Dialysers vary in design and performance but all work on the principle of a semipermeable membrane separating blood from dialysis fluid. Haemodialysis is undertaken two to three times a week for 4 to 6 hours a session. *Peritoneal dialysis* uses the peritoneal lining as a semipermeable membrane. Approximately 2 litres of sterile fluid is run into the peritoneum through the permanent indwelling catheter, is left for 3 to 4 hours, and the cycle is repeated three to four times per day. Most patients undertake continuous ambulatory peritoneal dialysis (CAPD), a few use a machine overnight (continuous cycling peritoneal dialysis, CCPD) which allows greater clearance of toxins. Disadvantages of haemodialysis include cardio-vascular instability, hypertension, bone disease, anaemia and development of periarticular amyloidosis (q.v.). Disadvantages of peritoneal dialysis include peritonitis, poor drainage of fluid and gradual loss of overall efficiency as endogenous renal function declines. Both haemodialysis and peritoneal dialysis carry a relatively high morbidity and the ideal treatment for patients with end-stage renal failure is successful *renal transplantion*.

DIAMORPHINE and DIACETYLMORPHINE are other names for heroin (q.v.).

DIAPHORESIS is another name for sweating. (See PERSPIRATION.)

DIAPHRAGM, or MIDRIFF, is the muscular partition which separates the cavity of the abdomen from that of the chest. It is very thin and is of a dome shape, extending up on the right side to the space beneath the fourth rib, on the left to that beneath the fifth. In contact with its lower surface are, on the right side, the liver, right kidney, and suprarenal body, and to the left the stomach, pancreas, left kidney, suprarenal body, and spleen; while upon its upper surface lies the heart, with a lung on either side. The diaphragm is attached by its edge to the lower margin of the chest all round, and consists of muscular fibres meeting round a trefoil-shaped piece of fibrous tissue in the centre. It completely shuts off the above-named cavities from one another, being pierced only by openings for the gullet, the aorta, and the inferior vena cava, with a few minute openings for nerves and small vessels. The diaphragm is of great importance in respiration, playing the chief part in filling the lungs. During deep respiration its movements are responsible for 60 per cent of the total amount of air breathed and in the horizontal posture, or in sleep, an even greater percentage.

The description 'diaphragm' is also used for the hemispherical rubber ('dutch') cap used in conjunction with a chemical spermicide as a contraceptive. It fits over the neck of the uterus (cervix) inside the vagina. (See CONTRACEPTION.)

DIAPHYSECTOMY is the operation whereby a part of the shaft of a long bone (e.g. humerus, femur) is excised.

DIAPHYSIS The shaft of a long bone.

DIAPULSE is a form of pulsed high-frequency electrical energy, consisting of pulsed short-wave bursts of energy of 1000 watts maximum, with an average input of 36 watts. It is used as a form of physiotherapy, particularly in the treatment of severe sprains.

DIARRHOEA or looseness of the bowels is increased frequency, fluidity or volume of bowel movements as compared to the person's customary pattern of bowel movements. Most people have occasional attacks of acute diarrhoea, usually caused by contaminated food or water. Such attacks normally clear up within a day or two, whether or not they are treated. Chronic diarrhoea, on the other hand, may be the result of a serious intestinal disorder or of more general disease.

The commonest cause of acute diarrhoea is food poisoning (q.v.), the organisms involved usually being staphylococcus, clostridium bacteria, salmonella or campylobacter. A person may also acquire infective diarrhoea as a result of droplet infections from adenoviruses or echoviruses. Interference with the bacterial flora of the intestine may cause acute diarrhoea: this often happens to someone who travels to another country and acquires unfamiliar intestinal bacteria. Other infections include bacillary dysentery, typhoid fever and paratyphoid fevers (see ENTERIC FEVERS). Drug toxicity, food allergy, food intolerance and anxiety may also cause acute diarrhoea, and habitual constipation may result in attacks of diarrhoea.

Treatment of diarrhoea in adults depends on the cause. The water and salts (see ELECTROLYTES) lost during a severe attack must be replaced to prevent dehydration. Ready-prepared mixtures of salts can be bought from a chemist. Antidiarrhoeal drugs such as codeine phosphate or loperamide should be used in infectious diarrhoea only if the symptoms are disabling. Antibacterial drugs may be used under medical direction. Persistent diarrhoea – longer than a week – or blood-stained diarrhoea must be investigated under medical supervision.

DIARRHOEA IN INFANTS is such a serious condition that it requires separate consideration. One of its features is that it is usually accompanied by vomiting. Some 10 per cent of the cases in this country are due to the dysentery organisms (q.v.) and will not be considered here. The remainder constitute the group of cases now usually referred to as infantile gastroenteritis. The condition is rare after the age of fifteen months, and the majority of cases occur between the ages of two and four months. The younger the infant, the higher the mortality rate. This is the type of diarrhoea which used to be known as 'summer diarrhoea' because of its high incidence in the late summer, but during recent years this seasonal incidence has tended to disappear. The precise cause is still obscure, but certain strains of the organism known as Escherichia coli (E. coli) are responsible for some cases, whilst in others a virus, often the rotavirus (q.v.), is the cause. One predisposing factor is artificial feeding. The condition is rare in breast-fed babies, and when it does occur in these it is usually less severe. The environment of the infant is also important. The condition is highly infectious and, if a case occurs in a maternity home or a children's hospital, it tends to spread quickly. This is why such an institution is closed to all further admissions if a case of infantile gastroenteritis occurs; and is not opened until the infection has been completely eradicated. A third factor is infection elsewhere in the body, particularly in the ear or the mastoid.

An infant with diarrhoea should not be fed milk but should be given an electrolyte mixture to replace lost water and salts. If the diarrhoea improves within 24 hours, milk can gradually be reintroduced. If diarrhoea continues beyond 36 to 48 hours, a doctor should be consulted. Any signs of dehydration require urgent medical attention; such signs include drowsiness, lack of response, loose skin, persistent crying, glazed eyes and a dry mouth and tongue.

DIASTASE is a mixture of enzymes obtained from malt. These enzymes have the property of converting starch into sugar. It is used in the preparation of predigested starchy foods, and in the treatment of dyspepsia, particularly that due to inability to digest starch adequately. It is also used for the conversion of starch to fermentable sugars in the brewing and fermentation industries.

DIASTASIS is a term applied to separation of the end of a growing bone from the shaft. The condition resembles a fracture, but is more serious because of the damage done to the growing cartilage through which the separation takes place, so that the future growth of the bone is considerably diminished.

DIASTOLE means the relaxation of a hollow organ. The term is applied in particular to the heart, to indicate the resting period between the beats (systole), while blood is flowing into the organ.

DIASTOLIC PRESSURE   The pressure exerted by the blood against the arterial wall during diastole. This is the lowest blood pressure in the cardiac cycle.

DIATHERMY is a process by which electric currents can be passed into the deeper parts of the body so as to produce internal warmth and relieve pain; or, by using powerful currents, to destroy tumours and diseased parts bloodlessly. The form of electricity used consists of high-frequency oscillations, the frequency of oscillation ranging from 10 million to 25,000 million oscillations per second. The current passes between two electrodes placed on the skin.

The so-called ultra-short-wave diathermy (or short-wave diathermy, as it is usually referred to) has replaced the original long-wave diathermy, as it is produced consistently at a stable wave-length (11 metres) and is easier to apply. In recent years microwave diathermy has been developed, which has a still higher oscillating current (25,000 million cycles per second, com-

pared with 500 million for short-wave diathermy).

When the current passes, a distinct sensation of increasing warmth is experienced and the temperature of the body gradually rises; the heart's action becomes quicker; there is sweating with increased excretion of waste products. The general blood-pressure is also distinctly lowered. The method is used in painful rheumatic conditions, both of muscles and joints, and in severe cases of neuritis, such as sciatica.

By concentrating the current in a small electrode, the heating effects immediately below this are very much increased. The diathermy knife utilizes this technique to cauterize blood vessels and abnormal tissue during surgery.

DIATHESIS is another name for constitution (q.v.).

DIAZEPAM (see TRANQUILLIZERS, BENZODIAZEPINES).

DIBUTYL PHTHALATE is an insect repellent. It is less effective than dimethyl phthalate (q.v.), but has the advantage of being harmless to clothing and resists washing better. When rubbed into clothing it may give protection for up to a fortnight.

DICEPHALUS is the term applied to a fetal 'monster' having two heads.

DICOPHANE is the official name for DDT (q.v.).

DICROTIC pulse is one in which at each heartbeat two impulses are felt by the finger. A dicrotic wave is naturally present in a tracing of any pulse as recorded by an instrument for the purpose, but in health it is imperceptible to the finger. In fevers, a dicrotic pulse indicates considerable prostration, in which the heart continues to beat violently while the small blood-vessels have lost their tone. (See PULSE.)

DIELDRIN is an effective insecticide toxic to a wide range of insects. It is more toxic to man than DDT, and must therefore be handled with care. Its use in the UK is restricted.

DIENOESTROL is a synthetic oestrogen closely related to stilboestrol (q.v.). It is not as potent as stilboestrol, but is less toxic and is used as a cream to treat vaginal dryness.

DIET is an environmental factor in the aetiology of several diseases. Variations in morbidity and mortality between population groups are believed to be due, in part, to differences in diet. A balanced diet was traditionally viewed as one which provided at least the minimum requirement of energy, protein, vitamins and minerals needed by the body. However, since nutritional deficiencies are no longer a major problem in developed countries, it seems more appropriate to consider a 'healthy' diet as being one which provides all essential nutrients in sufficient quantities to prevent deficiencies but which also avoids health problems associated with nutrient excesses.

Major diet-related health problems in prosperous communities tend to be the result of dietary excesses, whereas in underdeveloped, poor communities problems associated with dietary deficiencies predominate. Excessive intakes of dietary energy, saturated fats, sugar, salt and alcohol, together with an inadequate intake of dietary fibre, have been linked to the high prevalence of obesity (q.v.), cardiovascular disease, dental caries, hypertension (q.v.), gall-stones (see GALL-BLADDER, DISEASES OF), non-insulin dependent diabetes mellitus (q.v.) and certain cancers (q.v.) (e.g. breast, endometrium, intestine and stomach) seen in developed nations. Health-promotion strategies in these countries generally advocate a reduction in the intake of fat, particularly saturated fat, and salt, the avoidance of excessive intakes of alcohol and simple sugars, an increased consumption of starch and fibre and the avoidance of obesity. A maximum level of dietary cholesterol is sometimes specified.

Under-nutrition, including protein-energy malnutrition and specific vitamin and mineral deficiencies, is an important cause of poor health in underdeveloped countries. Priorities here centre on ensuring that the diet provides enough nutrients to maintain health.

In healthy people, dietary requirements depend on age, sex and level of physical activity. Pregnancy and lactation further alter requirements. The presence of infections, fever, burns, fractures and surgery all increase dietary energy and protein requirements and can precipitate under-nutrition in previously well-nourished people.

In addition to disease prevention, diet has a role in the treatment of certain clinical disorders, e.g. obesity, diabetes mellitus, hyperlipidaemias, inborn errors of metabolism, food intolerances and hepatic and renal diseases. Therapeutic diets increase or restrict the amount and/or change the type of fat, carbohydrate, protein, fibre, vitamins, minerals and/or water in the diet according to clinical indications. Additionally, the consistency of the food eaten may need to be altered. A commercially available or 'homemade' liquid diet can be used to provide all or some of a patient's nutritional needs if necessary. Although the enteral (by mouth) route is the preferred route for feeding and can be used for most patients, parenteral or intravenous feeding is occasionally required in a minority of patients whose gastrointestinal tract is unavailable or unreliable over a period of time.

DIETETICS Dietitians apply dietetics, the science of nutrition, to the feeding of groups and individuals in health and disease. Their training requires a degree course in the nutritional and biological sciences. The role of the dietitian can be divided as follows.

PREVENTIVE By liaising with health education departments, schools and various groups in the community. They plan and provide nutrition education programs including in- service training and the production of educational material in nutrition. They are encouraged to plan and participate in food surveys and research projects which involve the assessment of nutritional status.

THERAPEUTIC They advise patients who require specific dietary therapy as all or part of their treatment. They teach patients in hospitals to manage their own dietary treatment and ensure a supportive follow-up so that they and their families can be seen to be coping with the diet. They advise catering departments on the adaptation of menus for individual diets and on the nutritional value of the food supplied to patients and staff. They advise Social Services departments so that meals-on-wheels provision has adequate nutritional value.

INDUSTRY The advice of dietitians is sought by industry in the production of product information literature, data sheets and professional leaflets for manufacturers of ordinary foods and specialist dietetic food. They give advice to the manufacturers on nutritional and dietetic requirements of their products.

DIETHYLCARBAMAZINE CITRATE is a derivative of piperazine, which is proving of value in the treatment of filariasis and other parasitic diseases.

DIFFERENTIAL DIAGNOSIS A list of the possible diagnoses that might explain a patient's symptoms and signs and from which the correct diagnosis will be extracted after further investigations.

DIGESTION, ABSORPTION, AND ASSIMILATION are the three processes by which food is incorporated in the living body. In digestion, the food is softened and converted into a form which is soluble in the watery fluids of the body, or, in the case of fat, into very minute globules. In absorption, the substances formed are taken up from the bowels and carried throughout the body by the blood. In assimilation, these substances, deposited from the blood, are united with the various tissues for their growth and repair. For the maintenance of health each of these must proceed in a regular manner. Transit time through the digestive tract in young and middle-aged people in Britain averages two to four days, all but twelve hours of this being in the colon. Transit time is probably longer in the elderly.

SALIVARY DIGESTION begins as soon as the food enters the mouth. Saliva runs from the minute orifices of the salivary gland ducts, and contains a ferment named ptyalin, which actively changes the starch of bread, potatoes, and the like, into sugar. The object of chewing is not only to bruise the food, and make it more permeable for the gastric juice, but also to mix the starchy parts thoroughly with saliva. This process goes on, after swallowing, for the first twenty minutes or half-hour that the food remains in the stomach, after which the action of the saliva is checked by the acid of the gastric juice.

GASTRIC DIGESTION begins a little time after the food enters the stomach, the gastric juice exuding rapidly from the openings of the minute glands with which the interior surface of this organ is covered. The gastric juice begins to be secreted even before the food enters the stomach, at the sight and smell of food (psychic secretion). This juice contains ferments or enzymes, named pepsins, which have the power to break down the proteins of food into smaller molecules containing fewer amino-acids and to clot milk. There are also present free hydrochloric acid, which aids the action of the pepsin and prevents putrefaction of the food, and acid salts, such as phosphate of soda, which have a similar action. The slow, churning movements which take place in the walls of the stomach have the effect of thoroughly mixing the food and gastric juice, and, to a slight extent, of breaking up the former. The main function of the stomach is to render the ingested food soluble, and mix it thoroughly with the gastric juice until it assumes a gruel-like consistency. This material, known as *chyme*, is then passed through the pylorus into the intestine. Very soon after soft food has been taken, waves of movement may be seen on X-ray examination, the orifice at the lower end of the stomach (pylorus) opens, and the food is squeezed quickly in small quantities into the bowel; but if any hard food comes in contact with the stomach wall near the exit the orifice at once closes. Gastric digestion of a simple meal of tea, bread, butter and jam should be complete in about an hour, a meal containing milk, eggs or light meat requires three or four hours, while a heavy dinner with soup, meat, fruit, and wine or beer is not entirely treated by the stomach till six or seven hours have elapsed. Hence the English plan of taking the heavy meal of the day (dinner) in the evening is a sound one, giving time during the night for the later stages of digestion.

INTESTINAL DIGESTION   The softened food, or chyme, which leaves the stomach is exposed in the bowels to the action of four factors: (*a*) bile, (*b*) pancreatic juice, (*c*) intestinal juice, (*d*) bacteria. Bile is collected from the liver and gall-bladder into the common bile-duct, which, together with the duct from the pancreas, opens into the duodenum a short distance from the exit of the stomach. The bile consists mainly of complex salts and pigments, which assist in digesting the fats of the food, and partly of waste products removed from the blood. The pancreatic juice contains four powerful ferments, which have the following effects: lipase breaks down fats into glycerol and fatty acids;

amylase completes the digestion of starch; and trypsin and chymotrypsin carry on the breaking down of proteins begun in the stomach. Intestinal juice contains small amounts of enzymes which (1) complete the breakdown of proteins into the constituent amino-acids; (2) act upon the disaccharides, maltose, sucrose and lactose, converting them into the monosaccharide glucose; (3) split fats into fatty acids and glycerin. Bacteria are normal inhabitants of both small and large intestine. In the former they have a fermentive, in the latter a putrefactive, action. In the former they act upon carbohydrate to produce acetic, butyric, and lactic acids. In the latter, bacteria decompose protein into such products as histamine, phenol, cresol, indole, skatole. These are no longer believed to be responsible for the ill-effects of constipation. The intestinal bacteria also play an important and valuable role in the manufacture of certain components of the vitamin B complex.

ABSORPTION   The only substance absorbed from the stomach to any extent is alcohol. Water is quickly passed from the stomach into the intestine, and considerable quantities are there absorbed in a few minutes. But it is only after subjection to digestion in the intestine for several hours that the bulk of the food is taken up into the system. The semi-solid chyme which leaves the stomach is converted into a yellowish fluid of creamy consistence called chyle by the action of bile and pancreatic fluid. From this the fats, in the form of a fine emulsion, are taken up by lymph vessels called lacteals, and ultimately reach the blood, while sugars, salts, and amino-acids formed from proteins pass directly into the small blood-vessels of the intestine. The process is facilitated by the extreme unevenness of the intestinal wall, which is folded into many ridges and pockets, while, in microscopic structure, the surface is covered by fine finger-like processes named villi, which are bathed in the fluids passing down the intestine. Further, absorption is probably assisted by the leucocytes, or white cells of the blood, wich are increased in numbers after a meal, and which have the power of wandering out of the blood-stream and taking up particles into their substance. Food materials are absorbed almost exclusively by the small intestine. The large intestine, or colon, absorbs water and salts. The food is passed down the intestine by the contractions of its muscular coat, and, finally, the indigestible residue, together with various waste substances excreted from the liver and intestinal walls, is cast out of the body in the stools.

ASSIMILATION takes place more slowly, the blood circulating through every organ, and each taking from it what is necessary for its own growth and repair. Thus the cells in the bones extract lime salts, muscles extract sugar and protein, and so forth. When the supply of food is much in excess of the immediate bodily requirements it is stored up for future use, fat being deposited in various sites, sugar being converted into glycogen in the liver. The greater bulk of nutriment is assimilated by the muscles for heat production and work, the sugar and amino-acids being built up into a substance which forms the permanent part of the muscle. The substance so formed undergoes chemical changes, and is broken down to form carbonic acid, lactic acid and other waste products as the muscle does work. Various hormones, such as insulin, which is an internal secretion of the pancreas, circulate in the blood and are concerned in these processes. For all these processes to function satisfactorily an adequate daily intake of water is necessary; about 1·5 litres (3 pints) are drunk or taken with the food and absorbed daily, a similar amount being discharged from the body in the urine, perspiration, and other excretions.

DIGITALIS is the leaf of the wild fox-glove, *Digitalis purpurea*, gathered when the flowers are at a certain stage, dried, and powdered. The leaf contains several active principles, which can be extracted in various ways. Its action is to strengthen involuntary muscular contraction, particularly that of the muscle fibres in the heart and blood-vessels. For many years it was used to treat heart disease associated with atrial fibrillation. Digitalis no longer appears in the *British National Formulary*; digoxin (q.v.) is used instead. Digitalis has the double action of increasing the strength of each beat and of lengthening each intervening pause (diastole), so that the muscle of the damaged organ obtains longer periods for rest and repair. It promotes the excretion of sodium by the kidney and so has a diuretic effect.

DIGOXIN One of a number of drugs known as cardiac glycosides. They increase myocardial contractility, depress the conducting tissue while increasing myocardial excitability, and increase activity of the vagus nerve (q.v.). It is usually given orally for the treatment of atrial fibrillation (q.v.) and heart failure. The adverse effects of overdosage (which occur more commonly in people with hypokalaemia, the elderly, and those with renal failure) are vomiting, dysrhythmias, muscle weakness, and visual disturbances. The electrocardiogram has a characteristic appearance.

DILATOR (1) A muscle which has the action of increasing the diameter of an organ or vessel. (2) A drug which usually acts by relaxing smooth muscle to increase the diameter of blood vessels, the bronchial tree, or other organs. (3) An instrument used to increase the diameter of an orifice or organ either to treat a stricture or allow surgical access.

DILTIAZEM (see CALCIUM-CHANNEL BLOCKERS).

DILUENTS are watery fluids of a non-irritating nature, which are given to increase the amount of perspiration or of urine, and carry solids with them from the system. Examples are water, milk, barley-water, and solutions of alkaline salts.

DIMENHYDRINATE, or DRAMAMINE, is a drug which is widely used, with considerable success, in the treatment of travel sickness.

DIMERCAPROL is the official name for BAL (British Anti-Lewisite), the antidote to lewisite poisoning which was discovered during the 1939–45 war. It was subsequently found to be an excellent antidote to poisoning with certain heavy metals, including arsenic, mercury and gold, and it is now widely used for this purpose.

DINOESTROL (see OESTROGEN).

DIOCTYL SODIUM SULPHOSUCCINATE is a faecal-softening agent that is proving useful in the treatment of constipation in old people.

DIODONE is a complex, organic, iodine-containing preparation. It is used primarily for contrast radiography of the kidney passages, but can also be used for contrast radiography of the biliary tract.

DIOPTRE is a term used in the measurement of the refractive or focusing power of lenses; one dioptre is the power of a lens with a focal distance of one metre and is the unit of refractive power. As a stronger lens has a greater refractive power, this means that the focal distance will be shorter. The strength in dioptres therefore is the reciprocal of the focal length expressed in metres.

DIPHENHYDRAMINE is a widely used antihistamine drug (q.v.).

DIPHENOXYLATE is a drug chemically related to pethidine that is proving of value in the treatment of travellers' diarrhoea by quietening down the gut. It has no anti-infective action.

DIPHTHERIA is an acute infectious disease of the respiratory tract. Rarely seen in the UK since the introduction of inoculation in 1940, it is still an important cause of disease in many parts of the world. The infection is caused by the *Corynebacterium diphtheriae*, of which there are three strains, and is spread by water droplets. It usually presents with a sore throat, and there is a slightly raised membrane on the tonsils surrounded by an inflammatory zone. There may be some swelling of the neck and lymph nodes, though the patient's temperature is seldom much raised. Occasionally the disease occurs in the eye or genital tract, or it may complicate lesions of the skin. More serious consequences follow the absorption of toxins (q.v.) which damage the heart muscle and the nervous system. The disease is notifiable, and has an average incubation period of two to four days. Patients are isolated until cultures from six daily nose and throat swabs are negative. Diphtheria may occur at all ages, though it is commonest in childhood. In the Schick test, a minute amount of toxin is injected into the skin of the arm, producing an area of inflammation in those with little resistance, who should then be immunized.

Treatment Provided the patient is not allergic to horse serum, an injection of the antitoxin is given immediately. A one-week course of penicillin is started (or erythromycin if the patient is allergic to penicillin). Diphtheria may cause temporary muscle weakness or paralysis, which should resolve without special treatment; if the respiratory muscles are involved, however, artificial respiration may be necessary.

DIPHYLLOBOTHRIUM LATUM is a fish tapeworm which infests man and may cause a form of megaloblastic anaemia. (See ANAEMIA.)

DIPLEGIA is extensive paralysis on both sides of the body. (See PARALYSIS.)

DIPLO- is a prefix meaning twofold.

DIPLOCOCCUS is a group of bacterial organisms which have a tendency to occur in pairs: e.g. pneumococci.

DIPLOË is the layer of spongy bone which intervenes between the compact outer and inner tables of the skull.

DIPLOPIA means double vision. It is due to some irregularity in action of the muscles which move the eyeballs, in consequence of which the eyes are placed so that rays of light from one object do not fall upon corresponding parts of the two retinae, and two images are produced. It is a symptom of several nervous diseases, and often a temporary attack follows an injury to the eye, intoxication, or some febrile disease like diphtheria.

DIPROSOPUS is the term applied to a fetus which has two faces instead of one.

DIPSOMANIA is a morbid and insatiable craving for alcohol. (See ALCOHOL.)

DIPYGUS is the term applied to a fetus which has a double pelvis.

DISABLED PERSONS in the United Kingdom have a range of services and financial support available to help them to lead as normal and active a life as possible. Officially, the disabled include those with significant impairment of any kind, including impairment of sight and hearing, learning difficulties, and chronic illness as well as disablement due to accidents and the like.

Social services are provided by local authority social services departments. They include: practical help in the home (usually through home helps or aids to daily living), assistance in taking advantage of available educational facilities, help with adaptations to the disabled person's house, provision of meals ('Meals on Wheels' or luncheon centres), and help in obtaining a telephone. Many of these facilities will involve the disabled person in some expense, but full details can be obtained from the local social services department which will, if necessary, send a social worker to discuss the matter in the disabled person's home. Owing to lack of funds and staff, many local authority social service departments are unable to provide the full range of services.

Aids to daily living There is now a wide range of aids for the disabled. Full details and addresses of local offices can be obtained from: Disabled Living Foundation; British Red Cross; National Demonstration Centre, Pinderfields General Hospital; and Disability Scotland, Information Department. See APPENDIX 2: ADDRESSES.

Aids to mobility and transport Some car manufacturers make specially equipped or adapted cars, and some have official systems for discounts. Details can be obtained from local dealers. Help can also be obtained from Motability, which provides advice (see APPENDIX 2: ADDRESSES).

DISARTICULATION is the amputation of a bone by cutting through the joint of which the bone forms a part.

DISC An anatomical term describing a rounded flattened structure. Examples are the cartilagenous disc positioned between two vertebrae (see SPINAL COLUMN) and the optic disc. (See EYE.)

DISCHARGE is the term applied to abnormal emissions from any part of the body. It usually applies to purulent material: e.g. the septic material which comes away from an infected ear, or nose.

DISCISSION is the term applied to an operation for destroying a structure by tearing it without removal: e.g. the operation of needling the lens of the eye for cataract.

DISEASE Any abnormality of bodily structure or function, other than those arising directly from physical injury.

DISINFECTION Processes by which vegetative organisms, excluding spores, are killed in order to prevent the items disinfected from passing on infection. Equipment, bedlinen and hard surfaces may all be disinfected – the method chosen will depend on the material and size of the object. One of the most important procedures in preventing the spread of infection is the careful washing of hands before handling equipment and between treating different patients. Sterilization is different from disinfection in that the methods used kill all living organisms and spores.

Methods of disinfection (1) Skin, wounds etc. – chlorhexidine (with detergent or spirit); iodine (with detergent or spirit); cetrimide; ethyl alcohol; all must stay in contact with the skin for long enough for bacteria to be killed. (2) Hard surfaces (floors, walls etc.) – hypochlorites (i.e. bleaches) with or without detergent; cetrimide; iodine-containing solutions; ethyl alcohol. (3) Equipment – wet or dry heat (e.g. boiling for more than five minutes); submersion in liquid disinfectants for the appropriate time (e.g. glutaraldehyde 2·5 per cent, chlorhexidine in spirit 70 per cent, formaldehyde (irritant), chlorhexidine 0·1 per cent aqueous), hypochlorites.

DISINFESTATION means the destruction of insect pests, especially lice, whether on the person or in dwelling-places.

DISLOCATIONS are injuries to joints of such a nature that the ends of the opposed bones are forced more or less out of connection with one another. Besides displacement of the bones, there is bruising of the tissues around them, and tearing of the ligaments which bind the bones together.

Dislocations, like fractures, are divided into simple and compound, the bone in the latter case being forced through the skin. This seldom occurs, since the round head of the bone has not the same power to wound as the sharp end of a broken bone. Dislocations are also divided according as they are (1) congenital, i.e. present at birth in consequence of some malformation, or (2) acquired at a later period in consequence of injury, the great majority falling into the latter class. The reduction of a dislocated joint is a skilled procedure and should be done by an appropriately trained professional.

DISODIUM CROMOGLYCATE is a drug used in the prophylactic treatment of allergic disorders, particularly asthma, conjunctivitis, nasal allergies, and food allergies, especially in children. Although inappropriate for the treatment of acute attacks of asthma, regular inhalations of the drug can reduce the incidence of asthma, and allow the dose of bronchodilators (q.v.) and oral corticosteroids (q.v.) to be cut.

DISORIENTATION Orientation in a clinical sense includes a person's awareness of time and place in relation to himself and others, the recognition of personal friends and familiar places and the ability to remember at least some past experience and to register new data. It is therefore dependent on the ability to recall all learned memories and make effective use of memory. Disorientation can be the presenting feature of both delirium (q.v.) (confusion) and dementia (q.v.); delirium is reversible, developing dramatically, and accompanied by evidence of systemic disease, dementia is a gradually evolving, irreversible condition.

DISPLACEMENT is a term used in psychological medicine to describe the mental process of attaching to one object painful emotions associated with another object.

DISSECTION (1) The cutting of tissue to separate the structural components for identification or removal during an operation or the study of anatomy. (2) Dissection of an artery involves tearing of the inner part of the wall allowing blood to track through the media occluding the origins of smaller arteries and often leading to vessel rupture.

DISSEMINATED Spread of disease from its original site throughout an organ or the body. Often used to describe the spread of cancer.

DISSEMINATED SCLEROSIS (see MULTIPLE SCLEROSIS).

DISTICHIASIS is the term applied to the condition in which there are two complete rows of eyelashes in one eyelid (or in both).

DISTOMA is a general term including various forms of trematodes, or fluke-worms, parasitic in the intestine, lung and other organs.

DISTRICT HEALTH AUTHORITY (see NATIONAL HEALTH SERVICE).

DISULFIRAM, the full chemical name of which is tetraethylthiuram disulphide, is used as an adjunct in the treatment of alcoholism. It is relatively non-toxic by itself, but when taken in conjunction with alcohol it produces most unpleasant effects: e.g. flushing of the face, palpitations, a sense of oppression and distress, and ultimately sickness and vomiting. The rationale of treatment therefore is to give the alcoholic subject a course of disulfiram and then demonstrate, by letting him take some alcoholic liquor, how unpleasant are the effects. If the patient is co-operative, the treatment may be effective, but there is some risk so it must be given under skilled medical supervision.

DISUSE ATROPHY The wasting of muscles after prolonged immobility. This can be seen after lengthy immobilization in a plaster cast and is particularly severe following paralysis of a limb through nerve injury. (See ATROPHY.)

DIURESIS An increase in the production of urine. This may result from increased fluid intake, decreased levels of antidiuretic hormone, renal disease, or the use of drugs (see DIURETICS).

DIURETICS Substances which increase urine and solute production by the kidney. They are used in the treatment of heart failure, hypertension, and sometimes for ascites secondary to liver failure. They may work by extra-renal or renal mechanisms.
EXTRA-RENAL (*a*) Inhibiting release of antidiuretic hormone, e.g. water, alcohol. (*b*) Increased renal blood flow, e.g. dopamine in renal doses.
RENAL (*a*) Osmotic diuretics act by 'holding' water in the renal tubules and preventing its reabsorption, e.g. mannitol. (*b*) Loop diuretics prevent sodium, and therefore water, reabsorption, e.g. frusemide. (*c*) Drugs acting on the cortical segment of the Loop of Henle prevent sodium reabsorption, but are 'weaker' than loop diuretics, e.g. thiazides. (*d*) Drugs acting on the distal tubule prevent sodium reabsorption by retaining potassium, e.g. spironalactone.
The potential side-effects of diuretics are hypokalaemia, dehydration, and gout (in susceptible individuals).

DIVERTICULAR DISEASE The presence of numerous diverticula (sacs or pouches) in the lining of the colon accompanied by spasmodic lower abdominal pain and erratic bowel movements. The sacs may become inflamed causing pain (diverticulitis).

DIVERTICULITIS is inflammation of diverticula (see DIVERTICULUM) in the large intestine. It is characterized by pain in the left lower side of the abdomen, which has been aptly described as 'left-sided appendicitis' as it resembles the pain of appendicitis but occurs in the opposite side of the abdomen. The onset is often sudden, with fever and constipation. It may, or may not, be preceded by diverticulosis (q.v.). Treatment consists of rest, no solid food but ample fluid, and the administration of tetracycline. Complications are unusual but include abscess formation, perforation of the colon, and severe bleeding.

DIVERTICULOSIS means the presence of diverticula (see DIVERTICULUM) or sacs in the large intestine. Such diverticula are not uncommon over the age of 40, increasing with age until over the age of 70 they may be present in one-third to one-half of the population. They mostly occur in the lower part of the colon, and are predominantly due to muscular hyperactivity of the bowel forcing the lining of the bowel through weak points in the bowel wall, just as the inner tube of a pneumatic tyre bulges through a defective tyre. There is increasing evidence that the low-residue diet of western civilization is a contributory cause. The condi-

tion may or may not produce symptoms. If it does, these consist of disturbance of the normal bowel function and pain in the left side in the lower abdomen. If it is causing symptoms, treatment consists of a high-residue diet (see CONSTIPATION) and an agar (q.v.) or methyl-cellulose (q.v.) preparation.

DIVERTICULUM means a pouch or pocket leading off a main cavity or tube. The term is especially applied to protrusions from the intestine, which may be present either at the time of birth as a developmental peculiarity, or which develop in numbers upon the large intestine during the course of life. The process of formation of these intestinal pockets is known as diverticulosis, and inflammation of them as diverticulitis.

DIZYGOTIC TWINS Two people born at the same time to the same parents after fertilization of two separate oocytes. They may be of different sexes and are no more likely to resemble each other than any other sibling pairs.

DIZZINESS is a vague symptom and it is important to establish what the individual means by dizziness. It may encompass a feeling of disequilibrium, it may be light-headedness, faintness, a sensation of swimming or floating, an imbalance or unsteadiness or episodes of mental confusion. It may be true vertigo which is an hallucination of movement (SEE VERTIGO). These symptoms may be due to diseases of the ear, eye, central nervous system, cardiovascular system, endocrine system or they may be a manifestation of psychiatric disease. It is a common symptom in the elderly and by the age of eighty two thirds of women and one third of men have suffered from the condition.

DNA is the abbreviation for deoxy-ribonucleic acid, one of the two types of nucleic acid (q.v.) that occur in nature. It is the fundamental genetic material of all cells, and is present in the nucleus of the cell (q.v.) where it forms part of the chromosome (q.v.) and acts as the carrier of genetic information. The molecule is very large, with a molecular weight of several millions, and consists of two single chains of nucleotides (see NUCLEIC ACID) which are twisted round each other to form a double helix (or spiral). The genetic information carried by DNA is encoded along one of these strands. A gene (q.v.), which represents the genetic information needed to form protein, is a stretch of DNA containing, on average, around 1000 nucleotides paired in these two strands.
To allow it to fulfil its vitally important function as the carrier of genetic information in living cells, DNA has the following properties. It is stable so that successive generations of species maintain their individual characteristics, but not so stable that evolutionary changes cannot take place. It must be able to store a vast

amount of information. For example, an animal cell contains genetic information for the synthesis of over a million proteins. It must be duplicated exactly before each cell division to ensure that both daughter cells contain an accurate copy of the genetic information of the parent cells (see CELLS; GENETIC CODE).

DOBUTAMINE is a drug which acts on sympathetic receptors in cardiac muscle and increases the contractility and hence improves the cardiac output but has little effect on the cardiac rate. It is particularly useful in cardiogenic shock. It must be given by intravenous infusion.

DOG BITES (see BITES AND STINGS; RABIES).

DOLICHOCEPHALIC means long-headed and is a term applied to skulls the breadth of which is less than four-fifths of the length.

DONOR INSEMINATION Use of the semen of an anonymous donor to produce fertilization in cases of infertility where the male partner has oligospermia or impotence. The donor is chosen for ethnic and physiognomic similarity to the male partner and is screened for transmissible diseases (e.g. HIV, syphilis, hepatitis, gonorrhoea, and genetic disorders). Insemination is performed at the time of ovulation by introducing the semen into the upper vagina. Semen may be fresh or have been stored frozen in liquid nitrogen. (See ARTIFICIAL INSEMINATION.)

DONORS People who donate parts of their bodies for use in other people. Many organs and tissues can be donated. The commonest is blood; but skin, corneas, kidneys, livers, and hearts can all be used. Combined heart and lung transplants are being increasingly used for patients with severe lung diseases, and, if the recipients have a condition such as cystic fibrosis in which the heart is normal, it is sometimes possible for them to receive a heart and lungs from one donor and to donate their own heart to someone else. Recent work has explored the possibility of using pancreatic transplants. Apart from blood, it is unusual for tissue to be taken from living donors. Skin, small pieces of liver, and a kidney can, in theory, be obtained from living donors, but the ethics of this are hotly debated and the situations under which it may be done are tightly controlled. Because transplanted organs are seen by the receiving body as 'foreign bodies', careful cross-matching before transplantation is necessary to avoid rejection.

There are strict regulations about how death should be diagnosed before organs can be removed for transplantation, and potential donors must satisfy the brain-stem death criteria (q.v.), performed twice by two doctors who are independent of the transplant team. There

is a great shortage of suitable organs for donation – partly because they must be in excellent condition if the operation is to be a success. Some medical conditions or modes of death make people unsuitable as organ donors. This makes it all the more important that people should be encouraged to donate their organs. People who wish to do so can carry a special card indicating their willingness to become donors in the event of their death. These cards can be obtained from various sources, including hospitals, GPs' surgeries and many public buildings such as libraries.

Information about becoming a blood donor can be obtained by telephoning 0345-711 711. Those who wish to bequeath their bodies for dissection purposes should get in touch with HM Inspector of Anatomy. Other would-be organ donors may contact the British Organ Donor Society. (See APPENDIX 2: ADDRESSES.)

DOPA A precursor of dopamine and noradrenaline. Levodopa is a drug used in the treatment of Parkinson's disease. It can cross the blood-brain barrier and increase the concentration of dopamine in the basal ganglia. It also inhibits prolactin secretion and may be used to treat galactorrhea.

DOPAMINE is a catecholamine (q.v.) and a precursor of noradrenaline (q.v.). Its highest concentration is in that portion of the brain known as the basal nuclei (see BRAIN) where its function is to convey inhibitory influences to the extrapyramidal system. There is good evidence that dopamine deficiency is one of the causative factors in Parkinsonism (q.v.).

DORSAL ROOT GANGLIA These are swellings on the dorsal roots of spinal nerves just proximal to the union of the dorsal and ventral nerve roots. They are situated in the intervertebral formanina and contain the cell bodies of sensory neurones. (See SPINAL COLUMN and SPINAL CORD.)

DORSUM The back or posterior part of an organ or structure. The dorsum of the hand is the opposite surface to the palm.

DOSAGE Many factors influence the activity with which drugs operate. Among the factors which affect the necessary quantity are age, weight, sex, idiosyncrasy, genetic disorders, habitual use, disease, fasting, combination with other drugs, the form in which the drug is given, and the route by which it is given. AGE is but one factor. Normally, a young child requires a smaller dose than an adult. There are, however, other factors to be taken into consideration. Thus, children are more susceptible than adults to some drugs such as morphine, whilst they are less sensitive to others such as atropine. Various methods have been introduced for calculating roughly and quickly appropriate doses. These may be based on age, body weight or body surface area, the latter being most reliable. For example, a formula based on the surface area of the child is:

$$\text{adult dose} \times \frac{\text{surface area in square metres}}{1 \cdot 82}$$

An approximate rule of thumb, based on children of average height and weight, and assuming an adult dose of 100 mg is:

Age	Average weight	Dose
years	kg	mg
1	10	25
7	25	50
12	40	75
Adult	70	100

Old people, too, often show an increased susceptibility to drugs. This is probably due to a variety of factors, such as decreased weight in many old people; diminished activity of the tissues and therefore diminished rate at which a drug is utilized; and diminished activity of the kidneys resulting in decreased rate of excretion of the drug.

WEIGHT AND SEX have both to be taken into consideration. Women require slightly smaller doses than men, probably because they tend to be lighter in weight. The effect of weight on dosage is partly dependent on the fact that much of the extra weight of a heavy individual is made up of fatty tissue which is not as active as other tissue of the body. In practice, the question of weight seldom makes much difference unless the individual is grossly overweight or underweight.

IDIOSYNCRASY occasionally causes drugs administered in the ordinary dose to produce unexpected effects. Thus, some people are but little affected by some drugs, whilst in others certain drugs, such as potassium iodide, or atropine, produce excessive symptoms in minute doses. In some cases this may be due to hypersensitiveness, or an allergic reaction, to the drug. This is a possibility that must always be borne in mind, particularly with penicillin. As a rule the individual has had the drug in question previously. An individual who is known to be allergic to penicillin is strongly recommended to carry a card to this effect.

HABITUAL USE of a drug is perhaps the influence that causes the greatest increase in the dose necessary to produce the requisite effect. The classical example of this is opium and its derivatives. Arsenic is another example that was often encountered in the days when arsenical drugs were one of the great stand-bys in the Pharmacopoeia.

DISEASE may modify the dose of medicines. This can occur in several ways. Thus, in serious illnesses the patient may be more susceptible to drugs, such as narcotics, that depress tissue activity, and therefore smaller doses must be given. Again, absorption of the drug from the gut may be slowed up by disease of the gut, or its effect may be enhanced if there is disease of

the kidneys, interfering with the excretion of the drug.

FASTING aids the rapidity of absorption of, and also makes the body more susceptible to the action of, drugs. Partly for this reason, as well as to avoid irritation of the stomach, it is usual to prescribe drugs to be taken after meals, and diluted with water.

COMBINATION OF DRUGS is to be avoided if possible as it is often difficult to assess what their combined effect may be. In some cases they may have a mutually antagonistic effect, which means that the patient will not obtain full benefit. Sometimes a combination may have a deleterious effect.

FORM, ROUTE AND FREQUENCY OF ADMINISTRATION are all important and doctors and pharmacists will advise a given patient on these. Drugs are now produced in many forms, though tablets are the most common and, usually, convenient. In Britain, medicines are given *by mouth* whenever possible, unless there is some degree of urgency, or because the drug is either destroyed in, or is not absorbed from, the gut. In these circumstances, it is given *intravenously*, *intramuscularly* or *subcutaneously*. In some cases, as in cases of asthma or bronchitis, the drug may be given in the form of an *inhalant* (q.v.), in order to get the maximum concentration at the point where it is wanted: that is, in the lungs. If a local effect is wanted, as in cases of diseases of the skin, the drug is applied *topically* to the skin. In some countries there is a tendency to give medicines in the form of a *suppository* which is inserted in the rectum.

Recent years have seen developments whereby the assimilation of drugs into the body can be more carefully controlled. These include, for example, what are known as transdermals, in which drugs are built into a plaster that is stuck on the skin, and the drug is then absorbed into the body at a controlled rate. This method is now being used for the administration of glyceryl trinitrate (q.v.) in the treatment of angina pectoris (q.v.), and of hyoscine hydrobromide in the treatment of motion sickness (q.v.). Another is a new class of implantable devices. These are tiny polymers infused with a drug and implanted just under the skin by injection. They can be tailored so as to deliver drugs at virtually any rate – from minutes to years. A modification of these polymers now being investigated is the incorporation of magnetic particles which allow an extra burst of the incorporated drug to be released in response to an oscillating magnetic field which is induced by a magnetic 'watch' worn by the patient. In this way the patient can switch on an extra dose of drug when this is needed: insulin, for instance, in the case of diabetics. In yet another new development, a core of drug is enclosed in a semi-permeable membrane and is released in the stomach at a given rate. (See also LIPOSOMES.)

DOTHIEPIN is a drug used in the treatment of depression, particularly when the patient needs sedation. (See ANTIDEPRESSANTS.)

DOUBLE BLIND TRIAL A scientific study in which neither the investigators assessing the outcome nor the subjects being treated know which treatment the subject is receiving. The results are analysed after all the data has been collected and the code has been broken.

DOUBLE VISION (see SQUINT).

DOUCHE An application to the body of a jet of fluid via a pipe or tube. It may be used to clean any part of the body but is used most commonly with reference to the vagina. (Although used as a method of contraception it is ineffective.)

DOWN'S (DOWN) SYNDROME (or MONGOLISM) is a genetic disorder in which the affected person usually carries an extra chromosome – 47 instead of the normal 46 – resulting in a characteristic flat facial look with slanting eyes, hence its original description of Mongolism. A large tongue, a small round skull and short thick hands and feet are other manifestations. Many victims have varying degrees of mental handicap. The palm print is distinctive and those with the syndrome may also have heart defects, intestinal malformations, deafness and squints. The condition was named after Dr J. L. H. Down, the London doctor who first described it in 1866.

The incidence is approximately 1 per 600 births, but the incidence in the community is lower than this, as many Down's syndrome victims die in infancy. This high death-rate is due partly to the fact that these children have a much higher incidence of other congenital deformities, such as malformations of the heart, than other children, and partly to their lower resistance to infection.

It is much commoner in children born to older women. Thus, the risk of having a Down's child in women over 45 is more than 1 in 60, compared with less than 1 in 1000 in women under 30. Forty per cent of children with Down's syndrome are born to mothers over 40, 30 per cent to those aged 35 to 40. For mothers who give birth to a Down's child when they are younger the chances of a subsequent child being affected is relatively high. Precise figures in this respect can be misleading, and the best advice for a young mother who has had a Down's child, and who wishes to know the risk of her having another, is to go and discuss the matter with her family doctor. Despite the low risk of recurrences, particularly in young couples, diagnostic amniocentesis (q.v.) is often advised in future pregnancies, especially if the mother is over 35. Other prenatal screening tests are chorionic villus sampling and the triple marker test. (See PRENATAL SCREENING.)

In 95 per cent of cases the cause is the presence of an extra chromosome (q.v.) in the ovum. The cause of this extra chromosome is not known. In the remaining cases the cause is a fault in the division of the germ cells known

as translocation. There is an extra chromosome (q.v.) in the no. 21 group, hence the disease is referred to as trisomy 21. It is usually caused by an unequal distribution of chromosomes in the production of the egg cells. Occasionally it results from chromosomal rearrangements, or abnormal mitosis in the fertilized egg cell.

The degree of mental backwardness varies considerably. Up to a third of all severely mentally handicapped children of school age have Down's syndrome. It has been estimated that 6 per cent of Down's children are probably capable of profiting appreciably from attendance at schools for the educationally handicapped. Practically all who survive to school age gain some benefit. Most eventually acquire some degree of speech, and about 5 per cent learn to read. They practically never learn to write. Most learn to wash, dress and feed themselves, and many are able to run simple errands.

Although there is no known cure for the condition, there is much that can be done for the children, especially if they can be kept at home rather than sent to an institution, and a number of societies are very helpful. Parents will naturally feel a combination of strong emotions, including anger and guilt, and vigorous counselling can be very valuable. Contact: The Down's Syndrome Association (see APPENDIX 2: ADDRESSES).

DOXORUBICIN is one of the most successful and widely used antitumour drugs. It is used in the treatment of acute leukaemia, lymphoma, and various forms of sarcoma and cancer, including cancer of the bladder. (See CYTOTOXIC.)

DOXYCYCLINE is a wide-spectrum, long-acting antibiotic of the tetracycline group (q.v.), which is active against a wide range of micro-organisms, including the causative organisms of scrub typhus, trachoma, psittacosis, Lyme disease and some influenzas.

DRACONTIASIS or DRACUNCULIASIS A nematode infection caused by *Dracunculus medinensis* (guinea-worm). Although mentioned in ancient writings from the Middle East (it is arguably the oldest parasitic disease to have been documented), it is now confined to west and central Africa, and western parts of India. Infection is acquired by drinking water containing water-fleas (*Cyclops* spp.) – freshwater crustaceans – which carry infected larvae. These are freed by digestive enzymes following ingestion, and migrate to the body cavities, where they mature. The female attains a length of 60–120 cm and, when gravid, migrates to subcutaneous tissues, usually in the feet and legs. Secretion of enzyme(s) produces a papular (bullous) lesion in which larvae are formed; this bursts in fresh water, discharging a milky fluid, containing numerous larvae. These are ingested by water-fleas, thus completing the cycle. The major clinical problem is secondary infection of the worm track, causing cellulitis, synovitis, epididymo-orchitis, periarticular fibrosis, and arthritis; tetanus is a potentially lethal complication. Chemotherapy is unsatisfactory; metronidazole, mebendazole, thiabendazole, and niridazole have been used with some success, but the time-honoured method of extracting the female adult by winding it around a matchstick remains in use. Surgical treatment may be necessary. Ultimate prevention consists of removing *Cyclops* spp. from drinking water (in this sense, dracontiasis is probably unique); the WHO is attempting to achieve this.

DRAMAMINE is the trade name for dimenhydrinate, a drug widely used in the treatment of travel sickness.

DRAUGHT, or DRAFT, is a small mixture intended to be taken at one dose. It consists generally of two or four tablespoonfuls of fluid.

DREAMS (see SLEEP).

DREPANOCYTOSIS is another term for sickle-cell anaemia (q.v.), which is characterized by the presence in the blood of red blood corpuscles sickle-like in shape. The anaemia is a severe one and afflicts black people.

DRESSINGS (see WOUNDS).

DROP ATTACKS are attacks, usually in a middle-aged woman, whose legs suddenly 'give way', so that she falls to the ground without any warning. There is no loss of consciousness. In some cases the loss of tone in the muscles, responsible for the fall, may persist for several hours. In such cases moving the patient or applying pressure to the soles of the feet may restore the tone to the muscles. In most cases, however, recovery is immediate. The cause is probably a temporary interference with the blood supply to the brain. In others there may be some disturbance of the vestibular apparatus which controls the balance of the body. (See EAR; TRANSIENT ISCHAEMIC ATTACK.)

DROP-FOOT This is the inability to dorsiflex the foot at the ankle. The foot hangs down and has to be swung clear of the ground while walking. It is commonly caused by damage to the lateral popliteal nerve or the peroneal muscles.

DROP WRIST This is the inability to extend the hand at the wrist. It is usually due to damage to the radial nerve which supplies the extensor muscles.

DROWNING (see APPENDIX 1: BASIC FIRST AID).

DRUG ABSORPTION Drugs are usually administered distant to their site of action in the body. They must then pass across cell membranes to reach their site of action. For example – drugs given by mouth must pass across the gut membrane to enter the blood stream and then pass through the endothelium of vessel walls to reach the site of action in the tissues. This process is called absorption and may depend on lipid diffusion, aqueous diffusion, active transport, or pinocytosis – a process in which a cell takes in small droplets of fluid by cytoplasmic engulfment.

DRUG ADDICTION or DEPENDENCE is the compulsion to take a drug repeatedly. (See ADDICTION.) Psychological dependence occurs when the drug user craves the drug's desirable effects. Physical dependence occurs when the user has to continue taking the drug to avoid distressing withdrawal or abstinence symptoms. Drug misuse and dependence are surprisingly common, occurring with widely used drugs such as alcohol, caffeine, and nicotine as well as with certain prescribed drugs such as benzodiazepine tranquillizers. Less socially acceptable but frequently misused drugs are described below.

Cannabis, derived from the plant *Cannabis sativa*, is a widely used but illegal recreational drug that does not seem to be addictive. Its two main forms are marijuana – known in the 1960s as 'pot' – which comes from the dried leaves, and hashish which comes from the resin. Cannabis may be used in food and drink but is usually smoked in cigarettes called 'joints' or 'reefers' to induce relaxation and a feeling of well-being. Heavy use can cause apathy and vagueness and may even cause psychosis. Whether or not cannabis leads people to using harder drugs is debatable.

About 1 in 10 of Britain's teenagers misuses volatile substances such as toluene at some time, but only about 1 in 40 does so regularly. These substances are given off by certain glues, solvents, varnishes, and liquid fuels, all of which can be bought cheaply in shops, although their sale to children under 16 is illegal. They are often inhaled from plastic bags held over the nose and mouth. Central-nervous-system excitation, with euphoria and disinhibition, is followed by depression and lethargy. Unpleasant effects include facial rash, nausea and vomiting, tremor, dizziness, and clumsiness. Death from coma and acute cardiac toxicity is a serious risk. Chronic heavy use can cause peripheral neuropathy and irreversible cerebellar damage. (See SOLVENT ABUSE.)

The hallucinogenic or psychedelic drugs include lysergic acid diethylamide (LSD or acid), magic mushrooms, ecstasy (MDMA), and phencyclidine (PCP or 'angel' dust, mainly used in the USA). These drugs have no medicinal uses. Taken by mouth, they produce vivid 'trips', with heightened emotions and perceptions and sometimes with hallucinations. They are not physically addictive but can cause nightmarish bad trips during use and flashbacks (vivid reruns of trips) after use, and can probably trigger psychosis.

Stimulant drugs such as amphetamine and cocaine act like adrenaline and speed up the central nervous system, making the user feel confident, energetic, and powerful for several hours. They can also cause severe insomnia, anxiety, paranoia, psychosis, and even sudden death due to convulsions or tachycardia. Depression may occur on withdrawal of these drugs, and in some users this is sufficiently deterrent to cause psychological dependence. Amphetamine ('speed') is mainly synthesized illegally and may be eaten, sniffed, or injected. Related drugs such as dexamphetamine sulphate (Dexedrine) and diethylpropion hydrochloride (Tenuate, Dospan) are prescribed pills that enter the black market. Cocaine and related drugs are used in medicine as local anaesthetics. Illegal supplies of cocaine ('snow' or 'ice') and its derivative, 'crack', come mainly from South America, where they are made from the plant *Erythroxylon coca*. Cocaine is usually sniffed ('snorted') or rubbed into the gums; crack is burnt and inhaled.

Opiate drugs are derived from the opium poppy, *Papaver somniferum*. They are described as narcotic because they induce sleep. Their main medical use is as potent oral or injectable analgesics such as morphine, diamorphine, pethidine, and codeine. The commonest illegal opiate is heroin, a powdered form of diamorphine that may be smoked, sniffed, or injected to induce euphoria and drowsiness. Regular opiate misuse leads to tolerance (the need to take ever larger doses to achieve the same effect) and marked dependence. The withdrawal syndrome is like a bout of severe gastric flu with painful abdominal cramps. A less addictive oral opiate, methadone, can be prescribed as a substitute that is easier to withdraw.

Some 75,000–150,000 Britons now misuse opiates and other drugs intravenously, and pose a huge public-health problem because injections with shared dirty needles can carry the blood-borne viruses that cause AIDS and hepatitis B. Many clinics now operate schemes to exchange old needles for clean ones, free of charge.

DRUG BINDING The process of attachment of a drug to a receptor or plasma protein, fat, mucopolysaccharide or other tissue component. This process may be reversible or irreversible.

DRUG CLEARANCE The volume of blood from which a drug is completely removed in one minute is known as clearance. Renal clearance of a drug is the amount of blood completely cleared of the drug by the kidney in one minute.

DRUG INTERACTIONS Many patients are on several prescribed drugs, and numerous medicines are available over the counter, so the potential for drug interaction is large. A drug may interact with another by inhibiting its action, potentiating its action, or by simple summation of effects.

The interaction may take place: (*a*) Prior to absorption or administration, e.g. antacids bind tetracycline in the gut and prevent absorption. (*b*) By interfering with protein binding – one drug may displace another from binding sites on plasma proteins. The action of the displaced drug will be increased because more drug is now available, e.g. anticoagulants are displaced by analgesics. (*c*) During metabolism or excretion of the drug – some drugs increase or decrease the activity of liver enzymes which metabolize drugs, thus affecting their rate of destruction, e.g. barbiturates, nicotine, and alcohol all activate hepatic enzymes. Altering the pH of urine will affect the excretion of drugs via the kidney. (*d*) At the drug receptor – one drug may displace another at the receptor affecting its efficacy or duration of action.

DRUG METABOLISM A process by which the body destroys and excretes drugs, so limiting their duration of action. Phase 1 metabolism consists of transformation by oxidation, reduction, or hydrolysis. In phase 2 this transformed product is conjugated (joined up) with another molecule to produce a water-soluble product which is easier to excrete.

DRUGS In Britain the supply of drugs is controlled by the Medicines Act. Some drugs are available only on prescription, some both on prescription and over the counter, and some are not available on NHS prescription. When enquiring about drugs that a patient is taking, it is essential to ask about all items bought over the counter and any herbal or traditional remedies that might be used, as these can interact with other prescribed drugs or affect the patient's presenting complaints. Each drug has a single generic name, but many will also have several proprietary (brand) names. It is often much cheaper to prescribe the generic form of a drug, and many doctors do so. Many hospitals and general practices in the United Kingdom now provide a list of suggested drugs for doctors to prescribe. If a doctor wishes to use a drug not on the list he has to give a valid reason.

Prescriptions for drugs should be written clearly in ink and signed and dated by the prescriber. They should include the patient's name, address and age (obligatory for children under 12), the name of the drug to be supplied, the dose and dose frequency, and the total quantity to be supplied. Any special instructions (e.g. 'after food') should be stated. There are special regulations about the prescription of drugs controlled under the Misuse of Drugs Regulations, 1985 (see CONTROLLED DRUGS). A pharmacist can advise about which drugs are available without prescription, and is able to recommend treatment for many minor complaints. Information about exemption from prescription charges in the NHS can be obtained from health visitors, general practitioners, or social security offices.

DRUGS IN PREGNANCY Unnecessary drugs during pregnancy should be avoided because of the adverse effect of some drugs on the fetus which have no harmful effect on the mother. Drugs may pass through the placenta and damage the fetus because their pharmacological effects are enhanced as the enzyme systems responsible for their degradation are undeveloped in the fetus. Thus, if the drug can pass through the placenta, the pharmacological effect on the fetus may be great whilst that on the mother is minimal. Warfarin may thus induce fetal and placental haemorrhage and thiazide administration may produce thrombocytopenia in the new born. Many progestogens have androgenic side effects and their administration to a mother for the purpose of preventing recurrent abortion may produce virilization of the female fetus. Tetracycline administered during the last trimester commonly stains the deciduous teeth of the child yellow.

The other dangers of administering drugs in pregnancy are the teratogenic effects. It is understandable that a drug may interfere with a mechanism essential for growth and result in arrested or distorted development of the fetus and yet cause no disturbance in the adult in whom these differentiation and organization processes have ceased to be relevant. Thus the effect of a drug upon a fetus may differ qualitatively as well as quantitatively from its effect on the mother. The susceptibility of the embryo will depend on the stage of development it has reached when the drug is given. The stage of early differentiation, that is from the beginning of the third week to the end of the tenth week of pregnancy, is the time of greatest susceptibility. After this time the risk of congenital malformation from drug treatment is less although the death of the fetus can occur at any time.

DRUNKENNESS (see ALCOHOL).

DUCHENNE MUSCULAR DYSTROPHY An inherited sex-linked recessive disorder characterized by progressive muscular weakness and wasting. It is the most common muscular dystrophy, occurring in 30 per 100,000 live male births. Spontaneous mutations are common. The calf muscles become bulky (pseudohypertrophy). Affected boys develop symptoms in early childhood and die in their teens or early twenties from respiratory infections. Female carriers may be identified by screening for abnormalities of muscle enzymes. Genetic research is pointing the way to possible treatments.

DUCT is the name applied to a passage leading from a gland into some hollow organ, or on to the surface of the body, by which the secretion of the gland is discharged: e.g. the pancreatic duct and the bile duct opening into the duodenum, and the sweat ducts opening on the skin surface.

DUCTLESS GLAND is the term applied to any one of certain glands in the body the secretion of which goes directly into the blood stream and so is carried to different parts of the body. These glands – the pituitary, thyroid, parathyroid, adrenal and reproductive – are also known as the ENDOCRINE GLANDS (q.v.). Some glands may be both duct glands and ductless glands. For example, the pancreas manufactures a digestive juice which passes by a duct into the small intestine. It also manufactures, by means of special cells, a substance called insulin which passes straight into the blood.

DUCTUS ARTERIOSUS is the blood-vessel in the fetus through which blood passes from the pulmonary artery to the aorta, thereby bypassing the lungs, which do not function during intra-uterine life. (See CIRCULATION OF THE BLOOD.) The ductus normally ceases to function soon after birth and within a few weeks is converted into a fibrous cord. Occasionally this obliteration does not occur: a condition known as patent ductus arteriosus. This is one of the more common congenital defects of the heart, and one which responds particularly well to surgical treatment. Closure of the duct can also be achieved in some cases by the administration of indomethacin. (See HEART DISEASES.)

DUCTUS DEFERENS, or VAS DEFERENS, is the tube which carries spermatozoa from the epidydimis to the seminal vesicles. (See TESTICLE.)

DUMBNESS (see SPEECH DISORDERS).

DUMPING SYNDROME A sensation of weakness and sweating after a meal in patients who have undergone gastrectomy (q.v.). Rapid emptying of the stomach and the drawing of fluid from the blood into the intestine has been blamed, but the exact cause is debated.

DUODENAL ILEUS is the term applied to dilatation of the duodenum due to chronic obstruction of the duodenum, caused by an abnormal position of arteries in the region of the duodenum pressing on it.

DUODENAL ULCER is related to gastric ulcer (see STOMACH, DISEASES OF), both being a form of chronic peptic ulcer. Although becoming less frequent in Western communities, peptic ulcers still affect around 10 per cent of the

UK population at some time. The incidence of peptic ulcer is increasing in many developing countries. Duodenal ulcers are 10–15 times more common than gastric ulcers, and occur in people from 20 years onwards; gastric ulcers generally occur in those over 40 years, and are rare in women until after the menopause. The male to female ratio for duodenal ulcer varies between 4:1 and 2:1 in different communities, while that for gastric ulcer is less than 2:1. Social class (q.v.) and blood groups (q.v.) are also influential, with duodenal ulcer being more common among the upper social classes, and those of blood group O.

Causes Until recently there was no general consensus of expert opinion as to the precise cause of peptic ulcers. What probably happens is that there is some abrasion, or break, in the lining membrane (or mucosa) of the stomach and/or duodenum, and that it is gradually eroded and deepened by the gastric juice. What was not known, however, was why this only occurred in some people. It is now known that the bacterium *Helicobacter pylori* (q.v.) is present in the antrum of the stomach of people with peptic ulcers and that the ulcers heal if *H. pylori* is eradicated. Mental stress is also a probable provocative factor. Smoking seems to accentuate, if not cause, duodenal ulcer, and the drinking of alcohol is probably harmful. The apparent association with a given blood group, and the fact that relatives of a patient with a peptic ulcer are unduly likely to develop such an ulcer suggest that there is some constitutional factor.

Symptoms and signs Peptic ulcers may present in different ways, but chronic, episodic pain lasting several months or years is most common. Occasionally, however, there may be an acute episode of bleeding or perforation, or obstruction of the gastric outlet, with little previous history. Most commonly, there is pain of varying intensity in the middle or upper right part of the abdomen. It tends to occur two or three hours after a meal, most commonly at night, and is relieved by some food, such as a glass of milk; untreated it may last up to an hour. Vomiting is unusual, but there is often tenderness and stiffness ('guarding') of the abdominal muscles. Confirmation of the diagnosis is made by radiological examination ('barium meal'), the ulcer appearing as a niche on the film, or direct endoscopic visualization of the ulcer (see FIBREOPTIC ENDOSCOPY). Chief complications are perforation of the ulcer, leading to the vomiting of blood, or haematemesis (q.v.); or less severe bleeding from the ulcer, the blood passing down the gut, resulting in dark, tarry stools (see MELAENA).

Treatment involves initial management of any complications, such as shock, haemorrhage, perforation, or gastric outlet obstruction, usually involving surgery and blood replacement. Attention is then focused on the patient's chronic complaint. While a period of rest, with regular meals and a milky diet, avoiding strong tea and coffee, and reducing intake of fried foods and alcohol are undoubtedly beneficial, the mainstay of treatment involves 4-to-6-week courses with drugs such as cimetidine and ranitidine. These are H_2 receptor antagonists (q.v.) which heal peptic ulcers by reducing gastric-acid output. Smoking should be avoided.

DUODENUM is the first part of the intestine immediately beyond the stomach, so named because its length is about twelve fingerbreadths. (See INTESTINE.)

DUPUYTREN'S CONTRACTURE A condition of unknown aetiology in which there is progressive thickening and contracture of the palmar fascia with adherence of the overlying skin. A clawing deformity of the fingers, particularly the little and ring fingers, develops. It is associated with liver disease, diabetes, epilepsy, and gout. Treatment is surgical to excise the affected fascia.

DURA MATER is the outermost and strongest of the three membranes or meninges which envelop the brain and spinal cord. In it run vessels which nourish the inner surface of the skull. (See BRAIN.)

DWARF, or DWARFISM, is a term applied to under-development of the body. The causes are either developmental or due to food insufficient in quantity or unsuitable in quality, or to defects in some of the body secretions which can be corrected. The first-named group includes pituitary dwarfism, the subjects being very small people with normally proportioned parts, also achondroplasic dwarfs (see ACHONDROPLASIA) with large globular head and shortened limbs and stumpy fingers. It is now known that in a certain proportion of children of short stature this can be remedied by administration of the growth hormone of pituitary gland (q.v.), provided this is given at an early enough age. All children who by the age of 5 years are at least what is technically known as 'three standard deviations below the mean' should be referred for examination by specialists to determine whether or not their lack of height is due to lack of growth hormone and therefore likely to respond to treatment with the hormone. Where dwarfism is attributable to a primary defect of the thyroid gland, the condition may be treatable. In this class are also included various forms of defective growth associated with defects in the secretions of the digestive organs, especially the pancreas; this type of defect, often known as pancreatic infantilism, is mainly confined to a retardation of physical development, while the mental changes are little marked. Another form of dwarfism, associated with a deformity of the bones, is produced by rickets in early life, such persons showing high forehead, great bending of the leg bones, and deformity of the chest. (See RICKETS.)

DYNAMOMETER is an elliptical ring of steel to which is attached a dial and moving index. It is used to test the strength of the muscles of the forearm, being squeezed in the hand, and registering the pressure in pounds or kilograms.

DYS- is a prefix meaning difficult or painful.

DYSARTHRIA is a general term applied when weakness or incoordination of the speech musculature prevents clear pronunciation of words. The individual's speech may sound as if it is slurred or weak. It may be due to damage affecting the centres in the brain which control movements of the speech muscles or damage to the muscles themselves.

Examples of dysarthria may be found in stroke illness, cerebral palsy and the latter stages of Parkinson's disease, multiple sclerosis and motor neurone disease. Whatever the cause a speech therapist can assess the extent of the dysarthria and suggest exercises or an alternative means of communication.

DYSCHEZIA is constipation due to retention of faeces in the rectum. This retention is the outcome of irregular habits, which damp down the normal reflex causing defaecation.

DYSDIADOKOKINESIA means loss of the ability to perform rapid alternate movements, such as winding up a watch. It is a sign of a lesion in the cerebellum. (See BRAIN.)

DYSENTERY A clinical state arising from invasive colo-rectal disease; it is accompanied by abdominal colic, diarrhoea, and passage of blood/mucus in the stool. It is accompanied by fever. It is common throughout the tropics and subtropics. Although the two major forms are caused by *Shigella* spp. (bacillary dysentery) and *Entamoeba histolytica* (amoebic dysentery), other organisms including enterohaemorrhagic *Escherichia coli* (serotypes) 0157:H7 and 026:H11) and *Campylobacter* spp. are also relevant. The condition(s) should be differentiated from inflammatory bowel disease (especially ulcerative colitis), which can present clinically for the first time in a traveller to a tropical/subtropical area. Other causes of dysentery include *Balantidium coli* and that caused by schistosomiasis (bilharzia) – *Schistosoma mansoni* and *S. japonicum* infection.

SHIGELLOSIS This form occurs both sporadically and endemically, and is usually caused by *Shigella dysenteriae*-1 (Shiga's bacillus), *Shigella flexneri*, *Shigella boydii*, and *Shigella sonnei*; the latter is the most benign and occurs in temperate climates also. It is transmitted by food and water contamination, direct contact, and by flies; the organisms thrive in the presence of overcrowding and insanitary conditions. The incubation is 1–7 days, and the severity of the clinical manifestations is depend-

ent on the responsible strain. Duration of illness varies from a few days to two weeks. Disease is particularly severe in young, old, and malnourished individuals. Complications include perforation and haemorrhage from the colo-rectum, the haemolytic uraemic syndrome (which includes renal failure), and Reiter's syndrome. Diagnosis is dependent on demonstration of *Shigella* spp. in a faecal sample(s) – before or usually after culture. If dehydration is present, this should be treated accordingly, usually with an oral rehydration technique. *Shigella* spp. responds to many antimicrobial compounds, the first used being sulphonamides; trimethoprim-sulphamethoxazole, trimethoprim, ampicillin, and amoxycillin have also been used extensively. Recently, a widespread resistance to broad-spectrum antibiotics has developed, especially in Asia and southern America, and the agent of such choice is a quinolone compound, e.g., ciprofloxacin; nalidixic acid is also effective. Prevention depends on improved hygiene and sanitation, careful protection of food from flies, fly destruction, and garbage disposal. A *Shigella* spp. carrier must not be allowed to handle food.

ENTAMOEBA HISTOLYTICA INFECTION Although most cases occur in the tropics and subtropics, this is not always the case. Dysentery may be accompanied by weight loss, anaemia, and occasionally dyspnoea. *E. histolytica* contaminates food, e.g., uncooked vegetables, or drinking water. After ingestion of the cyst-stage, and following the action of digestive enzymes, the motile trophozoite emerges in the colon causing local invasive disease (amoebic colitis). On entering the portal system, these organisms may gain access to the liver, causing invasive hepatic disease (amoebic liver 'abscess'). Other sites of 'abscess' formation include the lungs (usually right) and brain. In the colo-rectum an amoeboma may be difficult to differentiate from a carcinoma. Clinical symptoms usually occur within a week, but can be delayed for months, or even years; onset may be acute – as for *Shigella* spp. infection. Perforation, colorectal haemorrhage, and appendicitis are unusual complications. Diagnosis is by demonstration of *E. histolytica* trophozoites in a fresh faecal sample; other amoebae affecting man do not invade tissues. Research techniques can be used to differentiate between pathogenic (*E. dysenteriae*) and non-pathogenic strains (*E. dispar*). Alternatively, several serological tests are of value in diagnosis, but only in the presence of invasive disease. Treatment consists of one of the 5-nitroimidazole compounds – metronidazole, tinidazole, and ornidazole; alcohol avoidance is important during their administration. A 5–10 day course should be followed by diloxanide furoate for 10 days. Other compounds – emetine, chloroquine, iodoquinol, and paromomycin – are now rarely used. Invasive disease involving the liver or other organ(s) usually responds favourably to a similar regimen; aspiration of a liver 'abscess' is now rarely indicated, as controlled trials have indicated a similar resolution rate whether this technique is used or not, provided a 5-nitro-imidazole compound is administered.

DYSIDROSIS means disturbance of sweat secretion.

DYSLEXIA is difficulty in reading or learning to read. It is always accompanied by difficulty in writing, and particularly by difficulties in spelling. Reading difficulties might be due to various factors, for example, a general learning problem, bad teaching or understimulation, or a perceptive problem such as poor eyesight. Specific dyslexia ('word blindness'), however, affects 4–8 per cent of otherwise normal children to some extent. It is three times more common in boys than in girls, and there is often a family history.

Support and advice may be obtained from the British Dyslexia Association (see APPENDIX 2: ADDRESSES).

DYSMENORRHOEA means painful menstruation. (See MENSTRUATION.)

DYSPAREUNIA means painful or difficult coitus.

DYSPEPSIA This is another name for indigestion. It describes a sensation of pain or discomfort in the upper abdomen or lower chest following eating. There may be additional symptoms of heartburn, flatulence, or nausea. There are many causes of dyspepsia including oesophagitis, peptic ulcer, gallstones, hiatus hernia, malignancy of the stomach or oesophagus, and hepatic or pancreatic disease. Occasionally it may be psychological in origin. Treatment depends on the underlying cause but, if there is no specific pathology, avoidance of precipitating foods may be helpful.

DYSPHAGIA is the medical term for difficulty in swallowing.

DYSPHASIA is the term used to describe the difficulties in understanding language and in self-expression, most frequently after stroke (see STROKE), or other brain damage. When there is a total loss in the ability to communicate through speech or writing, it is known as *global aphasia*. Many more individuals have a partial understanding of what is said to them. They are also able to put their own thoughts into words to some extent. The general term for this less severe condition is *dysphasia*. Individuals vary widely, but in general there are two main types of dysphasia. Some people may have a good understanding of spoken language but have difficulty in self-expression; this is called *expressive* or *motor dysphasia*. Others may have a very poor ability to understand speech, but will have a considerable spoken output consisting of jargon words; this is

known as *receptive* or *sensory dysphasia*. Similar difficulties may occur with reading, and this is called *dyslexia* (a term more commonly encountered in the different context of children's reading disability). Adults who have suffered a stroke or another form of brain damage may also have difficulty in writing, or *dysgraphia*. The speech therapist can assess the finer diagnostic points. (See SPEECH THERAPY.)

No case is too severe or too mild to be referred to a speech therapist for an assessment. The victim, his relatives and other visitors may be anxious about the effects of the stroke and may find it helpful to have the details of the dysphasic problem explained to them. The speech therapist can help them adjust to the effects of the stroke on communication. Treatment may be conducted on an individual or group basis according to the needs of the individual. It is important for people who come into contact with the dysphasic person to treat him just as they would have done before the stroke: to be patient rather than patronizing.

Dysphasia may come on suddenly and last only for a few hours or days, being due to a temporary block in the circulation of blood to the brain. The effects may be permanent, but although the individual may have difficulty in understanding language and expressing himself, he will be quite aware of his surroundings and may be very frustrated by his inability to communicate with others.

Further information may be obtained from Action for Dysphasic Adults. (See APPENDIX 2: ADDRESSES.)

DYSPNOEA means difficulty in breathing (see BREATHLESSNESS; ORTHOPNOEA).

DYSTOCIA means slow or painful birth of a child.

DYSTONIA refers to a type of involuntary movement characterized by a sustained muscle contraction, frequently causing twisting and repetitive movements or abnormal postures, and caused by inappropriate instructions from the brain. It is sometimes called torsion spasm, and may be synonymous with athetosis when the extremities are involved. Often the condition is of unknown cause (idiopathic), but an inherited predisposition is increasingly recognized among some cases. Others may be associated with known pathology of the brain such as cerebral palsy or Wilson's disease. The presentation of dystonia may be focal (usually in adults) causing blepharospasm (forceful eye closure), oromandibular dystonia (spasms of the tongue and jaw), cranial dystonia/Meige syndrome/Brueghel's syndrome (eyes and jaw both involved), spastic or spasmodic dysphonia/laryngeal dystonia (strained or whispering speech), spasmodic dysphagia (difficulty swallowing), spasmodic torti/latero/ante/retrocollis (rotation, sideways, forward or backward tilting of the neck), dystonic writer's cramp or axial dystonia (spasms deviating the torso). Foot dystonia occurs almost exclusively in children and adolescents. In adults, the condition usually remains focal or involves at most an adjacent body part. In children, it may spread to become generalized. The condition has always been considered rare, but commonly is either not diagnosed or mistakenly thought to be of psychological origin. It may, in fact, be half as common as multiple sclerosis. Similar features can occur in some subjects treated with major tranquillizing drugs, in whom a predisposition to develop dystonia may be present.

DYSTROPHIA MYOTONICA is a type of muscular dystrophy (see MYOPATHY) in which the affected person has weakness and wasting of the muscles, particularly those in the face and neck. Other effects are cataract (q.v.), ptosis (see EYE DISEASES), baldness and malfunctioning of the endocrine system (q.v.). Both sexes may be affected by this inherited disorder.

DYSTROPHY means defective or faulty nutrition, and is a term applied to a group of developmental changes occurring in the muscles, independently of the nervous system (see MYOPATHY). The best-known form is progressive muscular dystrophy, a group of hereditary disorders characterized by symmetrical wasting and weakness, with no sensory loss. There are three types: Duchenne (q.v.) (usually occurring in boys within the first three years of life), limb girdle (occurring in either sex in the second or third decade), and facio-scapulo-humeral (either sex, any age). The three types have different prognoses, but may lead to severe disability and premature death, often from respiratory failure. The third type progresses very slowly, however, and is compatible with a long life.

Diagnosis may be confirmed by electromyography (EMG) or muscle biopsy. Although genetic research is pointing to possible treatment or prevention, at present no effective treatment is known, and deterioration may occur with excessive confinement to bed. Physiotherapeutic and orthopaedic measures may be necessary to counteract deformities and contractures, and may help in coping with some disabilities.

DYSURIA means difficulty or pain in urination.

E

EAR   The ear is concerned with two functions. The more evident is that of the sense of hearing; the other is the sense of equilibration and of motion. The organ is divided into three parts: (*a*) the external ear, consisting of the auricle on the surface of the head, and the tube which leads inwards to the drum; (*b*) the middle ear, separated from the former by the tympanic membrane or drum, and from the internal ear by two other membranes, but communicating with the throat by the Eustachian tube; and (*c*) the internal ear, comprising the complicated labyrinth from which runs the vestibulocochlear nerve into the brain.

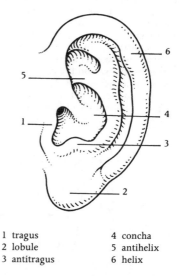

1 tragus	4 concha
2 lobule	5 antihelix
3 antitragus	6 helix

The auricle or pinna of the ear.

EXTERNAL EAR   The auricle or pinna, shaped in man something like a crumpled-up funnel, is not essential to the sense of hearing, although in animals it appears to play an important part. It consists of a framework of elastic cartilage covered by skin, the lobule at the lower end being a small mass of fat. From the bottom of the concha the external auditory (or acoustic) meatus runs inwards for 25 mm (1 inch), to end blindly at the drum. This passage is short in young children, in whom the drum is almost at the surface, and it lengthens as the skull bones develop. The outer half of the passage is surrounded by cartilage, lined by skin, on which are placed fine hairs pointing outwards, and glands secreting a small amount of wax. In the inner half, the skin is smooth and lies directly upon the temporal bone, in the substance of which the whole hearing apparatus is enclosed. The two parts meet at a slight angle, so as to give the whole passage a curve, which can be straightened by pulling the auricle upwards and backwards, when the drum can often be clearly seen by a good light.

MIDDLE EAR   The tympanic membrane, forming the drum, is stretched completely across the end of the passage, being placed rather obliquely, so that it makes an angle of about 60° with the floor. It is about 8 mm (one-third of an inch) across, very thin, and white or pale pink in colour, so that it is partly transparent, and some of the contents of the middle ear shine through it. From this description it can be readily understood how easily it is torn, and how dangerous are blows on the side of the head, and rough manipulations to remove wax. The cavity of the middle ear is about 8 mm (one-third of an inch) wide and 4 mm (one-sixth of an inch) in depth from the tympanic membrane to the inner wall of bone. Although important structures, like the facial nerve which runs down behind it, lie close around, its only important contents are three small bones, the malleus (hammer), incus (anvil), and stapes (stirrup), collectively known as the auditory ossicles, with two minute muscles which regulate their movements, and the chorda tympani nerve which runs across the cavity. The auditory ossicles are of great importance. The malleus has a long spicule of bone, the handle,

embedded in the substance of the drum, while its head is in contact with the incus. The incus, suspended by one process of bone, has another affixed to the stapes, and the latter fits, by what would in a real stirrup be the footpiece, into one (fenestra vestibuli) of the two openings which lead through the inner wall of the middle ear into the internal ear. Accordingly these three bones form a chain across the middle ear, connecting the drum with the internal ear. Their function is to convert the air-waves, which strike upon the drum, into mechanical movements which can affect the fluid in the inner ear, because air-waves produce little effect upon fluid directly.

The middle ear has two connections which are of great importance as regards disease: in front, it communicates by a passage 37 mm (1½ inches) long, the Eustachian (or auditory) tube, with the upper part of the throat, behind the nose; behind and above, it opens into a cavity known as the mastoid antrum. The Eustachian tube admits air from the throat, and so keeps the pressure on both sides of the drum fairly equal. Serious deafness is produced by its closure, and it also, unfortunately, forms a channel by which acute inflammation, as in measles, can and does spread to the ear. The antrum occupies the interior of the projecting mass of bone, the mastoid process, which is felt

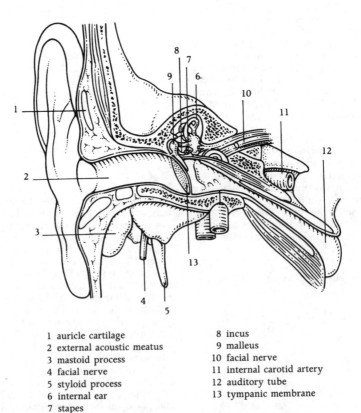

1 auricle cartilage	8 incus
2 external acoustic meatus	9 malleus
3 mastoid process	10 facial nerve
4 facial nerve	11 internal carotid artery
5 styloid process	12 auditory tube
6 internal ear	13 tympanic membrane
7 stapes	

External and middle parts of the right ear from the front.

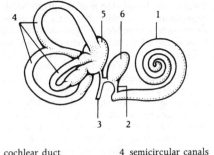

1 cochlear duct   4 semicircular canals
2 ductus reuniens   5 utricle
3 ductus endolymphaticus   6 saccule

The membranous labyrinth of inner ear.

on the surface of the head behind the ear; this cavity, along with the middle ear, is separated from the interior of the skull only by a thin plate of bone about the thickness of a playing card. INTERNAL EAR This consists of a complex system of hollows in the substance of the temporal bone enclosing a membranous duplicate. Between the membrane and the bone is a fluid known as perilymph, while the membrane is distended by another collection of fluid known as endolymph. This membranous labyrinth, as it is called, consists of two parts. The hinder part, comprising a sac, the utricle, and three short semicircular canals opening at each end into it, is the part concerned with the balancing sense; the forward part consists of another small bag, the saccule, and of a still more important part, the cochlear duct, and is the part concerned in hearing. In the cochlear duct is placed the spiral organ of Corti, on which the sound-waves are finally received and by which the sounds are communicated to the cochlear nerve, a branch of the vestibulocochlear nerve, which ends in filaments to this organ of Corti. The essential parts in the organ of Corti are a double row of rods and several rows of cells furnished with fine hairs of varying length. Different musical notes are perhaps appreciated by different rods and hair cells. THE ACT OF HEARING When sound-waves in the air reach the ear, the drum is alternately pressed in and pulled out, in consequence of which a to-and-fro movement is communicated to the chain of ossicles. The foot of the stapes communicates these movements to the perilymph. Finally these motions reach the delicate filaments placed in the organ of Corti, and so affect the nerve of hearing, which conveys impressions to the centre in the brain. There are two theories of hearing. The first is that of Helmholtz, who compared the organ of Corti to a piano and presumed that each sound caused a vibration of a corresponding part of Corti's organ. The second and later theory assumes that the entire organ of Corti is thrown into vibration by sounds, and that the nature of the sound is analysed and perceived by the hearing-centre in the brain.

EAR, DISEASES OF Diseases may affect the ear alone or as part of a more generalized condition. The disease may affect the outer, middle or inner ear or a combination of these. A full assessment, including detailed examination, is essential to enable the correct choice of treatment to be made.
EXAMINATION of the ear includes inspection of the external ear. An auriscope is used to examine the external ear canal and the ear drum. As the auriscope is inserted, the auricle is pulled gently upwards and backwards to straighten the ear canal and allow a better view of the ear drum. If a more detailed inspection is required, a microscope may be used to improve illumination and magnification.
TUNING-FORK TESTS are routinely performed to identify the presence of deafness. They also help to differentiate between conductive and nerve deafness.
HEARING TESTS are carried out to determine the level of hearing. An audiometer is used to deliver a series of short tones of varying frequency to the ear, either through a pair of headphones or via a sound transducer applied directly to the skull. The intensity of the sound is gradually reduced until it is no longer heard and this represents the threshold of hearing, at that frequency, through air and bone respectively. It may be necessary to play a masking noise into the opposite ear to prevent that ear from hearing the tones, enabling each ear to be tested independently.
General symptoms The following are some of the chief symptoms of ear disease:
DEAFNESS (SEE DEAFNESS).
EARACHE is most commonly due to acute inflammation of the middle ear, but may also be due to acute or chronic inflammation of the external ear or neuralgia affecting the outer ear. Perceived pain in this region may be referred from other areas, such as the earache commonly experienced after tonsillectomy or that caused by carious teeth. The treatment will depend on the underlying cause.
RINGING in the ear, or TINNITUS, is very common and is sometimes the only symptom of ear disease. It is often extremely annoying and can be the cause of severe depression. It may be described as hissing, buzzing, the sound of the sea, or of bells. The intensity of the tinnitus usually fluctuates, sometimes disappearing altogether, but is often most noticeable in quiet surroundings. It may occur in almost any form of ear disease, but is particularly troublesome in nerve deafness due to ageing and in noise-induced deafness. It may be a symptom of general diseases such as anaemia, high blood pressure and arterial disease, in which cases it is often synchronous with the pulse, and may also be caused by drugs such as quinine (q.v.), salicylates and certain antibiotics (q.v.). Treatment of the underlying ear or generalized disease may reduce or even cure the tinnitus, but unfortunately in many cases the noises persist. Reassurance and treatment of any depression often help to reduce the annoyance of the symptom.

WAX is produced by specialized glands in the outer part of the ear canal only. Impacted wax within the ear canal can cause deafness, tinnitis and sometimes disturbance of balance. It is removed, in most cases, by syringing with either warm (37 °C) saline or a solution of sodium bicarbonate. In some cases, prior to syringing, it may be necessary to use sodium bicarbonate or olive oil drops for several days in order to soften the wax sufficiently. If a perforation of the drum is suspected, the removal of wax should be carried out by a specialist.

FOREIGN BODIES, such as peas, beads or buttons, may be found in the external ear canal, especially in children who have usually introduced them themselves. Live insects may also be trapped in the external canal causing intense irritation and noise, and in such cases spirit drops are first instilled into the ear to kill the insect. Except in foreign bodies of vegetable origin, where swelling and pain may occur, syringing may be used to remove some foreign bodies, but often removal by a specialist using suitable instrumentation and an operating microscope is required. In children a general anaesthetic may be needed.

BOILS or FURUNCLES in the skin lining the outer ear canal are caused by a bacterial infection of hair follicles and give rise to intense pain, aggravated by movement of the auricle. This pain is relieved by packing the ear lightly with a piece of gauze soaked either in a 10-per-cent solution of ichthammol glycerin, or in 8-percent aluminium acetate. Treatment with an appropriate antibiotic is essential for at least five days.

ECZEMA is an allergic dermatitis (q.v.), which may affect the external ear canal. It causes redness, crusting and cracking of the skin, often with a watery discharge and intense irritation. It occurs as a result of skin sensitivity which may be infective in origin or due to contact with an irritating substance such as hair lotions, cosmetics and more commonly to certain antibiotic ear drops. Treatment includes identification and avoidance of the underlying allergic cause and the use of steroid ointments applied to the inflamed part.

TUMOURS of the ear can arise in the skin of the auricle often as a result of exposure to sunlight and can be benign or malignant. Within the ear canal itself, the commonest tumours are benign outgrowths from the surrounding bone, said to occur in swimmers as a result of repeated exposure to cold water. Polyps may result from chronic infection of the ear canal and drum, particularly in the presence of a perforation. These polyps are soft and may be large enough to fill the ear canal, but may shrink considerably after treatment of the associated infection.

Diseases of the middle ear

OTITIS MEDIA, or infection of the middle ear, usually occurs, in its acute form, as a result of infection spreading up the Eustachian tubes from the nose, throat or sinuses. It may occur following a cold, tonsilitis or sinusitis, and may also be caused by swimming and diving where water and infected secretions are forced up the Eustachian tube into the middle ear. Primarily it is a disease of children with as many as 1.5 million cases occurring in Britain every year. Pain is always present and it may be intense and throbbing or sharp in character. It is accompanied by deafness, fever and often tinnitus (q.v.). In infants, crying may be the only sign that something is wrong, though this is usually accompanied by some localizing manifestation such as rubbing or pulling at the ear. Examination of the ear usually reveals redness, and sometimes bulging, of the ear drum. In the early stages there is no discharge, but in the later stages there may be a discharge from perforation of the ear drum as a result of the pressure created in the middle ear by the accumulated pus. This is usually accompanied by an immediate reduction in pain.

Treatment consists of the immediate administration of an antibiotic, usually one of the penicillins, e.g. amoxycillin. In the majority of cases, no further treatment is required, but if this does not quickly bring relief, then it may be necessary to perform a myringotomy, or incision of the ear drum, to drain pus from the middle ear. When otitis media is treated immediately with sufficient dosage of the appropriate antibiotic, the chances of any permanent damage to the ear or to hearing are reduced to a negligible degree, as is the risk of any complications such as mastoiditis (discussed later in this section).

OTITIS MEDIA WITH EFFUSION, or GLUE EAR, is the commonest inflammatory condition of the middle ear in children, to the extent that one in four children in the UK entering school has had an episode of 'glue ear'. It is characterized by a persistent sticky fluid in the middle ear (hence the name 'glue ear') which causes a conductive-type deafness (see DEAFNESS). It may be associated with enlarged adenoids which impair the function of the Eustachian tube. If the hearing impairment is persistent and causes problems, drainage of the fluid and insertion of ventilation tubes or grommets may be needed, possibly in conjunction with removal of the adenoids.

MASTOIDITIS is a serious complication of inflammation of the middle ear, the incidence of which has been dramatically reduced by the introduction of penicillin. Inflammation in this cavity usually arises by direct spread of acute or chronic inflammation from the middle ear. The signs of this condition include swelling and tenderness of the skin behind the ear, redness and swelling inside the ear, pain in the side of the head, high fever, and a discharge from the ear. The management of this condition in the first instance is with antibiotics, usually given intravenously but, if the condition fails to improve, surgical treatment is necessary. This involves draining any pus from the middle ear and mastoid, and removing diseased lining and bone from the mastoid.

Diseases of the inner ear

MENIERE'S DISEASE is a common disorder characterized by the triad of episodic vertigo with deafness and tinnitus. The aetiology is unknown and usually one ear only is affected at first, but eventually the opposite ear is affected in approximately 50 per cent of cases. The onset of dizziness is often sudden and lasts for up to 24 hours. The hearing loss is temporary in the early stages, but with each attack there may be a progressive nerve deafness. Nausea and vomiting often occur. Treatment during the attacks includes rest and drugs to control sickness. Surgical treatment is sometimes required if crippling attacks of dizziness persist despite these measures.

OTOSCLEROSIS is a condition in which new bone grows in the middle ear to cause fixation of the stapes bone leading to impairment of the transmission of sound. The conductive-hearing loss is usually progressive, but may be partially overcome by a hearing aid. Surgical treatment involves bypassing the fixed bone with an artificial prosthesis.

EATING DISORDERS covers the terms obesity (q.v.), feeding problems in childhood, anorexia nervosa, and bulimia nervosa, of which the latter two are described here.

ANOREXIA NERVOSA, often called the slimmer's disease, is a syndrome characterized by loss of at least a quarter of normal weight, by fear of normal weight and, in women, by amenorrhea. An individual's body image may be distorted so that the sufferer cannot judge real weight and wants to diet even when already very thin.

Anorexia nervosa usually begins in adolescence, affecting about 1–2 per cent of teenagers and college students at any time. It is ten times commoner among women than men and is commonest among daughters of professional couples. Up to 10 per cent of sufferers' sisters also have the syndrome.

The symptoms result from secretive self-starvation, usually with excessive exercise, self-induced vomiting, and misuse of laxatives. An anorexic (or anorectic) person may wear layers of baggy clothes to keep warm and to hide the figure. Fine facial hair called lanugo may grow, perhaps as heat insulation. Starvation can cause serious problems such as anaemia, low blood pressure, slow heart rate, swollen ankles, and osteoporosis. Sudden death from heart arrythmias may occur, particularly if the sufferer misuses diuretic tablets to lose weight and also depletes the body's level of potassium.

There is probably no single cause of anorexia nervosa. Social pressure to be thin seems to be an important factor and has increased over the past 20–30 years, along with the incidence of the syndrome. Psychological theories include fear of adulthood and fear of losing parents' attention.

Treatment should start with the general practitioner who should first rule out other illnesses causing similar signs and symptoms. These include depression and disorders of the bowel, pituitary gland, thyroid gland, and ovaries.

If the diagnosis is clearly anorexia nervosa, the general practitioner may refer the sufferer to a psychiatrist or psychologist. Moderately ill sufferers can be treated by cognitive behaviour therapy. A simple form of this is to agree targets for daily calorie intake and for acceptable body weight. The sufferer and the therapist (the general practitioner or a member of the psychiatric team) then monitor progress towards both targets by keeping a diary of food intake and measuring weight regularly. Counselling or more intensely personal psychotherapy may help too. Severe life-threatening complications will need urgent medical treatment in hospital, including rehydration and feeding using a nasogastric tube or an intravenous drip.

About half of anorectic sufferers recover fully within four years, a quarter improve, and a quarter remain severely underweight with menstrual abnormalities. Recovery after ten years is rare and about 3 per cent die within that period, half of them by suicide.

BULIMIA NERVOSA is a syndrome characterized by binge eating, self-induced vomiting and laxative misuse, and fear of fatness. There is some overlap between anorexia nervosa and bulimia but, unlike the former, bulimia may start at any age from about 16 to 40 and is probably more directly linked with ordinary dieting. Bulimic sufferers say that, although they feel depressed and guilty after binges, the 'buzz' and relief after vomiting and purging are addictive. They often respond well to cognitive behaviour therapy.

Bulimia nervosa does not necessarily cause weight loss because the binges – for example of a loaf of bread, a packet of cereal, and several cans of cold baked beans at one sitting – are cancelled out by purging and by brief episodes of starvation. The full syndrome has been found in about 1 per cent of women but mild forms may be much commoner. In one survey of female college students 13 per cent admitted to having had bulimic symptoms.

Bulimia nervosa rarely leads to serious physical illness or death. But repeated vomiting can cause oesophageal burns, salivary gland infections, small tears in the stomach, and occasionally dehydration and chemical imbalances in the blood. Inducing vomiting using fingers may produce two tell-tale signs – bite marks on the knuckles and rotten, pitted teeth.

Those suffering from this condition may obtain advice from the Eating Disorders Association, (see APPENDIX 2: ADDRESSES).

EBOLA VIRUS DISEASE is another name for VIRAL HAEMORRHAGIC FEVER (q.v.). The ebola virus is one of the most virulent microorganisms known. Like the Marburg virus (q.v.), it belongs to the filavirus group which originates in Africa.

EBURNATION is a process of hardening and polishing which takes place at the ends of bones, giving them an ivory-like appearance. It is caused by the wearing away, in consequence of osteoarthrosis, of the smooth plates of cartilage which in health cover the ends of the bones.

ECCHYMOSIS means the discoloured patch resulting from escape of blood into the tissues just under the skin, often from bruising.

ECG (See ELECTROCARDIOGRAM.)

ECHINOCOCCUS is the immature form of a small tapeworm, *Taenia echinococcus*, found in dogs, wolves, and jackals from which human beings become infected, so that they harbour the immature parasite in the form known as hydatid cyst. (See TAENIASIS.)

ECHOCARDIOGRAPHY is the use of ultra-sonics (see ULTRASOUND) for the purpose of examining the heart. By thus recording the echo (hence the name) from the heart of ultra-sound waves it is possible to study, for example, the movements of the heart valves (see HEART), as well as the state of the interior of the heart.

ECHOLALIA is the meaningless repetition, by a person suffering from mental degeneration, of words and phrases addressed to him.

ECHOVIRUSES, of which there are more than 30 known types, occur in all parts of the world. Their full name is Enteric Cytopathogenic Human Orphan (hence the abbreviation, ECHO). They owe their cumbersome full name to the fact that they were originally found in the stools of children without disease. Practically all of them, however, have now been identified with definite diseases. They are more common in children than in adults, and have been responsible for outbreaks of meningitis, common-cold-like illnesses, gastro-intestinal infections, and infections of the respiratory tract. They are particularly dangerous when they infect premature infants, and there have been several outbreaks of such infection in neonatal units, in which premature infants and other seriously ill small babies are nursed. The virus is introduced to such units by mothers, staff and visitors who are unaware that they are carriers of the virus.

ECLAMPSIA is the name applied to convulsions arising in pregnancy. This condition is said to occur in around 50 out of every 100,000 cases of pregnancy. It occurs especially in the later months and at the time of delivery, but a certain proportion of cases occur only after delivery has taken place. The cause is not known although cerebral oedema is thought to occur. In practically all cases the kidneys are profoundly affected.
Symptoms There are several warning symptoms, such as dizziness, headache, vomiting, and the secretion of albumin in the urine. These pre-eclamptic symptoms may be present for some days or weeks before the seizure takes place, and, if a woman is found to have these during antenatal care, preventive measures must be taken. The seizure consists of rigidity

of the body, with unconsciousness, followed by twitching in the face and limbs lasting for one or two minutes and then passing into a state of deep unconsciousness with stertorous breathing. In mild cases there are a few fits at long intervals and the patient recovers consciousness between them, but in severer cases the fits succeed one another so rapidly that there is no appreciable interval. In cases which progress to a fatal termination, the pulse and temperature rise, and cerebral haemorrhage, uraemia or pneumonia may supervene, or the breathing may gradually cease. It accounts for 1 in 12 of all maternal deaths.
Treatment The treatment of the seizures is that generally applicable to convulsions of any kind, with appropriate sedatives given which may include thiopentone sodium (q.v.) given intravenously. Alternatively a combination of chlorpromazine (q.v.) and pethidine (q.v.) may be used. Magnesium sulphate given intra-muscularly sometimes helps to control the fits. The baby's condition should be monitored throughout.

A common presentation of eclampsia is an epileptic fit in the home. The patient should be turned on her side and the airway cleared. The most effective drugs to control eclampsia are intravenous diazepam given slowly or chlormethiazole intravenously, slowly. When the patient is in hospital she should be kept quiet as any stimulus, be it auditory, visual or tactile, may provoke a further epileptiform convulsion. The hypertension should be controlled and urgent Caesarean section undertaken.

ECSTASY refers to a morbid mental condition, associated with an extreme sense of well-being, with a feeling of rapture, and temporary loss of self-control. It often presents as a form of religious insanity, with a feeling of direct communication with God, saintly voices and images being perceived. The patient has a rapt, intense look, and in severe cases is completely incommunicative and absorbed in the experience, unlike the interfering hyperactivity of the manic patient. In milder cases the patient may preach in a high-flown way, as though with a divine mission to help others. Ecstasy may occur in happiness psychosis, schizophrenia, certain forms of epilepsy, and abnormal personalities with appropriate religious training.

The term is also used to refer to a group of hallucinogenic drugs (also known as magic mushrooms, MDMA; see DRUG ADDICTION).

ECT (See ELECTROCONVULSIVE THERAPY.)

ECTHYMA is the term applied to a pustular eruption accompanied by surrounding inflammation. The pustules burst and discharge, leaving pigmented scars.

ECTO- is a prefix meaning on the outside.

ECTOPIC means out of the usual place. For example, in congenital displacement of the heart outside the thoracic cavity it is said to be ectopic, while an 'ectopic gestation' means a pregnancy outside of the womb.

ECTOPIC BEAT A heart muscle contraction that is outside the normal sequence of the cardiac cycle. The impulse is generated outside the usual focus of the sinoatrial node (q.v.). Also known as extrasystoles, ectopic beats are called ventricular if they arise from a focus in the ventricles (q.v.) and supraventricular if they arise in the atria (q.v.). They may cause no symptoms and the affected subject may be unaware of them. The beat may, however, be the result of heart disease or may be caused by nicotine or caffeine. If persistent, the individual may suffer from irregular rhythm or ventricular fibrillation and need treatment with anti-arrhythmic drugs.

ECTROMELIA means the absence of a limb or limbs, from congenital causes.

ECTROPION (see EYE DISEASES).

ECZEMA (see DERMATITIS).

EDENTULOUS Lacking teeth: this may be because teeth have not developed or because they have been removed or fallen out.

EDTA Ethylenediamine tetraacetic acid is used to treat poisoning with metals such as lead and strontium. A chelating agent EDTA is used in the form of sodium or calcium salts. The stable chelate compounds resulting from the treatment are excreted in the urine.

EEG (See ELECTRO-ENCEPHALOGRAPHY.)

EFFERENT is the term applied to vessels which convey away blood or a secretion from a part, or to nerves which carry nerve impulses outwards from the nerve-centres.

EFFLEURAGE is a form of massage by gentle stroking movements.

EFFORT SYNDROME, also known as Da Costa's syndrome, is a condition in which symptoms occur, such as palpitations and shortness of breath, which are attributed by the patient to disorder of the heart. There is no evidence, however, of heart disease, and psychological factors are thought to be of importance. (See PSYCHOSOMATIC DISEASES.)

EFFUSION means a pouring out of fluid from the vessels in which it is naturally enclosed into the substance of the organs, or into cavities of the body, as a result of inflammation or of injury: for example, pleurisy with effusion, effusions into joints, and effusion of blood.

EGG is a term applied to any animal ovum.

EISENMENGER REACTION A condition in which the subject suffers from a defect in one of the dividing walls (septum) of the heart and this is accompanied by pulmonary hypertension (q.v.). The defect allows blood low in oxygen to flow from the right to the left side of the heart and be pumped into the aorta, which normally carries oxygenated blood to the body. The patient suffers from cyanosis and has a dusky blue appearance. There is an increase in red blood cells as the body attempts to compensate for the lowered oxygen delivery. The condition requires early surgical repair of the septal defect.

EJACULATION The expulsion of semen from the penis during orgasm. The stimulation of sexual intercourse or masturbation produces a spinal reflex action that causes ejaculation. The semen comprises several constituents arising from Cowper's gland, the prostate gland, the testicles, and the seminal vesicles and these are discharged in sequence. (See also PREMATURE EJACULATION.)

ELBOW is the joint formed between the humerus above and the radius and ulna below. The humerus has at its lower end a rounded surface, against which the head of the radius moves, and a deep groove to which a saddle-shaped surface at the upper end of the ulna fits. The head of the radius rests upon a projection of the ulna and is bound to it by a stout annular ligament, within which it can rotate. Two important movements take place at this joint: a flail-like backward and forward movement of the radius and ulna moving together upon the humerus, and a rotary movement of the radius on the ulna, by which the lower end of the radius is crossed over the ulna and again brought side by side with it, according as the hand is turned palm downwards and palm upwards. The joint is secured at the sides by strong lateral ligaments, and at the back and front is covered by powerful muscles. The ulnar nerve as it passes down to the forearm has an exposed position behind the inner edge of the humerus at its lower end; this is popularly known as the 'funny- bone'. The elbow is seldom dislocated, but a not uncommon accident consists in the chipping off, through a fall on the elbow, of the olecranon process which forms the point behind the joint.

ELECTRICAL INJURIES are usually caused by the passage through the body of an electric current of high voltage owing to accidental contact with a live wire or to a discharge of lightning. The general effects produced are included under the term electric shock, but vary greatly in degree. The local effects include spasmodic contraction of muscles, fracture of bones, and in severe cases more or less widespread destruction of tissues which may amount simply to burns of the skin or may include necrosis of masses of muscle and internal organs. Fright due to unexpectedness of the shock and pain due to the sudden cramp of muscles are the commonest symptoms and in most cases pass off in a few minutes or less. In more severe cases, especially when the person has remained in contact with a live wire for some time or has been unable to let go of the electrical contact owing to spasmodic contraction of his muscles, the effects are more pronounced and may be those of concussion of the brain or of compression of the brain. (See BRAIN, DISEASES OF.) In still severer cases, death may ensue either from paralysis of the respiration or stoppage of the heart's action. In either instance, the condition may be at first one of suspended animation, and death may not ensue if prompt measures are taken for treatment.

In Britain there are an average of 110 deaths a year from electrocution, half of these occurring in the home.)

Treatment No electrical apparatus or switch should be touched by anyone who is in metallic contact with the ground, such as through a metal pipe, especially, for example, from a bath. The first action is to break the current. This can sometimes be done by turning off a switch. If the victim is grasping or in contact with a live wire, the contact may be severed with safety only by someone wearing rubber gloves or rubber boots, but as these are not likely to be immediately available, his hands may be protected by a thick wrapping of dry cloth, or the live wire may be hooked or pushed out of the way with a long wooden stick. If the injured person is unconscious, and especially if breathing has stopped, *artificial respiration should be applied* as described in APPENDIX: BASIC FIRST AID, Electrocution. When the patient begins to breathe again, he must be treated for shock and professional help obtained urgently.

ELECTROCARDIOGRAM (ECG) is a record of the variations in electric potential which occur in the heart as it contracts and relaxes. Any muscle in use produces an electric current, but when an individual is at rest the main muscular current in the body is that produced by the heart. This can be recorded by connecting the outside of the body by electrodes with an instrument known as an electrocardiograph. The patient is connected to the electrocardiograph by leads from either the arms and legs or different points on the chest. The normal electrocardiogram of each heart-beat shows one wave corresponding to the activity of the atria and four waves corresponding to the phases of each ventricular beat (see illustration). Various readily recognizable changes are seen in cases in which the heart is acting in an

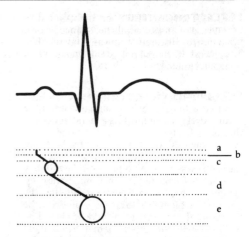

(a) origin of the sinus impulse
(b) conduction through the sino-atrial junction
(c) atrial activation
(d) conduction through the atrioventricular junction
(e) spread of activation within the ventricles

Tracing of normal electrical impulse that initiates heartbeat (after *The Cardiac Arrhythmias Pocket Book*, Boehrringer, Ingelheim).

abnormal manner, or in which one or other side of the heart is hypertrophied. This record therefore forms a useful aid in many cases of heart disease. The main applications of the electrocardiogram are in the diagnosis of myocardial infarction and of cardiac arrhythmias.

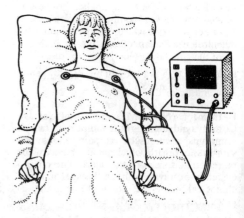

Patient connected via electrodes on chest to electrocardiograph (heart-monitoring machine).

ELECTROCAUTERY or GALVANOCAUTERY. The use of an electrically heated needle or loop to destroy diseased or unwanted tissue. Benign growths, warts and polyps can be removed with this technique.

ELECTROCOCHLEOGRAPHY is a method of recording the activity of the cochlea, the part of the inner ear concerned with hearing. (See EAR.)

ELECTROCONVULSIVE THERAPY ECT is a controversial treatment for severe depression. Electrical shocks are administered by electrodes placed on the skull to induce seizures of the brain. The patient is given a general anaesthetic and muscle relaxants. Up to 12 treatments may be given over a month and improvement usually shows after the third treatment. Amnesia is often a side-effect of ECT. Widely used at one time, the treatment is now given only to carefully selected patients.

ELECTRO-ENCEPHALOGRAPHY (EEG) In the brain there is a regular, rhythmical change of electric potential, due to the rhythmic discharge of energy by nerve cells. These changes can be recorded graphically and the 'brain waves' examined. These records – electro-encephalograms – are useful in diagnosis. For example, the abnormal electro-encephalogram occurring in epilepsy is characteristic of this disease. The normal waves, known as alpha waves, occur with a frequency of 10 per second. Abnormal waves, with a frequency of 7 or less per second, are known as delta waves and occur in the region of cerebral tumours and in the brains of epileptics.

ELECTROLYTES Substances, for example, potassium chloride, whose molecules split into their constituent electrically charged particles, known as ions, when dissolved in fluid. In medicine the term is customarily used to describe the ion itself. The description 'serum electrolyte concentration' means the amounts of separate ions – for example, sodium and chloride in the case of salt – present in the serum of the circulating blood. Various diseases alter the amounts of electrolytes in the blood, either because more than normal are lost through vomiting or diarrhoea, or electrolytes may be retained because the kidney is not excreting them properly. Measurements of electrolytes are valuable clues to the type of disease and provide a means of monitoring a course of treatment. Electrolyte imbalances can be corrected by administering appropriate substances orally or intravenously or by dialysis (q.v.).

ELECTROMYOGRAPHY The recording of electrical activity in a muscle using electrodes placed in the fibres. The procedure is used to diagnose muscle and nerve disorders and to assess recovery in certain types of paralysis.

ELECTRON is one of the subatomic particles. (See RADIOTHERAPY.)

ELECTRO-OCULOGRAPHY is a method of recording movements of the eyes, which is proving of value in assessing the function of the retina (see EYE.)

ELECTROPHORESIS means the migration of charged particles between electrodes. A simple method of electrophoresis, known as paper electrophoresis, has been introduced which is proving of value in examining the proteins in body fluids. This method consists in applying the protein-containing solution as a spot or a streak to a strip of filter paper which has been soaked in buffer solution and across the ends of which a potential difference is then applied for some hours.

ELECTRORETINOGRAM An electroretinogram is the record of an electrical response of visual receptors in the retina (see EYE), which can be measured with corneal electrodes.

ELEPHANTIASIS is a clinical state characterized by chronically oedematous and thickened tissue, especially involving the lower extremities and genitalia, regardless of the cause. It arises from repeated attacks of inflammation of the skin and subcutaneous tissue, with concurrent obstruction of lymphatic vessels. In a tropical country, the usual cause is lymphatic filariasis; however, podoconiosis (resulting from silica particles which penetrate the intact skin of the feet) – which has a more limited geographical distribution – should also be considered.
FILARIAL ELEPHANTIASIS *Wuchereria bancrofti* and *Brugia malayi* are conveyed to man by a mosquito bite. Patrick Manson first delineated the man–mosquito component in the life-cycle at Amoy, China in 1875–9; G. C. Low (1900) was responsible for elucidation of the mosquito–man cycle. Resultant lymphatic obstruction gives rise to enlargement and disfiguration, with thickening of the skin (resembling that of an elephant) in one or both lower limbs and occasionally genitalia (involving particularly the scrotum). Elephantiasis affecting an upper limb is unusual; when it occurs, it is usually associated with *B. malayi* infection. Concurrent involvement of the abdominal lymphatics can give rise to chyluria. By the time the condition is clinically manifest, lymphatic damage is invariably irreversible, and evidence (including serology) of an active filarial infection is usually absent. However, where evidence of continuing activity exists, a course of diethylcarbamazine should be administered (see FILARIASIS). Relief can be obtained by using elastic bandaging, massage, rest, and elevation of the affected limb. Surgery is sometimes indicated. In prevention, destruction of mosquitoes is important.

ELISA (See ENZYME-LINKED IMMUNO-SORBENT ASSAY.)

ELIXIR is a liquid preparation of a potent or nauseous drug made pleasant to the taste by the addition of aromatic substances and sugar. The name was specially applied to several preparations greatly used in the Middle Ages, which had the effect of acting as a tonic to the stomach and relieving constipation, and which were known, for example, as the elixir of Paracelsus, the elixir of long life. The main constituent of all of these was tincture of aloes.

EMACIATION means pronounced wasting, and is a common symptom of many diseases, particularly of those which are associated with a prolonged or repeated rise of temperature, such as tuberculosis. It is also associated with diseases of the alimentary system in which digestion is inefficient, or in which the food is not fully absorbed: for example, in diarrhoea of long-standing, whatever its cause. It is also a marked feature of malignant disease.

EMBALMING (see DEAD, DISPOSAL OF THE).

EMBOLECTOMY Surgical removal of a clot or embolus to clear an obstruction in an artery. The obstruction may be cleared by inserting a balloon (Fogarty) catheter into the blood vessel or by surgical incision through the arterial wall. Embolectomy may be a life-saving operation when a patient has a pulmonary embolism (q.v.).

EMBOLISM means the plugging of a small blood-vessel by material which has been carried through the larger vessels by the blood stream. It is due usually to fragments of a clot which has formed in some vessel, or to small portions carried off from the edge of a heart-valve when this organ is diseased; but the plug may also be a small mass of bacteria, or a fragment of a tumour, or even a mass of air bubbles sucked into the veins during operations on the neck. The result is usually more or less destruction of the organ or part of an organ supplied by the obstructed vessel. This is particularly the case in the brain, where softening of the brain, with aphasia or apoplexy, may be the result. If the plug is a fragment of malignant tumour, a new growth develops at the spot; and if it is a mass of bacteria, an abscess forms there. Air-embolism occasionally causes sudden death in the case of wounds in the neck, the air bubbles completely stopping the flow of blood. Fat-embolism is a condition which has been known to cause death, masses of fat, in consequence of such an injury as a fractured bone, finding their way into the circulation and stopping the blood in its passage through the lungs. (See also PULMONARY EMBOLISM.)

EMBROCATIONS are mixtures, usually of an oily nature, intended for external application in cases of rheumatism, sprains, and other painful conditions. Their action is due partly to the massage employed in rubbing in the embrocations, partly to the counter-irritant action of the drugs which they contain. (See LINIMENTS.)

EMBRYO means the fetus in the womb prior to the end of the second month. (See FETUS.)

EMBRYO TRANSFER is the process whereby the initial stages of procreation are produced outside the human body and completed in the uterus or womb. The procedure is also known as EMBRYO TRANSPLANTATION and IN VITRO FERTILIZATION. It consists of extracting an ovum (or egg) from the prospective mother's body and placing this in a dish where it is mixed with the male partner's semen and special nutrient fluids. After the ovum is fertilized by the sperm it is transferred to another dish containing a special nutrient solution. Here it is left for several days while the normal early stages of development (see FETUS) take place. The early embryo (q.v.) as it has then become, is then implanted in the mother's uterus, where it 'takes root' and develops as a normal fetus.

The first 'test-tube baby', to use the popular, and widely used, term for such a child was born by Caesarean section in England on 25 July 1978. Many other children, conceived in this manner, have since been born, and, though only 10 per cent of women conceive at the first attempt, the overall success rate is improving. Embryo transplantation and research are controversial procedures and in many countries are controlled by legislation.

EMESIS means vomiting (q.v.).

EMETICS are drugs or other means which produce vomiting.
Varieties Emetics are divided into two important classes: (1) direct emetics, which, being taken by the mouth, irritate the stomach and so cause vomiting, and (2) indirect emetics, which will cause vomiting, even when injected into the blood, by action upon the centre in the brain controlling the act of vomiting. Examples of the first type are sulphate of zinc, mustard in water, alum, sal volatile, copper sulphate, and even copious draughts of warm salt water. In the second class we have apomorphine, ipecacuanha, and tartar emetic; to this class also belong such means as tickling the throat, or presenting evil-smelling substances to the nose.
Uses Emetics are now rarely used and are contraindicated for several types of poison. They must only be given if the victim is conscious, one drink of salty water, containing sodium chloride (common salt), or a dose of Ipecacuanha Syrup USP: 15 millilitres followed by 200 millilitres (a tumblerful) of water, should be given. Medical advice should be sought before using emetics for the treatment of poison-

ing. Emetics in doses too small to produce vomiting are often used in cough mixtures to render the secretions in the bronchial tubes more fluid and therefore more easy to cough up. Wine of ipecacuanha is used for this purpose.

EMETINE is one of the active principles of ipecacuanha. (See IPECACUANHA.)

EMMETROPIA is a term applied to the normal condition of the eye as regards refraction of light rays. In this state when the muscles in the eyeball are completely relaxed the focusing power is accurately adjusted for parallel rays, so that vision is perfect for distant objects.

EMOLLIENTS are substances which have a softening and soothing effect upon the skin. They include dusting powders such as French chalk, oils such as olive oil and almond oil, and fats such as the various pharmacopoeial preparations of paraffin, suet, and lard. Glycerin is also an excellent emollient.
Uses They are used in various inflammatory conditions such as eczema, when the skin becomes hard, cracked, and painful. They may be used in the form of a dusting powder, an oil or an ointment.

EMPHYSEMA means an abnormal presence of air in certain parts of the body. In its restricted sense, however, it is generally employed to designate an affection of the lungs, of which there are two forms. In one of these there is over-distension of the air-cells of these organs, and in parts destruction of their walls, giving rise to the formation of large sacs, from the rupture and running together of a number of contiguous air-vesicles. This is much the more common of the two forms and is the one which is usually meant when the term 'emphysema' is used. In the other form the air is infiltrated into the connective tissue beneath the pleura and between the pulmonary air-cells, constituting what is known as *acute interstitial emphysema*.
Causes Where a portion of the lung has become wasted, or its vesicular structure permanently obliterated by disease, without corresponding falling-in of the chest wall, the neighbouring air-vesicles, or some of them, undergo dilatation to fill the vacuum.
    In cases of bronchitis, and especially of bronchial asthma, where numbers of the smaller bronchial tubes become obstructed, the air in the pulmonary vesicles remains imprisoned, the force of expiration being insufficient to expel it; on the other hand, the stronger force of inspiration being adequate to overcome the resistance, the air-cells tend to become more and more distended, and permanent alterations in their structure, including emphysema, are the result.
    Emphysema also arises from exertion involving expiratory efforts, during which the glottis is constricted, as in paroxysms of coughing, in straining, and in lifting heavy weights. Whooping-cough is well known as an exciting cause of emphysema.
    Smoking is an important cause of emphysema. According to the United States Surgeon General's 1984 report, cigarette smoking is the major cause of chronic obstructive lung disease morbidity and 80 to 90 per cent of cases are attributable to smoking.
Symptoms In the affected portions of the lungs there are loss of the natural elasticity of the air-cells, destruction of many of the pulmonary capillary blood-vessels, and diminution of aerating surface for the blood. As a consequence there is a strain on the heart and the venous system generally, leading to dilatation of the right side of the heart, and so to oedema. The chief symptom in this complaint is shortness of breath, more or less constant but greatly aggravated by exertion, and by attacks of bronchitis, to which people suffering from emphysema are specially liable. The respiration is of a wheezy character. In severe forms of the disease the patient comes to acquire a peculiar bluish and bloated appearance, and the configuration of the chest is altered, assuming the character known as the *barrel-shaped chest*.
Treatment The patient's general health should be improved and he or she should stop smoking and avoid polluted environments. Regular physiotherapy to drain the lungs of fluid and improve breathing is of great help. Emphysematous patients are prone to infection of the lungs and they should have annual immunization against influenza. During attacks of urgent breathlessness anti-spasmodic remedies should be given, while inhalation of oxygen will often afford marked and speedy relief.
SURGICAL EMPHYSEMA is the term applied when air is present under the skin. It may get there, for example, if the lungs are wounded through the chest wall, or if the wind-pipe is pierced at any point in its path.

EMPIRICAL treatment is that school of treatment which is founded simply on experience. Because a given remedy has been successful in the treatment of a certain group of symptoms, it is assumed, by those who uphold this principle, that it will be successful in the treatment of other cases presenting similar groups of symptoms, without any inquiry as to the cause of the symptoms or reason underlying the action of the remedy. It is the contrary of 'rational' or 'scientific' treatment. Sometimes a course of treatment must perforce be empirical for want of knowledge.

EMPROSTHOTONOS is the term applied to the spasm of the belly muscles that occurs in tetanus, making the body arch forwards.

EMPYEMA is an accumulation of pus within a cavity, the term being generally reserved for collections of pus within one of the pleural cavities. Since the advent of antibiotics, the condition is relatively uncommon in developed countries. The condition is virtually an abscess, and therefore gives rise to the general symptoms accompanying that condition; but, on account of the thick unyielding wall of the chest, it is unlikely to burst through the surface, and therefore it is of particular importance that the condition should be recognized early, and, as a rule, treated surgically.

The condition most commonly follows an attack of pneumonia. It may also occur in the advanced stage of pulmonary tuberculosis. Empyema also occurs at times through infection from some serious disease in neighbouring organs, such as cancer of the gullet, or follows upon wounds penetrating the chest wall.

EMULSIONS are mixtures containing oily substances in a state of very fine division. The division is effected and the oil kept suspended in the fluid by means of alkalis and sticky ingredients such as albumin, glycerin, or mucilage. Milk is an example of a perfect emulsion of fat globules each surrounded by an envelope of albumin. The various preparations of cod-liver oil are usually emulsified by the aid of glycerin. The oil is not only rendered more devoid of taste, but digestion and absorption are also rendered easier by emulsification.

ENALAPRIL A drug introduced in 1986 and used to treat hypertension (see ESSENTIAL HYPERTENSION). It reduces the action of angiotensin (q.v.) and this reduces blood vessel constriction.

ENAMEL (see TEETH).

ENCEPHALITIS means inflammation or infection of the brain, usually caused by a virus. It occurs throughout the world and affects all racial groups and ages. Rarely it occurs as a complication of common viral disease such as measles, mumps, glandular fever, or chickenpox. It may occur with no evidence of infection elsewhere such as herpes simplex encephalitis, the most common form seen in Europe and America. Rabies is another form of viral encephalitis, and the HIV virus which causes AIDS invades the brain to cause another form of encephalitis. In some countries – North and South America, Japan and east Asia and Russia – there may be epidemics spread by the bite of mosquitoes or ticks.

The clinical features begin with symptoms like influenza – aches, temperature and wretchedness; then the patient develops a headache with drowsiness, confusion, and neck stiffness. Severely ill patients develop changes in behaviour, abnormalities of speech and deterioration to come with epileptic seizures. Some develop paralysis and memory loss. CT and MRI brain scans shows brain swelling, and damage to the temporal lobes if the herpes virus is involved. Electroencephalography, which records the

brainwaves, is abnormal. Diagnosis is possible by an examination of the blood or other body fluids for antibody reaction to the virus, and modern laboratory techniques are very specific.

In general, drugs are not effective against viruses – antibiotics are of no use. Herpes encephalitis does respond to treatment with the anti-viral agent, acyclovir. Treatment is supportive: patients should be given painkillers, fluid replacement drugs to reduce brain swelling and to counter epilepsy if it occurs. Fortunately, most sufferers from encephalitis make a complete recovery but some are left severely disabled with physical defects, personality and memory disturbance and epileptic fits. Rabies is always fatal and the changes found in patients with AIDS are almost always progressive. Except in very specific circumstances, it is not possible to be immunized against encephalitis.

ENCEPHALOID is the name applied to a form of cancer which, to the naked eye, resembles the tissue of the brain.

ENCEPHALOMYELITIS means inflammation of the substance of both brain and spinal cord.

ENCEPHALOPATHY is the term used to describe certain conditions in which there are signs of cerebral irritation without any localized lesion to account for them. The two best examples are *hypertensive encephalopathy* and *lead encephalopathy*. In the former, which occurs in the later stages of chronic glomerulonephritis, or uraemia (q.v.), the headache, convulsions, and delirium which constitute the main symptoms are supposed to be due to a deficient blood-supply to the brain. In the latter the symptoms are probably due to spasm of the arteries in the brain.

ENCHONDROMA means a tumour formed of cartilage. (See TUMOUR.)

ENCYSTED means enclosed within a bladder-like wall. The term is applied to parasites, collections of pus, etc., which are shut off from surrounding tissues by a membrane or by adhesions.

ENDARTERITIS means inflammation of the inner coat of an artery. (See ARTERIES, DISEASES OF.)

ENDEMIC is a term applied to diseases which exist in particular localities or among certain races. Some diseases, which are at times epidemic over wide districts, have a restricted area where they are always endemic, and from which they spread. For example, both cholera and plague are endemic in certain parts of Asia.

ENDO- is a prefix meaning situated inside.

ENDOCARDITIS Inflammation of the lining, valves and muscle of the heart. The main causes are bacterial and virus infections and rheumatic fever and the condition occurs most often in patients whose endocardium is already damaged by congenital deformities or whose immune system has been suppressed by drugs. Infection may be introduced into the bloodstream during dental treatment or surgical procedures, especially on the heart or on the gastrointestinal system. Treatment is with large doses of antibiotic drugs.

ENDOCRINE GLANDS are organs whose function is to secrete into the blood or lymph substances known as hormones which play an important part in general chemical changes or the activities of other organs at a distance. Some organs have a double function, such as the pancreas, which pours digestive secretions by a duct into the intestine, and, at the same time, has an endocrine or internal secretion (insulin) which is secreted direct into the blood. Various diseases arise as the result of defects or excess in the internal secretions of the different glands. The chief endocrine glands are the thyroid, adrenal, pituitary, parathyroid, pancreas, ovaries, and testicles.

THYROID GLAND   This gland, situated in front of the neck, produces a secretion which has an important effect in regulating the general metabolism of the body. When it is defective, the conditions known as myxoedema and cretinism result; whilst excess of the secretion is associated with thyrotoxicosis. The active principle of this secretion is thyroxine and this is used in patients in whom the secretion is defective.

ADRENAL GLANDS   These two glands, also known AS SUPRARENAL GLANDS, lie immediately above the kidneys. The central or medullary portion of the glands forms the secretions known as adrenaline or epinephrine, and noradrenaline. Adrenaline acts upon structures innervated by sympathetic nerves; its action is therefore said to be sympathomimetic. Briefly, the blood-vessels of the skin and of the abdominal viscera (except the intestines) are constricted, and at the same time the arteries of the muscles and the coronary arteries are dilated; systolic blood-pressure rises; blood-sugar increases; the metabolic rate rises; muscle fatigue is diminished. Adrenaline can be synthetically prepared in the laboratory. This substance is widely used in medicine in 1 in 1000 solutions, for the purpose of checking bleeding, relieving congestion of mucous membranes, for the relief of asthma, and in the treatment of anaphylactic shock. The superficial or cortical part of the glands produce a series of chemical substances which have as their basis a complicated steroid nucleus. The best known of these are aldosterone, cortisone, hydrocortisone, and deoxycortone acetate. These substances are essential for the maintenance of life. It is the absence of these substances, due to atrophy or destruction of the suprarenal cortex, that is responsible for the condition known as Addison's disease (q.v.).

PITUITARY GLAND   This gland is attached to the base of the brain and rests in a hollow on the base of the skull immediately above the hinder part of the throat. The pituitary gland is the most important of all endocrine glands and has been called the conductor of the endocrine orchestra. It consists of two embryologically and functionally distinct lobes. The function of the anterior lobe depends on the secretion by the hypothalamus (q.v.) of certain 'neuro-hormones' which are carried down the infundibular stalk in the hypophyseal portal system. These neuro-hormones are secreted into the portal venous system flowing from the median eminence of the hypothalamus to the anterior lobe of the pituitary gland and control the secretion of the pituitary trophic hormones. The hypothalamic centres involved in the control of specific pituitary hormones appear to be anatomically separate. Through the pituitary trophic hormones the activity of the thyroid, adrenal cortex and the sex glands is controlled. A reciprocal relationship between the anterior pituitary and the target glands exists. The liberation of trophic hormones is inhibited by a rising concentration of the circulating hormone of the target gland and stimulated by a fall in its concentration. Six trophic hormones are formed by the anterior pituitary. Growth hormone and prolactin are simple proteins formed in the acidophil cells. Follicle-stimulating hormone, luteinizing hormone and thyroid-stimulating hormone are glycoproteins formed in the basophil cells. Adrenocorticotrophic hormone (ACTH), although a polypeptide, is derived from basophil cells. The chromophobe cell, once thought to be inactive, is in fact the stem cell and 50 per cent of chromophobe adenomas secrete prolactin.

All these pituitary hormones are polypeptides. When used therapeutically they cannot be given by mouth, as they would be digested in the gastro-intestinal tract. They are therefore prepared in powder form for intramuscular injection. The powder should be dissolved carefully, and after injection the site should be massaged to ensure efficient absorption.

The posterior pituitary lobe, or neuro-hypophysis, is closely connected with the hypothalamus by the hypothalmic-hypophyseal tracts. It is concerned with the production or storage of oxytocin and vasopressin (the anti-diuretic hormone).

PITUITARY HORMONES   Rapid advances have taken place in the past decade in the methods of assay of pituitary hormones and in the production and preparation of these hormones for clinical use. Growth hormone, gonadotrophic hormone, adrenocorticotrophic hormone and thyrotrophic hormones can be assayed in blood or urine by radio-immuno-assay techniques. Growth hormone extracted from human pituitary glands obtained at autopsy was available for clinical use until 1985 when it was withdrawn as it is believed to carry the virus responsible for Creutzfeldt-Jakob disease. However growth hormone produced by DNA recombinant techniques is now available as Somatonorm.

Human pituitary gonadotrophins are readily obtained from post-menopausal urine. Commercial extracts from this source are available and are effective for treatment of infertility due to gonadotrophin insufficiency.

The adrenocorticotrophic hormone is extracted from animal pituitary glands and has been available therapeutically for many years. It is used as a test of adrenal function, and, under certain circumstances, in conditions for which cortico-steroid therapy is indicated. The pharmacologically active polypeptide of ACTH has now been synthesized. It is called tetracosactrin, and as it is a pure substance it is prescribed by weight. Thyrotrophic hormone is also available but it has no therapeutic application. Melanocyte-stimulating hormone (MSH) does not occur in the human pituitary.

HYPOTHALAMIC RELEASING HORMONES which affect the release of each of the six anterior pituitary hormones have been identified. Their blood levels are only one- thousandth of those of the pituitary trophic hormones. The release of thyrotrophin, adrenocorticotrophin, growth hormone, follicle-stimulating hormone and luteinizing hormone is stimulated whilst release of prolactin is inhibited. The structure of the releasing hormones for TSH, FSH-LH, GH and, most recently, ACTH is known and they have all been synthesized. Thyrotrophin-releasing hormone (TRH) is already in clinical use as a diagnostic test of thyroid function but it has no therapeutic application. FSH-LH-releasing hormone provides a useful diagnostic test of gonadotrophine reserve in patients with pituitary disease and is now used in the treatment of infertility and amenorrhoea in patients with functional hypothalamic disturbance. As this is the commonest variety of secondary amenorrhoea the potential use is great. The therapeutic use of GH-releasing hormone and corticotrophin releasing hormone has yet to be established. Most cases of congenital deficiency of GH, FSH, LH and ACTH are due to defects in the hypothalamic production of releasing hormone and are not a primary pituitary defect, so that the therapeutic implication of this recently synthesized group of releasing hormones is considerable.

Galactorrhoea (q.v.) is frequently due to a microadenoma of the pituitary and less frequently results from impairment of the tonic inhibition exerted on the pituitary by the hypothalamus. Dopamine is the prolactin-release inhibiting hormone. Its duration of action is short so its therapeutic value is limited. However, bromocriptine is a dopamine agonist with a more prolonged action and is effective treatment for galactorrhoea whether this is due to a prolactin-secreting adenoma or to impairment of the tonic inhibition exerted by the prolactin-release inhibiting hormone.

PARATHYROID GLANDS   These are four minute glands lying at the side of, or behind, the thyroid. They have a certain effect in controlling the absorption of lime salts by the bones and other tissues. When their secretion is defective, tetany occurs.

PANCREAS   This gland is situated in the upper part of the abdomen and, in addition to the digestive ferments which it produces, a substance known as insulin is absorbed from it into the circulating blood. This has the effect of adapting sugary foods for incorporation in the muscles and other tissues that particularly require such foodstuffs. Lack of it is followed by the production of the disease known as diabetes mellitus.

OVARIES AND TESTICLES   In addition to their main function of producing reproductive cells, these organs secrete substances which have a general effect upon the other bodily tissues.

The ovary secretes at least two hormones, known, respectively, as oestradiol (follicular hormone) and progesterone (corpus luteum hormone). Oestradiol develops (under the stimulus of the anterior pituitary lobe) each time an ovum in the ovary becomes mature, causes extensive proliferation of the endometrium lining the uterus, a stage ending with shedding of the ovum about 14 days before the onset of menstruation. The corpus luteum, which then forms, secretes both progesterone and oestradiol. Progesterone brings about great activity of the glands in the endometrium. The uterus is now ready for the nesting of the ovum if it is fertilized. If fertilization does not occur, the corpus luteum degenerates, the hormones cease acting, and menstruation takes place.

The hormone secreted by the testicles is known as testosterone. It is responsible for the growth of the male secondary sex characteristics.

ENDOCRINOLOGY   The study of the endocrine system, the substances (hormones) it secretes and its disorders (see ENDOCRINE GLANDS.)

ENDOGENOUS   Coming from within the body. Endogenous depression, for instance, occurs as a result of causes inside a person.

ENDOMETRIOSIS is the condition in which the endometrium (i.e. the cells lining the interior of the uterus) is found in other parts of the body. The most common site of such misplaced endometrium is the muscle of the uterus. The next most common site is the ovary, followed by the peritoneum (q.v.) lining the pelvis (q.v.), but it also occurs anywhere in the bowel. The cause is not known. It never occurs before puberty and seldom after the menopause. The main symptoms it produces are menorrhagia (q.v.), dyspareunia (q.v.), painful menstruation and pelvic pain. Treatment is usually by removal of the affected area, but in some cases satisfactory results are obtained from the administration of progestogens (q.v.) such as norethisterone (q.v.), norethynodrel (q.v.) and danazol (q.v.).

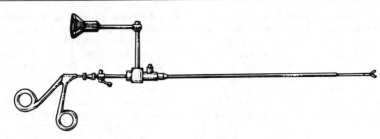

Percutaneous nephroscope and stone forceps.

ENDOMETRITIS means inflammation of the mucous membrane lining the womb. (See UTERUS, DISEASES OF.)

ENDOMETRIUM is the mucous membrane which lines the interior of the uterus.

END ORGAN A structure at the end of a peripheral nerve that acts as receptor for a sensation. For example, the olfactory nerves have end organs that pick up smells.

ENDORPHINS are peptides (q.v.) produced in the brain which have a pain-relieving action. Hence their alternative name of opiate peptides. Their name is derived from *endo*genous mor*phine*. They have been defined as endogenous opiates or any naturally occurring substances in the brain with pharmacological actions resembling opiate alkaloids such as morphine. There is some evidence that the pain-relieving action of acupuncture (q.v.) may be due to the release of these opiate peptides. It has also been suggested that they may have an anti-psychotic action and therefore of value in the treatment of major psychotic illnesses such as schizophrenia.

ENDOSCOPE A tube-shaped instrument inserted into a cavity in the body to investigate and treat disorders. It is flexible and equipped with lenses and a light source. Examples of endoscopes are the cystoscope for use in the bladder, the gastroscope for examining the stomach and the arthroscope for looking into joints. (See FIBREOPTIC ENDOSCOPY.)

ENDOTHELIUM is the membrane lining various vessels and cavities of the body, such as the pleura, pericardium, peritoneum, lymphatic vessels, blood-vessels, and joints. It consists of a fibrous layer covered with thin flat cells, which render the surface perfectly smooth and secrete the fluid for its lubrication.

ENDOTOXIN A poison produced by certain bacteria that is released after the micro-organisms die. Endotoxins can cause fever and shock, the latter by rendering the walls of blood vessels permeable so that fluid leaks into the tissues, with a consequent sharp fall in blood pressure.

ENDOTRACHEAL INTUBATION Insertion of a rubber or plastic tube through the nose or mouth into the trachea. The tube often has a cuff at its lower end which, when inflated, provides an airtight seal. This allows an anaesthetist to supply oxygen or anaesthetic gases to the lungs and know exactly how much the patient is receiving. Endotracheal intubation is necessary to undertake artificial ventilation of a patient.

ENEMA means an injection of fluid into the bowel.
Uses PURGATIVE ENEMAS are given generally in large bulk, so as to distend the rectum; they also contain various stimulating substances. For an adult, 450 to 900 ml (1 to 2 pints) are slowly and carefully injected, for a young child about 170 ml (6 ounces). Enemas are best given by a professional or by a carer or parent who has been shown how to do it.

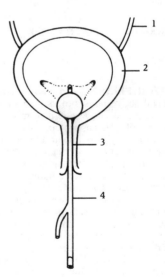

1 ureter
2 bladder
3 urethra
4 cystoscope

Cystoscope: an endoscope for examining inside the bladder.

DISPOSABLE ENEMAS are largely supplanting the traditional soap-and-water enemas – largely on account of their convenience. The ingredients, usually sodium diphosphate and sodium phosphate in the case of a purgative enema, are contained in around 100 ml of solution in a small plastic bag with tube and plug.

MINIATURE ENEMAS are in increasing use. Their great advantage is that they are of a much smaller volume – only 2 millilitres, and therefore much more comfortable for the patient. They are also prepared much more easily and are supplied ready made up in a plastic container with a soft nozzle. They may be self-administered. As a rule, a movement of the bowels occurs within fifteen minutes. A widely used formula for such a miniature enema is: 5 mg of bisacodyl; 0·5 millilitre of glycerin; made up to 2 millilitres with Sulphated Castor Oil BPC.

ENGAGEMENT   The event during pregnancy when the presenting part of the baby, usually the head, moves down into the mother's pelvis.

ENKEPHALINS are peptides that have a pain-killing effect similar to that of endorphins (q.v.). Produced by certain nerve endings and in the brain, enkephalins (also spelt encephalins) are also believed to act as a sedative and mood changer.

ENOPHTHALMOS is a term applied to abnormal retraction of the eye into its socket: for example, when the sympathetic nerve in the neck is paralysed.

ENSURE (see ENTERAL FEEDING).

ENTAMOEBA (see AMOEBA).

ENTERAL FEEDING   In severely ill patients the metabolic responses to tissue damage may be sufficient to cause a reduction of muscle mass and of plasma proteins. This state of catabolism may also impair the immune response to infection and delay the healing of wounds. It is probable that as many as one half of patients who have had a major operation a week previously show evidence of protein malnutrition. This can be detected clinically by a loss of weight and a reduction in the skinfold thickness and arm circumference. Biochemically the serum albumin concentration falls as does the lymphocyte count. The protein reserves of the body fall even more dramatically when there are sepsis, burns, acute pancreatitis or renal failure.

The purpose of enteral feeding is to give a liquid, low residue food through a naso-gastric feeding tube. It has the advantage over parenteral nutrition that the septic complications of insertion of catheters into veins are avoided. It is also much cheaper. Enteral feeding may either take the form of intermittent feeding through a large-bore naso-gastric tube or continuous gravity feeding through a fine-bore tube.

A number of proprietary enteral foods are available and these avoid the necessity of nursing or dietetic staff making up the preparations. Some of these proprietary feeds contain whole protein as the nitrogen source. Others, and these are called elemental diets, contain free amino acids. Diarrhoea is the most common problem with enteral feeding and it tends to occur when enteral feeding is introduced too rapidly or with too strong a preparation.

ENTERALGIA is another name for colic.

ENTERIC-COATED   A description of tablets covered in material that allows them to pass through the stomach and enter the intestine unaltered. Drugs coated in this way are those whose action is reduced or stopped by acid in the stomach.

ENTERIC FEVER   Enteric fever is caused by bacterial infection with either *Salmonella typhi* or *Salmonella paratyphi* A, B or C. These infections are called typhoid fever, or paratyphoid fever respectively. Unlike other salmonellas, *S. typhi* and *S. paratyphi* are primarily human pathogens – infections that attack humans – and humans are the main reservoir from person to person. Transmission usually occurs by ingestion of water or food that has been contaminated with human faeces, for example, by drinking water contaminated with sewage, or foods prepared by a cook infected with or carrying the organisms. Enteric fever is endemic (q.v.) in many areas of the world, including Africa, Central and South America, the Indian subcontinent and southeast Asia. Infection occasionally occurs in southern and eastern Europe, particularly with *S. paratyphi* B. However, in northern and western Europe and North America most cases are imported.

Clinical course   The incubation period of enteric fever is 7–21 days. During this time ingested organisms penetrate the wall of the small intestine and replicate in local lymph nodes before invading the blood stream. They are dispersed around the body, settling particularly in the reticulo-endothelial tissue (q.v.) of the liver, spleen and bone marrow, and also the gall bladder. Early symptoms include headache, malaise, dry cough, constipation and a slowly rising fever. Despite the fever the patient's pulse rate is often slow and he or she may have an enlarged spleen. In the second week of illness organisms invade the blood stream again and symptoms progress. In general, symptoms of typhoid fever are more severe than those of paratyphoid fever. Increasing mental slowness and confusion are common, and a more sustained high fever is present. In some individuals discrete red spots appear on the upper trunk (rose spots). By the third week of illness the patient may become severely toxic, with marked confusion and delirium, abdominal distension, myocarditis (q.v.), and occasionally intestinal haemorrage and/or perforation. Such complications may be fatal, although are unusual if prompt treatment is given. Subsequently symptoms improve slowly into the fourth and fifth weeks, although may relapse.

Diagnosis Enteric fever should be considered in any traveller or resident in an endemic area presenting with a febrile illness. The most common differential diagnosis is malaria. Diagnosis is usually made by isolation of the organism from cultures of blood in the first two weeks of illness. Later the organisms are found in the stools and urine. Serological tests for antibodies (q.v.) against *Salmonella typhi* antigens (q.v.) (the Widal test) are less useful due to cross-reactions with antigens on other bacteria, and difficulties with interpretation in individuals immunized with typhoid vaccines.

Treatment Where facilities are available hospital admission is required. Antibiotic therapy with chloramphenicol, cotrimoxazole or amoxycillin is effective. However, widespread resistance to these agents has emerged, and quinolone antibiotics, such as ciprofloxacin, are now recommended initial therapy for enteric fever in the UK and in areas where resistance is common. A few individuals become chronic carriers of the organisms after they have recovered from the symptoms. These people are a potential source of spread to others and should be excluded from occupations handling food or drinking water. Prolonged courses of antibiotic therapy may be required to eradicate carriage.

Prevention Worldwide, the most important preventive measure is improvement of sanitation and maintenance of clean water supplies. Vaccination is available for travellers to endemic areas.

ENTERITIS means inflammation of the intestines. (See DIARRHOEA; INTESTINE, DISEASES OF.)

ENTEROBIASIS is infection with *Enterobius vermicularis*, the threadworm, or pinworm as it is known in the USA. It is the most common of all the intestinal parasites in Britain and the least harmful. The male is about 6 mm (¼ inch) in length and the female about 12 mm (½ inch) in length. Each resembles a little piece of thread. These worms live in considerable numbers in the lower bowel, affecting children particularly. They cause great irritation round the anus, especially in the evening when the female worm emerges from the anus to lay its eggs and then die. Apart from this irritation around the anus, they seldom cause any symptoms. The most effective form of treatment is either viprynium embonate or piperazine citrate.

ENTEROCELE means a hernia of the bowel. (See HERNIA.)

ENTEROGASTRONE is a hormone derived from the mucosal lining of the small intestine which inhibits the movements and secretion of the stomach.

ENTEROKINASE is the enzyme (q.v.) secreted in the duodenum (q.v.) and jejunum (see INTESTINE) which converts the enzyme, trypsinogen, secreted by the pancreas (q.v.) into trypsin (q.v.). (See also DIGESTION.)

ENTEROPTOSIS means a condition in which, owing to a lax condition of the mesenteries and ligaments which support the bowels, the latter descend into the lower part of the abdominal cavity.

ENTEROSTOMY means an operation by which an artificial opening is formed into the intestine.

ENTEROVIRUSES are a family of viruses which include the poliomyelitis, coxsackie and echo groups of viruses. Their importance lies in their tendency to invade the central nervous system. They receive their name from the fact that their mode of entry into the body is through the gut.

ENTOMOPHOBIA is excessive fear of insects, particularly spiders, mites and other anthropods.

ENTONOX A proprietary analgesic drug taken by inhalation and comprising half nitrous oxide and half oxygen. It is valuable in providing relief to casualties who are in pain as it provides analgesia without making them unconscious. Entonox is also used in obstetric practice.

ENTROPION (see EYE DISEASES).

ENURESIS means the unconscious or involuntary passage of urine. (See NOCTURNAL ENURESIS.)

ENZYME is the name applied to a chemical ferment produced by living cells. The first enzyme was obtained in a reasonably pure state in 1926 and shown to be a protein. Since then several hundred enzymes have been obtained in pure crystalline form. Many more have been purified to less exacting standards and all have been proved to be proteins. They are present in the digestive fluids and in many of the tissues, and are capable of producing in small amount the transformation on a large scale of various compounds. Indeed, they are an integral, essential component of what might be described as the *modus operandi* of the body. Examples of enzymes are found in the ptyalin of saliva and diastase of pancreatic juice which split up starch into sugar, the pepsin of the gastric juice and the trypsin of pancreatic juice which break proteins into simpler molecules and eventually into the constituent amino-acids, the thrombin of the blood which causes coagulation.

ENZYME-LINKED IMMUNOSORBENT ASSAY (ELISA) This is a sensitive, safe and cheap method for measuring the quantity of a substance. An antibody to the substance is prepared along with an enzyme which binds to the antibody and which can be accurately measured using colour changes that occur as a result of the chemical reaction.

EOSINOPHIL is any cell in the body with granules in its substance that stain easily with the dye eosin. About 2 per cent of the white cells of the blood are eosinophils.

EOSINOPHILIA means an abnormal increase in the number of eosinophils in the blood. It occurs in Hodgkin's disease, in asthma and hay fever, in some skin diseases, and in parasitic infestation.

EPHEDRINE is an alkaloid derived from a species of *Ephedra* or prepared synthetically. A broncho-dilator, it was once widely used to treat asthma but its side-effects and the arrival of the more effective beta$_2$-adrenoceptor stimulants has greatly restricted its use.

EPHELIS is a freckle (q.v.). *Ephelis ab igne* is the dark-brown pigmentation produced on the legs by constant exposure of them to a fire. A similar discoloration of the skin of the abdomen may be produced by constant use of a hot-water bottle.

EPI- is a prefix meaning situated on or outside of.

EPICANTHIC FOLD A vertical skinfold that runs from the upper eyelid to the side of the nose. These folds are normal in oriental races but uncommon in others, although babies may have a temporary fold that disappears. Folds are present in people with Down's Syndrome.

EPIDEMIC is a term applied to a disease which affects a large number of people in a particular locality at one time. The term is, in a sense, opposed to endemic, which means a disease always found in the locality in question. A disease may, however, be endemic as a rule – for example, malaria in swampy districts, and may become at times epidemic, when an unusually large number of people are affected.

An epidemic disease is usually infectious from person to person, but not necessarily so since many persons in a locality may simply be exposed to the same cause at one time; for example, outbreaks of lead-poisoning are epidemic in this sense.

The laws which govern the outbreak of epidemics are ill understood. Infected food supplies, such as drinking water contaminated by waste from people with cholera or typhoid fever, milk infected with tubercle bacillus, or 'fast food' products contaminated with salmonella. The migrations of certain animals, such as rats, are in some cases responsible for the spread of plague, from which these animals die in great numbers. Certain epidemics occur at certain seasons: for example, whooping-cough occurs in spring, whereas measles produces two epidemics, as a rule, one in winter and one in March. Influenza, the common cold, and other infections of the upper respiratory tract, such as sore throat, occur predominantly in the winter.

There is another variation, both as regards the number of persons affected and the number who die in successive epidemics: the severity of successive epidemics rising and falling over periods of five or ten years.

EPIDEMIC ENCEPHALITIS is another term for ENCEPHALITIS LETHARGICA (see ENCEPHALITIS).

EPIDEMIOLOGY The study of disease as it affects groups of people. Originating in the study of epidemics of diseases like cholera, plague and smallpox, epidemiology is an important discipline which contributes to the control not only of infectious diseases but also of conditions such as heart disease and cancer. Their distributions in populations can provide important pointers to possible causes. The relation between the environment and disease is an essential part of epidemiology.

EPIDERMIS The outer layer of the skin, which forms the protective covering of the body. Comprising four layers, the epidermis constantly renews itself, with the bottom or germinative layer producing new cells and the top layer, stratum corneum, made up of dead cells which are regularly worn off. The cells of the two intermediate layers are gradually impregnated with keratin, a horny substance which gives the epidermis its toughness.

EPIDURAL ANAESTHESIA (see ANAESTHESIA).

EPIDYDIMIS is an oblong body attached to the upper part of each testicle, composed of convoluted vessels and ducts. It is liable to be the seat of tuberculous and other inflammation. (See TESTICLE.)

EPIGASTRIUM is the region lying in the middle of the abdomen over the stomach.

EPIGLOTTIS is a leaf-like piece of elastic cartilage covered with mucous membrane, which stands upright between the back of the tongue and the glottis, or entrance to the larynx. In the act of swallowing, it prevents fluids and solids from passing off the back of the tongue into the larynx.

EPIGLOTTITIS Acute epiglottitis is an acute inflammatory oedema of the epiglottis, due to *Haemophilus influenzae*, which causes laryngeal obstruction due to swelling and immobilization of the epiglottis. It is a disease predominantly of children, occurs usually in the winter, and may prove rapidly fatal.

EPIGNATHUS is a mal-development of the fetus in which the deformed remains of one twin are united to the upper jaw of the other.

EPILATION means the removal of hair by the roots. (See DEPILATION.)

EPILEPSY (FITS, SEIZURES) Epilepsy is a common symptom with a prevalence of 1 in 200 (0·5 per cent) of the population and an incidence of about 50/100,000 per year. In childhood up to 5 per cent of individuals have one or more fits before the age of 12, but in many children the prognosis is good.

It is a recurrent and paroxysmal disorder starting suddenly and ceasing spontaneously due to occasional sudden excessive rapid and local discharge of the nerve cells in the grey matter (cortex) of the brain. Epilepsy always arises as a disorder of the brain, commonly of microscopic size, but it is not itself a disease. Epilepsy should be diagnosed by the clinical symptoms based on the observations of witnesses. Its cause is established by laboratory tests, and brain scanning. Fits can be the first sign of a tumour, or follow a stroke, brain injury or infection.

A single epileptic fit is not epilepsy. Of those people who have a single seizure, a significant minority (20 per cent) have no further attacks. By definition, they are *not* epileptic.

MAJOR (GENERALIZED) SEIZURES The salient features are a sudden, often unprovoked onset; the patient emits a cry, then falls to the ground, rigid, blue, and then twitching or jerking both sides of the body: the tonic-clonic convulsion. Drowsiness and confusion may last for some hours after recovering consciousness. Some experience a momentary warning (aura): a smell, or sensation in the head or abdomen, vision, or *déjà vu*.

PARTIAL SEIZURES: FOCAL MOTOR (JACKSONIAN) begin with twitching of the angle of the mouth, the thumb, or the big toe. If the seizure discharge then spreads, the twitching or jerking spreads gradually through the limbs. Consciousness is preserved unless the seizure spreads to produce a secondary generalized fit. In some attacks the eyes and head may turn, the arm may rise, and the body may turn, whilst some patients feel tingling in the limbs.

In TEMPORAL LOBE SEIZURES (COMPLEX PARTIAL SEIZURES) the patient usually appears blank, vacant and may be unable to talk or may mumble or chatter, though later he often has no memory of this period. He may be able to carry out complex tasks, taking off gloves or clothes and may smack his lips or, rub repeatedly on one limb (*automatisms*). A sense of strangeness supervenes: unreality, or a feeling of having experienced it all before (*déjà vu*). There may be a sense of panic. Strange unpleasant smells and tastes are olfactory and gustatory hallucinations. The visual hallucinations evoke complex scenes. An initial *rising* sense of warmth or discomfort in the stomach, or 'speeding-up' of thoughts are common psychomotor symptoms. All these strange symptoms are brief, disappearing within a few seconds or up to 3 or 4 minutes.

PETIT MAL attacks start in childhood. They last a few seconds. The child ceases what he is doing, stares, looks a little pale, and may flutter the eyelids. The head may drop forwards. Attacks are commonly provoked by overbreathing. The child and parents may be unaware of the attacks – 'just daydreaming'. Major fits develop in one third of subjects. By contrast with other types of epilepsy, the electroencephalogram (EEG) is diagnostic.

Precautions Children with epilepsy should take normal school exercises and games, and can swim under strict supervision. Adults must avoid working at heights, with exposed dangerous machinery and driving vehicles on public roads. Current legislation allows driving after two years' complete freedom from attacks during waking hours; those who for more than three years have had a history of attacks only whilst asleep may also drive.

Treatment identifies, and avoids where possible, any factors (such as shortage of sleep or excessive fluids) which aggravate or trigger attacks. Antiepileptic drugs are usually necessary for several years under medical supervision. Carbamazepine, phenytoin and sodium valproate are the most frequently prescribed. The dose is governed by the degree of control of fits and some drug levels can be monitored by blood tests. Strict adherence to the drug schedule gives a good chance of total suppression of fits, especially in younger patients whose fits have started recently. The table summarizes anticonvulsant drugs in use.

	Therapeutic Range	Indications†
First-choice drugs:		
Ethosuximide	40–100 mg/l	PM, JME
Phenobarbitone	15–30 mg/l	M, P
Phenytoin	10–20 mg/l (40–80μ mol/l)	M, P, CP
Carbamazepine	3–10 mg/l	M, P, CP
Valproate	none*	M, PM, JME
Second-line drugs:		
Primidone	5–12 mg/l	M, P, CP
Clobazam	none*	M, CP
Vigabatrin	none*	M, CP, P
Lamotrigine	none*	M, CP, P
Gabapentin	none*	M, CP, P

* Serum levels have no useful correlation with efficacy.
† M = major generalized tonic-clonic; P = partial or focal; CP = complex partial (temporal lobe); PM = petit mal; JME = juvenile myoclonic epilepsy.

Anticonvulsant drugs

Patients with epilepsy and their relatives can obtain further advice and information from the British Epilepsy Association or the Epilepsy Association of Scotland (see APPENDIX 2: ADDRESSES).

EPILOIA (see TUBEROSE SCLEROSIS).

EPIPHORA Inadequate drainage of tears in the eyes with the result that they 'overflow' down the cheeks. The condition is caused by an abnormality of the tear ducts which drain away the normal secretions that keep the eyeball moist.

EPIPHYSIS means the spongy extremity of a bone, attached to it for the purpose of forming a joint with the similar process of another bone. An epiphysis is covered on its surface by cartilage, is developed from a distinct centre of ossification, and in a young person is connected with the shaft of the bone by a plate of cartilage that disappears in the adult. Separation of an epiphysis is a form of fracture which sometimes occurs in children, and is apt to be more serious than a break through bony tissue because it involves damage to the plate of growing cartilage, so that, although union takes place readily, the subsequent growth of the bone may be interfered with and the full growth of the limb may afterwards fail to be attained.

EPIPHYSITIS means inflammation of an epiphysis.

EPISCLERA The most superficial layer of the sclera of the eye (see EYE). It sometimes becomes inflamed (episcleritis) but the condition usually clears without treatment.

EPISIOTOMY is the operation of cutting the outlet of the vagina in childbirth so as to facilitate the birth of the child.

EPISTAXIS means bleeding from the nose. (See HAEMORRHAGE.)

EPITHELIOMA is a tumour of malignant nature arising in the epithelium covering the surface of the body. (See CANCER.)

EPITHELIUM is the cellular layer which forms the epidermis on the skin, covers the inner surface of the bowels, and forms the lining of ducts and hollow organs, like the bladder. It consists of one or more layers of cells which adhere to one another, and is one of the simplest tissues of the body. It is of several forms: for example, the epidermis is formed of scaly epithelium, the cells being in several layers and more or less flattened. (See SKIN.) The bowels are lined by a single layer of columnar epithelium, the cells being long and narrow in

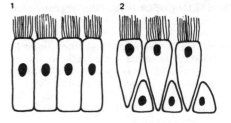

Diagram of ciliated epithelium (1) and pseudostratified columnar ciliated epithelium (2).

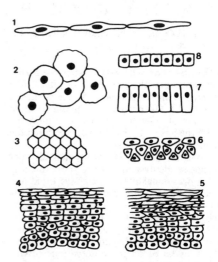

1 squamous epithelium seen in section
2 squamous epithelium seen in face view
3 cuboidal and columnar epithelium in face view
4 stratified, squamous, non-keratinized epithelium
5 stratified, squamous, keratinized epithelium
6 transitional epithelium
7 columnar epithelium
8 cuboid epithelium

Diagram of various types of epithelium.

shape. The air passages are lined by ciliated epithelium: that is to say, each cell is provided with lashes which drive the fluid upon the surface of the passages gradually upwards.

EPIZOÖTIC is a term applied to any disease in animals which diffuses itself widely. The term corresponds to the word epidemic as applied to human beings. In plague, for example, an epizoötic in rats usually precedes the epidemic in human beings.

EPSOM SALTS is the popular name for magnesium sulphate, which is perhaps the most commonly used saline purgative.

EPSTEIN BARR VIRUS The virus that causes GLANDULAR FEVER or infectious mononucleosis. It is similar to the viruses that cause herpes and is associated with Burkitt's Lymphoma (q.v.).

EPULIS is a term applied to any tumour connected with the jaws. (See MOUTH, DISEASES OF.)

EQUINE OESTROGENS (see OESTROGEN).

ERB'S PARALYSIS is a form of paralysis of the arm due to stretching or tearing of the fibres of the brachial nerve plexus. Such damage to the brachial plexus may occur during birth, and it is found that the arm lies by the side of the body with elbow extended, forearm pronated, and the fingers flexed. The infant is unable to raise the arm.

ERECTION The rigid state of the penis when it responds to sexual stimulus. An erection is necessary for satisfactory intercourse to occur. As a result of sexual arousal the three cylinders of erectile tissue in the penis become engorged with blood, lengthening, raising and hardening the penis. Muscles surrounding the blood vessels contract and retain the blood in the penis. Erections also occur during sleep and in young boys. Inability to have or maintain an erection is one cause of impotence.

ERETHISM is the psychic disturbance that is one of the manifestations of chronic mercury poisoning (see MERCURY). It is characterized by irritability, self-consciousness, shyness, timidity, embarrassment, lack of concentration, depression and resentment of criticism. It was this condition that gave rise to the phrase, 'mad as a hatter', as chronic mercurial poisoning used to be one of the occupational hazards of the hat-making industry.

ERGOMETRINE is one of the active constituents of ergot (q.v.). It has a powerful action in controlling the excessive bleeding from the womb which may occur after childbirth. The official *British Pharmacopoeia* preparation is Ergometrine Maleate.

ERGOSTEROL is a sterol found in yeasts and fungi and in plant and animal fat. Under the action of sunlight or ultra-violet rays it produces vitamin D_2. The substance produced in this way is known as calciferol, and is used for the prevention and cure of rickets and osteomalacia. A similar change in the ergosterol of the skin is produced when the body is freely exposed to sunlight. Calciferol is probably not so active as, and differs chemically from, the vitamin D occurring in fish-liver oils.

ERGOT is the spawn of *Claviceps purpurea*, a fungus which grows in the grain of rye. It contains several active principles, including the alkaloids, ergometrine, ergotoxine and ergotamine. Ergot causes prolonged contraction of unstriped muscle fibres all over the body, particularly the muscle fibres of the blood-vessels and of the womb. This action on the womb has made the drug of great value in midwifery since the 16th century until replaced by ergometrine (q.v.).

ERGOTAMINE is one of the alkaloids in ergot. In the form of ergotamine tartrate it is most effective in the treatment of migraine (q.v.). It is usually given by mouth. Its continued use is not without risk so should only be used under medical supervision.

ERGOT POISONING or ERGOTISM occasionally results from eating bread made from diseased rye. Several terrible epidemics (*St Anthony's Fire*), characterized by intense pain and hallucinations, occurred in France and Germany during the Middle Ages (cf ERYSIPELAS). Its symptoms are the occurrence of spasmodic muscular contractions, and the gradual production of gangrene in parts like the fingers, toes and tips of the ears.

EROSION means a process of gradual wearing down of structures in the body. The term is applied to the effect of tumours, when they cause destruction of tissue in their neighbourhood without actually growing into the latter: for example, an aneurysm may erode bones in its neighbourhood. The term is also applied to minute ulcers, for example, erosions of the stomach, caused by extreme acidity of the gastric juice.
DENTAL EROSION is the loss of tooth substance due to a cause other than decay or trauma. This is usually due to the presence of acid, e.g. frequent vomiting or the excessive intake of citrus fruits. The teeth appear very smooth and later develop saucer-shaped depressions.

ERUCTATION, or belching, is the sudden escape of gas or of portions of half-digested food from the stomach up into the mouth.

ERUPTION or RASH, means an outbreak, in a scattered form, upon the surface of the skin, usually raised and red, or it may be covered with scales, or crusts, or vesicles containing fluid. The appearance of an eruption depends, to a certain extent, upon the nature of the disease, or other source of irritation, which causes it: for example, the eruption of measles is always distinguishable from that of chicken-pox. But the same disease may also produce different eruptions in different people or in the same person in different states of health, or even on different parts of the body at one time.
Eruptions may be acute or chronic. Most of

the acute eruptions belong to the exanthemata (q.v.): i.e. they are bright in colour and burst out suddenly like a flower. These are the eruptions of scarlet fever, measles, German measles, smallpox and chickenpox. In general the severity of these diseases can be measured by the amount of eruption, but in cases in which the eruption is suppressed, or, as it is popularly termed, 'goes in', the disease is apt to be serious.

Some eruptions are very transitory, like nettle-rash, appearing and vanishing again in the course of a few hours.

(For chronic eruptions see SKIN DISEASES.)

ERYSIPELAS (synonyms, *the Rose, St Anthony's Fire*) is a streptococcal infection of the skin, characterized by unilateral, clear-cut lesions, usually on the face or a leg. It usually occurs in people over 40 years.

Signs and symptoms The organism enters the skin via a minor abrasion and infects the superficial lymphatic vessels. It presents as a bright red, swollen patch, painful and tender, associated with fever, malaise, and leucocytosis (q.v.). Initially circumscribed, erysipelas tends to spread, until most of the leg or one side of the face may become involved.

Treatment should be started immediately with full doses of penicillin. In those allergic to penicillin, erythromycin is substituted. No topical therapy is required, and a prompt response to the antibiotic can be expected.

ERYTHEMA is a general term signifying several conditions in which areas of the skin become congested with blood, and consequently a red eruption appears. The eruption is accompanied by tingling, and often by itching and pain.

Causes It may be due to heat, such as exposure to the sun, or the constant exposure, by cooks or iron-workers, of the face, hands or legs to a blazing fire. *Erythema ab igne* is the reddening of the skin of the leg producing a net-like pattern that is found in people who sit huddled over the fire. Another form, known as *erythema pernio*, is due to exposure to cold and wet. (See CHILBLAINS.) A variety, which appears, usually on the front of the legs, in the form of red or livid, tender swellings, often over 2·5 cm in breadth, is known as *erythema nodosum*, and is a hypersensitivity reaction to infection with the streptococcus or mycobacterium tuberculosis. It is also a manifestation of sarcoidosis and may be an allergic reaction to the sulphonamide drugs. Children and young adults, especially women, may also suffer from a severer form, which begins as red blotches on the hands, and, spreading up the arms to the body, produces lumps and vesicles, or even large blebs full of fluid. This form, on account of the diversity of the appearances in different parts, is known as *erythema multiforme*. The cause in some cases is a virus. It also occurs as a drug-rash from the use of such drugs as sulphonamides and barbiturates. *Erythema infectiosum*, or slapped cheek disease, is characterized by a fiery red rash on the cheeks: hence its alternative name. It occurs in children, in the spring. The rash, which spreads to the rest of the body, lasts for up to three weeks. Although highly infectious, the causative organism, probably a virus, has not been discovered.

ERYTHRASMA is a reddish-brown macular eruption of the skin, caused by a micro-organism known as *Nocardia minutissima*.

ERYTHROBLASTOSIS FETALIS (see HAEMOLYTIC DISEASE OF THE NEW-BORN).

ERYTHROBLASTS A series of nucleated cells in the bone marrow that go through various stages of development until they form erythrocytes (q.v.). They may appear in the blood in certain diseases.

ERYTHROCYTES are the biconcave red blood cells that carry oxygen from the lungs to the tissues, and return carbon dioxide. They have an excess of membrane, some of which may be lost in various disorders, as a result of which they become progressively more spherical and rigid. Erythrocytes, which have no nuclei, are formed during erythropoesis (q.v.) from erythroblast (q.v.) cells in the bone marrow (q.v.) and each cubic mm^3 of blood contains 5 million of them. They are by far the largest constituent among the blood cells and they contain large amounts of the oxygen carrier haemoglobin. They have a life of about 120 days after which they are absorbed by macrophages (q.v.), the blood's scavenging cells. Most components of the erythrocytes including the red pigment haemoglobin (q.v.) are reused, though some of the pigment is broken down to the waste product bilirubin (q.v.).

ERYTHROCYTE SEDIMENTATION RATE (see ESR).

ERYTHRODERMA An abnormal inflammation, thickening and flaking of the skin of the body. Also called exfoliative dermatitis, this condition occurs most commonly after the age of 50 and affects men more often than women, sometimes developing from a previously existing skin disease such as eczema or psoriasis. About two-thirds of patients recover after two or three months, a few develop chronic erythroderma and some patients die from complications.

ERYTHROEDEMA Other terms for this condition are ACRODYNIA and PINK DISEASE. This is a disease of infants with the following features: restlessness, weakness, neuritis and swelling and redness of the face, fingers and toes. In the vast majority of cases it is a manifestation of mercurial poisoning, often due to the infant's having been given teething powders containing a mercurial laxative.

ERYTHROMELALGIA, or RED NEURALGIA, is a condition in which the fingers or toes, or even larger portions of the limbs, become purple, bloated in appearance, and very painful. In people suffering from the condition, which is not a common one, the attacks come and go, being worse in summer (unlike chilblains), and worse on exertion or when the affected parts are warmed or allowed to hang down. The condition may appear without apparent cause, but is often associated with vascular diseases, such as hypertension and polycythaemia vera. It aso occurs in association with certain diseases of the central nervous system, and in cases of metallic poisoning: e.g. arsenic, mercury and thallium. Treatment is unsatisfactory. Residence in a moderate climate, the wearing of light-weight stockings or socks, and sandals, and the avoidance of excessive heat help to relieve the discomfort. Aspirin also gives marked relief.

ERYTHROMYCIN is an antibiotic derived from *Streptomyces erythreus*. Its antibacterial range of activity is comparable to that of penicillin, being especially effective against Gram-negative bacteria, and it is effective when taken by mouth.

ERYTHROPOEISIS The process by which erythrocytes or red blood cells are produced. The initiating cell is the haemopoietic stem cell from which an identifiable proerythroblast develops. This goes through several stages as a normoblast before losing its nucleus to become an erythrocyte. This process takes place in the blood-forming bone-marrow tissue.

ERYTHROPOIETIN is the protein, produced mainly in the kidney, that is the major stimulus for the production of erythrocytes, or red blood corpuscles. (See BLOOD.)

ESCHAR is a piece of the body killed by heat or caustics.

ESCHERICHIA is the generic name given to the group of gram-negative, rod-shaped bacteria found as normal inhabitants of the lower bowel: e.g. *Escherichia coli*.

ESERINE is another name for physostigmine (q.v.).

ESMARCH'S BANDAGE is a rubber bandage which is applied to a limb from below upwards in order to drive blood from it. The bandage is used when operating on a limb as it reduces bleeding.

ESR The ESR or erythrocyte sedimentation rate is a test that measures the rate at which red blood cells settle out of suspension in blood plasma. In certain diseases, such as infection and malignancy, the amount of proteins in the plasma increases; the result is that red cells settle out more quickly and this test is used to show whether disease is present.

ESSENTIAL AMINO ACIDS are amino acids that are essential for the body to grow and develop normally but which the body is unable to produce. Nine essential amino acids exist – histidine, isoleucine, leucine, lysine, methionine, phenylalanine, threonine, tryptophan, and valine (qq.v.) – and they are present in foods rich in protein: dairy products, eggs, meat, and liver.

ESSENTIAL FATTY ACIDS Three acids – arachidonic, linolenic and tinoleic – essential for life which the body cannot produce. They are found in natural vegetable and fish oils and their functions are varied. EFAs have a vital function in fat metabolism and transfer and they are also precursors of prostaglandins (q.v.).

ESSENTIAL HYPERTENSION or BENIGN HYPERTENSION is the traditional name for the disorder which affects most people with high blood pressure. As many as 20 per cent of middle-aged people in the United Kingdom probably have hypertension. The systolic pressure of those with essential hypertension is raised but they have no other classic signs of high blood pressure – for example, changes in the fundus of the eye or protein in the urine. Research has not shown any identifiable cause but, untreated, the condition can lead to complications including malignant and accelerated-phase hypertension (see HYPERTENSION).

ESTER is an organic compound formed from an alcohol and an acid by the removal of water.

ETHACRYNIC ACID is a potent diuretic (q.v.), with a rapid onset, and a short duration (4 to 6 hours), of action. (See BENZOTHIADIAZINES, DIURETICS.)

ETHAMBUTOL is a synthetic drug, often included in the treatment regimen of tuberculosis (q.v.). The main side-effects are visual disturbances, chiefly loss of acuity and colour blindness. Such toxic effects are more common when excessive dosages are used, or the patient has some renal impairment, in which case the drug should be avoided, as it should be in young children.

ETHAMIVAN is chemically similar to nikethamide (q.v.) and has a similar action in stimulating the respiratory centre.

ETHANOL is another name for ethyl alcohol. (See ALCOHOL.)

ETHER is a colourless, volatile, highly inflammable liquid formed by the action of sulphuric acid upon alcohol, with the aid of heat. Ether boils below the body temperature, and so, when sprayed over the skin, rapidly evaporates. It dissolves many substances, such as fats, oils and resins, better than alcohol or water, and is accordingly used in the preparation of many drugs.

Uses Externally it is used as a cleansing agent before operations. By inhalation it is used as a general anaesthetic. (See ANAESTHESIA.) Internally it is used occasionally for relieving pain such as colic.

ETHICS A degree of trust between patients and doctors is vital, and some regulation of the latter is necessary in order to ensure that doctors do not abuse their power. These have ranged from the Hippocratic Oath (4th century BC) to the modern-day professional conduct and medical ethics committees (q.v.). The rapid advances in medical science in the latter half of the 19th century and early 20th century, together with the changing attitudes of society, necessitated modification of the Hippocratic Oath. This need was met by the Declaration of Geneva, formulated by the World Medical Association in 1947. Since then, ethical issues in the UK have been guided by the General Medical Council and British Medical Association.

ETHICS COMMITTEES It is now generally agreed that research investigations on human beings should be governed by codes, such as those of the World Medical Association (Declaration of Helsinki) and of the Medical Research Council of Britain. Ethics committees developed in this country when the Royal College of Physicians, in 1967, recommended that clinical research investigations should be the subject of ethical review. The Medical Research Council requires ethical review of projects prior to making a grant and some scientific journals require it as a condition of publication. The objectives of ethics committees are to facilitate medical research in the interest of society, to protect subjects of research from possible harm, to preserve their rights and to provide reassurance to the public that this is being done. Ethics committees comprise medical, nursing and lay members. Ethics committees have now been established in most health authorities in this country. Adequate information should be provided to all committees to allow the ethics of the research proposal to be evaluated, as well as the scientific merit.

ETHINYLOESTRADIOL is a highly active oestrogen (q.v.), which is about twenty times as active as stilboestrol (q.v.). It is active when given by mouth. (See OESTROGEN.)

ETHISTERONE is the name approved by the *British Pharmacopoeia* for the orally active analogue of progesterone. It is given in certain cases of menorrhagia and habitual abortion, where a deficient secretion of the corpus luteum is suspected. (See PROGESTERONE.)

ETHMOID is a bone in the base of the skull which separates the cavity of the nose from the membranes of the brain. It is a spongy bone with numerous cavities or sinuses.

Suppuration in the ethmoidal sinuses is sometimes responsible for inflammation in neighbouring parts such as the eye.

ETHOSUXIMIDE is a drug used in the treatment of the form of epilepsy known as petit mal. (See EPILEPSY.)

ETHYL CHLORIDE is a gas at ordinary temperatures and pressures, but is liquefied by slight compression. It is extremely volatile, and rapidly produces freezing of the surface, when sprayed upon it. Accordingly it is used to produce insensibility to pain for small and short operations. It is put up in graduated glass or metal tubes, with a fine nozzle. The tube is warmed by the hand and the liquid jets out in a fine spray which evaporates at once and so freezes the skin upon which it is sprayed. At one time it was used by inhalation to produce general anaesthesia for very brief operations, and to induce anaesthesia in patients in whom the anaesthesia is subsequently to be maintained by some other anaesthetic such as nitrous oxide or ether, but is seldom used now for this purpose.

ETHYLENE is a colourless inflammable gas used as an anaesthetic.

ETHYLOESTRENOL (see ANABOLIC STEROIDS).

ETIDRONATE is one of a group of substances known as diphosphonates which are proving of value in the treatment of Paget's disease of bone (q.v.). One of its practical advantages is that it is taken by mouth, and not by injection as is the case with calcitonin.

ETIOLOGY, or AETIOLOGY, means the group of conditions which form the cause of any disease.

EU- is a prefix meaning satisfactory or beneficial.

EUCALYPTUS, or BLUE-GUM (*Eucalyptus globulus*), is a tree, originally a native of Australia, and now grown all over the world. Its important constituent, oil of eucalyptus, is an oil of pleasant smell and spicy taste, which is obtained by distillation from the leaves of the tree. Similar oils are obtained in varying amount from most species of gum-trees, some of which have peculiar and fragrant odours. Groves of eucalyptus trees exert a marked influence upon the soil and air in their neighbourhood. The trees, which reach a great size, and have wide-spreading roots, remove much moisture from the soil, and have accordingly a powerful action in drying up swampy ground. The oil constantly exhaled from the leaves has the power of oxidizing and destroying large quantities of the foul gases which emanate from swamps, and of checking to some extent the growth of microbes. Accordingly these trees have a beneficial influence upon unhealthy districts in which they are planted.

Uses The oil is used as a disinfectant and deodorant. It is also used as an inhalation or internally in bronchitis and in coryza.

EUGENICS is the study and cultivation of conditions that may improve the human race, in particular the detection and elimination of genetic disease.

EUSOL, which stands for Edinburgh University Solution, is a solution of 12·5 g of boric acid and 12·5 g of chlorinated lime in 1 litre of water. It was introduced during the 1914–18 War as an antiseptic for the treatment of wounds, and proved to be one of the most valuable antiseptics then available. It is now largely replaced by modern antiseptics, and the introduction of the sulphonamides (q.v.) and antibiotics.

EUPHORIA A feeling of well-being. This may occur normally, for instance, when someone has passed an examination. In some neurological or psychiatric conditions, however, patients may have an exaggerated and quite unjustified feeling of euphoria. This is then a symptom of the underlying condition. Euphoria may also be drug induced – by drugs of addiction or by therapeutic drugs such as corticosteroids.

EUPHORIANTS are drugs which induce a state of euphoria or well-being.

EUSTACHIAN TUBES are the passages, one on each side, leading from the throat to the middle ear. Each is about 38 mm (1½ inches) long and is large at either end, though at its narrowest part it only admits a fine probe. The tubes open widely in the act of swallowing or yawning. The opening into the throat is situated just behind the lower part of the nose, so that a catheter can be passed through the corresponding nostril into the tube for inflation of the middle ear. (See also EAR; NOSE.)

EUTHANASIA means the procuring of an easy and painless death. It has been advocated in some quarters that a medical practicioner should have the power to put to death painlessly, by means of such drugs as morphine, any person suffering from a painful, distressing and incurable disease the outcome of which is inevitably fatal, the patient or his relatives consenting. Various legal safeguards have been proposed, but there are obvious moral and religious – not to mention medical – objections to the recognition of such a procedure. The possible introduction of euthanasia, including arguments about whether some doctors occasionally practise it, is a burning medical, legal and moral topic in many Western countries.

EVACUANT is a name for a purgative medicine.

EWING'S SARCOMA An uncommon but very malignant cancer of the bone in children and young adults, the condition was first identified as different from osteosarcoma (q.v.) by Dr J. Ewing in 1921. It usually occurs in the limbs or pelvis and soon spreads to other parts of the body. Treatment is radiotherapy and anticancer drugs. Since the use of the latter the number of patients who survive for five years or more has much improved.

EXANTHEMATA is an old name used to classify the acute infectious diseases distinguished by a characteristic eruption. (See ERUPTION.)

EXCHANGE TRANSFUSION A method of treating new-born infants with haemolytic disease (q.v.). blood is taken out of the baby through the *umbilical* vein and is replaced with the same quantity of blood from a donor that is compatible with the mother's blood. The procedure is repeated several times to get rid of damaged cells while maintaining the infant's blood volume and keeping its red cell (erythrocyte) count constant.

EXCIPIENT means any more or less inert substance added to a prescription in order to make the remedy as prescribed more suitable in bulk, consistence, or form for administration.

EXCISION means literally a cutting out, and is a term applied to the removal of any structure from the body, when such removal necessitates a certain amount of separation from surrounding parts. For example, one speaks of the excision of a tumour, of a gland, of a joint. When an opening is simply made into the body the term incision is used. When a limb, or part of one, is removed, the term amputation is employed.

EXCITEMENT (see DELIRIUM; HYSTERIA; MENTAL ILLNESS).

EXCORIATION means the destruction of small pieces of the surface of skin or mucous membrane. (See CHAFING OF THE SKIN.)

EXCRETA Waste substances discharged from the body, in particular faeces.

EXERCISE is an important activity for everyone. It helps keep the weight down, it is an important form of relaxation, stimulates the cardiovascular system, and is particularly important for diabetics, and those normally engaged in sedentary occupations.
EFFECTS OF EXERCISE The right amount of the right type of exercise results in all parts of the body working at their best. The muscles are firm in tone, strong and working at maximum efficiency, so that the onset of fatigue, with its accompanying aching and soreness, is postponed. The heart, too, works more efficiently, pumping more blood round the body. For instance, when an individual is resting, the output of the heart per minute is 5 litres. When running at 12 km (7½ miles) per hour, this shoots up to around 25 litres: a five-fold increase. This increased volume of blood dealt with by the heart per minute is achieved with increasing efficiency, as is shown by the fact that at each contraction the heart expels 150 millilitres, compared with 70 millilitres at rest. The lungs also function more efficiently. Again taking the example of the individual running at 12 km (7½ miles an hour), the amount of oxygen used up increases twelvefold, although the output of the heart has only increased five-fold. The digestive tract, including the liver, also functions better, partly because it is not being overloaded by unnecessary food. The increased expenditure of energy involved in exercise ensures that the food eaten is metabolized, or used up, immediately to cope with the increased energy demands. The nervous system also works more efficiently, reflexes becoming brisker and the muscles thereby being able to respond more promptly and more effectively to any special stress or strain.
LACK OF EXERCISE Failure to take adequate exercise affects the body adversely at all ages. In children it may lead to faulty posture and flabby muscles. In adult life, and particularly in middle age, lack of exercise leads to the putting on of weight, with consequential hazards to health (see OBESITY). Of even more serious import is an increased tendency to atherosclerosis (q.v.) and coronary thrombosis (q.v.).
OVER-EXERCISE rarely causes permanent harm except in the rapidly growing adolescent and in the old, provided the individual is healthy. However, should there be any undetected disease of the heart, then undue exercise may be harmful. This is why a careful medical examination is an essential preliminary to any severe form of exercise. This is particularly important for school children. Older people can do moderate exercise but should use common sense and not overdo it.
In the case of adolescents and young adults, the wise rule is to ensure that the individual, and particularly his heart, is sound. They would be wise to train regularly before doing any demanding exercise such as competitive running, swimming, rowing or football.

EXFOLIATION means the separation, in layers, of pieces of dead bone or skin.

EXOCRINE GLAND A gland that secretes its products through a duct to the surface of the body or of an organ. The sweat glands in the skin and the salivary glands in the mouth are examples. The secretion is set off by a hormone (q.v.) or a neurotransmitter (q.v.).

EXOGENOUS Arising outside the body. For example, exogenous depression is an illness caused by an outside factor such as the death of a close relative. Or an illness may occur because of something eaten in the diet.

EXOMPHALOS is the term applied to a hernia formed by the projection of abdominal organs through the umbilicus.

EXOPHTHALMIC GOITRE is a disease in which there is overactivity of the thyroid gland, protrusion of the eyes, and other symptoms. (See GOITRE.)

EXOPHTHALMOS, or PROPTOSIS, refers to forward displacement of the eyeball and must be distinguished from retraction of the eyelids, which causes an illusion of exophthalmos. Lid retraction usually results from activation of the autonomic nervous sytem. Exophthalmos is a more serious disorder caused by inflammatory and infiltrative changes in the retro-orbital tissues and is essentially a feature of Graves' disease (q.v.), though it has been described in chronic thyroiditis. Exophthalmos commonly starts shortly after the development of thyrotoxicosis but may occur months or even years after hyperthyroidism has been successfully treated. Only 3 per cent of patients with Graves' disease develop severe exophthalmos. The degree of exophthalmos is not correlated with the severity of hyperthyroidism even when their onset is simultaneous. Some of the worst examples of endocrine exophthalmos occur in the euthyroid state and may appear in patients who have never had thyrotoxicosis; this disorder is named ophthalmic Graves' disease. The exophthalmos of Graves' disease is due to autoimmunity. Antibodies to surface antigens on the eye muscles are produced and this causes an inflammatory reaction in the muscle and retro-orbital tissues.
Exophthalmos may also occur as a result of a tumour at the back of the eye, pushing the eyeball forwards. In this situation it is always unilateral.

EXOSTOSIS means an outgrowth from a bone; it may be due to chronic inflammation, constant pressure or tension on the bone, or tumour-formation. (See BONE, DISEASES OF.)

EXPECTANT is a form of treatment in which the cure of the patient is left mainly to nature, while the physician simply watches for any unsatisfactory developments or symptoms, and relieves them if they occur.

EXPECTORANTS are drugs which are claimed to help the removal of secretions from the air passages. There is, however, no clear evidence that they do this. A simple expectorant may, however, be a useful placebo. Most preparations are available without a doctor's prescription and pharmacists will advise on which might be helpful for particular patients with dry or congestive coughs.

EXPECTORATION means either material brought up from the chest by the air passages, or the act by which it is brought up.

EXPIRATION (1) Breathing out air from the lungs. (2) The act of dying.

EXSANGUINATE The removal of blood from the body. This may occur as the result of a serious accident in which the victim bleeds extensively. Rarely it may happen that bleeding becomes uncontrollable during an operation.

EXTENSION is the process of straightening or stretching a limb. When used in the natural sense, it involves the contraction of the muscles opposing those used in flexion (q.v.). In cases of fractured limbs, extension is employed during the application of splints, in order to reduce the displacement caused by the fracture, and prevent movement of the broken ends of bone. It is effected by gently and steadily pulling upon the part of the limb beyond the fracture. Extension of a more permanent type is used in the after-treatment of some fractures, as well as in diseases of the spine, by placing the patient upon an inclined bed and affixing weights to his lower limbs or to his head by means of adhesive plaster or of straps.

EXTRA- is the Latin prefix meaning outside of, or in addition, such as extra-capsular, meaning outside the capsule of a joint, and extrasystole, meaning an additional contraction of the heart.

EXTRACTS are preparations, usually of a semi-solid consistence, containing the active parts of various plants extracted in one of several ways. In the case of some extracts the juice of the fresh plant is simply pressed out and purified; in the case of others the active principles are dissolved out in water, which is then to a great extent driven off by evaporation; other extracts are similarly made by the help of alcohol, and in some cases ether is the solvent.

EXTRADURAL Outside the dura mater (q.v.), the outermost of the three membranes that cover the brain and spinal cord (qq.v.). The extradural or epidural space is the space between the vertebral canal and the dura mater of the spinal cord (see ANAESTHESIA: epidural).

EXTRAPYRAMIDAL SYSTEM This is a complex part of the nervous system, extending from the cortex to the medulla, in the brain, from which emerge descending spinal pathways which influence voluntary motor activity throughout the body. Although the normal functions of the system are ill understood, there are characteristic signs of an extrapyramidal lesion. These include disturbance of voluntary movements, notably slowness and 'poverty' of movement; disturbance of muscular tone, which may be increased or decreased; and involuntary movements, such as a tremor, irregular jerking movements, or slow writhing movements.
Diseases There are several diseases that result from lesions to the extrapyramidal system, of which the most common is parkinsonism (q.v.). Others include Wilson's disease (q.v.), kernicterus (q.v.), chorea (q.v.), ballism, and athetosis (q.v.).

EXTRASYSTOLE is a term applied to premature contraction of one or more of the chambers of the heart. A beat of the heart occurs sooner than it should do in the ordinary rhythm and is followed by a longer rest than usual before the next beat. In an extrasystole the stimulus to contraction arises in a part of the heart other than the usual. Extrasystoles often give rise to an unpleasant sensation as of the heart stumbling over a beat, but their occurrence is not usually serious. (See HEART.)

EXTRAVASATION means an escape of fluid from the vessels or passages which ought to contain it. Extravasation of blood due to tearing of vessel walls is found in apoplexy, and in the commoner condition known as a bruise. Extravasation of urine takes place when the bladder or the urethra is ruptured by a blow on the abdomen or on the crutch (or perineum), or torn in a fracture of the pelvis.

EXTRINSIC (1) Originating outside the body. (2) Extrinisc muscle is one whose origin is some way from the part of the body it acts on – for example, the muscles controlling the movement of the eyeball which are attached to the bony orbit in which the eye sits.

EXUDATION means the process in which some of the constituents of the blood pass slowly through the walls of the small vessels in the course of inflammation, and also means the accumulation resulting from this process. For example, in pleurisy the solid, rough material deposited on the surface of the lung is an exudation.

EYE The eye is the sensory organ of sight. It is an elaborate photoreceptor detecting information, in the form of light, from the environment and transmitting this information by a series of electro-chemical changes to the brain. The visual cortex is the part of the brain that processes this information (i.e. the visual cortex is what 'sees' the environment). There are two eyes, each a roughly spherical hollow organ held within a bony cavity (the orbit). Each orbit is situated on the front of the skull, one on each side of the nose. The eye consists of an outer wall of three main layers and a central cavity divided into three.

The outer coat consists of the opaque *sclera* posteriorly and the clear *cornea* anteriorly; their junction is called the *limbus*.

(a) SCLERA   This is white, opaque, and constitutes the posterior five-sixths of the outer layer. It is made of dense fibrous tissue. The sclera is visible anteriorly, between the eyelids, as the 'white of the eye'. Posteriorly and anteriorly it is covered by Tenons capsule, which in turn is covered by transparent conjunctiva. There is a hole in the sclera medial to the posterior pole of the eye through which nerve fibres from the retina leave the eye in the optic nerve. Other smaller nerve fibres and blood vessels also pass through the sclera at different points.

(b) CORNEA   This constitutes the transparent colourless anterior one-sixth of the eye. It is transparent in order to allow light into the eye and is more steeply curved than the sclera. Viewed from in front, the cornea is roughly circular. Most of the focusing power of the eye is provided by the cornea (the lens acts as the 'fine adjustment'). It has an outer *epithelium*, a central *stroma* and an inner *endothelium*. The cornea is supplied with very fine nerve fibres which make it exquisitely sensitive to pain. The central cornea has no blood supply – it relies mainly on aqueous humour for nutrition. Blood vessels and large nerve fibres in the cornea would prevent light entering the eye.

(c) LIMBUS is the junction between cornea and sclera. It contains the *trabecular meshwork*, a sieve-like structure through which aqueous humour leaves the eye.

The middle coat (uveal tract) consists of the *choroid, ciliary body* and *iris*.

(a) CHOROID   A highly vascular sheet of tissue lining the posterior two-thirds of the sclera. The network of vessels provides the blood supply for the outer half of the retina. The blood supply of the choroid is derived from numerous *ciliary vessels* which pierce the sclera in front and behind.

(b) CILIARY BODY   A ring of tissue extending 6 mm back from the anterior limitation of the sclera. The various muscles of the ciliary body by their contractions and relaxations are responsible for changing the shape of the lens during accommodation. The ciliary body is lined by cells that secrete aqueous humour. Posteriorly the ciliary body is continuous with the choroid, anteriorly it is continuous with the iris.

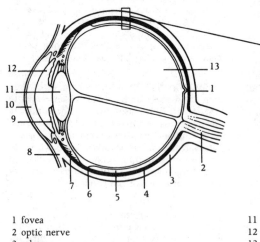

1 fovea	11 lens
2 optic nerve	12 anterior chamber
3 sclera	13 vitreous humour
4 choroid	14 pigment cells
5 retina	15 cone
6 ora serrata	16 rod
7 ciliary muscle	17 felt-work of dendrons
8 conjunctiva	18 axon
9 iris	19 ganglion cells
10 cornea	20 axon to optic nerve

(Left) Horizontal section through the right eye. (Right) Cross-section of the retina of eye.

(c) IRIS A flattened muscular diaphragm that is attached at its periphery to the ciliary body and has a round central opening, the *pupil*. By contraction and relaxation of the muscles of the iris the pupil can be dilated or constricted (dilated in the dark or when aroused, constricted in bright light and for close work). The iris forms a partial division between the *anterior chamber* and the *posterior chamber* of the eye. It lies in front of the lens and forms the back wall of the anterior chamber. The iris is visible from in front, through the transparent cornea, as the 'coloured part of the eye'. The amount and distribution of iris pigment determine the colour of the iris. The pupil is merely a hole in the centre of the iris and appears black.

The inner layer The RETINA is a multi-layered tissue (ten layers in all) which extends from the edges of the optic nerve to line the inner surface of the choroid up to the junction of ciliary body and choroid. Here the true retina ends at the *ora serrata*. The retina contains light sensitive cells of two types: (i) *cones*: Cells that operate at high and medium levels of illumination. They subserve fine discrimination of vision and colour vision. (ii) *rods*: Cells that function best at low light intensity and subserve black and white vision.

The retina contains about 6 million cones and about 100 million rods. Information from them is conveyed by the nerve fibres which are in the inner part of the retina to leave the eye in the optic nerve. There are no photoreceptors at the optic disc (the point where the optic nerve leaves the eye) and therefore there is no light perception from this small area. The optic disc thus produces a physiological blind spot in the visual field.

The retina can be subdivided into several areas: (a) PERIPHERAL RETINA contains mainly rods and a few scattered cones. Visual acuity from this area is fairly coarse. (b) MACULA LUTEA, so called because histologically it looks like a yellow spot. It occupies an area 4·5 mm in diameter lateral to the optic disc. This area of specialized retina can produce a high level of visual acuity. Cones are abundant here but there are few rods. (c) FOVEA CENTRALIS: A small central depression at the centre of the macula. Here the cones are tightly packed, rods are absent. It is responsible for the highest levels of visual acuity.

The chambers of the eye There are three, *anterior* and *posterior chambers* and the *vitreous cavity*. The ANTERIOR CHAMBER is limited in front by the inner surface of the cornea, behind by the iris and pupil. It contains a transparent clear watery fluid, the *aqueous humour*. This is constantly being produced by cells of the ciliary body and constantly drained away through the trabecular meshwork. The trabecular meshwork lies in the angle between the iris and inner surface of the cornea. The POSTERIOR CHAMBER: A narrow space between the iris and pupil in front and the lens behind. It too contains aqueous humour in transit from the ciliary epithelium to the anterior chamber, via the pupil. The VITREOUS CAVITY: The largest cavity of the eye. In front it is bounded by the lens

and behind by the retina. It contains *vitreous humour*. The *lens* is transparent, elastic and biconvex in cross section. It lies behind the iris and in front of the vitreous cavity. Viewed from the front it is roughly circular and about 10 mm in diameter. The diameter and thickness of the lens vary with its accommodative state. The lens consists of (a) *capsule*: a thin transparent membrane surrounding the cortex and nucleus; (b) *cortex*: This is made up of newly made lens fibres that are relatively soft. It separates the capsule on the outside from the nucleus at the centre of the lens; (c) *nucleus*: The dense central area of old lens fibres that have become compacted by new lens fibres laid down over them. The *zonule* consists of numerous radially arranged fibres attached between the ciliary body and the lens around its circumference. Tension in these zonular fibres can be adjusted by the muscles of the ciliary body, thus changing the shape of the lens and altering its power of accommodation. The *vitreous humour* is a transparent clear jellylike structure made up of a network of collagen fibres suspended in a viscid fluid. Its shape conforms to that of the vitreous cavity within which it is contained, i.e. it is spherical except for a shallow concave depression on its anterior surface. The lens lies in this depression.

Eyelids These are multilayered curtains of tissue whose functions include spreading of the tear film over the front of the eye to prevent desiccation, protection from injury or external irritation and to some extent to control light entering the eye. Each eye has an upper and lower lid which form an elliptical opening (the *palpebral fissure*) when the eyes are open. The lids meet at the *medial canthus* and *lateral canthus* respectively. The inner medial canthus is fixed, the lateral canthus is more mobile. An *epicanthus* is a fold of skin which covers the medial canthus in oriental races. Each lid consists of several layers. From front to back they are: very thin skin, a sheet of muscle (*orbicularis oculi* whose fibres are concentric around the palpebral fissure and which produce closure of the eyelids), the orbital septum (modified near the lid margin to form the *tarsal plates*) and, finally, lining the back surface of the lid, the conjunctiva (known here as *tarsal conjunctiva*). At the free margin of each lid are the eyelashes, the openings of tear glands which lie within the lid and the *lacrimal punctum*. Toward the medial edge of each lid in an elevation known as the *papilla*. The lacrimal punctum opens into this papilla. The punctum forms the open end of the *cannaliculus*, part of the tear-drainage mechanism.

Orbit The bony cavity within which the eye is held. The orbits lie one on either side of the nose, on the front of the skull. They afford considerable protection for the eye. Each is roughly pyramidal in shape, with the apex pointing backwards and the base forming the open anterior part of the orbit. The bone of the anterior orbital margin is thickened to protect the eye from injury. There are various openings into the posterior part of the orbit, namely the *optic canal* which allows the optic nerve to leave the orbit en route for the brain, the *superior orbital fissure* and *inferior orbital fissure* which allow passage of nerves and blood vessels to and from the orbit. The most important structures holding the eye within the orbit are the *extra-ocular muscles*, a *suspensory ligament* of connective tissue that forms a hammock on which the eye rests and which is slung between the medial and lateral walls of the orbit. Finally, the *orbital septum*, a sheet of connective tissue extending from the anterior margin of the orbit into the lids, helps keep the eye in place. A pad of fat fills in the orbit behind the eye and acts as a cushion for the eye.

Conjunctiva A transparent mucous membrane that extends from the limbus over the anterior sclera or 'white of the eye'. This is the *bulbar* conjunctiva. The conjunctiva does not cover the cornea. Conjunctiva passes from the eye on to the inner surface of the eyelid at the *fornices* and is continuous with the *tarsal* conjunctiva. The *semilunar fold* is the vertical crescent of conjunctiva at the medial aspect of the palpebral fissure. The *caruncle* is a piece of modified skin just within the inner canthus.

Eye muscles (extra ocular muscles) There are six in all, the four rectus muscles (superior, inferior, medial and lateral rectus muscles) and two oblique muscles (superior and inferior oblique muscles). The muscles are attached at various points between the bony orbit and the eyeball. By their combined action they move the eye in horizontal and vertical gaze. They also produce torsional movement of the eye (i.e. clockwise or anticlockwise movements when viewed from the front).

Lacrimal apparatus There are two components, a tear production system, namely the lacrimal gland and accessory lacrimal glands, and a drainage system.

LACRIMAL GLAND is located below a small depression in the bony roof of the orbit. Numerous tear ducts open from it into predominantly the upper lid. *Accessory lacrimal glands* are found in the conjunctiva and within the eyelids. The former open directly on to the surface of the conjunctiva, the latter on to the eyelid margin.

LACRIMAL DRAINAGE SYSTEM consists of (a) *Punctum*: an elevated opening toward the medial aspect of each lid. Each punctum opens into a cannaliculus. (b) *Cannaliculus*: a fine tube- like structure running within the lid, parallel to the lid margin. The cannaliculus from upper and lower lid join to form a common cannaliculus which opens into the lacrimal sac. (c) *Lacrimal sac*: a small sac on the side of the nose which opens into the nasolacrimal duct. During blinking the sac sucks tears into itself from the cannaliculus. Tears then drain by gravity down the nasolacrimal duct. (d) *Nasolacrimal duct*: A tubular structure which runs down through the wall of the nose and opens into the nasal cavity.

Tears keep the front of the eye moist; they also contain nutrients and various components to protect the eye from infection. Crying results from excess tear production. The drainage system cannot cope with the excess and therefore tears overflow on to the face. Newborn babies do not produce tears for the first three months of life.

Visual pathway Light stimulates the rods and cones of the retina. Electrochemical messages are then passed to nerve fibres in the retina and then via the *optic nerve* to the *optic chiasm*. Here information from the temporal (outer) half of each retina continues to the same side of the brain. Information from the nasal (inner) half of each retina crosses to the other side within the optic chiasm. The rearranged nerve fibres then pass through the *optic tract* to the *lateral geniculate body*, then the *optic radiation* to reach the *visual cortex* in the occipital lobe of the brain.

EYE DISEASES *Arcus senilis* The white ring or crescent which tends to form at the edge of the cornea with age. It is uncommon in the young when it may be associated with high levels of blood lipids.

Blepharitis A chronic inflammation of the lid margins. Seborrhoea (q.v.) and staphylococcal infection (q.v.) are likely contributors. The eyes are typically intermittently red, sore and gritty over months or years. Treatment is difficult and prone to fail. Measures to reduce debris on the lid margins, intermittent courses of topical antibiotics, steroids or systemic antibiotics may help the sufferer.

Blepharospasm Involuntary closure of the eye. This may accompany irritation but may also occur without an apparent cause. It may be severe enough to interfere with vision. Treatment involves removing the source of irritation, if present. Severe and persistent cases may respond to injection of Botulinum toxin into the orbicularis muscle.

Chalazion A firm lump in the eyelid relating to a blocked meibomian (q.v.) gland, felt deep within the lid. Treatment is not always necessary. A proportion spontaneously resolve. There can be associated infection when the lid becomes red and painful requiring antibiotic treatment. If troublesome, the chalazion can be incised under local anaesthetic.

Conjunctivitis Inflammation of the conjunctiva which may affect one or both eyes. Typically the eye is red, itchy, sticky and gritty but is not usually painful. Redness is not always present. Conjunctivitis can occasionally be painful, particularly if there is an associated keratitis (see below) (e.g. adenovirus infection, herpetic infection). The cause can be infective (bacteria, viruses or chlamydia (q.v.)) chemical (e.g. acids, alkalis) or allergic (e.g. in hay-fever). Conjunctivitis may be caused by contact lenses. Preservatives in eye drops or even the drugs in eye drops may cause conjunctival inflammation. Conjunctivitis may also occur in association with other illnesses, e.g. with upper-respiratory-tract infection, Stevens–Johnson syndrome (q.v.), Reiter's syndrome (q.v.). The treatment depends on the cause.

In many patients acute conjunctivitis is self-limiting.

Dacryocystitis Inflammation of the lacrimal sac. This may present acutely as a red, painful swelling between the nose and the lower lid. An abscess may form which points through the skin or may need to be drained by incision. Systemic antibiotics may be necessary. Chronic dacryocystitis may occur with recurrent discharge from the openings of the tear ducts and recurrent swelling of the lacrimal sac. Obstruction of the tear duct is accompanied by watering of the eye. If the symptoms are troublesome, the patient's tear passageways need to be surgically reconstructed.

Ectropion The lid margin is everted, usually the lower lid. Ectropion is most commonly associated with ageing, when the tissues of the lid become lax. It can also be caused by shortening of the skin of the lids such as happens with scarring or mechanical factors – e.g., a tumour pulling the skin of the lower lid downwards. Ectropion tends to cause watering and an unsightly appearance. The treatment is surgical.

Entropion The lid margin is inverted, usually the lower lid. Entropion is most commonly associated with ageing, when the tissues of the lid become lax. It can also be caused by shortening of the inner surfaces of the lids due to scarring – e.g., trachoma or chemical burns. The inwardly directed lashes cause irritation and can abrade the cornea. The treatment is surgical.

Episcleritis Inflammation of the episclera (q.v.). There is usually no apparent cause. The inflammation may be diffuse or localized and may affect one or both eyes. It sometimes recurs. The affected area is usually red and moderately painful. Episcleritis is generally not thought to be as painful as scleritis and does not lead to the same complications. Treatment is generally directed at improving the patient's symptoms. The inflammation may respond to non-steroidal anti-inflammatory drugs or topical corticosteroids.

Keratitis Inflammation of the cornea which is a response to a variety of insults – viral, bacterial, chemical, radiation, or mechanical trauma. Keratitis may be superficial or involve the deeper layers, the latter being generally more serious. The eye is usually red, painful and photophobic. Treatment is directed at the cause.

Nystagmus Involuntary rhythmic oscillation of one or both eyes. There are several causes including nervous disorders, vestibular disorders, eye disorders and certain drugs including alcohol.

Pinguecula A benign degenerative change in the connective tissue at the nasal or temporal limbus. This is visible as a small flattened yellow-white lump adjacent to the cornea.

Pterygium Overgrowth of the conjunctival tissues at the limbus on to the cornea. This usually occurs on the nasal side and is associated with exposure to sunlight. The pterygium is surgically removed for cosmetic reasons or if it is thought to be advancing towards the visual axis.

Ptosis Drooping of the upper lid. May occur because of a defect in the muscles which raise the lid (levator complex), sometimes the result of ageing or trauma. Other causes include Horner's syndrome (q.v.), third cranial nerve palsy, myasthenia gravis (q.v.), and dystrophia myotonica (q.v.). The cause needs to be determined and treated if possible. The treatment for a severely drooping lid is surgical, but other measures can be used to prop up the lid with varying success.

Scleritis Inflammation of the sclera. This can be localized or diffuse, can affect the anterior or the posterior sclera and can affect one or both eyes. The affected eye is usually red and painful. Scleritis can lead to thinning and even perforation of the sclera. This can happen sometimes with little sign of inflammation. Posterior scleritis in particular may cause impaired vision and require emergency treatment. There is often no apparent cause, but there are some associated conditions, for example, herpes zoster ophthalmicus (q.v.), rheumatoid arthritis (q.v.), gout , and an autoimmune disease affecting the nasal passages and lungs called Wegener's granulomatosis. Treatment depends on severity but may involve non-steroidal anti-inflammatory drugs, topical corticosteroids or systemic immunosuppressive (q.v.) drugs.

Stye Infection of a lash follicle. This presents as a painful small red lump at the lid margin. It often resolves spontaneously but may require antibiotic treatment if it persists or recurs.

Sub-conjunctival haemorrhage Haemorrhage between the conjunctiva and the underlying episclera. It is painless. There is usually no apparent cause and it resolves spontaneously.

Trichiasis Inward misdirection of lashes. Trichiasis occurs due to inflammation of or trauma to the lid margin. Treatment involves removal of the patient's lashes. Re-growth may be prevented by electrolysis or cryotherapy (q.v.) to the lid margin or possible surgery.

For the subject of *artificial* eyes see under PROSTHESES; CATARACT, GLAUCOMA, RETINA, DISORDERS OF, SQUINT, and UVEITIS are dealt with under these headings.

EYE DROPS (AND OINTMENT) are used extensively in the treatment of eye disease. They should be used as instructed by the prescribing physician. Most can be used for one month after the bottle has been opened but should then be discarded and a repeat prescription obtained if necessary. Any eye drops or ointment can have side effects and any difficulty with them should be referred to the prescribing physician.

EYE INJURIES *Blunt injuries* Blunt injuries may cause haemorrhage inside the eye, cataract, retinal detachment or even rupture of the eye. Injuries from large blunt objects – for example, a squash ball – may also cause a 'blow-out fracture' of the orbital floor causing double vision. Surgical treatment may be required depnding on the patient's specific problems.

Chemical burns Most chemical splashes cause conjunctivitis and superficial keratitis in the victim; both conditions are self-limiting. Alkalis are, however, more likely to penetrate deeper into the eye and cause permanent damage, particularly to the cornea. Prompt irrigation is important. Further treatment may involve testing the pH (q.v.) of the tears, topical antibiotics and corticosteroids and vitamin C (drops or tablets), depending on the nature of the injury.

Corneal abrasion Loss of corneal epithelium (outermost layer). Almost any sort of injury to the eye may cause this. The affected eye is usually very painful. In the absence of other problems the epithelium heals very rapidly. Small defects may close within 24 hours. Treatment conventionally consists of antibiotic ointment and sometimes a pad over the injured eye.

Foreign bodies Most foreign bodies which hit the eye are small and are found in the conjunctival sac or on the cornea; most are superficial and can be easily removed. A few foreign bodies penetrate deeper and may cause infection, cataract, retinal detachment or haemorrhage within the eye. The foreign body is usually removed and the damage repaired; nevertheless the victim's sight may have been permanently damaged. Particularly dangerous activities include hammering or chiselling on metal or stone and people carrying out these activities and others such as hedge cutting and grass strimming should wear protective goggles.

EYE STRAIN (see REFRACTION).

F

FACE is that part of the head extending from the forehead to the chin. It is supported by 14 bones: 2 nasal bones. 2 superior maxillae which carry the upper teeth. 2 lacrimal bones, 2 zygomatic bones, 2 palatine bones, 2 nasal bones at the sides of the nose, the vomer, forming a partition between the nostrils, and the mandible carrying the lower teeth. The lower jaw forms a joint of hinge-shape with the temporal bones of the skull, whilst the other bones of the face are firmly fixed together by sutures. The face in man is relatively small, as compared with that in lower animals, on account of the development of the cranium containing the brain. For the same reason, the face has an almost vertical direction instead of being sloped backwards as in animals.

The general character of the features depends chiefly upon the presence of air spaces in the frontal bone, situated immediately behind the eyebrows and in the upper jaw-bones. The varying expressions which are connected with the emotions and the general expression denoting character are chiefly due to the action of numerous thin muscles situated around the openings of the eyes, nose, and mouth. (See MUSCLE.) These are controlled by the 7th cranial nerve, which springs from the back part of the brain, passes through the skull to the ear, and, emerging immediately below the latter, passes forward on to the face round the edge of the lower jaw. In this position it is vulnerable to damage. Injury may result in a flat and expressionless appearance of one side of the face known as *Bell's palsy* (or *paralysis*) or *facial paralysis*. (See BELL'S PALSY.) The sensory nerve of the face is the 5th cranial nerve, which originates from the neighbouring part of the brain and within the skull divides into three portions called, respectively, ophthalmic, maxillary, and mandibular divisions. Each of these sends branches on to the face through a notch that can be felt near the inner end of the eyebrow, through an opening immediately beneath the eye, and through another opening near the middle of the chin. On their way to the face these nerves supply the parts about the eye, the teeth, and the muscles which move the lower jaw in chewing. The various parts of this nerve are subject to a particularly painful form of neuralgia, known sometimes as tic douloureux. (See NEURALGIA.)

FACIAL NERVE is the seventh cranial nerve, and supplies the muscles of expression in the face, being purely a motor nerve. It enters the face immediately below the ear after splitting up into several branches. (See BELL'S PALSY.)

FACIES is a term applied to the expression or appearance of the face.

FAECES is another name for the stools. (See CONSTIPATION; DIARRHOEA; STOOLS.)

FAINTING, or SYNCOPE, is a temporary loss of consciousness caused by inadequate brain perfusion. It may be preceded by nausea, sweating, loss of vision, and ringing in the ears. It is most often caused by pooling of blood in the extremities, which reduces venous return and thus cardiac output. This may be caused by hot weather or prolonged standing. Occasionally fainting on standing occurs in people with low blood pressure, autonomic neuropathy (in which normal vasomotor reflexes are absent), or those taking antihypertensive drugs. A prolonged rise in intrathoracic pressure caused by coughing, micturition, or the valsalva manoeuvre also impedes venous return and may cause fainting. Hypovolaemia (q.v.) produced by bleeding, prolonged diarrhoea, or vomiting may also cause fainting. Fainting is also produced by severe pain or emotional upset. Cardiac causes, such as severe stenotic valve disease or rhythm disturbances (particularly complete heart block or very rapid tachycardias), may result in fainting. Treatment must be directed towards the underlying cause, but immediate first aid consists of laying the patient down and elevating the legs.

FALLING SICKNESS is an old name for epilepsy. (See EPILEPSY.)

FALLOPIAN TUBES, or UTERINE TUBES, are tubes, one on each side, which are attached at one end to the womb, and have the other unattached but lying close to the ovary. Each is between 10 to 12·5 cm (4 to 5 inches) long, large at the end next the ovary, but communicating with the womb by an opening which admits only a bristle. These tubes conduct the ova from the ovaries to the interior of the womb. Blockage of them by a chronic inflammatory process resulting from infection is a not uncommon cause of infertility in women. (See REPRODUCTIVE SYSTEM.)

FALLOT'S TETRALOGY A hereditary defect of the heart in which intraventricular septal defect, pulmonary stenosis, right ventricular hypertrophy and a wrongly positioned aorta occur. It is usually treatable by surgery.

FALSE MEMBRANE is the name given to the deposit which forms upon the walls of the air passages in cases of diphtheria. It consists partly of fibrin derived from the blood, partly of the destroyed surface of the mucous membrane upon which it rests, and it contains bacteria in enormous numbers. If it is removed, it leaves a raw and bleeding surface upon which new membrane quickly forms.

FAMILY HEALTH SERVICES AUTHORITY An appointed committee that is responsible for the provision of local medical, dental, pharmaceutical and ophthalmic services in the NATIONAL HEALTH SERVICE in England and Wales. Its functions and organization are undergoing change as a result of the ongoing reforms of the NHS, which will result in the amalgamation of FHSAs with district health authorities.

FANSIDAR is a combination of pyrimethamine (q.v.) and sulfadoxine (q.v.) which is being used for the prevention of malaria (q.v.). It has the advantage of needing to be taken only once a week, or even only once a fortnight. It should not be taken by pregnant women, nor by those hypersensitive to sulphonamides.

FARMER'S LUNG is a form of external allergic alveolitis (see ALVEOLITIS) caused by the inhalation of dust from mouldy hay or straw.

FASCIA is the name applied to sheets or bands of fibrous tissue which enclose and connect the muscles.

FASCIITIS is inflammation of fascia (q.v.). The commonest site for it is the sole of the foot where it is known as plantar fasciitis. It is characterized by gnawing pain. There is no specific treatment, but it usually clears up spontaneously though over a considerable time.

FASCIOLIASIS is the disease caused by the liver fluke, *Fasciola hepatica*. This is found in sheep, cattle and other herbivorous animals, in which it is the cause of the condition known as liver rot. It measures about 35 × 13 mm, and is transmitted to man from the infected animals by snails. In Britain it is the commonest disease found in animal slaughterhouses. The danger to man is in eating vegetables, particularly wild watercress, that have been infected by snails. There have been several outbreaks of fascioliasis in Britain due to eating contaminated wild watercress. Much larger outbreaks of fascioliasis due to eating wild watercress have also been reported in France. The disease is characterized by fever, dyspepsia, heavy sweating, loss of appetite, abdominal pain, urticaria, and a troublesome cough. In the more serious cases there may be severe damage to the liver with or without jaundice. The diagnosis is clinched by the finding of the eggs of the fluke in the stools. The two drugs used in treatment are bithionol and chloroquine. Even though many cases are quite mild and recover spontaneously, prevention is particularly important. This consists primarily of never eating wild watercress, as this is the main cause of infestation. Lettuces have also been found to be infested.

FASTIGIUM means the highest temperature reached in a feverish state or the period when a disease process reaches its peak. It also describes the top of the roof of the fourth ventricle of the BRAIN.

FASTING is the abstention from, or deprivation of, food and drink. It may result from a genuine desire to lose weight – in an attempt to improve one's health or appearance – or may result from a mental illness (q.v.). such as depression, or an eating disorder (q.v.). Certain religious customs and practices may demand periods of fasting. Forced fasting, often extended, has been used for many years as an effective means of torture.

Without food and drink the body rapidly becomes thinner and lighter as it draws upon its stored energy reserves, initially mainly fat. The temperature gradually falls, and muscle is progressively broken down as the body struggles to maintain its vital functions. Dehydration, leading to cardiovascular collapse, inevitably follows unless a basic amount of water is taken, particularly if the body's fluid output is high, such as may occur with excessive sweating.

After prolonged fasting the return to food should be gradual, with careful monitoring of blood-pressure levels and concentrations of serum electrolytes (q.v.). Feeding should consist mainly of liquids and light foods at first, with no heavy meals being taken for several days.

FAT as a food has more energy-producing power weight for weight than any other food. Animal fat is a mixture in varying proportions of stearic, palmitic, and oleic acids combined with glycerin. Butter contains about 80 per cent of fat, ordinary cream contains 20 per cent fat, and rich cream 40 per cent, whilst olive oil is practically a pure form of fat. Fat requires, when taken to a large extent in the diet, to be combined with a certain proportion of either carbohydrate or protein in order that it may be completely consumed, otherwise harmful products, known as ketones, are apt to be formed in the blood. Each gram of fat has an energy-producing equivalent of 9·3 Calories.

From the medical point of view, fats are divided into saturated fats, that is, animal fats and dairy produce, and unsaturated fats which include vegetable oils from soya bean, maize and sunflower, and marine oils from fish (eg. cod-liver oil). (See ADIPOSE TISSUE; LIPID; OBESITY.)

FATIGUE is brought about in two ways. In the first place muscles become fatigued by the lactic acid accumulating in them as the result of their activity. For the removal of lactic acid in the recovery phase of muscular contraction oxygen is needed. If the supply of oxygen is not plentiful enough, or cannot keep pace with the work the muscle is doing, then lactic acid accumulates and fatigue results. There is also a nervous element in muscular fatigue: it is diminished by stimulation of the sympathetic nervous system. (See MUSCLE.)

Chronic fatigue is a symptom of some illnesses such as anaemia (q.v.), hypothyroidism (q.v.), motor neurone disease (q.v.), myasthenia gravis (q.v.), myalgic encephalitis (ME) (q.v.) and others. Some drugs may also produce a feeling of fatigue.

FAT NECROSIS In injury to, or inflammation of, the pancreas the fat-splitting enzyme in it may escape into the abdominal cavity, causing death of fat-containing cells.

FATTY DEGENERATION As a result of anaemia, interference with blood or nerve supply, or because of the action of various poisons, body cells may undergo abnormal changes accompanied by the appearance in their substance of fat droplets.

FAUCES is the somewhat narrowed opening between the mouth and throat. It is bounded above by the soft palate, below by the tongue, and on either side by the tonsil. In front of, and behind, the tonsil are two ridges of mucous membrane, the anterior and posterior pillars of the fauces.

FAVISM is a haemolytic anaemia, attacks of which occur within an hour or two of eating broad beans (*Vicia fava*). It is a hereditary disease due to lack of an essential enzyme called glucose-6-phosphate dehydrogenase which plays an important part in the metabolism of glucose and is necessary for the continued integrity of the red cell. This defect is inherited as a sex-linked dominant trait, and the red cells of patients with this abnormality have a normal life span until challenged by certain drugs or fava beans when the older cells are rapidly destroyed, resulting in haemolytic anaemia. Fourteen per cent of American Negroes are affected and 60 per cent of Yemenite Jews in Israel. The perpetuation of the gene is due to the greater resistance against malaria that it carries. Severe and even fatal haemolysis has followed the administration of the antimalarial compounds pamaquine and primaquine in sensitive individuals. These red cells are sensitive not only to fava beans and primaquine but also to sulphonamides, acetanilide, phenacetin, para-aminosalicyclic acid, nitrofurantoin, probenecid and vitamin K analogues.

FAVUS is another name for honeycomb ringworm. (See RINGWORM.)

FEBRILE Having a fever. Describes a patient whose body temperature is greater than normal (36·9–37·8 °C).

FEMINIZATION The development of a feminine appearance in a man, often the result of an imbalance in the sex hormones. Castration, especially before puberty, causes feminization as may the use of hormones to treat an enlarged prostate gland (q.v.).

FEMORAL Appertaining to the femur or the region of the thigh. Thus named are the femoral nerve, artery, vein, and canal.

FEMUR is the bone of the thigh, and is the longest and strongest bone in the body. As the upper end is set at an angle of about 120 degrees to the rest of the bone, and since the weight of the body is entirely borne by the two femora, fracture of one of these bones close to its upper end is a common accident in old people, whose bones are becoming brittle. The femur fits, at its upper end, into the acetabulum of the pelvis, forming the hip-joint, and, at its lower end, meets the tibia and patella in the knee-joint.

FENBUFEN (see NON-STEROIDAL ANTI-INFLAMMATORY DRUGS).

FENESTRATION is the operation whereby a new opening is made into the labyrinth of the ear. It has proved most valuable in restoring hearing to patients with otosclerosis (q.v.), particularly in young people with this disease.

FENFLURAMINE is an anorexiant drug, introduced to *aid* the slimming process by suppressing or reducing appetite. Although less likely to become a drug of addiction than some of the other anorexiant drugs, it is not without its risks and must only be used under skilled medical supervision. One of its disadvantages is that in some people it induces an increased frequency of dreaming or even nightmares.

FENNEL is the seed-like fruit of *Foeniculum vulgare* used as a carminative: i.e. to relieve griping, flatulence, and distension of the stomach. Fennel water used to be a popular remedy for griping.

FENOTEROL is a drug that is proving useful by inhalation in the treatment of asthma.

FERRUM is the Latin name for iron.

FERTILIZATION The process by which male and female gametes (spermatozoa and oöcytes respectively) fuse to form a zygote which develops by a complex process of cell division and differentiation into a new individual of the species. In humans fertilization occurs in the fallopian tubes. Sperm deposited in the upper vagina traverse the cervix and uterus to enter the fallopian tube. Many sperm attempt to penetrate the zona pellucida surrounding the oöcyte, but only one is able to penetrate the oöcyte proper and this prevents any other sperm entering. Once the sperm has entered the oöcyte, their nuclei fuse before the zygote begins to divide.

FESTER is a popular term used to mean any collection or formation of pus. It is applied to both abscesses and ulcers. (See ABSCESS; ULCER; WHITLOW.)

FESTINATION is the term applied to the involuntary quickening of gait seen in some nervous diseases, especially in PARKINSONISM (q.v.).

FETISHISM This is a form of sexual deviation in which the person becomes sexually stimulated by parts of the body, such as the feet, which are not usually regarded as erotogenic.

FETUS is the name given to the unborn child after the eight week of development. The human being, like the young of all animals, begins as a single cell, the *ovum*, in the ovary. After fertilization with a spermatozoon the ovum becomes embedded in the mucous membrane of the uterus, its covering being known as the decidua. Increase in size is rapid, and development of complexity is still more marked. The original cell divides again and again to form new cells, and these become arranged in three layers, known as the ectoderm, mesoderm, and endoderm. From the first are produced the skin, the brain and spinal cord, and the nerves; from the second the bones, muscles, blood-vessels, and connective tissues; while the third develops into the lining of the digestive system and the various glands attached to it.

The ovum produces not only the fetus but several membranes and appendages which serve it till birth, and are then cast away. The embryo develops upon one side of the ovum, its first appearance consisting of a groove, the edges of which grow up and join to form a tube, which in turn develops into the brain and spinal cord. At the same time, a part of the ovum beneath this is becoming pinched off to form the body, and within this the endoderm forms a second tube, which in time is changed in shape and lengthened to form the digestive canal. From the gut there grows out very early a process called the allantois, which attaches itself to the wall of the womb, forming later on the navel-string and afterbirth, by which nourishment is gained for growth. (See PLACENTA.)

The remainder of the ovum, which within two weeks of conception has increased to about 2 mm (1/12 inch) in size, splits into an outer and inner shell, from the outer of which are developed two covering membranes, the chorion and amnion, while the inner constitutes the yolk sac, attached by a pedicle to the developing gut of the embryo. From two weeks after conception onward, the various organs and limbs appear and grow, the name of *embryo* being applied to the developing being while almost indistinguishable in appearance from the embryo of other animals, till the middle of the second month, when it begins to show a distinctly human form. After this stage it is called the *fetus*. The property of 'life' is present from the very beginning, although the movements of the fetus are not felt by the mother till the fifth month.

During the first few days after conception the eye begins to be formed, beginning as a cup-shaped outgrowth from the mid-brain, its lens being formed as a thickening in the skin. It is very soon followed by the beginnings of the nose and ear, both of which arise as pits on the surface, which increase in complexity, and are joined by nerves that grow outward from the brain. These three organs of sense have practically their final appearance as early as the beginning of the second month.

As already stated, the body closes in from behind forward, the sides growing forward from the spinal region. In the neck, the growth takes the form of five arches, similar to those which bear gills in fishes. From the first of these the lower jaw is formed, from the second the hyoid bone, all the arches uniting, and the gaps between them closing up by the end of the

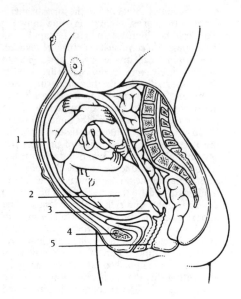

1 uterus
2 fetal head in position for normal delivery
3 cervix
4 symphysis pubis
5 vagina
6 superior vena cava
7 fetal liver

8 placental vein
9 placenta
10 fetal lungs
11 fetal heart ventricles
12 fetal aorta
13 inferior vena cava
14 placental arteries

(Left) Vertical section of mother's abdomen with fetus in the womb (viewed from the left side). (Right) Diagram of fetal circulation.

second month. At this time the head and neck have assumed quite a human appearance.

The digestive canal begins as a simple tube running from end to end of the embryo, but it grows in length and becomes twisted in various directions to form the stomach and bowels. From this tube also the lungs and the liver arise as two little buds, which quickly increase in size and complexity. The kidneys also appear very early, but go through several changes before their final form is reached.

The genital organs appear late. The swellings, which form the ovary in the female and the testicle (or testis) in the male, are produced in the region of the loins, and gradually descend to their final positions. The outward organs are exactly similar in the two sexes till the end of the third month, and the sex is not clearly distinguishable till late in the fourth month.

The blood-vessels appear in the ovum even before the embryo. The heart, originally double, forms as a dilatation upon the arteries which later produce the aorta. These two hearts later fuse into one. (For the circulation in the fetus, see CIRCULATION OF BLOOD.)

The limbs appear about the end of the third week as buds which increase quickly in length and split at their ends into five parts, for fingers or toes. The bones at first are formed of cartilage, in which true bone begins to appear during the third month.

The following table gives the average size and weight of the fetus at different periods:

Age	Length	Weight
4 weeks	5 mm	1·3 grams
3 months	8 to 9 cm	30 to 60 grams
5 months	15 to 25 cm	170 to 340 grams
7 months	32 to 35 cm	1360 to 1820 grams
Birth	45 to 60 cm	3200 grams

Approximate length and weight of the fetus at different periods.

FEVER, or PYREXIA, is the abnormal rise in body temperature that frequently accompanies disease in general.

Causes   The cause of fever is the release of an endogenous pyrogen by phagocytic cells called monocytes and macrophages. The cause of the fever is a small protein which is produced in response to a variety of infectious, immunological and neoplastic stimuli. The lymphocytes play a part in fever production because they recognize the antigen and release substances called lymphokines and these lymphokines promote the production of endogenous pyrogen.

The pyrogen then acts on the thermo-regulatory centre in the hypothalamus and this results in an increase in heat generation and a reduction in heat loss, resulting in a rise in body temperature.

In considering the general subject of fever, regard must be had in particular to the two main features of the febrile process: the abnormal elevation of temperature, and the changes affecting the tissues of the body.

The average temperature of the body in health ranges between 36·9 and 37·5 °C (98·4 and 99·5 °F). It is liable to slight variations from such causes as the ingestion of food, the amount of exercise, the menstrual cycle, and the temperature of the surrounding atmosphere. There are, moreover, certain appreciable daily variations, the lowest temperature being between the hours of 01.00 and 07.00 hours, and the highest between 16.00 and 21.00 hours, with trifling fluctuations during these periods. (See TEMPERATURE.)

The development and maintenance of heat within the body are generally regarded as depending on the destructive oxidation of all its tissues, consequent on the changes continually taking place in the processes of nutrition. In health this constant tissue disintegration is exactly counterbalanced by the introduction of food, whilst the uniform normal temperature is maintained by the due adjustment of the heat thus developed, and of the processes of exhalation and cooling which take place, especially from the lungs and skin. In the febrile state this relationship is no longer preserved, the tissue waste being greatly in excess of the food supply, while the so-called 'law of temperature' is in abeyance. In this condition the body wastes rapidly, the loss to the system being chiefly in the form of nitrogen compounds (e.g. urea). In the early stage of fever a patient excretes about three times the amount of urea that he would excrete on the same diet if he were in health – the difference being that in the latter condition he discharges a quantity of nitrogen equal to that taken in with the food, whilst in the fevered state he wastes the store of nitrogen contained in the tissues and the blood. The amount of fever is estimated by the degree of elevation of the temperature above the normal standard. When it reaches as high a point as 41·1 °C (106 °F) the term hyperpyrexia (excessive fever), is applied, and is regarded as indicating a condition of danger; while, if it exceeds 41·7 or 42·2 °C (107 or 108 °F) for any length of time, death almost always results.

The body's temperature will also rise if exposed too long to a high ambient temperature. (See HEAT STROKE.)

Symptoms The onset of a fever is usually marked by a rigor or shivering, which may exist only as a slight but persistent feeling of chilliness, or, on the other hand, be of a violent character, and, as occasionally happens with children, find expression in the form of well-marked convulsions. The skin feels hot and dry, and the raised temperature will often be found to show daily variations – namely, a rise toward evening, and a fall in the morning. There is a relative increase in the rate of the pulse and quickness of breathing. The tongue is dry and furred; the thirst is intense, while the appetite is gone; the urine is scanty, of high specific gravity, containing a large quantity of solid matter, particularly urea.

The decline of the fever takes place either by the occurrence of a *crisis*, i.e. a sudden termination of the symptoms, or by a more gradual subsidence of the temperature, technically termed a *lysis*. If death ensues, this is due to failure of the vital centres in the brain or of the heart, as a result of either the infection or hyperpyrexia.

Fever may be continuous as in typhoid fever; relapsing as in *Borrelia* infection; intermittent as in malaria; remittent as in some tropical diseases.

Treatment Fever is a symptom, and the correct treatment is therefore that of the underlying condition. Occasionally, however, it is also necessary to reduce the temperature by more direct methods: physical cooling by, for example, tepid sponging, and the use of antipyretic drugs such as aspirin.

FEVERFEW The leaf of *Chrysanthemum parthenium* which is an old herbal treatment for the relief of fever. It has also been used for the prevention of migraine (q.v.). Its side-effects are not common, but include itching, mouth ulcers and indigestion. It should not be taken by pregnant women.

FIBRE, DIETARY (see ROUGHAGE).

FIBREOPTIC ENDOSCOPY has transformed the management of gastro-intestinal disease. In chest disease fibreoptic bronchoscopy has now replaced the rigid wide-bore metal tube which was previously used for examination of the tracheo-bronchial tree. The principle of fibreoptics is that a light from a cold light source passes down a bundle of quartz fibres to illuminate the lumen of the gastro-intestinal tract or the bronchi. The reflected light is returned to the observer's eye via the image bundle which may contain up to 20,000 fibres. The tip of the instrument can be angulated in both directions and finger-tip controls are provided for suction, air insufflation and for water injection to clear the lens or the mucosa. The oesophagus, stomach and duodenum can be visualized. Furthermore, visualization of the pancreatic duct and direct endoscopic cannulation is now possible, as is visualization of the bile duct. Fibreoptic colonoscopy can visualize the entire length of the colon and it is now possible to biopsy polyps or suspected carcinomas and to perform polypectomy. The flexible smaller fibreoptic bronchoscope has many advantages over the rigid tube and extends the range of view to all segmental bronchi and enables biopsy of pulmonary parenchyma itself. A biopsy forceps can be directed well beyond the tip of the bronchoscope itself and the more flexible fibreoptic instrument causes less discomfort to the patient. (See ENDOSCOPE, BRONCHOSCOPE, LARYNGOSCOPE, LAPHROSCOPE, COLPOSCOPE, COLONOSCOPE.)

Fibreoptic laparoscopy is a valuable technique that allows the direct vizualisation of the female pelvic organs, in order to detect the presence of suspected lesions (and, in certain cases, their subsequent removal), to check on the development and position of the fetus, and to test the patency of the Fallopian tubes.

FIBRILLATION is a term applied to rapid contraction or tremor of muscles, especially to a form of abnormal action of the heart muscle in which individual bundles of fibres take up independent action. It is believed to be due to a state of excessive excitability in the muscle associated with the stretching which occurs in dilatation of the heart. Fibrillation is distinguished as atrial or ventricular, according as the muscle of the atria or of the ventricles is affected. In atrial fibrillation the heart beats and the pulse become extremely irregular, both as regards time and force. When the atrium is fibrillating there is no significant contraction of the atrial muscle but the cardiac output is maintained by ventricular contraction. In ventricular fibrillation there is no significant contractile force so that there is no cardiac output and the patient is essentially dead. If the ventricular fibrillation takes place in hospital resuscitation and de-fibrillation can be applied and the normal cardiac function restored.

FIBRIN is a substance formed in the blood as it clots. Its formation indeed causes clotting. The substance is produced in threads. After the threads have formed a close meshwork through the blood, they contract, and produce a dense felted mass. The substance is formed not only from shed blood but also from lymph which exudes from the lymph-vessels. Thus fibrin is found in all inflammatory conditions within serous cavities like the pleura, peritoneum, and pericardium, and forms a thick coat upon the surface of the inflamed membranes. It is also found in inflamed joints, and in the lung as a result of pneumonia. (See COAGULATION.)

FIBRIN FOAM is one of a series of absorbable haemostatics introduced into surgical use. A haemostatic is a preparation which arrests bleeding, and the great advantage of an absorbable haemostatic is that it produces no irritation in the tissues into which it is introduced and that it does not need to be removed after the bleeding is arrested, but is gradually absorbed by the tissues. Fibrin foam is a spongy material which is soaked in a solution of thrombin immediately before use. Other absorbable haemostatics now in use include oxidized cellulose which is prepared as a gauze, and calcium alginate (derived from seaweed) which is prepared as a gauze and as wool. These absorbable haemostatics, which constitute a great advance in surgery, are of particular value

in operations on the brain and in operations on blood-vessels and nerves.

FIBRINOGEN is the soluble protein in the blood which is the precursor of fibrin (q.v.), the substance in blood-clot.

FIBROADENOMA A benign tumour of glandular epithelium containing fibrous elements. The commonest benign tumour of the breast, often occurring in young women.

FIBROCYSTIC DISEASE OF THE PANCREAS (see CYSTIC FIBROSIS).

FIBROID, or fibromyoma, is the commonest form of tumour of the uterus (see UTERUS, DISEASES OF), and one of the most common tumours of the human body. It is composed of a mixture of muscular and fibrous tissue.

FIBROMA is a tumour, consisting mainly of fibrous tissue, and most commonly occuring on the skin. In association with the skin disease tuberose sclerosis (q.v.), two forms of fibromata are seen: periungal – multiple nodules around the nails, and perivascular – raised, red nodules on the face, mainly around the nose. Considerable cosmetic improvement may be achieved by diathermy (q.v.) or surgical removal of the latter.

FIBROSING ALVEOLITIS In this disease there is diffuse fibrosis of the alveolar wall. This causes loss of lung volume with both forced expiratory volume and vital capacity affected but the ratio between them remaining normal. The patient complains of cough and progressive dyspnoea. Typically the patient will be cyanosed, clubbed, and have crackles in the mid and lower lung fields. Blood gases will reveal hypoxia and, in early disease, hypocapnia (due to hyperventilation). There is an association with rheumatoid arthritis (q.v.) (about ⅛ cases). Systemic lupus erythamatosis, and systemic sclerosis. Certain drugs, e.g., bleomycin, busulphan, hexamethonium, high concentrations of oxygen, and inhalation of cadmium fumes may also cause this condition.

FIBROSIS means the formation of fibrous or scar tissue, which is usually due to either infection or deficient blood supply.

FIBROSITIS, also known as MUSCULAR RHEUMATISM describes pain and muscular stiffness and inflammation affecting the soft tissues of the arm, legs and trunk. The cause is unknown but may include immunological factors, muscular strain and psychological stress. Treatment is usually palliative.

FIBROUS DYSPLASIA is a rare disease in which areas of bone are replaced by fibrous tissue (q.v.). This renders the bone fragile and liable to fracture. It may involve only one bone, usually the thigh bone, or femur (q.v.), or several bones. This latter form of the disease may be accompanied by pigmentation of the skin and the early onset of puberty. There is another form of the disease known as cherubism because of the appearance it gives to the face, in which the abnormality of bone is confined to the upper and lower jaw-bones (the maxilla and mandible). The cause of the disease is not known.

FIBROUS TISSUE is one of the most abundant tissues throughout the body. White fibrous tissue consists of fibres of a substance known as collagen, which yields gelatine on being boiled. Between these fibres lie flattened or star-shaped cells, by which the fibres are produced. The fibres, like the cells, are of microscopic size, and are grouped into bundles which are held together by other fibres running round them. Yellow fibrous tissue is a rarer form, and consists of bundles of long yellow fibres, formed from a substance known as elastin. White fibrous tissue is very unyielding and forms sinews, ligaments, the material which binds muscle fibres together, the substance of the true skin. It is also the tissue which is laid down in the repair of wounds, or as a result of inflammation, and so forms the tissue composing a scar. It has the property of contracting and becoming denser as time goes on, and hence the puckering seen in scars, and the contraction resulting from burns and inflammation. Yellow fibrous tissue is highly elastic, and so is found in the walls of arteries, and in ligaments, like that on the back of the neck, which are often stretched. (See also ADHESION; SCAR; WOUNDS.)

FIBULA is the slender bone upon the outer side of the leg.

FILARIASIS is the term used to describe several clinical entities caused by one or other of the nematode filariae; these include *Wuchereria bancrofti/Brugia malayi, Onchocerca volvulus, Loa loa, Dracunculus medinensis* (dracontiasis or guinea-worm disease), *Mansonella perstans*, etc. These organisms have widely differing geographical distributions. Whereas lymphatic filariasis is present throughout much of the tropics and subtropics, onchocerciasis (river blindness) is largely confined to west and central Africa and southern America, loaiasis is an infection of west and central Africa, and dracontiasis involves west and central Africa and western India only. Clinically, the lymphatic filariases characteristically cause elephantiasis (lymphoedema); onchocerciasis gives rise to ophthalmic complications (river blindness), rashes and subcutaneous nodules; loaiasis causes subcutaneous 'Calabar swellings' and subconjunctival involvement; and dracontiasis predisposes to secondary bacterial infections (usually involving the lower limbs). Diagnosis is by finding the relevant filarial nematode, either in blood (day and night films should be examined), or one or other of the body fluids. An eosinophilia is often present in peripheral blood. Serological diagnosis is also of value. In onchocerciasis, skin-snips and the Mazotti reaction are valuable adjuncts to diagnosis. The mainstay of chemotherapy consists of diethylcarbamazine (aimed predominantly at the larval stage of the parasite). However, ivermectin has recently proved of value in onchocerciasis, and metronidazole or one of the benzimidazole compounds have limited value in dracontiasis. Suramin has been used to kill adult filarial worms. Prevention consists of eradication of the relevant insect vector.

FINASTERIDE is a drug which inhibits the enzyme that metabolizes testosterone (q.v.) into the more potent androgen (q.v.) dihydrotestosterone, This action results in a reduction of prostate tissue. The drug is used to treat enlarged prostate glands (q.v.), thus improving urinary flow. Its side-effects include reduced libido and impotence. Finasteride offers an alternative to prostatectomy for some men but a significant minority do not improve.

FINGERS consist of three bones called phalanges united by hinge-joints and strong ligaments. The thumb, like the great toe, differs from the others in having only two bones. These are bent or flexed, and straightened or extended by powerful sinews, two in front and two behind, which are brought into action by the contraction of muscles in the forearm. The sinews are enveloped in complicated synovial sheaths, through which they slide without friction, and are attached to the bases of the middle and end phalanges, back and front.

Running up each side of each finger are two small arteries and two small nerves, which supply the various structures and especially the overlying skin. The skin of the fingers is specially strong and particularly sensitive, and the end of the finger has a highly specialized part, the nail (see SKIN). Each finger is set upon a bone, the metacarpal, which lies in the substance of the hand between the finger and the carpus or wrist.

FIRST AID Emergency procedures to help an ill or injured person before he or she receives expert medical attention or is admitted to hospital. Courses of instruction in first aid comprise six to twelve sessions, each of about two hours' duration. Syllabuses of instruction are published by various organizations, the principal ones being the British Red Cross, the St John Ambulance Association, and the St Andrew's Ambulance Association. (See APPENDIX 1: FIRST AID and APPENDIX 2: ADDRESSES.)

FISSURE is a term applied both to clefts of normal anatomical structure and also to small narrow ulcers occurring in skin and mucous membrane. The latter type of fissure occurs especially at the corners of the mouth and at the anus. (See LIPS; RECTUM, DISEASES OF.)

FISTULA is an unnatural, narrow channel, leading from some natural cavity, such as the duct of a gland, or the interior of the bowels, to the surface. Or it may be a communication between two such cavities, where none should exist, as, for example, a direct communication between the bladder and bowel.

Cause Sometimes a child is born with a fistula, as a result of some defect in development, for example, a fistula from the thyroid gland to the surface; but, as a rule, the cause of the formation is either disease or injury. Often, the blockage of the duct of a gland leads to a fistula and the escape of the secretion from the gland on to the surface. Thus a salivary fistula may form on the face as a result of blockage by a concretion of the salivary duct in the cheek, and saliva then runs out on the cheek instead of into the mouth. Injury may also be the cause. For example, if the pelvis is fractured, the urethra may be torn across, so that urine, instead of being properly voided, passes among the tissues, and, by a process of suppuration, gradually bursts its way out through the skin, forming a permanent urinary fistula. A fistula from the bowel or bladder occasionally arises in women as a result of injury during protracted child-birth. Disease is another cause; thus an abscess may form at the side of the lower end of the bowel, and, bursting into the bowel on one side, and through the skin on the other, forms a fistula. This fistula in ano, as it is known, forms the most important variety of fistula. The abscess which produces the fistula may be tuberculous or an acute abscess due to other micro-organisms. (See ABSCESS, ACUTE.) Sometimes a fish-bone or pin, which has been swallowed, travels through the whole digestive canal without doing damage, till it reaches this point, where it lodges and produces a fistula.

Treatment As a rule, a fistula is extremely difficult to close, especially after it has persisted for some time. The treatment consists in an operation to restore the natural channel, be it salivary duct, or urethra, or bowel. This is effected by appropriate means in each locality, and when it is attained the fistula heals quickly under simple dressings.

Fistula in ano is a very troublesome condition, and is kept from healing by the constant entrance into it of material from the bowel. It is only to be cured by dividing the tissues which separate it from the bowel, and, each day, after the bowels move, packing the wound in such a way as to compel it to heal gradually from its deepest part. The process of healing is therefore a tedious one.

FIT is a popular name for a sudden convulsive seizure, although the term is also extended to include sudden seizures of every sort. During the occurrence of a fit of any sort the chief object should be to prevent the patient from doing any harm to himself by the convulsive movements. The person should therefore be laid flat, and the head supported on a pillow or other soft material. To prevent the tongue from being bitten, some object of moderate hardness may be placed between the teeth. (See CONVULSIONS; ECLAMPSIA; EPILEPSY; FAINTING; HYSTERIA; STROKE; URAEMIA.)

FLACCID Relaxed or lacking in stiffness. Used to describe muscles that are not contracting (or following denervation) and organs, e.g. the penis, that are lying loose, empty, or with wrinkles. The opposite of firm or erect.

FLAIL CHEST (see FRACTURES).

FLAP A section of tissue (usually skin) separated from underlying structures but still attached to its distal end by a pedicle through which it receives its blood supply. The free end may then be sutured into a new position to cover a defect caused by trauma or excision of diseased tissue. A free flap involves detachment of a section of tissue, often including bone and muscle, to a distant site where the artery and vein supplying it are anastomosed to adjacent vessels and the tissue is sutured into place.

FLAT-FOOT, or PES PLANUS, is a deformity of the foot in which its arch sinks down so that the inner edge of the foot comes to rest upon the ground.

Causes Most cases occur in young people in whom the ligaments which support the arch are still soft. It also tends to develop in obese middle-aged individuals who have to stand about a great deal without actually exercising the muscles.

Symptoms There is pain along the instep and beneath the outer ankle, the foot is stiff and broad, walking is tiresome, and the toes turn far out.

Treatment Change of occupation to one which allows sitting is sometimes necessary. In early cases the leg muscles may be strengthened by tiptoe exercises performed for ten minutes night and morning. A pad to support the arch may have to be worn inside the shoe. In severe cases surgical correction may be necessary.

FLATULENCE means a collection of gas in the stomach or bowels. In the former case the gas is expelled from time to time in noisy eructations by the mouth; in the latter case it may produce unpleasant rumblings in the bowels, or be expelled from the anus.

Causes When gas is found in large amount in the bowels its production is usually due to fermentation set up by bacteria. Marsh gas and hydrogen are formed from the cellulose of vegetables, sulphuretted hydrogen and carbon disulphide from eggs, peas, and other articles of diet containing much sulphur. Many cases of flatulence are much aggravated by a habit of gulping mouthfuls of air.

Treatment Flatulence in the stomach is treated by relieving the dyspepsia which causes it. It may also be relieved, or eased, by the administration of carminatives (q.v.). In many cases the flatulence is aggravated by an anxiety condition. If the flatulence is due to, or aggravated by, the habit of swallowing air, the patient must try and break the habit. In cases of intestinal flatulence, articles of diet which tend to decompose, e.g. green vegetables and starchy foods, should be avoided, and the food should be light and quickly digestible.

FLAVINE (see ANTISEPTICS).

FLEAS (see INSECTS IN RELATION TO DISEASE).

FLEXIBILITAS CEREA is an abnormal state in which the limbs remain in any position into which they are moved.

FLEXION is the bending of a joint in the sagittal (q.v.) plane. Usually an anterior movement, it is occasionally posterior, as in the case of the knee joint. Lateral flexion refers to the bending of the spine in the coronal plane, that is, from side to side.

FLEXOR A muscle that causes bending of a limb or other body part.

FLEXURE A bend in an organ or body part. The term is used, for example, to describe the skin on the inner aspect of the elbow or knee as in the 'hepatic flexure' of the colon.

FLIES (see INSECTS IN RELATION TO DISEASE).

FLOODING is a popular name for an excessive blood-stained discharge from the womb. (See MENSTRUATION.) In the majority of cases flooding is the sign of a miscarriage. (See ABORTION.)

FLUCLOXACILLIN (see PENICILLIN, ANTIBIOTIC).

FLUCTUATION is a sign obtained from collections of fluid by laying the fingers of one hand upon one side of the swelling, and, with those of the other, tapping or pressing suddenly on a distant point of the swelling. The thrill communicated from one hand to the other through the fluid is one of the most important signs of the presence of an abscess, or of effusion of fluid into joints or into the peritoneal cavity.

FLUCYTOSINE is a drug that is proving of value in the treatment of certain fungal infec-

tions such as candidiasis (see CANDIDA) and cryptococcosis (q.v.).

FLUFENAMIC ACID is a drug with analgesic, anti-inflammatory and anti-pyretic actions used in the treatment of osteoarthrosis and rheumatoid arthritis.

FLUKES are a variety of parasitic worms. (See FASCIOLIASIS.)

FLUOCINOLONE is a corticosteroid for application to the skin as a cream, lotion or ointment. It is more potent than hydrocortisone. It must not be given by mouth.

FLUORESCEIN is a dye which has the special property of absorbing blue-light energy and emitting this energy as green light. This property is made use of in examining the cornea for scratches or ulceration and it is also used to detect abnormally permeable (or leaking) blood vessels in the retina and iris – especially in diabetic retinopathy and diseases of the macula.

FLUORINE, one of the halogen series of elements. In the form of fluoride it is one of the constituents of bone and teeth. Supplementing the daily intake of fluorine diminishes the incidence of dental caries. American and British evidence indicates that people who, throughout their lives, have drunk water with a natural fluorine content of 1 part per million, have less dental caries than those whose drinking water is fluorine free. All the available evidence indicates that this is the most satisfactory way of giving fluorine, and that if the concentration of fluorine in drinking water does not exceed 1 part per million, there are no toxic effects.

FLUOROSCOPE is an apparatus for rendering X-rays visible after they have passed through the body by projecting them on a screen of calcium tungstate. The technique of using it is known as FLUOROSCOPY. It provides a method of being able to watch, for instance, the beating of the heart, or the movements of the intestine after the administration of a barium meal. (See X-RAYS.)

FLUOROURACIL is a drug that is proving of value when given intravenously, in the treatment of recurrent and inoperable carcinoma of the colon and rectum, as well as secondaries from cancer of the breast. (See CYTOTOXIC.)

FLUOXETINE is one of a group of antidepressant drugs that produce their effect by inhibiting the reuptake of serotonin (q.v.). Termed selective serotonin-reuptake inhibitors (SSRIs), these drugs seem to be effective in alleviating depressive illness. Their sedative effects are less than those of the tricyclic antidepressive drugs and they have few antimuscarinic effects.

Withdrawal of fluoxetine and other SSRIs should be done slowly, and they interact with some other antidepressive drugs. A large number of side-effects have been reported with the use of fluoxetine (trade name Prozac), including allergic reactions, dyspnoea, nausea, anorexia and anxiety.

FLUPENTHIXOL is a tranquillizer used in the treatment of schizophrenia (see MENTAL ILLNESS).

FLUPHENAZINE is one of the phenothiazine derivatives of value as an anti-psychotic drug. (See NEUROLEPTICS.)

FLURAZEPAM (see BENZODIAZEPINES).

FLURBIPROFEN is a drug that is proving of value in the treatment of rheumatoid arthritis and ankylosing spondylitis. (See NON-STEROIDAL ANTI-INFLAMMATORY DRUGS.)

FLUSPIRILENE is a tranquillizer that is used in the treatment of schizophrenia (see MENTAL ILLNESS). It is given by intramuscular injection, and the effect of one injection lasts for six to fifteen days.

FLUTTER, or ATRIAL FLUTTER, is the term applied to a form of abnormal cardiac rhythm, in which the atria contract at a rate of between 200 and 400 beats a minute, and the ventricles more slowly. The abnormal rhythm is the result of a diseased heart.

FOETOR OF THE BREATH (see BREATH, DISORDERS OF).

FOETUS (see FETUS)

FOLIC ACID, one of the constituents of the vitamin B complex, derives its name from the fact that it is found in many green leaves, including spinach and grass. It has also been obtained from liver, kidney, and yeasts. In 1945 it was synthesized by American workers, who proposed that the chemical name should be pteroylglutamic acid. It has proved of value in the treatment of macrocytic anaemias, particularly those associated with sprue and nutritional deficiencies.

FOLIUM is the latin term for leaf: e.g. digitalis folium is digitalis leaf. (Plural: folia.)

FOLLICLE is the term applied to a very small sac or gland: e.g. small collections of adenoid tissue in the throat and the small digestive glands on the mucous membrane of the intestine.

FOLLICLE-STIMULATING HORMONE A hormone produced by the anterior pituitary gland (see PITUITARY BODY) which stimulates the formation of follicles in the ovary each menstrual cycle and of spermatocytes in the testis. It is under hypothalamic control and in the female there is feedback inhibition by oestrogens from the developing follicle.

FOLLICULAR HORMONE (see OESTRADIOL).

FOMENTATION (see also POULTICES) is any warm application to the surface of the body in the form of a cloth. Usually the fomentation cloth is heated by being wrung out of hot water, but the term is also applied to dry applications and to hot cloths upon which various drugs are sprinkled.

FOMITES is a term used to include all articles which have been brought into sufficiently close contact with a person sick of some infectious disease to retain the infective material and spread the disease. For example, clothes, bedding, carpets, toys, books, may all be fomites till disinfected.

FONTANELLE is the term applied to areas on the head on which bone has not yet formed. The chief of these is the anterior fontanelle, situated on the top of the head between the frontal and two parietal bones. In shape it is four-sided, about 25 mm (1 inch) square at the time of birth, gradually diminishing until it is completely covered by bone, which should happen by the age of 18 months. The pulsations of the brain can be readily felt through it. Delay in its closure is particularly found in cases of rickets, as well as in other states of defective development. The fontanelle becomes more tense than usual in acute fevers, whooping-cough, and bronchitis, and tends to bulge in cases of hydrocephalus. It becomes unusually depressed in all cases of diminished vitality, such as that due to diarrhoea or wasting from any cause.

FOOD INTOLERANCE Most cases of food intolerance are not due to allergy. The most common cause of an aversion to food is psychological. Patients with a history of neurotic ill health may develop an obsessional aversion first to one food and then to another. Other cases of food intolerance are due to idiosyncrasy, that is a genetic defect in the patient, such as alactasia, where the intestine lacks the enzyme that digests milk sugar with the result that individuals so affected develop diarrhoea when they drink milk. Intolerance to specific foods, as distinct from allergy, is probably quite common and may be an important factor in the aetiology of the irritable bowel syndrome.

For the diagnosis of true food allergy it is necessary to demonstrate that there is a reproducible intolerance to a specific food and then that there is evidence of an abnormal immunological reaction to it. Occasionally the allergic response may not be to the food itself but to food contaminants such as penicillin, or to food additives such as tartrazine. There may also be reactions to foods which have pharmacological effects, such as caffeine in strong coffee or histamine in fermented cheese, or such reactions may be due to the irritant effect on the intestinal mucosa, especially if it is already diseased, by highly spiced curries. Of those patients who believe that their symptoms are provoked by food, probably only two out of every ten can be shown to have a true food intolerance and one in ten to have an immunological basis which would justify the diagnosis of food allergy.

FOOD POISONING is characterized by vomiting, diarrhoea, and abdominal pain and results from eating food contaminated with metallic or chemical poisons, or certain micro-organisms, or microbial products. Alternatively, the foods may contain natural poisons (for examples, undercooked red kidney beans or fish of the scrombroid family (mackerel and tuna)). Food poisoning caused by chemical or metallic substances usually occurs rapidly, within minutes or a few hours of eating. Among micro-organisms, bacteria are the leading cause of food poisoning, particularly *Staphylococcus aureus*, *Clostridium perfringens* (formerly *Cl. welchii*), *Salmonella* spp. and *Campylobacter jejuni*.

Staphylococcal food poisoning occurs after food such as meat products, cold meats, milk, custard, and egg products become contaminated before or after cooking, usually through incorrect handling by humans who carry *S. aureus*. In the food the bacteria produce an enterotoxin, which causes the symptoms of food poisoning one to eight hours after ingestion. The toxin can withstand heat; thus subsequent cooking of contaminated food will not prevent illness.

Heat-resistant strains of *Cl. perfringens* cause food poisoning associated with meat dishes, soups, or gravy that results when dishes cooked in bulk are left unrefrigerated for prolonged periods before consumption. The bacteria are anaerobes and form spores; the anaerobic conditions in these cooked foods allow the germinated spores to multiply rapidly during cooling, resulting in heavy contamination. Once ingested, the bacteria produce enterotoxin in the intestine, causing symptoms within eight to twenty-four hours.

Many different types of Salmonella (about 2000) cause food poisoning or enteritis, from eight hours to three days after ingestion of food in which they have multiplied. *S. brendeny, S. enteritidis, S. heidelberg, S. newport* and *S. thompson* are among those commonly causing enteritis. Salmonella infections are common in domesticated animals such as cows, pigs and poultry, whose meat and milk may be infected, although the animals may show no symptoms.

Duck eggs may harbour Salmonella (usually *S. typhimurium*), arising from surface contamination with the bird's faeces, and foods containing uncooked or lightly cooked hen's eggs, such as mayonnaise, have been associated with outbreaks of enteritis. The incidence of human *S. enteritidis* infection has been increasing (fifteenfold in England and Wales, from 1,101 to 31,000 cases annually between 1982 and 1993), with a sharp rise in phage type-4 isolates. A serious source of infection seems to be poultry meat and hen's eggs.

Although Salmonella are mostly killed by heating at 60 °C for 15 minutes, contaminated food requires considerably longer cooking and, if frozen, must be completely thawed beforehand, to allow even heating at a sufficient temperature.

Enteritis due to *Campylobacter jejuni* is usually self limiting, lasting one to three days. Since reporting of the disease began in 1977, in England and Wales its incidence has increased from 1,349 reports initially to 12,822 in 1982 to over 34,000 in the early 1990s. Outbreaks have been associated with unpasteurized milk: the main source seems to be infected poultry.

Food poisoning associated with fried or boiled rice is due to *Bacillus cereus*, whose heat-resistant spores survive cooking. An enterotoxin is responsible for the symptoms, which occur two to eight hours after ingestion and resolve after eight to twenty-four hours.

Viruses are emerging as an increasing cause of some outbreaks of food poisoning from shellfish (cockles, mussels, and oysters).

Public-health measures to control the incidence of food poisoning include agricultural aspects of food production, implementing standards of hygiene in abattoirs, and regulating the environment and process of industrial food production, handling, transportation, and storage.

FOOT is that portion of the lower limb situated below the ankle-joint. Its structure is similar to that of the hand. There are seven tarsal bones, of which the talus, supporting the leg bones, and the calcaneus, forming the heel, are the largest. The others are the navicular, three cuneiform, and the cuboid bones. Then comes a row of five metatarsal bones (known together as the metatarsus), and finally fourteen phalanges contained in the toes, the great toe having two only, while each of the others has three. The arrangement of the arteries and nerves is similar to the found in the hand and fingers.

The arch of the foot is a most important structure. The bones are so arranged that the sole is hollow both from before back and from side to side. In walking, the outer edge only, at the middle of the sole, should touch the ground. The arch is further supported by a short plantar ligament situated in the hollow of the arch, running from the calcaneus to the cuboid bone, and by a long plantar ligament situated nearer the surface. It is also slung up by two sinews on either side, coming from muscles in the leg, the two tibial muscles on the inner side, and the two peroneal muscles on the outer side. When this arch gives way, flat-foot (q.v.) is the result.

For diseases of the foot see BONE, DISEASES OF; CHAFING OF THE SKIN; CHILBLAIN; CLAW-FOOT; CLEFT-FOOT; CLUB-FOOT; CORNS AND BUNIONS; DROP-FOOT; FLAT-FOOT; GOUT; HALLUX RIGIDUS; HALLUX VALGUS; MALLET TOE; METATARSUS for metatarsus varus; METATARSALGIA; NAILS, DISEASES OF.

FORAMEN is the Latin term for a hole. It is especially applied to natural openings in bones, such as the foramen magnum, the large opening in the base of the skull through which the brain and spinal cord are continuous.

FORCED DIURESIS A means of encouraging the renal excretion of a compound by altering the pH and increasing the volume of the urine. Occasionally used after drug overdoses, but potentially dangerous, and so only suitable where proper intensive monitoring of the patient is possible. Excretion of acid compounds, such as salicylates, can be encouraged by raising the pH of the urine to $7 \cdot 5 – 8 \cdot 5$ by the administration of an alkali such as bicarbonate (forced alkali diuresis) and that of bases, such as amphetamines (q.v.), by lowering the pH of the urine to $5 \cdot 5 – 6 \cdot 5$ by giving an acid such as ammonium chloride (forced acid diuresis).

FORCED FEEDING (see ENTERAL FEEDING).

FORCEPS Surgical instruments with a pincerlike action which are used for grasping objects firmly. There are many different designs for different uses. Obstetric forceps are designed to fit around the infant's head and allow traction to be applied to aid its delivery.

FORENSIC MEDICINE That branch of medicine concerned with matters of law and the solving of crimes, for example, by determining the cause of a death in suspicious circumstances or identifying a criminal by examining tissue found at the scene of a crime.

FORESKIN (see PREPUCE).

FORMALDEHYDE The *British Pharmacopoeia* preparation, Formaldehyde Solution, also known as FORMALIN, contains 34 to 38 per cent formaldehyde in water. It is a powerful antiseptic, and has also the power of hardening the tissues. The vapour is very irritating to the eyes and nose.

Uses For disinfection it is largely used in the form of a spray. It can also be vaporized by heat. One of its advantages is that it does not damage metals or fabrics. In 3 per cent solution in water it is used for the treatment of warts on the palms of the hands and the soles of the feet.

FORMULARY A list of formulae used as drugs and other medical preparations.

FOSSA is a term applied to various depressions or holes, both on the surface of the body and in internal parts, such as the iliac fossa in each lower corner of the abdomen, and the fossae within the skull which lodge the different parts of the brain.

FOVEA A small depression. In the eye this is an area near the fundus which contains predominantly cones and is the area with greatest visual acuity (see EYE; VISION).

FOXGLOVE (see DIGITALIS).

FRACTURES occur when there is a break in the continuity of the bone. This happens either as a result of violence or because the bone is unhealthy and unable to withstand normal stresses.

Simple fracture refer to fractures where the skin remains intact or merely grazed. *Compound fractures* have at least one wound which is in communication with the fracture which means that bacteria can enter the fracture site and cause infection. A compound fracture is also more serious because there is greater potential for blood loss. Compound fractures usually need hospital admission, antibiotics and careful reduction of the fracture. Debridement (cleaning and excising dead tissue) in a sterile theatre may also be necessary.

The type of fracture depends on the force which has caused it. Direct violence occurs when an object hits the bone often causing a transverse break – which means the break runs horizontally across the bone.

Indirect violence occurs when a twisting injury to the ankle, for example, breaks the calf bone (the tibia) higher up. The break may be more oblique. A fall on the outstretched hand may cause a break at the wrist, in the humerus or at the collar-bone depending on the force of impact and age of the person.

Fatigue fractures occur after the bone has been under recurrent stress. A typical example is the March fracture of the second toe which army recruits suffer from after long marches.

Pathological fractures occur in bone which is already diseased, for example, by osteoporosis in post-menopausal women. A woman has a one-in-two chance of suffering from an osteoporotic fracture in her lifetime. These fractures are typically crush fractures of the vertebrae, fractures of the neck of the femur, and Colles fractures (wrist). Pathological fractures also occur in bone which has secondary-tumour deposits.

Greenstick fractures occur in young children whose bones are soft and bend in response to stress rather than break. The bone tends to buckle on the side opposite to the force. These fractures heal quickly but still need any deformity corrected and plaster of Paris to maintain the correction.

Complicated fractures involve damage to important soft tissue such as nerves, blood vessels or internal organs. In these cases the soft-tissue damage needs as much attention as the fracture site.

Comminuted fractures occur when a fracture has more than two fragments. It usually means the injury was more violent and that there is more risk of vessels and nerves' being damaged. These fractures are unstable and take longer to unite. Rehabilitation tends to be protracted.

Depressed fractures are most commonly found in skull fractures. A fragment of bone is forced inwards so that it lies lower than the level of the bone surrounding it. It may damage the brain beneath it.

Hair-line fractures occur when the bone is broken but the force has not been severe enough to cause visible displacement. These fractures may be easily missed.

Symptoms and signs The fracture site is usually painful, swollen and deformed. There is asymmetry of contour between limbs. The limb is held uselessly. If the fracture is in the upper limb, the arm is usually supported by the patient, if it is in the lower limb the patient is not able to bear weight on it. The limb may appear short because of muscle spasm.

Examination may reveal crepitus – a bony grating – at the fracture site. The diagnosis is confirmed by radiography.

Healing of fractures (union) begins with the bruise around the fracture's being resorbed and new bone-producing cells and blood vessels migrating into the area. Within a couple of days they form a bridge of primitive bone across the fracture. This is called *callus*.

The callus is replaced by woven bone which gradually matures as the new bone remodels itself. Treatment of fractures is designed to ensure this process occurs with minimal residual deformity to the bone involved.

Treatment is initially to relieve pain and may involve temporary splinting of the fracture site. Reducing the fracture means restoring the bones to their normal position and this is particularly important at the site of joints where any small displacement may limit movement considerably. A Potts fracture at the ankle joint, for example, may also lead to early osteoarthritis if the congruity of the joint is not fully restored.

In children it is possible to accept a higher degree of deformity at the fracture site because childrens' bones re-model so well.

Reduction may be done under a general anaesthetic which relaxes muscles and makes manipulation easier. Traction, which means sustained but controlled pulling on the bone, then restores the fragments of the fracture into their normal position. They are then kept in position with plaster of Paris. If closed traction does not work, then open reduction of the fracture may be needed. This may involve fixing the fracture with internal-fixation methods, using metal plates, wires or screws.

This holds the fracture site in a rigid position with the two ends closely opposed. The system developed by the Association for the Study of Internal Fixation (ASIF) has changed the philosophy of fracture healing by encouraging early mobilization after fractures.

External fixators are usually metal devices applied to the outside of the limb to support the fracture site. They are useful in compound fractures where internal fixators are at risk of becoming infected.

Consolidation of a fracture means that repair is complete. The time taken for this depends on the age of the patient, the bone and the type of fracture. A wrist fracture may take six weeks, a femoral fracture three to six months in an adult.

Complications of fractures are fairly common. In *non-union* the fracture does not unite usually because there has been too much mobility around the fracture site. Treatment may involve internal fixation. *Mal-union* means that the bone has healed with a persistent deformity and the adjacent joint may then develop early osteoarthritis. Sudeck's atrophy typically occurs after the plaster of Paris cast has been removed from Colles fractures of the wrist. The fingers remain swollen and the wrist is tender. It tends to resolve after six months.

Myositis ossificans commonly occurs at the elbow after a fracture. A big mass of calcified material develops round the fracture site which restricts elbow movements. Late surgical removal (after six to twelve months) is recommended.

Fractured neck of femur (q.v.) typically affects elderly women after a trivial injury. The

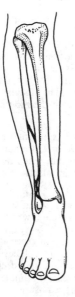

Right leg showing a simple spiral fracture of the fibula (top) and comminuted fracture of the fibula (bottom).

bone is usually osteoporotic. The leg appears short and is rotated outwards. Usually the patient is unable to put any weight on the affected leg and is in extreme pain. The fractures are classified under Garden's classification which identifies the fractures most likely to result in cutting off the blood supply to the femoral head. Most of these fractures of the neck of femur need fixing by metal plates or hip replacements as immobility in this age group has a mortality of nearly 100 per cent.

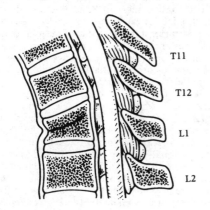

T11
T12
L1
L2

T11 Thoracic 11
T12 Thoractic 12
L1   Lumbar 1
L2   Lumbar 2

Injury to the spine: compression fracture of first lumbar vertebra with no damage to spinal cord

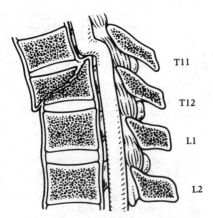

T11
T12
L1
L2

T11 Thoracic 11
T12 Thoracic 12
L1   Lumbar 1
L2   Lumbar 2

Injury to the spine: fracture/dislocation of twelfth thoracic vertebra with damage to spinal cord.

In fractures of the *spinal column* (q.v.) mere damage to the bone, as in the case of the so-called compression fracture, in which there is no damage to the spinal cord, is not necessarily serious. If, however, the spinal cord is damaged, as in the so-called fracture dislocation, the accident may be a very serious one, the usual result being paralysis of the parts of the body below the level of the injury. Therefore the higher up the spine is fractured, the more serious the consequences. The injured person should not be moved till skilled assistance is at hand, or, if he must be removed, this should be done on a rigid shutter or door, not on a canvas stretcher or rug, and there should be no lifting which necessitates bending of the back. In such an injury an operation designed to remove a displaced piece of bone and free the spinal cord from pressure is often necessary and successful in relieving the paralysis. Dislocation or subluxation (q.v.) of the spine is not uncommon in certain sports, particularly rugby. Anyone who has had such an injury in the cervical spine (i.e. in the neck) should be strongly advised not to return to any form of body-contact sport or vehicular sport.

Simple fissured fractures and depressed fractures of the skull often follow blows or falls on the head, and may not be serious, though there is always a risk of damage which is potentially serious to the brain at the same time.

Compound fractures may result in infection within the skull, and if the skull is extensively broken and depressed, surgery is usually required to check any intercranial bleeding or to relieve pressure on the brain. Another risk of fracture is that some of the small arteries on the inner surface of the skull may be torn and may bleed, thus causing compression of the brain. For this reason also the skull is often trephined (q.v.).

JAW The lower jaw is often fractured by a blow on the face. There is generally bleeding from the mouth, the gum being torn. Also there are pain and grating sensations on chewing, and unevenness in the line of the teeth. The treatment is simple, the line of teeth in the upper jaw forming a splint, against which the lower jaw is bound, with the mouth closed.

FRAMYCETIN is an antibiotic derived from *Streptomyces decaris*. It is active against a wide range of organisms, when taken by mouth or applied locally in infections of the skin.

FRECKLES, or SUMMER-SPOTS, are small yellow or brown spots which appear on the exposed parts of the body during hot or windy weather. They appear especially in people with fair skin and red hair. They consist of small pigmented areas in the deeper part of the epidermis, which are stimulated to increased development by exposure.

FREMITUS is a sensation which is communicated to the hand of an observer when it is laid upon the chest in certain diseases of the lungs and heart. Friction fremitus is a grating feeling communicated to the hand by the movements of lungs or heart when the membrane covering them is roughened, as in pleurisy or pericarditis. Vocal fremitus means the sensation felt by the hand when a person speaks; it is increased when the lung is more solid than usual. The 'thrills' felt over a heart affected by valvular disease are also varieties of fremitus.

FREUD'S THEORY is the term applied to a theory that emotional and allied diseases are due to a psychic injury or trauma, generally of a sexual nature, which did not produce an adequate reaction when it was received and therefore remains as a subconscious or 'affect' memory to trouble the patient's mind. As an extension of this theory Freudian treatment consists in encouraging the patient to tell everything that happens to be associated with trains of thought which lead up to this memory, thus securing a 'purging' of the mind from the original 'affect memory' which is the cause of the symptoms. This form of treatment is also called psychocatharsis or abreaction. The general term, psychoanalysis, is applied, in the first place, to the *method* of helping the patient to recover buried memories by free association of thoughts. In the second place, the term is applied to the body of psychological knowledge and theory accumulated and devised by Sigmund Freud (1856–1939) and his followers. The term 'psychoanalyst' should be applied only to those who have had a strict Freudian training, not to anyone who happens to practise psychotherapy. Freud's ideas are being increasingly questioned by some modern psychiatrists.

FRIARS' BALSAM (see BALSAMS).

FRICTION is the name given either to the fremitus felt, or to the grating noise heard, when two rough surfaces of the body move over one another. It is characteristically obtained over the chest in cases of dry pleurisy.

FRIEDREICH'S ATAXIA is a hereditary disease resembling locomotor ataxia, and due to degenerative changes in nerve tracts and nerve cells of the spinal cord and the brain. It occurs usually in children, or at any rate before the twentieth year of life, and affects often several brothers and sisters. Its chief symptoms are unsteadiness of gait, with loss of the knee jerks, followed later by difficulties of speech, tremors of the hands, head, and eyes, deformity of the feet, and curvature of the spine. There is often associated heart disease. The sufferer gets gradually worse, but may live, more or less helpless, for twenty or thirty years.

FRÖHLICH'S SYNDROME is a condition in children characterized by obesity, physical sluggishness, and retarded sexual development. It is the result of disturbed pituitary function.

FRONTAL BONE is the bone which forms the forehead and protects the frontal lobes of the brain. Before birth, the frontal bone consists of two halves, and this division may persist throughout life, a deep groove remaining down the centre of the forehead. Above each eye is a heavy ridge in the bone, most marked in men, and, behind this, in the substance of the bone, is a cavity on each side, the frontal sinus, which communicates with the nose. Catarrh in these cavities produces the frontal headache characteristic of a 'cold in the head', and suppuration may occur in them, producing discharge from the nose. (See NOSE, DISEASES OF.)

FRONTAL LOBE The anterior part of the cerebral hemisphere as far back as the central sulcus. It contains the motor cortex and the parts of the brain concerned with personality, behaviour and learning. (See BRAIN.)

FROSTBITE results from the action of extreme cold (below 0 °C) on the skin. Vasoconstriction (q.v.) results in the reduced blood – and hence, oxygen supply – leading to necrosis of the skin and, in severe cases, the underlying tissues. Chiefly affecting exposed parts of the body, such as the face, and the limbs, it occurs especially in people exercising at high altitudes, or in those at risk of peripheral vascular disease, such as diabetics, who should take particular care of their fingers and toes when in cold situations.

In mild cases, the condition sometimes known as frostnip, the skin on exposed parts of the body, such as the cheeks or nose, becomes white and numb with a sudden and complete cessation of cold and discomfort. In more severe cases blisters develop on the frozen part, and the skin then gradually hardens and turns black until the frozen part, such as a finger, is covered with a black shell of dead tissue. Swelling of the underlying tissue occurs and this is accompanied by throbbing and aching. If, as is often the case, only the skin and the tissues immediately under it are frozen, then in a matter of months the dead tissue peels off. In the most severe cases of all, muscles, bone and tendon are also frozen, and the affected part becomes cold, swollen, mottled and blue or grey. There may be no blistering in these severe cases. At first there is no pain, but in time shooting and throbbing pains usually develop.

Prevention This consists of wearing the right clothing and never venturing on even quite short expeditions in cold weather, particularly on mountains, without taking expert advice as to what should be worn.

Treatment Frostnip is the only form of frostbite that should be treated on the spot. As it usually occurs on exposed parts, such as the face, each member of the party should be on the look out for it in the other. The moment whitening of the skin is seen, the individual should seek shelter and warm the affected part by covering it with his warm hand or a glove until the normal colour and consistency of the affected part are restored. In more severe cases treatment should only be given in hospital or a well-equipped camp. In essentials this consists of warming the affected part, preferably in warm water, against a warm part of the body or warm air. Rewarming should be done for spells of twenty minutes at a time. The affected part should never be placed near an open fire. Generalized warming of the whole body may also be necessary, using hot drinks, and putting the victim in a sleeping bag.

FROZEN SHOULDER is a painful condition of the shoulder accompanied by stiffness and considerable limitation of movement. The usual age-incidence is between 50 and 70. The cause is not known. There is no specific treatment, but there is practically always complete recovery, even though this may take twelve to eighteen months.

FRUCTOSE is another name for laevulose, or fruit sugar, which is found along with glucose in most sweet fruits. It is sweeter than sucrose (cane or beet sugar) and this has led to its use as a sweetener.

FRUSEMIDE is a potent diuretic (q.v.) with a rapid onset (30 minutes), and short duration, of action. (See BENZOTHIADIAZINES, DIURETICS.)

FUGUE literally means flight and it is used to describe the mental condition in which an individual is suddenly seized with an unconscious motivation to flee from some intolerable reality of everyday existence. This usually involves some agonizing interpersonal relationship. As a rule, it lasts for a matter of hours or days, but may go on for weeks or even months. During the fugue the individual seldom behaves in a particularly odd manner though he may be considered somewhat eccentric. When it is over there is no remembrance of events during the fugue.

FUMIGATION is a means of disinfection by the vapour of powerful antiseptics. (See DISINFECTION).

FUNCTIONAL DISEASES (see PSYCHOSOMATIC DISEASES).

FUNDUS (1) The base of an organ or that part remote from its opening. (2) Point on the retina opposite the pupil through which nerve fibres and blood vessels traverse the retina (see EYE).

FUNGAL INFECTIONS Two main groups of fungi infect man. Most common is the candida (q.v.) group of yeasts, followed by the dermatophytes (q.v.), which cause athlete's foot and nail infections. Dermatophyte skin infections are characterized by ring-like lesions

– hence the old term, ringworm. Usually superficial, they tend to occur in moist, warm situations. Generalized systemic infections with candida are rare, and are usually associated with intense immunosuppression (q.v.) or antibiotic therapy.
Treatment Confirmation of a suspected diagnosis is obtained by swabbing the lesion. Treatment is usually topical, using nystatin (q.v.) for candida, or miconazole (q.v.) cream or powder for either. Persistent, or severe dermatophyte skin and nail infections require oral anti-fungal therapy with terbinafine (see FUNGUS; MICROBIOLOGY).

FUNGUS A simple plant that is parasitic on other plants and animals. Included in this group are mildews, moulds, mushrooms, toadstools and yeasts. Unlike other plants they do not contain the green pigment chlorophyll. Most of the world's 100,000 different species are harmless or even beneficial to humans. Yeasts are used in the preparation of food and drinks and antibiotics are obtained from some fungi. A few, however, can cause fatal disease and illness in humans.

FUNGUS-POISONING About 2000 mushrooms (toadstools) grow in England, of which 200 are edible and a dozen are classified as poisonous. Not all the poisonous ones are dangerous. It is obviously better to prevent mushroom poisoning by ensuring correct identification of those that are edible and books and charts are available.

Muscarine is the poisonous constituent of some species. Within two hours of ingesting it, the victim starts salivating and sweating, has visual disturbances, vomiting, stomach cramps, diarrhoea, vertigo, confusion, hallucinations and coma, the severity of symptoms depending on the amount eaten and type of mushroom. Untreated, a few people may die but most recover in 24 hours with treatment.

Death from mushrooms is nearly always due to phallotoxins and amatoxins – which interfere with cell metabolism – found in the death cap mushroom (*Amanita Phalloides*) and related species. Symptoms develop 6 to 24 hours after ingestion and the gastrointestinal upsets that occur are similar to those induced by the muscarine-containing mushrooms. In addition, the victim's urine output fails (oliguria) or may even stop (anuria); jaundice (q.v.) is also common. Some people recover but around 50 per cent may die within 8 days.

Symptoms of mushroom poisoning may vary within the same species or at different times of the growing season. Alcohol may precipitate or worsen symptoms.
Treatment If possible, early lavage should be carried out in all cases of suspected poisoning; an emetic (q.v.) may be used. Apomorphine (q.v.) is given *once* to induce vomiting. A strong saline drink can help. Identification of the mushroom species is a valuable guide to treatment. For muscarine poisoning, atropine (q.v.)

is a specific antidote. In phalloidine poisoning, a high carbohydrate diet and intravenous administration of dextrose and sodium choride counter the hypoglycaemia caused by any damage to the liver. Hospital treatment, with parenteral fluids, intensive care and haemodialysis (q.v.), is necessary in cases of severe poisoning.

FURUNCLE is another name for a boil. (See BOILS.)

FUSIDIC ACID is an antibiotic derived from the fermentation products of the fungus, *Fusidium coccineum*. It is particularly active against staphylococci, including those which are resistant to penicillin.

G

GABA Gamma aminobutyric acid is an amino acid that occurs in the central nervous system, mainly in the brain tissue. It is a chemical substance that transmits inhibitory impulses from nerve endings across synapses to other nerves or tissues.

GAG A device that when placed between a person's teeth keeps the mouth open.

GAIT, the way in which an individual walks, is an important sign of health and disease both physical and psychological. Children, as a rule, begin to walk between the ages of twelve and eighteen months, having learned to stand before the end of the first year. If a normal-sized child shows no ability to make movements by this time the possibility of his being mentally retarded must be borne in mind, and if the power of walking is not gained by the time the child is a year and a half old, rickets, cerebral palsy, or a malformation of the hip-joint must be excluded. (See RICKETS; PARALYSIS.)

In *hemiplegia*, or paralysis down one side of the body following a stroke (q.v.), the person drags the paralysed leg.

Steppage gait occurs in certain cases of alcoholic neuritis, tertiary syphilis (tabes) and other conditions where the muscles that raise the foot are weak and the toes in consequence droop. The person bends the knee and lifts the foot high, so that the toes may clear obstacles on the ground. (See DROP-FOOT.)

In *locomotor ataxia* (q.v.) or tabes dorsalis the sensations derived from the lower limbs are blunted, and consequently the movements of the legs are uncertain and the heels planted on the ground with unnecessary force. When the person tries to turn or stands with the eyes shut

he may fall over. When he walks he feels for the ground with a stick or keeps his eyes constantly fixed upon it.

In *spastic paralysis* the limbs are moved with jerks. The foot first of all clings to the ground and then leaves it with a spasmodic movement, being raised much higher than necessary.

In Parkinsonism (q.v.) the movements are tremulous, and as the person takes very short steps, he has the peculiarity of appearing constantly to fall forward, or to be chasing himself.

In *chorea* (q.v.) the walk is bizarre and jerky, the affected child often seeming to leave one leg a step behind him, and then, with a screwing movement on the other heel, go on again.

Hysterical disorders of gait are usually of a striking nature, quite different from those occuring in any neurological conditions. They tend to draw attention to the patient, and are worse when he or she is observed.

GALACTOCELE is a cyst-like swelling in the breast which forms as a result of obstruction in the milk-duct draining the swollen area.

GALACTORRHOEA is a recurrent or persisting discharge of milk from the breast.

GALACTOSAEMIA is a very rare, recessively inherited disease, with an incidence of around 1 in 75,000 births. Its importance lies in the disastrous consequences of being overlooked. It results from the deficiency of an enzyme, essential for the metabolism of galactose (q.v.). Normal at birth, affected infants soon develop jaundice, vomiting, diarrhoea, and fail to thrive on starting milk feeds. If the disorder remains unrecognized, liver disease, cataracts, and mental retardation result. Treatment consists of a lactose-free diet, and special lactose-free milks are now available.

GALACTOSE A constituent of lactose, galactose is a simple sugar that is changed in the liver to glucose. A rare genetic metabolic disease, galactosaemia (q.v.), results in infants' being unable to do this conversion because the enzyme necessary for the reaction is absent.

GALL is another name for bile. (See BILE.)

GALL-BLADDER (see LIVER).

GALL-BLADDER, DISEASES OF The gall-bladder rests on the underside of the liver and joins the common hepatic duct via the cystic duct to form the common bile duct. The gall-bladder acts as a reservoir and concentrator of bile, alterations in the composition of which may result in the formation of gall-stones, the commonest disease of the gall-bladder.

Gall-stones affect 22 per cent of women and 11 per cent of men. The incidence increases with age, but only about 30 per cent of those with gall-stones undergo treatment as the majority of cases are asymptomatic. There are three types of stone: cholesterol, pigment and mixed, depending upon their composition; stones are usually mixed and may contain calcium deposits. The cause of most cases is not clear but sometimes gall-stones will form around a 'foreign body' within the bile ducts or gall-bladder, such as suture material or the corpse of a parasite.

In *biliary colic* muscle fibres in the biliary system contract around a stone in the cystic duct or common bile duct producing pain in the right upper quarter of the abdomen, with nausea and occasionally vomiting. Gall-stones small enough to enter the common bile duct may block the flow of bile and cause *jaundice*. Blockage of the cystic duct may lead to *acute cholecystitis*; the gall-bladder wall becomes inflamed resulting in pain in the right upper quarter of the abdomen, fever and an increase in the white blood cell count. There is characteristically tenderness over the tip of the right ninth rib on deep inhalation (Murphy's sign). Infection of the gall-bladder may accompany the acute inflammation and occasionally an empyema of the gall-bladder may result. The elderly are particularly prone to complications of acute cholecystitis, including perforation of the gall-bladder and the formation of an abnormal connection with the small intestine (fistula). *Chronic cholecystitis* is a more insidious form of gall-bladder inflammation, producing non-specific symptoms of abdominal pain, nausea and flatulence which may be worse after a fatty meal.

Diagnosis of gall-stones is usually on the basis of the patients' reported symptoms, although asymptomatic gall-stones are often an incidental finding when investigating another complaint. Confirmatory investigations include abdominal radiography – although many gall-stones are not calcified and thus do not show up on these images; ultrasound scanning (see ULTRASOUND), oral cholecystography, which entails a patient's swallowing a substance opaque to X-rays which is concentrated in the gall-bladder, and endoscopic retrograde cholangio-pancreatography (ERCP) – a technique in which an endoscope (q.v.) is passed into the duodenum and a contrast medium injected into the biliary duct.

Treatment of gall-stone disease is now available in several forms. Biliary colic is treated conservatively with bed rest and injection of morphine-like analgesics. Once the pain has subsided, the patient may then be referred for further treatment as outlined below. Acute cholecystitis is treated by surgical removal of the gall-bladder within 2–3 days of admission to hospital. There are two techniques available for this procedure; firstly, conventional cholecystectomy in which the abdomen is opened and the gall-bladder cut out and, secondly, laparoscopic cholecystectomy in which fibreoptic instruments called endoscopes (see FIBREOPTIC ENDOSCOPY) are introduced into the abdominal cavity via several small incisions. Laparoscopic surgery has the advantage of reducing the patient's recovery time. Gall-stones may be removed during ERCP, they can be dissolved using ultrasound waves (lithotripsy) or tablet therapy (dissolution chemotherapy), Pigment stones, calcified stones or stones larger than 15 mm in diameter are not suitable for this treatment, which is also less likely to succeed in the overweight patient. Drug treatment is prolonged but stones can disappear completely after two years. Stones may reform on stopping therapy. The drugs used are derivatives of bile salts, particularly chenodeoxycholic acid; side-effects include diarrhoea and liver damage.

Other disorders of the gall-bladder are rare. *Polyps* may form and, if symptomatic, should be removed. Malignant change is rare. *Carcinoma* of the gall-bladder is a disease of the elderly and is almost exclusively associated with gall-stones. By the time such a cancer has produced symptoms, the prognosis is bleak: 80 per cent of these patients die within one year of diagnosis. If the tumour is discovered early, 60 per cent of patients will survive five years.

GALL-STONES (see GALL-BLADDER, DISEASES OF.)

GAMETE is a sexual or germ cell: for example, an ovum (q.v.) or spermatozoon (q.v.).

GAMETE INTRAFALLOPIAN TRANSFER (GIFT) (see ARTIFICIAL INSEMINATION).

GAMGEE TISSUE is a surgical dressing composed of a thick layer of cotton-wool between two layers of absorbent gauze, introduced by the Birmingham surgeon, Sampson Gamgee (1828–1886). (Gamgee Tissue has been a registered trade mark since 1911.)

GAMMA BENZENE HEXACHLORIDE is a drug that is used in the treatment of pediculosis (q.v.) and scabies (q.v.).

GAMMA-GLOBULIN describes a group of proteins present in the blood plasma (q.v.). They are characterized by their rate of movement in an electrical field and can be separated by the process of electrophoresis (q.v.). Most gamma-globulins are immunoglobulins. Gamma-globulin injection provides passive or active immunity against Hepatitis A (q.v.). (See GLOBULIN, IMMUNITY and IMMUNOLOGY.)

GAMMA RAYS Short-wavelength penetrating electromagnetic rays produced by some radioactive compounds. More powerful than X-rays, they are used in certain radiotherapy (q.v.) treatments and to sterilize some materials.

GAMMEXANE is the proprietary name for a synthetic insecticide which is a formulation of benzene hexachloride. It is active against a large range of insects and pests, including mosquitoes, fleas, lice, cockroaches, houseflies, clothes moths, bed-bugs, ants, and grain pests.

GANGLION is a term used in two senses. In anatomy, it means an aggregation of nerve-cells found in the course of certain nerves (see NERVES). In surgery, it means an enlargement of the sheath of a tendon, containing fluid. The latter occurs particularly in connection with the sinews in front of, and behind, the wrist.

Causes The cause of these dilatations on the tendon-sheaths is either some irregular growth of the synovial membrane which lines them and secretes the fluid that lubricates their movements, or the forcing out of a small pouch of this membrane through the sheath in consequence of a strain. In either case a bag-like swelling forms, whose connection with the synovial sheath becomes cut off, so that synovial fluid collects in it and distends it more and more.

Symptoms A soft, elastic, movable swelling forms, most often on the back of the wrist. When noticed first it is perhaps the size of a pea, and its connection with a tendon can easily be made out. It may remain this size for many years and occasion no trouble at all, but generally a ganglion gives a peculiar feeling of weakness to the wrist, and on account of its size or position it may be very inconvenient. A ganglion which forms in connection with the flexor tendons in front of the wrist sometimes attains a large size, and extends down the sinews to form another swelling in the palm of the hand.

Treatment Sudden pressure with the thumbs may often burst a ganglion and disperse its contents beneath the skin, after which it should be prevented from refilling by bandaging the part tightly, a very efficient pad being made by wrapping up a large coin in a piece of lint. If it cannot be burst, there only remains the opening of the ganglion, with scraping of its interior. As the ganglion may disappear spontaneously there should be no rush to remove it unless it is causing inconvenience or pain.

GANGRENE, is the death and decay of body tissues caused by a deficiency or cessation of the blood supply. There are two types, dry and moist. The former is a process of mummification, with the blood supply of the affected area of tissue stopping the tissue withering up. Moist gangrene is characterized by death and putrefactive tissue decay caused by bacterial infection. The dead part, when formed of soft tissues, is called a slough and, when part of a bone, is called a sequestrum.

Causes These include injury – especially injuries caused in war – disease, frostbite, severe burns, atheroma (q.v.) in large blood vessels and diseases, such as diabetes mellitus (q.v.) and Raynaud's disease (q.v.). Gas gangrene is a form that occurs when injuries are infected with soil contaminated with gas-producing bacilli such as *Clostridium welchii*, which are found in well-cultivated ground.

Treatment Dry gangrene must be kept dry and amputation of the dead tissue done when a clear demarcation line with healthy tissue has formed. Wet gangrene requires urgent surgery and prompt use of appropriate antibiotics.

GARGLES Gargling is a process by which various substances in solution are brought in contact with the throat without being swallowed. The watery solutions used for the purpose are called gargles. Gargles are used in the treatment of infections of the throat: i.e. 'sore throat', pharyngitis, and tonsillitis.

GARGOYLISM, or HURLER'S SYNDROME, is a rare condition due to lack of a specific enzyme (q.v.). It is a progressive disorder usually leading to death before the age of 10 years. The affected child is usually normal during the first few months of life. Mental and physical deterioration then set in. The characteristic features include coarse facial features (hence the name of the condition), dwarfism, chest deformity, stiff joints, clouding of the cornea, enlargement of the liver and spleen, deafness, and heart murmurs, with mental deterioration. It occurs in about 1 in 100,000 births.

GAS (see ANAESTHESIA; CARBON MONOXIDE; NITROUS OXIDE GAS).

GAS GANGRENE (see GANGRENE).

GASTRECTOMY is an operation for removal of the whole or part of the stomach. The main indication is in the treatment of peptic ulcers (see STOMACH, DISEASES OF) when complications – especially malignant change – supervene. The two varieties of operation most commonly performed are the Billroth 1 gastrectomy, for removal of gastric ulcer, and the Polya gastrectomy. Although most patients are satisfied with the final result, several unpleasant post-gastrectomy syndromes may occur.

GASTRIC means anything connected with the stomach, such as gastric ulcer.

GASTRIC LAVAGE A technique of washing out the stomach with warm water or saline to remove the contents. It is usually done when a person, often a child, has eaten something such as poisonous berries that are potentially harmful. It is also used for treating people who have taken an overdose of drugs. The procedure should be done only by an experienced nurse or doctor.

GASTRIC ULCER (see STOMACH, DISEASES OF).

GASTRIN A hormone produced by the mucous membrane (q.v.) in the pyloric part of the stomach (q.v.). The arrival of food stimulates production of the hormone which in turn stimulates the production of gastric juice.

GASTRITIS is inflammation of the stomach. (See DYSPEPSIA.)

GASTROCNEMIUS is the large double muscle which forms the chief bulk of the calf, and ends below in the tendo calcaneus.

GASTROENTERITIS is inflammation of the stomach and intestines, usually resulting from an acute bacterial or viral infection. Although generally a mild disease in western countries, it is still reputed to be the fifth commonest cause of death in the UK in children under 1 year, with epidemics of *E. coli* gastroenteritis being particularly serious in neonatal units. The main symptoms are diarrhoea and vomiting, often accompanied by fever and – especially in infants – dehydration. These represent an enormous health problem in developing countries, with over 1·5 million children dying annually from the disease in India – a situation exacerbated by early weaning and malnutrition. Complications may include convulsions, kidney failure, and, in severe cases, brain damage.
Treatment This involves the urgent correction of dehydration, using intravenous saline and dextrose feeds initially, with continuing replacement as required. Antibiotics are not indicated unless systemic spread of bacterial infection is likely.

GASTROENTEROSTOMY is an operation performed usually in order to relieve some obstruction to the outlet from the stomach, and consists in making one opening in the lower part of the stomach, another in a neighbouring loop of the small intestine, and stitching the two together.

GASTROSCOPE is an instrument for viewing the interior of the stomach, by means of a special arrangement of light and mirrors attached to a hollow tube, which is introduced into the stomach via the mouth and gullet. A special camera attachment makes it possible to photograph the interior of the stomach. The modern instruments are fully flexible, transmitting an image through a fibreoptic bundle or by a small videocamera. The operator can see and photograph all areas of the stomach and also take biopsy specimens when required. (See FIBREOPTIC ENDOSCOPY.)

GASTROSTOMY is an operation on the stomach by which, when the gullet is blocked by a tumour or other cause, an opening is made from the front of the abdomen into the stomach, so that fluid food can be passed into the organ.

GAUCHER'S DISEASE is a disease characterized by abnormal storage of lipoids, particularly in the spleen, bone marrow, and liver. This results in enlargement of the spleen and the liver, particularly the former, and anaemia. It runs a chronic course. There is no curative treatment, but splenectomy (removal of the spleen) is often helpful.

GEL is the term applied to a colloid substance which is firm in consistence although it contains much water: e.g ordinary gelatin.

GELATIN is derived from collagen (q.v.), the chief constituent of connective tissue. It is a colourless transparent substance which dissolves in boiling water, and on cooling sets into a jelly. Such a jelly is a pleasant addition to the invalid diet, especially when suitably flavoured, but it is of relatively little nutritive value as not more than 1 ounce can be taken in the day: i.e. the amount required to make one pint of jelly. Although it is a protein, it is lacking in several of the vital amino-acids. The ordinary household 'stock' made from boiling bones contains gelatin. Mixed with about two and a half times its weight of glycerin, gelatin forms a soft substance used as the basis for many pastilles and suppositories.

GENERAL PARALYSIS OF THE INSANE, also known as GPI OR DEMENTIA PARALYTICA, is a late manifestation of syphilis (q.v.), usually occurring 5 to 15 years after the primary infection. It is much commoner among men than women, and occasionally it is found in adolescents, when it is due to congenital syphilis.
Signs and symptoms It may present with physical or mental degeneration, though the main pathological changes are seen in the brain. The most characteristic feature is dementia (q.v.), usually insidious in onset and slow in progression. Mild physical signs such as tremors of the tongue and facial muscles, and transient paralysis of the eye muscles, are often present, though tend to be masked by the great emotionalism and delusions of grandeur (see MENTAL ILLNESS). Less common features include epileptic fits and transient episodes of focal cerebral disturbance.
Treatment Early recognition of the disease is vital, and the most effective form of treatment is penicillin. Early institution of treatment may prolong life to ten years or more, while, unrecognized, the disease rarely lasts more than two or three years.

GENERAL PRACTITIONER is the doctor who provides primary medical care and is also responsible for community health-care programmes such as vaccination (q.v.). As the initial health service contact in the United Kingdom for those seeking medical advice or treatment – or merely reassurance – it is vital that the general practitioner establishes a close relationship with his or her patients, with a high degree of trust and confidence. In the National Health Service the general practitioner (GP) or family doctor provides 90 per cent of the medical care for the population. Most illnesses are treated by the GP and, except when emergency patients go direct to hospital, he or she advises whether a patient should see a specialist. This gatekeeper function in the NHS helps to ensure that expensive hospital facilities are used only by those patients who really need them. GPs usually see patients in their surgeries but will also visit them at home when necessary. Around 70 per cent of GPs, of whom there are over 33,000 in the United Kingdom, work in partnerships of two or more, covering each other's work, and on average they each look after 1,900 patients. They are responsible to local family health service authorities (q.v.) and are paid in part by capitation fees according to the number of patients registered with them and in part by item of service fees. Almost every person in the country is registered with a GP, who is also allowed to do private practice. General-practitioner training in the UK normally consists of a three-year course, comprising four six-month periods as a junior hospital doctor, working in specialties such as paediatrics, geriatrics, psychiatry and accident and emergency medicine, followed by an apprenticeship spent working in a general practitioner's surgery.

GENERIC DRUG   A medicinal drug that is sold under its official (generic) name instead of its proprietary (patented brand) name. NHS doctors are advised to prescribe generic drugs where possible as this enables any suitable drug to be dispensed, saving delay to the patient and the sometimes expense to the NHS.

GENES, of which there are between 50,000 and 100,000, in humans are the biological units of heredity. They are arranged along the length of the 23 pairs of chromosomes and, like the chromosomes (q.v.), therefore come in pairs (see GENETIC CODE). Human beings have 46 chromosomes, comprising 2 sex chromosomes and 44 autosomes, but there is also a mitochondrial (q.v.) chromosome outside the cell nucleus which is inherited from the mother.

GENETIC CODE is the message set out sequentially along the human chromosomes. So far only part of the code has been translated and this is the part that occurs in the genes. Genes are responsible for the protein (q.v.) synthesis of the cell. They instruct the cell how to make a particular polypeptide chain for a particular protein.

Genes carry in coded form the detailed specifications for the thousands of kinds of protein molecules the cell requires for its existence, for its enzymes (q.v.), for its repair work and for its reproduction. These proteins are synthesized from the 20 natural amino-acids,

which are uniform throughout nature and which exist in the cell cytoplasm (q.v.) as part of the metabolic pool. The protein molecule consists of amino-acids (q.v.) joined end to end to form long polypeptide chains. An average chain contains 100 to 300 amino-acids. The sequence of bases in the nucleic acid chain of the gene corresponds in some fundamental way to the sequence of amino-acids in the protein molecule, and hence it determines the structure of the particular protein. This is the genetic code. Deoxyribonucleic acid (DNA) (q.v.) is the bearer of this genetic information.

DNA has a long backbone made up of repeating groups of phosphate and sugar deoxyribose. To this backbone four bases are attached as side groups at regular intervals. These four bases are the four letters used to spell out the genetic message. They are adenine, thymine, guanine and cystosine. The molecule of the DNA is made up of two chains coiled round a common axis to form what is called a double helix. The two chains are held together by hydrogen bonds between pairs of bases. Since adenine only pairs with thymine, and guanine only with cystosine, the sequences of bases in one chain fixes the sequence in the other. Several hundred bases would be contained in the length of DNA of a typical gene. If the message of the DNA-based sequences is a continuous succession of thymine, the ribosome (q.v.) will link together a series of the amino-acid phenylalanine. If the base sequence is a succession of cytosine, the ribosome will link up a series of prolines. Thus each amino-acid has its own particular code of bases. In fact each amino-acid is coded by a word consisting of three adjacent bases. In addition to carrying genetic information, DNA is able to synthesize or replicate itself and so pass its information on to daughter cells.

All DNA is part of the chromosome and so it remains confined to the nucleus of the cell (except in the mitochondrial DNA). Proteins are synthesized by the ribosomes which are in the cytoplasm. DNA achieves control over protein production in the cytoplasm by directing the synthesis of ribonucleic acid (RNA) (q.v.). Most of the DNA in a cell is inactive, otherwise the cell would synthesize simultaneously every protein that the individual was capable of forming. When part of the DNA structure becomes 'active', it acts as a template for the ribonucleic acid which itself acts as a template for protein synthesis when it becomes attached to the ribosome. Ribonucleic acid exists in three forms. First 'messenger RNA' carries the necessary 'message' for the synthesis of a specific protein, from the nucleus to the ribosome. Second, 'transfer RNA' collects the individual amino-acids which exist in the cytoplasm as part of the metabolic pool and carries them to the ribosome. Third, there is RNA in the ribosome itself. RNA has a similar structure to DNA but the sugar is ribose instead of deoxyribose and uracil replaces the base thymine. Before the ribosome can produce the proteins, the amino-acids must be lined up in the correct order on the messenger RNA template. This alignment is carried out by transfer RNA, of which there is a specific form for each individual amino-acid. Transfer RNA can not only recognize its specific amino-acid, but also identify the position it is required to occupy on the messenger RNA template. This is because each transfer RNA has its own sequence of bases and recognizes its site on the messenger RNA by pairing bases with it. The ribosome then travels along the chain of messenger RNA and links the amino-acids, which have thus been arranged in the requisite order, by peptide bonds and protein is released. Proteins are important for two main reasons. First, all the enzymes of living cells are made of protein. One gene is responsible for one enzyme. Genes thus control all the biochemical processes of the body and are responsible for the inborn difference between human beings. Second, proteins also fulfil a structural role in the cell so that genes controlling the synthesis of structural proteins are responsible for morphological differences between human beings.

GENETIC COUNSELLING is the procedure whereby advice is given about the risks of a genetic disorder and the various options that are open to the individual at risk. This may often involve establishing the diagnosis in the family, as this would be a prerequisite before giving any detailed advice. Risks can be calculated from simple Mendelian inheritance (see MENDELISM) in many genetic disorders. However, in many disorders with a genetic element such as cleft lip or palate, the risk of recurrence is obtained from population studies. Risks include not only the likelihood of having a child who is congenitally affected by a disorder, but also, for adults, that of being vulnerable to an adult-onset disease. The options for individuals would include taking no action, modifying their behaviour, or taking some form of direct action. For those at risk of having an affected child, where prenatal diagnosis is available, this would involve either carrying on with reproduction regardless of risk, deciding not to have children, or deciding to go ahead to have children, but opting for prenatal diagnosis. For an adult-onset disorder such as a predisposition to ovarian cancer, an individual may choose to take no action, to take preventive measures such as use of the oral contraceptive pill, to have screening of the ovaries with measures such as ultrasound, or to take direct action such as removing the ovaries to prevent ovarian cancer occurring.

There are now regional genetics centres throughout the United Kingdom, and patients can be referred through their family doctor or specialists.

GENETIC DISORDERS are caused when there are mutations or other abnormalities which disrupt the code of a gene or set of genes. These are divided into autosomal dominant,

autosomal recessive, sex-linked and polygenic disorders.

DOMINANT GENES   A dominant characteristic is an effect which is produced whenever a gene or gene defect is present. If a disease is due to a dominant gene, those affected are heterozygous, that is they only carry a fault in the gene on the one of the pair of chromosomes concerned. Affected people married to normal individuals transmit the gene directly to one half of the children, although this is a random event just like tossing a coin. Huntington's chorea (q.v.) is due to the inheritance of a dominant gene, as is neurofibromatosis and familial adenomatous polyposis of the colon. Achondroplasia is an example of a disorder in which there is a high frequency of a new dominant mutation, for the majority of affected people have normal parents and siblings. However, the chances of the children of a parent with achondroplasia (q.v.) being affected are one in two, as with any other dominant characteristic. Other diseases inherited as dominant characteristics include spherocytosis, haemorrhagic telangiectasia and adult polycystic kidney disease.

RECESSIVE GENES   If a disease is due to a recessive gene, those affected must have the faulty gene on both copies of the chromosome pair (i.e. be homozygous). The possession of a single recessive gene does not result in overt disease, and the bearer usually carries this potentially unfavourable gene without knowing it. If that person marries another carrier of the same recessive gene, there is a one-in-four chance that their children will receive the gene in a double dose, and so have the disease. If an individual sufferer from a recessive disease marries an apparently normal person who is a heterozygous carrier of the same gene, one half of the children will be affected and the other half will be carriers of the disease. The commonest of such recessive conditions in Britain is cystic fibrosis (q.v.), which affects about one child in 2,000. Approximately 5 per cent of the population carry a faulty copy of the gene. Most of the inborn errors of metabolism, such as phenylketonuria (q.v.), galactosaemia (q.v.) and congenital adrenal hyperplasia (see ADRENOGENITAL SYNDROME), are due to recessive genes.

There are characteristics which may be incompletely recessive, that is, neither completely dominant nor completely recessive and the heterozygotus person, who bears the gene in a single dose, may have a slight defect, whilst the homozygotus, with a double dose of the gene, has a severe illness. The sickle-cell trait (q.v.) is a result of the sickle-cell gene in single dose, and sickle-cell anaemia is the consequence of a double dose.

SEX-LINKED GENES   If a condition is sex-linked, affected males are homozygous for the mutated gene as they carry it on their single X chromosome. The X chromosome carries many genes, while the Y chromosome bears few genes, if any, other than those determining masculinity. The genes on the X chromosome of the male are thus not matched by corresponding genes on the Y chromosome. There is thus no chance of the Y chromosome neutralizing any recessive trait on the X chromosome. A recessive gene can therefore produce disease since it will not be suppressed by the normal gene of the homologous chromosome. The same recessive gene on the X chromosome of the female will be suppressed by the normal gene on the other X chromosome. Such sex-linked conditions include haemophilia (q.v.), Christmas disease (q.v.), Duchenne (q.v.) type of muscular dystrophy (see MYOPATHY) and nephrogenic diabetes insipidus (q.v.). If the mother of an affected child has another male relative affected, she is a heterozygote carrier; half her sons will have the disease and half her daughters will be carriers. The sister of a haemophiliac thus has a 50-per-cent chance of being a carrier. An affected male cannot transmit the gene to his son because the X chromosome of the son must come from the mother; all his daughters, however, will be carriers as the X chromosome for the father must be transmitted to all his daughters. Hence sex-linked recessive characteristics cannot be passed from father to son. Sporadic cases may be the result of a new mutation, in which case the mother is not the carrier and is not likely to have further affected children. It is probable that one third of haemophiliacs arise as a result of fresh mutations and these patients will be the first in the families to be affected. Sometimes the carrier of a sex-linked recessive gene can be identified. The sex-linked variety of retinitis pigmentosa (see RETINA, DISORDERS OF) can often be detected by ophthalmoscopic examination.

A few rare disorders are due to dominant genes carried on the X chromosome. An example of such a condition is familial hypophosphataemia with vitamin-D-resistant rickets.

POLYGENIC INHERITANCE In many inherited conditions the disease is due to the combined action of several genes and the genetic element is then called multi-factorial or polygenic. In this situation there would be an increased incidence of the disease in the families concerned, but it will not follow the Mendelian (see MENDELISM, GENETIC CODE) ratio. The greater the number of independent genes involved in determining a certain disease, the more complicated will be the pattern of inheritance. Furthermore, many inherited disorders are the result of a combination of genetic and environmental influences. Diabetes mellitus is the most familiar of such multi-factorial inheritance. The predisposition to develop diabetes is an inherited characteristic, although the gene is not always able to express itself: this is called incomplete penetrance. Whether or not the individual with a genetic predisposition towards the disease actually develops diabetes will also depend on environmental factors. Diabetes is more common in the relatives of diabetic patients, and even more so amongst identical twins. Non-genetic factors which are important in precipitating overt disease are obesity, excessive intake of carbohydrate foods and pregnancy.

Schizophrenia is another example of the combined effects of genetic and environmental influences in precipitating disease. The risk of schizophrenia in a child, one of whose parents has the disease, is one in ten, but this figure is modified by the early environment of the child.

GENETIC ENGINEERING, or RECOMBINANT DNA TECHNOLOGY, has only developed in the past decade or so; it is the process of changing the genetic material of a cell. Genes from one cell, for example a human cell, can be inserted into another cell, usually a bacterium, and made to function. It is now possible to insert the gene responsible for the production of human insulin, human growth hormone and interferon from a human cell into a bacterium. Segments of DNA for insertion can be prepared by breaking long chains into smaller pieces by the use of restriction enzymes. The segments are then inserted into the affecting organism, usually the bacteria *Eschericia coli* (q.v.) by using plasmids (q.v.) and bacteriophages (q.v.). Plasmids are small packets of DNA that are found within bacteria and can be passed from one bacterium to another. Already genetic engineering is contributing to easing the problems of diagnosis. DNA analysis and production of monoclonal antibodies (q.v.) are other applications of genetic engineering. Genetic engineering has significantly contributed to horticulture and agriculture with certain characteristics of one organism or variant of a species being transfected into another. This has given rise to higher-yield crops and to alteration in colouring and size in produce. Genetic engineering is also contributing to our knowledge of how human genes function as these can be transfected into mice and other animals which can then act as models for genetic therapy. Studying the effects of inherited mutations derived from human DNA in these animal models is thus a very important and much faster way of learning about human disease.

GENETIC FINGERPRINTING This technique shows the relationships between individuals. For example, it can be used to prove maternity or paternity of a child. The procedure is also used in forensic medicine whereby any tissue left behind by a criminal at the scene of a crime can be compared genetically with the tissue of a suspect. DNA (q.v.), the genetic material in living cells, can be extracted from blood, semen, and other body tissues. The technique, pioneered in Britain in 1984, is now widely used.

GENETICS is the science which deals with the origin of the characteristics of an individual or the study of heredity.

GENETIC SCREENING A screening procedure that tests whether a person has a genetic make-up that is linked with a particular disease. If so, the person may either develop the disease or pass it on to his or her offspring. When an individual has been found to carry a genetically linked disease, he or she should receive genetic counselling (q.v.) from an expert in inherited diseases. (See GENES; GENETIC DISORDERS.)

GENITALIA are the external organs of reproduction.

GENITO-URINARY MEDICINE the branch of medicine that deals with sexually transmitted diseases (see VENEREAL DISEASES).

GENITO-URINARY TRACT consists of the kidneys, ureters, bladder, and urethra and, in the male, the genital organs.

GENOME is a complete set of chromosomes derived from one parent, or the total gene complement of a set of chromosomes. An international study is well under way to produce a complete map of the human genome.

GENOTYPE All of an individual's genetic information that is encoded in his or her chromosomes (q.v.). It also means the genetic information carried by a pair of alleles which controls a particular characteristic. (See GENES.)

GENTAMICIN is an antibiotic derived from a species of micro-organisms, *Micromonospora purpurea*. Its main value is that it is active against certain micro-organisms such as *Pseudomonas pyocyanea, E. coli* and *Aerobacter aerogenes* which are not affected by other antibiotics, as well as staphylococci which have become resistant to penicillin.

GENTIAN VIOLET, or CRYSTAL VIOLET, is a dye belonging to the rosaniline group. Gentian violet is a good superficial antiseptic. It is used in the treatment of burns, either alone or in conjunction with brilliant green and proflavine. Applied to a burn, gentian violet forms a tough pliable film.

GENU VALGUM is the medical term for knock-knee (q.v.).

GENU VARUM is the medical term for bow leg (q.v.).

GERIATRICS is that branch of medicine which treats of the disorders and diseases associated with old age.

GERMAN MEASLES, or RUBELLA, is an acute infectious disease of a mild type, which may sometimes be difficult to differentiate from mild forms of measles and scarlet fever.

Cause The cause of infection is a virus. It is spread by close contact with infected individuals, and is infectious for a week before the rash appears and at least four days afterwards. It occurs in epidemics every three years or so, predominantly in the winter and spring. Children are more likely to be affected than infants. One attack gives permanent immunity. The incubation period is usually 14 to 21 days.

Symptoms are very mild, and the disease is not at all serious. On the day of onset there may be shivering, headache, slight catarrh with sneezing, coughing and sore throat, very slight fever, not above 37·8 °C (100 °F), and at the same time the glands of the neck become enlarged. These symptoms are usually slight. Within 24 hours of the onset a pink, slightly raised eruption appears, first on the face or neck, then on the chest, and the second day spreads all over the body.

An attack of German measles during the early months of pregnancy may be responsible for congenital defects in the fetus. The incidence of such defects is not precisely known, but probably around 20 per cent of children, whose mothers have had German measles in the first three months of the pregnancy, are born with congenital defects. These defects take a variety of forms, but the most important ones are: low birth weight with retarded physical development; malformations of the heart; cataract, and deafness.

Treatment The only treatment necessary is confinement to bed so long as there are any symptoms. Infectivity ceases within four days provided there are no symptoms. Children who develop the disease should not return to school until they have recovered, and in any case not before four days have passed from the onset of the rash. In view of the mildness of the disease, contacts are seldom kept in quarantine, but they should be carefully watched from the tenth to the twenty-first day from exposure to infection.

In view of the possible effect of the disease upon the fetus, particular care should be taken to isolate pregnant mothers from contact with infected subjects. As the risk to the fetus is particularly high during the first sixteen weeks of pregnancy, any pregnant mother exposed to infection during this period should be given an intramuscular injection of gamma-globulin (q.v.). A vaccine is available to protect an individual against rubella. In the United Kingdom it is official policy for all children to have the combined measles, mumps and rubella (MMR) vaccine (q.v.), subject to parental consent. All women of childbearing age, who have been shown by a simple laboratory test not to have had the disease, should be vaccinated, provided the woman is not pregnant at the time and has not been exposed to the risk of pregnancy during the previous eight weeks.

GERMS (see MICROBIOLOGY).

GESTATION is another name for pregnancy.

GIARDIASIS is a condition caused by a parasitic organism known as *Giardia lamblia*, which is found in the duodenum (see INTESTINE) and the upper part of the small intestine. This organism is usually harmless, but is sometimes responsible for causing diarrhoea. Over 3000 cases a year are reported in Britain. In most of these the infection has been acquired from drinking untreated water in the Middle East or Russia. The illness develops one or two weeks after exposure to infection, and usually starts as an explosive diarrhoea, with the passage of pale fatty stools, abdominal pain and nausea. It responds well to metronidazole or mepacrine.

GIDDINESS (see VERTIGO).

GIGANTISM (see ACROMEGALY).

GINGIVITIS means inflammation of the gums. (See TEETH, DISEASES OF.)

GLANDERS, or EQUINIA, is a specific infectious disease to which certain animals, chiefly those with an undivided hoof – such as horses, asses, and mules – are liable, and communicable by them to man, but this is rare. The cause of glanders is a short rod-shaped organism, known as the *Loefflerella mallei*. It has been eradicated from Britain, but still occurs in Eastern Europe and Asia. Untreated, the acute form of disease may be fatal in humans. About half of those with the chronic form survive without treatment. Antibiotics are the treatment of choice.

GLANDS are divisible into several classes. In the first place, the term is applied to organs like the liver, pancreas, and kidneys, which produce a secretion; but in general the term is limited to smaller structures concerned in the production of some excretion from the body, or of some substance needful to its working. These latter are divided into two quite distinct groups: (1) glands which produce some form of secretion or excretion; (2) lymphatic glands.

(1) SECRETING AND EXCRETING GLANDS comprise glands in almost all parts of the body, which vary much in appearance, in size, and in the character of the substances they produce. The skin, for example, is richly supplied with sebaceous glands, which secrete an oily material, and with sweat glands, which are placed in rows whose openings can be seen with a weak magnifying lens upon the ridges of the palms and soles. The lining membrane of the stomach is made up of long tubular glands set closely side by side, and in these the gastric juice is formed. The structure of the mucous membrane in the intestine is much the same. In all these mucous membranes there are situated other glands, generally formed each of a small mass of twisted tubes, which secrete a clear shining fluid known as mucus, that gives to these membranes their soft, smooth appearance and their name. The glands so far mentioned are all of microscopic size, but there are many of large dimensions. The parotid gland, situated just in front of the ear, the submaxillary gland, which can be easily felt, of the size of a chestnut beneath the jaw, and the sublingual gland, which can be seen beneath the tongue, are occupied in producing saliva, and known as salivary glands. The breasts or mammary glands are a pair of large glands situated in the skin over the front of the chest, and secrete milk. The thyroid gland, situated in front of the neck, has no outlet to the exterior, but produces an important secretion which is absorbed by the blood and carried throughout the body. The adrenal (suprarenal) glands situated immediately above the kidneys act under similar conditions. Many of the glands which have an outlet through which one secretion comes, such as the pancreas and testes, also produce what is called an internal secretion that is absorbed by the blood, and exerts a profound effect upon general nutrition and metabolism.

Glands which produce an internal secretion are known as endocrine glands. (See ENDOCRINE GLANDS.)

(2) LYMPHATIC GLANDS are scattered all through the body in connection with the system of lymphatic vessels. They vary much in size, from that of microscopic masses to that of large beans, but they have essentially the same structure everywhere. Round each gland is a fibrous tissue capsule, from which partitions and bands run into the gland to join one another and give it cohesion. In the meshes of these lie enormous numbers of lymph corpuscles in the circulating blood. These corpuscles are arranged in masses round which the lymph circulates freely. Numbers of lymph-vessels (afferent vessels) pierce the capsule of the gland, and the lymph, after passing from them, percolates through the gland and leaves its central part, carrying with it many corpuscles, by a few larger lymph-vessels (efferent vessels). The vessels leaving one gland pass on to enter another, the glands being, as a rule, arranged in chains.

In the limbs the lymph-vessels pass from the foot and hand up to the knee and elbow, respectively, before they encounter glands. A few glands are situated in the bend of each of these joints, and the vessels passing from these reach large chains of glands in the groin and armpit, respectively. The chains of glands beneath the jaw and down each side of the neck are known to everyone from the frequency with which they become inflamed and swollen. Inside the abdomen small lymph vessels known as lacteals collect certain parts of the food from the intestine, and pass their contents through mesenteric glands, situated deep in the abdominal cavity. Deep in the chest, too, lie many large bronchial glands, receiving lymphatics from the lungs. The lymph-vessels from the lower limbs and abdomen, after passing through numerous glands, unite into a single trunk, about the size of a quill, called the thoracic duct, which passes upwards through the chest, collecting the lymphatics of the chest, left arm, and left side

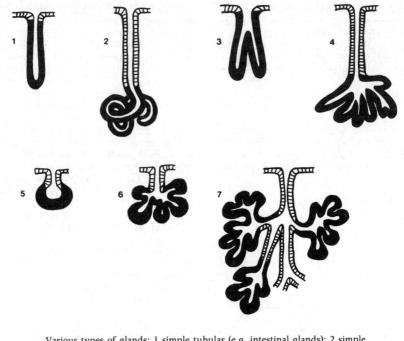

Various types of glands; 1 simple tubular (e.g. intestinal glands); 2 simple coiled tubular (e.g. sweat glands); 3, 4 simple branched tubular (e.g. gastric glands); 5 simple alveolar; 6 simple branched alveolar (e.g. sebaceous glands); 7 compound (e.g. salivary and mammary glands). The secretory part of the gland is black.

of the neck, to open into the veins on the left side of the neck. A shorter lymphatic vessel collects the lymphatics from the right side of the chest, right arm, and right side of the neck, opening into the veins of the right side. The point where the lymphatic system on each side opens into the venous system is at or close to the point of union of the subclavian vein with the internal jugular vein. By means of these connections the lymph corpuscles formed in the glands may reach the blood. Beyond forming these corpuscles, the glands have another function, acting as a species of filters upon the lymph circulation, and keeping back micro-organisms and other dangerous impurities from entering the blood circulation.

GLANDULAR FEVER (see MONONUCLEOSIS).

GLANS The term applied to the ends of the penis (q.v.) and the clitoris (q.v.). In the penis the glans is the distal helmet-shaped part that is formed by the bulbous corpus spongiosum (erectile tissue). In an uncircumcised man the glans is covered by the foreskin or prepuce when the penis is flaccid.

GLASGOW COMA SCALE A method developed by two doctors in Glasgow that is used to assess the depth of coma or unconsciousness suffered by an individual. The scale is split into

three groups: eye opening, motor response, and verbal response, with the level of activity within each group given a score. A person's total score is the sum of the numbers scored in each group and this provides a reasonably objective assessment of the patient's coma state.

GLAUCOMA is a term used to describe a group of disorders characterized by the intra-ocular pressure being so high as to damage the nerve fibres in the retina and optic nerve as it leaves the eye. Glaucoma is usually classified as being either open-angle glaucoma or narrow-angle glaucoma. *Open-angle glaucoma* is a chronic, slowly progressive, usually bilateral disorder. It occurs in 1 in 200 of people over 40 and amounts for 20 per cent of those registered blind in Great Britain. Symptoms are virtually non-existent until well into the disease, when the patient may experience visual problems. It is not painful. The characteristic findings are that the intra-ocular pressure is raised (normal pressure is up to 21 mm Hg) causing cupping of the optic disc and a glaucomatous visual-field loss. The angle between the iris and the cornea remains open. Treatment is aimed at decreasing the intra-ocular pressure initially by drops and tablets. Surgery may be required later. A *trabeculectomy* is an operation to create a channel through which fluid can drain from the eye in a controlled fashion in order to bring the pressure down. *Narrow-angle glaucoma* affects

1 in 1000 people over 40 years of age and is more common in women. Symptoms may start with coloured haloes around street lights at night. These may then be followed by rapid onset of severe pain in and around the eye accompanied by a rapid fall in vision. One eye is usually affected first; this alerts the surgeon so that action can be taken to prevent a similar attack in the other eye. Treatment must be started as an emergency with intensive drops and tablets to bring the pressure down. This is followed by surgery to prevent recurrence. Acute narrow-angle glaucoma occurs because the peripheral iris is pushed against the back of the cornea. This closes off the angle between iris and cornea through which aqueous humour drains out of the eye. Since the aqueous humour cannot drain away, it builds up inside the eye causing a rapid increase in pressure.

GLEET means a chronic form of gonorrhoea (q.v.).

GLENOID is the term applied to the shallow socket on the shoulder-blade into which the humerus fits, forming the shoulder-joint.

GLIBENCLAMIDE is a drug which stimulates the beta cells of the pancreas to liberate insulin, and is thereby proving of value in some cases of diabetes mellitus (q.v.). (See SULPHONYLUREAS.)

GLICLAZIDE (see SULPHONYLUREAS).

GLIOMA is a tumour which forms in the brain or spinal cord, composed of neuroglia, which is the special connective tissue that in these organs supports the nerve-cells and nerve-fibres.

GLIPIZIDE (see SULPHONYLUREAS).

GLIQUIDONE (see SULPHONYLUREAS).

GLOBIN A protein which when it combines with haem forms haemoglobin (q.v.), the molecule found in the red blood cell that carries oxygen and carbon dioxide.

GLOBULIN is a class of proteins which are insoluble in water and alcohol and soluble in weak salt solution. (See also GAMMA-GLOBULIN.)

GLOBUS is a term applied generally to any structures of ball shape, but especially to the sensation of a ball in the throat causing choking, which forms a common symptom of hysteria.

GLOMERULAR FILTRATION RATE The kidney filters a large volume of blood – 25 per cent of cardiac output or around 1300 ml – through its two million glomeruli (q.v.) every minute. The glomeruli filter out cell, protein, and fat-free fluid which, after reabsorption of certain chemicals, is excreted as urine. The rate of this ultrafiltration process, which in health is remarkably constant, is called the glomerular filtration rate (GFR). Each day nearly 180 litres of water plus some small molecular-weight constituents of blood are filtrated. The GFR is thus an indicator of kidney function. The most widely used measurement is creatinine (q.v.) clearance and this is assessed by measuring the amount of creatinine in a 24-hour sample of urine and the amount of creatinine in the plasma; a formula is applied that gives the GFR.

GLOMERULONEPHRITIS (see KIDNEYS, DISEASES OF)

GLOMERULUS is a small knot of blood-vessels about the size of a sand grain, of which around 1,000,000 are found in each kidney, and from which the excretion of fluid out of the blood into the tubules of the kidney takes place.

GLOSSITIS means inflammation of the tongue.

GLOSSOPHARYNGEAL nerve is the ninth cranial nerve, which in the main is a sensory nerve, being the nerve of taste in the posterior third of the tongue and the nerve of general sensation for the whole upper part of the throat and middle ear. It also supplies the parotid gland and one of the muscles on the side of the throat.

GLOTTIS is the narrow opening at the upper end of the larynx. The glottis is made up of the true vocal cords. (See AIR PASSAGES; CHOKING; LARYNX.)

GLUCAGON is a hormone secreted by the alpha cells of the islets of Langerhans in the pancreas, which increases the amount of glucose in the blood. This it does by promoting the breakdown of liver glycogen (glycogenolysis). It is secreted in response to a lowered blood sugar and is used therapeutically to treat hypoglycaemia (q.v.).

GLUCOCORTICOIDS is the group of steroid hormones produced by the adrenal cortex, which includes cortisol and cortisone (q.v.), and which particularly affect protein, fat and carbohydrate metabolism.

GLUCONEOGENESIS means the formation of sugar from amino-acids in the liver.

GLUCOSE (DEXTROSE; GRAPE SUGAR) is the form of sugar found in honey and in grapes and some other fruits. It is also the form of sugar circulating in the blood stream and the form into which all sugars and starches are converted in the small intestine before being absorbed. Glucose is a yellowish-white crystalline substance soluble in water and having the property of turning the ray of polarized light to the right. It is often given to patients as an easily assimilated form of carbohydrate. It has the further practical advantage in this context of not being nearly as sweet-tasting as cane sugar and therefore relatively large amounts can be consumed without sickening the patient. For patients unable to take food by the mouth, glucose is sometimes administered in the form of an enema consisting of 5 per cent of glucose in normal saline fluid, or 28·5 grams (1 ounce) of glucose to 570 ml (1 pint) of water. The same fluid, when carefully sterilized, may be injected beneath the skin or directly into the veins, and is quickly absorbed. (See SUGAR; URINE.)

GLUCOSE-TOLERANCE TEST A way of assessing the body's efficiency at metabolizing glucose (q.v.). The test is used in diagnosing diabetes mellitus (q.v.). The patient is starved for up to 16 hours after which he is fed glucose by mouth. The concentrations of glucose in the blood and urine are then measured at half-hour intervals over two hours.

GLUCOSIDE is a glycoside (q.v.) formed from glucose.

GLUE EAR is another name for secretory otitis media. (See EAR, DISEASES OF.)

GLUE SNIFFING (see SOLVENT ABUSE).

GLUTEAL is the name applied to the region of the buttock and the structures situated in it, such as the gluteal muscles, arteries, and nerves.

GLUTEN is the constituent of wheat-flour which forms an adhesive substance on addition of water, and allows the 'raising' of bread. It can be separated from the starch of flour, and being of a protein nature is used to make bread for those diabetics who are debarred from starchy and sugary foods.

It is also responsible for certain forms of what is now known as the malabsorption syndrome (q.v.). In these cases an essential part of treatment is a gluten-free diet.

GLUTETHIMIDE is a non-barbiturate hypnotic, which induces sleep fairly rapidly, and whose effects last about six hours.

GLUTEUS Three gluteal muscles form each buttock. The gluteus maximus is the large powerful muscle that gives the buttocks their rounded shape. The remaining two muscles are the gluteus medius and gluteus minimus and together the three muscles are responsible for moving the thigh.

GLYCERIN, or GLYCEROL, is an alcohol, $C_3H_8O_3$, which occurs naturally in combination with organic acids in the form of fats or triglycerides. It is a clear, colourless, thick liquid of sweet taste. It dissolves many substances, and it has a great power of absorbing water.

Uses Glycerin has many varied uses. Numerous substances, such as carbolic acid, tannic acid, alum, borax, boric acid, starch, are dissolved in it for application to the body. It is frequently applied along with other remedies to inflamed areas for its action in extracting fluid and thus diminishing inflammation.

Mixed with an equal quantity of water it forms a useful mouth-wash when the tongue and gums are furred or dry, and, as a spray, is one of the best ways of relieving the discomfort of laryngitis. It is also useful for application to the skin in order to prevent chapping in cold weather, and to protect and heal all sorts of small abrasions.

Internally, pure glycerin, in doses of 1 or 2 teaspoonfuls, acts as a laxative, administered either by the mouth or as an enema. For its pleasant taste it is added to various medicines. It is mixed with gelatin to form a basis for pastilles. (See GELATIN.)

GLYCEROL is another name for glycerin (q.v.).

GLYCERYL TRINITRATE, also known as trinitrin and nitroglycerin, is a drug of explosive properties, which is used in the treatment of angina pectoris (q.v.). It is normally given as a sublingual tablet or spray, though percutaneous preparations may be useful in the prophylaxis of angina, particularly for patients who suffer attacks at rest, especially at night. Sublingually it provides rapid symptomatic relief of angina, but is only effective for 20–30 minutes. It is a potent vasodilator, and this may lead to unwanted side-effects such as flushing, headache, and postural hypotension (q.v.). Its anti-spasmodic effects are also valuable in the treatment of asthma (q.v.), biliary and renal colic (q.v.), and certain cases of vomiting (q.v.).

GLYCO- is a prefix meaning of the nature of, or containing, sugar.

GLYCOGEN, or ANIMAL STARCH, is a carbohydrate substance found specially in the liver, as well as in other tissues. It is the form in which carbohydrates taken in the food are stored in the liver and muscles before they are converted into glucose as the needs of the body require.

GLYCOSIDE is a compound of a sugar and a non-sugar unit. Glycosides are widespread throughout nature and include many important drugs such as digoxin.

GLYCOSOLATED HAEMOGLOBIN (HbA1) is a small proportion of the total haemoglobin (q.v.) in the blood. It differs from the major component, HbA, in that it has a glucose group attached. The rate of synthesis of HbA1 is a function of the blood-glucose concentration, and since it accumulates throughout the life span of the red blood cell – normally 120 days – the concentration of HbA1 is related to the mean blood-glucose concentration over the past 3–4 months. It is thus a useful indicator of medium-term diabetic control (see DIABETES MELLITUS) – a good target range would be a concentration of 5 to 8 per cent. When interpreting the HbA1 level, however, it is important to remember that wide fluctuations in blood-glucose concentration, together with anaemia (q.v.) or a reduced erythrocyte life span, may give misleading results.

GLYCOSURIA means the presence of sugar in the urine. By far the most common cause of glycosuria is diabetes mellitus, but it may also occur as a result of a lowered renal threshold for sugar when it is called renal glycosuria, and is not indicative of disease.

GOBLET CELL A columnar secretory cell occurring in the epithelium of the respiratory and intestinal tracts. The cells produce the main constituents of mucus (q.v.).

GOITRE is a term applied to a swelling in the front of the neck caused by an enlargement of the thyroid gland. The thyroid lies between the skin and the front of the windpipe and in health is not large enough to be seen. The four main varieties of goitre are the simple goitre, the nodular, the lymphadenoid goitre and the toxic goitre.
SIMPLE GOITRE is a benign enlargement of the thyroid gland with normal production of hormone. It is a physiological response to maintain the synthesis of thyroid hormone. It may occur sporadically, but in certain geographical areas of the world it is found more frequently and it is then referred to as 'endemic'. It may be the result of a deficiency of iodine, which is essential for thyroid hormone production. If iodine intake is deficient and the production of thyroid hormone is threatened, the anterior pituitary secretes increased amounts of thyrotrophic hormone with consequent hyperplasia of the thyroid gland. The prevalence of endemic goitre can be, and has been, reduced by the iodinization of domestic salt in many countries. Simple goitres commonly occur at puberty, during pregnancy and at the menopause, which are times of increased demand for thyroid hormone. They may also result from defective utilization of iodine in the synthesis of thyroxine. The immediate cause of simple goitre is increased production of thyrotrophic hormone by the pituitary. The only effective treament is thyroid replacement therapy to suppress the enhanced production of thyrotrophic hormone.

NODULAR GOITRES do not respond as well as the diffuse goitres to thyroxine treatment. They are usually the result of alternating episodes of hyperplasia and involution which lead to permanent thyroid enlargment. The only effective way of curing a nodular goitre is to excise it and thyroidectomy should be recommended if the goitre is causing pressure symptoms or if there is a suspicion of malignancy.
LYMPHADENOID GOITRES are due to the production of antibodies against antigens in the thyroid gland. They are an example of an auto-immune disease. They tend to occur in the 3rd and 4th decade and the gland is much firmer than the softer gland of a simple goitre. Lymphadenoid goitres respond to treatment with thyroxine.
TOXIC GOITRES are usually the result of Graves' disease (q.v.), though much less frequently autonomous nodules of a nodular goitre may be responsible for the increased production of thyroxine and render the patient hyperthyroid (toxic). Graves' disease is also an auto-immune disease in which an antibody is produced that stimulates the thyroid to produce excessive amounts of hormone, making the patient thyrotoxic.

GOLD SALTS are used in the treatment of rheumatoid arthritis. Gold may be administered in various forms, such as sodium aurothiomalate. It is injected in very small doses intramuscularly and produces a reaction in the affected tissues which leads to their scarring and healing. If gold is administered in too large quantities skin eruptions, albuminuria, metallic taste in the mouth, jaundice, and feverishness may be produced, so that it is necessary to prolong a course of this remedy over many months in minute doses. Routine blood and urine tests are also necessary in order to detect any adverse or toxic effect at an early stage.

GOLFER'S ELBOW is a term applied to a condition comparable to tennis elbow. It is not uncommon in the left elbow of right-handed golfers who catch the head of their club in the ground when making a duff shot. (See ELBOW.)

GONAD is a gland which produces a gamete; an ovary or a testis. There are four stages of sexual development: (1) gonadal differentiation, (2) development of internal genitalia, (3) external genital differentiation, (4) puberty.
The testis and ovary both develop from the undifferentiated gonad which appears in the fourth week of gestation. This indifferent gonad has a cortex and a medulla. In the presence of a Y chromosome the medulla of this structure evolves into a testis and the cortex regresses. In the presence of two X chromosomes the cortex differentiates into an ovary and the medulla regresses. (See GENETIC CODE.)
The internal genitalia also develop from separate primitive structures that transiently

co-exist in embryos of both sexes. In the male the Wolffian ducts give rise to the vas deferens, the seminal vesicles and the epididymus, and the Mullerian ducts regress (the prostatic utricle is a remnant). In the female the Mullerian ducts fuse to produce the Fallopian tubes, the uterus and the upper vagina, and the Wolffian ducts regress. The development of the Wolffian ducts and the suppression of the Mullerian ducts requires the presence of a functioning fetal testis from which an 'inducer' diffuses locally to both suppress the Mullerian ducts and stimulate the development of the Wolffian ducts. This inducer is not androgen which is unable to suppress the Wolffian ducts. In the absence of this substance the duct system differentiates along feminine lines irrespective of the genetic sex. Thus if there is no gonad, as in gonadal agenesis, the ducts will develop along female lines. Jost showed in 1947 that surgical castration of the animal fetus before the time of sexual differentiation prevented masculinization and all the litters grew up as apparent females. The developing testis was thus essential for masculinity but the ovary was not essential for feminity. The female form, both internal and external, was that of the neuter sex.

The third stage of sexual development, namely the differentiation of the external genitalia, also involves development from primitive structures common to both sexes. In the female the genital folds become the labia minora, the genital swellings the labia majora and the genital tubercule the clitoris, whilst in the male under the influence of androgens the shaft of the penis, the glans penis and the scrotum are respectively developed. Failure of the genital folds to fuse correctly in the male results in hypospadias. Thus both in the development of the internal genitalia and the external genitalia differentiation to the male form requires a positive influence, otherwise development follows the female pattern.

The final stage of sexual development is puberty when pituitary gonadotrophin production increases to adult levels, and secondary sex characteristics appear.

GONADOTROPHINS, or GONADOTROPHIC HORMONES, are hormones that control the activity of the gonads (i.e. the testes and ovaries). In the male they stimulate the secretion of testosterone and the production of spermatozoa. In the female they stimulate the production of ova and the secretion of oestrogen (q.v.) and progesterone (q.v.). There are two gonadotrophins produced by the pituitary gland. *Chorionic gonadotrophin* is produced in the placenta and excreted in the urine.

GONORRHOEA is an inflammatory disease affecting especially the mucous membrane of the urethra in the male and that of the vagina in the female, but spreading also to other parts. It is the most common of the venereal diseases (q.v.). According to the World Health Organization, 200 million new cases are notified annually in the world. In England in 1992, there were over 14,500 cases.

Causes The disease is directly contagious from another person already suffering in this manner, usually by sexual intercourse, but occasionally it is conveyed by the discharge on sponges, towels or clothing as well as by actual contact. The infecting agent is the gonococcus or *Neisseria gonorrhoeae*. This is found in the discharge expressed from the urethra, which may be spread as a film on a glass slide, suitably stained, and examined under the microscope; or a culture from the discharge may be made on certain bacteriological media and films from this, similarly examined under the microscope. Since discharges resembling that of gonorrhoea accompany other forms of inflammation, the identification of the organism is of great importance.

Symptoms These differ considerably, according to whether the disease is in an acute or a chronic stage. In *men*, after an incubation period of between two and ten days, irritation in the urethra, scalding pain on passing water, and a viscid yellowish-white discharge appear; the glands in the groin often enlarge and may suppurate. The urine when passed is hazy and is often found to contain yellowish threads of pus visible to the eye. After some weeks, if the condition has become chronic, the discharge is clear and viscid, there may be irritation in passing urine, and various forms of inflammation in neighbouring organs may appear, the testicle, prostate gland and bladder becoming affected. At a still later stage the inflammation of the urethra is apt to lead to gradual formation of fibrous tissue around this channel. This contracts and produces narrowing, so that the passage of water becomes difficult or may be stopped for a time altogether (the condition known as stricture). Inflammation of some of the joints is a common complication in the early stage, the knee, ankle, wrist, and elbow being the joints most frequently affected, and this form of 'rheumatism' is very intractable and liable to lead to permanent stiffness. The fibrous tissues elsewhere may also develop inflammatory changes, causing lumbago, pain in the foot, etc. In occasional cases, during the acute stage, a general blood-poisoning results, with inflammation of the heart-valves (endocarditis) and abscesses in various parts of the body. The infective matter occasionally is inoculated accidentally into the eye producing a very severe form of conjunctivitis. In the newly born child this is known as *ophthalmia neonatorum* and until recently was one of the chief causes of blindness. (See EYE DISEASES.)

In women the course and complications of the disease are somewhat different. It begins with a yellow vaginal discharge, pain on passing water, and very often inflammation or abscess of the Bartholin's glands, situated close to the vulva or opening of the vagina. The chief seriousness, however, of the disease is due to the spread of inflammation to neighbouring organs, the uterus, Fallopian tubes, and ovaries, causing permanent destructive changes in these,

and leading occasionally to peritonitis through the Fallopian tube, with a fatal result. Many cases of prolonged ill-health and sterility or recurring miscarriages are due to these changes.
Treatment The chances of cure are better the earlier treatment is instituted. The treatment of gonorrhoea was revolutionized by the introduction of the sulphonamides. These, in turn, have now been replaced by the antibiotics. Penicillin is now the antibiotic of choice: a single injection of 2·4 or 4·8 mega units of procaine penicillin. Unfortunately, the gonococcus is liable to become resistant to penicillin. In patients who are infected with penicillin-resistant organisms, one of the other antibiotics is used. In all cases it is essential that bacteriological investigation should be carried out at weekly intervals for three or four weeks, to make sure that the patient is cured.

GOUT is a term used to describe several disorders associated with a raised concentration of uric acid in the blood, of which various forms of inflammatory arthritis (q.v.) and kidney disease (q.v.) are the most important. The condition has an overall prevalence in the UK of around 0·6 per cent.
Causes The cardinal feature of gout is the presence of an excessive amount of uric acid, and its deposition in the joints in the form of sodium monourate. The cause of this excess of uric acid is not known. Uric acid is formed in the system in the processes of nutrition, and is excreted by the kidneys, the amount passing off in the urine being 0·1 to 2 grams daily. In the healthy human subject the blood contains 3 to 6 mg per 100 millilitres, but in gout it is increased, both before and during the acute attack, while in chronic gout the amount in the blood and elsewhere in the body is always above the normal level.

Gout is in a marked degree hereditary. A family history of the disease is obtained in from 50 to 80 per cent of cases. Gout is said to affect the sedentary more readily than the active, but this cannot be taken as a constant rule. On the other hand, inadequate exercise, habitual over-indulgence in animal food and rich dishes, and especially in alcoholic drinks, are undoubtedly important precipitating factors in the production of the disease. These, however, are no more than precipitating factors, and the disease can occur in vegetarians and teetotallers.

Gout is more common in mature age than in the earlier years of life, being infrequent before the age of 40, but it may occasionally affect very young people in whom there is a strong family history. About 95 per cent of patients are males. In women it most often appears after the cessation of the menses.
Symptoms An attack of gout may appear without warning, or there may be premonitory symptoms.

The affected joint is swollen and of a deep red hue. The skin is tense and glistening, and the surrounding veins are more or less distended. After a few hours there is a remission of the pain, slight perspiration takes place, and the patient may fall asleep. The pain, however, returns next night, and these nocturnal exacerbations occur with greater or less severity during the continuance of the attack, which generally lasts for a week or ten days. As the symptoms decline, the swelling and tenderness of the affected joint abate. Attacks usually recur, initially in the same joints, although in advanced cases scarcely any joint escapes, and the disease becomes chronic. Chalk-stones, or tophi, are gradually formed round the affected joints. These deposits, which are highly characteristic of gout, at first occur in the form of a semi-fluid material, consisting for the most part of bi-urate of soda, which gradually becomes more dense, and ultimately quite hard.

A variety of urinary calculus – the uric acid stone – formed by concretions of this substance in the kidneys is a not infrequent occurrence in connection with gout; hence the well-known association of this disease and gravel (q.v.).
Treatment and prevention Non-steroidal anti-inflammatory drugs (q.v.) sych as indomethacin, naproxen, or phenylbutazone should be started as soon as possible, and given in adequate doses, to treat an acute attack. After the attack subsides, a lower dose should be continued for at least a week. Salicylates (such as aspirin) and diuretics should be avoided.

In patients prone to recurrent or particularly severe attacks, long-term prophylaxis with allopurinol (q.v.) is indicated, especially when associated with kidney disease. This drug, which has few side-effects, lowers the serum urate concentration by preventing the formation of uric acid. Although there is no need for severe dietary restrictions, an excessively rich diet is best avoided, and alcohol intake should be reduced. Gradual weight loss should be encouraged. Blood pressure and renal function should be monitored regularly.

GRAFT is the term applied to a piece of tissue removed from one person or animal and implanted in another, or the same, individual in order by its growth to remedy some defect. Skin grafts are commonly used. Bone grafts are also used to replace bone which has been lost by disease: for example, a portion of rib is sometimes removed in order to furnish support for a spine weakened by disease, after the disease has been removed. Also, the bone of young animals is used to afford additional growth and strength to a limb bone which it has been necessary to remove in part on account of disease or injury. Vein grafts are used to replace stretches of arteries which have become blocked, particularly in the heart and lower limbs. The veins most commonly used for this purpose are the saphenous veins of the individual in question provided they are healthy. An alternative is specially treated umbilical vein. (See SKIN-GRAFTING.)

GRAFT VERSUS HOST DISEASE (GVHD)
A condition that is a common complication of

bone marrow transplant. It results from certain lymphocytes (q.v.) in the transplanted marrow attacking the transplant recipient's tissues, which they identify as 'foreign'. GVHD may appear soon after a transplant or develop several months later. The condition, which is fatal in about a third of victims, may be prevented by immuno-suppressant drugs such as cyclosporin (see IMMUNO-SUPPRESSION).

GRAM, or GRAMME, is the unit of weight in the metric system and is equal to a little over 15·4 grains. For purposes of weighing food, 30 grams are usually taken as approximately equal to 1 ounce.

GRAM'S STAIN, named after the bacteriologist, H. C. J. Gram, who first described it in 1884, is one of the most valuable methods of differentiating certain micro-organisms. The principle involved depends upon the fact that certain bacteria, when treated with a dye such as gentian violet and then with iodine, fix the dye, whereas other bacteria do not. Those bacteria, such as the pneumococcus, that fix the dye are known as Gram-positive, whilst those that do not fix it, e.g. the gonococcus, are said to be Gram-negative.

GRAND MAL is the name applied to a convulsive epileptic attack, also known as a tonic-clonic seizure in contrast to petit mal, which includes the milder forms of epilepsy (q.v.).

GRANULATIONS are small masses of formative cells containing loops of newly formed blood-vessels which spring up over any raw surface, as the first step in the process of healing of wounds. (See ULCER; WOUNDS.)

GRANULOCYTE White blood cells which, when stained with Romanowsky stains containing thiazine dyes and eosin, are found to contain granules in their cytoplasm. The colour of the granules enables the cells to be further classified as basophils, eosinophils, and neutrophils (qq.v.).

GRANULOMA is a tumour or new growth made up of granulation tissue. This is caused by various forms of chronic inflammation, such as syphilis and tuberculosis.

GRAVEL is the name applied to any sediment which falls down in the urine, but particularly to small masses of uric acid. It produces various unpleasant symptoms. (See URINARY BLADDER, DISEASES OF; GOUT; URINE.)

GRAVES' DISEASE or THYROTOXICOSIS is the commonest form of hyperthyroidism (q.v.). It is a syndrome consisting of diffuse goitre (swollen thyroid gland, q.v.), overactivity of the thyroid gland and exophthalmos (protruding eyes, q.v.). Patients lose weight and develop an increased appetite, heat intolerance and sweating. They are anxious, irritable, hyperactive and sometimes depressed. Their heart rate rises and they may suffer from palpitations and breathlessness as well as muscle weakness. The hyperthyroidism is due to the production of antibodies to the TSH receptor which stimulate the receptor with resultant production of excess thyroid hormones. The goitre is due to antibodies that stimulate the growth of the thyroid gland. The exophthalmos is due to another immunoglobulin called the ophthalmopathic immunoglobulin which is an antibody to a retro-orbital antigen on the surface of the retro-orbital eye muscles. This provokes inflammation in the retro-orbital tissues which is associated with the accumulation of water and mucopolysaccharide which fills the orbit and causes the eye to protrude forwards.

Although Graves' disease may affect any age group the peak incidence is in the 3rd decade. Females are affected ten times as often as males. The prevalence in females is one in 500. As with many other auto-immune diseases, there is an increased prevalence of auto-immune thyroid disease in the relatives of patients with Graves' disease. Some of these patients may have hypothyroidism and others thyrotoxicosis. Patients with Graves' disease may present with a goitre or with the eye signs or, most commonly, with the symptoms of excess thyroid hormone production. Thyroid hormone controls the metabolic rate of the body so that the symptoms of hyperthyroidism are those of excess metabolism.

The diagnosis of Graves' disease is confirmed by the measurement of the circulating levels of the two thyroid hormones, thyroxine and tri-iodothyronine.

Treatment There are several effective treatments for Graves' disease. (1) Antithyroid drugs: these drugs inhibit the iodination of tyrosine and hence the formation of the thyroid hormones. The most commonly used drugs are the thiourea compounds carbimazole, propylthiouricil and methimazole. They will control the excess production of thyroid hormones in virtually all cases. Once the patient has been rendered euthyroid the dose can be reduced to a maintenance dose and is usually continued for two years. The disadvantage of antithyroid drugs is that even after two years' treatment nearly half the patients will relapse and will then require more definitive therapy.

(2) Partial thyroidectomy: removal of three-quarters of the thyroid gland is effective treatment of the hyperthyroidism of Graves' disease. It is the treatment of choice in those patients with large goitres. The patient must however be rendered euthyroid before surgery is undertaken, or thyroid crisis and arrhythmias may complicate the operation.

(3) Radioactive iodine therapy: this has been in use for many years. It is an effective means of controlling hyperthyroidism. One of the disadvantages of radioactive iodine is that the incidence of hypothyroidism is much greater

than with other forms of treatment. However the management of hypothyroidism is simple and requires only the taking of thyroxine tablets, so that, provided the patients are followed up and the hypothyroidism is diagnosed, this presents little problem. There is no evidence of any increased incidence of cancer of the thyroid or leukaemia following radio-iodine therapy. It has been the pattern in Britain to reserve radio-iodine treatment to those over the age of 35 or those whose prognosis is unlikely to be more than 30 years as a result of cardiac or respiratory disease. Radioactive iodine treatment should not be given to a seriously thyrotoxic patient.

(4) The beta-adrenoceptor-blocking drugs (q.v.), usually propranolol (q.v.), are useful for symptomatic treatment during the first 4 to 8 weeks until the longer-term drugs have reduced thyroid activity.

GRAVID means pregnant.

GREENSTICK FRACTURE is an incomplete fracture, in which the bone is not completely broken across. It occurs in the long bones of children and is usually due to indirect violence. (See FRACTURES.)

GREY MATTER Those parts of the brain and spinal cord that comprise mainly the interconnected and tightly packed nuclei of nerve cells. The tissue is darker than that of the white matter, which is made of *axons* from the nerve cells. In the brain grey matter is mainly found in the outer layers of the cerebrum, which is the zone responsible for advanced mental functions. The inner core of the spinal cord is made up of grey matter.

GRIPES is a popular name for the colic of infants, generally due to irregular feeding. (See COLIC.)

GRISEOFULVIN is an antibiotic obtained from *Penicillium griseofulvum Dierckse*, which is proving of value in the treatment of various forms of ringworm.

GROIN is the region which includes the upper part of the front of the thigh and lower part of the abdomen. A deep groove runs obliquely across it, which corresponds to the inguinal ligament, and divides the thigh from the abdomen. The principal diseased conditions in this region are enlarged glands (see GLANDS), and hernia (q.v.).

GROMMET is a small bobbin-shaped tube used to keep open the incision made in the ear drum in the treatment of secretory otitis media. It acts as a ventilation tube by allowing the Eustachian tube to recover its normal function. (See EAR, DISEASES OF; EUSTACHIAN TUBES.)

GROUP THERAPY Psychotherapy in which at least two, but more commonly up to ten patients as well as the therapist, take part. The therapist encourages the patients to analyse their own and the others' emotional and psychological difficulties. Group therapy is also used to help patients with the same condition, for instance, alcoholism or compulsive gambling. They discuss their problems for perhaps an hour twice a week and explore ways of resolving them.

GROWTH is a popular term applied to any new formation in any part of the body. (See CANCER; CYSTS; GANGLION; TUMOUR.) For growth of children, see WEIGHT AND HEIGHT.

GROWTH HORMONE A product of the anterior part of the pituitary gland that promotes normal growth and development in the body by changing the chemical activity in the cells. The hormone activates protein production in the muscle cells as well as the release of energy from the metabolism of fats. Its release is controlled by the contrasting actions of growth-hormone releasing factor and somatostatin. If the body produces too much growth hormone before puberty gigantism (q.v.) results; in adulthood the result is acromegaly (q.v.). Lack of growth hormone in children causes dwarfism (q.v.).

GUANETHIDINE is one of a group of adrenergic neurone-blocking drugs. Occasionally necessary in combination with other drugs in the treatment of resistant hypertension, it causes several side-effects, notably postural hypotension (q.v.), and is rarely used nowadays.

GUINEA-WORM (see DRACUNCULIASIS).

GULLET, or OESOPHAGUS, is the tube down which food passes from the throat to the stomach. (See OESOPHAGUS.)

GUM is a complex viscid substance which exudes from the stems and branches of various trees, and consists principally of arabin or bassorin. The two best-known gums are gum acacia and gum tragacanth. Gum-resins such as asafoetida, galbanum, and myrrh also contain resin.

GUMBOIL is a painful condition of inflammation, ending sometimes as an abscess, situated about the root of a carious tooth.

GUMMA is a hard swelling, or granuloma (q.v.), characteristic of tertiary syphilis (q.v.). It normally develops in the skin or subcutaneous tissue, mucous membranes or sub-mucosa, and the long bones. Although often painless, it may produce marked symptoms by interfering with the brain or other internal organs in which it may be located. Treatment with penicillin (or tetracycline if the patient is allergic) usually ensures a rapid disappearance of the gumma.

GUMS, DISEASES OF (see MOUTH, DISEASES OF; TEETH, DISEASES OF).

GYNAECOLOGY is that branch of medicine dealing with the female pelvic and uro-genital organs, in both the normal and diseased states. It encompasses aspects of contraception, abortion, and in-vitro fertilization (q.v.). Covering the full age range, it is closely related to obstetrics, while involving aspects of both surgery and psychiatry.

GYNAECOMASTIA is the term used for describing an abnormal increase in size of the male breast.

GYRUS is the term applied to a convolution of the brain.

H

H₂ RECEPTOR ANTAGONISTS are drugs that block the action of histamine (q.v.) at the H_2 receptor (which mediates the gastric and some of the cardiovascular effects of histamine). By reducing the production of acid by the stomach, these drugs – chiefly cimetidine, ranitidine, and the newer ones, famotidine and nizatidine – are valuable in the treatment of peptic ulcers (healing when used in high dose, preventing relapse when used as maintenance therapy in reduced dose), reflux oesophagitis (see OESOPHAGUS, DISEASES OF), and the Zollinger-Ellison syndrome (q.v.).

HAEMANGIOMA is a benign tumour composed of tortuous dilated blood-vessels.

HAEMARTHROSIS is the process of bleeding into, or the presence of blood in, a joint. It may occur as a result of major trauma (for example, fracture of the patella may lead to bleeding into the knee joint), or, more commonly, following minor trauma, or even spontaneously, in cases of haemophilia (q.v.) or other disorders of blood clotting. If repeated several times it may lead to fibrosis of the joint lining and inflammation of the cartilage, causing marked stiffness and deformity.

HAEMATEMESIS means vomiting of blood. Blood brought up from the stomach is generally dark in colour, and is often so far digested

as to form small brown granules resembling coffee grounds. Vomiting of blood is one of the chief symptoms of peptic ulcer, but it may also occur in gastritis, especially when this is due to the action of irritant poisons or alcohol, and cancer of the stomach. It should always be remembered that the blood may come from the nose or throat, and, after being swallowed, provoke vomiting. (See HAEMORRHAGE.)

HAEMATIN is an organic growth factor. As an intravenous infusion it is increasingly being used as an effective treatment for acute attacks of porphyria (q.v.); early use may prevent the chronic neuropathy sometimes associated with this condition.

HAEMATINIC is a drug that raises the quantity of haemoglobin (q.v.) in the blood. Ferrous sulphate is a common example of iron-containing compounds given to anaemic patients whose condition is due to iron deficiency. Traditionally haematinics have been used to prevent anaemia in pregnant women.

HAEMATOCOELE means a cavity containing blood. Generally as the result of an injury which ruptures blood-vessels, blood is effused into one of the natural cavities of the body, or among loose cellular tissue, producing a haematocoele.

HAEMATOCOLPOS is the condition in which menstrual blood is held up in the vagina as a result of an imperforate hymen.

HAEMATOCRIT Also known as packed cell volume, this is an expression of the fraction of blood volume occupied by the red cells. It is determined by centrifuging a sample of blood in a capillary tube and measuring the height of the resulting packed cells as a percentage of the total sample height.

Normal values: males 42–53%
or 0.42–0.53 mL/dL
females 32–48%
or 0.36–0.48 mL/dL

HAEMATOGENOUS is an adjective applied to a biological process which produces blood or to an agent produced in or coming from blood. For example, a haematogenous infection is one resulting from contact with blood that contains a virus or bacterium responsible for the infection.

HAEMATOLOGY is the study of diseases of the blood.

HAEMATOMA means a collection of blood forming a definite swelling. It is found often upon the head of new-born children after a protracted and difficult labour. It may occur as the result of any injury or operation.

HAEMATOXYLON, or LOGWOOD, is the wood of *Haematoxylon campechianum*, which is used as a dye in staining tissues in histology. As it has a mildly astringent action, it is used for checking diarrhoea.

HAEMATURIA means the condition of blood in the urine. (See URINE.) The blood may come from any part of the urinary tract. When the blood comes from the kidney or upper part of the urinary tract, it is usually mixed throughout the urine, giving the latter a brownish or smoky tinge. This condition is usually the result of glomerulonephritis, or it may be present in persons suffering from high blood-pressure or pyelitis (q.v.). Blood may also appear in the urine when a stone or gravel is present in the pelvis of the kidney setting up irritation, especially after exercise. The blood may also originate from a bladder that is inflamed or infected or which contains benign (papilloma) or malignant growths. Inflammation or injury to the urethra can also cause haematuria. Someone with haematuria should seek medical advice.

HAEMIC MURMUR is a term applied to unusual sounds heard over the heart and large blood-vessels in severe cases of anaemia. They disappear as the condition is recovered from. Murmurs of this type are to be distinguished from 'organic murmurs', which are due to some disease of the heart-valves or vessel walls.

HAEMOCHROMATOSIS, or BRONZED DIABETES, is a disease in which cirrhosis of the liver, enlargement of the spleen, pigmentation of the skin, and diabetes mellitus are associated with the abnormal and excessive deposit in the organs of the body of the iron-containing pigment, haemosiderin.

HAEMOCYTOMETER is an instrument for counting corpuscles in the blood.

HAEMODIALYSIS is the principle used in the artificial kidney (see KIDNEY, ARTIFICIAL), whereby the patient's blood is circulated through a cellophane tube, on the other side of which is a dialysing solution containing electrolytes in the concentration they should be in normal blood. This technique for removing waste materials or poisons from the blood is used in patients whose kidneys are malfunctioning. Haemodialysis restores the blood to its normal state, but the process usually has to be repeated at regular intervals. (See also DIALYSIS.)

HAEMOFILTRATION A means of removing excess fluid, electrolytes and some waste products from the blood in patients with acute renal failure. The filter usually consists of a cylinder containing a large number of microtubules which are made from a membrane which is permeable to water and small molecules (molecular weight<12,000). Blood from the patient is passed through the cylinder where water and solutes pass out of the blood and through the membrane by convection before the blood is returned to the patient. The process is continuous via an extracorporeal (outside the body) circulation. As the system removes large volumes of water and electrolytes from blood, these are replaced by intravenous infusion of a balanced salt solution (the volume is calculated to produce an overall negative, positive or static fluid balance each day).

HAEMOGLOBIN is the colouring material which produces the red colour of blood. It is a chromoprotein, made up of a protein called globin and the iron-containing pigment, haemin. When separated from the red blood corpuscles, each of which contains about 600 million haemoglobin molecules, it is crystalline in form. It exists in two forms: simple haemoglobin, found in venous blood, and oxyhaemoglobin, which is a loose compound with oxygen, found in arterial blood after the blood has come in contact with the air in the lungs. This oxyhaemoglobin is again broken down as the blood passes through the tissues, which take up the oxygen for their own use. This is the main function of haemoglobin: to act as a carrier of oxygen from the lungs to all the tissues of the body. When the haemoglobin leaves the lungs it is 97 per cent saturated with oxygen. When it comes back to the lungs in the venous blood it is 70 per cent saturated. The oxygen content of 100 millilitres of blood leaving the lungs is 19·5 millilitres, and that of venous blood returning to the lungs is 14·5 millilitres. Thus each 100 millilitres of blood delivers 5 millilitres of oxygen to the tissues of the body. Human male blood contains 13 to 18 grams of haemoglobin per 100 millilitres. In women, there are 12 to 16 grams per 100 millilitres. A man weighing 70 kilograms (154 pounds) has around 770 grams of haemoglobin circulating in his red blood corpuscles.

HAEMOGLOBINOPATHIES Haemoglobin (q.v.) is a pigment composed of an iron protoporphyrin complex combined with a protein globin. It is the globin portion which varies in different types of haemoglobin. Impairment of adult haemoglobin formation is the characteristic abnormality of the haemoglobinopathies, which are hereditary haemolytic anaemias, genetically determined and related to race. The haemoglobin may be abnormal because: (1) there is a defect in the synthesis of normal adult haemoglobin and this occurs in thalassaemia when there may be an absence of one or both of the polypeptide chains characteristic of normal adult haemoglobin, or (2) an abnormal form of haemoglobin such as haemoglobin S, that of sickle-cell disease, is formed instead of adult haemoglobin. This abnormality may involve as little as one amino acid of the 300 in the haemoglobin molecule. In sickle-cell haemoglobin one single amino acid molecule, that of glutamic acid, is replaced by another, that of valine, and this results in such a deficient end product that the ensuing disease is frequently rapidly fatal.

HAEMOGLOBINURIA means the presence of blood pigment in the urine caused by the destruction of blood corpuscles in the blood-vessels or in the urinary passages. It produces in the urine a dark red or brown colour. In some people this condition, known as intermittent haemoglobinuria, occurs from time to time, especially on exposure to cold. It is also produced by various poisonous substances taken in the food. It occurs in malarious districts in the form of one of the most fatal forms of malaria: blackwater fever (q.v.). (See also MARCH HAEMOGLOBINURIA.)

HAEMOLYSIS means the breaking up of blood corpuscles by the action of poisonous substances, usually of a protein nature, circulating in the blood, or by certain chemicals. It occurs, for example, gradually in some forms of anaemia and rapidly in poisoning by snake venom.

HAEMOLYTIC DISEASE OF THE NEW-BORN A serious disease of the new-born characterized by haemolytic anaemia and jaundice (qq.v.). It may be associated with oedema, and if there is a great deal of fluid in the PERICARDIAL, PLEURAL, and PERITONEAL cavities the condition is known as Hydrops fetalis. If jaundice appears within 24 hours of birth it is likely to be due to blood-group incompatibility between the mother and baby. The commonest cause of haemolytic disease of the new-born is rhesus incompatibility (see BLOOD GROUPS) – a previously sensitized rhesus-negative mother produces antibodies which cause haemolysis (destruction of the blood cells) in her rhesus-positive baby.

The infant's serum bilirubin (q.v.) concentration should be plotted regularly so that treatment can be given before levels likely to cause brain damage occur. Safe bilirubin concentrations depend on the age of the child, and reference charts should always be used.

High bilirubin concentrations may be treated with phototherapy. The infant, with its eyes suitably protected, is nursed under ultraviolet light. Extra fluid is given to prevent dehydration and to improve bilirubin excretion by shortening the gut transit time. Severe jaundice and anaemia may require exchange transfusion (see TRANSFUSION OF BLOOD). Haemolytic disease of the new-born secondary to rhesus incompatibility has become less common since the introduction of anti-D. This antibody should be given to all rhesus-negative women at any risk of a fetomaternal transfusion, to prevent

them from mounting an antibody response. Anti-D is given routinely to rhesus-negative mothers after the birth of a rhesus-positive baby, but doctors should also remember to give it after threatened abortions, antepartum haemorrhages, miscarriages, and terminations of pregnancy.

HAEMOLYTIC URAEMIC SYNDROME A disease of children resulting in acute oliguric (q.v.) renal failure. A febrile illness of the gastrointestinal or respiratory tracts is followed by intravascular coagulation of blood which results in haemolysis (q.v.), anaemia (q.v.), thrombocytopaenia (q.v.) and renal failure (resulting from fibrin deposition in renal arterioles and glomerular capillaries).

The death rate is 2–10 per cent and the majority of patients survive without renal failure. The longer the period of oliguria the greater the risk of chronic renal failure.

Treatment is supportive with replacement of blood and clotting factors, control of hypertension (q.v.) and careful observance of fluid balance.

HAEMOPHILIA An inherited disorder of blood coagulation which results in prolonged bleeding even after minor injury. There is a deficiency of Factor VIII, an essential clotting factor in the coagulation cascade – the complex series of biochemical events that lead from injury of the wall of a blood vessel to the formation of a blood clot that checks bleeding. It is a sex- linked recessive disorder (though a small number of cases arise by spontaneous mutation) so that females carry the disease, half their sons will be affected and half their daughters will be carriers. The sons of haemophiliacs are unaffected but half their daughters will be carriers. Haemophilia affects approximately 1:4,000 of the UK population but only 1:20,000 is severely affected. Severity of the disease depends upon the percentage, compared with normal, of Factor VIII activity present. Less than 1 per cent and there will be spontaneous bleeding into joints and muscles; 1–5 per cent and there will be occasional spontaneous bleeding and severe bleeding after minor injury; 5–25 per cent and there will only be severe bleeding after major injury. Before treatment was available, severe haemophiliacs suffered from severe pain and deformity from bleeds into joints and muscles. Bleeding also occurred into the gut, kidney and brain and few survived past adolescence.

Freeze-dried Factor VIII may be kept in domestic refrigerators. Haemophiliacs can use it to abort minor bleeds by reconstituting it and injecting it intravenously. More major bleeding or preparation for surgery involves raising Factor VIII levels to 30–100 per cent by giving cryoprecipitate.

With treatment most haemophiliacs lead normal lives, though obviously dangerous or contact sports should be avoided.

There is a National Haemophilia Register

and each registered sufferer carries a card with details about his condition. Information may also be obtained from NHS haemophilia centres and the Haemophilia Society (see APPENDIX 2: ADDRESSES).

HAEMOPHILUS A genus of the heterogeneous group of Parvobacteria, which contains several important human (and animal) pathogens. They are Gram-negative (see GRAM'S STAIN), rod-like, aerobic, non-sporing and non-motile, parasitic bacteria. Mostly found in the respiratory tract, they may be part of the normal flora, but may also be responsible for several diseases. The main pathogenic species of haemophilus is *H. influezae*, which may cause severe exacerbations of chronic bronchitis (q.v.), as well as meningitis, epiglottitis, sinusitis, and otitis media. Other species may cause conjunctivitis (see EYE DISEASES) or chancroid (q.v.). Haemophilus species are sensitive to a wide range of antibiotics, though generally resistant to penicillin.

HAEMOPOIESIS The formation of blood.

HAEMOPTYSIS means the spitting up of blood from the lower air passages. The blood is usually coughed or gently hawked up, it may be in mouthfuls at a time, and is bright red and frothy, thus differing from the blood brought up from the stomach. Generally the condition results from some disease of the heart or lungs. It should be remembered, however, that in elderly people haemoptysis may be due to a varicose condition of the small veins in the throat, not to haemorrhage in the lungs; while in young people this condition is often due to bleeding from the nose, in which, owing to the position of the head, the blood happens to run backwards instead of forwards through the nostrils. (See HAEMORRHAGE; TUBERCULOSIS.)

HAEMORRHAGE is the escape of blood from any of the blood vessels, normally in response to some trauma, or as a result of a clotting disorder such as haemophilia (q.v.). The bleeding may be external, for example, following a skin laceration, or internal, for example, haematemesis (bleeding into the stomach), haemoptysis (bleeding from the lungs), haematuria (bleeding from the kidneys or urinary tract). Bleeding into or around the brain is a major concern following serious head injuries, or in newborn infants following a difficult labour. Haemorrhage is classified as arterial – the most serious type, in which the blood is bright red and appears in spurts (in severe cases the patient may bleed to death in a few minutes); venous, less serious (unless from torn varicose veins) and easily checked, in which the blood is dark and wells up gradually into the wound; and capillary, in which the blood slowly oozes out of the surface of the wound, and soon stops spontaneously.

Haemorrhage is also classified as primary, reactionary, and secondary (see WOUNDS). Severe haemorrhage causes shock (q.v.) and anaemia (q.v.), and blood transfusion is often required.

Natural arrest When a small artery is cut across, the bleeding stops in consequence of changes in the wall of the artery on the one hand, and in the constitution of the blood on the other. Every artery is surrounded by a fibrous sheath, and when cut, the vessel retracts some little distance within this sheath, in consequence of the shortening of its muscle fibres; and further, by the same process the end contracts so as to form an opening of smaller size than the rest of the vessel. In the space between the end of the vessel and its sheath, and afterwards for some distance up the interior of the narrowed artery, blood-clot quickly forms by the following process, and rapidly blocks the open end of the vessel. When blood is shed so as to come in contact with any surface other than the smooth lining of blood-vessels, the fibrinogen which is dissolved in its fluid becomes converted into threads of fibrin through combination with the lime salts of the blood, and the action of a chemical given off probably by the blood platelets. These threads of fibrin slowly contract and develop into a dense felt-work, in the meshes of which the corpuscles are held, and in this way a blood-clot of increasing hardness is produced, within and round the ends of the injured vessels. This chain of events is called the coagulation cascade (see COAGULATION).

Four main principles are applicable in the control of a severe external haemorrhage: (*a*) direct pressure on the bleeding point or points; (*b*) elevation of the wounded part; (*c*) pressure on the main artery of supply to the part; and (*d*) application of substances known as styptics, which contract the vessels or aid the coagulation of the blood.

Control of internal haemorrhage is more difficult than for external bleeding. First-aid measures should be taken while professional help is sought. The patient should be laid down with legs raised. He or she should be reassured and kept warm. The mouth may be kept moist but no fluids should be given. (See APPENDIX 1: FIRST AID.)

HAEMORRHOIDS (see PILES).

HAEMOSTASIS The process by which bleeding stops. It involves constriction of blood vessels, the formation of a platelet plug, and blood clotting. The term is also used for surgical interventions to stop bleeding, e.g. the use of diathermy. (See HAEMORRHAGE.)

HAEMOSTATICS are any means, whether of the nature of mechanical appliances or drugs, used to control bleeding. (See FIBRIN FOAM; HAEMORRHAGE.)

HAEMOTHORAX means an effusion of blood into the pleural cavity.

HAIR (see SKIN; WHITE HAIR).

HAIR, REMOVAL OF (see DEPILATION).

HALF LIFE: The time taken for the plasma concentration of a drug to decline by half from redistribution, metabolism and excretion.

HALIBUT-LIVER OIL is the oil expressed from fresh, or suitably preserved, halibut liver. It is a particularly rich source of vitamin A (30,000 international units per gram), and also contains vitamin D (2300 to 2500 units per gram). Because of the relatively small volume required, it is often used as a means of giving vitamin D: either as drops of the oil or in capsules. Care must be taken to ensure that the child is receiving at least 700 international units of vitamin D daily. (See VITAMIN.)

HALITOSIS is another term for bad breath. (See BREATH, DISORDERS OF.)

HALLUCINATIONS are false perceptions arising without an adequate external stimulus, as opposed to illusions, which are misinterpretations of stimuli arising from an external object. Hallucinations come from 'within', although the affected individual may see them as coming from 'without'. Nevertheless, they may occur at the same time as real perceptions, and may affect any sense (vision, hearing, smell, taste, touch, etc.).
Causes They may be the result of intense emotion or suggestion, sensory deprivation (for example, overwork or lack of sleep), disorders of sense organs, or disorders of the central nervous system. Although hallucinations may occur in perfectly sane people, they are more commonly an indication of a mental illness (q.v.). They may be deliberately induced by the use of hallucinogens (q.v.).

HALLUCINOGENS are compounds characterized by their ability to produce distortions of perception, emotional changes, depersonalization, and a variety of effects on memory and learned behaviour. They include lysergic acid diethylamide (q.v.) and mescaline (q.v.). (See also DRUG ADDICTION.)

HALLUX is the anatomical name of the great toe.

HALLUX RIGIDUS is stiffness of the joint between the great toe and the foot which induces pain on walking. It is usually due to a crush injury or stubbing of the toe. Such stubbing is liable to occur in adolescents with a congenitally long toe. If troublesome it is treated by an operation to create a false joint.

HALLUX VALGUS is outward displacement of the great toe and is always associated with a bunion. It is due to the pressure of footwear on an unduly broad foot. In adolescents this broad foot is inherited; in adults it is due to splaying of the foot as a result of loss of muscle tone. The bunion is produced by pressure of the footwear on the protruding base of the toe. In mild cases the wearing of comfortable shoes may be all that is needed. In more severe cases the bunion may need to be removed, while in the most severe the operation of arthroplasty (q.v.) may be needed. (See also CORNS AND BUNIONS.)

HALO is a coloured circle seen round a bright light in some eye conditions. When accompanied by headache it is specially likely to be caused by glaucoma (q.v.).

HALOPERIDOL is one of the butyrophenone group of drugs that is proving useful in the treatment of mania and schizophrenic excitement. It is also of value in some cases of stuttering, intractable hiccups and uncontrollable sneezing.

HALOTHANE is a non-inflammable gaseous anaesthetic, the chemical formula of which is $CF_3CHClBr$. Patients recover rapidly from its effects. (See ANAESTHESIA.)

HALOTHANE HEPATITIS A very rare form of hepatitis following exposure to halothane during anaesthesia (1:35,000 halothane anaesthetics). Jaundice develops three to four days after exposure and will occasionally develop into a fatal massive hepatic necrosis. It is of unknown aetiology but probably has an immunological basis. It is more common following multiple exposures in a short time (less than 28 days), and in obesity, middle age and females. It is rare in children.

HAMARTOMA These are benign tumours, usually in the lung, containing normal components of pulmonary tissue such as smooth muscle and connective tissue.

HAMMER-TOE is the deformity in which there is permanent flexion, or bending of the middle joint of the toe. The condition may affect all the toes as in claw-foot (q.v.). More commonly it affects one toe, usually the second. It is due to a relatively long toe and the pressure on it of the footwear. A painful bunion usually develops on it. In mild cases relief is obtained by protecting the toe with adhesive pads. If this does not suffice operation is necessary. (See CORNS AND BUNIONS.)

HAMSTRINGS is the name given to the tendons at the back of the knee, two on the inner side and one on the outer side, which bend this joint. They are attached to the tibia below.

HAND is the section of the upper limb below the wrist. The hand of man is more highly developed in its structure and in its nervous connections than the corresponding part in any other animal. Indeed the possession of a thumb which can be 'opposed' to the other fingers for grasping objects is one of the distinguishing features of the human race that has contributed to its evolutionary success. Of all the parts of the body, the hand, which is connected with a large area on the surface of the brain, is capable of the highest degree of education.

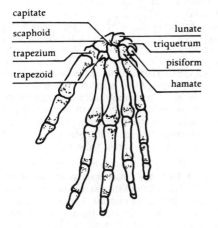

capitate
scaphoid
lunate
triquetrum
trapezium
pisiform
trapezoid
hamate

The bones of the hand and wrist, anterior view.

In structure, the hand has a bony basis of eight small carpal bones in the wrist, five metacarpal bones in the fleshy part of the hand, and three phalanges in each finger, two only in the thumb. From the muscles of the forearm twelve strong tendons or sinews run in front of the wrist. Of these, nine go to the fingers and thumb and are bound down by a strong band, the flexor retinaculum, in front of the wrist. They are enclosed in a complicated synovial sheath, and pass through the palm and down the fingers. (See FINGERS.) Behind the wrist twelve tendons likewise cross from forearm to hand.

Forming the ball of the thumb and that of the little finger, and filling up the gaps between the metacarpal bones, are other muscles, which act to separate and bring together the fingers, and to bend them at their first joints (knuckles).

Deep in the palm the ulnar artery makes an arch across the hand, giving off branches which run down the sides of the fingers; while the radial artery makes an arch across at a still deeper level, lying in close contact with the bones.

The skin of the hand is richly supplied with nerve filaments, in accordance with its highly specialized sense of touch, the outer three and a half digits being supplied in front by the median, behind by the radial nerve, whilst the inner one and a half fingers have their nerve supply both back and front from the ulnar nerve.

HAND, FOOT AND MOUTH DISEASE is a disease characterized by an eruption of blisters on the palms of the hands, on the feet (often the toes) and in the mouth. It is most common in children and is due to infection with coxsackie A16 virus. The incubation period is three to five days.

HANGING is a form of death due to suspension of the body from the neck, either suddenly, as in judicial hanging, so as to damage the spinal column and cord, or in such a way as to constrict the air passages and the blood-vessels to the brain. Death is, in any case, speedy, resulting in two or three minutes, if not instantaneous, although in bygone days criminals who were shored-up, or supported by their friends, have come round after half-an-hour's suspension. The mark of the noose on the neck is oblique in hanging, which serves to distinguish this form of death from strangling, in which the mark is circular. Apart from judicial hanging, and in the absence of any signs of a struggle, hanging is usually due to suicide. The resuscitation of people found hanging is similar to that for drowning. (See APPENDIX 1: BASIC FIRST AID, cardiac/respiratory arrest.)

HANG-NAIL means a splitting of the skin at the side of the finger nail. Usually caused by some form of trauma, physical or chemical, it occurs most often in manual workers, though occasionally it forms part of a generalized ischaemic syndrome (see ISCHAEMIA). It is often a very tender condition, especially if it becomes infected and inflamed. Treatment consists of reducing trauma to the finger, together with emollients (q.v.), and antibiotics if necessary.

HARDNESS is a term applied to water that contains a large amount of calcium and magnesium salts (lime salts) which form an insoluble curd with soap and thus interfere with the use of the water for purposes of washing. Hard water is especially found in districts where the soil is chalky. Temporary hardness, which is due mainly to the presence of bicarbonates of lime, can be remedied by boiling, when the lime is precipitated as carbonate of lime. Permanent hardness is not remedied by boiling, and is due to the presence of a large amount of sulphate of lime. It may be removed by the addition of sodium carbonate (washing soda) or by the Permutit process which involves the use of various combinations of silicate of alumina and soda. In the past hard water was often blamed for many ills – without any convincing evidence. Today medical statisticians are suggesting that the drinking of soft water may lead to heart disease.

HARE-LIP (see PALATE, MALFORMATIONS OF).

HARTMANN'S SOLUTION is a solution commonly used as a means of fluid replacement in dehydrated patients. Each litre contains 3·1 grams of sodium lactate, 6 grams of sodium chloride, 0·4 gram of potassium chloride, and 0·7 gram of calcium chloride.

HASHIMOTO'S DISEASE is a condition in which the whole of the thyroid gland is diffusely enlarged and firm. It is one of the diseases produced by auto-immunity (q.v.). The enlargement is due, not to increase of colloid, but to diffuse infiltration of lymphocytes and increase of fibrous tissue. This form of goitre appears in middle-aged women, does not give rise to symptoms of thyrotoxicosis, and tends to produce myxoedema.

HAVERSIAN CANALS are the fine canals in bone which carry the blood-vessels, lymphatics, and nerves necessary for the maintenance and repair of bone. (See BONE.)

HAY FEVER, this is caused by an allergy (q.v.) to the pollen of grasses, trees and other plants. Contact with the particular pollen that the sufferer is allergic to causes histamine (q.v.) release resulting in a blocked, runny nose and itchy watering eyes. It affects approximately 3 million people each year in the UK.

The mainstays of treatment are antihistamines (q.v.) and the use of steroid nasal spray and eyedrops. Occasionally desensitization may work if the particular allergen is known.

HEAD (see BRAIN; FACE; SCALP; SKULL).

HEADACHE is a very common condition which may vary considerably in severity and type. Its significance and cause may vary tremendously, at one extreme indicating the presence of a tumour or meningitis, while at the other extreme it may merely indicate a common cold or tiredness. Even so, persistent or recurrent headaches should always be taken seriously. Although the brain itself is insensitive to pain, the surrounding membranes – meninges – are very sensitive, and changes in intracranial arteries, or spasm of the neck or scalp muscles, which may occur for various reasons, may cause considerable pain. In most cases a clinical diagnosis should be possible; further investigations should only be necessary following head injury, if headaches recur or if neurological signs such as drowsiness, vomiting, confusion, seizures, or focal signs, develop.

Some of the more common causes of headaches are as follows. Anxiety is probably the most common cause of headache and, where possible, the reason for the anxiety – overwork, family problems, unemployment, financial difficulties, etc. – should be tackled. Some people are more prone to anxiety than others. An unpleasant environment such as traffic pollution, badly ventilated or overcrowded working conditions, excessive smoking, etc., may provoke headaches in some people. Migraine (q.v.) is a characteristic and often disabling type of headache. High blood pressure may cause headaches. Occasionally refractive errors of the eyes are associated with headaches. Sinus infections are often characterized by frontal headaches. Rheumatism in the muscles of the neck and scalp produce headaches. Fever is commonly accompanied by a headache, and sunstroke and heatstroke customarily result in headaches. Finally, as already stated, diseases in the brain such as meningitis, tumours and haemorrhage may first manifest themselves as persistent or recurrent headaches.

Treatment Obtaining a reliable diagnosis – with the help of further investigations when indicated – should always be the initial aim; treatment in most cases should then be aimed at the underlying condition. This same principle applies whether the cause is physical or stress induced. Used sensibly, a low dose of aspirin or paracetamol, for a limited period, may be helpful. In many cases of stress-induced headache, however, the most effective treatment is relaxation, possibly aided initially with a little alcohol or a mild sedative.

HEAD INJURY Any injury to the head, whether associated with a skull fracture or not. Patients with head injuries should be assessed for signs of neurological damage, which may not develop at once. Patients with drowsiness, vomiting, confusion, or any focal neurological signs after a head injury should be seen by a doctor.

People suffering the results of such injuries and their relatives can obtain help and advice from Headway (National Head Injuries Association) (see APPENDIX 2: ADDRESSES).

HEALING (see WOUNDS).

HEALTH The state of health implies much more than freedom from disease, and good health may be defined as the attainment and maintenance of the highest state of mental and bodily vigour of which any given individual is capable. Environment, including living and working conditions, plays an important part in determining a person's health. The UK government is now placing much greater emphasis on health promotion and the prevention of disease and has published national targets for reducing the incidence of some major diseases.

HEALTH AND SAFETY EXECUTIVE The statutory body in Britain responsible for the health and safety of workers. The address of the HSE can be found in APPENDIX 2: ADDRESSES.

HEALTH CENTRE An imprecise term that may refer to a group of doctors and supporting staff operating from one building owned or leased by the doctors, or a building owned or leased by a district health authority that contains staff or services from one or more sections of the National Health Service.

HEALTH EDUCATION   The process of educating the public to adopt a healthy lifestyle and abandon dangerous or unhealthy behaviour. Information on all aspects of health education in the United Kingdom can be obtained from the Health Education Authority (see APPENDIX 2: ADDRESSES).

HEALTH SERVICE COMMISSIONER   An official, responsible to the United Kingdom's parliament, appointed to protect the interests of National Health Service patients in matters concerning the administration of the health service. Known colloquially as the health ombudsman, the commissioner presents regular reports on the complaints dealt with.

HEALTH VISITORS are nurses with a special training who form an important part of the primary health care team. Working in close conjunction with general practitioners (q.v.), they are primarily responsible for the health care of children and elderly people in the community. Health education and general promotion of health are an important part of their role. Contact the Health Visitors' Association (see APPENDIX 2: ADDRESSES).

HEARING (see DEAFNESS; EAR).

HEARING AIDS   Nearly two-thirds of people aged over 70 have some degree of hearing impairment (see DEAFNESS). Hearing aids are no substitute for definitive treatment of the underlying cause of poor hearing, so examination by an ear, nose and throat surgeon is sensible before a hearing aid is issued (and is essential before one can be given through the NHS). The choice of aid depends on the age, manipulative skills, and degree of hearing impairment of the patient and the underlying cause of the deafness. The choice of hearing aid for a deaf child is particularly important as impaired hearing can hinder speech development.

Ear trumpets, although old fashioned, may occasionally help an elderly person who is unable to manage an electronic aid.

Electronic aids consist, essentially, of a microphone, an amplifier, and an earphone. In postaural aids the microphone and amplifier are contained in a small box worn behind the ear or attached to spectacles. The earphone is on a specially moulded earpiece. Some patients find it difficult to manipulate the controls of an aid worn behind the ear, and they may be better off with a device worn on the body. Some hearing aids are worn entirely within the ear and are very discreet. They are particularly useful for people who have to wear protective headgear such as helmets.

All types have a volume control and a special setting for use with telephone and in rooms fitted with an inductive coupler that screens out background noise.

In making a choice therefore from the large range of effective hearing aids now available, the expert advice of an ear specialist must be obtained. The RNID (Royal National Institute for Deaf People) (see APPENDIX 2: ADDRESSES), provides a list of clinics where such a specialist can be consulted. It also gives reliable advice concerning the purchase and use of hearing aids.

HEART is a hollow muscular pump with four cavities, each provided at its outlet with a valve, whose function is to maintain the circulation of the blood. The two upper cavities are known as atria, the two lower ones as ventricles. The term auricle is applied to the ear-shaped tip of the atrium on each side.

Position   The heart lies in the chest between the two lungs, but projecting more to the left side than to the right. On the left side its apex reaches out in the adult between 8 and 9 cm (3½ and 4 inches), almost to the nipple, and lies beneath the fifth rib, while its right border extends only a short distance, at most 2·4 cm, beyond the margin of the breast-bone. Its lower border rests upon the diaphragm, by which it is separated from the liver and stomach, and this close connection has an important influence upon the heart in several disorders of the stomach. Above, the heart extends to the level of the second rib, where the great vessels, the aorta on the right side and the pulmonary artery on the left, lie behind the breast-bone.

Shape and size   The heart of any individual was described by Laennec as, roughly, of the size and shape of the clenched fist. Its weight in the male varies from 280 to 340 grams, and in the female from 230 to 280 grams. It continues to increase in weight and size up to a ripe old age, more so in men than in women. One end of the heart is pointed (apex), the other is broad (base), and is deeply cleft at the division between the two atria. One groove running down the front and up the back shows the division between the two ventricles; a circular, deeper groove marks off the atria above from the ventricles below. The capacity of each cavity is somewhere between 90 and 180 ml.

Structure   The heart lies within a strong fibrous bag, known as the pericardium, and since the inner surface of this bag and the outer surface of the heart are both covered with a smooth, glistening membrane faced with flat cells and lubricated by a little serous fluid (around 20 millilitres), the movements of the heart are accomplished almost without friction. The main thickness of the heart wall consists of bundles of muscle fibres, which run, some in circles right round the heart, others in loops, first round one cavity, then round the corresponding cavity of the other side. Within all the cavities is a smooth lining membrane, continuous with that lining the vessels which open into the heart. The investing smooth membrane is

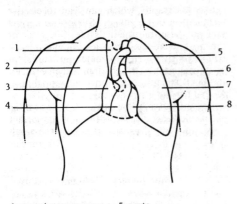

1 superior vena cava   5 aorta
2 right lung   6 pulmonary artery
3 right atrium   7 left lung
4 right ventricle   8 left ventricle

Diagram of the heart as seen on X-ray film.

Valves As stated above, there are four valves. The mitral valve consists of two triangular cusps, the tricuspid valve of three smaller cusps. The aortic and pulmonary valves each consist of three semilunar-shaped segments. The structure of a valve is a double layer of the lining membrane of the heart (endocardium) strengthened by fibrous tissue between. Two valves are placed at the openings leading from atrium into ventricle, the tricuspid valve on the right side, the mitral valve on the left, so as completely to prevent blood from running back into the atrium when the ventricle contracts. Two more, the pulmonary valve and the aortic valve, are at the entrance to these arteries, and prevent regurgitation into the ventricles of blood which

known as epicardium, the muscular substance as myocardium, and the smooth lining membrane as endocardium.

For the regulation of the heart's action there are important nervous connections, especially with the vagus nerve and with the sympathetic system. In the hinder part of the atria lies a collection of nerve cells and connecting fibres, known as the sinuatrial node, which forms the starting-point for the impulses that initiate the beats of the heart. Hence its alternative name of the pacemaker of the heart. In the groove between the ventricles and the atria lies another collection of similar nerve tissue, known as the atrioventricular node. From it there runs downwards into the septum between the two ventricles a band of special muscle fibres, known as the atrioventricular bundle, or the bundle of His. This splits up into a right and a left branch for the two ventricles, and the fibres of these distribute themselves throughout the muscular wall of the ventricles and control their contraction. (For illustrations of the heart and its blood vessels see CIRCULATION.)

Openings There is no direct communication between the cavities on the right side and those on the left; but the right atrium opens into the right ventricle by a large circular opening, and similarly the left atrium into the left ventricle. Into the right atrium open two large veins, the superior and inferior venae cavae, with some smaller veins from the wall of the heart itself, and into the left atrium open two pulmonary veins from each lung. One opening leads out of each ventricle, to the aorta in the case of the left ventricle, to the pulmonary artery from the right.

Prior to birth there is an opening (*foramen ovale*) from the right into the left atrium through which the blood passes; but when the child first draws air into his lungs this opening closes and is represented in the adult only by a depression (*fossa ovalis*). (For illustration of internal anatomy of heart see CIRCULATION.)

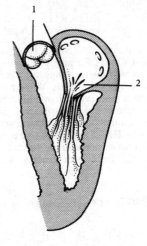

1 aortic valve
2 mitral valve

Interior of the left ventricle, showing structure of mitral and aortic valves.

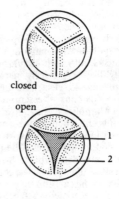

closed

open

1 cavity of left ventricle
2 valve cusp

Aortic valve, a semilunar-type valve. The pulmonary valve is also of this type.

has been driven from them into the arteries. The noises made by these valves in closing constitute the greater part of what are known as the heart sounds, and can be heard by anyone who applies his ear to the front of a person's chest. Murmurs heard accompanying these sounds indicate defects in the valves, and form one of the chief signs of heart disease.

Action At each heart-beat the two atria contract and expel their contents into the ventricles, which at the same time they stimulate to contract together, so that the blood is driven into the arteries, to be returned again to the atria after having completed a circuit in about fifteen seconds through the body or lungs as the case may be. The heart beats from sixty to ninety times a minute, the rate in any given healthy person being about four times that of the respirations. The heart is to some extent regulated by a nerve centre in the medulla, closely connected with those centres which govern the lungs and stomach, and nerve fibres pass to it in the vagus nerve. By some of these fibres its rate and force can be diminished, by others increased, according to the needs of the various organs of the body. If this nerve centre is injured or poisoned, for example, by lack of oxygen, the heart stops beating in human beings, although in some of the lower animals – e.g. frogs, fishes, and reptiles – the heart may under favourable conditions go on beating for hours even after its entire removal from the body.

HEARTBURN means a burning sensation experienced in the region of the heart and up the back to the throat. It is caused by an excessive acidity of the gastric juice, and is relieved temporarily by taking alkaline substances, such as 1·2 grams of bicarbonate of soda or a similar amount of bismuth carbonate or carbonate of magnesia in water. It is also relieved by the chewing of aluminium-containing antacid tablets such as Aluminium Hydroxide Tablets, BP.

HEART DISEASES: The heart is essentially a muscle pump which receives its own nutrient supply through the coronary arteries. It contains four valves which are designed to direct blood flow and the heart itself sits in a silky sac known as the pericardium. The action of the heart is determined by a sophisticated electric circuit known as the conducting system (see HEART).

Heart disease can affect any of the structures and more than one at a time.

CONGENITAL HEART DISEASE accounts for 1–2 per cent of all cases of organic heart disease. It may be inherited, present at birth for no obvious reason or in rare cases related to German measles (q.v.) in the mother or to drugs taken in pregnancy. The commonest forms are holes in the heart (atrial septal defect, ventricular septal defect (see SEPTAL DEFECT), a patent ductus arteriosus (q.v.) and coarctation of the aorta (q.v.). Many complex forms also exist and can be diagnosed in the womb by fetal

echocardiography which can lead to elective termination of pregnancy. Surgery to correct many of these abnormalities is feasible, even for the most severe abnormalities, but may only be palliative giving rise to major difficulties of management as the children become older. Heart transplantation is now increasingly employed for the uncorrectable lesions.

CORONARY ARTERY DISEASE, also known as ischaemic heart disease, is the most important cause of symptoms and death in the adult population. It may present for the first time as sudden death but more usually it causes angina pectoris (q.v.), myocardial infarction (heart attack) or heart failure. It can also lead to a disturbance of heart rhythm. Its cause is not fully known but factors associated with an increased risk of developing coronary artery disease include male sex, increasing age, diabetes, cigarette smoking, high blood pressure and a raised concentration of cholesterol in the blood. Around 146,000 people died of coronary-artery disease in England and Wales in 1992; it was the biggest single cause of death.

HEART MUSCLE DISEASE or cardiomyopathy usually indicates a weakness of the left ventricle which secondarily affects the right ventricle. The efficiency of the pump deteriorates, the heart attempts to compensate by increasing muscle thickness (hypertrophy) and by dilating (enlarged heart), but after a variable time it fails, leading to the symptoms of breathlessness due to fluid accumulation in the lungs (pulmonary oedema). With a failure to pump efficiently the output falls and fatigue becomes a problem. When more advanced, fluid distends the liver and the ankles may become swollen.

Cardiomyopathy may be secondary to coronary artery disease, present in the absence of coronary artery disease and of no obvious cause, due to an inflammation of the heart muscle (myocarditis) most commonly caused by a virus infection or due to excessive consumption of alcohol. Myocarditis may resolve, as may cardiomyopathy due to excessive alcohol consumption if drinking is stopped, but most forms of cardiomyopathy are progressive, needing regular medication to maintain quality and quantity of life.

VALVULAR HEART DISEASE primarily affects the mitral and aortic valves which can become narrowed (stenosis) or leaking (incompetence). Pulmonary valve problems are usually congenital (stenosis) and the tricuspid valve is sometimes involved when rheumatic heart disease primarily affects the mitral or aortic valves. Rheumatic fever (q.v.), usually in childhood, remains a common cause of chronic valvular heart disease causing stenosis, incompetence or both of the aortic and mitral valves, but each valve has other separate causes for malfunction.

AORTIC VALVE DISEASE is more common with increasing age. When narrowed the heart hypertrophies and may later fail. Symptoms of angina or breathlessness are common and dizziness or blackouts (syncope) also occur.

Replacing the valve is a very effective treatment, even with advancing age. Aortic stenosis may be caused by degeneration (senile calcific), inheriting two leaflets instead of the usual three (bicuspid valve) or rheumatic fever. Aortic incompetence again leads to hypertrophy, but dilatation is more common as blood leaks back into the ventricle. Breathlessness is the more common complaint. The causes are the same as stenosis but also include inflammatory conditions such as syphilis (q.v.) or ankylosing spondylitis (q.v.) and other disorders of connective tissue. The valve may also leak if the aorta dilates stretching the valve ring as with hypertension (q.v.), aortic aneurysm (q.v.) and Marfans Syndrome – an inherited disorder of connective tissue that causes heart defects. Infection (endocarditis) can worsen acutely or chronically destroy the valve and sometimes lead to abnormal outgrowths on the valve (vegetations) which may break free and cause devastating damage such as a stroke or blocked circulation to the bowel or leg.

MITRAL VALVE DISEASE leading to stenosis is rheumatic in origin. Mitral incompetence may be rheumatic but in the absence of stenosis can be due to ischaemia (q.v.), infarction (q.v.), inflammation, infection and a congenital weakness (prolapse). The valve may also leak if stretched by a dilating ventricle (functional incompetence). Infection (endocarditis) may affect the valve in a similar way to aortic disease. Mitral symptoms are predominantly breathlessness which may lead to wheezing or waking at night breathless and needing to sit up or stand for relief. They are made worse when the heart rhythm changes (atrial fibrillation) which is frequent as the disease becomes more severe. This leads to a loss of efficiency of up to 25 per cent and a predisposition to clot formation as blood stagnates rather than leaves the heart efficiently. Mitral incompetence may remain mild and be of no trouble for many years but infection must be guarded against (endocarditis prophylaxis).

ENDOCARDITIS is an infection of the heart which may acutely destroy a valve or lead to chronic destruction. Bacteria settle usually on a mild lesion. Antibiotics taken at vulnerable times can prevent this happening (antibiotic prophylaxis); one of the most common occasions is before dental treatment. If established, vigorous intravenous antibiotic therapy is needed and surgery is often necessary. The mortality is 30 per cent but may be higher if the infection settles on a replaced valve (prosthetic endocarditis). Complications include heart failure, shock, embolization (generation of small clots in the blood) and cerebral (mental) confusion.

PERICARDITIS is an inflammation of the sac covering the outside of the heart. The sac becomes roughened and pain occurs as the heart and sac rub together. This is heard by stethoscope as a scratching noise (pericardial rub). Fever is often present and a virus the main cause. It may also occur with rheumatic fever, kidney failure, tuberculosis or from an adjacent lung problem such as pneumonia or cancer. The inflammation may cause fluid to accumulate between the sac and the heart (effusion) which may compress the heart causing a fall in blood pressure, a weak pulse and circulatory failure (tamponade). This can be relieved by aspirating the fluid. The treatment is then directed at the underlying cause.

DISTURBANCES OF RHYTHM are common and of several types. Many do not reflect underlying disease. Usually the patient becomes aware of his heart beat (palpitations) which may be fast or appear to miss a beat or kick. Stress or stimulants such as caffeine or alcohol are a frequent cause. Occasionally the disturbance can be troublesome, even though not dangerous, and merit treatment, but drugs should be avoided if no obvious disease exists.

Disturbances reflecting disease may lead to the heart's going fast or slow or both intermittently.

ATRIAL FIBRILLATION may occur without obvious disease but usually presents when there is coronary artery disease, cardiomyopathy, high blood pressure or mitral valve disease. The rhythm is very irregular and may lead to rapid poorly co-ordinated contractions of the ventricle leading to heart failure. It predisposes to clots' forming in the heart. Treatment may be directed to converting the heart back to normal (sinus) rhythm by drugs or electric shock treatment or to controlling the speed with drugs such as digoxin (q.v.). It is a serious irregularity. Blood-thinning medication such as warfarin (q.v.) is often prescribed.

EXTRASYSTOLES are very common and usually perceived as missed beats or extra beats (a kick or thump). They are not usually serious but they may, however, complicate coronary artery disease or heart muscle disease when certain forms need specialized therapy.

HEART BLOCK refers to a failure to conduct normally through the electric circuit of the heart. There are three types; 1st degree which can be a normal variation and does not cause slowing; 2nd degree which causes intermittent slowing and 3rd degree or complete block where there is no electrical connection and heart beats are slow and unpredictable leading to blackouts (Stokes-Adams attacks) and/or heart failure. For most 2nd degree and all complete cases a pacemaker relieves symptoms and improves life expectancy.

SINUS NODE DISEASE The main electrical control of the heart is the sinus node. If this is diseased or inherits a malfunction, the heart may develop rapid, slow or both rapid and slow rhythms. Often a tape recording for 24 hours (Holter) is used to document the irregularities. The heart itself may well be normal but these electrical disturbances can be very symptomatic. Treatment may include drugs, a cardiac pacemaker (q.v.) or both.

MISCELLANEOUS There are many infrequent causes of heart problems which for the affected individual are a cause of debility. These include a problem of heart muscle thickening (hypertrophic cardiomyopathy), which can cause angina, irregular heart beats and sudden death, and Wolf Parkinson White Syndrome which causes the heart to race due to an extra fast conducting section in the circuit. This may induce pain, dizziness and blackouts. Some electrical conditions of the heart merit specific study known as electrophysiology (EPS) which allows the abnormality to be mapped out, thus facilitating drug or intervention treatment (ablation) to stop abnormal conduction.

HEAT-CRAMPS are painful cramps in the muscles occurring in workers, such as stokers, who labour in hot conditions. The cramps are the result of loss of salt in the sweat, and can be cured by giving salty water to drink. (See HEAT-STROKE.)

HEAT SPOTS is a vague term applied to small inflamed and congested areas which appear especially upon the skin of the face, neck, and chest or other parts of the body in warm weather.

HEATSTROKE A condition resulting from environmental temperatures which are too high for compensation by the body's thermo-regulatory mechanism(s). It is characterized by hyperpyrexia, nausea, headache, thirst, confusion, and dry skin. If untreated, coma and death ensue. Its occurence is sporadic; whereas a single individual may be affected (occasionally with fatal consequences), his or her colleagues may remain unaffected. Predisposing factors include unsatisfactory living or working conditions, inadequate acclimatization to tropical conditions, unsuitable clothing, underlying poor health, and possibly dietetic or alcoholic indiscretions. It can be a major problem during pilgrimages, e.g., the Hadj. Four clinical syndromes are recognized: (1) HEAT COLLAPSE is characterized by fatigue, giddiness, and temporary loss of consciousness. It is accompanied by hypotension and bradycardia; there may be vomiting and muscular cramps. Urinary volume is diminished. Recovery is usual. (2) HEAT EXHAUSTION is characterized by increasing weakness, dizziness, and insomnia; in the majority, sweating is defective; there are few, if any, signs of dehydration. Pulse rate is normal, and urinary output good. Body temperature is usually 37·8–38·3 °C. (3) HEAT CRAMPS (usually in the legs, arms, or back and occasionally involving the abdominal muscles) are associated with hard physical work at a high temperature. Sweating, pallor, headache, giddiness, and intense anxiety are present. Body temperature is only mildly raised. (4) HEAT HYPERPYREXIA is heralded by energy loss and irritability; this is followed by mental confusion and diminution of sweating. The individual rapidly becomes restless, comatose, and body temperature rises to 41–42 °C or even higher. The condition is fatal unless expertly treated as a matter of urgency.
Treatment With syndromes 1–2, the affected individual must be removed immediately to a cool place, and isotonic saline administered, intravenously in a severe case. Syndrome 4 is a medical emergency. The patient should be placed in the shade, stripped, and drenched with water; fanning should be instigated. He or she should be wrapped in a sheet soaked in cool water and fanning continued. When rectal temperature has fallen to 39 °C the patient is wrapped in a dry blanket. Immediately after consciousness returns, normal saline should be given orally; this usually provokes sweating. The risk of circulatory collapse exists. Convalescence may be protracted and the patient should be repatriated to a cool climate. Prophylactically, personnel intended for work in a tropical climate must be very carefully selected. Adequate acclimatization is also essential; severe physical exertion must be avoided for several weeks. Light clothes should be worn. The diet should be light but nourishing, and fluid intake adequate. Those performing hard physical work at a very high ambient temperature should receive sodium chloride supplements. Attention to ventilation and air-conditioning is essential; fans are also of value.

HEBEPHRENIA is a form of mental disorder coming on in youth and marked by depression and gradual failure of mental faculties with egotistic and self-centred delusions. It is one of the forms of schizophrenia.

HEBERDEN'S NODES are little hard knobs which appear at the sides of the last phalanges of the fingers in people who are the subject of osteoarthrosis.

HEEL is the hinder part of the foot formed by the calcaneus and the specially thick skin covering it. It is not subject to many diseases. Severe pain in the heel is sometimes a sign of gout or rheumatism.

HEIGHT (see WEIGHT AND HEIGHT).

HELICOBACTER PYLORI is a bacterium that colonizes the human stomach causing inflammation called type B gastritis. Strongly associated with peptic ulceration, the bacterium is also linked with gastric cancer. In the developed world most people are infected by the age of 10. Spontaneous eradication of *H. pylori* is rare and the infection usually persists for many years.

HELIUM is the lightest gas known, with the exception of hydrogen. This property renders it of value in anaesthesia (q.v.), as its addition to the anaesthetic means that it can be inhaled with less effort by the patient. Thus it can be used in the presence of any obstruction to the entry of air to the lungs.

HELMINTHS is a name for worms.

HEMIANAESTHESIA means loss of touch-sense down one side of the body.

HEMIANOPIA, HEMIANOPSIA, and HEMIOPIA are terms meaning loss of half the usual area of vision. The affected person may see everything clearly to the left or to the right, the field of vision stopping abruptly at the middle line, or he may see things only when straight in front of him, or thirdly, he may see objects far out on both sides, although there is a wide area straight in front for which he is quite blind. The position of the blind area is important in localizing the position in the brain of the disease responsible for the condition.

HEMIATROPHY is atrophy of one side of the body, or of part of the body on one side: for example, facial hemiatrophy, in which one-half of the face is smaller than the other either in the course of development or as a result of some nervous disorder.

HEMIBALLISMUS are involuntary movements similar to choreiform movements but of much greater amplitude and force. They are violent throwing movements of the limbs which are usually unilateral. They tend to occur acutely as a result of vascular damage to the mid-brain.

HEMICOLECTOMY An operation to remove the right or left half of the colon, usually with end-to-end anastomosis of the remaining portion of the intestine. This is often used for the treatment of malignant or inflammatory diseases of the colon.

HEMICRANIA means a headache limited to one side of the head. (See MIGRAINE.)

HEMIMELIA This consists of defects in the distal part of the extremities such as the absence of a forearm or hands. This is a congenital defect and large numbers of cases resulted from the administration of Thalidomide during pregnancy.

HEMIPARESIS Paralysis affecting the muscles of one side of the body. This most commonly follows a stroke and occurs when parts of the brain serving motor function on the opposite side of the body are damaged.

HEMIPLEGIA means paralysis limited to one side of the body. (See PARALYSIS.)

HENLE, LOOP OF That part of the nephron (see KIDNEYS) between the proximal and distal convoluted tubules. It extends into the renal medulla as a hairpin-shaped loop. The ascending link of the loop actively transports sodium from the lumen of the tube to the interstitium,

and this, combined with the 'counter-current' flow of fluid through the two limbs of the loop, plays a part in concentrating the urine.

HEPARIN is a naturally produced anticoagulant (q.v.) with a rapid effect and is thought to act by neutralizing thrombin (see COAGULATION). Inactive when taken orally, it is normally given intravenously – it may be given for a few days, combined with an oral anticoagulant such as warfarin, to initiate anticoagulation. Low-dose heparin may be given by subcutaneous injection for longer periods, for the prophylaxis of deep-vein thrombosis or pulmonary embolism in 'high-risk' patients, such as those with obesity or a history of thrombosis, or postoperatively. If haemorrhage occurs, withdrawal of heparin is usually sufficient, but protamine sulphate is a rapidly active and specific antidote. Prolonged treatment with heparin may cause osteoporosis.

HEPATECTOMY is the operation for removal of the liver, or part of it.

HEPATITIS Hepatitis, or inflammation of liver cells (see LIVER), may be acute or chronic and symptoms may be absent or non-specific. *Acute* hepatitis causes jaundice (q.v.), itching, abdominal pain and liver tenderness, malaise, anorexia (q.v.), fever and nausea. Treatment consists of bed-rest and relief of symptoms. All unnecessary drugs must be stopped and alcohol should be avoided. *Chronic* hepatitis can cause any of the symptoms above, but they tend to be more insidious in onset.

Diagnostic investigations include blood tests to assess liver function, liver biopsy to classify the type and cause of hepatitis and ultrasound scanning (see ULTRASOUND).

There are many causes; some agents can produce both acute and chronic hepatitis. Alcohol abuse is the commonest cause in Great Britain.

VIRAL HEPATITIS classically refers to infection with one of the so-called hepatitis viruses, of which there are at least five: A, B, C, D and E. Many other virus infections produce liver inflammation and these include glandular fever and HIV. Treatment with many drugs causes hepatitis as a side-effect; halothane general anaesthesia (q.v.), methyl dopa and paracetamol in overdose are examples. Autoimmune diseases such as rheumatoid arthritis (q.v.) may exhibit associated chronic hepatitis.

FULMINANT HEPATITIS is the severest form of liver inflammation; there is massive destruction of liver cells resulting in liver failure with severe jaundice, impaired consciousness, fluid retention and a bleeding tendency. Kidney failure may follow. Causes include alcohol abuse, acute viral hepatitis and paracetamol overdose. Liver transplantation has dramatically improved the outlook of this condition.

INFECTIOUS HEPATITIS is caused by hepatitis A virus. It is transmitted by eating food contaminated with faecal material from an infected individual, particularly seafood, and it is common in areas where standards of hygiene are poor. In temperate climates it tends to occur in late summer; in the tropics there is no seasonal variation. Incubation period is 15 to 45 days. Patients should not return to work until at least 7 days after complete clinical recovery, when the prognosis is good and there is no risk of chronic infection. Hepatitis E virus is similar to Hepatitis A, except that in pregnancy the mortality rate of the former may be as high as 20 per cent.

SERUM HEPATITIS is due to infection with viruses B, C or D. They share the same routes of infection – through transfusion of infected blood, sharing needles for injection of drugs, tattooing or through sexual intercourse with an infected individual – and tend to have a longer incubation period, up to 180 days in the case of virus B. These virus infections carry a much higher mortality rate (1–3 per cent in hepatitis B and C, up to 20 per cent in virus D) and the viruses may remain in the blood for many years, causing chronic carrier status (such individuals remain an infectious risk to others) and chronic hepatitis. Diagnosis of these various types of viral infection is by the demonstration of specific antibodies (q.v.) and antigens (q.v.) in the blood. Following the discovery of the responsible virus, non-A non-B hepatitis is now known as hepatitis C.

Persistence of hepatitis B virus in the blood with hepatic inflammation lasting more than 6 months after hepatitis B infection is defined as chronic type-B hepatitis. Hepatocellular carcinoma is common in areas of the world where hepatitis-B carrier status is frequent and chronic hepatitis – of any cause – may result in cirrhosis. Therefore much effort has gone into finding treatments for chronic type-B hepatitis, the most successful of which has been antiviral chemotherapy with interferon (q.v.). The response to this treatment may be disappointing with a high rate of relapse.

HEPATOLENTICULAR DEGENERATION
(see WILSON'S DISEASE).

HEPATOMA
A primary malignant tumour of liver cells. It has marked geographical variation, being most common in parts of Africa and the Far East. It is more common in men and with those who have pre-existing cirrhosis (q.v.).

HEPATOMEGALY
Enlargement of the liver. This may be caused by congestion (e.g. in heart failure), infection (e.g. hepatitis), malignancy, inflammation, or early cirrhosis (q.v.).

HEREDITY
is the principle on which various peculiarities of bodily form or structure, or of physical or mental activity are transmitted from parents to offspring. (See GENES.)

HERMAPHRODITE is an individual in whom both ovarian and testicular tissue is present. Hermaphrodites may have a testis on one side and an ovary on the other, or an ovotestis on one side and an ovary or testis on the other, or there may be an ovotestis on both sides. Both gonads are usually intra-abdominal. The true hermaphrodite usually has a uterus and at least one fallopian tube on the side of the ovary. On the side of the testis there is usually a vas deferens. Most true hermaphrodites are raised as males but external virilization is not usually complete. Even when significant phallic development is present hypospadias and cryptorchism are common. At puberty gynaecomastia develops and menstruation is common, as ovarian function is usually more nearly normal than testicular function.

HERNIA is the protrusion of an organ, or part of an organ through the wall of the cavity that normally contains it. The most common types of hernia involve the organs of the abdomen which can herniate externally through the abdominal wall, or internally usually through a defect in the diaphragm. External hernias appear as a swelling, covered with skin, which bulge out on coughing or straining but which can normally be made to disappear with gentle pressure.

Types The commonest hernia is the inguinal hernia, which appears in the groin at the site of inguinal canal, which contains the spermatic chord in males. Less common is the femoral hernia which appears just below the groin, passing through a defect close to the main blood vessels of the leg. The inguinal hernia is commoner in males and the femoral hernia in females. Other common types of abdominal hernia include an incisional hernia, through a defect in any abdominal surgical scar, a paraumbilical hernia arising just to the side of the umbilicus and an epigastric hernia in the mid line above the umbilicus. In children, herniation may occur through the umbilicus itself, which is a natural weak spot. The commonest internal hernia is a hiatus hernia, when

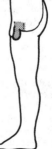

Site of inguinal hernia (shaded).

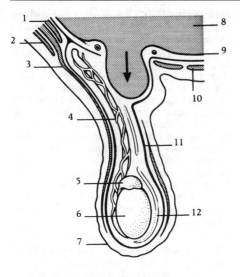

1 transverse abdominis muscle
2 external oblique muscle
3 internal oblique muscle
4 spermatic cord
5 epidydimis
6 testis
7 scrotum
8 abdominal contents
9 abdominal peritoneum
10 rectus femoris
11 internal spermatic fascia
12 tunica vaginalis

Anatomy of indirect inguinal hernia: arrow shows direction of displaced loop of intestine moving into scrotum.

part of the stomach slips upwards into the chest through the diaphragm (q.v.).
Causes Hernias may be due to a defect present at birth (congenital), or may develop later in life (acquired). Acquired hernias arise due to the development of a defect or injury of the abdominal wall or due to increased pressure within the abdominal cavity, which forces the organ through a potential weakness. Such causes include chronic coughing or excessive straining due to constipation.
Complications Small hernias may cause no problems at all. However, some may be large and cumbersome, or may give rise to a dragging sensation or even pain.

Although most hernias will reduce spontaneously under the effects of gravity or gentle pressure, any organs that may have been displaced inside some hernias may become stuck, when they are said to be irreducible. If the contents become so trapped that their blood supply is cut off, then strangulation occurs. This is a surgical emergency because the strangulated organs will soon die or rupture. When strangulation does occur, the hernia becomes irreducible, red, and very painful. If the hernia

contains bowel, then the bowel may also become obstructed.
Treatment Conservative treatment with a compression belt, or truss, is now less popular than in previous eras. Surgical repair is the preferred option whenever possible, and consists of returning the herniated organs to their proper place, and then repairing the defect through which the hernia occurred. This may be done safely under local or general anaesthetic, often as a day-case procedure, and most operative repairs result in a permanent cure.

HEROIN, also known as diacetyl morphine, is a drug of the opiate type, which includes morphine, codeine, pethidine, and methadone. It is a powerful analgesic and cough suppressant, but its capacity to produce euphoria rapidly induces dependence. Popular with addicts, its mostly pleasant effects soon produce tolerance, and the need to inject the drug, with associated risks of HIV infection, is decreasing its popularity (see DRUG ADDICTION). Withdrawal symptoms include restlessness, insomnia, muscle cramps, vomiting, and diarrhoea; signs include dilated pupils, raised pulse rate, and disturbed temperature control. Although rarely life threatening, they may cause great distress; for this reason methadone, which has a slower and less severe withdrawal syndrome, is commonly used when weaning addicts off heroin. Legally still available to doctors in the UK, heroin is normally only used in patients with severe pain, or to comfort the dying.

HERPANGINA is a short febrile illness in which minute vesicles or punched-out ulcers develop in the posterior parts of the mouth. It is due to infection with the group A Coxsackie viruses (q.v.).

HERPES GENITALIS or genital herpes is a vesicular infection of the genitals caused by the *Herpes simplex* virus (q.v.) and transmitted by sexual intercourse.

HERPES SIMPLEX is an acute infectious disease, characterized by the development of groups of superficial vesicles, or blebs, in the skin and mucous membrane. It is due to a virus, and infection can occur at any time from birth onwards, but the usual time for primary infection is between the second and fifteenth year. Once an individual is infected, the virus persists in the body for the rest of the individual's life. It is one of the causes of scrum-pox (q.v.).
Symptoms The symptoms vary with the age of infection. In young infants it may cause a generalized infection which may prove fatal. In young children the infection is usually in the mouth, and this may be associated with enlargement of the glands in the neck, general irritability and fever. The condition usually settles in seven to ten days. In adults the vesicles may occur anywhere in the skin or mucous membranes. The more common sites are the

lips, mouth and face where they are known as cold sores. The vesicles may also appear on the genitalia, when it is known as *Herpes genitalis* (q.v.), or in the conjunctiva or cornea and the brain may be infected, causing encephalitis (q.v.) or meningitis. The first sign is the appearance of small painful swellings. These quickly develop into vesicles (q.v.), containing clear fluid, and surrounded by a reddened area of skin. Some people are particularly liable to recurrent attacks, and these often tend to be associated with some debilitating condition or infection, such as pneumonia.

Except in the case of herpes of the cornea, the eruption clears completely unless it becomes contaminated with some other organism. In the case of the cornea, there may be residual scarring, which may impair vision.

Treatment A local treatment which may help, if the skin is involved, is idoxuridine. Should the eye be involved the patient must be referred immediately to an eye specialist. An antiviral agent such as acyclovir may be of help in treating the disease.

HERPES ZOSTER, or SHINGLES, is a skin eruption of acute nature, closely related to chickenpox, consisting in the appearance of small yellow vesicles (q.v.), which spread over an area, dry up, and heal by scabbing. It receives its name from the Greek word, for a 'circingle' or girdle, because it spreads in a zone-like manner round half the chest. Herpes of the face also occurs, particularly on the brow and round the eye.

Causes It is due to a virus identical with that of chickenpox. This invades the ganglia of the nerves, particularly the spinal nerves of the chest and the fifth cranial nerve which supplies the face. In spite of its being due to the same virus as chickenpox, it is rare for herpes zoster to occur as a result of contact with a case of chickenpox. On the other hand, it is not unusual for a patient with herpes zoster to infect a child with chickenpox. It is a disease of adults rather than children, and the older the person the more likely is he to develop the disease. Thus in adults under 50 the incidence is around 2·5 per 1000 people a year. Between 50 and 60 it is around 5 per 1000, whilst in octogenarians it is 10 per 1000. Most adults who acquire the disease have had chickenpox in child-hood. Occasionally it may be associated with some serious underlying disease such as leukaemia, lymphadenoma, or multiple myeloma.

Symptoms The first symptoms of herpes are much like those of any feverish attack. The person feels unwell for some days, has a slight rise of temperature, and vague pain in the side or in various other parts. The pain finally settles at a point in the side, and, two or three days after the first symptoms, the rash appears. Minute yellow blebs or vesicles as they are known are seen on the skin of the back, of the side, or of the front of the chest, or simultaneously on all three, the points corresponding to the space between one pair of ribs right round.

These blebs increase in number for some days, and spread till there is often a complete half girdle round one side of the chest. The pain in this stage is severe, but it appears to vary a good deal with age, being slight in children and very severe in old people, in whom indeed herpes sometimes forms a serious illness. After one or two weeks, most of the vesicles have dried up and formed scabs. The pain may not pass off when the eruption disappears, but may remain for weeks or even months: a condition known as post-herpetic neuralgia. Old people are prone to develop this condition.

Treatment In the very early stage, before the vesicles have formed, cocaine or atropine ointment rubbed into the side eases the pain and seems to prevent to some extent the outbreak of the eruption. Later, when the vesicles have formed and are discharging, a dusting-powder of starch, zinc oxide, and bismuth subnitrate gives much relief.

Should post-herpetic neuralgia persist, the administration of analgesics is essential. Acupuncture is also said to be helpful.

HERTZ is the SI (International System of Units) unit of frequency. It indicates the number of cycles per second (c/s). The abbreviation for hertz is Hz.

HETEROGRAFT is a transplant from one animal to another of a different species. It is also known as a xenograft.

HETEROSEXUAL Concerning sexual relationships between members of opposite sexes.

HETEROZYGOUS An individual having dissimilar members of the pair of genes coding for a given characteristic (see GENES).

HEXACHLOROPHANE is a widely used antiseptic which is active against a range of microorganisms, including Gram-positive and Gram-negative organisms, *Shigella dysenteriae*, and *Salmonella typhi*. One of its advantages is that it retains its activity in the presence of soap, and it is therefore often used in soaps and creams in a concentration of 1 to 2 per cent. It must be used with caution in babies as it can be absorbed through the skin and prove harmful.

HEXAMINE is a substance which, when excreted by the kidneys, sets free formaldehyde, that has an antiseptic action. It is given in cases of cystitis when the urine decomposes within the bladder, and it exerts its beneficial action very speedily. It acts only in urine with an acid reaction, and, if the urine is alkaline, acid phosphate of soda is usually taken along with the hexamine. The dose of each of these is 0·6 to 2 grams several times daily.

HEXOESTROL (see OESTROGENS).

Hg The chemical symbol for mercury. Blood pressure (q.v.) is traditionally measured in millimetres (mm) of mercury using a sphygmomanometer (q.v.) consisting of an inflatable cuff (usually wrapped round the upper arm) connected by a rubber tube to a column of mercury calibrated in mm of mercury.

HIATUS HERNIA is a displacement of a portion of the stomach through the opening in the diaphragm through which the oesophagus passes from the chest to the abdominal cavity.

HICCUP An involuntary spasmodic contraction of the diaphragm (q.v.) which produces an indrawing of breath during which there is a sudden closure of the vocal cords. This results in the well-known sound and sensation.

It is usually of benign cause (e.g. indigestion) but may be a symptom of medullary brain damage, uraemia, typhoid fever or encephalitis lethargica.

There are many folk remedies for hiccups but most subside spontaneously. Prolonged hiccups due to disease may respond to treatment with chlorpromazine.

HILUM is a term applied to the depression on organs such as the lung, kidney, and spleen, at which the vessels and nerves enter it and round which the lymphatic glands cluster. The hilum of the lung is also known as its root.

HIP That part of the body on each side of the pelvis where it articulates with the head of the femur (thigh bone).

HIP-JOINT is the joint formed by the head of the thigh-bone and the deep cup-shaped hollow on the side of the pelvis which receives it (acetabulum). The joint is of the ball-and-socket variety, is dislocated only by very great violence, and is correspondingly difficult to reduce to its natural state after dislocation. The joint is enclosed by a capsule of fibrous tissue, strengthened by several bands, of which the principal is the ilio-femoral or Y-shaped ligament placed in front of the joint. A round ligament also unites the head of the thigh-bone to the margin of the acetabulum.

For hip-joint disease see under JOINTS, DISEASES OF.

HIPPOCRATIC OATH An oath traditionally taken by doctors on qualification that sets out the moral precepts of their profession and binds them to a code of behaviour and practice. It is named after Hippocrates (460–370 BC), the Greek 'father of medicine'.

HIPPUS is a tremor of the iris which produces alternating contraction and dilatation of the pupil. This is often a sign of hysteria.

HIRSCHSPRUNG'S DISEASE, or MEGA-COLON, is a condition in childhood which is characterized by great hypertrophy and dilatation of the colon.

HIRSUTISM, or HYPERTRICHOSIS, is the growth of hair of the male type and distribution in women. It is either due to the excess production of androgens or to undue sensitivity of the hair follicle to normal female levels of circulating androgens. The latter is called idiopathic because the cause is unknown. The increased production of androgens in the female may come from the ovary and be due to the polycystic ovary syndrome or an ovarian tumour, or the excess androgen may come from the adrenal cortex and be the result of congenital adrenal hyperplasia, an adrenal tumour or Cushing's syndrome. However there is a wide range of normality in the distribution of female body hair. It varies with different racial groups. The Mediterranean races have more body hair than Nordic women and the Chinese and Japanese have little body hair. Many normal women, especially those with dark hair, have hair apparent on the upper lip and a few coarse hairs on the chin and around the nipples are not uncommon. Extension of the pubic hair towards the umbilicus is frequently found in normal women. Dark hair is much more apparent than fair hair and this is why bleaching is of considerable benefit in the management of hirsutism.

The treatment of hirsutism is that of the primary cause. When it is idiopathic hirsutism it must be managed by simple measures such as bleaching the hair and the use of depilatory waxes and creams. Coarse facial hairs can be removed by electrolysis, although this is time consuming. Shaving is often the most effective remedy and neither increases the rate of hair growth nor causes the hairs to become coarser.

HISTAMINE is an amine (q.v.) derived from histidine (q.v.). It is widely distributed in the tissues of plants and animals, including man. It is a powerful stimulant of gastric juice, a constrictor of smooth muscle including that of the bronchi, and a dilator of arterioles and capillaries. It is this last action which is responsible for the eruption of urticaria (q.v.).

HISTIDINE is an amino-acid from which histamine is derived by bacterial decomposition.

HISTOLOGY is the study of the minute structure of the tissues.

HISTOPLASMOSIS is a disease due to a yeast-like fungus known as *Histoplasma capsulatum*. Most cases have been reported from USA. In infants it is characterized by fever, anaemia, enlargement of the liver and spleen, and involvement of the lungs and gastro-intestinal tract. In older children it may resemble pulmonary tuberculosis, whilst in adults it may be confined to involvement of the skin.

HIV Human immunodeficiency virus: the virus that is responsible for AIDS. It is one of the family of human T-cell lymphocytotrophic viruses, others of which may cause lymphomas in man. (See AIDS/HIV INFECTION.)

HIVES is a popular term applied to eruptions of the nature of urticaria (q.v.).

HLA SYSTEM The major histocompatibility complex, or human leucocyte antigen (HLA) region, consists of genetically determined antigens, situated on chromosome 6. Found in most tissues, though to a differing extent, the four gene loci are known as A, B, C, D, while the individual alleles at each locus are numbered 1, 2, 3, etc. The number of possible combinations is thus enormous, and the chance of two unrelated people being identical for HLA is very low. HLA incompatibility causes the immune response, or rejection reaction, that occurs with unmatched tissue grafts. Strong associations between HLA and susceptibility to certain diseases – notably the autoimmune diseases such as rheumatoid arthritis, insulin-dependent diabetes, and thyrotoxicosis – have been described. Certain HLA antigens occur together more frequently than would be expected by chance (linkage disequilibrium), and may have a protective effect, conferring resistance to a disease.

HODGKIN'S DISEASE, so called after Thomas Hodgkin (1798–1866), the Guy's Hospital pathologist who first described it, or LYMPHADENOMA, is a condition in which the lymphatic glands all over the body undergo a gradually progressive enlargement. The cause is not known. The glands affected may reach a great size. The male:female ratio is 1·4:1 and the disease is rare before 10, peaking in the twenties and late middle age. The patient often runs a characteristic form of fever (Pel-Ebstein fever), in which bouts of fever alternate with several days with no fever. Along with these changes a considerable degree of anaemia arises, and the affected person becomes gradually weaker. Treatment consists of radiotherapy when the disease is relatively localized. When it is more widespread, however, chemotherapy is the treatment of choice. This is now given in the form of a combination of drugs, rather than one single drug. Drugs used include doxorubicin, lomustine, mustine, vinblastine, vincristine, procarbazine and prednisolone. The results of treatment are now such that over 80 per cent treated by radiotherapy, and 78 per cent of those treated by combined chemotherapy, are still alive after five years.

HOLISTIC A method of medical care in which patients are treated as a whole and which takes into account their physical and mental state as well as social background rather than just treating the disease alone.

HOMATROPINE is an alkaloid derived from atropine, which is used to produce dilatation of the pupil and to paralyse accommodation temporarily for the purpose of examining the interior of the eye. It is used in 1 per cent solution, and its effects pass away in the course of a few hours.

HOMOCYSTINURIA is a congenital disease due to the inability of the affected individual to metabolize, or utilize properly one of the essential amino-acids (q.v.) known as methionine. The main features of the condition are abnormality of the lens of the eye, mental retardation, fair complexion and fair hair and a high cheek colour.

HOMOEOPATHY is a system of medicine founded by Hahnemann at the end of the eighteenth century. It is based upon the theory that diseases are curable by those drugs which produce effects on the body similar to symptoms caused by the disease (*similia similibus curantur*). In administering drugs, the theory is also held that their effect is increased by giving them in minute doses obtained by diluting them to an extreme degree.

HOMOGRAFT is a piece of tissue or an organ, such as a kidney, transplanted from one animal to another of the same species: e.g. from man to man. It is also known as an allograft.

HOMOSEXUALITY is sexual activity with a member of the same sex. There has been considerable debate among psychiatrists as to whether homosexuality should be regarded as a normal sexual variant or as a psycho-pathological development or deviation. Although homosexuality is found in virtually every society and culture there is no society in which it is the predominant or preferred mode of sexual activity. Various attempts have been made to link homosexuality to hormonal factors, particularly lowered testosterone levels, or to find a genetic explanation, but there is no evidence for either. Psycho-analytic theories link homosexuality to early child-rearing influences, in particular the close binding and intimate mother.

The number of homosexual men in the UK is unknown. There has never been a representative population survey. Re-analysis of the Kinsey report suggests that only 3 per cent of adult men have exclusively homosexual leanings and a further 3 per cent have extensive homosexual and heterosexual experience. Homosexuality seems to be less common among women. Homosexual intercourse (and penetration) is a well-known means of transmission of the HIV virus.

There are still differences in the way homosexuals and heterosexuals are treated in British law. The age of consent for homosexuals is 18, while for heterosexuals it is 16.

HOMOZYGOUS An individual having identical members of the pair of genes coding for a given characteristic, (see GENES).

HONKING is the term applied to a persistent cough of emotional origin which occurs in emotionally disturbed children. It is of an explosive brassy character and has been compared to the call of the Canada goose. When coughing the child grimaces and tends to hold the chin close to the chest. One of its major characteristics is that it never occurs at night. Quite often it follows on a cold or sore throat. No specific treatment is needed. It disappears when the cause of the emotional upset, such as, for example, difficulties at school, is dealt with and removed.

HOOKWORM (see ANCYLOSTOMIASIS).

HORMONE REPLACEMENT THERAPY (see MENOPAUSE).

HORMONES These are 'chemical messengers' that are dispersed by the blood and act on target organs to produce effects distant from their point of release. The main organs involved in hormone production are the pituitary, pancreas, ovary, testis, thyroid, and adrenal (qq.v.). The release of many hormones is, ultimately, under the control of the central nervous system via a series of inhibiting and releasing factors from the hypothalamus (q.v.). Hormones are involved in maintaining homeostasis: e.g. insulin regulates the concentration of glucose in the blood. They also participate in growth and maturation: e.g. growth hormone promotes growth and helps to regulate fat, carbohydrate, and protein metabolism; and the sex hormones promote sexual maturation and reproduction. (See ENDOCRINE GLANDS.)

HORNER'S SYNDROME This is the description given to a combination of changes resulting from paralysis of the sympathetic nerve in the neck. They are: small pupil, a drooping upper lid and an apparently (though not actually) sunken eye.

HORRIPILATION is another term for gooseflesh, due to contraction of the small muscles in the skin which make the hairs erect.

HORSESHOE KIDNEY (see KIDNEYS, DISEASES OF).

HOSPICE A hospital that cares only for the terminally ill and dying. The emphasis is on providing quality of life and special care is taken in providing pain relief by whichever methods are deemed best suited to the person's needs. In the United Kingdom hospice care has been greatly developed, in particular with the leadership of Dr (Dame) Cicely Saunders.

HOSPITAL An institution providing treatment for sick and injured persons. This may be done on an inpatient or outpatient basis. It provides investigative and therapeutic services which are not available on a domiciliary basis. Hospitals are broadly divided into general hospitals (available in each district in the United Kingdom) and hospitals specializing in particular ailments (e.g. ophthalmology, ear, nose and throat, neurology, etc.). In addition there are teaching hospitals which have the dual function of patient care and the education of medical staff.

HOST An organism on which a parasite lives.

HOUR-GLASS STOMACH is the term given to the X-ray appearance of a stomach which is constricted in its middle part because of either spasm of the stomach muscle or contraction of scar tissue from a gastric ulcer.

HOUSEMAID'S KNEE is an inflammation of the bursa in front of the knee-cap, often mistaken for some disease in the joint itself (see BURSITIS).

HUMAN CHORIONIC GONADOTROPHIN A glycoprotein hormone secreted by the placenta (see PLACENTA) in early pregnancy which stimulates the corpus luteum (q.v.) within the ovary (q.v.) to secrete oestrogen (q.v.), progesterone (q.v.), and relaxin. It is essential for the maintenance of pregnancy up to about 6–8 weeks of gestation. A radio-immuno assay (q.v.) can be used to detect it and pregnancy can be diagnosed as early as six days after conception by testing for it in the urine. Some tumours also secrete human chorionic gonadotrophin, particularly hydatidiform moles (q.v.), which produce large amounts.

HUMAN IMMUNODEFICIENCY VIRUS (see AIDS/HIV infection).

HUMAN LEUCOCYTE ANTIGEN (see HLA SYSTEM).

HUMERUS is the bone of the upper arm. It has a rounded head, which helps to form the shoulder joint, and at its lower end presents a wide pulley-like surface for union with the radius and ulna. Its epicondyles form the prominences at the sides of the elbow.

HUMIDIFICATION of the air we breathe is essential for the efficient working of the lungs.

(See RESPIRATION.) This is achieved largely by the nose (q.v.) which acts as an air-conditioner, warming, moistening, and filtering the 10,000 litres of air which we inhale daily, in the process of which, incidentally, it produces around 1·5 litres of secretion daily. Humidity is expressed as relative humidity (RH). This is the amount of moisture in the air expressed as a percentage of the maximum possible at that temperature. If the temperature of a room is raised without increasing the moisture content, the RH falls. The average outdoor RH in Britain is around 70 to 80 per cent. With central heating it may drop to 25 per cent or lower.

This is why humidification, as it is known, of the air is essential in buildings heated by modern heating systems. The aim should be to keep the RH around 30 to 50 per cent. In houses this may be achieved quite satisfactorily by having a jug or basin of water in the room, or some receptacle that can be attached to the heater. In offices some more elaborate form of humidifier is necessary. Those suffering from chronic bronchitis are particularly susceptible to dry air. (See also VENTILATION.)

HUMIDIFIER FEVER is a form of alveolitis (q.v.) caused by contamination of the water used to humidify, or moisten, the air in air-conditioning plants. The breathing of the contaminated air results in infection of the lung, which is characterized by fever, cough, shortness of breath and malaise, worse on Monday and tending to improve during the course of the week. (See also LEGIONNAIRE'S DISEASE.)

HUMOUR is a term applied to any fluid or semi-fluid tissue of the body: e.g. the aqueous and vitreous humours in the eye. The term, humour, is also associated with a theory regarding the causation of disease, which originated with Pythagoras and lasted in a modified form until the early part of the nineteenth century. According to this theory diseases are due to an improper mixture in the body of blood, bile, phlegm and black bile.

HUNGER is a craving for food or other substance necessary to bodily activity. Hunger for food is supposed to be directly produced by strong contractions of the stomach which occur when it is empty or nearly so. (See also THIRST.) AIR HUNGER is an instinctive craving for oxygen resulting in breathlessness, either when a person ascends to great heights where the pressure of air is low, or in some diseases such as pneumonia and diabetes mellitus.

HUNTINGTON'S CHOREA is a hereditary disease characterized by involuntary movements and dementia. Each child of a parent with the disease has a 50:50 chance of developing it. The usual time of onset is between 35 and 45, but 10 per cent of cases occur under the age of 20. Some patients show more severe mental disturbance, others more severe disturbances of

movement, but in all it pursues an inexorable downward course over a period of ten to twenty years to a terminal state of physical and mental helplessness. It is estimated that there are around 6000 cases in Britain. The cause is not known and there is no effective treatment. Genetic counselling of affected families is very important. People with Huntington's chorea and their relatives can obtain help and guidance from Huntington's Disease Association (see APPENDIX 2: ADDRESSES).

HURLER'S SYNDROME (see GARGOYLISM).

HUTCHINSON'S TEETH is the term applied to the narrowed and notched permanent incisor teeth which occur in congenital syphilis. They are so named after Sir Jonathan Hutchinson (1828–1913), the London physician who first described them.

HYALINE   Tissue material that has a glass-like appearance when stained and viewed under the microscope. It occurs in a variety of tissues and diseases, particularly Respiratory Distress Syndrome (see ADULT RESPIRATORY DISTRESS SYNDROME), hyaline degeneration of arterioles and alcoholic liver disease.

HYALINE MEMBRANE DISEASE is a condition found in premature infants and infants born by Caesarean section, characterized by the onset of difficulty in breathing a few hours after birth. About half the affected babies die, death usually occurring before the third day. At post-mortem examination the alveoli and finer bronchioles of the lungs are found to be lined with a dense membrane. The cause of the condition is obscure. (See ADULT RESPIRATORY DISTRESS SYNDROME.)

HYALURONIDASE is an enzyme (q.v.) which hydrolyses hyaluronic acid. The latter is a gel-like substance which is widely distributed throughout the body and which helps to bind together the tissue cells and also acts as a lubricant in joints. By virtue of its action in hydrolysing hyaluronic acid, hyaluronidase is now used in subcutaneous injections of fluid as it facilitates the spread of the injected fluid and therefore its absorption.

HYDATID is a cyst produced by the growth of immature forms of a tapeworm. (See TAENIASIS.)

HYDATIDIFORM MOLE, or VESICULAR MOLE as it is sometimes known, is a rare complication of pregnancy, in which there is tremendous proliferation of the epithelium of the chorion (the outer of the two fetal membranes). It seldom occurs during a first pregnancy. Treatment consists of immediate evacuation of the womb.

HYDRADENITIS SUPPURATIVA is a chronic inflammatory disease of the apocrine sweat glands (see PERSPIRATION). It is more common in women, in whom it usually occurs in the armpit, than in men in whom it is most common in the perineum of the drivers of lorries and taxis. It occurs in the form of painful, tender lumps underneath the skin, which burst often in a week or so. Treatment consists of removal by operation.

HYDRALAZINE is a hypotensive drug, useful as an adjunct to other treatment for hypertension (q.v.).

HYDRAMNIOS is the condition characterized by excess of fluid in the amniotic cavity. (See AMNION.)

HYDROCEPHALUS is the condition in which there is abnormal accumulation of cerebrospinal fluid within the skull. It is due to one or more of three main causes: (i) excessive production of spinal fluid (see CEREBROSPINAL FLUID); (ii) defective absorption of cerebrospinal fluid; (iii) blockage to the circulation of cerebrospinal fluid. The causes of these disturbances of circulation of cerebrospinal fluid may be congenital (most commonly associated with spina bifida (q.v.), meningitis, or a tumour.
Symptoms In children the chief symptoms observed are the gradual increase in size of the upper part of the head, out of all proportion to the face or the rest of the body. The head is globular, with a wide anterior fontanelle and separation of the bones at the sutures. The veins in the scalp are prominent, and there is a 'crackpot' note on percussion. The normal infant's head should not grow more than 2·5 cm (1 inch) in each of the first two months of life and much more slowly subsequently. Growth beyond this rate should arouse suspicions of hydrocephalus. Another useful rule is that the circumference of the head should not exceed that of the chest. In chronic hydrocephalus, the head of an infant 3 months old has been known to measure 72·5 cm (29 inches); and in the case of the man, Cardinal, who died in Guy's Hospital, the head measured 82·5 cm (33 inches).
The cerebral ventricles are widely distended, and the convolutions of the brain flattened, while occasionally the fluid escapes into the cavity of the cranium, which it fills, pressing down the brain to the base of the skull. As a consequence of such changes, the functions of the brain are interfered with, and in general the mental condition of the patient is impaired. The child is dull and listless, irritable and sometimes suffers from severe mental subnormality. The special senses become affected as the disease advances, especially vision, and sight is often lost, as is also hearing. Towards the end paralysis is apt to occur.
The outlook for children with hydrocephalus is not as gloomy as was at one time thought to be the case. Such a child has a 50 per cent chance of survival with the disease arrested. He then has a 75 per cent chance of being educable. Almost one-third of arrested cases can be expected to enjoy normal intelligence with little or no physical disability.
Treatment Numerous ingenious operations have been devised for the treatment of hydrocephalus. The most satisfactory of these utilize the Holter or Pudenz unidirectional valves, whereby the cerebrospinal fluid is by-passed into the right atrium of the heart or the peritoneal cavity, but it is only in a proportion of affected children that these operations produce a satisfactory result. The choice of operation and of the children likely to benefit is a highly skilled one that can only be made by an experienced surgeon.

HYDROCHLORIC ACID A colourless, pungent, fuming liquid. Secreted by the parietal cells in the lining of the stomach, it aids in the digestion of the food.

HYDROCHLOROTHIAZIDE (see BENZO-THIADIAZINES).

HYDROCOELE is a collection of fluid connected with the testis or spermatic cord. When there is no obvious cause, it is classified as primary. Such hydrocoeles are usually large and tense, and are commonly found in middle-aged and younger men, presenting as a large, painless scrotal swelling. Congenital hydrocoeles may occur in infants, when they are often associated with a hernial sac. Hydrocoele of the cord is rare. Secondary hydrocoele is generally smaller and lax; it is usually secondary to a tumour or inflammation of the underlying testis or epididymis.
Treatment Congenital hydrocoeles usually disappear spontaneously and may be safely watched; surgery is only indicated when there is a hernia, or if it persists after the first year. Hydrocoeles in adults should be tapped and the testis palpated to exclude primary lesions. Primary hydrocoeles may be managed by intermittent tapping, or preferably, by surgical removal. Secondary hydrocoeles require treatment of the underlying condition.

HYDROCORTISONE, or compound F, has the chemical formula, 17-hydroxycorticosterone. It is closely allied to cortisone (q.v.) both in its structure (cortisone is an oxidation product of hydrocortisone) and in its action. Available in tablet, topical or injection form, hydrocortisone is used in adrenocortical insufficiency, for the suppression of local and systemic inflammatory and allergic disorders and in the treatment of shock. Its mineralocorticoid effects mean that the drug should not be used long term.

HYDROGEN PEROXIDE has the chemical formula H_2O_2 and is a thick colourless liquid. It is available in solution with water in concentrations of 3, 6 and 27 per cent and as a cream. It is readily reduced to water giving up oxygen in the process, which causes the characteristic frothing seen when used. The frothing helps to dislodge adherent discharges or dead tissue and it also has antiseptic and deodorizing properties. Thus it is used as a mouthwash, to clean wounds and ulcers and occasionally to disinfect body cavities at operation. It is also a bleach.

HYDRONEPHROSIS is a chronic disease in which the kidney becomes greatly distended with fluid. It is caused by obstruction to the flow of urine at the pelvi-ureteric junction. If the ureter is obstructed the ureter proximal to the obstruction will dilate and pressure will be transmitted back to the kidney to cause hydronephrosis. Obstruction may occur at the bladder neck or in the urethra itself. Enlargement of the prostate is a common cause of bladder-neck obstruction. This would give rise to hypertrophy of the bladder muscle and both dilatation of the ureter and hydronephrosis. If the obstruction is not relieved progressive destruction of renal tissue will occur. As a result of the stagnation of the urine infection is probable and cystitis and pyelonephritis may occur.

HYDROPHOBIA is another name for RABIES (q.v.).

HYDROPS FETALIS (see HAEMOLYTIC DISEASE OF THE NEW-BORN).

HYDROTHERAPY Treatment using water in the form baths, douches, etc.

HYDROTHORAX means a collection of fluid in the pleural cavities.

HYDROXOCOBALAMIN, or vitamin B_{12}, has now replaced cyanocobalamin (q.v.) in the treatment of pernicious anaemia. (See ANAEMIA.) It has the practical advantage that fewer injections are required than in the case of cyanocobalamin. Like cyanocobalamin it belongs to the group of substances known as cobalamins which have an enzyme (q.v.) action in practically every metabolic system in the body and are essential for normal growth and nutrition.

HYDROXYUREA is a drug that is proving of value in the treatment of chronic myeloid leukaemia.

HYDROXYZINE HYDROCHLORIDE is a tranquillizer that is proving of value in the treatment of anxiety states. (See BENZODIAZEPINES.)

HYGIENE is the science of preserving health.

HYMEN is the thin membranous fold partially closing the lower end of the virginal vagina.

HYOID is a U-shaped bone at the root of the tongue. It can be felt from the front of the neck, lying about 2·5 cm above the prominence of the thyroid cartilage.

HYOSCINE   An alkaloid (q.v.) obtained from the plant henbane (hyoscyamus). It is an anticholinergic drug (q.v.) sometimes used as a premedicant in patients undergoing anaesthesia for its sedative and antiemetic effects and its ability to reduce saliva production. It may cause confusion in the elderly.

HYPERACUSIS means an abnormally acute sense of hearing.

HYPERAEMIA means congestion or presence of an excessive amount of blood in a part.

HYPERAESTHESIA means over-sensitiveness of a part, as found, for example, in certain nervous diseases. (See TOUCH.)

HYPERALGESIA means excessive sensitiveness to pain. (See PAIN; TOUCH.)

HYPERCALCAEMIA is a state in which the plasma calcium concentration is significantly raised. The most important causes are hyperparathyroidism (q.v.), malignant bone disease and other (non-metastatic) cancers, and chronic renal failure. Less common causes include sarcoidosis, myelomatosis, vitamin D overdosage, hyperthyroidism, and immobilization.
Signs and symptoms   A general malaise and depression are common, with generalized muscular weakness, anorexia and vomiting. Disturbed renal function causes increased urine output and thirst, with calcium deposits eventually leading to renal stones. Primary bone disease may cause pain and weakness, with an increased incidence of fractures, and there may be gritty deposits of calcium in the eyes. Severe hypercalcaemia produces anuria, with confusion and coma leading to death.
Treatment   The patient should be rehydrated and a diuretic, such as frusemide, given. Attention should then be focused on the underlying cause – usually a parathyroid adenoma or bone tumour – and surgical removal should produce complete clinical cure, provided advanced renal disease is not already present.

HYPERCALCIURIA means an abnormally large amount of calcium in the urine. It is the most common single cause of stones in the kidneys in Britain.

HYPERCAPNIA means an abnormal increase in the amount of carbon dioxide in the blood or in the lungs (see BLOOD GASES). It may be caused by a reduced respiratory rate or effort, diseases of the chest wall and lung (affecting breathing) and cyanotic heart disease.

HYPERCHLORHYDRIA is the condition in which there is an excessive production of hydrochloric acid in the stomach. It is a characteristic finding in certain forms of dyspepsia, particularly that associated with a duodenal ulcer. It causes heartburn (q.v.) and waterbrash (q.v.). (See DUODENAL ULCER; DYSPEPSIA; STOMACH, DISEASES OF.)

HYPERCHOLESTEROLAEMIA (see CHOLESTEROL and HYPERLIPIDAEMIA).

HYPEREMESIS GRAVIDARUM A rare condition (less than 0·2 per cent) of pregnancies in which there is severe vomiting. If untreated it can result in severe dehydration, ketoacidosis (an excess of ketone (q.v.) acids) and liver damage. More common in multiple pregnancy it may recur in subsequent pregnancies.

HYPERGLYCAEMIA means excess of sugar in the blood, the condition accompanying diabetes mellitus. The amount of sugar normally present in the blood is dependent upon how much sugar has been consumed, but in the fasting state it runs around 80 to 100 milligrams per 100 millilitres of blood. A fasting blood level of sugar above this is regarded as hyperglycaemia; in diabetes mellitus (q.v.) the sugar may rise to four or five times that amount.

HYPERIDROSIS, or HYPERHIDROSIS, means excessive sweating. (See PERSPIRATION.)

HYPERKALAEMIA A serum potassium (q.v.) concentration above the normal range. Often caused by renal failure or excessive intake of potassium, perhaps in a drug. It may be complicated by cardiac dysrhythmias (abnormal rhythm of the heart).

HYPERKINETIC SYNDROME A disorder of children characterized by excessive activity and impaired ability to learn. The child has a short attention span and may be aggressive. There is an association with mental subnormality. Treatment involves behaviour therapy (q.v.), drugs (such as amphetamines) and family therapy.

HYPERLIPIDAEMIA means an excess of fat in the blood. The two most important fats circulating in the blood are cholesterol and triglycerides. Raised blood levels of cholesterol predispose to atheroma and coronary artery disease and raised triglycerides predispose to pancreatitis. Some of the hyperlipidaemias are familial and some are secondary to other diseases such as hypothyroidism, diabetes mellitus, nephrotic syndrome and alcoholism. There is evidence that therapy which lowers the lipid concentration reduces the progression of premature atheroma, particularly in those who suffer from the familial disorder. There are a number of drugs available for lowering the lipid content of the plasma but these should be reserved for patients in whom severe hyperlipidaemia is inadequately controlled by weight reduction. Clofibrate, bezafibrate, nicotinic acid and nicofuranose lower plasma cholesterol and plasma triglyceride concentration through their effect on reducing the hepatic production of lipoproteins. Cholestyramine and colestipol, both of which are resins, bind bile salts in the gut and so decrease the absorption of the cholesterol that these bile salts contain and hence lower plasma cholesterol concentrations. Probucol lowers plasma cholesterol concentrations by increasing the metabolism of low-density lipoproteins.

HYPERMETROPIA or HYPEROPIA, is a term applied to long- sightedness, in which the eye is too flat from front to back and rays of light are brought to a focus behind the retina. (See VISION; SPECTACLES.)

HYPERNATRAEMIA A serum sodium concentration above normal. It is usually caused by dehydration (either from inadequate intake or excessive loss of water). Occasionally it may be caused by excessive sodium intake and rarely by a raised level of aldosterone hormone.

HYPERNEPHROMA is a term applied to a malignant tumour resembling the tissue of the suprarenal gland and occurring in the kidney.

HYPERPARATHYROIDISM Increased activity of the parathyroid gland. Parathyroid hormone increases serum calcium. Hyperparathyroidism may be primary (due to an adenoma or hyperplasia of the gland), secondary (in response to hypocalcaemia) or tertiary (when secondary hyperparathyroidism causes the development of an autonomous adenoma).

HYPERPITUITARISM Overactivity of the anterior lobe of the pituitary (q.v.) causing acromegaly (q.v.) (gigantism).

HYPERPLASIA means an abnormal increase in the number of cells in a tissue.

HYPERPYREXIA means an excessive degree of fever. (See FEVER; TEMPERATURE.)

HYPERSENSITIVITY is the abnormal immunological reaction produced in certain individuals when re-exposed to antigens that are innocuous to normal individuals. An antigen or allergen stimulates an allergic response. This produces a state of altered re-activity or an allergic state. Such a state of altered re-activity may be beneficial to the host, as in establishing a state of immunity, or it may be harmful to the host and produce a state of disease. Hypersensitivity is thus an allergic reaction in an individual sensitized by previous exposure to the antigen and in whom the allergic process constitutes the disease.

HYPERTENSION   This may be defined as a blood pressure above 160/90 mm Hg. Some people's blood pressure, particularly the systolic measurement, may vary with daily activity, rising with exercise or anxiety. Circadian variations also occur. Systolic blood pressure also rises with age in people living in the developed world.

Hypertension can be divided into primary and secondary types.

PRIMARY HYPERTENSION can be characterized as: labile (as in opening paragraph); isolated systolic due to arteriosclerotic changes in the elderly; essential or benign (q.v.); malignant or accelerated phase (q.v.) due to breakdown in the tissues and nervous control of the blood vessels; and hypertension in pregnancy, which may lead to pre-eclampsia and eclampsia (q.v.).

SECONDARY HYPERTENSION is a consequence of disease elsewhere in the body, for example, chronic renal failure, endocrine disorders, such as phaeochromocytomas (q.v.), congenital defects, and rare disorders such as porphyria (q.v.), and lead poisoning. Drugs given for other disorders – for example, arthritis – can also cause a rise in blood pressure.

Treatment   This varies according to the type of hypertension and careful investigation is often needed to decide the correct diagnosis and treatment. Attention to risk factors is important. Those affected should not smoke and should control their alcohol intake. A low-fat and low-salt diet is advisable, and obese patients should lose weight. Moderate exercise and avoidance of stress may help to reduce blood pressure, as may relaxation therapy. Such changes should be done after medical advice. Drugs being given for other conditions – for example, arthritis – may have to be stopped.

If these measures fail then drug treatment will probably be necessary. Drug regimens will depend on the type and severity of hypertension and they need careful monitoring. Among the commonly used drugs, sometimes given in combination, are: diuretics (q.v.); calcium antagonist or channel blockers (q.v.); beta-adrenoreceptor blockers (q.v.) and angiotensin-converting enzyme (ACE) inhibitors.

Hypertension in pregnancy requires skilled treatment, often in hospital. Malignant hypertension, a potentially fatal condition, may require urgent hospital admission with bed rest and a combination of drug regimens prescribed. Surgery may be necessary to treat hypertension due to a phaeochromocytoma,

the abnormal adrenal gland (q.v.) being removed.

HYPERTHERMIA means abnormally high body temperature. It is also the name given to the treatment of disease by the artificial production of fever. This can be achieved by various methods, such as radiation heat cabinets boosted with radio frequency (RF); immersion in a hot wax bath; heated suits or blankets; techniques using electromagnetic waves (e.g. RF, microwaves (q.v.)); ultrasound (q.v.) of appropriate frequencies. It is sometimes of help as an adjunct to surgery, chemotherapy, or radiotherapy in the treatment of cancer.

HYPERTHYROIDISM is excessive activity of the thyroid gland. It is a common disorder affecting between 2 and 5 per cent of all females at some time in their lives. Most cases are the result of disease of the thyroid gland. The commonest cause is Graves' disease (q.v.), also called thyrotoxicosis. Single or multiple adenomas (q.v.) or nodules in the thyroid also cause hyperthyroidism. There are several other rare causes, including inflammation caused by a virus, autoimmune reactions and cancer. The symptoms of hyperthyroidism affect many of the body's system as a consequence of the much increased metabolic rate: these include the cardiovascular, nervous, alimentary and musculoskeletal systems.

HYPERTONIC   (1) Referring to one solution which has a greater osmotic pressure than another. Physiologically it is used to describe solutions which have a greater osmotic pressure than body fluids. (2) Muscles with abnormally increased tone (e.g. following a stroke).

HYPERTROPHY means the increase in size which takes place in an organ as the result of an increased amount of work demanded of it by the bodily economy. For example, when valvular disease of the heart is present, compensation occurs by an increase in thickness of the heart-muscle, and the organ, by beating more powerfully, is able to overtake the strain thrown upon it. Similarly, if one kidney is removed, the other hypertrophies or grows larger to overtake the double work.

HYPERVENTILATION   An abnormally rapid resting respiratory rate. If voluntary it causes lightheadedness and then unconsciousness by lowering the blood tension of carbon dioxide. It is a manifestation of chest and heart diseases which raise carbon dioxide tension or cause hypoxia (q.v.) (e.g. severe chronic obstructive pulmonary disease or pulmonary oedema). Mechanically ventilated patients may be hyperventilated to lower carbon dioxide tension in order to reduce intracranial (q.v.) pressure.

HYPERVOLAEMIA An increase in the volume of circulating blood above the normal range.

HYPNOTICS are drugs that induce sleep (q.v.). Before a hypnotic is prescribed, it is important to establish – and, where possible, treat – the cause of the insomnia. They are most often needed to help an acutely distressed patient, for example, following bereavement, or in cases of jet lag, or in shift workers. They may be required in states of chronic distress, whether induced by disease or environment; in these cases it is especially important to limit their use in order to prevent undue reliance on the drugs, and not to allow the use of hypnotics and sedatives to become a means of evading the patient's real problem. In many cases, such as chronic depression, overwork, and alcohol abuse, hypnotics are quite inappropriate; some form of counselling and relaxation therapy is often preferable.

Hypnotics should always be chosen and prescribed with care, bearing in mind the patient's full circumstances. They are generally best avoided in the elderly (confusion is a common problem), and in children – apart from special cases. The most commonly used hypnotics are the benzodiazepines (q.v.) such as nitrazepam and temazepam; chloral derivatives, while useful in children, are generally second choice. They should be used in the lowest possible dose for the minimum period. Side-effects include daytime drowsiness – which may interfere with driving and other skilled tasks – and insomnia following withdrawal, especially after prolonged use, is a hazard.

HYPNOTISM is the process of producing a state of mind known as hypnosis. Although a process which has been known for hundreds of years, its precise nature is still unknown. One modern writer has defined hypnosis as 'a temporary condition of altered attention, the most striking feature of which is greatly increased suggestibility'. There is no evidence, as has been claimed, that women can be more easily hypnotized than men. Children and young adults are the more easily hypnotized, middle-aged people being more resistant. There are various methods of induction of hypnosis, but the basis of them is some rhythmic stimulus accompanied by the repetition of carefully worded suggestions. The most commonly used method is to ask the patient to fix his eye on a given spot, or light, and then keep on repeating to him, in a quiet soothing voice, that his eyes will gradually become tired and that he will want to close them. There are various levels of hypnosis, usually classified as light, medium, and deep, and it has been estimated that 10 per cent of people cannot be hypnotized, 35 per cent can be taken into light hypnosis, 35 per cent into medium hypnosis, and 20 per cent into deep hypnosis.

Hypnosis can be used as a treatment in psychiatric patients and in some people with psychosomatic conditions in which emotional or psychological disturbances precipitate physical disorders such as skin lesions or headaches. Hypnosis may help to relieve pain in childbirth; asthma may also respond to it. Some people may find hypnosis of help 'in overcoming addictions to smoking, alcohol or gambling. Hypnosis has risks and its use in treatment should be by doctors trained in the technique.

HYPOCALCAEMIA A serum concentration of calcium below the normal range (9–11 mg of calcium per 100 ml of serum). This may cause tetany (q.v.), acutely, and chronically may give rise to rickets, osteomalacia or osteoporosis (qq.v.). It may be caused by hypoparathyroidism (q.v.), vitamin D deficiency, malabsorption, renal failure or acute pancreatitis (see PANCREAS, DISEASES OF).

HYPOCAPNIA A blood tension of carbon dioxide below normal. It is produced by hyperventilation which may be voluntary, mechanical (if the patient is on a ventilator) or in response to a physiological insult such as metabolic acidosis or brain injury.

HYPOCHLORHYDRIA means an insufficient secretion of hydrochloric acid from the digestive cells of the stomach lining.

HYPOCHONDRIASIS is a delusion (q.v.) of ill health, often severe, such that patients may believe they have a brain tumour or incurable insanity. Furthermore, patients may believe that they have infected others, or that their children have inherited the condition. It is a characteristic feature of depression, but may also occur in schizophrenia, when the delusions may be secondary to bodily hallucinations (q.v.), and a sense of subjective change. Chronic hypochondriasis may be the result of an abnormal personality development, for example, the insecure, bodily conscious person. Delusional preoccupations with the body – usually the face – may occur, such that the patient is convinced that his or her face is twisted, or disfigured with acne.

Treatment Hypochondriacal patients may also develop physical illness, and any new symptoms must always be carefully evaluated. In most patients the condition is secondary, and treatment should be directed to the underlying depression or schizophrenia. In the rare cases of primary hypochondriasis, supportive measures are the mainstay of treatment.

HYPODERMIC means of, or pertaining to, the region immediately under the skin. Thus, a hypodermic injection is an injection given underneath the skin. A hypodermic syringe is a small syringe which, fitted with a fine needle, is used to give such injections. A hypodermic injection is given for one of three main reasons: (1) because the substance administered cannot be given by mouth on account of its being destroyed in the stomach before it can be absorbed, e.g. insulin; (2) because it is not possible or it is inadvisable to give anything by mouth to the patient, e.g. because of vomiting; (3) because a quick action is necessary, e.g. morphine in cases of severe pain.

HYPOGASTRIC means pertaining to the lower middle part of the abdomen just above the pubis.

HYPOGLOSSAL NERVE is the twelfth cranial nerve, and supplies the muscles of the tongue, together with some others lying near it.

HYPOGLYCAEMIA is a deficiency of glucose in the blood – the normal range being 3·5–7·5 mmol/l (see DIABETES MELLITUS). It most commonly occurs in diabetic patients, for example, after an excessive dose of insulin, heavy exercise, particularly with inadequate or delayed meals. It may also occur in non-diabetic people, however, for example, in very cold situations or after periods of starvation. Hypoglycaemia is normally indicated by characteristic warning signs and symptoms – particularly if the blood-glucose concentration is falling rapidly. These include anxiety, tremor, sweating, breathlessness, raised pulse rate, blurred vision, often with reduced concentration, leading – in severe cases – to unconsciousness. These may be relieved by taking some sugar, some sweet biscuits or drink. In emergencies, such as when the patient is comatose, an intramuscular injection of glucagon (q.v.), or intravenous glucose should be given. Early treatment is vital, since prolonged hypoglycaemia, by starving the brain cells of glucose, may lead to irreversible brain damage.

HYPOGLYCAEMIC AGENTS There are two groups of oral hypoglycaemic drugs, the sulphonylureas and the biguanides. Both have been used in the treatment of diabetes for about 30 years. The sulphonylureas act on the beta cell to stimulate insulin release and on peripheral tissues to increase sensitivity, though the latter is a less important action. Chlorpropamide (q.v.) and glibenclamide (q.v.) have a higher ceiling of potency than tolbutamide and this is associated with a considerably longer half life in the body. A newer arrival, gliquidone, claims to have the hypoglycaemic power of the second generation and the short biological half life of tolbutamide and may therefore be more suitable for those who require protection from nocturnal hypoglycaemia. The biguanides reduce carbohydrate absorption and facilitate the action of insulin on peripheral tissues. In the obese diabetic in whom increased insulin production is better avoided metformin alone may be used to reinforce the dietary treatment.

HYPOGONADISM is the condition characterized by deficient production of the hormones secreted by the gonads: that is, the ovaries and testes.

HYPOMANIA is a slight degree of mania.

HYPONATRAEMIA A serum concentration of sodium below the normal range. It may be produced by dilution of blood (giving large volumes of salt-poor solutions intravenously), excessive water retention (inappropriate secretion of antidiuretic hormone), excessive sodium loss, and, rarely, by inadequate salt intake.

HYPOPARATHYROIDISM Underactivity of the parathyroid glands (q.v.). Thus there is a lack of parathyroid hormone resulting in hypocalcaemia (q.v.). It may be caused by inadvertent removal of the glands when the thyroid gland is surgically removed or by failure of the glands because of autoimmune disease.

HYPOPHYSECTOMY means surgical excision of the pituitary gland.

HYPOPHYSIS is another name for the pituitary gland.

HYPOPIESIS is the condition, or state, characterized by abnormally low blood-pressure.

HYPOPITUITARISM Underactivity of the pituitary gland. It can cause dwarfism (see DWARF), delayed puberty, impotence, infertility, amenorrhoea, hypothyroidism (q.v.), and hypoadrenalism. Causes include tumours, irradiation of the gland, sarcoidosis, and necrosis associated with postpartum haemorrhage (Sheehan's syndrome).

HYPOPLASIA means excessive smallness of an organ or part, arising from imperfect development.

HYPOSPADIAS is a developmental abnormality in the male, in which the urethra opens on the under-surface of the penis or in the perineum (q.v.).

HYPOSTASIS is the term applied to the condition in which blood accumulates in a dependent part as a result of a feeble circulation. Congestion of the base of the lungs in old people from this cause, and infection, is called hypostatic pneumonia.

HYPOTENSION means abnormally low blood-pressure. *Postural hypotension* is the abnormal fall in blood-pressure which may occur on suddenly standing up. It is more liable to occur in old folk.

HYPOTHALAMUS is that part of the forebrain situated beneath and linked with the thalamus on each side and forming the floor of the third ventricle. Also linked to the pituitary gland beneath it, the hypothalamus contains collections of nerve cells believed to form the controlling centres of (1) the sympathetic and (2) the parasympathetic nervous systems. The hypothalamus is the nervous centre for primitive physical and emotional behaviour. It contains nerve centres for the regulation of certain vital processes: the metabolism of fat, carbohydrate and water; sleep; body temperature and genital functions.

HYPOTHERMIA   A core body temperature of less than 35 °C. As the temperature of the body falls, there is increasing dysfunction of all the organs, particularly the central nervous and cardiovascular systems. The patient becomes listless and confused, with onset of unconsciousness between 33–28 °C. Cardiac output at first rises with shivering but then falls progressively, as do the oxygen requirements of the tissues. Below 17–26 °C cardiac output is insufficient even to supply this reduced demand for oxygen by the tissues. The heart is susceptible to spontaneous ventricular fibrillation below 28 °C. Metabolism is disturbed and the concentration of blood glucose (q.v.) and potassium (q.v.) rise as the temperature falls. Cooling of the kidneys produces a diuresis (q.v.) and further fluid loss from the circulation to the tissues causes hypovolaemia (q.v.).

Severe hypothermia is sometimes complicated by gastric erosions and haemorrhage and pancreatitis. Infants and the elderly are less efficient at regulating temperature and conserving heat than other age groups and are therefore more at risk from accidental hypothermia during cold weather, if their accommodation is not warm enough. Approximately half a million elderly people are at risk in Britain each winter from hypothermia. The other major cause of accidental hypothermia is near drowning in icy water. Deliberate hypothermia is sometimes used to reduce metabolic rate so that prolonged periods of cardiac arrest may occur without tissue hypoxia developing. This technique is used for some cardiac and neurosurgical operations and is produced by immersion of the anaesthetized patient in iced water or by cooling an extracorporeal circulation.

Treatment of hypothermia is by warming the patient and treating any complications that arise. Passive warming is usual with conservation of the patient's own body heat with insulating blankets. If the core temperature is below 28 °C, then active rewarming should be instituted by means of warm peritoneal, gastric or bladder lavage or using an extracorporeal circulation. Care must be taken in moving hypothermic patients as a sudden rush of cold peripheral blood to the heart can precipitate

ventricular fibrillation. Prevention of hypothermia in the elderly is important. Special attention must be paid to diet, heating the home and adequate clothing in several layers to limit heat loss.

HYPOTHYROIDISM means the condition produced by defective action of the thyroid gland. (See MYXOEDEMA.)

HYPOTONIC   (1) Referring to a solution which has a lower osmotic pressure (see OSMOSIS) than another. Physiologically it describes a solution with a lower osmotic pressure than body fluids. (2) Muscles with abnormally reduced tone.

HYPOVENTILATION   Shallow and/or slow breathing, often caused by the effects of injury or drugs on the respiratory centre. It causes hypercapnia and hypoxia (qq.v.).

HYPOVOLAEMIA   A reduced circulating blood volume. Acutely it is caused by unreplaced losses from bleeding, sweating, diarrhoea, vomiting or diuresis. Chronically it may be caused by inadequate fluid intake.

HYPOXIA   A low blood tension of oxygen. It may be caused by low inspired concentration of oxygen, an abnormal breathing pattern, lung disease or heart disease. If severe and prolonged it will cause organ damage and death as cellular function is dependent on oxygen.

HYSTERECTOMY is the operation of removing the uterus. HYSTERO-OOPHORECTOMY is the term applied to removal of the uterus and ovaries.

HYSTERIA is a traditional description for a symptom (or symptoms) with no obvious organic cause, which is an unconscious reaction and from which the person may benefit. It is now recognized as a dissociative disorder. Such disorders – amnesia (q.v.), fugues (q.v.), multiple personality states (q.v.) and trancelike conditions – are powerful defence mechanisms against severe stress of someone's inability to cope with life. Mass hysteria is a phenomenon characterized by extreme suggestibility in a group of often emotionally charged people.

The name originates from the idea that hysteria – a Greek-based word for 'uterus' – was in some way associated with the womb. Hence the old-fashioned – and sometimes modern – association of hysteria with women and supposed sexual disturbances. Doctors should eliminate a diagnosis of physical disease before diagnosing a dissociative disorder. Most hysterial conversion reactions subside spontaneously. If not, the individual needs psychiatric advice. Treatment is difficult. Reasons for stress should be explored and, if possible, resolved. Hypnosis to help the person to relive stressful episodes – known as abreaction (q.v.) – may be of value.

HYSTEROSCOPY is the direct visualization of the interior of the uterus using fibreoptic endoscopy (q.v.). The technique, which allows minor surgical procedures to be carried out at the same time, has transformed the management of uterine disorders.

HYSTEROTOMY An operation in which the uterus (q.v.) is opened to remove a fetus (q.v.) before 28 weeks' gestation. After 28 weeks it would be called a Caesarean section (q.v.). It is now seldom used as a means of abortion.

I

IATRIC means anything pertaining to a physician.

IATROGENIC DISEASE is disease induced by a physician: essentially a drug-induced disease.

IBUPROFEN is a drug which is of value as an anti-inflammatory agent and as an analgesic in the treatment of rheumatoid arthritis and other forms of rheumatism. (See NON-STEROIDAL ANTI-INFLAMMATORY DRUGS.)

ICD See INTERNATIONAL CLASSIFICATION OF DISEASE.

ICHTHAMMOL, ICHTHYOL, is ammonium ichthosulphonate, an almost black, thick liquid of fishy smell, prepared from a bituminous shale. It is used in several chronic skin diseases.

ICHTHYOSIS is a bullous skin disease in which the surface is very rough and presents a dry, cracked appearance, resembling fish-scales. The disorder, which has several forms, is generally hereditary, and persists through life, the skin being permanently hard, and deficient in oily material. The appearances differ considerably according to the part affected. There is no cure for the disease but the skin can be softened by application of an emollient such as plain petroleum jelly or mineral oil. Some types of ichthyosis respond to 6-per-cent salicylic acid in a gel comprising propylene glycol, hydroxypropylene cellulose, ethyl alcohol and water.

ICTERUS is another name for jaundice (q.v.).

ICTUS is another term for a stroke.

IDIOPATHIC is a term applied to diseases to indicate that their cause is unknown.

IDIOSYNCRASY implies an inherent abnormal qualitative reaction to a drug that is primarily the result of a constitutional defect in the patient. The abnormal sensitivity of patients with porphyria to barbiturates and sulphonamides is an example. Hereditary biochemical defects of red blood cells are responsible for many drug-induced haemolytic anaemias and for favism. Drug-sensitive red cells are deficient in the enzyme glucose phosphate dehydrogenase which plays an important part in the metabolism of glucose and is necessary for the continued integrity of the cell. When patients with porphyria are given certain drugs, particularly barbiturates and sulphonamides, they are liable to develop acute neurological episodes with peripheral and respiratory paralysis which may result in death. Porphyria variegata, the South African variety of porphyria, is an example of an inborn error of metabolism which was without serious symptoms until the advent of barbiturate drugs. Taking these drugs can precipitate total paralysis and death.

IDOXURIDINE An iodine containing antiviral agent still widely used in the treatment of cases of herpes simplex involvement of the cornea of the eye (see EYE DISEASE).

IFOSFAMIDE (see CYTOTOXIC).

ILEITIS means inflammation of the ileum. It may be caused by Crohn's disease (q.v.), typhoid (q.v.), tuberculosis (q.v.) or the bacterium *Yersinia enterocolitica*. Ileitis may also accompany ulcerative colitis (see COLITIS).

Patients and their relatives can obtain help and guidance from the National Association for Colitis and Crohn's Disease (see APPENDIX 2: ADDRESSES).

ILEO-CAECAL is the term applied to the region of the junction between the small and large intestines in the right lower corner of the abdomen. The ileo-caecal valve is a structure which allows the contents of the intestine to pass onwards from the small to the large intestine, but, in the great majority of cases, prevents their passage in the opposite direction.

ILEOSTOMY is the operation by which an artificial opening is made into the ileum and brought through the abdominal wall to create an artificial opening or stoma. It is most often performed as part of the operation for cancer of the rectum, in which the rectum has usually to be removed. An ileostomy is then performed which acts as an artificial anus, to which a bag is attached to collect the waste matter. Distressing though this may at first be, the vast majority of people with an ileostomy learn to lead a fully active and normal life. Help and advice in adjusting to what can be described as an 'ileostomy life' can be obtained from the Ileostomy Association of Great Britain and Ireland (see APPENDIX 2: ADDRESSES). (See STOMA.)

ILEUM is the lower part of the small intestine. (See INTESTINE.)

ILEUS is a paralysis of the bowel muscle. (See INTESTINE, DISEASES OF.)

ILIUM is the uppermost of the three bones forming each side of the pelvis. (See BONE; PELVIS.)

ILLUSIONS (see HALLUCINATIONS).

IMIPRAMINE is one of the so-called tricyclic antidepressants which is proving of value in the treatment of depression. (See ANTIDEPRESSANTS.)

IMMERSION FOOT is the term applied to a condition which develops as a result of prolonged immersion of the feet in cold or cool water. It was a condition commonly seen during the 1939–45 War in shipwrecked sailors and airmen who had crashed in the sea and spent long periods before being rescued. Such prolonged exposure results in vasoconstriction of the smaller arteries in the feet, leading to coldness and blueness of the feet, and finally, in severe cases, to ulceration and gangrene.

IMMUNE SYSTEM (see IMMUNITY).

IMMUNITY is the body's defence against foreign substances. Its major function is to combat infectious micro-organisms (bacteria, viruses and parasites) but it also protects against drugs, toxins, and cancer cells. Immunity is partly non-specific since it does not depend on previous exposure to the foreign substance. For example, micro-organisms are engulfed and inactivated by polymorphonuclear leucocytes as a first line of defence before specific immunity has developed. Acquired immunity depends on specific recognition of the foreign substance and is the usual outcome of natural infection or prophylactic immunization. Foreign substances which provoke an immune response are termed 'antigens'. These are usually proteins but smaller molecules such as drugs and chemicals can also induce an immune response. Proteins are taken up and processed by specialized cells called 'antigen presenting cells', strategically sited where microbial infection may enter the body. The complex protein molecules are broken down into short amino-acid chains (peptides) and transported to the

cell surface where they are presented by structures called HLA antigens. These antigens are the human form of histocompatibility antigens which confer individuality on the cells of most mammalian species.

Foreign peptides presented by human leucocyte antigen (HLA) molecules (q.v.) are recognized by cells called T lymphocytes. These originate in the bone marrow and migrate to the thymus where they are educated to distinguish between foreign peptides which elicit a primary immune response and self-antigens which do not. Non-responsiveness to self-antigens is termed 'tolerance' (see AUTO-IMMUNITY). Each population or clone of T cells is uniquely responsive to a single peptide sequence because it expresses a surface molecule ('receptor') which fits only that peptide. The responsive T cell clone induces a specific response in other T and B lymphocyte populations. Cytotoxic T cells penetrate infected tissues and kill cells which express peptides derived from invading micro-organisms, thereby helping to eliminate the infection.

B lymphocytes secrete antibodies which are collectively termed gamma-globulins or immunoglobulins (Ig). Each B cell population (clone) secretes antibody uniquely specific for antigens encountered in the blood, extracellular space, and the lumen of organs such as the respiratory passages and gastrointestinal tract. Antibodies belong to different Ig classes; IgM antibodies are initially synthesized followed by smaller and therefore more penetrative IgG molecules. IgA antibodies are adapted to cross the surfaces of mucosal tissues so that they can adhere to organisms in the gut, upper and lower respiratory passages, thereby preventing their attachment to the mucosal surface. IgE antibodies also contribute to mucosal defence but are implicated in many allergic reactions (see ALLERGY).

Antibodies are composed of constant portions, which distinguish antibodies of different class, and variable portions, which confer unique antigen-binding properties on the product of each B cell clone. In order to match the vast range of antigens the immune system has to combat, the variable portions are synthesized under the instructions of a large number of encoding genes whose products are assembled to make the final antibody. The antibody produced by a single B cell clone is called a monoclonal antibody (q.v.); monoclonal antibodies are synthesized *in vivo* and *in vitro* for diagnostic and therapeutic purposes. Primary immune responses induce memory for the initiating antigen which persists in selected lymphocytes. Further challenge with the same antigen stimulates an accelerated, more vigorous secondary response by both T and B lymphocytes. Priming the immune system in this manner forms the physiological basis for immunization programmes.

Populations of lymphocytes with different functions and other cells engaged in immune responses carry distinctive protein markers. By convention these are classified and enumerated by their 'CD' markers, using monoclonal antibodies specific for each marker.

Immune responses are influenced by cytokines which function as hormones acting over a short range to accelerate the activation and proliferation of other cell populations contributing to the immune response. Specific immune responses collaborate with non-specific defence mechanisms. These include the complement system (q.v.), a protein cascade reaction designed to eliminate antigens neutralized by antibodies and to recruit cell populations which kill micro-organisms.

Immunization (q.v.) is the introduction of antigens into a body (by injection, orally or via a nasal spray) to provoke immunity usually against infectious diseases such as whooping-cough, measles and poliomyelitis.

IMMUNIZATION The introduction of antigens (q.v.) into a body to produce immunity (q.v.). See table below.

IMMUNO-ASSAY Procedures which measure the concentration of any antigenic material to which an antibody can be created. The amount of antigen bound to this antibody is proportional to the parent substance. Enzymes (ELISA (q.v.)) or radioactive labels ('radio-immuno assay' (q.v.)) are used to measure the concentration of antigenic material.

IMMUNOGLOBULINS are a group of naturally occurring proteins that act as antibodies (q.v.). They are structurally related, their differences determining their biological behaviour.

Man has 5 types of immunoglobulin with different protective functions: IgA, IgD, IgE, IgG and IgM. In the laboratory they are separated and identified by a chemical process called electrophoresis. Most antibodies have a molecular weight of 160,000.

Certain immunoglobulins can be used in the active or passive immunity of people against infectious diseases such as rabies and viral hepatitis (see IMMUNITY and GAMMA-GLOBULIN).

IMMUNODEFICIENCY Impaired immunity resulting from inherited or acquired abnormalities of the immune system. This leads to increased vulnerability to infection (see IMMUNITY). Important inherited examples of immunodeficiency are defects in function of granulocytes (q.v.) and the complement system (q.v.). Common acquired forms of immunodeficiency are defective function of B-type lymphocytes (q.v.) and hence antibody deficiency in 'common variable hypogammaglobulinaemia' and grossly deficient CD4 T-cell function – malfunctioning T-type lymphocytes (q.v.) – in AIDS (see AIDS), secondary to HIV infection.

IMMUNOLOGY The study of immune responses to the environment. Its main clinical applications include improving resistance to microbial infections (see IMMUNITY), combating the effects of impaired immunity (see IMMUNODEFICIENCY), controlling harmful immune reactions (see ALLERGY), and manipulating immune responses (see IMMUNOSUPPRESSION and IMMUNOTHERAPY) to prevent harmful immunological responses such as graft rejection

Age	Disease and mode of administration
3 days	BCG (Bacille Calmette-Guerin) by injection if tuberculosis in family in past 6 months.
2 months	Poliomyelitis (oral); diphtheria, whooping-cough (pertussis)[1] and tetanus[2] (given together by injection); HIb injection[3]
3 months	Poliomyelitis (oral); diphtheria, whooping-cough (pertussis)[1] and tetanus[2] (given together by injection); HIb injection[3]
4 months	Poliomyelitis (oral); diphtheria, whooping-cough (pertussis)[1] and tetanus[2] (given together by injection); HIb injection[3]
12–18 months	Measles, mumps, and rubella (German measles)[4] (given together by injection)

SCHOOL ENTRY

4–5 years	Poliomyelitis (oral); diphtheria and tetanus (given together by injection); give MMR vaccine if not already given at 12–18 months
10–14 females	Rubella (by injection) if they have missed MMR
10–14	BCG (Bacille Calmette-Guerin) by injection to tuberculin-negative children to prevent tuberculosis
15–18	Poliomyelitis (oral); tetanus (by injection)

1 Pertussis may be excluded in certain susceptible individuals.
2 Known as DPT or triple vaccine.
3 *Haemophilus influenzae* immunization (type B) is being introduced to be given at same time, but different limb.
4 Known as MMR vaccine.

Recommended immunization schedules in the United Kingdom

and auto-immune diseases (see AUTOIMMUNITY). The clinical study of disordered immunity now forms the allied discipline of clinical immunology, which is closely linked to the laboratory-based discipline of immunopathology.

IMMUNOSUPPRESSION The suppression of harmful immune responses. The prevention of organ rejection by recipients of kidney, heart, and bone-marrow transplants is the most clear-cut application. Immunosuppression is also necessary in many diseases mediated in whole or in part by abnormal immune reactions (see ALLERGY and AUTOIMMUNITY). Most immunosuppressive drugs in current clinical practice are non-specific since they inhibit protective immunity and not just the harmful immune reaction. Corticosteroids are most commonly used. The anti-proliferative drugs azathioprine and methotrexate are also widely employed. The introduction of more selective drugs such as cyclosporine and biological agents (see IMMUNOTHERAPY) promises to improve the situation.

IMMUNOTHERAPY The manipulation of immunity by immunological means to reduce harmful reactions or to boost beneficial responses. Severe allergy to wasp or bee stings is often treated by a course of injections with allergen purified from insect venom. There are current attempts to treat autoimmune diseases with monoclonal antibodies to the T-cell populations or cytokines implicated in the immunopathogenesis of the disorder (see AUTOIMMUNITY and IMMUNITY).

Strategies are also being evaluated for treating cancer by boosting the patient's own immunity to cancer cells. One approach is immunization with cancer cells manipulated *in vivo* to increase a T-lymphocyte attack on antigens expressed by tumour cells. Another method is to manipulate the cytokine network into encouraging an immune attack on or self-destruction ('apoptosis') of malignant cells.

However immunotherapy is a developing science and its place in the routine treatment of immunological and malignant diseases has yet to be established.

IMPACTION is a term applied to a condition in which two things are firmly lodged together. For example, when after a fracture one piece of bone is driven within the other, this is known as an impacted fracture; when a tooth is firmly lodged in its socket so that its eruption is prevented, this is known as dental impaction.

IMPETIGO is an infectious skin disease caused usually by the *Staphylococcus aureus*. It consists of vesicles which appear particularly on the face, and dry up, leaving yellowish-brown scabs from which the discharge is infectious. These scabs fall off, leaving no scars, but the disease spreads from place to place over the skin, and may last for months if untreated.

When it occurs in very young children, it is liable to run a severe course unless treatment is initiated immediately. This form of the disease is known as pemphigus neonatorum (see PEMPHIGUS) because of the marked blistering of the skin that tends to occur.

Treatment Infected crusts are removed by washing with saline or cetrimide lotion. Infection can be caused by *Staphylococcus aureus* or *Streptococcus* and both are sensitive to cloxacillin or cephalosporin given systematically. Topical application of mupirocin ointment may be effective. (See PEDICULOSIS.)

IMPOTENCE is the inability to perform the sexual act. It may be partial or complete, temporary or permanent. Of the many classifications of this quite common condition, the most satisfactory is probably that which divides it into two main groups: *organic* and *psychological*. Among organic causes are lesions of the external genitalia, e.g. a tight foreskin; disturbances of the endocrine glands, such as diminished activity of the gonads, thyroid gland or pituitary gland; diseases of the central nervous system, e.g. tabes dorsalis; any severe disturbance of health, such as diabetes mellitus, addiction to alcohol and the like. Psychological factors are the commonest cause and these are anxiety, ignorance, fear, guilt, weakness of sexual desire or abnormality of such desire. Counselling or sex therapy, preferably with the partner, has a 50-per-cent chance of helping to cure long-term impotence of psychological origin.

INCIDENCE One of the main ways to measure the frequency of a disease in a particular population; the incidence of a disease is the number of new cases that occur during a particular time. Prevalence, the other measure, is the total number of cases of disease present at any one time and covers both old and new cases.

INCISION means a cut or wound and is a term specially applied to surgical openings.

INCISOR is the name applied to the four front teeth of each jaw. (See TEETH.)

INCOMPATIBILITY is a term applied to unsuitability in a prescription owing to the fact that its different contents either cannot be mixed, or that when mixed they undergo chemical changes, or that their actions are opposed to one another.

INCOMPETENCE is a term applied to the valves of the heart when, as a result of disease in the valves or alterations in size of the chambers of the heart, the valves become unable to close the orifices which they should protect. (See HEART DISEASES.)

INCONTINENCE URINARY INCONTINENCE is the involuntary loss of urine. This distressing condition affects 5 per cent of the population, 8 per cent of women and 3 per cent of men. The two main groups of urinary incontinence are urge and stress incontinence.

URGE INCONTINENCE This is the involuntary loss of urine associated with the strong desire to void, and is the result of bladder dysfunction. Urge incontinence may be the result of overactive motor nerves to the bladder, which may be due to spinal problems such as multiple sclerosis (q.v.), nerve problems such as diabetes (q.v.) or secondary to bladder outflow obstruction as a result of prostate disease (q.v.), or idiopathic (q.v.) causes. Similarly urge incontinence may be the result of overactive sensory nerves, which is associated with cystitis, bladder stones, or bladder tumours.

STRESS INCONTINENCE This is the involuntary loss of urine during activities, such as coughing, exercise, or lifting. Caused by weakness in the urethral muscle which holds the urine in the bladder, stress incontinence is usually the result of obesity, childbirth or, in men, a broken pelvis, or an operation on the prostate gland.

Investigations These would include, in women, a vaginal examination to look for prolapse (q.v.), a urine test to exclude any infections, and specific tests to assess the function of the bladder known as urodynamics.

Treatment Urge incontinence can be treated by bladder-training measures, by the use of drugs to calm the bladder, or by distending the bladder under an anaesthetic. Stress incontinence is treated by the individual's performing pelvic-floor exercises, which can be supplemented by stimulation of the pelvic floor. An operation designed to raise and support the bladder and urethra may also be effective.

FAECAL INCONTINENCE is the inability to control bowel movements and may be due to local disease or to injury or disease of the spinal cord or nervous supply to rectum and anal muscles. Those with the symptom need investigation.

INCOORDINATION is a term applied to irregularity of movements produced either by loss of the sensations by which they are governed or by defects in the muscles themselves or their nerves.

INCUBATION means the period elapsing between the time when a person becomes infected by some agent and the first appearance of the symptoms of the disease. Most acute infectious diseases have fairly definite periods of incubation, and it is of great importance that people who have run the risk of infection should know the length of time which must elapse before they can be sure whether or not they are to contract the disease in question. A person who has been exposed to infection is, during the incubation period, technically known as a contact. By isolating and watching contact

cases medical officers can often successfully check a threatened epidemic. It must be noted that diseases are not communicated to others by a person while passing through the stage of incubation. Some diseases, however, such as measles, become infectious as soon as the first symptoms set in after the incubation period is over; others, like scarlet fever and smallpox, are not so infectious then as in their later stages. The incubation period for any given disease is remarkably constant, although in the case of a severe attack the incubation is usually slightly shortened, and if the oncoming attack be a mild one, the period may be lengthened. All of these may, however, take a few days longer than the time stated to show themselves. (See INFECTION.) Several also, and especially whooping-cough, may be difficult to recognize in their early stages.

	days
Chickenpox	14–21
Diphtheria	2–5
German measles	14–21
Measles	10–15
Mumps	18–21
Poliomyelitis	3–21
Smallpox	10–16
Typhoid fever	7–21
Whooping-cough	7–10

Incubation periods of the commoner infectious diseases.

INDIAN HEMP (see CANNABIS INDICA).

INDIGESTION (see DYSPEPSIA).

INDOMETHACIN is a non-steroidal anti-inflammatory drug used in the treatment of gout and rheumatoid arthritis. It is said to be of particular value in the relief of night pain and morning stiffness. It is also used to treat the congenital abnormality of the heart known as patent ductus arteriosus. (See DUCTUS ARTERIOSUS.)

INDORAMIN is an alpha-adreno-receptor-blocking drug which is proving of value in the treatment of high blood-pressure. (See ADRENERGIC RECEPTORS.)

INDUCTION Bringing about a particular event, for example, the induction or starting of labour; the induction of anaesthesia.

INDURATION The pathological hardening of a tissue or organ. This may occur when a tissue is infected or when it is invaded by cancer.

INDUSTRIAL DISEASES (see OCCUPATIONAL DISEASES).

INFANT A baby who is under 1 year old.

INFANT FEEDING The new-born infant may be fed naturally from the breast or artificially from a bottle.

BREAST-FEEDING Unless there is a genuine contra-indication, every baby should be breast-fed. The nutritional components of human milk are in the ideal proportions to promote the healthy growth of the human new-born. The mother's milk, especially colostrum (the fluid secreted before full lactation is established) contains immune cells and antibodies that increase the baby's resistance to infection. In addition, breast milk does not require elaborate and expensive preparation rituals. From the mother's point of view, breast-feeding helps the womb to return to its normal size and helps her to lose excess body fat gained during pregnancy. Most importantly, breast-feeding promotes intimate contact between mother and baby. A final point to be borne in mind, however, is that drugs taken by a mother can be excreted in her milk. These include antibiotics, sedatives, tranquillizers, alcohol, nicotine and high-dose steroids or vitamins.

ARTIFICIAL FEEDING Unmodified cows' milk is not a satisfactory food for the human new-born and may cause dangerous metabolic imbalance. If breast-feeding is not feasible, one of the many commerciallly available formula milks should be used. Most of these are made from cows' milk which has been modified to reflect the composition of human milk as nearly as possible. For the rare infant who develops cows'-milk-protein intolerance, a milk based on soya-bean protein is indicated.

FEEDING AND WEIGHT GAIN The main guide as to whether an infant is being adequately fed is the weight. During the first days of life a healthy infant loses weight, but, however, by the end of the second week, should return to birth weight. From then on, weight gain should be approximately 6oz. (170g) each week.

The timing of feeds reflects social convention rather than natural feeding patterns. Among the most primitive hunter-gatherer tribes of South America, babies are carried next to the breast and allowed to suckle at will. Fortunately for developed society, however, babies can be conditioned to intermittent feedings. As each bottle feed requires considerable preparation, it has been expedient to define rigid feeding guidelines. Whilst these are a useful starting point, they should not be viewed in the same light as the Ten Commandments, and allowance should be made for each baby's individual temperament.

As the timing of breast-feeding is more flexible, little or no preparation time being required, mothers can feed their babies on demand. Far from spoiling the baby, demand feeding is likely to lead to a contented infant. The only necessary caution being that a crying baby is not always a hungry baby.

In general, a new-born will require feeding every two to four hours and, if well, is unlikely to sleep for more than six hours. After the first months, a few lucky parents will find their infant sleeping through the night.

WEANING Weaning on to solid foods is again a matter of some individuality. Most babies will become dissatisfied with a milk-only diet round about six months and develop enthusiasm for cereal-based weaning foods. Introduction of solids before the age of four months is unusual and, unless really necessary to quell an apparently insatiable appetite, should be avoided. Similarly, delaying the commencement of weaning beyond nine months is nutritionally undesirable. As weaning progresses, the infant's diet requires less milk. Once established on a varied solid diet, breast and formula milks can be safely replaced with cows' milk. There is, however, no nutritional contra-indication to continued breast-feeding until the mother wishes to stop.

It is during weaning that infants realize that they can arouse extreme maternal anxiety by refusing to eat. This can lead to force-feeding and battles of will which may culminate in a breakdown of the mother–child relationship. To avoid this, parents must resist the temptation to coax the child to eat. If the child refuses solid food, the meal should be taken away with a minimum of fuss. Children's appetites reflect their individual genetic structure and a well child will eat enough to grow and maintain satisfactory weight gain. If a child is not eating properly, weight gain will be inadequate over a prolonged period and an underlying illness is the most likely cause. Indeed, failure to thrive is the paediatrician's best clue to chronic illness.

ADVICE ON FEEDING Many sources of conflicting advice are available to new parents. It is impossible to satisfy everyone and ultimately it is the well-being of the mother and infant and the closeness of their relationship that matter. In general, mothers should be wary of people who give rigid advice, as this suggests that their understanding of infant nutrition may be rather limited. An experienced midwife, health visitor or well-baby-clinic nursing sister are among the most reliable sources of information.

	Protein per cent	Fat per cent	Sugar per cent	Calories per cent
Human milk	1·1	4·2	7·0	70
Cow's milk	3·5	3·9	4·6	66

Composition of human and cow's milk

INFANTILE PARALYSIS is an old name for POLIOMYELITIS (q.v.).

INFANTILISM is the condition characterized by imperfect sexual development at puberty. It may or may not be associated with small stature. It may be due to lack of development of certain of the endocrine glands: i.e. the gonads (q.v.), pituitary gland or the adrenal glands. In other cases it may be associated with a generalized disease such as diabetes mellitus, asthma, ulcerative colitis and rheumatoid arthritis.

INFANT MORTALITY is the number of deaths of infants under one year of age. The infant mortality rate in any given year is calculated as the number of deaths in the first year of life in proportion to every 1000 registered live births in that year. Along with perinatal mortality (q.v.), it is accepted as one of the most important criteria for assessing the health of the community and the standard of the social conditions of a country.

The improvement in the infant mortality rate has occurred mainly in the period from the second month of life. There has been much less improvement in the neonatal mortality rate: i.e. the number of infants dying during the first four weeks of life, expressed as a proportion of every 1000 live births. During the first week of life the main causes of death are asphyxia, prematurity, birth injuries and congenital abnormalities. After the first week the main cause of death is infection.

Social conditions also play an important rôle in infant mortality. In England and Wales the infant mortality rate in 1930–32 was: Social Class I (professional), 32·7; Social Class III (skilled workers), 57·6; Social Class V (unskilled workers), 77·1. The comparable figures for Scotland for 1939–45 were: Class I, 30·9; Class III, 53·4; Class V, 78·6. Many factors come into play in producing these social variations, but overcrowding is undoubtedly one of the most important. For instance, in 1936 the infant mortality rate in Bournemouth, where only 0·3 per cent of working-class families were overcrowded, was 78 per cent of that for the entire country, compared with 145 per cent in Newcastle-upon-Tyne where 10·7 per cent of working-class families were overcrowded. The same discrepancy persists to the present day as shown by a comparison of the Standardized Mortality Ratios in the areas covered by the North Western (which includes Lancashire) and the East Anglian Regional Health Authorities. In 1976–78 for children under the age of 1 year these were 110·2 for boys and 110·7 for girls in the former and 86 for boys, and 69·5 for girls in East Anglia.

1838–39	146	1951–55	26·9
1841–50	153	1956–60	22·6
1851–60	154	1961–65	20·6
1861–70	154	1968	18·3
1871–80	149	1970	18·2
1881–90	142	1971	17·5
1891–1900	153	1972	17·2
1901–05	138	1973	16·9
1906–10	117·1	1974	16·3
1911–15	108·1	1975	15·7
1916–20	90·9	1976	14·2
1921–25	74·9	1977	13·7
1926–30	67·9	1978	13·1
1931–35	62·2	1979	12·7
1936–40	55·3	1980	12·0
1941–45	49·8	1990	7·9
1946–50	36·4	1992	6·5

Infant mortality rate in England and Wales (1838–1968) and England 1970–92.

It is thus evident that for a reduction of the infant mortality rate to the minimum figure the following conditions must be met. The mothers and potential mothers of the country must be housed adequately amid surroundings which permit adequate fresh air and healthy exercise. The pregnant and nursing mother must be ensured an adequate diet. Effective antenatal supervision must be available to every mother, as well as skilled supervision during labour. The new-born infant must be adequately nursed and adequately fed and mothers encouraged to breast feed. Adequate environmental and public-health measures must be taken to ensure adequate housing, a clean milk supply and full availability of such protective measures as immunization against diphtheria, measles, poliomyelitis and whooping-cough. (See also PERINATAL MORTALITY.)

INFARCTION means the changes which take place in an organ when an artery is suddenly blocked, leading to the formation of a dense, wedge-shaped mass in the part of the organ supplied by the artery. It occurs as the result of embolism or of thrombosis. (See EMBOLISM.)

INFECTION is the process by which a disease is communicated via micro-organisms from one person to another. All diseases so communicable are called infectious. This micro-organism may be a bacterium, a Rickettsia, a virus, a protozoon, or a metazoon. Invasion of the body by a metazoon (e.g. by an intestinal worm) is more often known as an infestation.

The skin is an important protection against micro-organisms entering the body tissues. A large measure of protection is afforded by the factors which ensure immunity against diseases. (See IMMUNITY.)

Modes of infection The infective material may be transmitted to the person by direct contact with a sick person, when the disease is said to be contagious, although such a distinction is purely artificial. Different diseases are specially infectious at different periods of their course; and the practical question of guarding against infection is rendered much more difficult by the fact that some diseases such as measles are infectious at a stage even before they are clearly recognizable.

Infection may be conveyed on dust, in drinking-water, food, particularly milk, the body's waste products and secretions, scabs from the infected person's body, or even clothes and linen which have been in contact with him.

In this connection what are termed carriers are of great importance. Some people who have suffered from a disease, or who have simply been in contact with an infectious case, harbour the germ of the disease. This is particularly the case in typhoid fever, the bacillus continuing to develop in the gall-bladder of some people, who have had the disease, maybe for years after the symptoms have disappeared. In the case of cholera, which is endemic in some localities of the East, 80 per cent or more of the population may harbour the bacillus and spread infection when other circumstances favour this. Similarly in the case of dysentery, people who have completely recovered may still be capable of infecting dust and drinking-water by their stools. Diphtheria and cerebrospinal meningitis, which is particularly liable to infect children, are other examples.

Flies can infect milk and other food with the organisms causing typhoid fever and food poisoning. Mosquitoes carry the infective agents of malaria and yellow fever, these undergoing part of their development in the body of the mosquito. Fleas convey the germ of plague from rat to man, lice are responsible for inoculating typhus fever and one form of relapsing fever by their bite. A tick is responsible for spreading another form of relapsing fever, and kala-azar (or leishmaniasis) is spread by the bites of sandflies.

Notifiable diseases Certain of the common and most serious infectious diseases are notifiable in the United Kingdom. A doctor diagnosing someone infected by a notifiable disease must inform the authorities. For the current list of notifiable infectious diseases in the UK see NOTIFIABLE DISEASES.

Prevention is an important aspect of the control of infectious diseases and various steps can be taken to check the spread of such infections as dysentery, tuberculosis, malaria and others. (See also IMMUNITY; INCUBATION.)

INFECTIOUS MONONUCLEOSIS (see MONONUCLEOSIS).

INFERTILITY is present when a couple have not achieved a pregnancy after one year of regular unprotected sexual intercourse. Between 15–20 per cent of couples have difficulties in conceiving. The 'fault' lies with the male partner in about a third of cases, with the female partner in about a third and with both partners in about a third. Couples should be investigated together efficiently and as quickly as possible to decrease the distress which is invariably associated with the diagnosis of infertility. In about 10–15 per cent of women suffering from infertility ovulation is disturbed. Mostly they will have either irregular periods or no periods at all.

Checking a hormone profile in the woman's blood will help in the diagnosis of ovulatory disorders like polycystic ovaries, an early menopause, anorexia or other endocrine illnesses. Ovulation itself is best assessed by ultrasound scan at mid-cycle or by a blood hormone progesterone level in the second half of the cycle.

The fallopian tubes may be damaged or blocked in 20–30 per cent of infertile women. This is usually caused by previous pelvic infection or endometriosis, where menstrual blood is thought to flow backwards through the fallopian tubes into the pelvis and seed with cells from the lining of the uterus in the pelvis. This process often leads to scarring of the pelvic tissues;

5–10 per cent of infertility is associated with endometriosis.

To assess the fallopian tubes adequately a procedure called laparoscopy is performed. A telescope is inserted through the umbilicus and at the same time a dye is pushed through the tubes to assess their patency. The procedure is performed under a general anaesthetic.

In a few cases the mucus around the cervix may be hostile to the partner's sperm and therefore prevents fertilization.

Defective sperm production is responsible for up to a quarter of infertility. It may result from the failure of the testes to descend in early life, from infections of the testes or previous surgery for testicular torsion. The semen is analysed to assess the numbers of sperm and their motility and to check for abnormal forms.

In a few cases the genetic make-up of one partner does not allow the couple ever to achieve a pregnancy naturally.

In about 25 per cent of couples no obvious cause can be found for their infertility.

Ovulation may be induced with drugs.

In some cases damaged fallopian tubes may be repaired by tubal surgery. If the tubes are destroyed beyond repair a pregnancy may be achieved with *in vitro* fertilization (q.v.).

Endometriosis may be treated either with drugs or laser therapy and pregnancy rates after both forms of treatment are between 40–50 per cent, depending on the severity of the disease.

Few options exist for treating male-factor infertility. These are artificial insemination by husband or donor and more recently in vitro fertilization. Drug treatment and surgical repair of varicoceles have disappointing results.

Following investigations between 30 and 40 per cent of infertile couples will achieve a pregnancy usually within two years.

INFESTATION is a term applied to the occurrence of animal parasites in the intestine, hair or clothing. (See INSECTS IN RELATION TO DISEASE.)

INFILTRATION The invasion of tissues or organs by cells or fluid that are not normally present. Local anaesthetic is infiltrated into an area of tissue to produce analgesia (q.v.) in a defined area.

INFLAMMATION is the reaction of the tissues to any injury, which may be the result of trauma, infection or chemicals. The victim feels pain and the affected tissue becomes hot, red and swollen. Inflammation also interferes with function. Local blood vessels dilate, thus increasing blood flow to the injured site. White blood cells invade the affected tissue engulfing bacteria or other foreign bodies; related cells consume any dead cells, thus producing pus after which the site starts to heal. If the infection is severe it may persist locally – chronic inflammation – or spread elsewhere in the body – systemic infection.

INFLUENZA is an acute infectious disease, characterized by a sudden onset, fever and generalized aches and pains, which usually occurs in epidemics and pandemics.
Cause The disease is caused by a virus of the influenza group. There are at least three types of influenza virus, known respectively as A, B and C. One of their most characteristic features is that infection with one type provides no protection against another type. Equally important is the ease with which the influenza virus can change its character. It is these two characteristics which explain why one attack of influenza provides little, if any, protection against a subsequent attack, and why it is so difficult to prepare an effective vaccine against the disease.

Epidemics of influenza due to virus A occur in Britain at two- to four-year intervals, and outbreaks of virus B influenza in less frequent cycles. Virus A influenza, for instance, was the prevalent infection in 1949, 1951, 1955 and 1956, whilst virus B influenza was epidemic in 1946, 1950, 1954 and, along with virus A, in 1958–59. The pandemic of 1957, which swept most of the world, though fortunately not in a severe form, was due to a new variant of virus A – the so-called Asian virus – and it has been suggested that it was this variant that was responsible for the pandemics of 1889 and 1918. Since 1957, variants of virus A have been the predominating causes of influenza accompanied on occasions by virus B.
Symptoms The incubation period of influenza A and B is two to three days and the disease is characterized by a sudden onset. In most cases this is followed by a short, sharp febrile illness of two to four days' duration, associated with headache, prostration, generalized aching and respiratory symptoms. In many cases the respiratory symptoms are restricted to the upper respiratory tract, and consist of signs of irritation of the nose, pharynx and larynx. There may be nose-bleeds, and a dry hacking cough is often a prominent and troublesome symptom. The fever is usually remittent and the temperature seldom exceeds 39·4 °C (103 °F), tending to fluctuate between 38·3 and 39·4 °C (101 and 103 °F).

The most serious complication is infection of the lungs. This infection is usually due to organisms other than the influenza virus. It is a complication which can have serious results in elderly people.

The very severe form which tends to occur during pandemics – and which was so common during the 1918–19 pandemic – is characterized by the rapid onset of broncho-pneumonia and severe prostration. Because of the toxic effect on the heart there is a particularly marked form of cyanosis, known as heliotrope cyanosis.

Convalescence following influenza tends to be prolonged. Even after an attack of average severity there tends to be a period of weakness and depression.
Treatment Expert opinion is still divided as to the real value of influenza vaccine in preventing

the disease. Part of the trouble is that, as already pointed out, there is no value in giving any vaccine until it is known which particular virus is causing the infection. As this varies from winter to winter, and as the protection given by vaccine does not exceed one year, it is obviously not worth while attempting to vaccinate the whole community. The general rule therefore is that, unless there is any evidence that a particularly virulent type of virus is responsible, only those should be vaccinated who are particularly vulnerable, such as children in boarding schools, elderly people, pregnant women, and people who suffer from chronic bronchitis. In the face of an epidemic, people in key positions, such as doctors, nurses and those concerned with public safety, transport and other public utilities should be vaccinated.

For an uncomplicated attack of influenza, treatment is symptomatic: that is, rest in bed, analgesics to relieve the pain, sedatives, and a light diet. A linctus is useful to sooth a troublesome cough. The best analgesic is aspirin – either alone, or combined with paracetamol and codeine. None of the sulphonamides or the known antibiotics has any effect on the influenza virus. On the other hand, should the lungs become infected, antibiotics should be given immediately, because, as has already been pointed out, such an infection is usually due to other organisms. If possible, a sample of sputum should be examined to determine which organisms are responsible for the lung infection. The choice of antibiotic then depends upon which antibiotic the organism is most sensitive to.

INFUNDIBULUM A funnel-shaped passage. The word is used specifically to describe the hollow conical stalk that links the hypothalmus (q.v.) to the posterior lobe of the pituitary gland (q.v.).

INFUSION is the intravenous or subcutaneous injection of one of a variety of therapeutic solutions, such as saline, glucose, or gum acacia, in the treatment of severe dehydration, hypoglycaemia, or other plasma electrolyte imbalance. Blood infusions may be given in cases of severe anaemia, for example, after heavy bleeding. Infusions may be given in intermittent amounts of around 570 ml (1 pint) at a time, or alternatively by continuous drip-feed over several hours.

INGESTION The act of taking fluid, food, or medicine into the stomach. The way in which a phagocytic cell surrounds and absorbs foreign substances such as bacteria in the blood.

INGUINAL HERNIA An extrusion of the abdominal peritoneum (q.v.), sometimes containing a loop of bowel, through natural openings in the region of either groin (see HERNIA).

INGUINAL REGION The groin, the area of the body where the lower part of the abdomen meets the upper thigh. The inguinal ligaments extend on each side from the superior spines of the iliac bones to the pubic bone. It is also called Poupart's ligament (see diagram of ABDOMEN).

INHALANTS Substances that can be inhaled into the body through the lungs. They may be delivered in traditional form dissolved in hot water and inhaled in the steam or as an aerosol, a suspension of very small liquid or solid particles in the air. The latter are now usually delivered by devices in which the aerosol is kept under pressure in a small hand-held cylinder and delivered in required doses by a release mechanism.

AEROSOLS Asthmatic patients find aerosol devices of value in controlling their attacks. They provide an effective and convenient way of applying drugs directly to the bronchi, thus reducing the risks of unwanted effects accompanying systemic therapy. They are of particular use in asthma. Broncho-dilator aerosols contain either a beta-sympathomimetic agent or ipratropium bromide which is an anticholinergic drug. Of the beta-adrenoceptor agonists isoprenaline was the first compound to be widely used as an aerosol. It did however stimulate beta$_1$ receptors in the heart as well as beta$_2$ receptors in the bronchi and so produced palpitations and even dangerous cardiac arrhythmias. Newer beta-adrenoceptor agonists are specific for the beta$_2$ receptors and thus have a greater safety margin. They include salbutamol, terbutaline, rimiterol, fenoterol and reproterol. Unwanted effects such as palpitations, tremor and restlessness are uncommon with these more specific preparations. In patients who get insufficient relief from the beta-adrenoreceptor agonist the drug ipratropium bromide is worth adding.

Patients must be taught carefully and observed while using their inhalers. It is important that patients should realize that if the aerosol no longer gives more than slight intransient relief they should not increase the dose but seek medical help.

INHALATION is a method of applying drugs in a finely divided or gaseous state, so that, when breathed in, they may come in contact with the nose, throat and lungs. There are two chief means by which drugs are mingled with the air and so taken in by breathing. These are traditional steam inhalations and modern aerosol devices which deliver a fine spray direct into the mouth.

INHIBITION means arrest or restraint of some process effected by nervous influence. The term is applied to the action of certain inhibitory nerves: e.g. the vagus nerve which contains fibres that inhibit or control the action of the heart. It is also applied generally to the mental processes by which instinctive but undesirable actions are checked by a process of self-control.

INJECTIONS (see ENEMA; HYPODERMIC).

INNER EAR This comprises three fluid-filled chambers or labyrinths situated in the bony temporal area that are concerned with identifying a person's position in space. Each chamber lies in a different plane and movement of fluid in it is picked up by sensory cells that transmit the information to the brain. Disease or damage to the inner ear upsets the sense of balance and causes vertigo. Motion sickness (q.v.) is caused by the inner ear's being unable to accommodate to the changes in position resulting from motion.

INNERVATION The nerve supply to a tissue, organ or part of the body. It carries motor impulses to and sensory impulses away from the part.

INOCULATION is the process by which infective material is brought into the system through a small wound in the skin or in a mucous membrane. Many infectious diseases and blood-poisoning are contracted by accidental inoculation of microbes. Inoculation is now used as a preventive measure against many infectious diseases. (See VACCINE.)

INOTROPIC Adjective describing anything that affects the force of muscle contraction. It is usually applied to the heart muscle and an inotrope is a drug that improves its contraction.

INPATIENT A person who stays in a bed in hospital for investigation or treatment.

INSANITY (see MENTAL ILLNESS).

INSECT REPELLENTS (See DIBUTYL PHTHALATE; DIMETHYL PHTHALATE.)

INSECTICIDES are substances which kill insects. Since the discovery of the insecticidal properties of DDT (q.v.) in 1940, a steady stream of new ones has been introduced, and their combined use has played an outstanding part in international public health campaigns, such as that of the World Health Organization for the eradication of malaria.

Unfortunately, insects are liable to become resistant to insecticides, just as bacteria are liable to become resistant to antibiotics, and it is for this reason that so much research work is being devoted to the discovery of new ones.

It is against this beneficial background that must be viewed the increasing evidence that the indiscriminate use of some of these potent preparations is having an adverse effect, not only upon human beings, but also upon the balance of nature.

Some such as DDT, the use of which is now banned in the UK, are very stable compounds that enter the food chain and may ultimately be lethal to many animals, including birds and fishes.

INSECTS IN RELATION TO DISEASE
Many insects play an important part in the transmission of infectious diseases. Thus, flies by their feet and their feeding habits carry the organisms which cause typhoid fever, the tsetse fly spreads sleeping sickness, mosquitoes transmit the germs of malaria and yellow fever, fleas convey plague germs and lice convey typhus fever and one form of relapsing fever. In addition, these creatures are nuisances as well as dangers.

HOUSE-FLY (*Musca domestica*) This fly lays its eggs in manure, or in moist, fermenting vegetable matter. The maggot is hatched in eight hours to two days, feeds on the manure, passes through the pupa stage in anything from a few days to four weeks, and, becoming a fly, is capable of egg-laying about three weeks from its own appearance as an egg. As 120 to 150 eggs are laid in a batch by each female fly, this fly is capable, under the most favourable conditions, of producing over half-a-million progeny within her life of three months. The fly gorges on fluid food which it sucks up by means of its proboscis, and it has the habit of repeatedly vomiting and re-swallowing the contents of its crop as it feeds. Its immense power to distribute disease germs over the surface of uncovered food is evident.

BLOW-FLY, or BLUE-BOTTLE (*Calliphora erythrocephala*), lays its eggs (450 to 600 in number) on meat, fish or decaying animal matter. The maggot hatches out within a day, passes through the pupa stage and becomes a full-grown fly in about three weeks. Its habits are similar to those of the house-fly, though in numbers it is much less plentiful.

Treatment of flies The most important measure is to destroy their breeding grounds near human dwellings. No kitchen refuse should be left exposed so that flies may deposit their eggs in it. Stable litter and manure must be disposed of, or kept covered and shut up in outhouses, not allowed to accumulate in the open air and sunshine near houses. Adult flies may be destroyed in a great extent by proper protection and storage of all food. An insecticide may be used as a powder, a spray or a paint, but care must be exercised that it does not come in contact with food or with surfaces on which food is prepared.

LICE There are three lice which infest man: the body louse (*Pediculus corporis*), the head louse (*Pediculus capitis*) and the crab louse (*Pediculus pubis*). The head louse is by far the most common in Britain. Infestation is most common in children under school age, but it is not unusual in adults. Head lice spread by close human contact. (See also PEDICULOSIS.)

As already noted, lice convey the causative micro-organisms of typhus fever, one form of relapsing fever, and trench fever, and it has been estimated that in this way the louse is responsible for more human deaths than any other insect barring the malaria mosquito (see RELAPSING FEVER; TRENCH FEVER; TYPHUS FEVER).

Treatment of lice In individuals infested with the body louse the clothing should be dusted with an insecticide, packed in a bag and then sent for washing or storing. A temperature of 54 °C (129 °F) is rapidly lethal to both lice and their eggs. At a temperature of −20 °C (−4 °F) lice are killed in half-an-hour and eggs are killed in five hours. As the lice tend to congregate into the seams, hot ironing these is a useful measure.

For body lice, the body should be coated with malathion cream or 1 per cent dusting powder. This may need to be repeated for several days. Calamine lotion containing 1 per cent phenol eases the itching. For crab, or pubic, lice, the affected area is rubbed with either Dicophane Application BPC, or Malathion dusting powder which is left on for two days, and the process then repeated. Alternatively, carbaryl or malathion may be used.

For head lice, a lotion containing 0·5 per cent Malathion in 10 ml should be rubbed with the fingers into the hair and its roots and left for twenty-four hours. The hair is then washed. This may need to be repeated twice or three times. The hair is then carefully combed with a fine comb to remove the nits. Removal may be easier if the hairs are rubbed previously with a swab soaked in vinegar. Unfortunately the head louse is becoming resistant to gamma benzene hexachloride, which is therefore being replaced by malathion (q.v.) or carbaryl. Malathion is applied in a 0·5-per-cent solution in spirit until the scalp is thoroughly moist. The hair is then allowed to dry naturally without the use of any heat. After twelve hours the hair is shampooed and combed with a fine metal comb while wet to remove the dead nits. Only one such treatment is usually necessary, but all close contacts including the parents of the infested child should be examined and treated forthwith with malathion if infested. Only in this way can the infestation be eradicated from the family. Carbaryl is available as a shampoo and a lotion. The lotion is the preparation of choice. It is rubbed gently into the hair. The hair is then left to dry naturally and washed with a shampoo the next day. After the shampoo, the hair, while still wet, is combed with a fine metal comb to remove the dead lice and eggs (nits).

FLEAS *Pulex irritans* is the common flea that afflicts mankind. *Xenopsylla cheopis* is the rat flea that conveys *Pasteurella pestis*, the causative organism of plague, from rat to man. The flea lays its eggs singly. They take two to four days in summer, two weeks in winter, to hatch into larvae which are fully grown in a fortnight. The larva then becomes a pupa from which the adult emerges two weeks later. The flea can survive for a long time without food.

Treatment of fleas Human beings vary tremendously in their susceptibility to flea bites. For those who are susceptible the best preventive is dimethyl phthallate sprayed on the trousers or socks where it is effective for several days. In the absence of dimethyl phthallate, alternative methods of prevention are the smearing of the skin with oil of pennyroyal, oil of lavender, or 10 per cent crotamiton cream or lotion, or dusting the socks and underclothing with pyrethrum powder, menthol or camphor. For disinfestation of buildings, a solution of insecticide in kerosene is effective. For bedding a powder containing 0·5-per-cent gamma benzene hexachloride is effective. Other anti-flea agents are pyrethrum, flaked naphthalene, or parachlorbenzene.

BED BUGS (*Cimex lectularius*) are best got rid of by a solution of insecticide in kerosene, with or without the addition of pyrethrum. (See BED BUG.)

MOSQUITOES One of these (*Anopheles gambiae*) is responsible for conveying the parasite of malaria, another (*Aedes aegypti*) for distributing the infection of yellow fever.

Treatment of mosquitoes See under MALARIA; YELLOW FEVER.

INSEMINATION The ejaculation of semen in the vagina in the act of sexual intercourse. In artificial insemination the semen is placed there by the use of an instrument.

INSIGHT A person's knowledge of him or herself. The description is especially relevant to a person's realization that he or she has psychological difficulties. Thus someone with a psychosis (q.v.) lacks insight. Insight also refers to an individual's concept of his or her personality and problems.

INSOLATION is a term applied both to treatment by exposure to the sun's rays and to fever caused by excessive heat (see HEAT-STROKE).

INSOMNIA (see SLEEP; HYPNOTICS).

INSPISSATION is the process of the drying or thickening of fluids or excretions by evaporation.

INSTITUTIONALIZATION A condition brought about by a prolonged stay in an impersonal institution. The individual becomes apathetic and listless as a result of inadequate stimulation in an uninteresting environment. The condition can occur in mental institutions or long-stay nursing homes; the affected person loses the ability to make any decisions.

INSUFFLATION means the blowing of powder or vapour into a cavity, especially through the air passages, for the treatment of disease.

INSULIN is the internal secretion of the pancreas formed by groups of cells called the islets of Langerhans in this organ. Its existence was indicated by Sharpey-Schafer in 1909, and it was successfully isolated in a pure form by McLeod, Banting and Best in 1921. It acts by enabling the muscles and other tissues which require sugar for their activity to take up this substance from the blood. When it is deficient, the sugar derived from the food accumulates in the blood and is wastefully excreted in the urine. Insulin is administered by hypodermic (subcutaneous) injection in cases of diabetes mellitus (q.v.), and thus enables the sugar in the circulation to be utilized so that its excretion in the urine ceases. Each unit of insulin administered to a diabetic patient enables him to utilize somewhere between one and two grams of additional carbohydrate material. The appropriate dose of insulin in any given case depends upon its severity.

Over 40 insulin preparations are listed in the *British National Formulary*. These differ in their speed of onset, and duration, of action.

Hitherto insulin has been obtained from the pancreas of oxen and pigs. Human insulin is now available. This is made either by genetic manipulation of the micro-organism, *Escherichia coli*, or by enzymatic manipulation (see ENZYME) of pig insulin. Beef, pig, and human insulin differ in the number of amino-acids (q.v.) they contain. Hitherto insulin was available in three strengths: of 20, 40 and 80 units per millilitre. These have now been replaced by one strength of 100 units per millilitre, known as U100 insulin.

INTELLIGENCE QUOTIENT, or IQ as it is usually known, is the ratio between the mental age and chronological age multiplied by 100. Thus, if a boy of 10 years of age is found to have a mental age of 12 years, his IQ will be: 120.

On the other hand, if he is found to have a mental age of 8 years his IQ will be: 80.

The mental age is established by various tests, the most widely used of which are the Stanford-Binet Scale, the Wechsler Adult Intelligence Scale, and the Mill Hill Vocabulary Test.

Average intelligence is represented by an IQ of 100, with a range of 85 to 115. For practical purposes it is taken that the intellectual level reached by the average 15-year-old is indistinguishable from that of an adult.

INTENSIVE THERAPY UNIT (ITU) A hospital unit in which patients undergo specialized resuscitation, monitoring and treatment procedures. People who have had severe injuries, heart attacks, or major operations – for example, cardiac surgery – are admitted to ITUs, which are staffed 24 hours a day with highly trained nurses, technicians and doctors and equipped with electronic monitoring devices that allow continuous assessment of vital body functions such as heart rate, blood pressure and blood chemistry.

INTERCOSTAL is the term applied to the nerves, vessels and muscles that lie between the ribs, as well as to diseases affecting these structures.

INTERFERON It has been known for many years that one virus will interfere with the growth of another. In 1957, workers at the National Institute for Medical Research in London isolated the factor that was responsible for the phenomenon. They gave it the name of interferon. There are now known to be three human interferons. They are glycoproteins and are released from cells infected with virus or exposed to stimuli which mimic virus infection. They not only inhibit the growth of viruses. They also inhibit the growth and reduplication of cells. This is the basis for their investigation as a means of treating cancer. Hitherto the major difficulty has been obtaining sufficient supplies, but methods have now been evolved which promise to provide adequate amounts of it. The most promising of these is by means of what is known as genetic engineering, or manipulation, whereby a portion of DNA (q.v.) from interferon is inserted into the microorganism known as *Escherichia coli* (see ESCHERICHIA) which thus becomes a source of almost unlimited amounts of interferon as it can be grown so easily. The evidence to date indicates that interferon is of value in treating certain virus infections, particularly different forms of herpes. The case for its value in the treatment of cancer is still not proven.

INTERLEUKINS Interleukins are lymphokines, that is polypeptides produced by activated lymphocytes. They are involved in signalling between cells of the immune system and are released by several cell types, including lymphocytes. They interact to control the immune response of cells and also participate in haemopoiesis. There are seven varieties, interleukins 1 to 7. For example, interleukin 1 is produced as a result of inflammation and it stimulates the proliferation of T and B lymphocytes. They enhance the immune response by stimulating other lymphocytes and activating dormant T cells. Interleukin 2 has anti-cancer effects as it is able to activate T lymphocytes to become killer cells which destroy foreign antigens such as cancer cells, and this anti-cancer effect is being developed for clinical use. The remaining interleukins have a range of properties in cell growth and differentiation.

INTERMITTENT is a term applied to fevers which continue for a time, subside completely and then return again. The name is also used in connection with a pulse in which occasional heart-beats are not felt, in consequence of irregular action of the heart.

INTERMITTENT CLAUDICATION is a condition occurring in middle-aged and elderly people, which is characterized by pain in the legs after walking a certain distance. The pain is relieved by resting for a short time. It is due to arteriosclerosis (see ARTERIES, DISEASES OF) of the arteries to the leg, which results in inadequate blood supply to the muscles. Drugs have little effect in easing the pain, but useful preventive measures are to stop smoking, reduce weight (if overweight) and to take as much exercise as possible within the limits imposed by the pain.

INTERN A doctor in training who carries out his duties and training in hospital and usually spends some of his time living in the hospital. The description is used mainly in North America. Alternative terms are house officer or resident which are used in the United Kingdom.

INTERNATIONAL CLASSIFICATION OF DISEASE A World Health Organization classification of all known diseases and syndromes. The diseases are divided according to system (respiratory, renal, cardiac, etc.) or type (accidents, malignant growth, etc.). Each of them is given a three-digit number to facilitate computerization. This classification allows mortality and morbidity rates to be compared nationally and regionally.

INTERSEXUALITY is a state of indeterminate sexuality of an individual, and may present in many different forms. A characteristic is that only one type of gonad – testis or ovary – is present; in hermaphrodites (q.v.) both types are present. Intersexuality may be due to a fault in the genetic mechanism of sex determination as early as conception, or to later errors in sexual differentiation of the embryo and fetus, or after birth. Some cases may result from abnormal metabolism of the sex hormones, or may be drug-induced (for example, women given androgens or progesterone for repeated miscarriages may give birth to girls with some genital virilization). Abnormalities of the sex chromosomes may be associated with delayed (or failure of) sexual development, so that the individual shows some of the characteristics (often underdeveloped) of both sexes. Some of the more common presentations of the condition include hypogonadism (q.v.), cryptorchidism (q.v.), and primary amenorrhoea (q.v.).

Intersexuality inevitably leads to considerable psychological disturbance as the child grows up. It is therefore important to reach an early decision as to the child's sex – or at least, the sex that he (or she) is to be brought up as. Surgical or hormonal means should then be employed, when appropriate, to develop the attributes of that sex and diminish those of the other, together with psychological counselling.

INTERSTITIAL is a term applied to indifferent tissue set among the proper active tissue of an organ. It is generally of a supporting character and formed of fibrous tissue. The term is also applied to the fluid always present in this in a small amount, and to diseases which specially affect this tissue, such as interstitial keratitis. (See EYE DISEASES.)

INTERTRIGO is a term applied to a chafed or abraded condition between two surfaces of skin that rub together: e.g. under the breast, between the toes, or the armpit. (See ATHLETE'S FOOT; CHAFING OF THE SKIN.)

INTERVERTEBRAL DISC The fibrous disc that acts as a cushion between the bony vertebrae, enabling them to rotate and bend one on another. The disc tends to degenerate with age and may get ruptured and displaced – prolapsed or slipped disc – as a result of sudden strenuous action. Prolapsed disc occurs mainly in the lower back and is more common in men than women and in the 30–40 age group.

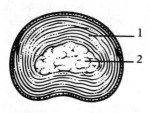

1 anulus fibrosus
2 nucleus pulposus

Cross-section of intervertebral disc.

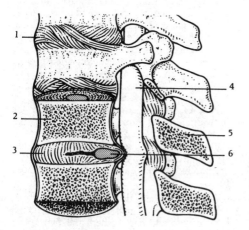

1 intervertebral disc
2 vertebral body
3 anulus fibrosus
4 spinal cord
5 vertebral spine
6 nucleus pulposus (protruding into spinal cord)

Lateral view of prolapsed intervertebral disc.

INTESTINE is the whole of the alimentary canal situated below the stomach. In it most digestion is carried on, and through its walls all the food material is absorbed into the blood and lymph streams. (See DIGESTION.) The length of the intestine in man is about 8·5 to 9 metres (28 to 30 feet), and it takes the form of one continuous tube suspended in loops in the abdominal cavity.

Divisions The intestine is divided into small intestine and large intestine. The former comprises that part of the tube which extends from the stomach onwards for 6·5 metres (22 feet) or thereabout, and at its broadest point is about 35 mm (1½ inches) in width. The large intestine is the second part of the tube, and though shorter (about 1·8 metres (6 feet) long) is much wider than the small intestine, reaching in places a width of 65 mm (2½ inches). The *small intestine* is divided rather arbitrarily into three parts: the *duodenum*, consisting of the first 25 or 30 cm (10 or 12 inches), into which the ducts of the liver and pancreas open; the *jejunum*, which is generally found empty after death, and comprises the next 2·4 or 2·7 metres (8 or 9 feet); and finally the *ileum*, which at its lower end opens into the large intestine.

The large intestine begins in the lower part of the abdomen on the right side. The first part is known as the caecum, and into this opens the appendix vermiformis. The appendix is a small tube, about the thickness of a quill, from 2 to 20 cm (average 9 cm) in length, which has much the same structure as the rest of the intestine. At one end it is closed, at the other it opens into the caecum, and although it appears to play little or no part in digestion, it is of great importance because of the frequency with which serious inflammation takes place in it. (See APPENDICITIS.) The caecum is continued into the colon. This is subdivided into: the ascending colon which ascends through the right flank to beneath the liver; the transverse colon which crosses the upper part of the abdomen transversely to the left side; the descending colon which bends downwards and descends through the left flank into the pelvis where it becomes the sigmoid colon. The last part of the large intestine is known as the rectum, which passes straight down through the back part of the pelvis, to open to the exterior through the anus.

Structure The intestine, both small and large, consists of four coats, which vary slightly in structure and arrangement at different points, but are of the same general nature throughout the entire length of the bowel. On the inner surface there is a mucous membrane; outside this is a loose submucous coat, in which blood-vessels run; next comes a muscular coat in two layers; and finally a tough, thin peritoneal membrane. The total thickness of all four coats amounts to about 3 mm.

MUCOUS COAT The interior of the bowel is completely lined by a single layer of pillar-like cells placed side by side. These rest upon a smooth, fine membrane, beneath which is a loose network of connective tissue and muscular fibres, richly supplied with blood-vessels

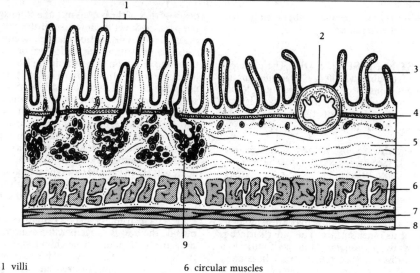

1 villi
2 lymph follicle
3 intestinal gland
4 muscularis mucosae
5 submucous coat

6 circular muscles
7 longitudinal muscles
8 peritoneum
9 duodenal gland

Longitudinal section of intestinal wall. (Left section) Duodenum;
(right section) small intestine.

and lymphatic-vessels. There are two arrangements by which the surface in the small intestine is much increased for the purposes of digestion and absorption. Countless ridges with deep furrows between them run across the upper part, and the whole surface is thickly studded with short hair-like processes called villi. As blood- and lymph-vessels run up to the end of these villi, the digested food passing slowly down the intestine is brought into very close relation with the circulation. Between the bases of the villi are set little openings, each of which leads into a simple, tubular gland lined by cells, which are similar to those covering the surface, and which produce a fluid with digestive powers. In the small intestine, cells here and there produce mucus, and, in the large intestine, a great number of cells are devoted to the production of this substance for lubricating the passage of the food through the bowel. A large number of minute masses, called lymph follicles, similar in structure to the tonsils and lymphatic glands, are scattered over the inner surface of the intestine. In the lower part of the small intestine these are grouped into patches of 2·5 square centimetres or thereabout in size, known as Peyer's patches, which are of special interest, because the inflammation and ulceration of the bowels that occur in typhoid fever are limited to them and to the scattered follicles. The large intestine is bare both of ridges and of villi, and, as already stated, its mucous membrane produces mucus in large amount.

SUBMUCOUS COAT   This consists of a loose connective tissue which allows the mucous membrane to play freely over the muscular coat. The blood-vessels and lymphatic-vessels which absorb the food in the villi pour their contents into a network of large vessels lying in this coat.

MUSCULAR COAT   The muscle in the small intestine is arranged in two definite layers, in the outer of which all the fibres run lengthwise with the bowel, whilst in the inner they pass circularly round it.

PERITONEAL COAT forms the outer covering for almost the whole intestine except parts of the duodenum and of the large intestine. It is a tough, fibrous membrane, covered upon its outer surface with a smooth layer of cells.

Support   The duodenum and greater part of the large intestine are covered only in front by the peritoneum which lines the abdominal cavity, and this tough membrane serves to bind these parts of the intestine firmly against the back wall of the abdomen. The jejunum and ileum, the transverse colon, and the first part of the rectum are not only completely surrounded by peritoneum, but a double layer of this membrane suspends these parts of the bowel at a distance of several inches from the lines on the back of the abdomen, where the two layers become continuous with the rest of the peritoneum. In this way freedom is given to the movements of these parts of the bowels. These suspending structures are known as mesenteries. That of the small intestine is the largest, being shaped like a fan, 200 mm (8 inches) long at its attached margin, and spreading out to 6·5 metres (22 feet) at its frilled border, where it meets the intestine. The vessels and nerves which supply the intestine run between the two layers of the mesentery.

INTESTINE, DISEASES OF   The principal signs of trouble which has its origin in the intestines consist of pain somewhere about the abdomen, sometimes vomiting, and irregularity in movement of the bowels in the direction either of stoppage or of excessive action.

Several diseases are treated under separate headings. (See APPENDICITIS; CHOLERA; COLITIS; CONSTIPATION; DIARRHOEA; DYSENTERY; ENTERIC FEVERS; HERNIA; ILEITIS; INTUSSUSCEPTION; IRRITABLE BOWEL SYNDROME; PERITONITIS; PILES; RECTUM, DISEASES OF.)

INFLAMMATION of the bowel may affect either its outer or its inner surface. The outer surface is covered by peritoneum, and peritonitis is a serious disease. (See PERITONITIS.) Inflammation of the inner surface is known generally as enteritis, inflammation of special parts receiving the names of colitis, appendicitis, and the like. Enteritis may form the chief symptom of certain infective diseases due to special organisms: for example in typhoid fever, cholera, dysentery. Again, it may be acute, though not connected with any definite organism, when, if severe, it is a very serious condition, particularly in young children. Or it may be chronic, especially as the result of dysentery, and then constitutes a less serious though very troublesome complaint.

PERFORATION of the bowel may take place as the result either of injury or of disease. Stabs and other wounds which penetrate the abdomen may damage the bowel, and severe blows or crushes may tear it without any external wound. Ulceration, as in typhoid fever, or, more rarely, in tuberculosis, may cause an opening in the bowel-wall also. Again, when the bowel is greatly distended above an obstruction, faecal material may accumulate and produce ulcers, which rupture with the ordinary movements of the bowels. Whatever the cause, the symptoms are much the same.

Symptoms   The contents of the bowel pass out through the perforation into the peritoneal cavity, and, making their way between the coils of intestine, set up a general peritonitis. In consequence, the abdomen is painful, and after a few hours becomes extremely tender to the touch, as a result of the peritonitis. The abdomen swells, particularly in its upper part, owing to gas having passed also into the cavity. Vomiting is a symptom, and the person passes into a state of collapse. Such a condition is almost invariably fatal in two, or at most three, days, if not promptly treated.

Treatment   All food should be withheld, because whatever is taken into the stomach is either vomited or is liable to pass out of the perforation into the peritoneal cavity. An operation is urgently necessary, the abdomen being opened in the middle line, the perforated portion of bowel found, and the perforation stitched up.

OBSTRUCTION of the bowels means a stoppage to the passage down the intestine of the partially digested food. Obstruction may be due either to some cause within the abdomen or to the thrusting of a loop of bowel through an opening in the wall of this cavity. The latter class of cases has been referred to under HERNIA. Obstruction may be acute when it comes on suddenly with intense symptoms, or it may be chronic, when the obstructing cause gradually increases and the bowel becomes slowly more narrow till it closes altogether, or when slight obstruction comes and goes till it ends in an acute attack. In chronic cases the symptoms are much the same as those of the acute variety, although they are milder in degree and more prolonged.

Causes   Obstruction may be due to causes outside the bowel altogether, for example, the pressure of tumours in neighbouring organs, the twisting round the bowel of bands produced by former peritonitis, or even the twisting of a coil of intestine round itself so as to cause a kink in its wall. Chronic and partial forms of obstruction are sometimes due to such kinks near the end of the small intestine, sometimes to the pressure of the mesentery on the upper end of the small intestine. Chronic causes of the obstruction may exist in the wall of the bowel itself: for example, a tumour, or the contracting scar of an old ulcer. The condition of intussusception (q.v.), where part of the bowel passes inside of the part beneath it, in the same way as one turns the finger of a glove outside in, causes obstruction and other symptoms. Finally some body, such as a concretion, or the stone of some large fruit, or even a mass of hardened faeces, may become jammed within the bowel and stop up its passage.

Symptoms   There are four chief symptoms of this condition, and any case in which these are combined demands immediate treatment. These are pain, vomiting, constipation and swelling of the abdomen.

Treatment   As a rule the surgeon opens the abdomen, finds the obstruction and relieves it or if possible removes it altogether.

TUMOURS are relatively uncommon in the small intestine and, when they do occur, they are usually benign. Conversely, they are relatively common in the large intestine where they are usually cancerous. The most common site for cancer of the large intestine is the rectum, with the sigmoid, caecum and ascending colon next in order of frequency. It is a disease of the older age-groups, and occurs with equal frequency in men and women. A history of altered bowel habit, in the form of increasing constipation or diarrhoea, or an alternation of these, or of bleeding from the anus, in a middle-aged person is an indication for taking medical advice. If the condition is cancer, then the sooner it is operated on, the better the result.

INTIMA is the innermost coat lining the arteries and the veins.

INTOLERANCE An adverse reaction of a patient to a drug or treatment.

INTOXICATION is a term applied to states of poisoning. The poison may be some chemical substance introduced from outside, e.g. alcohol (see ALCOHOL), or it may be due to the products of bacterial action, the bacteria either being introduced from outside or developing within the body. The term auto-intoxication is applied in the latter case.

INTRACRANIAL is the term applied to structures, diseases, and the like, contained in or rising within the head.

INTRACRANIAL PRESSURE This is the pressure that is maintained by the brain tissue, intracellular and extracellular fluid, cerebrospinal fluid and blood. An increase in intracranial pressure may occur as a result of inflammation, injury, haemorrhage, or tumour in the brain tissue as well as of some congenital conditions. The pressure is measured by lumbar puncture in which a syringe attached to a mamometer (pressure-measuring device) is inserted into the cerebrospinal fluid surrounding the lower part of the spinal cord.

INTRATHECAL means within the membranes or meninges which envelop the spinal cord. The intrathecal space, between the arachnoid and the pia mater, contains the cerebrospinal fluid.

INTRAUTERINE CONTRACEPTIVE DEVICE (IUD) A mechanical device, commonly a coil, inserted into the uterus to prevent conception. For many, though not all, women IUDs are an effective and acceptable form of contraception, though only about 10 per cent of women in the UK use them. The devices are of various shapes and made of plastic or copper; most have a string that passes through the cervix and rests in the vagina. (See CONTRACEPTION.)

INTRAVENOUS A term which means inside a vein. An intravenous injection is one that is given into a vein. Blood transfusions are given intravenously, as are other infusions of fluid.

INTRAVENOUS UROGRAM A procedure for getting X-ray pictures of the urinary tract. A radio-opaque medium is injected into a vein and, when it is excreted by the kidneys, the substance can be identified on X-rays. Any abnormalities in structure or foreign bodies such as calculi are outlined by the dye.

INTROSPECTION is the observation of one's own thoughts or feelings. It is generally applied to this process when it occurs to an abnormal extent in association with melancholia.

INTUBATION is a simple operation consisting in the introduction, through the mouth into the larynx, of a tube designed to keep the air passage open at this point.

INTUITION The immediate understanding of a situation by someone without the customary mental process of reasoning.

INTUSSUSCEPTION is a form of obstruction of the bowels in which part of the intestine enters within that part immediately beneath it. This can best be understood by observing what takes place in the fingers of a tightly fitting glove as they turn outside in when the glove is pulled off the hand. The people affected are almost always infants. The cause is not known. The point at which it most often occurs is the junction between the small and the large intestines, the former passing within the latter. The symptoms are those of intestinal obstruction in general, and in addition there is often a discharge of blood-stained mucus from the bowel. The treatment consists – unless the symptoms rapidly subside, when it may be assumed that the bowel has righted itself – of either hydrostatic reduction by means of a barium enema, or an operation. At operation the intussusception is either reduced or, if this not possible, the obstructed part is cut out and the ends of the intestine then stitched together. If treated adequately and in time, the mortality is now reduced to around 1 per cent.

INVASION The entry of bacteria into the body. The spread of cancer into normal, nearby tissues or organs.

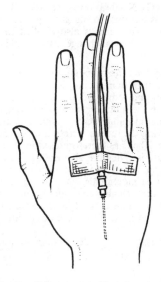

Position of intravenous needle inserted into vein on back of hand for administration of intravenous fluid or blood transfusion.

IN VITRO is a term commonly used in medical research and experimental biology. Literally 'in a glass', it refers to observations made outside the body: e.g. on the action of drugs on bacteria. The opposite term is IN VIVO, which refers to observations of processes in the body.

IN VITRO FERTILIZATION (IVF) Fertilization of the egg outside the body. The fertilized ovum is then incubated until the blastocyst stage develops when it is implanted into the uterus. The procedure was developed in Britain and the first successful in vitro baby, a girl, was born in 1978. IVF is used when a woman has blocked fallopian tubes or when the sperm and ovum are unable to fuse in the reproductive tract. Hormone treatment results in the potential mother's producing several mature ova, some of which are removed from the ovary using a laparoscope and fertilized with her partner's semen.

IN VIVO A Latin term to describe biological events that take place inside the bodies of living organisms.

INVOLUCRUM is the term applied to the sheath of new bone which is formed round a piece of dead bone in, for example, osteomyelitis.

INVOLUNTARY MUSCLE Muscle that does not operate under a person's conscious control. Involuntary muscle, also called smooth muscle because the cells do not contain the striations that occur in voluntary muscle (q.v.), is found in blood vessels, the heart, stomach, and intestines.

INVOLUTION is the process of change whereby the uterus returns to its resting size after parturition. The term is also applied to any retrograde biological change, as in senility.

IODIDES are salts of iodine, those which are especially used in medicine being the iodide of potassium and iodide of sodium. Iodides are excreted in the mucus secretions, as well as in the urine, saliva and sweat, and have an action in liquefying the mucus secretion of the bronchial tree. They are therefore used in expectorant mixtures. They are also used to assist in providing a supply of iodine in patients with goitre, or in individuals who live in an area where goitre is liable to occur because of a deficiency of iodine in the drinking water. They may be given in the form of iodized salt. (See GOITRE.)

Over-dosage of iodides results in iodism (q.v.).

IODINE is a non-metallic element which is found largely in seaweed. The body contains about 30 mg, largely concentrated in the thryoid gland where it is used to synthesize thyroid hormones. Iodine has a highly irritating action and when applied to the skin, stains the latter dark brown and causes it to peel off in flakes, while internally it is a violent irritant poison in large doses.

Externally iodine is used as an antiseptic. Its drawback is that it is fixed by protein, which reduces its antiseptic efficiency in open wounds. Its main use in this sphere therefore is for sterilizing the unbroken skin, as before an operation. Radioactive iodine is used for diagnosing and treating disease of the thyroid gland.

IODISM is the condition which is produced by an over-dose of iodides, but in some susceptible individuals iodism may be produced by very small amounts of iodides. It is characterized by running of the eyes and nose, sore throat, a heavy, dull feeling over the eyes, increased secretion of saliva and a typical skin eruption. These manifestations usually disappear rapidly upon the drugs being withdrawn.

ION EXCHANGE RESINS are synthetic organic substances, capable of exchanging ions – cationic or anionic – from the contents of the intestine. Originally used in the prevention of oedema (q.v.), they have been superseded in this role by the modern diuretics (q.v.), and are now used chiefly in the treatment of hyperkalaemia (q.v.). They are usually taken by mouth or as an enema.

IONIZATION means the breaking up of a substance in solution into its constituent ions.

IPECACUANHA, IPECAC, or HIPPO, is the root of *Cephaëlis ipecacuanha*, a Brazilian shrub. It contains an alkaloid, emetine, which acts as an irritant when brought in contact with the interior of the stomach, producing vomiting. This effect is also brought about after its absorption into the blood by its action on the vomiting centre in the brain. In small doses it acts, not as an irritant, but as a gentle stimulant to the mucous membrane of the stomach, bowels and respiratory passages. Emetine was for long the great stand-by in the treatment of amoebic dysentery.

Uses Ipecacuanha is a constituent of many expectorant mixtures given in the treatment of bronchitis. It is of value in this connection because of its action in liquefying the thick mucous secretion which occurs in bronchitis. Syrup of ipecacuanha is the treatment of choice for evacuating the stomach in young children who have swallowed a poison.

IPRATROPIUM is a bronchodilator drug of value in the treatment of asthma, bronchitis and rhinitis.

IRIDECTOMY The operation by which a hole is made in the iris, as, for example, in the treatment of glaucoma (q.v.) or as part of cataract surgery (q.v.).

IRIDENCLEISIS was an operation formerly used in the treatment of glaucoma. It has now been replaced by trabeculectomy (see GLAUCOMA).

IRIDOLOGY is the study of the iris (see EYE). It is an old practice dating back to the days of Aristotle, which has been revived in recent days as one of the more exotic branches of what is popularly known as 'fringe medicine'. By its exponents it is defined as 'diagnosis through photography of the iris', and extravagant, as yet unsupported, claims are made for its validity.

IRIS (see EYE).

IRITIS (see UVEITIS).

IRON is a metal which is an essential constituent of the red blood corpuscles, where it is present in the form of haemoglobin. It is also present in muscle, myoglobin, and in certain respiratory pigments which are essential to the life of many tissues in the body. Iron is absorbed principally in the upper part of the small intestine. It is then stored: mainly in the liver; to a lesser extent in the spleen and kidneys, where it is available, when required, for use in the bone marrow to form the haemoglobin in red blood corpuscles. The daily iron requirement of an adult is 15 to 20 milligrams. This requirement is increased during pregnancy. Iron salts also have an astringent action, especially the chloride, and this property is sometimes made use of when it is used as a styptic to check bleeding.
Uses The main use of iron is in the treatment of iron-deficiency anaemias. (See ANAEMIA.) The main form in which it is used is ferrous sulphate. Iron preparations sometimes cause irritation of the gastro-intestinal tract, and should therefore always be taken after meals. They sometimes produce a tendency towards constipation. Whenever possible, iron preparations should be given by mouth. It is a very small proportion indeed of cases of iron-deficiency anaemia which will not respond satisfactorily to iron given by mouth. For the occasional cases in which oral administration is not suitable, a preparation of iron is now available which can be given intravenously.

IRRADIATION is treatment by various forms of light and radiant activity.

IRRIGATION is the method of washing out wounds, or cavities of the body, like the bladder and bowels. (See DOUCHE; ENEMA.)

IRRITABLE BOWEL SYNDROME is a motility disorder of the gut. It is not confined to the large intestine so that the terms spastic colon or irritable colon are inaccurate. Some of the symptoms of the irritable bowel syndrome affect more than 10 per cent of the normal adult population, but most people accept these symptoms as a minor nuisance. Only those with severe symptoms or those who worry about their symptoms consult a doctor.
Symptoms Abdominal pain is the commonest symptom and it frequently moves from one area of the abdomen into another. A disturbed bowel habit is also common and this may alternate between diarrhoea and constipation. A feeling of abdominal distension is common, as is heartburn. Some patients suffer from painless, watery diarrhoea. The symptoms are either due to abnormal motility of the gut or to increased intestinal sensitivity to distension. The pain can, in fact, often be produced in patients by balloon inflation within the colon or other parts of the gut. The symptoms frequently start after an acute intestinal infection, and acute psychological stresses can also influence the activity of the bowel.
Treatment requires reassurance and explanation of the functional nature of the disorder. Anticholinergic drugs inhibit colonic motor activity and mebeverine has a direct relaxant effect on intestinal smooth muscle. Antidiarrhoeal drugs such as codeine phosphate reduce the frequency and urgency of defaecation. Lomotil is an effective alternative. Bulking agents speed colonic transit and allow the passage of softer, bulkier motions. High-fibre diets are beneficial.

ISCHAEMIA means bloodlessness of a part of the body, due to contraction, spasm, constriction or blocking (by embolus or by thrombus) of the arteries: for example, of the heart.

ISCHAEMIC HEART DISEASE (see CORONARY THROMBOSIS).

ISCHIO-RECTAL ABSCESS is an abscess arising in the space between the rectum and ischial bone and often resulting in a fistula.

ISCHIUM is the bone which forms the lower and hinder part of the pelvis. It bears the weight of the body in sitting.

ISHIHARA'S TEST A test for colour vision, introduced by a Japanese doctor, comprising several plates with round dots of different colours and sizes. It is also the name of a type of blood test for syphilis.

ISLETS OF LANGERHANS: Groups of specialized cells distributed throughout the pancreas (q.v.), that produce three hormones, insulin (q.v.), glucagon, and somatostatin.

ISOCARBOXAZID is a monoamine-oxidase inhibitor antidepressive drug. (See ANTIDEPRESSANTS).

ISO-IMMUNIZATION is the immunization of one member of a species by an antigen lacking in himself but present naturally in other members of the species, as, for example, the immunization of an Rh-negative mother by an Rh-positive fetus, the mother as a result producing anti-Rh agglutinins which injure the fetus. (See also HAEMOLYTIC DISEASE OF THE NEW-BORN; BLOOD GROUPS.)

ISOLATION in infectious diseases is an important procedure, applied both to people who are themselves sick and to those who have come in contact with them, technically known as contacts or suspects, and who may later develop the disease. (See INCUBATION; INFECTION; QUARANTINE.)

ISOLEUCINE One of the essential aminoacids, which are fundamental components of all proteins. It cannot be synthesized by the body and so must be obtained from the diet.

ISOMETRIC Of similar measurement. Isometric exercises are based on the isometric contraction of the muscles. Fibres are provoked into working by pushing or pulling an immovable object but this technique prevents them from shortening in length. These exercises improve a person's fitness and builds up his or her muscle strength.

ISONIAZID is one of the anti-tuberculous drugs. It has the advantages of being relatively non-toxic and of being active when taken by mouth. Unfortunately, like streptomycin, it may render the *Mycobacterium tuberculosis* resistant to its action. This tendency to produce resistance is considerably reduced if it is given in conjunction with streptomycin and/or para-aminosalicylic acid.

ISOPRENALINE is an inotropic sympathomimetic drug which is used as a short-term emergency treatment of heart block (q.v.) or severe bradycardia (q.v.).

ISOTONIC is a term applied to solutions which have the same power of diffusion as one another. An isotonic solution used in medicine is one which can be mixed with body fluids without causing any disturbance. An isotonic *saline solution* for injection into the blood, so that it may possess the same osmotic pressure as the blood serum, is one of 0·9-per-cent strength or containing 9 grams of sodium chloride to 1 litre of water. This is also known as *normal* or *physiological salt solution*. An isotonic solution of *bicarbonate of soda* for injection into the blood is one of 1·35-per-cent strength in water. An isotonic solution of *glucose* for injection into the blood is one of 5-per-cent strength in water.

Solutions which are weaker, or stronger than, the fluids of the body with which they are intended to be mixed are known as hypotonic and hypertonic, respectively.

ISOTOPE This is a form of a chemical element with the same chemical properties as other forms but which has a different atomic mass. It contains an identical number of positively charged particles called protons, in the nucleus, giving it the same atomic number, but the numbers of neutrons differ. A radioactive isotope is one that decays into other isotopes and in doing so emits alpha, beta or gamma radiation.

Applications of radioactive isotopes to diagnosis The use of radioactive isotopes in diagnosis is based on the fact that it is possible to tag many of the substances normally present in the body with a radioactive label. Because it is possible to detect minute quantities of radioactive material, only very small doses may be given. The body pool of the material is therefore not appreciably altered, and metabolism is not disturbed. Thus in studies of iodine metabolism the ratio of radioactive atoms administered to stable atoms in the body pool is of the order of 1 to 1,000 million. By measuring radioactivity in the body, in blood samples, or in the excreta it is possible to gain information about the fate of the labelled substance, and hence of the chemically identical inactive material. Hence it is theoretically possible to trace the absorption, distribution and the excretion of any substance normally present in the body, provided that it can be tagged with a suitable radioactive label.

If the investigation necessitates tracing the path of the material through the body by means of external counting over the body surface it is obviously essential to use an isotope that emits gamma radiation or positrons. If, however, only measurements on blood sample or excreta are required it is possible to use pure beta emitters. Whole-body counters measure the total radioactivity in the body, and these are of great value in absorption studies.

Five main groups of diagnostic uses may be defined:

(1) METABOLIC STUDIES The use of radioactive materials in metabolic studies is based on the fundamental property that all isotopes of an element are chemically identical. The radioactive isotope is used as a true isotope tracer – that is, when introduced into the body (in whatever form) it behaves in the same way as the inactive element. For example, isotopes of iodine are used to measure thyroid function, and isotopes of calcium enable kinetic studies of bone formation and destruction to be performed.

(2) ABSORPTION AND DISTRIBUTION STUDIES The fate of labelled substances given by mouth can be followed to assess their absorption, utilization and excretion. In most of these studies the

isotope is a true isotope tracer. For example, iron absorption can be measured with radioactive iron; vitamin-B_{12} absorption may be investigated with vitamin B_{12} tagged with radioactive cobalt.

(3) BODY COMPOSITION BY DILUTION STUDIES   By introducing an isotope into a compartment, such as the blood or extracellular space, it is possible to measure the volume of that compartment by determining the dilution of radioactivity when equilibrium has been reached.

(4) PHYSICAL TRACING STUDIES   In this type of study the isotope is not necessarily used as a true isotopic tracer. In other words, it does not trace the path of the corresponding inactive isotope. For example, xenon-133 is used in measurements of blood flow in muscles, and in lung-function studies; krypton-85 is used to detect intracardiac shunts. Neither of these elements is normally present in the body. The survival of red cells may be followed and the organ of sequestration revealed by labelling red cells with radioactive chromium.

(5) SCANNING OF ORGANS AND TISSUES   Scanning is a technique which is used to determine the distribution of radioactive isotopes within the body or within one particular organ. In the conventional scanner the radiation detector, which is a scintillation counter, 'sees' only a small cross-sectional area of the body at a time. The activity 'seen' at each point is registered, and a 'map' of the activity seen over the scanned area is recorded. Various methods of presentation have been used, and the recently improved display systems present the information gathered by the scanner more effectively. More recent developments are stationary detectors such as the gamma camera, auto-fluoroscope, and other devices which can view the whole of the area simultaneously. Thus when selective concentration of an isotope in a tissue occurs it is possible to examine the distribution of that isotope by means of scanning. A toxic nodule in the thyroid may be identified by its selective concentration of iodine-131. Areas of absent function on the radioactive scan ('cold' areas) suggest the presence of tumours, abscesses, and similar lesions. Iodine-131 may be used to localize tumours of the thyroid, and chlormerodrin labelled with mercury-197 to delineate tumours of the kidneys. Of even greater practical application is the localizing of brain tumours with human serum albumin labelled with iodine-131 or with radioactive technetium.

Treatment   Radioactive isotopes are also used in medical treatment. The overactivity of the thyroid gland in thyrotoxicosis can be treated by the ingestion of radioactive iodine. The ingested iodine is taken up by the thyroid gland where local irradiation of the gland takes place, reducing its activity. Radioactive phosphorus is used in the treatment of polycythemia rubra vera. It is largely taken up in bone as this is the main source of body phosphate and irradiation of the bone marrow results, controlling the overactivity that is characteristic of polycythemia

rubra vera. In cobalt teletherapy the isotope cobalt 60 is used to deliver 1·2–1·3-million-volt radiation which is equivalent to X-rays generated at a peak voltage of 3–4-million-volts. (See RADIOTHERAPY.)

ISSUE is an old term for a suppurating sore.

ITCH is a popular name for scabies (q.v.).

ITCHING, or PRURITUS, is a common and unpleasant condition of the skin, which induces scratching. It may be localized, in which case the cause is often easily identified, or generalized, when the diagnosis may be much harder. In all cases a careful history and appropriate investigations should be taken, to exclude both easily treated exogenous causes, such as occupational or domestic irritants, or scabies, and more serious systemic conditions, such as diabetes mellitus (q.v.), thyroid dysfunction, or liver disease (q.v.). Kidney disease (q.v.) and polycythaemia should be considered; infections such as threadworm should be sought in cases of pruritus ani (itching around the anus), and vaginal infections such as candidiasis or trichomonas in pruritus vulvae (vaginal itching). Fungal infections (q.v.) such as athlete's foot, often aggravated by a warm, moist atmosphere, should be considered, and the importance of psychological factors should not be forgotten.

Treatment   After the identification and removal of any exogenous causes, using antibiotics if appropriate, attention should be focused on any underlying systemic disease; improved diabetic control has a remarkable antipruritic effect. Otherwise, the mainstay of treatment is one of increased hygiene, and the use of soothing applications such as calamine lotion and emulsifying ointment. Soap should be used as little as possible, and after washing careful drying and application of talcum powder are helpful. In persistent or severe cases, weak topical corticosteroids (q.v.) may offer some relief.

-ITIS is a suffix added to the name of an organ to signify any diseased condition of that organ.

IVORY, or DENTINE, is the hard material which forms the chief bulk of the teeth. (See TEETH.)

J

JACKSONIAN EPILEPSY (see EPILEPSY).

JAUNDICE is a yellow discoloration of the skin due to the deposition of bile pigment in its deeper layers. (See also HEPATITIS.)

Causes Jaundice is caused by four broad categories of disease: prehepatic (unconjugated hyperbilirubinaemia); hepatitis (caused by various viruses); intra- or extrahepatic obstructive jaundice; chronic liver disease. Poisons and some drugs may also cause jaundice. Prehepatic causes of jaundice are haemolytic – resulting from the pathological breakdown of red blood cells – and defects in the processing of bilirubin (bile pigment).

When the bile cannot escape into the intestine in the usual way, it is absorbed by the blood- and lymph-vessels, and some of its constituents are deposited in the various tissues throughout the body. Some obstruction to the outflow of bile is therefore a necessary condition, and this obstruction may either exist in the bile-ducts, which convey the bile from liver to intestine, or it may be caused by some disorganization in the liver (e.g. hepatitis) which prevents the bile, formed by the liver-cells, from finding its way to the bile-ducts at all. The tint of the jaundice has not necessarily any direct relation to the severity of the cause. Obstruction may be due to gall-stones, and the resulting jaundice is then a symptom of this condition. (See GALL-BLADDER, DISEASES OF.) Obstruction may be due to some cause quite outside the liver and bile-ducts, for example, enlarged glands lying near the liver or cancer of the pancreas, the seriousness of the jaundice depending then upon the seriousness of the disease responsible for the pressure. Cirrhosis of the liver, in which the small branches of the bile-duct become compressed by the formation of fibrous tissue, may also be a cause of chronic jaundice. (See CIRRHOSIS.)

Viral hepatitis is a loosely used term to describe infection with one of the hepatotropic viruses. These are hepatitis A (HAV), B (HBV), Delta (HDV) and C (HCV) (see HEPATITIS). Among other viruses that can cause hepatitis are Epstein-Barr virus (q.v.), cytomegalovirus (q.v.) and some 'tropical viruses'.

Neonatal jaundice is a form of jaundice not uncommon in the newborn infant. It is due to temporary inability to deal with the normal metabolism of bilirubin and usually passes off in a few days. If it should persist, however, or become severe, it requires treatment. (See also BILIRUBIN; HAEMOLYTIC DISEASE OF THE NEWBORN; KERNICTERUS.)

Symptoms Yellowness, appearing first in the whites of the eyes and later over the whole skin, is the symptom that attracts notice. This tint varies from a pale sulphur-yellow through all gradations to a deep olive or bronze colour, according to the completeness of the obstruction and the length of time the jaundice has lasted. The urine passed is of a dark greenish-brown colour, owing to the excretion of bile by the kidneys. Various digestive disturbances are present: the tongue is furred, the appetite poor, and a feeling of sickness is often felt, and is aggravated by eating fats. The stools are of a grey or white colour, owing to the want of bile in the intestine.

Treatment The first essential is to treat the underlying cause if possible: for instance, gallstones, if these be the cause of the jaundice. Comprehensive laboratory investigations may be necessary. Supportive measures are required, but traditional measures such as bed rest and special diets do not seem to help.

JAW is the name applied to the bones that carry the teeth. The two upper jaw-bones, the maxillae, are firmly fixed to the other bones of the face. The lower jaw, the mandible, is shaped somewhat like a horseshoe, and, after the first year of life, consists of a single bone. It forms a hinge-joint with the squamous part of the temporal bone, immediately in front of the ear. Both upper and lower jaw-bones possess deep sockets, known as alveoli, which contain the roots of the teeth. (See DISLOCATIONS; FRACTURES; GUMBOIL; MOUTH; TEETH.)

JEJUNUM is part of the small intestine. (See INTESTINE.)

JELLY (see GELATIN).

JERK A sudden involuntary movement. The term is often used to describe the tendon reflexes.

JOINT-MOUSE is a popular term for a loose body in a joint. It is found especially in the knee. (See JOINTS, DISEASES OF.)

JOINTS A joint or articulation is the meeting-place between different parts of the skeleton, whether bones or cartilages.

Structure The great division of joints is into those which are fixed or relatively fixed (*fibrous* and *cartilaginous joints*), and those at which free movement can take place (*synovial joints*). In the former, a layer of cartilage or of fibrous tissue intervenes between the bones and binds them firmly together. This type of joint is exemplified by the sutures between the bones that make up the skull. Among these fixed joints, some have a thick disc of fibro-cartilage between the bones, so that, although the individual joint is really capable of very little movement, a series of these, like the joints between the bodies of the vertebrae, gives to the spinal column, as a whole, a flexible character (amphiarthrodial joint).

All movable joints involve four structures. These are the bones whose junction forms the

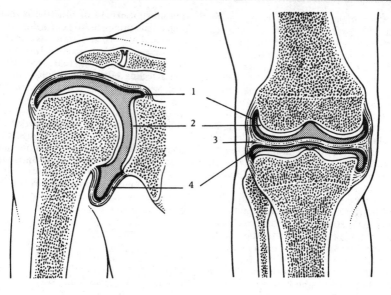

1 synovial membrane
2 articular cartilage
3 articular disc
4 capsule

Diagram of synovial joints. (Left) A right shoulder joint (simple synovial) from the front. (Right) Right knee joint (synovial with articular disc) from the front.

joint; a layer of cartilage covering the end of each of these and rendering the ends smooth; a sheath of fibrous tissue known as the capsule, thickened at various points into bands or ligaments, which hold the bones together; and, finally, a membrane known as synovial membrane, which lines this capsule and produces a synovial fluid to lubricate the movements of the joint. Further, the bones are kept in position at the joints by the various muscles passing over them and by atmospheric pressure. This type of joint is known as a synovial joint.

Some joints possess subsidiary structures, such as discs of fibro-cartilage, which adapt the ends of the bones more perfectly to one another in places where these do not quite correspond. In others, movable pads of fat under the synovial membrane fill up larger cavities and afford additional protection to the joint.

Varieties Apart from the main division of joints into those which are fixed and those which are movable, the movable joints fall into several groups. Gliding joints are those in which, like the wrist and ankle, the bones have flat surfaces capable of only a limited amount of movement. In hinge-joints, like the elbow and knee, the chief movement takes place round one axis. The ball-and-socket type is exemplified by the shoulder and hip, in which free movement is possible in any direction. There are other subsidiary varieties, named according to the shape of the bones which enter into the joint.

JOINTS, DISEASES OF 'Rheumatism' describes the non-specific symptoms arising from the tissue of the musculoskeletal system, comprising joints, ligaments, tendons and muscles. 'Arthritis' means pathological disorder of the system. Sprains of ligaments, strains of tendons and muscle, bursitis (q.v.), tendinitis (q.v.) and non-specific back pain are very common: for example, at any time about 20 per cent of people will have back pain and 80 per cent will have it at some time in their lives. Rheumatic symptoms may arise from over-use of healthy tissues (sports injuries) or from normal tissue being subjected to unusual strain; the 'weekend professional' problem of relatively unfit individuals lifting awkwardly. Back disorders are not well understood; chronic back pain in particular is linked to emotional problems such as stress and depression. The intervertebral disc has a soft centre, the nucleus pulposus, which may prolapse through an acquired defect in the ring of fibrous cartilage around it. Over the age of about 40 this nucleus is firmer and less likely to prolapse, so 'slipped disc' is really a young adult's problem. However, once the disc has prolapsed, the segment of the back is never quite the same again, as degeneration (osteoarthritis) develops in the adjacent facet joints. The segment will be stiffer and possibly painful, perhaps many years later. 'Sciatica' means pain radiating down the leg in the line of the sciatic nerve. Its rarer analogue at the front of the leg is cruralgia, radiating down the femoral nerve. Leg pain with back pain may not be true nerve pain but be referred from arthritis in the spinal facet joints. In all, only about 5 per cent of cases of back pain are accompanied by true sciatica and spinal surgery is most successful (about 85 per cent) in this group. It is much less successful when the complaint is of pain alone. Manipulation by properly trained practitioners, whether doctors, physiotherapists, osteopaths or chiropractors, can relieve symptoms temporarily and this may be sufficient to shorten the period of disability, but makes little difference to the ultimate outcome. Sprains and strains are treated effectively by rest, cold compresses and progressive rehabilitation.

DEGENERATIVE ARTHRITIS, more specifically called osteoarthritis (OA), rarely starts before the age of 40, but affects 80 per cent of the population by the age of 80. It consists of alteration in the structure and function of the articular cartilage, but also affects the collagenous matrix – the main structural substance – of tendons and ligaments. It is not purely 'wear and tear'. There are various sub-groups with a genetic component. Localized alteration in anatomy, such as a fracture or infection of a joint, will precipitate early OA. Reactive new bone growth, causing sclerosis beneath the joint and osteophytes – outgrowth of bone – at the margins of the joint is characteristic. The first metatarsal (great toe) joint, spinal facet joints, the knee, the base of the thumb and the terminal finger joints (Heberden's nodes) are the commonest sites.

The course of OA is slow but variable, with periods of pain and low-grade inflammation. Acute inflammation, especially of the knee, can be due to release of crystals of a chemical called pyrophosphate, causing *pseudo-gout*.

URATE GOUT is caused by uric acid (q.v.) crystallizing out in joints, against a background of hyperuricaemia – a high concentration of uric acid in the blood – which is contributed to by a mixture of genetic and environmental influences, such as excess dietary purines (compounds containing nitrogen), alcohol or diuretic drugs.

INFLAMMATORY ARTHRITIS is much less common, but potentially much more serious. There are several types:

Spondylarthritis This tends to affect younger men, with involvement of spinal and lower limb joints but especially with inflammation and often eventual ossification of the enthesis, which is where ligaments and tendons are inserted into the bone around joints. There is an association with skin (especially psoriasis), bowel and genitourinary inflammation and, in some instances, actual infection in the latter organs (such as dysentery). The syndromes most clearly delineated are ankylosing (see SPINE AND SPINAL CORD, DISEASES AND INJURIES OF), psoriatic or colitic spondylitis and Reiter's syndrome (q.v.). The diagnosis is made clinically and radiologically. There is no association with autoantibodies (q.v.). The clearest genetic association is in ankylosing spondylitis, for which a particular gene locus, HLA B27, has been identified. Psoriasis can also be associated with a characteristic peripheral arthritis.

SYSTEMIC AUTOIMMUNE RHEUMATIC DISEASES The commonest is *Rheumatoid arthritis (RA)*, characterized by lymphoid synovitis, which causes acute inflammation and also chronic erosion of the cartilage and associated bone of joints and soft tissues. Fibrosis follows, causing deformity. Autoantibodies against immunoglobulins (see IMMUNITY) are universal, of which the best known is IgM-anti-IgG (Rheumatoid Factor). Genetic factors are important in allowing the disease to be chronic and severe. RA can be complicated by Sjogren's syndrome, with inflammation of mucosal glands, producing, for example, dry mouth and eyes.

Systemic lupus erythematosus (SLE) (q.v.) and *systemic sclerosis* (diffuse scleroderma and localized sclerodactyly), *dermatomyositis* and various *overlap syndromes* Autoantibodies against nuclear proteins such as DNA (q.v.) are involved in inflammation caused by deposits of immune complexes and vasculitis (q.v.) in various tissues, such as kidney, brain, skin and lungs. There is a wide variety of resulting symptoms and sometimes organ failure.

Juvenile chronic arthritis The commonest form is juvenile chronic pauciarticular arthritis, which is relatively limited and benign, but systemic Still's disease, juvenile rheumatoid arthritis, psoriatic arthritis and dermatomyositis (q.v.) are all potentially crippling and may be fatal..

INFECTIVE ARTHRITIS includes *septic arthritis*, an uncommon, but potentially fatal disease if not diagnosed and treated early with appropriate antibiotics. Causative organisms include tubercle bacilli (q.v.) and staphylococci (q.v.). Susceptible people include the immunologically vulnerable such as children, the elderly, patients with RA and people taking corticosteroids. *Infection-associated arthritis* Rheumatic fever is the best known of this group but is now rare in Western countries. It is characterized by a migratory arthritis, rash and cardiac involvement. It is caused by a reaction to a streptococcal infection (q.v.). Other infections which are associated with arthritis include rubella (q.v.), parvovirus (q.v.) and Lyme disease (q.v.).

Treatment The only type of arthritis that can be cured is septic arthritis. The principles of treatment for the others are to reduce risk factors (such as hyperuricaemia); to suppress inflammation; to restore function with physiotherapy, and, in the event of joint failure, to perform surgical arthroplasty. Non-steroidal anti-inflammatory drugs (NSAIDs) (q.v.) include aspirin, indomethacin and many other more recently developed ones. They all carry a risk of toxicity, such as renal dysfunction or gastro-intestinal irritation, with haemorrhage, especially in the elderly. More powerful suppression of inflammation requires corticosteroids and cytotoxic drugs (q.v.) such as azathioprine, or cyclophosphamide. Current research promises more specific and perhaps less toxic control of inflammatory mediators (compounds which are involved in the process of inflammation) such as the cytokines.

JOULE is the unit of energy in the International System of Units. The official abbreviation is J. 4186·8 J = 1 Calorie (or kilocalorie). (See also CALORIE; APPENDIX 6: WEIGHTS AND MEASURES.)

JUGULAR is a general name for any structure in the neck, but is especially applied to three large veins, the anterior, external and internal jugular veins, which convey blood from the head and neck regions to the interior of the chest.

K

KALA-AZAR is another name for visceral leishmaniasis. (See LEISHMANIASIS.)

KANAMYCIN is an antibiotic derived from *Streptomyces kanamyceticus*. It is active against a wide range of organisms, including *Staphylococcus aureus* and *Mycobacterium tuberculosis*.

KAOLIN or CHINA CLAY, is a smooth white powder consisting of natural white aluminium silicate resulting from the decomposition of minerals containing felspar. It is used as a dusting powder for eczema and other forms of irritation in the skin. It is also used internally in cases of diarrhoea. The dose is 10 ml of Kaolin Mixture, BPC, best taken in water or milk before meals. Talc, French chalk and Fuller's earth are similar silicates.
  Kaolin poultice contains kaolin, boric acid, glycerin and various aromatic substances.

KAOLINOSIS is a form of pneumoconiosis (q.v.) caused by the inhaling of clay dust.

KAPOSI'S SARCOMA Once a very rare disease in Western countries, though more common in Africa, it is now a feature of AIDS (q.v.). It is a condition in which malignant skin tumours develop, originating from the blood vessels. The tumours form purple lumps which customarily start on the feet and ankles, then spread up the legs and develop on the arm and hands. In AIDS the sarcoma appears in the respiratory tract and gut and it causes serious bleeding. Radiotherapy normally cures mild cases of Kaposi's sarcoma but severely affected patients will need anti-cancer drugs to check the tumour's growth.

KAWASAKI DISEASE is a disease of childhood of unknown origin, which was first described in Japan but has now spread to Europe. It most commonly occurs between the ages of 6 months and 2 years, and is characterized by high fever, conjunctivitis (see EYE DISEASES), skin rashes, and swelling of the glands in the neck. In most cases there is complete and spontaneous recovery. Arteritis is however a common complication and results in the development of coronary artery aneurysms in 20 to 60 per cent of cases. These aneurysms and myocardial infarction are commonly detected after the second week of the illness.

KELOID is an overgrowth of fibrous tissue, usually on the site or scar of a previous injury. The chest and neck are susceptible and keloids may have a genetic basis as it is more common in negroid people. It gets its name from its claw-like off-shoots which pucker up the surrounding skin. It is sometimes painful, sometimes painless. It is much commoner in coloured than in white people. The most effective form of treatment is by injection of corticosteroids (q.v.) directly into the abnormal tissue. Radiotherapy may help. If this fails, surgical excision may be required, though not always successful.

KERATIN is the substance of which horn and the surface layer of the skin are composed.

KERATITIS (see EYE DISEASES).

KERATOMALACIA Softening of the cornea due to a severe vitamin A deficiency (see EYE DISEASES).

KERATOPLASTY Technical term for corneal graft.

KERATOSIS is a disease of the skin characterized by overgrowth of the horny layer of the skin (q.v.). It is induced by exposure to sunshine and in temperate climates usually develops in older people. In sunnier areas it may develop much earlier particularly in sun-bathing enthusiasts who repeatedly over-expose their skin to the sun. It takes the form of firm, dry adherent scales with redness of the surrounding skin and patchy pigmentation of the skin exposed to sunlight. Treatment, and prevention, consist of avoiding over-exposure to the sun.

KERION is a suppurating form of ringworm (q.v.).

KERNICTERUS is the staining with bile of the basal nuclei of the brain, with toxic degeneration of the nerve cells, which sometimes occurs in HAEMOLYTIC DISEASE OF THE NEWBORN (q.v.).

KERNIG'S SIGN is a sign found in cases of meningitis, consisting in the fact that, whereas a healthy person's thigh can be bent to a right angle with the body when the knee is straight, in cases of meningitis the knee cannot be straightened when the thigh is thus bent, or intense pain is caused to the patient by doing so.

KETOCONAZOLE is an imidazole antifungal drug available for both oral and topical use. It also has an anti-androgen effect which may give rise to gynaecomastia and impotence in men. In view of its potential hepatotoxicity it should not be given orally for trivial infections but reserved for systemic fungal infections.

KETOGENESIS The production of ketones (q.v.) in the body. Abnormal ketogenesis may result in ketosis (q.v.).

KETOGENIC DIET is one containing such an excess of fats that acetone and other *ketone bodies* appear in the urine. It is sometimes used in the treatment of epilepsy and chronic infections of the urinary tract by *Escherichia coli*. In this diet, butter, cream, eggs and fat meat are allowed, whilst sugar, bread and other carbohydrates are cut out as far as possible.

KETONE is another name for acetone or dimethyl ketone. The term, ketone bodies, is applied to a group of substances closely allied to acetone, especially beta-hydroxybutyric acid and acetoacetic acid. These are produced in the body from imperfect oxidation of fats and protein foods, and are found in specially large amount in severe cases of diabetes mellitus. KETONURIA is the term applied to the presence of these bodies in the urine.

KETOPROFEN (see NON-STEROIDAL ANTI-INFLAMMATORY DRUGS).

KETOSIS A condition in which an excessive amount of ketones (q.v.) are produced by the body and these accumulate in the blood stream. The affected person becomes drowsy, suffers a headache, breathes deeply, and may lapse into a coma. The condition results from an unbalanced metabolism of fat, which may occur in diabetes mellitus (q.v.) or starvation.

KEYHOLE SURGERY (see MINIMALLY INVASIVE SURGERY).

KIDNEY, ARTIFICIAL (see DIALYSIS).

KIDNEYS are a pair of glands situated close to the spine in the upper part of the abdomen. They are on a level with the last dorsal and upper two lumbar vertebrae, and each is, to a great extent, covered behind by the twelfth rib of its own side. They are kept in this position by a quantity of fat and loose connective tissue, in which they are embedded, by the large vessels which supply them with blood, and by the peritoneal membrane stretched over their front surface.

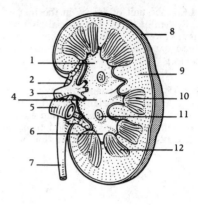

1 calyx minor	7 ureter
2 hilum	8 fibrous capsule
3 renal artery	9 cortex
4 pelvis	10 pyramid
5 renal vein	11 papilla
6 calyx major	12 medulla

Vertical section through the kidney

Structure In size each is about 10 cm (4 inches) long, 6·5 cm (2½ inches) wide, 5 cm (1½ inches) thick and weighs around 140 grams (5 ounces). The size, however, varies a good deal with the development, and probably with the habits of the individual. Kidney mass maintains a remarkably constant ratio to body weight. The left kidney is slightly longer and narrower, and lies a trifle higher in the abdomen than the right.

The kidney in adults presents a smooth exterior, although in early life (as in many animals) it is divided up into distinct lobes, corresponding to the pyramids found in the interior. Enveloping it is a tough fibrous coat, which, in the healthy state, is bound to the kidney only by loose fibrous tissue and by a few blood-vessels that pass between it and the kidney. The outer margin of the kidney is convex, the inner is concave, presenting a deep depression, known as the hilum, where the vessels enter its substance. At the hilum the renal vein lies in front of the renal artery, the former joining the inferior vena cava, and the latter springing from the aorta almost at a right angle. Here, too, is attached the ureter, which conveys urine down to the bladder. The ureter is spread out into an expanded, funnel-like end, known as the pelvis, to which the capsule of the kidney is firmly attached, and which further divides into little funnels known as the calyces. On splitting open a kidney, one finds it to consist of two distinct parts: a layer on the surface, about 4 mm thick, known as the cortex, and a part towards the hilum known as the medulla. The latter consists of pyramids, arranged side by side, with their base on the cortex and their apex projecting into the calyces of the ureter. The apex of each pyramid, of which there are about twelve, is studded with

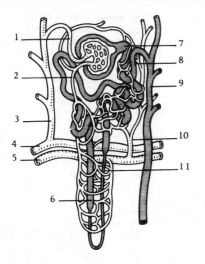

1 afferent arteriole
2 efferent arteriole
3 interlobular artery
4 arcuate artery
5 arcuate vein
6 descending limb of Henle's loop
7 proximal convoluted tubule
8 distal convoluted tubule
9 collecting tubule
10 interlobular vein
11 ascending limb of Henle's loop

Diagram of renal tubules and blood supply of the
kidney.

minute holes, which are the openings of the microscopic uriniferous tubes.

Each pyramid is, in effect, taken together with the portion of cortex lying along its base, an independent little kidney. About a score of small tubes open on the surface of each pyramid, and these, if traced up into its substance, divide again and again so as to form bundles of convoluted tubules, known as medullary rays, passing up towards the cortex. If one of these is traced still further back, it is found, after a very tortuous course, to end in a small rounded body: the Malpighian corpuscle or glomerulus. Each glomerulus and its convoluted tubule is known as a nephron, which constitutes the functional unit of the kidney. Each kidney contains around one million nephrons.

If the blood-vessels are now traced through the kidney their course is found to be as follows. The renal artery splits up into branches, which form arches at the line of junction of cortex and medulla, and from these again spring vessels that run up through the cortex, giving off small branches in every direction. Each of these last ends in a little tuft of capillaries enclosed in a capsule (Bowman's capsule) that forms the end of the uriniferous tubule just described, and capillaries with capsule are known as a glomerulus. After circulating in the glomerulus, the blood emerges by a small vein, which again

splits up into capillaries on the walls of the uriniferous tubules. From these it is collected finally into the renal veins and by them leaves the kidney. By means of the double circulation, first through the glomerulus and then around the tubule, a large amount of fluid is removed from the blood in the glomerulus, and then the concentrated blood passes on to the uriniferous tubule for removal of parts of its solid contents. Other straight arteries come off from the arches mentioned above and supply the medulla direct, the blood from these passing through another set of capillaries and also finally into the renal veins. Although the circulation just described is confined entirely to the kidney, it has certain small connections both by arteries and veins which pass through the capsule and, joining the lumbar vessels, communicate direct with the aorta.

Function The chief function of the kidneys is to separate fluid and certain solids from the blood. Briefly, the glomeruli filter from the blood the non-protein portion of the plasma. As this filtrate passes through the convoluted tubules, varying parts of it are reabsorbed. It is estimated that in 24 hours the total human glomeruli will filter between 150 and 200 litres, 99 per cent of which is reabsorbed by the tubules. The constituents of the filtrate may be grouped according to the extent to which they are reabsorbed by the tubules: (1) substances actively reabsorbed, such as amino-acids, glucose, sodium, potassium, calcium, magnesium and chlorine; (2) substances passing through the tubular epithelium by a simple process of diffusion when their concentration in the filtrate exceeds that in the plasma, such as urea, uric acid, phosphates; (3) substances not returned to the blood from the tubular fluid: e.g. creatine.

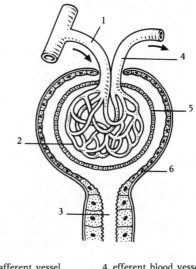

1 afferent vessel   4 efferent blood vessel
2 capillary tuft   5 glomerular capsule
3 tubule   6 capsule

Diagram of glomerulus.

When the kidneys are diseased and the number of glomeruli and tubules decreased in consequence, this alternating action is not so readily carried out, and therefore the work of the diseased kidney becomes increasingly embarrassed. When the blood-vessels of the kidney are partially closed by disease (arteriosclerosis), the general blood-pressure rises with the object of forcing more blood through the kidneys; in consequence, marked changes are produced upon the heart in this type of renal disease.

When the kidneys fail to act, these solid waste substances accumulate in the blood. The general 'poisoning' resulting from failure of renal functions produces the clinical condition known as uraemia (q.v.).

KIDNEYS, DISEASES OF   Diseases of the kidneys may be divided into medical conditions, such as pyelonephritis and glomerulonephritis requiring drugs and supportive treatment, and surgical problems, such as stones and malignancies.

Symptoms suggestive of kidney problems include loin pain associated with obstruction (renal colic) or due to infection, fevers, swelling (oedema), usually of the legs but occasionally including the face and arms, blood in the urine (haematuria), excess quantities of urine (polyuria), including at night (nocturia) due to failure of normal mechanisms in the kidney for concentrating urine. Patients with chronic renal failure often have very diffuse symptoms including nausea and vomiting, tiredness due to anaemia, shortness of breath, skin irritation, pins and needles (paraesthesia) due to damage of the peripheral nerves (peripheral neuropathy) and eventually (rarely seen nowadays) clouding of consciousness leading to coma and death. Many patients with kidney disorders do not have any symptoms, even when the condition is quite advanced.

Signs of kidney disease include loin tenderness, enlarged kidneys, signs of fluid retention, high blood pressure and, in patients with end-stage renal failure, pallor, pigmentation and a variety of neurological signs including absent reflexes, reduced sensation, a coarse flapping tremor (asterixis) due to severe disturbance of the body's normal metabolism and, as noted above, clouded consciousness, often with acidotic breathing, generalized convulsions and coma.

Acute medical conditions include *acute pyelonephritis* caused by direct bacterial invasion of the kidney, presenting with loin pain, fever, an infected urine and occasionally bacteraemia (q.v.) or septicaemia (q.v.). Causative organisms include Gram-negative bacilli (e.g. *E. coli* (q.v.)) or, less likely, a Gram-positive coccus (e.g. micrococcus). Acute pyelonephritis may occur in pregnancy or as a result of a structural abnormality of the urinary tract. Treatment consists of a 10-day course of a broad-spectrum antibiotic to which the organism is sensitive.

In contrast to acute pyelonephritis, *acute glomerulonephritis* is an immune-complex disorder due to entrapment within glomerular capillaries of antigen (usually derived from B haemolytic streptococci) antibody complexes initiating an acute inflammatory response (see IMMUNITY). The disease affects children and young adults, classically presents with a sore throat followed two weeks later by a fall in urine output (oliguria), haematuria, hypertension (q.v.) and mildly abnormal renal function. The disease is self limiting with 90 per cent of patients spontaneously recovering. Treatment consists of control of blood pressure, reduced fluid and salt intake, occasional diuretics (q.v.) and penicillin (q.v.).

Chronic renal conditions include *chronic pyelonephritis* due to chronic bacterial infection of the kidney and *chronic glomerulonephritis* due to immunological renal problems and best classified by taking a renal biopsy. Although chronic renal bacterial infection can occur, for example, secondary to stones or obstruction, the term chronic pyelonephritis is best replaced by *reflux nephropathy* which is defined radiologically (clubbing of calyx (q.v.) of kidney with overlying scar), a condition which develops in childhood due to reflux of urine from bladder to kidney and which leads, if extensive and bilateral, to proteinuria (q.v.), hypertension and renal failure. Reflux nephropathy can be complicated by urinary-tract infections at any stage. The condition is much more common in girls than boys, is the commonest cause of renal failure in children but is a less common cause of renal failure in adults compared with glomerulonephritis, hypertension or diabetes (q.v.) (see below, *Chronic renal failure*). *Chronic glomerulonephritis* may be subdivided into various histological varieties as determined by renal biopsy and includes *minimal change glomerulonephritis, focal and segmental glomerulosclerosis, membranous glomerulonephritis* and *glomerulonephritis associated with crescents on biopsy*. Proteinuria of various degrees is present in all these conditions but the clinical presentation varies greatly from one condition to another. *Minimal-change glomerulonphritis* (normal appearance on light microscopy) is the commonest cause of the nephrotic syndrome (proteinuria, hypoalbuminaemia and oedema) in children. Renal function is usually normal. The condition responds to steroids (q.v.) in short courses but may relapse. Patients with frequent relapses may be treated with the cytotoxic drug cyclophosphomide or the immunosuppressant, cyclosporin. The prognosis is usually excellent even in patients who relapse frequently. The cause of condition is unknown. *Focal glomerulosclerosis* may be initially confused with minimal-change glomerulonephritis since the histological lesions may resemble each other, but later the characteristic glomerular sclerotic lesions appear. The disease affects children and young adults who present with the nephrotic syndrome, often resistant to steroids and progressing into renal failure. The cause is unknown and this condition may recur after renal transplantation. *Focal and segmental glomerulonephritis* (focal nephritis) is the commonest renal histological lesion in adults associated with proteinuria and haematuria. The condition is often discovered coincidentally, e.g., during examination for medical insurance purposes. The histological lesion is characterized by deposits of immunoglobulin A (IgA) (q.v.) in a part of the glomerulus (q.v.) (hence 'IgA nephropathy'). Renal function and blood pressure are usually normal; no treatment has proved of benefit and the prognosis, in the main, is excellent. *Membranous glomerulonephritis* is another histological variety of glomerulonephritis with immune complexes deposited in the glomerulus. Patients present with proteinuria and nephrotic syndrome or rarely, renal failure. The precise cause is unknown but there is an association in a few patients with certain drugs (e.g. gold and penicillamine), infections (e.g. hepatitis B) or malignancies. Treatment of idiopathic membranous glomerulonephritis is controversial: steroids with or without cytotoxic (q.v.) drugs have been given.

Familial renal disorders include autosomal dominant inherited *polycystic kidney disease* and sex-linked *familial nephropathy*. Polycystic kidney disease is an important cause of renal failure in the UK. Patients, usually aged 30 to 50, present with haematuria, hypertension, loin or abdominal discomfort or, rarely, urinary-tract infection. Examination may show hypertension and enlarged kidneys. Diagnosis is based on ultrasound examination of the abdomen. Complications include renal failure, hepatic cysts and, rarely, subarachnoid haemorrhage (q.v.). No specific treatment is available. *Familial nephropathy* occurs more often in boys than girls and commonly presents as Alport's syndrome (familial nephritis with nerve deafness) with proteinuria, haematuria, progressing to renal failure and deafness. The cause of the disease lies in an absence of a specific antigen in a part of the glomerulus. The treatment is conservative, with most patients eventually requiring dialysis or transplantation.

Acute renal failure The origins of this are multiple and the disease most commonly occurs in a hospital setting, often secondary to severe sepsis and hypotension (q.v.) (septic shock (q.v.)) with multiple organ damage including kidneys, liver, lungs and brain. Other causes include severe hypotension secondary to blood loss, muscle damage (rhabdomyolysis), mismatched blood transfusions and certain drugs, notably aminoglycoside antibiotics, cisplatinum or rarely non-steroidal anti-inflammatory drugs. Severely ill patients need to be treated in an intensive-care unit with ventilation and continuous haemodialysis or haemofiltration. Less severely ill patients may be treated with conservative measures only. Despite advances in therapeutic agents, dialysis and mechanical ventilation, the mortality for the more severely ill patients remains around 50 per cent.

Chronic renal failure may result from any renal disorder but common causes include glomerulonephritis, diabetes, polycystic kidney disease, obstruction, hypertension including bilateral renal artery stenosis, reflux nephropathy, systemic lupus erythematosus (q.v.), vasculitis (q.v.) and renal calculus disease. Symptoms include loss of appetite, lassitude, shortness of breath, lethargy, polyuria, ultimately progressing in untreated patients to coma and death. End-stage renal failure develops in approximately 100 patients (aged 20 to 80) per million per year but is higher in certain ethnic populations. Treatment includes control of blood pressure, dietary restriction of protein, potassium and phosphate, control of salt and water balance, acidosis, and secondary hyper-parathyroidism. In most patients, renal failure gradually deteriorates and dialysis or kidney transplantation is needed once the glomerular filtration rate drops to 5 ml/minute or less.

Surgical kidney disease includes stones (calculi) and malignancies. Renal calculi may be formed from calcium phosphate or oxalate, urate, cystine or a combination of calcium, magnesium and ammonium phosphate (triple phosphate or struvite stones). Predisposing factors to stone formation include hyper-parathyroidism (q.v.) and excess excretion of calcium (hypercalciuria), excess ingestion of dietary calcium or protein and inadequate water intake resulting in concentrated urine. *Cystinuria* is an inherited metabolic defect in the renal tubular reabsorption of cystine, ornithine, lysine and arginine. Cystine precipitates in an alkaline urine to form cystine stones. Triple phosphate stones are associated with infection and may develop into a very large branching calculi (staghorn calculi). Stones present as renal or ureteric pain, or as an infection. Treatment has undergone considerable change with the introduction of minimal invasive surgery (q.v.) and the destruction of stone by sound waves (lithotripsy (q.v.)).

The commonest renal malignancy is a *hypernephroma* (q.v.) presenting as haematuria, abdominal or loin pain or as metastatic disease. Tumours of the lining of the pelvicalyceal system (*uroepithelioma*) are much less common but may be a consequence of long-term analgesic abuse. *Nephroblastoma* (Wilms' tumour) occurs in infants and children and may grow to a large size before recognition. Hypernephromas are treated by nephrectomy, uroepitheliomas by either local or more radical resection and radiotherapy, and Wilms' tumour by nephrectomy, radiotherapy and chemotherapy.

KINAESTHETIC SENSATIONS is a term used to describe those sensations which underlie muscle tension and position of joint and muscle. These sensations send impulses along nerves to the brain, and thus inform it of the position of the limb in space and of the relative position to each other of individual muscles and muscle-groups and of joints.

KININS are substances present in the body which are powerful vasodilators (q.v.). They also induce pain and are probably involved in the production of the headache of migraine. In addition, they play a part in the production of allergy (q.v.) and anaphylaxis (q.v.).

KISS OF LIFE (see APPENDIX 1: BASIC FIRST AID).

KLEBSIELLA A Gram-negative bacteria found in the intestinal, respiratory, and urogenital tracts of man and animals. Varieties of the bacteria, which are rod shaped and non-motile, can cause pneumonia and urinary infections.

KLEPTOMANIA is a psychological disorder in which the person afflicted has an irresistible compulsion to steal things, without necessarily having any need for the object stolen.

KLINEFELTER'S SYNDROME The original syndrome described by Klinefelter consisted of gynaecomastia, testicular atrophy and infertility. Intelligence was unimpaired. Cases have been described with associated mental defects and striking tallness of stature but the only constant feature of the syndrome is testicular atrophy with resulting azoospermia and infertility. The atrophy of the testis is the result of a peritubular fibrosis which begins to appear in childhood and progresses until all the seminiferous tubules are replaced by fibrous tissue. Gynaecomastia, mental retardation and eunuchoidism may be associated but the first is inconstant and the two last are infrequent. Most patients with Klinefelter's syndrome have 47 chromosomes instead of the normal 46. The extra chromosome is an X chromosome so that the sex chromosome constitution is XXY instead of XY. Klinefelter's syndrome is one of the most common chromosome abnormalities and occurs in 1 in 300 of the male population. Patients with this syndrome show that the Y chromosome is strongly sex determining. Thus a patient who has an XXY chromosome constitution may have the appearance of a normal male and the only incapacity is infertility. However the loss of a Y chromosome leads to the development of a bodily form which is essentially feminine (see TURNER'S SYNDROME).

KLUMPKE'S PARALYSIS Injury as a result of the stretching of a baby's brachial plexus during its birth may cause partial paralysis of the arm with atrophy of the muscles of the forearm and hand.

KNEE is the joint formed by the femur, tibia and patella (knee-cap). It belongs to the class of hinge-joints, although movements are much more complex than the simple motion of a hinge, the condyles of the femur partly rolling, partly sliding over the flat surfaces on the upper end of the tibia, and the acts of straightening and of bending the limb being finished and begun, respectively, by a certain amount of rotation. The cavity of the joint is very intricate: it consists really of three joints fused into one, but separated in part by ligaments and folds of the synovial membrane. The ligaments which bind the bones together are extremely strong, and include the popliteal and the collateral ligaments, a very strong patellar ligament uniting the patella to the front of the tibia, two cruciate ligaments in the interior of the joint, and two fibro-cartilages which are interposed between the surfaces of tibia and femur at their edge. All these structures give to the knee-joint great strength, so that it is seldom dislocated.

A troublesome condition often found in the knee consists of the loosening of one of the fibro-cartilages lying at the head of the tibia, especially of that on the inner side of the joint. The cartilage may either be loosened from its attachment and tend to slip beyond the edges of the bones, or it may become folded on itself. In either case, it tends to cause locking of the joint when sudden movements are made. This causes temporary inability to use the joint until the cartilage is replaced by forcible straightening, and the accident is apt to be followed by an attack of synovitis, which may last some weeks, causing a certain amount of lameness with pain and tenderness especially felt at a point on the inner side of the knee. This condition can be relieved by an operation – sometimes by key-hole surgery (see MINIMALLY INVASIVE SURGERY) – to remove the loose portion of the cartilage. Patients whose knees are severely affected by osteoarthritis or rheumatoid arthritis which cause pain and stiffness can now have the joint replaced with an artificial one. (See also JOINTS, DISEASES OF.)

KNEE JERK (See REFLEX ACTION).

KNOCK-KNEE, or GENU VALGUM, is a deformity of the lower limbs in such a direction that when the limbs are straightened the legs diverge from one another. As a result, in walking the knees knock against each other. The amount of knock-knee is measured by the distance between the medial malleoli of the ankles, with the inner surfaces of the knee touching and the knee-caps facing forwards. The condition is so common in children between the ages of 2 to 6 years that it may almost be regarded as a normal phase in childhood. When marked, or persisting into later childhood, it can be corrected by surgery (osteotomy).

KOCH'S BACILLUS The original name for *Mycobacterium tuberculosis*, which causes tuberculosis (q.v.) It stems from the name of the German doctor who first identified the bacillus.

KOILONYCHIA is the term applied to nails that are hollow and depressed like a spoon, a condition sometimes associated with chronic iron deficiency.

KOPLIK SPOTS are bluish-white spots appearing on the mucous membrane of the mouth in cases of measles about the third day, and forming the first part of the rash in this disease.

KORSAKOW'S SYNDROME is a form of mental disturbance occurring in chronic alcoholism and other toxic states, such as uraemia, lead poisoning and cerebral syphilis. Its special features are talkativeness with delusions in regard to time and place, the patient, although clear in other matters, imagining that he has recently made journeys or been in distant places.

KREBS CYCLE A series of cellular reactions starting and ending with oxaloacetic acid. Also called the citric acid or tricarboxylic acid cycle, it produces energy in the form of adenosine triphosphate and is the last stage in the biological oxidation of fats, proteins, and carbohydrates. Named after Sir Hans Kreb, a German biochemist working in England in 1900, who won the Nobel Prize for his discovery.

KUPFFER CELLS are the star-shaped cells present in the blood- sinuses of the liver (q.v.). They form part of the reticulo-endothelial system (q.v.) and are to a large extent responsible for the breakdown of haemoglobin into the bile pigments.

KURU is a slowly progressive fatal disease due to spongiform degeneration in the central nervous system, particularly the cerebellum (see BRAIN). It is confined to the Fore people in the Eastern Highlands of New Guinea. It is believed to be due to a slow virus infection acquired from the cannibalistic rite of eating the organs, particularly the brains, of deceased relatives (out of respect). This origin of the disease was suggested by the fact that originally it was a disease of women and children, and it was they who practised this rite. Since the rite was given up, the disease has largely disappeared in children, but still occurs in women as it has an incubation period of up to 20 years.

KWASHIORKOR is one of the most important causes of ill health and death among children in the tropics. It is predominantly a deficiency disease due to a diet deficient in protein. There is also some evidence that there may also be a lack of the so-called essential fatty acids. It affects typically the small child weaned from the breast and not yet able to cope with an adult diet, or for whom an adequate amount of first-class protein is not available, and it is mainly found in the less well-developed countries.

The onset of the disease is characterized by loss of appetite, often with diarrhoea and loss of weight. The child is flabby, the skin is dry, and the hair is depigmented, dry, sparse and brittle. At a later stage oedema develops and the liver is often enlarged. In the early stages the condition responds rapidly to a diet containing adequate first-class protein, but in the later stages this must be supplemented by careful nursing, especially as the child is very liable to infection.

KYPHOSCOLIOSIS: A combination of scoliosis and kyphosis (qq.v.) in which the spine is abnormally curved sideways and forwards. The condition may be the result of several diseases affecting the spinal muscles and vertebrae or it may happen during development for no obvious reason. Although braces may reduce the deformity, an operation may be necessary to correct it.

KYPHOSIS is the term applied to curvature of the spine in which the concavity of the curve is directed forwards. (See SPINE AND SPINAL CORD, DISEASES AND INJURIES OF.)

L

LABETALOL is an alpha- and beta-adrenoceptor blocker (see ADRENERGIC RECEPTORS) which is proving of value in the treatment of high blood-pressure.

LABIA Lips. The labia majora and labia minora are the outer and inner lip-like folds of skin surrounding the entrance to the vagina (see diagrams in REPRODUCTIVE SYSTEM).

LABIUM is the Latin word for a lip or lip-shaped organ.

LABORATORY ANIMAL ALLERGY (see ALLERGY).

LABOUR, or PARTURITION is the process by which the products of conception, normally a fully developed baby, are expelled from the mother's body by regular contractions of the uterus. The onset of labour is difficult to pinpoint accurately, but any one of the following suggests that labour may start soon: the protective mucus plug comes away from the cervix (q.v.) and the mother passes a small amount of blood-stained mucus vaginally – a 'show'. The membranes around the fetus rupture and the mother loses amniotic fluid vaginally. The mother becomes aware of painful contractions of the uterus. When these become regular, labour is said to be 'established'.

Labour is divided into three stages: the first stage is from the onset of labour to full (10 cm) dilation of the opening of the neck of the womb (cervical os). The duration of the first stage is very variable. During the first stage the strength and frequency of the uterine contractions are often measured and the fetal heart rate is monitored frequently. Abnormal responses of the fetal heart during labour can indicate that the baby is suffering from the effects of labour and may need expert assistance to be delivered safely.

The second stage is from full cervical dilation to delivery of the baby. At the onset of this stage the mother usually experiences an irresistible urge to push and a combination of strong co-ordinated uterine contractions and maternal effort gradually moves the baby down the birth canal. The duration of the second stage is variable. The mother can become exhausted by the effort of pushing and, if the second stage is very long, she may need expert assistance from the doctor or midwife. This may mean enlarging the vaginal opening with an episiotomy (cutting the outlet) or applying special obstetric forceps to the baby's head to allow the baby to be pulled out. Sometimes, if no progress is being made in the second stage because the baby's position is unsatisfactory or because the baby is becoming distressed, a Caesarian section (q.v.) may be necessary.

The third stage of labour is from delivery of the baby to delivery of the placenta. This usually occurs within a few contractions. The birth attendant must check that the placenta and membranes are complete as any retained products of conception can lead to serious bleeding or infection later.

LABYRINTH A convoluted system of structures forming the inner ear and involved in hearing and balance.

LACERATION A wound to the skin or surface of an organ which results in a cut with irregular edges (cf. an incision produced with a knife which has smooth, regular edges).

LACHESINE is a mydriatic: i.e. it dilates the pupil of the eye. It is sometimes used for this purpose instead of atropine, as its action is of shorter duration.

LACRIMAL Gland, duct, apparatus (see EYE DISEASES).

LACTATION is the period during which an infant is suckled on the mother's breast. (See BREASTS, DISEASES OF; INFANT FEEDING.)

LACTEAL is a lymphatic vessel that transmits chyle (q.v.) from the intestine. (See LYMPH.)

LACTIC ACID is a colourless, syrupy, sour liquid, which is produced by the action of a bacterium upon lactose. The growth of this organism and consequent formation of lactic acid cause the souring of milk, and the same change takes place to a limited extent when food is long retained in the stomach.

Lactic acid ($CH_3.CHOH.COOH$) is produced in the body during muscular activity, the lactic acid being derived from the breakdown of glycogen. Muscle fatigue is associated with an accumulation of lactic acid in the muscle. Recovery follows when enough oxygen gets to the muscle, part of the lactic acid being oxidized and most of it then being built up once more into glycogen.

LACTIC ACID BACILLI were introduced by Metchnikoff to prepare milk as a special article of diet. The bacilli, which are issued in various forms, are added to fresh milk, allowed to act on it in a warm place for several hours (according to the degree of sourness desired), and the milk is then consumed with the active bacilli. These, after a course of such treatment, come to replace the bacteria naturally found in the intestines, and are supposed to be less injurious to the system. The bacilli, which are harmless, have, in some cases of intestinal disease or of rheumatism, a beneficial action. Buttermilk has a similar effect. (See YOGHURT.)

LACTOSE is the official name for sugar of milk. (See SUGAR.)

LACTOSE INTOLERANCE is a form of indigestion which is much more common in certain coloured races than in white races. It is due to lack in the intestine of the enzyme (q.v.) known as lactase which is responsible for the digestion of lactose, the sugar in milk. In individuals the taking of milk is followed by nausea, a sensation of bloating, or distension, in the gut, abdominal pain and diarrhoea. Such disturbances after taking milk may also be due to the individual's being allergic to milk. Treatment is by means of a low-lactose diet. Foodstuffs high in lactose, such as fresh or powdered milk, and milk puddings should be avoided. Most people subject to it can tolerate fermented milk products and the small amounts of milk used in baking and added to margarine and sausages. In Britain it is said to occur in up to 80 per cent of non-Caucasian adults but only 5 per cent of Caucasian adults.

LACUNA means a small pit or depression.

LAEVULOSE is a sugar which forms one of the constituents of invert sugar. (See SUGAR.)

LAMBLIA (see GIARDIASIS).

LAMELLA is a small disc of glycerin jelly, 3 mm (⅛ inch) in diameter, containing an active drug for application to the eye. It is applied by insertion behind the lower lid.

LAMINECTOMY is an operation in which the arches of one or more vertebrae are removed so as to expose a portion of the spinal cord for removal of a tumour, relief of pressure due to a fracture, or disc protrusion.

LANOLIN is a fat derived from the wool of the common sheep. It is much used for ointments and can occasionally cause local dermatitis. It is very sticky, and for use is mixed generally with an equal quantity of petroleum jelly to make it softer. Lanolin also possesses the valuable property of being able to mix with and absorb water.

LANUGO Soft fine hair covering the fetus. It disappears by the ninth month of gestation and is therefore only seen on premature babies.

LAPAROSCOPE An instrument, consisting, essentially, of a cylinder, an eyepiece and a light source, which is inserted through a small incision into the abdominal cavity (which has already been distended with carbon dioxode gas). The laparoscope allows the contents of the abdominal cavity to be examined without performing a laparotomy (q.v.). Some operations may be performed using the laparoscope to guide the manipulation of instruments inserted through another small incision (e.g. sterilization, cholecystectomy). (See ENDOSCOPE.)

LAPAROSCOPY is a technique by which the contents of the abdomen may be examined, biopsies taken, and minor surgical procedures carried out, by the insertion of a tube through a small hole made in the abdominal wall (see LAPAROSCOPE; ENDOSCOPE). The advances of fibreoptic endoscopy (q.v.) have transformed the management of abdominal disease, particularly gastrointestinal problems.

LAPAROTOMY is a general term applied to any operation in which the abdominal cavity is opened.

LARVA The pre-adult stage in insects and nematodes occurring between the egg and the sexually mature adult.

LARYNGECTOMY is the operation for removal of the larynx. (See APPENDIX 2: ADDRESSES.)

LARYNGITIS, or inflammation of the mucous membrane of the larynx, may be either acute or chronic. This may be due to an infectious cause, most commonly viral but also bacterial, or may be due to voice abuse.
ACUTE LARYNGITIS **Causes** This complaint is usually a concommitant feature of an upper-respiratory-tract infection, usually viral in origin. It may accompany any form of infection of the upper respiratory tract. Excessive use of the

voice, as in loud and prolonged speaking, singing or shouting, may also produce an acute laryngitis. Inhalation of irritating particles in vapours may also lead to acute laryngitis.
Symptoms The main sympton is of hoarseness but there may also be pain in the throat. If there is marked swelling this may narrow the channel for the entrance of air leading to a noisy form of breathing called stridor. There may be some constitutional disturbance in the form of fever, malaise, generalized aches and pains and there may also be some difficulty in swallowing. A cough is a common accompanying symptom. The cough may be dry or may be productive of purulent sputum. The voice is hoarse and the breathing stridulous. The majority of cases of acute laryngitis require early voice rest, perhaps some steam inhalation and symptomatic treatment. Antibiotics are seldom necessary, although these would be prescribed if a bacterial infection were thought to supervene. Acute airway obstruction is an unusual event following laryngitis but, if the airway becomes threatened in any way, immediate specialist referral should be sought.
Treatment Bed rest may be indicated if severe constitutional symptoms are present. The voice should be rested and smoking forbidden. Steam inhalations and warm gargles are often soothing and help reduce mucosal oedema or swelling. Antibiotics should be prescribed if indicated. Some form of airway intervention, either endotracheal intubation or tracheostomy may have to be performed on rare occasions if severe obstruction results.
CHRONIC LARYNGITIS This may occur as a result of repeated attacks of acute laryngitis, excessive use of the voice, tumours, or be secondary to diseases such as tuberculosis and syphilis. The latter two complications are rare but are sometimes manifest as ulceration of the vocal chords and larynx.
Treatment Voice rest is essential. Any aggravating factors should be removed. Antibiotics are indicated if bacterial infection has supervened. Speech therapy is helpful. Patients should stop smoking and avoid polluted environments.
TUBERCULOUS LARYNGITIS is fortunately a rare disease in developed countries and the treatment involves the administration of anti-tuberculous drugs.
TUMOURS may be benign or malignant. Benign tumours or small nodules, such as singer's nodules, may be dealt with by speech therapy or may be removed at the operation of direct laryngoscopy. This is usually performed under general anaesthetic. Cancer of the larynx may be treated either by radiotherapy or by surgery, depending on the extent of the disease. Hoarseness may indeed be the only symptom of vocal cord disturbance or of carcinoma of the larynx and any case of hoarseness which has lasted for 6 weeks should be referred for a specialist opinion. The earlier the diagnosis is made, the more successful the results of treatment are. Laryngectomy clubs are now being established throughout the country to advise and help

patients who have had laryngectomy. Details of these can be obtained from the National Association of Laryngectomee Clubs (see APPENDIX 2: ADDRESSES). An important feature of patients who have undergone laryngectomy is the rehabilitation of their speech and the assistance of a speech therapist is essential.

Other abnormalities of voice may be caused by paralysis of either of the vocal cords. This may be a congenital problem or may be the result of pressure upon the recurrent laryngeal nerve by aneurysm or tumour or the nerve may be damaged in operations on the chest and neck. The symptom in this condition is one of weakness of the voice rather than actual hoarseness. *Aphonia* is a condition in which there is no voice at all. This is usually of psychological origin and the diagnosis is made after excluding any local pathology. Once again, the assistance of a speech therapist is invaluable.

LARYNGOLOGY is that branch of medical science concerned with disorders and diseases of the larynx.

LARYNGOSCOPE: Examination of the larynx may be performed indirectly with use of a laryngeal mirror, or directly by use of a laryngoscope. The direct examination is usually performed under general anaesthetic.

LARYNGO-TRACHEO-BRONCHITIS (CROUP) is an acute infection of the respiratory tract in infants and young children. It is usually a virus infection or may be caused by *Haemophilus influenzae*. The onset is variable but the croupy cough and stridulous breathing usually occur a few days after the onset of a viral upper-respiratory-tract infection. The harsh barking cough is typical of the condition. The majority of children with this condition can be treated with humidification and antibiotics if necessary, but they should always be referred for specialist assessment and hospitalization is preferable in all cases. Rarely, some form of intervention is necessary and this will either be in the form of endotracheal intubation or of a tracheostomy.

LARYNX is the organ of voice and also forms one of the higher parts of the air passages. It is placed high up in the front of the neck and there forms a considerable prominence on the surface. It is covered in front by the skin, a layer of fibrous tissue and a thin layer of muscles, whilst its sides are protected by the lateral lobes of the thyroid gland and by the large sternocleidomastoid muscles.

The larynx is almost 5 cm or 2 inches in height and forms a sort of box, well protected in front by cartilages, rather more open behind and communicating above with the pharynx at the root of the tongue and below the windpipe or trachea. The larynx is enclosed by five large cartilages: the thyroid cartilage, whose prominent pointed front forms the Adam's apple; the

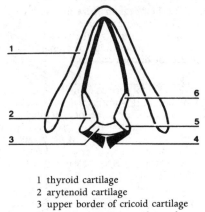

1 thyroid cartilage
2 arytenoid cartilage
3 upper border of cricoid cartilage
4 posterior cricoarytenoid muscles
5 muscular processes
6 vocal processes

Diagram of the opening of the larynx to show the action of the muscles. A horizontal section has been made at the level of the true vocal cords. The two cords are widely separated by the action of 4.

cricoid cartilage, a ring placed below it; the epiglottis, a leaf-like cartilage projecting above the thyroid cartilage into the interior of the throat at the root of the tongue; and a pair of arytenoid cartilages jointed to the top edge of the cricoid cartilage behind, where the thyroid cartilage is deficient. There are also four small nodules of cartilage above the arytenoids. The edges of the laryngeal cartilages do not fit closely together, and the spaces between are filled up by membranes. Certain of the ligaments which bind the cartilages together are of great importance. These pass along each side of the larynx, from the arytenoid cartilage behind

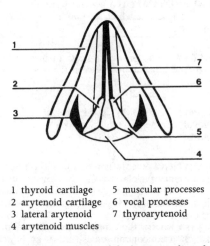

1 thyroid cartilage   5 muscular processes
2 arytenoid cartilage   6 vocal processes
3 lateral arytenoid   7 thyroarytenoid
4 arytenoid muscles

Diagram of the opening of the larynx to show the action of the muscles. The cords are now held together by the action of 3, 4 and 7.

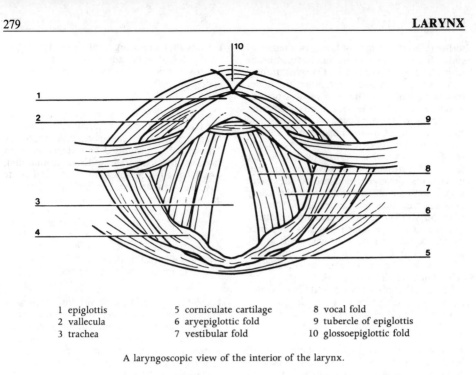

1 epiglottis	5 corniculate cartilage	8 vocal fold
2 vallecula	6 aryepiglottic fold	9 tubercle of epiglottis
3 trachea	7 vestibular fold	10 glossoepiglottic fold

A laryngoscopic view of the interior of the larynx.

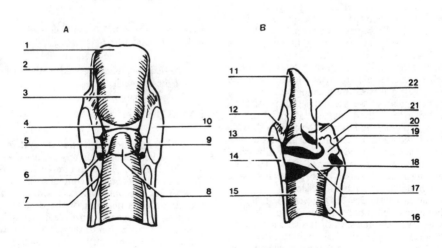

1 epiglottis	9 ventricle of larynx	16 cricoid cartilage
2 aryepiglottic fold	10 thyroid cartilage	17 vocal cord
3 tubercle	11 epiglottis	18 respiratory glottis
4 ventricular fold	12 adipose tissue	19 arytenoideus muscle
5 vocal fold	13 ventricle	20 corniculate cartilage
6 interior thyroarytenoid muscle	14 thyroid cartilage	21 cuneiform cartilage
7 cricoid membrane	15 cricothyroid membrane	22 false vocal cord
8 cricothyroid membrane		

Vertical section of larynx: (A) from behind, (B) from left side.

to the thyroid cartilage in front, two bands of elastic fibres covered by the mucous membrane which lines the whole larynx. One pair of these bands lies directly above the other, the upper pair being known as the false vocal cords; the lower pair are the true vocal cords. The latter are capable of various degrees of tenseness and slackness and of approximation and separation, these results being achieved by several small muscles, which are attached to the arytenoid cartilages and governed in their movements through branches of the vagus nerves. Between the true and false cord is a deep depression on each side known as the ventricle of the larynx. The larynx is lined throughout by mucous membrane, which generally is covered by ciliated cells; but over the true cords, which are subject to much friction in the production of the voice, the surface consists of flattened cells similar to those of the skin.

The vocal cords vibrating in different notes, according to their tenseness and the like, produce the sounds of voice and speech (q.v.).

LASER stands for Light Amplification by Stimulated Emission of Radiation. The light produced by a laser is of a single wavelength and all the waves are in phase with each other, allowing a very high level of energy to be projected as a parallel beam or focused on to a small spot. Various gases, liquids and solids will emit light when they are suitably stimulated. A gassed laser is pumped by the ionizing effect of a high voltage current. This is the same process as that used in a fluorescent tube. Each type of laser has a different effect on biological tissues and this is related to the wavelength of the light produced. The wavelength determines the degree of energy absorption by different tissues and because of this different lasers are needed for different tasks. The argon laser produces light in the visible green wavelength which is selectively absorbed by haemoglobin. It heats and coagulates tissues and it is thus possible to seal bleeding blood vessels and to selectively destroy pigmented lesions. The carbon-dioxide laser is the standard laser for cutting tissue. The infra-red beam it produces is strongly absorbed by water and so vaporizes cells. Thus by moving a finely focused beam across the tissue it is possible to make an incision.

The two main uses of the laser in surgery are the endoscopic photocoagulation of bleeding vessels and the incision of tissue. Lasers have important applications in ophthalmology in the treatment of such disorders of detachment of the retina and the diabetic complication of proliferative retinopathy. Lasers also have several important applications in dermatology. They are used in the treatment of pigmented lesions such as lentigo, in the obliteration of port-wine stains, in the removal of small, benign tumours such as verucas, and finally in the removal of tattoos.

The three great advantages of lasers are their potency, their speed of action, and the ability to focus on an extremely small area. For these reasons they are being used increasingly, and have allowed great advances to be made in microsurgery, and particularly fibreoptic endoscopy (q.v.).

LASSA FEVER, which derives its name from the fact that it was first reported in Lassa in Nigeria, is a disease due to an arenavirus (q.v.). This may be transmitted by rodents or direct from an infected person to those around him. The incubation period is three to twenty-one days. It is characterized by headache, lethargy and severe muscular pains, and there is often a rash due to bleeding into the skin and mucous membranes. Sore throat is often present. It may carry a high mortality rate, particularly in pregnant women. As it is a virus infection, there is no specific treatment, and all that can be done is careful nursing, with rest in bed.

LASSAR'S PASTE, officially known as Zinc and Salicylic Acid Paste, BP, is a preparation used as a remedy for eczema. It has a combined softening, antiseptic, astringent, and soothing action. It is made up of zinc oxide 24 grams; salicylic acid 2 grams; starch 24 grams; white soft paraffin 100 grams.

LATERAL Referring to the sides of an organ or the body or that part furthest from the midline or median plane.

LAUDANUM is the traditional name for tincture of opium. (See OPIUM.)

LAUGHING-GAS is a popular name for nitrous oxide gas (q.v.).

LAVAGE is the name applied to the washing out of the stomach.

LAXATIVES (see PURGATIVES).

LEAD has no action itself upon the system, but its salts, when absorbed in any quantity, or for any length of time, have very important effects. When a lead salt comes in contact with a wound or with any mucous surface, it combines with the albuminous material of the discharge or secretion to form a whitish glaze, which affords a degree of protection to the surface. Further, the lead salt has an astringent action upon the blood-vessels, and therefore helps to stop bleeding or relieve the congestion of inflammation. If one of the soluble lead salts is taken internally, in large amount, it has an irritant action, and the acetate (sugar of lead), subacetate, and nitrate of lead are irritant poisons when taken into the stomach, although their action is comparatively feeble.

LEAD POISONING Acute lead poisoning is rare but chronic lead poisoning is a common occurrence. Occupational lead poisoning is a notifiable disease in Britain. People who work with lead are protected by strict government regulations. Most incidents of lead poisoning occur in smelting workers and those working in scrap yards. Lead poisoning in a domestic environment usually affects children who ingest lead-based paints in the house or from old toys or cots. Lead water pipes may cause poisoning, though these are being phased out. Sometimes people are poisoned by the fluid from lead-based car batteries.

Clinical signs and symptoms of lead poisoning include: a blue line on the gums, loss of appetite, nausea, sickness, abdominal colic, constipation, anaemia, peripheral nerve damage and encephalopathy (q.v.). Concentrations of lead in the blood should be measured: more than 800 $\mu g/L^{-1}$ are dangerous.

The most important part of treatment is to remove the source of lead poisoning. The patient is given a lead chelator (q.v.) of which succimer, also known as DMSA, is the latest. Others include penicillamine and edetate calcium disodium (CaEDTA).

Sodium calciumedetate intramuscularly or intravenously, together with penicillamine, are the drugs of choice in acute cases. Oral penicillamine may then be substituted until the blood lead concentration falls, after which a low calcium diet allows mobilization from the bone, and elimination in the urine. (See POISONS and APPENDIX 2: ADDRESSES.)

LEARNING DISABILITY is a generalized, though often not uniform, intellectual, developmental and social impairment, deriving from brain dysfunction, requiring additional support, supervision and attention to enable an affected person to live as normal a life as possible. It is an administrative term, defined for its educational, social, physical and mental health implications for a condition which merits medical investigation. The consequences impair life prognoses and there may be genetic implications.

In the United Kingdom the 1993 Education Act uses 'learning difficulties': generalized (severe or moderate), or specific (e.g. dyslexia (q.v.), dyspraxia (or apraxia (q.v.)), language disorder). The 1991 Social Security (Disability Living Allowance) Regulations use the term 'severely mentally impaired' if a person suffers from a state of arrested development or incomplete physical development of the brain which results in severe impairment of intelligence and social functioning. This is distinct from the consequences of dementia. Though 'mental handicap' is widely used, 'learning disability' is preferred by the Department of Health.

Originally 'handicap' referred to weights in horse racing. Now distinction is drawn between impairment (a biological deficit), disability (the functional consequence) and handicap (the social consequence).

People with profound learning disability are unable to walk or talk, have multiple disabili-ties and are dependent on others for care and mobility. Children with severe learning disability develop at up to half the rate of normal children of the same age and, as adults, reach the average level of a child of 3–8 years. Some achieve basic functional literacy (recognition of name, common signs) and numeracy (some understanding of money) but most have a life-long dependency for aspects of self-care (some fastenings for clothes, preparation of meals, menstrual hygiene, shaving) and need supervision for outdoor mobility.

Children with moderate learning disability develop at between half and three-quarters of the normal rate and reach the standard of an average child of 8–11 years. They become independent for self-care and public transport unless they have associated disabilities. Most are capable of supervised or sheltered employment. Living independently and raising a family may be possible.

Occurrence Profound learning disability affects about 1 person per thousand, severe learning disability 3 per thousand and moderate learning disability requiring special service 1 per cent. With improved health care, survival of people with profound or severe learning disability is increasing.

Causation Most children with profound or severe learning disability have a diagnosable biological brain disorder. Forty per cent have a chromosome disorder (three quarters of whom have Down's syndrome (q.v.)). A further 15 per cent have other genetic causes, brain malformations or recognizable syndromes. About 10 per cent suffered brain damage during pregnancy (e.g. from cytomegalovirus infection (q.v.)). A similar proportion suffer post-natal brain damage from head injury, accidental or not, near-miss cot death or drowning, cardiac arrest, brain infection (encephalitis (q.v.) or meningitis (q.v.)) or in association with severe seizure disorders.

Explanations for moderate learning disability include Fragile X or other chromosome abnormalities in a tenth, neurofibromatosis (q.v.), fetal alcohol syndrome and other causes of intra-uterine growth retardation. Genetic counselling should be considered for children with learning disability. Prenatal diagnosis is sometimes possible.

Medical complications Epilepsy (q.v.) affects 1 in 20 with moderate, 1 in 3 with severe and 2 in 3 with profound learning disability, though only 1 in 50 with Down's syndrome is affected. One in 5 with severe or profound learning disability has cerebral palsy, many being difficult to feed in early years. Dental treatment is difficult also. Impairments of vision and/or hearing are common. Those with Down's syndrome are prone to heart and bowel malformations, thyroid insufficiency, glue ear (q.v.), myeloid leukaemia (q.v.) and Alzheimer's disease (q.v.).

Psychological and psychiatric needs Over half of the people with profound or severe and many with moderate learning disability show psychiatric or behavioural problems, especially in early years or adolescence. Symptoms may be atypical and hard to assess. Psychiatric disorders include autistic behaviour (q.v.) and schizophrenia (see MENTAL ILLNESS). Emotional problems include anxiety, dependence and depression. Behavioural problems include tantrums, hyperactivity, self-injury, passivity, masturbation in public and resistance to being shaved or helped with menstrual hygiene. There is greater vulnerability to abuse with its behavioural consequences.

Respite and care needs Respite care is arranged with link families for children or staffed family homes for adults where possible. Responsibility for care lies with social services departments which can advise also about benefits.

Education Special educational needs should be met in the least restrictive environment available to allow access to the national curriculum with appropriate modification and support. For older children with learning disability and for young children with severe or profound learning disability this may be in a special day or boarding school. Some children can be provided for in mainstream schools with extra classroom support. The 1993 Education Act lays down stages of assessment and support up to a written statement of special educational needs with annual reviews.

Pupils with learning disability are entitled to remain at school till aged 19 and most with severe or profound learning disability do so. Usually those with moderate learning disability move to further education after the age of 16.

Advice is available from the Mental Health Foundation, the British Institute of Learning Disabilities, Mencap (Royal Society for Mentally Handicapped Children and Adults), and the Scottish Society for the Mentally Handicapped (see APPENDIX 2: ADDRESSES).

LEBER'S DISEASE, or HEREDITARY OPTIC ATROPHY, is a hereditary disease in which blindness comes on at about the age of twenty.

LECITHIN is a very complex fat found in various tissues of the body, but particularly in the brain and nerves, of which it forms a large part. It is also found in large quantities in the yolk of an egg.

LEECHES are animals belonging to the class Vermes, provided with suckers and living a semi-parasitic life, their food being mainly derived from the blood of other animals. They abstract blood by means of a sucker surrounding the mouth, which is provided with several large sharp teeth. The medicinal leech, *Hirudo medicinalis*, was formerly employed for the abstraction of small quantities of blood in inflammatory and other conditions.

LEG This term is generally applied to the whole lower extremity but, properly speaking, includes that part between the knee and ankle

joints. The lower limb is attached to the pelvic bones by strong muscles, especially the gluteal and hamstring muscles behind and the abductor muscles on the inner side of the thigh. The head of the femur, or thigh bone, lies in a deep cup-shaped hollow, the acetabulum, on the outer side of the pelvis. The femur, which is the longest and strongest bone in the body, forms at its lower end the joint of the knee with the tibia. The knee-joint is protected in front by the patella or knee-cap. Along the outer side of the tibia lies the smaller fibula, which does not extend up to the knee but which, along with the tibia, forms the ankle joint. The two prominences on the ankle (*malleoli*) are formed by the tibia on the inner side and the fibula on the outer side. Seven tarsal bones comprise the hinder part of the foot, of which the talus takes the weight of the body from the tibia and fibula. There are five metatarsal bones in the front portion of the foot and each toe has three phalangeal bones, excepting the great toe which has two. The powerful quadriceps extensor muscle in front of the thigh is attached to the knee-cap, which in turn is attached to the front of the tibia by the patellar ligament. This muscle straightens the knee and keeps the body in an erect posture. Below the knee the muscles of the calf, attached to the heel through the tendo calcaneus, or tendon of Achilles, raise the heel off the ground in walking. In front of and to the outside of the leg lie the tibial and peroneal muscles, which bend the ankle upwards and raise the toes. In the sole of the foot are a number of small muscles which bend the toes downwards. The arch of the foot is a very important structure. (See FOOT.)

Most of the blood supply to the lower limb is carried by the femoral artery, which issues from the abdomen in the middle of the groin where its pulse can be felt. This passes down the inner side of the thigh to reach the middle of the back of the knee where it is known as the popliteal artery. Below the knee it divides into anterior and posterior tibial vessels. The former of these runs down the front of the leg and upper surface of the foot, and the latter, which is the larger, passes behind the inner ankle where its pulse can be felt about a finger's breadth behind the bony prominence. The blood returns from the leg partly by deep veins lying alongside the arteries, but to a large extent by the great saphenous vein, which can be seen or felt under the skin for most of the distance from the ankle up the inside of the leg and thigh to the inner side of the groin, where it joins the femoral vein.

The chief nerve in the lower limb is the sciatic nerve which runs down the middle of the back of the thigh deeply embedded in muscles. Above the knee it divides into two parts: the tibial and common peroneal nerves. The former of these runs down the back of the leg, deeply embedded in muscles, to the foot, and the latter passes round the upper end of the fibula on the outer side of the leg, where it can be felt and is liable to be damaged.

The arch of the foot is liable to give way,

especially in debilitated or overworked people, thus producing flat foot. The ankle joint is liable to sprains which consist of tearing of the ligaments, especially on the inner side. The fibula is liable to be fractured near its lower end (a common accident in professional soccer players), either by twists of the foot or by a blow on the outer side of the leg. Fracture of the tibia is also a common accident and, as the tibia lies immediately beneath the skin, this fracture is in danger of becoming compound. The knee-joint, by reason of its great strength, is seldom dislocated, but the partial displacement of a cartilage in the knee is a common occurrence. Fracture of the femur is a serious accident, requiring a period of several months for complete union of the bone. The long and poorly supported vein on the inner side of the leg and thigh is very apt to become distended along with its branches, producing the condition known as varicose veins with resultant eczema and ulcer. The bursa in front of the knee-cap, in people who kneel a lot, readily becomes inflamed and thickened in the condition known as 'housemaid's knee'. (See also FOOT; FRACTURES; JOINTS; KNEE; LIMBS; VEINS.)

LEGIONNAIRE'S DISEASE is a form of pneumonia due to a bacterium known as *Legionella pneumophila*. The bacterium is widely distributed in nature and is commonly found in surface water and soil. Legionnellae are ubiquitous in water. Stationary water and sludge in water tanks provide favourable conditions for primary multiplication. Inhalation of water aerosols seems the most likely way that people acquire the disease. The organism is able to multiply at water outlets. Some rubber outlets in showers and taps are able to support the growth of legionnellae so that high concentrations of the organism are released when the tap is first used in the morning. In the presence of the disease the treatment of infected water systems is essential by cleaning, chlorination or heating or a combination of all three.

The pneumonia caused by legionnellae has no distinctive clinical or radiological features, so that the diagnosis is based on laboratory findings. This depends on the detection of antibodies by the indirect fluorescent antibody test. There is no evidence that the disease is transmitted directly from person to person. The predominant root of infection is by inhalation. The incubation period is two to ten days. The disease starts with aches and pains followed rapidly by a rise in temperature, shivering attacks, cough and shortness of breath. The X-ray tends to show patchy areas of consolidation in the lungs. The assessment of treatment is still hampered by the lack of proper clinical trials but it does seem that erythromycin and rifampicin are the most useful antibiotics. Rifampicin, however, should never be given alone because of the rapid development of drug resistance. In England in 1984 there were 151 cases reported to the Public Health Surveillance unit. Between 1985 and 1987 200 cases were

reported each year; in 1990 the total in England and Wales had fallen to 179, with a ratio of three men to one woman's being affected. In 1993 60 cases were identified.

LEIOMYOMA is a tumour made up of unstriped or involuntary muscle fibres.

LEISHMANIASIS A group of infections caused by flagellate protozoan parasites of the genus *Leishmania* spp., transmitted to man by sandfly species of the genera *Phlebotomus* (Old World leishmaniasis) and *Lutzomiya* (New World leishmaniasis). The causative organism(s) was first visualized by Leishman and Donovan in 1903 and 1904 respectively.

VISCERAL LEISHMANIASIS (KALA-AZAR) A systemic infection caused by *Leishmania donovani* which occurs in tropical and subtropical Africa, Asia, the Mediterranean littoral (and some islands), and in tropical South America. Several mammals, including dogs, can act as zoonotic reservoirs of infection. In the Mediterranean region it is predominantly a disease of infants; in Africa, it occurs more commonly in adolescents and young adults. It constitutes an opportunistic infection in the presence of HIV (AIDS) infection. Onset is frequently insidious; incubation period is 2–6 months. Enlargement of spleen and liver may be gross; fever, anaemia, and generalized lymphadenopathy are usually present. Diagnosis is usually made from a bone-marrow specimen, splenic-aspirate, or liver-biopsy specimen; amastigotes (Leishman-Donovan bodies) of *L. donovani* can be visualized. Several serological tests are of value in diagnosis. Untreated, the infection is fatal within two years, in approximately 70 per cent of patients. Treatment traditionally involved sodium stibogluconate (a pentavalent antimonial compound). Other chemotherapeutic agents (including allupurinol, ketoconazole, and immunotherapy) are now in use, the most recently used being liposomal amphotericin B. Although immunointact persons usually respond satisfactorily, they usually relapse if they have HIV infection. Response to chemotherapy varies geographically, longer courses being required in India compared with the Mediterranean area.

CUTANEOUS LEISHMANIASIS This form is caused by infection with *L. tropica*, *L. major*, *L. aethiopica*, and other species. The disease is widely distributed in the Mediterranean region, Middle East, Asia, Africa, Central and South America, and the former Soviet Union; it is less common than formerly in northern Australia. It is characterized by localized cutaneous ulcers – usually situated on exposed areas of the body. There is no visceral involvement. Diagnosis is by demonstration of the causative organism in a skin biopsy-specimen; the leishmanin skin test is of value. Most patients respond to sodium stibogluconate (see above); local heat therapy is also used. Recently, paromomycin cream has been successfully applied locally.

MUCOCUTANEOUS LEISHMANIASIS This form is

caused by *L. braziliensis* and rarely *L. mexicana.* It is present in Central and South America, particularly the Amazon basin. It is characterized by highly destructive, ulcerative, granulomatous lesions of the skin and mucus membranes, especially involving the mucocutaneous junctions of the mouth, nasopharynx, genitalia, and rectum. Infection is usually via a superficial skin lesion at the site of a sandfly bite. However, spread is by haematogenous routes (usually after several years) to a mucocutaneous location. Diagnosis and treatment are the same as for cutaneous leishmaniasis.

LEMON is used in the form of the fresh peel, tincture, syrup, and oil. Its main value, however, is as a source of vitamin C (or ascorbic acid), the average content of ascorbic acid in the juice being 45 mg per 100 grams. (See also CITRIC ACID; VITAMIN.)

LENS OF THE EYE (see EYE).

LENTIGO is another name for freckles (q.v.).

LEPROSY A chronic bacterial infection caused by *Mycobacterium leprae* affecting the skin, mucous membranes, and nerves. *M. leprae* (demonstrated by Hansen in Norway in 1873) is taxonomically related to *M. tuberculosis*; it also possesses an acid-fast staining reaction. Although widespread in northern Europe and other temperature areas in the past (in medieval times it was a major problem in England and Scandinavia), infection is now almost confined to tropical and subtropical countries, mostly in Africa and India. A suggestion is that underlying tuberculosis protects against leprosy, but the reverse is clearly supported in the published literature. There is no clear evidence that underlying HIV infection predisposes to the disease. There are two distinct (polarized) clinical forms: *tuberculoid* and *lepromatous*. The former usually takes a benign course and is frequently self-limiting, whereas the latter is relentlessly progressive; between these two polar forms lies an intermediate/dimorphous group. It is very unusual in childhood. Susceptibility may be increased by malnutrition. Nasal secretions (especially in lepromatous disease) are teeming with *M. leprae* and constitute the main source of infection; however, living in close proximity to an infected individual seems necessary for someone to contract the disease. *M. leprae* can also be transmitted in breast milk from an infected mother. Only a small minority of those exposed to *M. leprae* develop the disease; those in contact with a lepromatous case are far more likely to contract it than is the case with the tuberculoid form. The incubation period is three to five years or longer. The major clinical manifestations involve skin and nerves. The former range from depigmented, often anaesthetic areas, to massive nodules. Nerve involvement ranges from localized nerve

swelling(s) to extensive areas of anaesthesia. Advanced nerve destruction gives rise to severe deformities: foot-drop, wrist-drop, claw-foot, extensive ulceration of the extremities with loss of fingers and toes, and bone changes. Eye involvement can produce blindness. Laryngeal lesions produce hoarseness and more serious sequelae. Clinical manifestations vary in different ethnic groups; whereas European and Mongoloid groups frequently acquire the lepromatous form, this is less often so in Indian and African groups. The diagnosis is essentially a clinical one; however, skin-smears, histological features and the lepromin skin-test help to confirm the diagnosis and to enable the form of disease to be graded. Introduction of the sulphone compound, dapsone, revolutionized management of the disease. More recently, rifampicin, clofazimine, minocycline, ofloxacin, and clarithromycin have been introduced; a number of regimens incorporating several of these compounds (multi-drug regimens – introduced in 1982) are now widely used. Dapsone-resistance is a major problem worldwide, but occurs less commonly when multi-drug regimens are used. Older compounds – ethionamide and prothionamide – are no longer used because they are severely toxic to the liver. Corticosteroids are sometimes required in patients with 'reversal reaction'. Thalidomide is occasionally used for severe *erythema nodosum leprosum* (an immune-complex reaction) in lepromatous disease. Supportive therapy includes physiotherapy; both plastic and orthopaedic surgery may be necessary in advanced stages of the disease. Improvement in socioeconomic conditions, and widespread use of BCG vaccination are of value as preventive strategies. Early diagnosis and prompt institution of chemotherapy should prevent long-term complications. The WHO objective is to eliminate the infection as a public health problem by the year 2000.

LEPTOMENINGITIS means inflammation of the inner and more delicate membranes of the brain or spinal cord.

LEPTOSPIRA is a group, or genus, of spiral micro-organisms, normally found in rodents and other small mammals in which they cause no harm. When transmitted to man by these animals, either directly or indirectly as through cows, they give rise to various forms of illness.

LEPTOSPIROSIS is the disease caused by infection with Leptospira. The three most common members of this group in the United Kingdom are *L. icterohaemorrhagiae*, *L. canicola*, and *L. hebiomadis*. It is an occupational hazard of farmers, sewage and abattoir workers, fish cutters and veterinary surgeons, but the infection can also be acquired from bathing in contaminated water. The disease varies in intensity from a mild influenza-like illness to a fatal form of jaundice due to severe liver disease. The kidneys are often involved and there may be meningitis. Penicillin or tetracycline are the usual treatment but unless they are given early in the disease their effect is limited. SPIROCHAETOSIS ICTEROHAEMORRHAGICA, or WEIL'S DISEASE, is the term applied to infection with the *Leptospira icterohaemorrhagiae* which is transmitted to man by rats, these animals excreting the organism in their urine; hence the liability of sewer workers to the disease. The condition is characterized by fever, jaundice, enlarged liver, nephritis, and bleeding from mucous membranes.

LESBIAN   A female homosexual (q.v.)

LESION meant originally an injury, but is now applied generally to all disease changes in organs and tissues.

LETHARGY or LASSITUDE means a loss of energy. It is a common presenting complaint to both the general practitioner and hospital consultant. It may have a physical cause or a psychological cause. It may be the result of inadequate rest, environmental noise, boredom, insomnia or recent illness. It may be the result of drugs, the most common of which are beta-blockers and diuretics. The common psycho-social problems producing lethargy are depression and anxiety. If the patient with lethargy runs a fever the differential diagnosis is that of a PUO (Pyrexia of unknown origin). Many patients with fatigue can establish the onset of the symptom to a febrile illness even though they no longer run a fever. The lethargy that follows glandular fever and other viral infections is well recognized. Some of these patients have a true depressive illness and their presentation and response to treatment is little different to sufferers from any other depressive illness. Organic causes of lethargy include anaemia, malnutrition, hypothyroidism, uraemia, alcoholism and diabetes mellitus.

LETTUCE is a green vegetable consisting of leaves of *Lactuca sativa*. It is a relatively rich source of vitamin A. The content of vitamin C is variable, ranging from 1 to 17 mg per 100 grams.

LEUCINE is one of the essential, or indispensable, amino-acids (q.v.). They are so called because they cannot be synthesized, or manufactured, in the body, and are therefore essential constituents of the diet.

LEUCO- (or LEUKO-) is a prefix meaning white.

LEUCOCYTE is the term applied to the white blood cells. Leucocytes differ from erythrocytes in that they contain no haemoglobin and are therefore colourless, and contain a well-formed nucleus. Most of them are larger than erythrocytes, being 8 to 15 micrometres in diameter,

and there are many fewer in the blood – usually about 8000 per cubic millimetre of blood. There are three main classes of white cells: granulocytes, lymphocytes, and monocytes. *Granulocytes*, or polymorphonuclear leucocytes as they are sometimes termed, which normally constitute 70 per cent of the white blood cells, have a lobed nucleus and a granular cytoplasm. They are divided into three groups according to the staining reactions of these granules: neutrophils, which stain with neutral dyes and constitute 65 to 70 per cent of all the white blood cells; eosinophils, which stain with acid dyes (e.g. eosin) and constitute 3 to 4 per cent of the total white blood cells; and basophils, which stain with basic dyes (e.g. methylene blue) and constitute about 0·5 per cent of the total white blood cells. *Lymphocytes*, which constitute 25 to 30 per cent of the white blood cells, have a clear non-granular cytoplasm and a relatively large nucleus which is only slightly indented. They are divided into two groups: small lymphocytes which are slightly larger than erythrocytes (about 8 micrometres in diameter); large lymphocytes, which are about 12 micrometres in diameter. *Monocytes*, which constitute about 5 per cent of the white blood cells, are 10 to 15 micrometres in diameter and differ from lymphocytes in having a rather smaller nucleus which tends to be more indented and to be placed more eccentrically. Monocytes are motile phagocytic cells that circulate in the blood and migrate into the tissues where they develop into various forms of macrophages such as tissue macrophages and Kupffer cells. They remove micro-organisms from the body and identify and present antigenic material to lymphocytes. The cytoplasm is non-granular. (See illustration, BLOOD.)
Site of origin   The granulocytes are formed in the red bone marrow. The lymphocytes are formed predominantly in lymphoid tissue. There is some controversy as to the site of origin of monocytes: some say they arise from lymphocytes, whilst others contend that they are derived from histiocytes: i.e. the reticuloendothelial system (q.v.).
Function   The leucocytes constitute one of the most important of the defence mechanisms against infection. This applies particularly to the neutrophil leucocytes. (See LEUCOCYTOSIS.) (See also ABSCESS; BLOOD; INFLAMMATION; PHAGOCYTOSIS; WOUNDS.)

LEUCOCYTOSIS means a temporary condition in which the polymorphonuclear leucocytes in the blood are increased in number. It occurs in many different circumstances, and forms a valuable means of diagnosis in certain diseases. It may occur, however, as a normal reaction in certain conditions: e.g. pregnancy, menstruation, and during muscular exercise. Apart from these conditions, leucocytosis is usually due to the presence of inflammatory processes. It is part of the body's defence mechanism against infection with micro-organisms, the purpose of the increase in the number of leucocytes being to help to destroy the invading bacteria. Thus, during many acute infective diseases, such as pneumonia, the number is greatly increased. In all suppurative conditions there is also a leucocytosis, and if it seems that an abscess is forming deep in the abdomen, or in some other site where it cannot be readily examined, as, for example, an abscess resulting from appendicitis, the examination of a drop of blood gives a valuable aid in the diagnosis, and may be sufficient, in the absence of other signs, to point out the urgent need of an operation. Typhoid fever constitutes the major exception to the statement that acute infective diseases show this increase of white corpuscles in the blood, and, accordingly, in the case of this disease, the presence of an increase is a specially reliable sign of abscess formation, or other severe complication.

Other infective conditions in which a leucocytosis does not occur include measles and influenza.

LEUCODERMA, or LEUCODERMIA, is a condition of the skin in which areas of it become white, as the result of various skin diseases.

LEUCOPENIA is a condition in which the white corpuscles of the blood are greatly reduced in numbers.

LEUCOPLAKIA (see LEUKOPLAKIA).

LEUCORRHOEA is a vaginal discharge that may be acute, when the discharge is thick and white, consisting mainly of pus, or more often chronic and catarrhal, when the discharge is usually thinner, sometimes of a clear mucous nature; in other cases acrid and offensive. The discharge may precede or follow the menstrual flow; in severer cases it continues throughout the whole intervening periods.

Causes Leucorrhoea may arise as a result of infection anywhere in the genital tract in women: i.e. in the uterus, cervix, or vagina. The commonest cause is some chronic inflammation of the womb following on childbirth, and associated with some laceration of its neck. Another important cause is gonorrhoea. In other cases is is due to infection of the vagina with the *Trichomonas vaginalis* (q.v.). A not uncommon cause is infection with *Candida albicans* resulting in the condition known as thrush. The condition may occur as a symptom of general debility. It may also be due to a tumour in the uterus or the cervix. An occasional cause of very offensive discharge is found in the irritation set up by the presence of a foreign body, such as a pessary that has been introduced for the support of a displaced womb, and then forgotten.

Treatment This depends upon the cause of the discharge. Thus, if it is due to infection with *Trichomonas vaginalis* (q.v.) metronidazole should be given. If it is due to gonorrhoea it is this that must be treated. (See GONORRHOEA.) If it is due to *Candida albicans* nystatin should be given. If it is due to an erosion of the cervix, or neck of the womb, this must be treated. In women past the menopause, or the change of life, the most effective treatment may be administration of an oestrogen (q.v.). (See also UTERUS, DISEASES OF.)

LEUCOTOMY (see PSYCHOSURGERY).

LEUKAEMIA, or LEUCOCYTHAEMIA, is a disease in which the number of white corpuscles in the blood is permanently increased. The disease is also characterized by great enlargement of the spleen, changes in the marrow of the bones, and by enlargement of the lymph glands all over the body. The condition may be either acute or chronic. According to the type of corpuscles chiefly present the acute form is called acute lymphoblastic leukaemia, or acute myeloid leukaemia. The names for the corresponding chronic forms of the disease are chronic lymphatic leukaemia, and chronic myeloid leukaemia. Acute lymphoblastic leukaemia is most common in the first five years of life, and rare after the age of 25. Acute myeloid leukaemia is most common in children and young adults, but may occur at any age. Chronic lymphatic leukaemia occurs at any age between 35 and 80, most commonly in the 60s, and is twice as common in men as in women. Chronic myeloid leukaemia is rare before the age of 25, and most common between 30 and 65. Men and women are equally affected. Each year over 5,000 new cases of leukaemia are diagnosed in the UK: around 4,000 people die from it.

Cause The cause of the disease is unknown.
Symptoms In the acute cases the patient shows pallor, occasional purpuric rash, and enlargement of the lymphatic glands and spleen. The temperature is raised, and the condition may be mistaken for an acute infection. Such cases usually run a rapid course, lasting a few weeks or months. In the chronic type of the disease the onset is gradual, and the first symptoms which occasion discomfort are either swelling of the abdomen and shortness of breath, due to painless enlargement of the spleen, or the enlargement of glands in the neck, armpits and elsewhere, or the pallor, palpitation, and other symptoms of anaemia which often accompany leukaemia. Occasional haemorrhages from the nose, stomach, gums, or bowels may occur, and may be severe. Generally, there is a slight fever. When the blood is examined microscopically, not only is there an enormous increase of the white corpuscles, which may be multiplied thirty- or sixty-fold, but various immature forms of corpuscles are found. In the lymphatic form of the disease the white corpuscles consist chiefly of corpuscles resembling in some measure the lymphocytes, which, in healthy blood, are present only in small numbers. In the myeloid form, myelocytes, or large immature corpuscles out of the bone-marrow, which are never present in healthy blood, appear in large

numbers, and there may also be large numbers of immature, nucleated, red blood corpuscles.

Although there is still no guaranteed cure, the outlook in both acute and chronic leukaemia has changed considerably for the better; particularly is this the case in the acute form of the disease. Thus, in those with acute lymphoblastic leukaemia, which accounts for around 85 per cent of all childhood leukaemias, the overall survival rate may be as high as 60 per cent, with the chance of inducing a remission reaching 90 per cent. The results in acute myeloid leukaemia are not nearly so satisfactory. In the case of chronic lymphatic leukaemia the average period from the time of diagnosis to death is around six years, although quite a number of cases, particularly the elderly, survive for ten years or more. In chronic myeloid leukaemia the average survival time is around three to four years, with 20 per cent surviving for more than five years.

Treatment Promising results are being obtained in the control of the disease using chemotherapy and bone-marrow transplantation. In the case of acute leukaemia the drugs now being used include mercaptopurine, methotrexate, cyclo-phosphamide, and vincristine. But cortisone and its derivatives sometimes produce dramatic temporary improvement. Blood transfusion plays an important part in controlling the condition during the period before the response to chemotherapy or hormone therapy can be expected. Chemotherapy has almost completely replaced radiotherapy in the treatment of chronic leukaemia. For the myeloid form busulphan is the most widely used drug, replaced by hydroxyurea, mercaptopurine, or one of the nitrogen mustard derivatives (q.v.) in the later stages of the disease. For the lymphatic form the drugs used are chlorambucil, cyclo-phosphamide, and the nitrogen mustard derivatives.

Prognosis Between 50 and 60 per cent of patients with acute lymphoblastic leukaemia may be cured; between 20 and 50 per cent of those with acute myeloid leukaemia have much improved survival rates. Prognosis of patients with chronic lymphocytic leukaemia is often good, depending on early diagnosis.

LEUKOPLAKIA A white plaque on mucous membranes caused by overgrowth of the tissues. It is occasionally a precancerous condition.

LEUKOTRIENES are a group of slow-reacting substances (SRSS) which have powerful smooth-muscle stimulating properties.

LEVALLORPHAN TARTRATE is an antidote to morphine. It is usually given intravenously. In opium poisoning the dose is 1 to 2 mg, repeated if necessary.

LEVAMISOLE is a drug that is proving of value in the treatment of ascariasis (q.v.). Its main advantage seems to be in mass treatment as one dose may prove effective. It is also being used in the treatment of a group of diseases of obscure origin including Crohn's disease (q.v.) and rheumatoid arthritis. The drug is unavailable in the UK.

LEVODOPA A drug used in the treatment of Parkinson's disease (q.v.). It is converted to dopamine in the brain, correcting the deficiency which causes the disorder. Carbidopa is often given with it to prevent its conversion to dopamine in the body before it reaches the brain. It may cause nausea, hypotension (q.v.) or cardiac dysrhythmias.

LEVORPHANOL is a synthetic derivative of morphine. It is an effective analgesic but, like morphine, is a drug of addiction.

LIBIDO is the desire for sexual intercourse. Lack of desire or diminished libido may occur in any general medical illness as well as in endocrine diseases when there is a lack of production of the sex hormones. It is frequently associated with psychiatric diseases and may be the result of certain drugs. It must be distinguished from impotence where the desire for intercourse is normal but the performance is defective due to the inability to achieve or maintain an erection.

LICE (see INSECTS IN RELATION TO DISEASE; PEDICULOSIS).

LICHEN is a term applied to a group of chronic skin diseases characterized by thickening and hardening of the skin, with the formation of papules (q.v.). *Lichen simplex* develops as a result of persistent scratching. The cause of the itching is often obscure. The disease is more common in women than in men. In women it occurs most commonly in the nape of the neck. It also occurs on the back of the forearm, the inner part of the thigh, the back of the knee and around the ankle. The skin becomes thickened, and has been compared in appearance to that of morocco leather, but there are no papules. Treatment consists of that of the underlying condition if this can be recognized, and the application of corticosteroid cream and emollients. *Lichen planus* begins on the wrists and then spreads to the body and legs. The eruption is characteristic, consisting of purplish, shiny papules with thickening of the surrounding skin. The papules are often found as well in the mouth. The cause is obscure. In some it is apparently nervous or emotional in origin. In some it is due to drugs, including the organic arsenical drugs, gold, mepacrine, chloroquine, and para-aminosalicylic acid (PAS). It usually persists for some three months, but occasionally it may last for years. Treatment consists of the corticosteroids (q.v.) given by mouth and applied locally.

LIGAMENTS are strong bands of fibrous tissue which serve to bind together the bones entering into a joint. They are, in some cases, cord-like, in others flattened bands, whilst most joints are surrounded by a fibrous capsule or capsular ligament. (See JOINTS.)

LIGATION Tying off – for example, a blood vessel – by completely encircling it with a tight band usually of catgut or some other suture material.

LIGATURE means a cord or thread used to tie round arteries in order to stop the circulation through them, or to prevent escape of blood from their cut ends. Ligatures are generally made of catgut or silk, and are tied with a reef-knot.

LIGHT REFLEX Pupillary constriction in the eye in response to light. The direct light reflex involves pupillary constriction in the eye into which a light is shone; the consensual light reflex is the pupillary constriction that occurs in the other eye. The afferent or inward pathway of the reflex is via the optic nerve (see EYE) and the efferent or outward pathway is via the occulomotor nerve.

LIGHTNING INJURIES are not uncommon – it is estimated that lightning strikes somewhere on the earth an average of 100 times a second, but the majority of those struck by lightning recover. A direct hit, however, means instantaneous death, with the clothes torn off, and the victim may be hurled quite a long distance. Even the individual who recovers falls unconscious the moment he is struck. Those who are a little farther away experience tingling of the skin and their hair may stand on end.

Preventive measures indoors during a lightning storm consist of keeping away from the fireplace, the main electrical switch, the bathroom, the kitchen sink and the television aerial. It is perfectly safe to use the telephone. There is no point in drawing the curtains, pulling down the blinds, covering mirrors or taking off metal-frame spectacles. Out of doors, solitary trees, walls, wire fences and other metallic structures such as sheds, park seats and tent-poles, ponds and river banks should be avoided. So also should flat open spaces, such as golf courses, where an individual may form the highest point. To use a metal-tipped umbrella or a golf club is asking for trouble. There is no risk inside a motor car, but it is wise to avoid moors or hills and make for the nearest low ground. If the storm is really severe, the safest thing is to lie down in a ditch. In Britain, there are around 10 deaths a year from lightning strikes.

Treatment of an individual struck by lightning consists of artificial respiration, which may need to be prolonged for several hours. (See APPENDIX 1: BASIC FIRST AID.)

LIGNOCAINE is a local anaesthetic. It is also used in the treatment of certain disorders of cardiac rhythm known as ventricular arrhythmias which may be particularly dangerous following a coronary thrombosis (q.v.).

LIMBS are outgrowths from the sides of the body, which, in man as in all the higher animals, number four. The limbs of all the higher animals, though differing much in outward appearance, are constructed on a similar plan, modified to suit the requirements of the owner, the fore-limb, for example, developing in birds into a wing, in seals into a flipper. In all, however, the various muscles, bones, and blood-vessels, though differing in size and shape, correspond in arrangement. Also, between the upper and lower limb, a strict comparison is possible, and the bones, muscles, and main arteries of the arm, forearm, and hand have all representatives in the thigh, leg, and foot. (See ARM; LEG.)

The union of the lower limb with the body is, however, more intimate than that of the upper limb. For, whilst the shoulder-blade and collar-bone of the upper limb are separated from the organs of the chest by the ribs and their muscles, the haunch-bone is applied on each side directly to the spine and forms the side of the pelvis.

In structure, each limb consists of four segments, the shoulder, arm, forearm, and hand in the case of the upper limb, corresponding to the haunch, thigh, leg, and foot in the lower limb. Upon the surface, the limb is enveloped by skin which, over the hand, is specially rich in its supply of sensory nerves. Beneath the skin is a layer of loose cellular tissue containing an amount of fat which varies with the corpulence of the individual. Next comes a strong layer of fibrous tissue, known as fascia, which provides a complete investment for the limb, and supplies a separate sheath for each muscle. The chief bulk of the limb is made up by the muscles or flesh. Finally, in the centre of the limb lie the bones which give it rigidity; and in general the large arteries and nerves are embedded among the muscles close to the bones.

The diseases affecting the limbs are those of the skin, muscles, bones, etc., forming them. (For injuries of the limbs see FRACTURES; HAEMORRHAGE; JOINTS, DISEASES AND INJURIES OF; WOUNDS.)

LIME-JUICE is a yellow liquid obtained by squeezing lime-fruit, *Citrus limetta*. In common with lemon-juice, it is a rich source of vitamin C (16·8 to 62·5 mg per 100 ml) and contains a large quantity of citric acid. It is used as a refreshing drink and as a preventive of, and remedy for, scurvy (q.v.). Lime-juice which has been boiled, or preserved for a prolonged period, loses its anti-scorbutic properties.

LINCTUS is a term applied to any thick syrupy medicine. Most of these are remedies for excessive coughing.

LINEA ALBA is the line of fibrous tissue stretching down the mid-line of the belly from the lower end of the sternum to the pubic bone. The linea alba gives attachment to the muscles of the belly wall.

LINEA NIGRA During pregnancy the linea alba (q.v.) becomes pigmented and appears as a dark line down the middle of the belly, and is called the linea nigra.

LINEAR ACCELERATOR (see RADIO-THERAPY).

LINGUAL Referring or related to the tongue: e.g. the lingual nerve supplied sensation to the tongue.

LINIMENTS, or embrocations (q.v.), are oily mixtures intended for external application by rubbing. Their chief use is in the production of pain relief, particularly in rheumatic conditions. They may be highly toxic if taken orally – a particular danger with children.

LINT was originally made of teased-out linen; now it consists of a loose cotton fabric, one side of which is fluffy, the other being smooth and applied next to the skin when the surface is broken. Marine lint consists of tow impregnated with tar, and is used where large quantities of some absorbent and deodorizing dressing are required. Cotton lint is impregnated with various substances, the most common being boracic lint. Lint containing perchloride of iron (15 per cent) is valuable as a styptic.

LIPAEMIA means the presence of an excessive amount of fat in the blood.

LIPASE is an enzyme widely distributed in plants, and present also in the liver and gastric and pancreatic juices, which breaks down fats to the constituent fatty acids and glycerol.

LIPID A substance which is insoluble in water, but soluble in fat solvents such as alcohol and ether. The main lipid groups are the triglycerides, phospholipids, and glycolipids. They play an important role in nutrition, health (particularly in the functioning of the cell membranes, and the immune response), and disease (notably cardiovascular disease). There is a strong correlation between the concentration of cholesterol in the blood (transported as lipoproteins) and the risk of developing atheroma and coronary heart disease. Lipoproteins are classified by their density and mobility, the chief groups being low-density (LDL) and high-density (HDL). High serum concentrations of LDL increase the risk of cardiovascular disease, while HDL is though to protect the vessel wall by removing cholesterol, and has an inverse relationship to risk. The various serum lipid abnormalities have been classified into five groups, according to the cause and particular lipoprotein raised. Most important are type II (increased LDL, genetically determined) and type IV (increased VLDL, associated with obesity, diabetes, and excess alcohol). Various lipid-lowering drugs are available, such as cholestyramine (q.v.) and clofibrate (q.v.), but any drug treatment must be combined with a strict diet, reduction of blood pressure, and cessation of smoking.

LIPODYSTROPHY is a congenital maldistribution of fat tissue. Subcutaneous fat is totally absent from a portion of the body and hypertrophied in the remainder. Another form of lipodystrophy occurs at the site of insulin injections. These are much less frequently seen nowadays as the new synthetic preparations of insulin are pure and unlikely to cause this reaction which was not uncommon with the older preparations. Occasionally the converse occurs at the site of insulin injections where the lipogenic action of insulin stimulates the fat cells to hypertrophy. This can also be disfiguring and usually results from using the same site for injections too frequently.

LIPOLYSIS The enzymatic breaking down of fat.

LIPOMA is a tumour mainly composed of fat. Such tumours arise in almost any part of the body, developing in fibrous tissues, particularly in that beneath the skin. They are simple in nature, and seldom give any trouble beyond that connected with their size and position. (See TUMOUR.)

LIPOSARCOMA A malignant tumour of adipose or fatty tissue. It occurs most frequently in the thighs, buttocks or retroperitoneum. The four main types are: well differentiated, myxoid, round cell and pleomorphic (variety of forms).

LIPOSOMES are essentially tiny oil droplets consisting of layers of fatty material known as phospholipid separated by aqueous compartments. Drugs can be incorporated into the liposomes, which are then injected into the bloodstream or into the muscles, or given by mouth. Using this method of giving drugs, it is possible to protect them from being broken down in the body before they reach the part of the body where their curative effect is required: for example, in the liver or in a tumour.

LIPS form a pair of curtains before the mouth, each composed of a layer of skin and of mucous membrane, between which lies a considerable amount of fat and of muscle fibres.

The diseases to which the lips are liable are not numerous. *Fissures*, coming on in cold weather, form a troublesome condition often difficult to get rid of. Such peeling and cracking of the vermilion of the lips is common in those exposed for long periods to wind and sunlight. Treatment consists of the application of aqueous cream BP. If the main cause is excessive exposure to sunlight, in which case the lower lip is mainly affected, the best application is mexenone cream BPC. Mexenone is also available as a proprietary lipstick (Uvistat). *Herpes*, in the form of what are known as 'cold sores', often develops on the lip as a result of a cold or other feverish condition, but quickly passes off. (See HERPES.) *Ulcers* may form on the inner surface of the lip, usually in consequence of bad teeth or of dyspepsia. Small *cysts* sometimes form on the inner surface of the lip, and are seen as little bluish swellings filled with mucus; they are of no importance. *Hare-lip* is a deformity sometimes present at birth. (See PALATE, MALFORMATIONS OF.) *Cancer* of the lip sometimes occurs, almost always in men, and usually on the lower lip. (See also MOUTH, DISEASES OF.)

LIQUOR (see SOLUTION).

LIQUORICE is the root of *Glycyrrhiza glabra*, a plant of southern Europe and Asia. It is a mild expectorant, but is mainly used to cover the taste of disagreeable and more powerful drugs. Solid and liquid extracts are made from it, but the most commonly used preparation is compound liquorice powder, which contains also senna and sulphur.

LISTERIOSIS is a rare disease, although the causal organism, *Listeria monocytogenes*, is widely distributed in soil, silage, water, and various animals, with consequent risk of food contamination. Neonates are the main age group affected – often as a result of a mild or inapparent infection in the pregnant mother. The disease presents in two main forms: meningo-encephalitis, or septicaemia with enlarged lymph glands. Elderly adults occasionally develop the first form, while younger adults are more likely to develop a mild or even inapparent form. The disease generally responds well to antibiotics such as ampicillin or chloramphenicol; nevertheless, the incidence rose over the past decade but seems to have levelled out, 102 cases being reported in 1993 compared to 106 in 1992.

LITHIASIS is a general name applied to the formation of calculi and concretions in tissues or organs: e.g. cholelithiasis means the formation of calculi in the gall-bladder.

LITHIUM CARBONATE is a drug widely used in the treatment of certain forms of mental illness. About one person in two thousand in Britain is said to be prescribed it. The major indication for its use is acute mania. It induces improvement or remission in over 70 per cent of such patients. In addition, it is effective in the treatment of manic-depressive patients, preventing both the manic and the depressive episodes. There is also evidence that it lessens aggression in prisoners who behave antisocially and in mentally retarded patients who mutilate themselves and have temper tantrums. It is not recommended for children. Because of its possible toxic effects it is a drug that must only be administered under medical supervision and with monitoring of the blood levels as the gap between therapeutic and toxic concentrations is narrow. Because of the risk of its damaging the unborn child, it should not be prescribed, unless absolutely necessary, during pregnancy, particularly in the first three months. Neither should mothers take it while breast feeding as it is excreted in the milk in high concentrations.

LITHOTOMY is the operation of cutting for stone in the bladder. The operation is of great historic interest, because more has probably been written about it in early times than about any other department of surgery, and because, for long, it formed almost the only operation in which the surgeon dared to attack diseases of the internal organs.

LITHOTRIPSY Extracorporeal shock-wave lithotripsy (ESWL) causes disintegration of renal and biliary stones without contact and is therefore an attractive procedure for patients and surgeons. Stones in the upper urinary tract are a common condition in the United Kingdom causing considerable morbidity and requiring large and lengthy operations with an extensive convalescent period. Percutaneous renal surgery has changed this picture but it requires at least puncture of the kidney and possibly open nephrolithotomy for large branched calculi. Extracorporeal shock-wave lithotripsy causes disintegration of the stone without contact and is therefore a far more attractive procedure.

The generation of shock waves as a form of treatment for urinary calculi was first described in 1955 by the Russian engineer Yutkin. Shock waves generated outside the body can be accurately focused with a reflector whilst the patient is suspended in water to facilitate transmission of the waves. These are focused on the calculus. The resultant fine fragments are passed spontaneously in the urine with minimal, if any, discomfort. The procedure has been shown to be safe, short and effective and is most acceptable to patients.

LITHOTRITY, or LITHOLAPAXY, is the term applied to the operation in which a stone in the bladder is crushed by an instrument introduced along the urethra, and the fragments washed out through a catheter.

LITMUS, which is prepared from several lichens, is a vegetable dye-substance, which on contact with alkaline fluids becomes blue, and on contact with acid fluids, red. Slips of paper, impregnated with litmus, form a valuable test for the acidity of the secretions and discharges.

LITTLE'S DISEASE is a form of cerebral palsy. (See CEREBRAL PALSY.)

LIVER The liver is a solid organ of dark-brown colour and the largest gland in the body. It discharges several functions, acting both as an excreting organ and as an elaborator and storehouse of nourishment.

Form The shape of the liver is generally described as that of a right-angled triangular prism, with the right angle rounded off. It has five surfaces, superior, anterior, right, posterior, and inferior, of which the anterior and posterior surfaces are triangular, with the base towards the right side and tapering off to the left. The surfaces are separated from one another by rounded margins, except in the case of the lower surface, which is divided from the right, front, and upper surfaces by a sharp edge. The organ is divided also into four lobes. The great bulk of it constitutes the right lobe; the left lobe is small and extends a little way into the left half of the abdomen, to end in a sharp left border, whilst the quadrate and caudate lobes are two small divisions upon the back and under surface. About the middle of the under surface, towards the back, is placed the porta hepatis, a transverse fissure, by which the hepatic artery and portal vein carry blood into the liver, and by which the right and left hepatic ducts emerge, carrying off the bile formed in the liver. The *gall-bladder* is attached to the under surface of the right lobe and projects from beneath the lower margin, where, if distended, it may be felt as a rounded swelling immediately beneath the end of the ninth rib. The connection of the gall-bladder – in which bile is stored – with the liver is rather complicated. The hepatic ducts emerge at the porta hepatis, one coming from the right and one from the left lobe. They immediately join to form the common hepatic duct, which is about 3 cm (1¼ inches) long, and joins the cystic duct, coming from the gall-bladder, at an acute angle. The hepatic and cystic ducts by their union form the bile duct, which is about 75 mm (3 inches) in length, and opens into the small intestine. Bile, which passes down from the liver by the hepatic duct, may either pass directly into the bile duct and so into the intestine, or it may pass upwards through the cystic duct into the gall-bladder, to be stored there, and later retraces its way through the cystic duct to the bile duct, and so to the intestine. The cystic duct and gall-bladder therefore together form a cul-de-sac in the bile passages.

Position The liver occupies the right-hand upper portion of the abdominal cavity. Its upper surface is in contact with the diaphragm, which also separates its right surface from the right lower ribs. About four-fifths of the organ lies to the right of the middle line of the body. As it is of a rounded shape it fills up the dome of the diaphragm, the lower part of the right lung being hollowed out to receive the liver, from which it is separated only by the diaphragm and pleural membrane. The liver, in turn, rests upon various abdominal organs, the right kidney and suprarenal gland, the large intestine, the duodenum, and the stomach all making impressions upon it. In addition, the liver is swung from the walls of the abdomen by five ligaments, four of which consist of thickened parts of the peritoneal membrane lining the whole abdominal cavity, and reflected from the upper part of the liver to its walls. These are the coronary ligament, right and left triangular ligaments, falciform ligament, and a dense fibrous cord, the round ligament, or ligamentum teres.

Dimensions The vertical thickness of the liver amounts, towards the right side, to over 12 cm (5 inches), and its extent from side to side is considerably more. Its weight is over 1·5 kg (50 ounces), varying with the size of the person, but making up about ¹/₄₀ or thereabout of the whole body weight. In young children it is relatively larger, accounting, to a large extent, for their protuberant abdomen, and making up about ¹/₁₈ of the weight of the whole body.

Vessels The blood supply of the organ differs from that of any other part of the body, in that the blood collected from the stomach and bowels into the portal vein does not pass directly to the heart, but is distributed to the

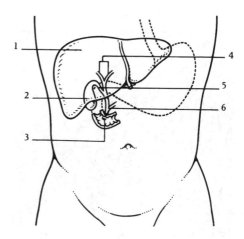

1 liver
2 gall-bladder
3 ampulla of Vater (leading into duodenum)
4 hepatic ducts
5 bile duct
6 common bile duct

Positions of liver, gall-bladder and connecting bile-ducts.

liver, in the substance of which the portal vein breaks up into capillary vessels. The effect of this is that some harmful substances, absorbed from the stomach and bowels, are abstracted from the blood-stream and destroyed, while various constituents of the food are stored up in the liver for gradual use. In addition, the liver receives a large hepatic artery from the coeliac axis, which also distributes branches to the stomach and pancreas, this blood supply serving to nourish the organ. After the blood has circulated through capillaries, it is collected together from both sources and emptied into the hepatic veins, which pass directly from the back surface of the liver into the inferior vena cava.

Minute structure The liver is enveloped in a capsule of fibrous tissue, Glisson's capsule, from which strands run along the vessels, and, penetrating to the furthest recesses of the organ, bind its structure together. The hepatic artery, portal vein, and bile-duct divide and sub-divide, the branches of each lying alongside corresponding divisions of the other two, till the finest divisions of artery, vein, and bile-duct, known as interlobular vessels, lie between the lobules, of which the whole gland is built up. These lobules, each about the size of a pin's head, form each in itself a complete secreting unit, and the liver is built up of many hundred thousands of such exactly similar lobules.

A lobule has the following structure: from the small vessels lying round its margin capillaries, or sinusoids, lined with stellate Kupffer cells (q.v.), are given off which run in towards the centre of the lobule, where they empty into

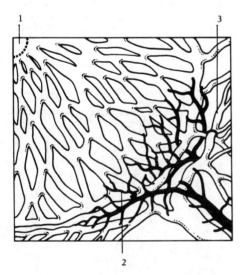

1 central vein connected by network of sinusoids with 2
2 interlobular bile-duct commencing in network of intercellular bile-canaliculi within the lobule
3 peripheral or interlobular veins

Diagram of liver lobule.

a small central vein. These central veins from neighbouring lobules collect together, and ultimately the blood passes into the hepatic veins, and so leaves the liver. Between the capillaries, which radiate from the central vein to the edge of the lobule, lie rows of large liver cells, these forming the distinctive tissue of the organ, upon which its activity depends. Between the rows of cells also lie fine bile capillaries, which collect the bile produced by the cells and discharge it into the bile-ducts lying along the margins of the lobules. The liver cells are among the largest cells in the body, and each contains one or two large, round nuclei. In the cells can often be seen droplets of fat or granules of glycogen, i.e. animal starch.

Functions The liver is a vast chemical factory. The heat produced by the chemical changes taking place in it forms an important contribution to the general warming of the body. The liver secretes bile, the chief constituents of which are the bile salts (sodium glycocholate and taurocholate), the bile pigments (bilirubin and biliverdin), cholesterol, and lecithin. The bile acids from which the salts are obtained are formed in the liver by the union of glycine and taurine with cholic acid. The bile salts are absorbed from the intestine and so find their way back to the liver again. The bile pigments are the iron-free and globin-free remnant of haemoglobin, being formed in the Kupffer cells of the liver. Bile pigments can, however, be formed in many other parts of the body: in the spleen, the lymph glands, bone-marrow, connective tissues (giving the colour to a bruise). Bile, then, serves to excrete pigment, the result of breakdown of old red blood corpuscles, and to aid the digestion of fat. Bile salts aid digestion of fat by emulsifying the fat, by activating pancreatic lipase, and by promoting fat absorption. Bile is necessary for the absorption of vitamins D and E.

In addition to forming bile the liver has a number of important functions. These are enumerated briefly: (1) In the embryo it forms red blood corpuscles, and in the adult stores vitamin B_{12}, a substance necessary for the proper functioning of the bone-marrow in the manufacture of red corpuscles. (2) It manufactures the fibrinogen of the blood, and also the albumin and globulin. (3) It stores iron and copper necessary for the manufacture of red corpuscles. (4) It produces heparin and, with the aid of vitamin K, prothrombin. (5) Its Kupffer cells in the liver blood-sinusoids are an important element in the reticulo-endothelial system, which breaks down red corpuscles, and probably manufactures antibodies. (6) It detoxicates noxious products made in the intestine and absorbed into the blood. (7) It stores carbohydrate in the form of glycogen, and maintains the two-way process: glucose glycogen. (8) It forms vitamin A from carotene and stores the B vitamins. (9) It splits up amino-acids and manufactures urea and uric acids. (10) It plays an essential part in the storage and metabolism of fat.

LIVER DISEASE IN THE TROPICS ACUTE
LIVER DISEASE Many viruses can be responsible for acute hepatocellular jaundice. The hepatitis viruses (A–F) are of paramount importance.
Hepatitis E (HEV), which causes a disease
overall very similar to HAV infection, often
produces acute hepatic failure in pregnant
women; extensive epidemics – transmitted by
contaminated drinking-water supplies – have
been documented at Delhi and Kashmir. HBV,
especially in association with HDV, also causes
acute liver failure in infected patients in several
tropical countries; however, the major importance of HBV is that the infection leads to
chronic liver disease (see below). Other
hepatotoxic viruses include the Epstein-Barr
virus, cytomegalovirus, yellow fever, Marburg/
Ebola viruses, etc. Acute liver disease also
occurs in the presence of several acute bacterial
infections, including *Salmonella typhi*, brucellosis, leptospirosis, syphilis, etc. Also, the complex type of jaundice associated with acute
systemic bacterial infection – especially
pneumococcal pneumonia and pyomiositis –
assumes a major importance in many tropical
countries, especially those in Africa and Papua
New Guinea. Of protozoan infections,
Plasmodium falciparum malaria, leishmaniasis,
and toxoplasmosis should be considered. *Ascaris
lumbricoides* (the roundworm) can produce
obstruction to the biliary system.
CHRONIC LIVER DISEASE Long-term disease is
dominated by sequelae of HBV and HCV
infections (often acquired during the neonatal
period), both of which can cause chronic active
hepatitis, cirrhosis, and hepatocellular carcinoma ('hepatoma'), one of the world's most
common malignancies. Chronic liver disease is
also caused by schistosomiasis (usually
Schistosoma mansoni and *S. japonicum*), and
acute and chronic alcohol ingestion. Furthermore, many local herbal remedies and also
orthodox chemotherapeutic compounds (e.g.
those used in tuberculosis and leprosy) can
result in chronic liver disease. Haemosiderosis
('Bantu siderosis') is a major problem in southern Africa. Hepatocytes contain excessive iron
– derived primarily from an excessive intake,
often present in locally brewed beer; however,
a genetic predisposition seems likely. Indian
childhood cirrhosis – associated with an excess
of copper – is a major problem in India and
surrounding countries. Epidemiological evidence shows that much of the copper is derived
from copper vessels used to store milk used
after weaning. Veno-occlusive disease was first
described in Jamaica. However, this disease,
which can present acutely, subacutely, chronically and is caused by pyrrolyzidine alkaloids
(present in bush-tea), including heliotropium, is
now known to occur far more widely. The
previously held view that severe malnutrition
predisposes to cirrhosis and other forms of
chronic liver disease can no longer be upheld.
Several HIV-associated 'opportunistic' infections can give rise to hepatic disease.
   A localized (focal) form of liver disease in all
tropical/subtropical countries results from in-

vasive *Entamoeba histolytica* infection (amoebic liver 'abscess'); serology and imaging techniques assist in diagnosis. This should be
differentiated form pyogenic liver abscess, which
usually occurs secondarily to another intra-
abdominal infection. Hydatidosis also causes
localized liver disease; one or more cysts usually
involve the right lobe of the liver. Serological
tests and imaging techniques are of value in
diagnosis. Whilst surgery formerly constituted
the sole method of management, prolonged
courses of albendazole and/or praziquantel
have now been shown to be effective; however,
surgical intervention is still required in some
cases.
   Hepato-biliary disease is also a problem in
many tropical/subtropical countries. In south-
east Asia, *Clonorchis sinensis* and *Opisthorchis
viverini* infections cause chronic biliary-tract
infection, complicated by adenocarcinoma of
the biliary system. Praziquantel is effective
chemotherapy before advanced disease ensues.
Fasciola hepatica (the liver fluke) is a further
hepato-biliary helminthic infection; treatment
is with bithionol or triclabendazole, praziquantel
being relatively ineffective.

LIVER DISEASES The liver may be extensively diseased without any very urgent symptoms, unless the circulation through it is impeded,
the outflow of bile checked, or neighbouring
organs implicated. Jaundice, which is a symptom of several liver disorders, is dealt with
elsewhere. Ascites, which may be caused by
interference with the circulation through the
portal vein of the liver, as well as by other
causes, is also considered separately. The presence of gall-stones is a complication of some
diseases connected with the liver, and is treated
under GALL-BLADDER, DISEASES OF. For hydatid
cyst of the liver see TAENIASIS. Liver diseases in
a tropical environment are dealt with later in
this section.
INFLAMMATION OF THE LIVER, or HEPATITIS, may
occur as part of a generalized infection or may
be a localized condition. Infectious hepatitis,
which is the result of infection with a virus, is
one of the most common forms of hepatitis.
(See HEPATITIS, ACUTE INFECTIVE.) There are
many other viruses that can cause hepatitis,
including that responsible for glandular fever
(q.v.). Certain spirochaetes may also be the
cause, particularly that responsible for
leptospirosis (q.v.), as can many drugs. Hepatitis may also occur if there is obstruction of the
bile duct, as by a gall-stone.
CIRRHOSIS OF THE LIVER The cause of cirrhosis
(q.v.) of the liver is still obscure. Experimentally
it has been shown that the condition can be
produced by a deficiency of certain of the
amino-acids found in protein, but this only
explains a small proportion of the cases found
in man. It is probable that in most cases three
factors are involved in varying degrees: a
nutritional deficiency, a toxic factor, and an
infective factor. Alcohol is the most common
cause of cirrhosis in the United Kingdom and

the USA. In Africa and many parts of Asia, infection with hepatitis B virus is a common cause. Certain drugs, for example, paracetamol, may damage the liver if taken in excess.

Symptoms In one form of cirrhosis the liver is much contracted (atrophic or coarse cirrhosis), its blood-vessels are pressed upon, and ascites results. In another form there is great enlargement of the organ (hypertrophic or biliary cirrhosis) and jaundice appears. In all cases there is loss of appetite and other signs of dyspepsia. There is a variable degree of anaemia. There may be a low-grade fever. In a certain number of cases, two characteristic signs may appear. One is so-called spider naevi (see NAEVUS). Each has a central red spot and may measure up to a centimetre in diameter. They rarely appear below the waist. The nosebleeds which occur in around 20 per cent of cases may be due to naevi in the nose. The other is so-called liver palms, or reddening of the palms of the hands, most marked on the ball of the thumb and the outer edge of the hand.

Treatment Nothing can be done to repair a cirrhosed organ, but the cause, if known, must be removed and further advance of the process thus prevented. In the case of the liver a high-protein, high-carbohydrate, low-fat diet is given, supplemented by liver extract and vitamins B and K. The consumption of alcohol should be banned. In patients with liver failure and a poor prognosis, liver transplantation is worthwhile but only after careful consideration. (See TRANSPLANTATION.)

ABSCESS OF THE LIVER   When an abscess develops in the liver, it is usually a manifestation of amoebic dysentery, appearing sometimes late in the disease, even after the diarrhoea is cured (see below). It may also follow upon inflammation of the liver due to other causes. In the case of an amoebic abscess treatment consists of oral metronidazole. Aspiration of the contents of the abscess is now rarely necessary.

ACUTE HEPATIC NECROSIS is a destructive and often fatal disease of the liver which is very rare. It may be due to chemical poisons, such as carbon tetrachloride, chloroform, phosphorus and industrial solvents derived from benzene. It may also be the cause of death in cases of poisoning with fungi. Very occasionally it may be a complication of acute infectious hepatitis.

CANCER OF THE LIVER is not uncommon, although it is rare for the disease to begin in the liver, the involvement of this organ being usually secondary to disease situated somewhere in the stomach or bowels. Cancer originating in the liver is more common in Asia and Africa. It usually arises in a fibrotic (or cirrhotic) liver and in carriers of the hepatitis B virus. There is great emaciation, which increases as the disease progresses. The liver is much enlarged, and its margin and surface are rough, being studded with hard cancer masses of varying size, which can often be felt through the abdominal wall. Pain may be present. Jaundice and oedema often appear.

LIVER-FLUKE is the popular name of *Fasciola hepatica*, a parasite which infests sheep, and which is occasionally found in the bile-passages and liver of man. (See FASCIOLIASIS.)

LIVER PILLS (see CHOLAGOGUES).

LIVER SPOT is a popular term applied to brownish marks which appear on the skin, especially of the face. This is sometimes caused by the growth of a parasite (*Tinea versicolor*) in the surface layers of the epidermis. It also frequently accompanies pregnancy or the presence of abdominal tumours. It may also be due simply to some long-continued form of local irritation.

LOBE is the term applied to the larger divisions of various organs, such as to the four lobes of the liver, the three lobes of the right and the two lobes of the left lung, which are separated by fissures from one another, and to the lobes or superficial areas into which the brain is divided. The term lobar is applied to structures which are connected with lobes of organs, or to diseases which have a tendency to be limited by the boundaries of lobes, such as lobar pneumonia.

LOBECTOMY is the operation of cutting out a lobe of the lung in such diseases as abscess of the lung and bronchiectasis.

LOBELIA, or INDIAN TOBACCO, is a traditional remedy for asthma. It consists of the leaves and tops of *Lobelia inflata*, a common weed in the United States. In large doses, it causes vomiting and paralyses the heart's action, being a dangerous poison, but in moderate doses it relieves the spasm to which asthma is due. It is a constituent of many burning powders made for smoking by asthmatics, but it is more commonly used in the form of tincture of lobelia combined with other drugs.

LOBOTOMY is the cutting of a lobe.

LOBULE is the term applied to a division of an organ smaller than a lobe: for example, the lobules of the lung are of the size of millet seeds, those of the liver slightly larger. Lobules form the smallest subdivisions or units of an organ, each lobule being similar to the others, of which there may be perhaps several hundred thousand in the organ.

LOCHIA is the discharge which takes place during the first week or two after child-birth. During the first four days it consists chiefly of blood; after the fifth day the colour should become paler, and after the first week the quantity should diminish and the appearance be creamy. There should at no time be any putrid odour, the presence of this being an indication of dangerous septic infection. The presence of blood after the second week indicates that the patient has been too active or that the natural absorptive changes are not duly taking place. (See PUERPERIUM.)

LOCKED-IN SYNDROME This describes a condition in which a patient is awake and retains the power of sense perception but is unable to communicate except by limited eye movements because the motor nervous system is paralysed. Several diseases can cause this syndrome which results from interruption of some of the nerve tracts between the mid brain and the pons (see BRAIN). Sometimes the syndrome is caused by severe damage to muscles or the nerves enervating them. Locked-in syndrome may sometimes be confused with a persistent vegetative state (q.v.).

LOCKJAW is a prominent symptom of tetanus (q.v.) and was once the popular name for this condition.

LOCOMOTOR ATAXIA The uncoordinated movements and unsteady lurching gait that occurs in the tertiary stage of untreated syphilis.

LOCUM TENENS A doctor who stands in for another.

LOFEPRAMINE is a tricyclic antidepressant drug (see ANTIDEPRESSANTS).

LOGORRHOEA is the technical term for garrulousness, a feature which may be exaggerated in certain states of mental instability.

LOIASIS is the disease caused by the filarial worm *Loa loa*, a thread-like worm which differs from *W. bancrofti* in that it is shorter and thicker, and it is found in the blood-stream during the day, not at night. It is transmitted by the mango fly, *Chrysops dimidiata*, but other flies of this genus can also transmit it. It is confined to West and Central Africa. The characteristic feature of the disease is the appearance of fugitive swellings which may arise anywhere in the body in the course of the worm's migration through the body. These are known as Calabar swellings. The worm is often found in the eye, hence the old name of the worm in Africa – the eye worm. Satisfactory results are being reported from the use of diethylcarbamazine in the treatment of this form of filariasis (q.v.).

LOIN is the name applied to the part of the back between the lower ribs and the pelvis. (For pain in the loins see BACKACHE; LUMBAGO.)

LONG-SIGHT (see REFRACTION).

LOPERAMIDE is a drug that reduces the motility of the gastrointestinal tract and is of limited use as an *adjunct* to fluid replacement in acute diarrhoea in adults and older children.

LORAZEPAM is a tranquillizer that is proving of value as a sedative for administration before operation. Its advantage, compared with other similar drugs, is that it stimulates, rather than depresses, breathing. It is used in the treatment of pre-eclampsia (q.v.) on the grounds that it has less of a depressant effect on the new-born child than other tranquillizers.

LORDOSIS means an unnatural curvature of the spine forwards. It occurs chiefly in the lumbar region, where the natural curve is forwards, as the result of muscular weakness, spinal disease, etc. (See SPINAL COLUMN.)

LOTIONS are fluid preparations intended for bringing in contact with, or for washing, the external surface of the body. Lotions are generally of a watery or alcoholic composition, and many of them are known as 'liquors'. Those external applications which are of an oily nature, and intended to be rubbed into the surface, are known as liniments.

LOUSE (see INSECTS IN RELATION TO DISEASE).

LOZENGES, also known as TROCHES, or TROCHISCI, consist of small tablets containing drugs mixed with sugar, gum, glycerin-jelly, or fruit-paste. They are used in various affections of the mouth and throat, being sucked and slowly dissolved by the saliva, which brings the drugs they contain in contact with the affected surface. Some of the substances used in lozenges are benzalkonium, benzocaine, betamethasone, bismuth, formaldehyde, hydrocortisone, liquorice, penicillin.

LSD (see LYSERGIC ACID).

LUGOL'S SOLUTION is a compound solution of iodine and potassium iodide.

LUMBAGO Pain in the lower (lumbar) region of the back. It may be muscular, skeletal or neurological in origin. A severe form associated with sciatica (q.v.) may be due to a prolapsed intervertebral disc. Less severe forms may be caused by osteoarthritis (q.v.) of the spine, a trapped nerve, inflammation of connective tissue or may follow an old injury.

The treatment will depend on the cause but mild lumbago will usually respond to non-steroidal anti-inflammatory drugs and the application of warmth.

LUMBAR is a term used to denote structures in, or diseases affecting, the region of the loins, as, for example, the lumbar vertebrae, lumbar abscess.

LUMBAR PUNCTURE is a procedure for removing cerebrospinal fluid from the spinal canal in the lumbar region in order: (1) to diagnose disease of the nervous system; (2) to introduce medicaments: spinal anaesthetics, or drugs, or serum.

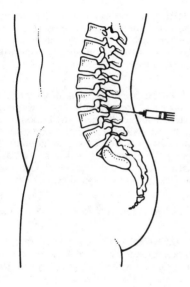

Site of lumbar puncture: between third and fourth lumbar vertebrae.

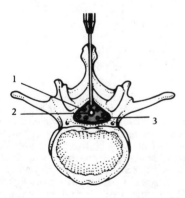

1 dura mater
2 filum terminale
3 cauda equina

Cross-section of lumbar vertebra to show needle in position in the cerebrospinal fluid.

LUMBAR SYMPATHECTOMY Destruction of the lumbar chain of sympathetic nerves by means of surgery, diathermy or injection of chemicals (phenol or alcohol). The technique is used to improve the blood flow to the leg in patients with peripheral vascular disease and to treat some types of chronic leg pain. The technique has only limited success.

LUMBAR VERTEBRA There are five lumbar vertabrae in the lower spinal column between the thoracic vertebrae and the sacrum (q.v. SPINAL COLUMN).

LUMBRICUS is a name sometimes applied to the roundworm or *Ascaris lumbricoides*. (See ASCARIASIS.)

LUMEN (1) The space enclosed by a tubular structure or hollow organ (e.g. the gastro-intestinal tract or bladder). (2) The SI unit of luminous flux (1 lumen (1m) = the amount of light emitted per second in a unit solid angle of 1 steradian by a 1-candela point source).

LUMPECTOMY An operation for breast cancer in which the tumour is removed from the breast rather than with it (see MASTECTOMY).

LUNAR CAUSTIC is another name for nitrate of silver.

LUNATIC is a general term applied to people of disordered mind, because lunacy was supposed at one time to be largely influenced by the moon. (See MENTAL ILLNESS.)

LUNGS The lungs form a pair of organs situated in the chest, and discharge the function of respiration. (See RESPIRATION.) Whilst this is their primary function, they also act as a filter for the blood. The air, which enters through the nose and passes down the throat, larynx, and windpipe in succession (see AIR PASSAGES), reaches the lungs by the right and left bronchial tubes, into which the windpipe divides within the chest, at the level of the second rib. The texture of the lungs is very highly elastic, so that when the chest is opened each lung collapses to about one-third of its natural bulk.
Form and position Each lung is roughly conical in shape, with an apex projecting into the neck, and a base resting upon the diaphragm. The rounded outer surface of each is in contact with the ribs of its own side, while the heart, lying between the lungs, hollows out the inner surface of each to some extent. There is an anterior border, along which the outer and inner surfaces meet, and the borders of the two lungs touch one another for a short distance behind the middle of the breast-bone. The apex, which is blunt, extends 35 mm (1½ inches) or more into the neck above the line of the collar-bone, being covered here by the muscles of the

neck. The base is deeply hollowed, in correspondence with the domed shape of the diaphragm, which is pushed up by the liver on the right side, and by the stomach and spleen on the left. The right lung is split by two deep fissures into three lobes; the left has two lobes divided by a single fissure. The weight of the two lungs together is about 1·1 kg, the right being rather heavier than the left. The lungs of men are heavier than those of women. There is a tendency for lung mass to increase throughout life. Each lung is enveloped in a membrane, the pleura or pleural membrane, in such a way that one layer of the membrane is closely adherent to the lung, from which indeed it cannot be separated, while the other layer lines the inner surface of one half of the chest. These two layers form a closed cavity, the pleural cavity, which everywhere surrounds the lung except at the point where the bronchi and vessels enter it. This cavity is, in the natural state, a merely potential space, the two layers of pleural membrane being separated only by a thin layer of fluid, which enables them to glide with very little friction over one another as the lung expands and retracts in breathing; but, in certain states, fluid collects in the pleural cavity, so that several pints of fluid may be effused there, compressing the lung. In some circumstances air escapes into the pleural cavity, and the lung then collapses temporarily upon its root, but air in the pleural cavity is usually absorbed, and the lung comes to occupy its original volume.

Colour In children, the colour of the lungs is rose-pink but, as life advances, they become more and more of a slaty hue, mottled with streaks and patches of dark grey and black, which are due to deposits in the lymph spaces of dust inhaled on the breath. Eskimos and others who live in an atmosphere free from dust retain the colour of childhood; on the other hand, the lungs of coal-miners become often of an almost uniform jet-black shade.

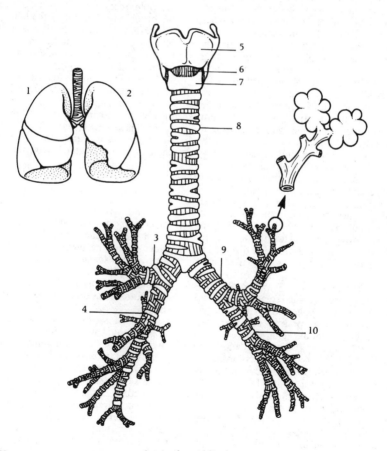

1 right lobes
2 left lobes
3 right bronchus
4 right hyparterial bronchus
5 thyroid cartilage
6 cricothyroid ligament
7 cricoid cartilage
8 trachea
9 left bronchus
10 left hyparterial bronchus

Lower air passages (centre) and their position relative to the lungs (left).
Respiratory bronchiole and alveolus (right).

Changes at birth Before birth, and in stillborn children, the lungs are of a yellowish colour, of solid gland-like appearance, and packed away in the back of the chest. Further, such lungs do not float in water, and their weight amounts to about $^1/_{70}$ of the whole body-weight. Immediately upon birth a remarkable change takes place: the tissue of the lungs expands, like the petals of an opening flower; the colour changes to rose-red, and the weight is suddenly doubled from the inrush of blood; the consistency becomes spongy, as air is drawn into the lungs, and if the child should die after drawing a few breaths, any portion of the lung which may be cut off floats in water. These changes are of importance, from the medico-legal point of view, in determining whether a dead infant was born alive or not.

Connections with heart Not only does the heart lie in contact with the two lungs, so that changes in the volume of the lungs cannot fail to have an effect upon the heart's action, but the heart is also connected by vessels with both lungs. The pulmonary artery passes from the right ventricle and divides into two branches, one of which runs straight outwards to each lung, entering its substance along with the bronchial tube at the hilum or root of the lung. From this point also emerge the pulmonary veins, which carry the blood purified in the lungs back to the left atrium.

Minute structure Each main bronchial tube, entering the lung at the root, divides into branches, which subdivide again and again, to be distributed all through the substance of the lung, till the finest tubes, known as respiratory bronchioles, have a width of only 0·25 mm ($^1/_{100}$ inch). In structure, all these tubes consist of a mucous membrane surrounded by a fibrous sheath. The windpipe as well as the larger and medium bronchi have in the fibrous layer large pieces of cartilage, which in the windpipe and largest bronchial tubes form regular hoops, and in the medium-sized tubes are disposed as irregular plates. These pieces of cartilage have the function of preventing the tubes from closing or being compressed, and so obstructing the passage of air. The larger and medium bronchi are richly supplied with glands secreting mucus, which is poured out upon the surface of the membrane. This surface is composed of columnar epithelial cells, which are provided with cilia. These have a co-ordinated beating action which sweeps mucus and bacteria upwards towards the throat. The wall of the bronchial tubes is rich in fibres of elastic tissue, and immediately beneath the mucous membrane is a layer of circularly placed unstriped muscle fibres, which is specially well developed in the smaller bronchi. This muscular layer plays an important role in the removal of mucus by coughing; it is also of great importance in connection with the causation of asthma. (See ASTHMA.)

The smallest divisions of the bronchial tubes, or bronchioles, divide into a number of tortuous tubes known as alveolar ducts and these branch into expanded passages known as atria, each of which leads into a terminal air saccule. The walls of the alveolar ducts, atria and air saccules are covered with minute sacs, known as alveoli, of which there are around 300 million. Each alveolus consists of a delicate membrane composed of flattened, plate-like cells, strengthened by a wide network of elastic fibres, to which the great elasticity of the lung is due; and in these thin-walled air-cells the important function of the lungs is carried on.

The branches of the pulmonary artery accompany the bronchial tubes to the furthest recesses of the lung, dividing like the latter into finer and finer branches, and ending in a dense network of capillaries, which lies everywhere between the air-vesicles, the capillaries being so closely placed that they occupy a much greater area than the spaces between them. The air in the air-vesicles is separated therefore from the blood only by two delicate membranes: the wall of the air-vesicle and the capillary wall, through which an exchange of gases readily takes place. The blood from the capillaries is collected by the pulmonary veins, which also accompany the bronchi to the root of the lung.

Another and much smaller set of bronchial blood-vessels runs actually upon the walls of the bronchial tubes, and these serve the purpose of nourishing the lung tissue.

There is in the lung also an important system of lymph vessels, which start in spaces situated between the air-vesicles, under the pleural membrane and in the walls of the bronchial tubes. These vessels leave the lung along with the blood-vessels, and are connected with a chain of bronchial glands lying near the end of the windpipe.

LUNGS, DISEASES OF The general symptoms and signs of chest diseases are mentioned under CHEST DISEASES and the chief affections to which these organs are liable are also treated under special headings. (See BRONCHIECTASIS; CHEST, DEFORMITIES OF; CHILLS AND COLDS; EMPHYSEMA; EXPECTORATION; HAEMOPTYSIS; HAEMORRHAGE; OCCUPATIONAL DISEASES; PLEURISY; PNEUMONIA; PULMONARY EMBOLISM; TUBERCULOSIS.)

INFLAMMATION OF THE LUNGS is generally known as pneumonia when it is due to infection, as alveolitis when the inflammation is immunological and as pneumonitis when it is due to physical or chemical agents. (See PNEUMONIA.) ABSCESS OF THE LUNG consists of a collection of pus within the lung tissue. Causes include inadequate treatment of pneumonia, inhalation of vomit, obstruction of the bronchial tubes by tumours and foreign bodies, pulmonary emboli and septic emboli. The patient becomes generally unwell with cough and fever. Bronchoscopy is frequently performed to detect any obstruction to the bronchi. Treatment is with a prolonged course of antibiotics. Rarely, surgery is necessary.

PULMONARY OEDEMA (CONGESTION OF THE LUNGS) is is due to accumulation of fluid in the pulmonary tissues and air spaces. This may occur due to cardiac disease (heart failure or disease of heart valves) or to an increase in the permeability of the pulmonary capillaries allowing leakage of fluid into the lung tissue (see ADULT RESPIRATORY DISTRESS SYNDROME).

Heart failure (left ventricular failure) is due to a weakness in the pumping action of the heart leading to an increase in back pressure forcing fluid out of the blood vessels into the lung tissue. Causes include heart attacks and hypertension (high blood pressure). Narrowed or leaking heart valves hinder the flow of blood through the heart; again, this produces an increase in back pressure increasing the capillary pressure in the pulmonary vessels followed by flooding of fluid into the interstitial spaces and alveoli. Accumulation of fluid in lung tissue produces breathlessness. Treatments include diuretics and other drugs to aid the pumping action of the heart. Surgical valve replacement may help when heart failure is due to valvular heart disease.

Adult Respiratory Distress Syndrome (ARDS) produces pulmonary congestion due to leakage of fluid through pulmonary capillaries. It complicates a variety of illnesses such as sepsis, trauma, aspiration of gastric contents and diffuse pneumonia. Treatment involves treating the cause and supporting the patient by providing oxygen.

COLLAPSE OF THE LUNG may occur due to blockage of a bronchial tube by tumour, foreign body or a plug of mucus which may occur in bronchitis or pneumonia. Air beyond the blockage is absorbed into the circulation causing the affected area of lung to collapse. Collapse may also occur when air is allowed into the pleural space – the space between the lining of the lung and the lining of the inside of the chest wall. This is called a pneumothorax and may occur following trauma, or spontaneously, for example when there is a rupture of a subpleural air pocket (such as a cyst) allowing a communication between the airways and the pleural space. Lung collapse by compression may occur when fluid collects in the pleural space (pleural effusion). When this fluid is blood it is known as a haemothorax. If it is due to pus it is known as an empyema.

TUMOURS OF THE LUNG are the most common cause of cancer in men and along with breast cancer are a major cause of cancer in women. In England and Wales in 1989 over 25,000 men and more than 11,500 women were diagnosed as having lung cancer. Its primary cause is cigarette smoking. A small proportion is curable by surgery. Other treatments include radiotherapy and chemotherapy.

WOUNDS OF THE LUNG may cause damage to the lung and by admitting air into the pleural cavity cause the lung to collapse with air in the pleural space (pneumothorax). This may require the insertion of a chest drain to remove the air from the pleural space and allow the lung to re-expand. The lung may be wounded by the end of a fractured rib or by some sharp body pushed between the ribs.

LUNG VOLUMES The volume of air within the lungs changes with the respiratory cycle. The volumes defined below can be measured and may be useful indicators of some pulmonary diseases.

Total lung capacity (TLC) The volume of air that can be held in the lungs at maximum inspiration.

Tidal volume (TV) The volume of air taken into and out of the lungs with each breath.

Inspiratory reserve volume (IRV) The volume of air that can still be inspired at the end of a normal quiet inspiration.

Expiratory reserve volume (ERV) The volume of air that can still be expired at the end of a normal quiet expiration.

Residual volume (RV) The volume of air remaining in the lungs after a maximal expiration.

Vital capacity (VC) The maximum amount of air that can be expired after a maximal inspiration.

Functional residual capacity (FRC) The volume of air left in the lungs at the end of a normal quiet expiration.

Normal values for a 60-kg man are:

	ml
TLC	5000–6000
TV	400–600
IRV	3300–3750
ERV	950–1200
RV	1200–1700
VC	3400–4800
FRC	2300–2600

LUPUS is a term used to designate a group of skin diseases of intractable character. There are two chief types of the disease: *Lupus vulgaris*, which is due to the *Mycobacterium tuberculosis*; and *Lupus erythematosus*, which is of unknown origin.

LUPUS VULGARIS begins most commonly before the age of 20, and, not infrequently, persists all through life, healing in one place to break out a short distance off. The nose, cheeks, brow, and sides of the neck are most commonly attacked, although the hands and the mucous membrane inside the nose and mouth are also common seats of the malady. The first sign of the disease is a small, soft nodule of yellowish transparent appearance, on this account often called an 'apple-jelly' nodule. No pain or itching accompanies the disease, but the skin gradually becomes thickened and discoloured, other nodules appear, and finally ulcers or small abscesses form. The disease progresses very slowly, but, after it has been in existence some years, the deformity produced may be very great.

Treatment Good results are obtained from the use of anti-tuberculous drugs. In certain cases it is still sometimes helpful to remove individual nodules by excision or by curettage, followed by the application of trichloracetic acid. The local application of intensive ultra-violet light is also sometimes of value.

LUPUS ERYTHEMATOSUS is a disease of unknown etiology. It occurs in two forms. The more common form, *discoid lupus erythematosus*, which is more common in women, involves only the skin and consists of rounded, red, and slightly raised patches, which are distributed most commonly on the nose and cheeks and which tend to fuse to give a characteristic butterfly appearance.

The second form, *systemic lupus erythematosus* (SLE), occurs predominantly in women in the proportion of nine women to one man. It is an auto-immune disease. There is some evidence that people who possess certain antigens (q.v.) are more vulnerable to it. It may be precipitated by a virus, exposure to sunlight, infection or the administration of sulphonamide drugs. Its manifestations vary considerably and include eruptions on the skin as in the discoid form, painful joints, involvement of the kidneys, alveolitis (q.v.), enlargement of the spleen, and fever. With adequate supervision the outlook is much better than was at one time thought to be the case, particularly if detected at an early stage. The disease usually responds dramatically to treatment with corticosteroids. Patients with systemic lupus erythematosus can obtain help and advice from Lupus U.K. (see APPENDIX 2: ADDRESSES).

LUTEINIZING HORMONE   A hormone secreted by the anterior pituitary which stimulates ovulation, maturation of the corpus luteum and the synthesis of progesterone by the ovary and testosterone by the testis.

LUX is the unit of illumination. The abbreviation is lx.

LUXATION is another word for dislocation. (See DISLOCATIONS.)

LYING-IN (see LABOUR).

LYME DISEASE   This comprises arthritis associated with skin rashes, fever and sometimes encephalitis (q.v.) or carditis (inflammation of the heart). It is caused by a spirochaete (q.v.) which is transmitted by tick bite. Treatment is with antibiotics.

LYMPH is the fluid which circulates in the lymphatic vessels of the body. It is a colourless fluid, like blood plasma in composition, only rather more watery. It contains salts similar to those of blood plasma, and the same proteins, though in smaller amount: fibrinogen, serum albumin, and serum globulin. It also contains colourless lymph corpuscles, or lymphocytes as they are known, derived from the glands. In certain of the lymphatic vessels, the lymph contains, after meals, a great amount of fat in the form of a fine milky emulsion. These are the vessels which absorb fat from the food passing

down the intestine, and convey it to the thoracic duct; they are called lacteals on account of the milky appearance of their contents. (See CHYLE.)

The lymph is derived, in the first place, from the blood, the watery constituents of which exude through the walls of the capillaries into the tissues, conveying material for the nourishment of the tissues and absorbing waste products.

The various gaps and chinks in the tissues communicate with lymph capillaries, which have a structure similar to that of the capillaries of the blood-vessel system, being composed of delicate flat cells joined edge to edge. These unite to form fine vessels, resembling minute veins in structure, to which the name of lymphatics is applied. These ramify all through the body, passing here and there through lymphatic glands, and ultimately discharge their contents into the blood circulation once more, by opening into the jugular veins in the root of the neck. Other lymph vessels commence in great numbers as minute openings on the surface of the pleura and peritoneum, and act as drains for these otherwise closed cavities. When fluid is effused into these cavities, as in a pleural effusion, for example, its absorption takes place through the lymphatic vessels. The course of these vessels is described under GLANDS.

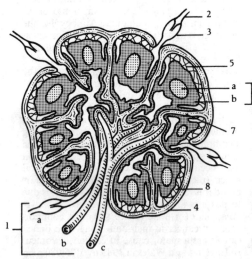

1 hilum: (a) efferent lymph vessel
           (b) venuole
           (c) arteriole
2 afferent lymph vessel
3 lymph valve
4 capsule
5 reticulin matrix
6 follicle: (a) lymphatic follicular node
            (b) medulla
7 trabecula
8 subscapula sinus

Structure of lymph node.

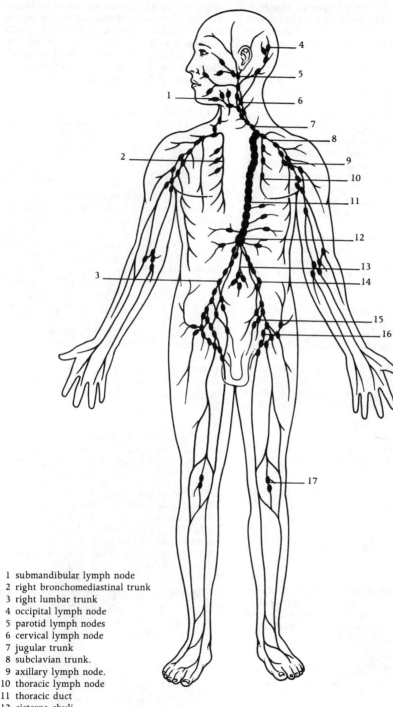

1 submandibular lymph node
2 right bronchomediastinal trunk
3 right lumbar trunk
4 occipital lymph node
5 parotid lymph nodes
6 cervical lymph node
7 jugular trunk
8 subclavian trunk.
9 axillary lymph node.
10 thoracic lymph node
11 thoracic duct
12 cisterna chyli
13 intestinal trunk
14 left lumbar trunk
15 iliac lymph node
16 inguinal lymph node
17 popliteal lymph node

Lymphatic system of body.

The circulation of the lymph is effected in some of the lower animals by lymph-hearts, which pump the lymph, just as the heart belonging to the blood-vessels keeps the blood in circulation. In man and most of the higher animals there is no heart for the lymph, which circulates partly by reason of the pressure at which it is driven through the walls of the blood capillaries, but mainly in consequence of incidental forces. The lymph capillaries and vessels are copiously provided with valves, which prevent any back flow of lymph, and every time these vessels are squeezed, as by the contraction of a muscle, or movement of a limb, the lymph moves on a little, leaving room for the exudation of fresh lymph. From this fact one can perceive the immense importance of regular exercise in maintaining the free circulation of lymph.

Lymph, like blood, possesses, in virtue of the fibrinogen which it contains, the power of clotting, forming, when it does so, a faintly yellow or colourless coagulum. This can be seen in the case of small wounds, after the blood has ceased to flow.

The term lymph is also applied to the serous fluid contained in the vesicles which develop as the result of vaccination, and used for the purpose of vaccinating other individuals. (See VACCINATION.)

The term lymph is also loosely applied to the layers and flakes of fibrin which are derived from the lymph and are found on the pleura and other serous membranes as the result of inflammation.

LYMPHADENITIS means inflammation of lymphatic glands. (See GLANDS, DISEASES OF.)

LYMPHADENOMA is another name for Hodgkin's disease (q.v.).

LYMPHANGIECTASIS means an abnormal dilatation of the lymph vessels, as in filariasis (q.v.).

LYMPHANGIOGRAPHY, or LYMPHOGRAPHY, is the procedure whereby the lymphatics (q.v.) and lymphatic glands can be rendered visible on X-ray films by means of the injection of radio-opaque substances.

LYMPHANGITIS means inflammation situated in the lymphatic vessels.

LYMPHATICS is the term applied to the vessels which convey the lymph (q.v.). (For an account of their arrangement, see GLANDS.)

LYMPH NODE Swellings which occur at various points in the lymphatic system through which lymph drains. They consist of a cortex, medulla and lymph sinuses and have two main functions: (1) The interception and removal of abnormal or foreign material from the lymph. (2) The production of immune responses. The lymph nodes become enlarged when the area of the body which they drain is the site of infection or as a manifestation of some systemic diseases. Occasionally they are the site of primary or metastatic malignant disease.

LYMPHOCYTE is a variety of white blood corpuscle produced in the lymphoid tissues and lymphatic glands of the body. It contains a simple rounded nucleus surrounded by protoplasm generally described as non-granular. Two varieties of lymphocyte are described, small lymphocytes and large lymphocytes, and together they form over 20 per cent of the white corpuscles of the blood. They play an important part in the production of antibodies (q.v.), and in the rejection of transplanted organs such as the heart. (See TRANSPLANTATION.) This they do in two different ways. What are known as B lymphocytes produce antibodies, while T lymphocytes attack and destroy antigens (q.v.) directly. They are known as T lymphocytes because they are produced by the thymus gland. Their numbers are increased in tuberculosis and certain other diseases. Such an increase is known as lymphocytosis.

LYMPHOCYTOSIS An increase in the number of lymphocytes (q.v.) in the blood, e.g. in response to infection or in chronic lymphocytic leukaemia (q.v.).

LYMPHOEDEMA means dropsical swelling of a part or organ due to obstruction to the lymph-vessels draining it.

LYMPHOGRANULOMA INGUINALE, LYMPHOGRANULOMA VENEREUM; PORADENITIS VENEREA; LYMPHOPATHIA VENEREUM, is a venereal disease in which the chief characteristic is enlargement of glands in the groin, the infecting agent being a virus. There were 17 cases in England in 1985.

LYMPHOID TISSUE Tissue involved in the formation of lymph, lymphocytes, and antibodies. It consists of the lymph nodes, thymus, tonsils and spleen.

LYMPHOKINES Lymphokines are polypeptides that are produced by lymphocytes as part of their immune response to an antigen and their function is to communicate with other cells of the immune system. Some lymphokines stimulate B cells to differentiate into antibody-producing plasma cells; others stimulate T lymphocytes to proliferate and other lymphokines become interferons.

LYMPHOMA is a malignant proliferation of lymphoid tissue classified into two main types: Hodgkin's and non-Hodgkin's. Another variety is found in children in Africa; sometimes called Burkitt's lymphoma after the surgeon who first described it. Because of its geographical distribution it is thought to be due to a virus which is transmitted by mosquitoes, but no virus has yet been definitely isolated from the tumour. Hodgkin's and non-Hodgkin's lymphomas present as enlarged lymph glands, mainly in the neck and axillae in the former and more generally in the latter variety. The difference rests in the histology of the enlarged glands. Radiotherapy and chemotherapy can be used for both types with more aggressive treatment needed for Hodgkin's lymphoma. Both types are graded according to severity and the grade is a guide to survival rates which are much improved with modern treatments.

LYMPHOSARCOMA is a malignant growth of the lymphoid elements of the body, and is characterized by generalized enlargement of the lymphatic glands, spleen, and liver. The majority of cases – about 55 per cent – occur in the 60 to 70 age-group, but it may occur at any age. The prognosis is poor, 80 per cent of cases dying within six years. Treatment is by means of irradiation or chemotherapy.

LYSERGIC ACID DIETHYLAMIDE (LSD) belongs to the ergot group of alkaloids (q.v.). It has various effects on the brain, notably analgesic and hallucinogenic, thought to be due to its antagonism of 5-hydroxytry tryptamine (5-HT). In small doses it induces psychic states, in which the individual may become aware of repressed memories. For this reason it may help in the treatment of certain anxiety states, if used under skilled supervision. LSD rapidly induces tolerance, however, and psychological dependence may occur, though not physical dependence. Serious side-effects include psychotic reactions, with an increased risk of suicide (see DRUG ADDICTION).

LYSINE An essential amino-acid, lysine was first isolated in 1889 from casein, the principal protein of milk. Like other essential amino-acids it ensures optimum growth in infants and balanced nitrogen metabolism in adults.

LYSIS means the gradual ending of a fever, and is opposed to crisis, which signifies the sudden ending of a fever. (See CRISIS.) It is also used to describe the process of dissolution of a blood-clot, or the loosening of adhesions.

LYSOFORM is a liquid soap containing formalin, which gives it a strong antiseptic power.

LYSOL is a brown, clear, oily fluid with antiseptic properties, made from coal-tar and containing 50 per cent cresol. When mixed with water it forms a clear soapy fluid. (See CRESOL.)

LYSOL POISONING When lysol is swallowed there is a sense of burning about the mouth and throat. There are signs of corrosion around and in the mouth, with brown discoloration, and the characteristic smell of lysol is very evident in the breath. If the lysol is not speedily removed, unconsciousness and stupor gradually come on and death may occur within 24 hours. Septic pneumonia is also liable to supervene, and may produce death at a later period.
Treatment If the skin has been contaminated with the lysol, it must be washed with water, and any lysol-contaminated clothing must be taken off. Large quantities of tepid water and salt may be given at once to dilute the lysol if it has been swallowed, and produce vomiting.

LYSOZYME is a bactericidal substance present in tears.

LYSSA is another term for rabies or hydrophobia.

M

McBURNEY'S POINT (see APPENDICITIS).

MACERATION is the softening of a solid by soaking in fluid.

MACROCYTE is an unusually large red blood corpuscle especially characteristic of the blood in pernicious anaemia.

MACROCYTOSIS This condition, present in certain anaemias, is characterized by the existence of abnormally large red cells in the blood. It is particularly associated with pernicious anaemia (q.v.).

MACROGLOSSIA means an abnormally large tongue.

MACROLIDES The original macrolide, erythromycin (q.v.), was discovered in the early 1950s and used successfully as an alternative to penicillin (q.v.). The name derives from the molecular structure of this group and two new drugs in the group have recently been introduced into the United Kingdom, clarithromycin and azithromycin. Macrolides check protein (q.v.) synthesis in bacteria (q.v.) and the latest ones are, like erythromycin, active against several bacterial species including Gram-positive cocci and rods. In addition they act against *Haemophilus influenzae*. Clarithromycin is potent against *Chlamydia trachomitis* (q.v.) and

Helicobacter pylori (q.v.). Azithromycin is efective against infections caused by *Legionella* spp. (see LEGIONNAIRE'S DISEASE), gonococci (q.v.) and *Mycoplasma pneumoniae* (q.v.).

MACROPHAGE A large phagocyte (q.v.) that forms part of the reticuloendothelial system. It is found in many organs and tissues, including connective tissues, bone marrow, lymph nodes, spleen, liver and central nervous system. Free macrophages move between cells and, using their scavenger properties, collect at infection sites to remove foreign bodies, including bacteria. Fixed macrophages are found in connective tissue.

MACROPSIA Condition in which objects appear larger than normal. It can be due to disease of the macula.

MACULA A spot or area of tissue that is different from surrounding tissue. An example is the macula letea, the yellow spot in the retina of the eye (see EYE).

MACULES are spots or stained areas of brown or purplish-brown colour in the skin. They may be due to old haemorrhages, sunburn, disease of internal organs, pregnancy, skin diseases such as eczema and psoriasis, syphilis, and burns.

MACULOPAPULAR A skin rash that is made up of macules (discoloration of the skin) and papules (raised abnormality of the skin).

MADURA FOOT is the name given to a disease found in the Tropics in which the foot becomes swollen and its bones and other tissues riddled by sinuses. It is caused by the presence of a fungus.

MAGNESIUM is a light metallic element. Magnesium is one of the essential mineral elements of the body, without which it cannot function properly. The adult body contains around 25 grams, the greater part of which is in the bones. More than two-thirds of our daily supply come from cereals and vegetables. As most other foods also contain useful amounts, there is thus seldom any difficulty in maintaining an adequate amount in the body. It is an essential constituent of several vital enzymes (q.v.). Deficiency leads to muscular weakness and interferes with the efficient working of the heart. The salts of magnesium used as drugs are the hydroxide of magnesium, the oxide of magnesium, generally known as 'magnesia', and the carbonate of magnesium, all of which have an antacid action; also the sulphate of magnesium generally known as 'Epsom salts', which acts as a purgative.

Uses Light and heavy carbonates of magnesia are used to correct hyperacidity of the stomach,

as are the hydroxide and the light oxide. They are also used as feeble laxatives. Cream of magnesia, the official *British Pharmacopoeia* name of which is Magnesium Hydroxide Mixture, is a widely used, effective antacid. In large doses it is a useful safe laxative.

Magnesium sulphate is a traditionally used saline purge. (See EPSOM SALTS.)

MAGNESIUM TRISILICATE A white powder with antacid properties. A mild antacid with prolonged action, it is used for treating peptic ulceration, commonly combined with quickly acting antacids. It has no side-effects so can be used in large doses.

MAGNETIC RESONANCE IMAGING (MRI) (see NUCLEAR MAGNETIC RESONANCE).

MALABSORPTION SYNDROME includes a multiplicity of diseases, all of which are characterized by faulty absorption from the intestine of essential foodstuffs, such as fat, vitamins and mineral salts. Among the conditions in this syndrome are coeliac disease (q.v.), sprue (q.v.), cystic fibrosis and pancreatis. Surgical removal of the small intestine also causes the syndrome. Symptoms include anaemia, diarrhoea, oedema, vitamin deficiencies, weight loss and, in severe cases, malnutrition.

MALACIA is a term applied to softening of a part or tissue in disease: e.g. osteomalacia or softening of the bones.

MALAISE means a vague feeling of feverishness, listlessness, and languor, which often precedes the onset of serious acute diseases, or accompanies passing derangements, such as dyspepsia, chills, and colds.

MALAR Anything relating to the cheek. For example, the malar (zygomatic) bone is also known as the cheek bone, and a malar flush is reddening of the cheeks.

MALARIA The term is derived from the Italian *mal aria*. Disease is caused by four species of *Plasmodium*: *P. falciparum*, *P. vivax*, *P. ovale*, and *P. malariae*. Clinically, malaria is characterized by recurrent febrile episodes, sometimes associated with rigors; enlargement of the spleen is common. *P. falciparum* infection can also be associated with several serious – often fatal – complications (see below); although other species cause chronic disease, acute mortality is unusual.

Malaria is a disease of great antiquity; one suggestion is that it contributed significantly to the fall of the Roman Empire. An association with marshes was recognized in ancient times, and an association with mosquitoes had been suggested on many occasions historically. However, it was not until 1897–8, that Ronald Ross working in India was able to establish clearly a host–mosquito–host cycle in avian malaria. Shortly afterwards the human–mosquito–human cycle was established beyond doubt; groups of British (led by Patrick Manson) and Italian (A. Bignami and others) researchers helped in this discovery.

The infection(s) is very widely distributed in tropical and subtropical countries; *P. falciparum* is, however, confined very largely to Africa, Asia, and South America. Not only are areas of transmission increasing, but *Plasmodium* spp. parasites are also increasingly developing resistance to various chemoprophylactic and chemotherapeutic agents. Malaria also constitutes a significant problem in travellers; so it is essential that travellers obtain sound advice on chemoprophylaxis before embarking on tropical trips (see APPENDIX 3: TRAVEL AND HEALTH), especially to a rural area where intense transmission can occur. Transmission has also been recorded at airports, and following blood transfusion.

During a bite by the female mosquito, one or more sporozoites (q.v.) are injected into the human circulaton; these are taken up by the hepatocytes (liver cells). Following division, merozoites (minute particles resulting from the division) are liberated into the bloodstream where they invade the erythrocytes. These in turn divide, releasing further merozoites. Merozoites are periodically liberated into the bloodstream, causing characteristic fevers, rigors, etc. To complete the life-cycle, sexual forms (gametocytes) are taken up during a further mosquito bite.

Diagnosis is by demonstration of trophozoites – a stage in the parasite's life-cycle that takes place in red blood cells – in thick/thin blood-films of peripheral blood. Serological tests are of value in deciding whether an individual has had a past infection, but are of no value in acute disease.

Various chemoprophylactic regimes are widely used. Those commmonly prescribed include: chloroquine + paludrine, mefloquine, and Maloprim (trimethoprim + dapsone); Fansidar (trimethoprim + sulphamethoxazole) has been shown to have significant side-effects, especially when used in conjunction with chloroquine, and is now rarely used. No chemotherapeutic regimen is totally effective so other preventive measures are again being used. These include people avoiding mosquito bites, covering exposed areas of the body between dusk and dawn, and using mosquito repellents.

Chemotherapy was for many years dominated by the synthetic agent chloroquine. However, with the widespread emergence of chloroquine-resistance, quinine is again the agent of choice. First introduced into Europe from South America as the 'bark' in the 17th century, it was first included in the *London Pharmacopoeia* (3rd edition) in 1677 as *Cortex Peruanus*. Quinine should be administered intravenously in a severe infection; the oral route is used subsequently and in minor cases. Other agents currently in use include mefloquine,

halofantrine, doxycycline, and the artemesinin alkaloids ('qinghaosu').

Complications of *P. falciparum* infection include cerebral involvement, due to adhesion of immature trophozoites on to the cerebral vascular endothelium; these lead to a high death rate when inadequately treated. Renal involvement (frequently resulting from haemoglobinuria), pulmonary oedema, hypotension, hypoglycaemia, and complications in pregnancy are also important. In complicated disease, haemodialysis and exchange transfusion have been used. No adequate controlled trial using the latter regimen has been carried out, however, and possible benefits must be weighed against numerous potential side-effects – for instance, the introduction of a wide range of infections, overloading the circulatory system with infused fluids and other complications.

P. vivax and *P. ovale* infections cause less severe disease, although overall there are many clinical similarities with *P. faciparum* infection; acute complications are unusual, but chronic anaemia is often present. Primaquine is necessary to eliminate the exoerythrocytic cycle in the hepatocyte (liver cell).

P. malariae usually produces a chronic infection, and chronic renal disease (nephrotic syndrome) is an occasional sequel, especially in tropical Africa.

Gross splenomegaly (hyperreactive malarious splenomegaly, or tropical splenomegaly syndrome) can complicate all four human *Plasmodium* spp. infections. The syndrome responds to long-term malarial chemoprophylaxis. Burkitt's lymphoma is found in geographical areas where malaria infection is endemic; the Epstein-Barr virus is aetiologically involved.

MALATHION is one of the less toxic organophosphorus insecticides (q.v.).

MALFORMATION (see DEFORMITIES).

MALIGNANT is a term applied in several ways to serious disorders. Tumours are called malignant when they grow rapidly, tend to infiltrate surrounding healthy tissues, and to spread to distant parts of the body, leading eventually to death. (See CANCER.) The term is also applied to types of disease which are much more serious than the usual form, such as malignant hypertension and malignant smallpox. Malignant pustule is another name for anthrax (q.v.).

MALIGNANT HYPERPYREXIA (see MALIGNANT HYPERTHERMIA).

MALIGNANT HYPERTENSION has nothing to do with cancer. It derives its name from the fact that, if untreated, it runs a rapidly fatal course. (See HYPERTENSION.)

MALIGNANT HYPERTHERMIA This disorder is a rare complication of general anaesthesia caused, it is believed, by a combination of an inhalation anaesthetic (usually halothane (q.v.)) and a muscle-relaxant drug (usually succinycholine). A life-endangering rise in temperature occurs, with muscular rigidity the first sign. Tachycardia (q.v.), arrythmia (q.v.), acidosis (q.v.) and shock (q.v.) usually occur. About 1:20,000 patients having general anaesthesia suffer from this disorder, which progresses rapidly and is often fatal. Surgery and anaesthesia must be stopped immediately and appropriate corrective measures taken, including the administration of dantrolene (q.v.) intravenously.

MALINGERING is a term applied to the feigning of illness. In the great majority of cases a person who feigns illness has a certain amount of disability, but exaggerates the illness or discomfort for some ulterior motive.

MALLEOLUS is the term applied to either of the two bony prominences at the ankle. (See LEG.)

MALLET FINGER is due to sudden forced flexion of the terminal joint of a finger, resulting in rupture of the tendon. As a result the individual is unable to extend the terminal part of the finger which remains bent forward. The middle, ring and little fingers are most commonly involved. Treatment is by splinting the finger. The end result is satisfactory provided the victim has sufficient patience.

MALLET TOE is the condition in which it is not possible to extend the terminal part of the toe. It is usually due to muscular imbalance but may be due to congenital absence of the extensor muscle. A callosity (q.v.) often forms on it which may be painful. Should this be troublesome, treatment consists of removal of the terminal phalanx.

MALLEUS The hammer-shaped lateral bone of the group of three that form the sound-transmitting ossicles in the middle ear. (See EAR.)

MALNUTRITION The condition arising from an inadequate or unbalanced diet. The causes may be a lack of one or more essential nutrients or inadequate absorption from the intestinal tracts. A diet that is deficient in carbohydrate usually contains inadequate protein, and this type of malnutrition occurs in Africa and Asia as a result of poverty, famine or war.

MALOPRIM is a combination of pyrimethamine (q.v.) and dapsone (q.v.) which is used for the prevention of malaria (q.v.). It has the advantage of only needing to be taken once weekly. It should not be taken by anyone hypersensitive to sulphonamides, and should not be used for the treatment of an acute attack.

MALPRACTICE Improper or inadequate medical treatment that fails to match the standards of skill and care that is reasonably expected from a qualified health care practitioner – usually a doctor or dentist.

MALPRESENTATION A situation during childbirth in which a baby is not in the customary head-first position before delivery. The result is usually a complicated labour in which a caesarean operation may be necessary to effect the birth.

MALT is a substance derived from barley by allowing a certain amount of growth to take place in the moistened grain, which is then dried and crushed. It contains an enzyme named diastase, together with a large amount of malt-sugar and dextrin, the latter constituents being still further developed from the starch of the barley by the action of the enzyme, when the malt is allowed to digest in water at a temperature approaching 40 °C (104 °F). Similarly, the enzyme will convert into sugar a large amount of the starch in flour mixed with malt, and so perform some of the functions of the saliva and pancreatic juice.

For these reasons malt is mixed with various proportions of flour to form some of the popular foods for children. It is also used in the form of malt extracts, 28 grams of which is equivalent to 80 Calories.

MALTA FEVER (see BRUCELLOSIS).

MAMMARY GLAND (see BREASTS).

MAMMILLA is the Latin term for the nipple.

MAMMOGRAPHY is the special technique whereby X-rays can be taken that reveal the structure of the breast. It is an effective way of distinguishing benign from malignant tumours. It can detect tumours that are not palpable. In a multi-centre study in the USA, called The Breast Cancer Detection Demonstration Project, which involved nearly 300,000 women in the 40–49 age group, 35 per cent of the tumours were found by mammography alone, 13 per cent by physical examination and 50 per cent by both methods. The optimum frequency of screening is debatable. The American College of Radiologists recommends a baseline mammogram at the age of 40 years with subsequent mammography at one to two year intervals up to the age of 50. Thereafter, annual mammography is recommended. In the United Kingdom a less intensive screening programme is in place with women over 50 being screened every three years. In 1991–2 1·4 million were invited for screening: 1·02 million accepted, among whom 6,605 cancers were identified. As breast cancer is the commonest malignancy in Western women and is increasing in frequency, the importance of screening for this form of cancer is obvious.

MANDELIC ACID is a non-toxic keto-acid used in the treatment of infections of the urinary tract, especially those due to the *Escherichia coli* and the *Streptococcus faecalis* or *Enterococcus*. It is administered in doses of 3 grams several times daily. As it is only effective in an acid urine, ammonium chloride must be taken at the same time.

MANDIBLE is the bone of the lower jaw.

MANGANESE is a metal, oxides of which are found abundantly in nature. Permanganate of potassium is a well-known disinfectant.

MANIA is a form of mental disorder characterized by great excitement. (See MENTAL ILLNESS.)

MANIC-DEPRESSIVE INSANITY, or CYCLOTHYMIA, is a form of madness characterized by alternate attacks of mania and depression. (See MENTAL ILLNESS.)

MANIPULATION is the passive movement – often forceful – of bones, joints, or soft tissues, carried out by orthopaedic surgeons, physiotherapists, osteopaths (q.v.) and chiropractors (q.v.) as an important part of treatment, often highly effective. It may be used for three chief reasons: correction of deformity (mainly the reduction of fractures and dislocations, or to overcome deformities such as congenital club foot (q.v.)); treatment of joint stiffness (particularly after an acute limb injury, or frozen shoulder (q.v.)); and relief of chronic pain (particularly when due to chronic strain, notably the spinal joints (see PROLAPSED INTERVERTEBRAL DISC)). Depending on the particular injury or deformity being treated, and the estimated force required, manipulation may be used with or without anaesthesia. Careful clinical and radiological examination, together with other appropriate investigations, should always be carried out before starting treatment, to reduce the risk of harm, or disasters such as fractures or the massive displacement of an intervertebral disc.

MANNITOL is an osmotic diuretic (q.v.) given intravenously. (See DIURETICS.)

MANOMETER is an instrument for measuring the pressure or tension of liquids or gases. (See BLOOD-PRESSURE.)

MANTOUX TEST, also known as MENDEL'S TEST, is a test for tuberculosis. It consists in injecting into the superficial layers of the skin (i.e. intradermally) a very small quantity of old tuberculin. A positive reaction of the skin – swelling and redness – shows that the person so reacting has been infected with the *Mycobacterium tuberculosis*. But it does not mean that such a person is suffering from active tuberculosis. (See TUBERCULIN.)

MANUBRIUM is the uppermost part of the breast-bone.

MARASMUS means progressive wasting, especially in young children, when there is no ascertainable cause. It is generally associated with defective feeding. (See ATROPHY; INFANT FEEDING.)

MARBURG DISEASE, also known as GREEN MONKEY DISEASE and VERVET MONKEY DISEASE because the first recorded cases acquired their infection from monkeys of this genus, is a highly dangerous viral infection with a high mortality rate. The incubation period is 4 to 9 days. The onset is sudden with marked nausea and severe headache. This is followed by rising temperature, diarrhoea, and vomiting. Towards the end of the first week a rash appears which persists for a week and is accompanied by internal bleeding. In those who recover convalescence is slow and prolonged. The world distribution of the causative virus is unknown, but apart from laboratory infections acquired through working with vervet monkeys, all the cases so far reported have occurred in Africa.

MARCH FRACTURE is a curious condition in which a fracture occurs of the second (rarely the third) metatarsal bone in the foot without any obvious cause. The usual story is that a pain suddenly developed in the foot while walking (hence the name) and that it has persisted ever since. The only treatment needed is immobilization of the foot and rest, and the fracture heals satisfactorily.

MARCH HAEMOGLOBINURIA is a complication of walking and running over long distances. It is due to damage to red blood cells in the blood-vessels of the sole of the feet. This results in haemoglobin (q.v.) being released into the bloodstream, which is then voided in the urine, the condition known as haemoglobinuria (q.v.). No treatment is required, but the complaint may be minimized by wearing shoes with resilient soles and, so far as possible, avoiding running on hard surfaces.

MARFAN'S SYNDROME An inherited disorder affecting about one person in 50,000 in which the connective tissue is abnormal. The result is defects of the heart, skeleton and eyes. The victims are unusually tall and thin with deformities of the chest and spine. They have spider-like hands and their joints and ligaments are weak. Orthopaedic intervention may help, as will drugs to control the heart problems. As affected individuals have a 50-per-cent chance of passing on the disease to their children, they should receive genetic counselling.

MARIJUANA is another term for CANNABIS INDICA, or hemp, or hashish. (See DRUG ADDICTION.)

MARRIAGE GUIDANCE (see RELATE MARRIAGE GUIDANCE).

MARROW (see BONE MARROW).

MARSH FEVER (see MALARIA).

MASOCHISM A condition in which a person gets pleasure from physical or emotional pain inflicted by others. The term is often used in the context of achieving sexual excitement through inflicted pain. Masochism may be a conscious or subconscious activity.

MASSAGE, or RUBBING, is a method of treatment in which the operator uses his hands, or occasionally other appliances, to rub the skin and deeper tissues of the person under treatment. It is often combined with (a) passive movements, in which the masseur moves the limbs in various ways, the person treated making no effort; or (b) active movements, which are performed with the combined assistance of masseur and patient. Massage is also often combined with baths and gymnastics in order to strengthen various muscles. Massage helps to improve circulation, prevent adhesions in injured tissues, relax muscular spasm, improve muscle tone and reduce any oedema. (See also CARDIAC MASSAGE.)

Massage for medical conditions is best done by trained practitioners. A complete list of members of the Chartered Society of Physiotherapy can be obtained on application to the Secretary of the Society (see APPENDIX 2: ADDRESSES).

MASSETER An important muscle of mastication that extends from the zygomatic arch in the cheek to the mandible or jaw bone. It acts by closing the jaw.

MASS HYSTERIA (see HYSTERIA).

MASS MINIATURE RADIOGRAPHY is a method of obtaining X-ray photographs of the chests of large numbers of people at about the rate of two per minute. It has been used on a large scale as a means of screening the population for pulmonary tuberculosis.

MASTALGIA is the term applied to pain in the breast.

MAST CELLS are round or oval cells found predominantly in the loose connective tissues. They contain histamine (q.v.) and heparin (q.v.), and carry immunoglobulin E, the antibody which plays a predominant part in allergic reactions. Although known to play a part in inflammatory reactions, allergy, and hypersensitivity, their precise function in health and disease is still not quite clear.

MASTECTOMY is the operation for removal of a breast. It is an operation that can cause considerable psychological disturbance. Those who find it difficult to adjust to the situation after the operation will obtain helpful advice from Breast Cancer Care (see APPENDIX 2: ADDRESSES).

MASTICATION is the act whereby, as a result of movements of the lower jaw, lips, tongue, and cheek, food is reduced to a condition in which it is ready to be acted on by the gastric juices in the process of digestion. Adequate mastication is an essential part of the digestive process. (See DIGESTION.)

MASTITIS is the term applied to inflammation of the breast. (See BREASTS, DISEASES OF.)

MASTOID PROCESS is the large process of the temporal bone of the skull which can be felt immediately behind the ear. It contains numerous cavities, one of which, the mastoid antrum, communicates with the middle ear, and is liable to suppurate when the middle ear is diseased. (See EAR, DISEASES OF.)

MASTURBATION is the production of an orgasm by self-manipulation of the penis or clitoris.

MAT BURN is a combination of a burn and an abrasion which occurs in wrestlers when the skin over the bony points is rubbed against the unyielding canvas mat. It is particularly liable to become infected. Treatment consists of thorough cleansing and the application of a dressing such as gauze and chlorhexidine covered by cotton-wool and firmly fixed by a bandage or elastoplast – depending on the extent of the injury.

MATCH-WORKERS' DISEASE (see PHOSPHORUS POISONING).

MATERIA MEDICA is that branch of medical study which deals with the sources, preparations, and uses of drugs.

MATERNITY AND CHILD WELFARE In the United Kingdom the proper care of pregnant women, mothers, infants and young children started largely on a voluntary basis early in the 20th century. With official backing it has now developed into an extensive network of clinics in NHS general practices, hospitals and local-authority premises, where skilled antenatal, postnatal and paediatric care is provided by consultants, general practitioners, midwives, health visitors and nurses. Local authorities also have certain responsibilities for the provision of appropriate accommodation for mothers with young children on low incomes. Various welfare benefits are available to young families, provided they meet official criteria. Day nurseries, some run by local authorities, others on a voluntary or privately funded basis are available in some areas to young mothers, especially those who are working. Efforts are being made to increase the numbers of such nurseries.

A recent official review of maternity and child health services called for substantial changes in professional practice to secure a 'woman-centred service'. The aim was greater acceptability and accessibility of maternity care founded on 'clinical practices of known effectiveness'.

MAXILLA is the name applied to the upper jaw-bones, which bear the teeth.

ME (see MYALGIC ENCEPHALOMYELITIS).

MEASLES, also known as MORBILLI, is an acute infectious disease occurring mostly in children and caused by an RNA paramyxovirus. The name, measles, comes from the teutonic root, *maes*, meaning a spot. Morbilli is a diminutive of morbus, a disease. It appears to have been known from an early period in the history of medicine, mention being made of it in the writings of Rhazes and others of the Arabian physicians in the tenth century. For long, however, its specific nature was not recognized, and it was held to be a variety of smallpox. Measles and scarlet fever were long confused with each other; and in the account given by Sydenham of epidemics of measles in London in 1670 and 1674, it is evident that even that accurate observer had not as yet clearly perceived their pathological distinction, although it would seem to have been made a century earlier by Ingrassia, a physician of Palermo. The disease known as German measles, or rubella, is a much milder disease than measles. Measles is compulsorily notifiable in Britain.

Causes Measles is a disease of the earlier years of childhood. Like most other infectious maladies, it is rare in infants under 6 months old on account of the antibodies that they have acquired from their mothers before birth. It is rare in adults because most have undergone an attack in early life, although second attacks can occur. The incubation period is 7 to 21 days.

There has been a dramatic fall in numbers from 1986 when over 80,000 cases were reported. This is due to the introduction in 1988 of the measles, mumps and rubella vaccine (MMR) (see IMMUNIZATION); 1990 was the first year in which no deaths from measles were reported. Even so, fears of side-effects of the vaccine against measles meant that some children in the UK were not immunized. Side-effects are, however, rare and the government is campaigning to raise the rate of immunization, with GPs being set targets for their practices.

There are few diseases so infectious as measles, and its rapid spread in epidemics is no doubt due to the fact that this viral infection is most potent in the earlier stages. Hence the difficulty of timely isolation and the readiness with which the disease is spread, which is mostly by infected droplets.

Symptoms Prodromal symptoms are catarrh, conjunctivitis (see EYE DISEASES), fever and a feeling of wretchedness. Then Koplik spots – a classic sign of measles – appear on the roof of the mouth and lining of the cheeks. The macular body rash, typical of measles, appears three to five days later.

Treatment Isolation of the patient and treatment of any secondary bacterial infection. Children usually run a high temperature which can be relieved with cool sponging and antipyretic drugs. Calamine lotion may alleviate any itching.

MEASURES (see APPENDIX 6: MEASUREMENTS IN MEDICINE).

MEAT (see PROTEIN).

MEATUS is a term applied to any passage or opening: e.g. external auditory meatus, the passage from the surface to the drum of the ear.

MECKEL'S DIVERTICULUM is a hollow process sometimes found attached to the small intestine. It is placed on the small intestine about 90 to 120 cm (3 or 4 feet) away from its junction with the large intestine, is several cms long, and ends blindly.

MECONIUM is the brown, semi-fluid material which collects in the bowels of a child prior to birth, and which should be discharged either at the time of birth or shortly afterwards. It consists partly of bile secreted by the liver before birth, partly of debris from the mucous membrane of the intestines.

MEDIA The middle layer of an organ or tissue, but more usually applied to the wall of an artery or vein, where the media comprises layers of elastic and smooth muscle fibres.

MEDIAL Near the middle of tissue, organ or body.

MEDIAL TIBIAL SYNDROME is the term applied by athletes to a condition characterized by pain over the inner border of the shin, which occurs in most runners and sometimes in joggers. The syndrome, also known as shin splints, is due to muscular swelling resulting in inadequate blood supply in the muscle: hence the pain. The disorder may be the result of compartment syndrome (build-up of pressure in the muscles), tendinitis, muscle or bone inflammation or damage to the muscle. It usually disappears within a few weeks, responding to rest and physiotherapy, with or without injections. In some cases, however, it becomes chronic and so severe that it occurs even at rest. If the cause is the compartment syndrome, relief is usually obtained by a simple operation to relieve the pressure in the affected muscles.

MEDIASTINUM is the space in the chest which lies between the two lungs. It contains the heart and great vessels, the gullet, the lower part of the windpipe, the thoracic duct, the phrenic nerves, as well as numerous structures of less importance.

MEDICATED Description of a substance that contains a medicinal drug, commonly applied to items such as sweets and soaps.

MEDULLA The inside part of an organ or tissue that is distinct from the outer part – for example, the marrow in the centre of a long bone or the inner portion of the kidneys or adrenal glands.

MEDULLA OBLONGATA is the hindmost part of the brain and is continued into the spinal cord. In it are situated several of the nerve-centres which are most essential to life, such as those governing breathing, the action of the heart, swallowing. (See BRAIN.)

MEFENAMIC ACID is a drug with pain-relieving, anti-inflammatory and antipyretic actions that is proving of value in the treatment of osteoarthritis and rheumatoid arthritis.

MEGA- and MEGALO- are prefixes denoting largeness.

MEGACOLON A greatly enlarged colon that may be present at birth or develop later. It can occur in all age groups and the condition is typified by severe chronic constipation. Megacolon is caused by obstruction of the colon which may be due to faulty innervation, or to psychological factors. Other causes are Hirschsprung's disease (q.v.) or ulcerative colitis (q.v.). In old people the persistent use of powerful laxative drugs may cause the condition.

MEGALOMANIA is a delusion of grandeur or an insane belief in a person's own extreme greatness, goodness, or power.

MEIBOMIAN GLANDS Numerous glands within the tarsal plates of the eyelids. Their secretions form part of the tears.

MEIOSIS or REDUCTION DIVISION is the form of cell division that only occurs in the gonads, that is the testis and the ovary, giving rise to the germ cells of the sperms and the ova. Two types of sperm cells are produced. One contains 22 autosomes and a Y sex chromosome and the other contains 22 autosomes and an X sex chromosome. All the ova, however, produced by normal meiosis have 22 autosomes and an X sex chromosome. Two divisions of the nucleus occur and only one division of the chromosomes, so that the number of chromosomes in the ova and sperms is half that of the somatic cells. Each chromosome pair divides so that the gametes receives only one member of each pair. The number of chromosomes is restored to full complement at fertilization so the the zygote has a complete set, each chromosome from the nucleus of the sperm pairing up with its corresponding partner from the ovum.

The first stage of meiosis involves the pairing of homologous chromosomes which join together and synapse lengthwise. The chromosomes then become doubled by splitting along their length and the chromatids so formed are held together by centromeres. As the homologous chromosomes, one of which has come from the mother and the other from the father, are lying together genetic interchange can take place between the chromatids and in this way new combinations of genes arise. All four chromatids are closely interwoven and recombination may take place between any maternal or any paternal chromatids. This process is known as crossing over or recombination. After this period of interchange homologous chromosomes move apart, one to each pole of the nucleus. The cell then divides and the nucleus of each new cell now contains 23 and not 46 chromosomes. The second meiotic division then occurs, the centromeres divide and the chromatids move apart to opposite poles of the nucleus so there are still 23 chromosomes in each of the daughter nuclei so formed. The cell divides again so that there are four gametes, each containing a half number (haploid) set of chromosomes. However, owing to the recombination or crossing over the genetic material is not identical with either parent or with other spermatozoa.

MELAENA means a condition of the stools in which dark, tarry masses are passed from the bowel. It is due to bleeding from the stomach or from the higher part of the bowel, the blood undergoing chemical changes under the action of the secretions, and being finally converted in large part into sulphide of iron.

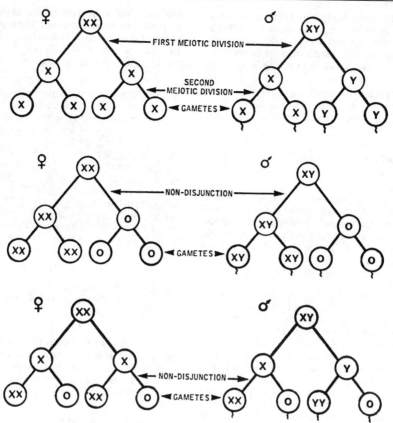

The formation of gametes. Top, normal meiosis. Centre, non-disjunction at
first meiotic division. Bottom, non-disjunction at second meiotic division.

MELANCHOLIA is a form of mental illness
characterized by great mental and physical
depression. (See MENTAL ILLNESS.)

MELANIN is the dark pigment found in the
skin and hair, as well as the choroid coat of the
eye. It is the amount of melanin which decides
the colour of the skin and hair. In white skin it
occurs as granules in cells known as melanocytes
situated in the stratum basale of the skin (q.v.).
On exposure to ultra-violet light these granules
are released and pass into the superficial layers
of the skin where they produce the brown
colour known as sun-tan which protects the
skin against the harmful effects of continued
exposure to the ultra-violet rays of the sun.
Genetic factors play an important role in
determining the distribution of melanin in the
skin and hence its colour. Thus in those with
genetically brown or black skin, as well as sun-
tanned white-skinned people, there is a widespread distribution of melanin in the more
superficial layers of the skin. This is due more
to increased activity of the melanocytes than to
an actual increase in their number. Melanin is
believed to play a role in maintaining the body's
natural circadian rhythms.

MELANOMA is a tumour arising from the
cells that produce melanin (q.v.). A highly
malignant form, known as malignant melanoma,
arises from the pigmented cells of moles (q.v.)
or naevi. Malignant melanoma, which requires
early excision to effect a cure, is much more
common in white people living in sunny climes
such as Australia, South Africa and parts of the
USA, but it can occur in the United Kingdom.
The hazards of ultra-violet light in causing
malignant melanoma cannot be ignored in the
British Isles, particularly in those who holiday
abroad. The incidence is steadily rising and will
continue to rise so long as our society remains
addicted to the sun. The prophylactic use of
sun-screening agents should be a routine for
people exposing themselves to the sun as the
reduction in the earth's protective ozone layer
is increasing the risk of sunburn. (See SUN-
BURN.)

MELATONIN A hormone that plays a key
role in the body's diurnal (night and day)
rhythms. Produced by the pineal gland (q.v.)
and derived from serotonin (q.v.), it acts on
receptors in an area of the brain above the
optic chiasma (q.v.), synchronizing them to the

diurnal rhythm. Melatonin is to be studied as a possible agent to treat insomnia in the elderly and in shift workers. It may also help people with seasonal affective disorder syndrome (q.v.) and those who suffer from jet lag.

MELPHALAN is one of the alkylating agents (q.v.) which is proving of value in the treatment of certain forms of malignant disease. (See CYTOTOXIC.)

MEMBRANES (see BRAIN; CROUP; DIPHTHERIA; LABOUR).

MEMORY is the capacity to remember. It is complex and probably occurs in many areas of the brain including the limbic system and the temporal lobes. Despite such poor knowledge of the anatomy of memory, research has revealed much about how the process works. There are three main steps: registration, storage, and recall.

During registration information from the sense organs and the cerebral cortex is put into codes for storage in the short-term memory system. The codes are usually acoustic (based on the sounds and words that would be used to describe the information) but may use any of the five senses. This system can take only a few chunks of information at a time. Research shows, for example, that only about seven longish numbers can be retained and recalled at once – the next new number displaces an earlier one that is then forgotten. And if a subject is asked to describe a person he has just met, he will recall only seven or so facts about that person. This depends on attention span and can be improved by concentration and rehearsal, for example, by reciting the list of things that must be remembered.

Material needing storage for several minutes stays in the short-term memory. More valuable information goes to the long-term memory where it can be kept for any period from a few minutes to a lifetime. Storage is more reliable if the information is in meaningful codes – it is much easier to remember people's names if their faces and personalities are memorable too. Using techniques such as mnemonics takes this into account.

The final stage is retrieval. Recognizing and recalling the required information involves searching the memory. In the short-term memory this takes about 40 thousandths of a second per item, a rate that is surprisingly consistent, even in people with disorders such as schizophrenia.

Most kinds of forgetting or amnesia occur during retrieval. Benign forgetfulness is usually caused by interference from similar items because the required information was not clearly coded and well organized. Retrieval can be improved by recreating the context in which the information was registered. This is why the police reconstruct scenes of crimes, and why revision for exams is more effective if facts are learnt in the form of answers to mock questions.

MENARCHE is the term applied to the beginning of the menstrual function. The average age at which it occurs in British girls is 12½ years. In London girls it is 13·1 years. There is considerable racial and geographical variation.

MENDELISM is the term applied to a law enunciated by G. J. Mendel that the offspring is not intermediate in type between its parents, but that the type of one or other parent is predominant. Characteristics are classed as either dominant or recessive. The offspring of the first generation tend to inherit the dominant characteristics, whilst the recessive characteristics remain latent and appear in some of the offspring of the second generation. If individuals possessing recessive characters unite, recessive characters then become dominant characters in succeeding generations. The law may be expressed by the following formula:

$$n(DD+2DR+RR)$$

in which DD represents dominant offspring, RR recessive offspring, and DR offspring with mixed characters.

MENDELSON SYNDROME Inhalation of regurgitated stomach contents, usually as a complication of general anaesthesia. It may cause death from anoxia or result in extensive lung damage.

MENIÈRE'S DISEASE, so called after the Frenchman, Prosper Menière, who first described it in 1861, is a disease characterized by tinnitus (q.v.), deafness and intermittent attacks of vertigo. It usually occurs in middle age, and is slightly more common in men than in women. The first manifestation is usually deafness on one side. Then, as a rule many months later, there is a sudden attack, without any warning, of intense vertigo. This often occurs during sleep, waking the patient up. It is soon followed by vomiting and sweating. The acute giddiness usually lasts for two to three hours but, after the attack, some unsteadiness persists for a few days. The time interval between attacks varies from a week to a few months. When they do recur, they tend to occur in clusters. The tinnitus, which tends to be high-pitched, comes on about the same time as the deafness. It is often described as being like rushing water or escaping steam. The deafness becomes gradually worse until it is complete. The condition is due to excessive fluid in the labyrinth of the ears (see EAR). The cause of this accumulation is not known, though it has been suggested that it might be a form of allergy, or might be due to spasm of the small blood-vessels.

Treatment Acute vertigo symptoms can sometimes be alleviated with drugs such as cyclizine or betahistine, and nicotinic acid, but the disorder is notoriously difficult to treat and no certain cure is available. Surgical decompression of the fluid in the ear's balancing mechanism may relieve vertigo and prevent the disease worsening. The vestibular nerve to the ear can also be cut to relieve vertigo while preserving hearing. (See TINNITUS.)

MENINGES are the membranes surrounding the brain and spinal cord. (See BRAIN.) The membranes include the dura mater, a tough, fibrous membrane closely applied to the inside of the skull; the arachnoid, a more delicate membrane, enveloping the brain but separated from its irregular surface by spaces containing fluid; and the pia mater, a delicate network of fibres containing blood-vessels and uniting the arachnoid to the brain. The two last are sometimes referred to as the pia-arachnoid. These membranes bear the blood-vessels which nourish the surface of the brain and the interior of the skull. Meningeal haemorrhage from these vessels forms one of the chief dangers arising from fracture of the skull.

MENINGISM is a condition with symptoms closely resembling those of meningitis, but due simply to a feverish state.

MENINGITIS is inflammation affecting the membranes of the brain (cerebral meningitis) or spinal cord (spinal meningitis) or, usually both. Meningitis may be caused by bacteria, viruses, fungi, malignant cells or blood (after subarachnoid haemorrhage (q.v.)). The term is, however, usually restricted to inflammation due to a bacterium or virus. Vital meningitis is normally a mild, self-limiting infection of a few days' duration. Bacterial meningitis is life threatening, and 70 per cent of cases of acute bacterial meningitis in the UK are caused by three bacteria: *Neisseria meningitidis* (meningococcus), *Haemophilus influenzae* (q.v.) and *Streptococcus pneumoniae* (pneumococcus). Other bacteria include *Escherichia coli* (q.v.), *Mycobacterium tuberculosis* (see TUBERCULOSIS), *Treponema pallidum* (see SYPHILIS) and staphylococci spp. (q.v.). Bacterial meningitis may occur by spread from nearby infected foci such as the nasopharynx, middle ear, mastoid and sinuses. Direct infection may be the result of penetrating injuries of the skull from accidents or gunshot wounds. Meningitis may also be a complication of neurosurgery despite careful aseptic precautions. Immunocompromised patients – those with AIDS or on cytoxic drugs – are vulnerable to infections. Bacterial meningitis is an emergency: the infection has a high mortality, even in the developed world. Untreated, it is fatal: the death rate among treated patients may be as high as 15 per cent.

First recognized in France in 1837, when there was an epidemic, bacterial meningitis has occurred in occasional epidemics in Europe and America since then. Spread is particularly likely in schools and similar communities. Many people harbour the meningococcus without developing meningitis. In recent years small clusters of cases, mainly in schoolchildren, have

occurred in Britain. In 1992 2,411 cases of meningitis were reported in England, 964 due to meningococcal infection.

Symptoms of meningitis are severe and rapidly developing malaise accompanied by fever, severe headache, photophobia (q.v.), vomiting, irritability, rigors, drowsiness and neurological disturbances. Neck stiffness and a positive Kernig's sign (q.v.) appearing within a few hours of infection are key diagnostic signs.

Diagnosis and treatment are urgent and, if bacterial meningitis is suspected, antibiotic treatment should be started even before laboratory confirmation of the infection. Analysis of the cerebrospinal fluid (q.v.) by means of a lumbar puncture (q.v.) is an essential step in diagnosis. The CSF is clear or turbid in viral meningitis, turbid or viscous in tuberculous infection and turbulent or purulent when meningococci or staphylococci are the infective agents. Cell counts and biochemical make-up of the CSF are other diagnostic pointers. Serological tests are done to identify possible syphilitic infection, which is now rare in Britain.

Patients with suspected meningitis should be admitted to hospital quickly. Meningococcal and pneumococcal infections are treated with large doses of intravenous penicillin; meningitis due to *H. influenzae* is treated with intravenous chloramphenicol (q.v.). Local infections such as sinusitis or middle-ear infection require treatment, and appropriate surgery for skull fractures or meningeal tears should be carried out as necessary. Tuberculous meningitis is treated for at least nine months with antituberculous drugs (see TUBERCULOSIS). If bacterial meningitis causes convulsions, these can be controlled with diazepam (q.v.) and analgesics will be required for the severe headache.

Treatment of close contacts such as family, school friends, medical and nursing staff is recommended if the patient has *H. influenzae* or *N. meningitidis*: rifampicin (q.v.) provides effective prophylaxis. Contacts of patients with pneumococcal infection do not need preventive treatment. Vaccines for meningococcal meningitis may be given to family members in small epidemics and to any contacts who are especially at risk such as infants, the elderly and immunocompromised individuals.

The outlook for a patient with bacterial meningitis depends on age – the young and old are vulnerable, speed of onset – sudden onset worsens the prognosis – and how quickly treatment is started, hence the urgency of diagnosis and admission to hospital.

MENINGOCELE is a protusion of the meninges of the brain through a defect in the skull. (See SPINA BIFIDA.)

MENINGOCOCCUS (see NEISSERIA).

MENINGOENCEPHALITIS is the term applied to infection of the membranes, or meninges, of the brain and the underlying brain matter. In practically all cases of meningitis (q.v.) there is some involvement of the underlying brain. It is when this involvement is considerable that the term, meningoencephalitis, is used. One form that has attracted attention in recent years is that caused by amoebae (q.v.), particularly that known as *Naegleria fowleri*, in which the infection is acquired through bathing in contaminated water. Effective chlorination of swimming baths kills this micro-organism.

MENINGOMYELOCELE is a protrusion of the meninges of the spinal cord through a defect in the spine. (See SPINA BIFIDA.)

MENISCUS is the term applied to a crescentic fibro-cartilage in a joint, such as the cartilages in the knee-joint.

MENOPAUSE is the term applied to the cessation of menstruation at the end of reproductive life. Usually it occurs between the ages of 45 and 50, although it may occur before the age of 30 or after the age of 50. It can be a psychologically disturbing experience which is quite often accompanied by physical manifestations. These include hot flushes, tiredness, irritability, lack of concentration, palpitations, aching joints and vaginal irritation. There may also be loss of libido. Most women can and do live happy, active lives through the menopause, the length of which varies considerably. The chauvinists would say that it was a natural event and it is those women that can accept it as such who are least likely to suffer from its manifestations. This is not true. The loss of oestrogen which occurs at the menopause causes atrophy of the genital tract. Vasomotor instability in the form of hot flushes, sweats and palpitations occur and can be very debilitating. The urinary urge, loss of libido and depression are not uncommon manifestations and are remediable with treatment.

One of the major problems of the menopause which does not give rise to symptoms until many years later is the osteoporosis which follows the cessation of menstruation. Osteoporosis is a metabolic bone disease characterised by a reduction in the total amount of bone but without any abnormality in the actual bone present. After the menopause 1 per cent of the bone is lost per annum to the end of life. This accounts for the frequency of fractures of the femur in elderly women as a result of osetoporosis but it can be prevented by hormone-replacement therapy. Oestrogens are more effective than tranquillizers or sedatives in relieving the short-term symptoms such as hot flushes, sweats and vaginal dryness. Atrophic vaginitis and vulvitis also usually respond to treatment with oestrogens. Oestrogen therapy reduces the demineralization of bone which normally occurs after the menopause and, if it is started early and continued for years, it may prevent the development of osteoporosis. Oestrogen is far more effective than calcium supplements

and has been shown greatly to reduce fractures affecting the spine, wrists and legs after the age of 50. Cyclical therapy is necessary to avoid abnormal bleeding in women who have reached the menopause. If oestrogens are given alone there is a slightly increased risk of endometrial hyperplasia which may proceed to endometrial cancer. This can be prevented by the administration of oestrogen-progestogen combinations. There is good evidence that a combination of oestrogen and a progestogen – known as hormone replacement therapy (HRT) – avoids the endometrial hyperstimulation produced by the oestrogen alone and relieves most of the symptoms of vasomotor instability of the menopause and prevents the bone loss associated with the menopause. It has been suggested there was a relationship between oestrogen treatment and breast tumours. However a study by the Boston Collaborative Drug Surveillance Program showed that there was no evidence of any association between oestrogen therapy and either benign or malignant breast tumours. There is good evidence that before the age of 50 men are a greater risk of developing myocardial infarction but in the post-menopausal women the risks are the same. It has thus been suggested that the secretion of oestrogens protects against cardiovascular disease in the reproductive years. Nevertheless there is no evidence that the administration of oestrogens in the menopause increases the risk of developing atherosclerotic vascular disease, breast cancer, thrombo-embolic disorders or hypertension.

MENORRHAGIA means an over-abundance of the menstrual discharge.

MENSTRUATION is a periodic change occurring in human beings and the higher apes, and consists chiefly in a flow of blood from the cavity of the womb, and associated with various slight constitutional disturbances. It begins between the ages of 12 and 15, as a rule, although its onset may be delayed till as late as 20, or it may begin as early as 10 or 11. Along with its first appearance the body develops the secondary sex characteristics of the sex: e.g. enlargement of the breasts, characteristic hair distribution. The duration of each menstrual period varies in different persons from two to eight days. It recurs in the great majority of cases with regularity, most commonly at intervals of twenty-eight days or thirty days, less often with intervals of twenty-one or twenty-seven days, ceasing only during pregnancy and lactation, till the age of 45 or 50 arrives, when it stops altogether, as a rule ceasing early if it has begun early, and vice versa. The final stoppage is known as the menopause (q.v.) or the climacteric (q.v.).

Menstruation depends upon a functioning ovary and this upon a healthy pituitary gland. The regular rhythm may depend upon a centre in the hypothalamus, which is in close connection with the pituitary. After menstruation the denuded uterine endometrium is regenerated under the influence of the follicular hormone, oestradiol. The epithelium of the endometrium proliferates, and about a fortnight after the beginning of menstruation great development of the endometrial glands takes place under the influence of progesterone, the hormone secreted by the corpus luteum. These changes are made for the reception of the fertilized ovum. In the absence of fertilization the uterine endometrium breaks down in the subsequent menstrual discharge.

Disorders of menstruation In the majority of healthy women, menstruation proceeds regularly for thirty years or more, with the exceptions connected with childbirth. In many persons, as the result either of general or local conditions, the process may be absent or excessive, or may be attended with great discomfort or pain. The term *amenorrhoea* is applied to cases in which menstruation is absent, *menorrhagia* and *metrorrhagia* to cases in which it is excessive, the former if the excess occurs at the regular periods, the latter if it is irregular, whilst *dysmenorrhoea* is the name given to cases in which the process is attended by pain.

AMENORRHOEA If menstruation has never occurred the amenorrhoea is termed *primary*. If it ceases after having once become established it is known as *secondary amenorrhoea*. The only value of these terms is that some patients with either chromosome abnormalities or malformations of the genital tract fall into the primary category. Otherwise the age of onset of symptoms is more important.

The causes of amenorrhoea are numerous and treatment requires dealing with the primary cause. The commonest cause is pregnancy. Hypothalamic disorders such as psychological stress or anorexia nervosa cause amenorrhoea. Poor nutrition or loss of weight by dieting may cause amenorrhoea and any serious underlying disease such as tuberculosis or malaria may also result in the cessation of periods. The excess secretion of prolactin, whether this is the result of a micro-adenoma of the pituitary gland or whether it is drug induced, will cause amenorrhoea and possibly galactorrhoea as well. Malfunction of the pituitary gland will result in a failure to produce the gonadotrophic hormones with consequent amenorrhoea. Excessive production of cortisol, as in Cushing's syndrome, or of androgens, as in the adreno-genital syndrome or the polycystic ovary syndrome, will result in amenorrhoea. Amenorrhoea occasionally follows use of the oral contraceptive pill and may be associated with both hypothyroidism and obesity. It is thus important to take a careful history with emphasis on psychological factors, weight fluctuations and the use of drugs that may stimulate the release of prolactin and it is also important to look for evidence of virilization. A gynaecological examination is necessary in primary amenorrhoea to exclude malformations of the genital tract. Estimations of the gonadotrophic hormone levels will reveal whether the amenorrhoea is primary ovarian failure or secondary to pituitary disease.

In view of the sometimes psychosomatic origins of amenorrhoea, reassurance of the patient is of great importance, in particular with reference to marriage and the ability to conceive. When weight loss is the cause of amenorrhoea, restoration of body weight alone can result in spontaneous menstruation. Patients with raised concentration of serum gonadotrophin hormones have primary ovarian failure. It is not amenable to treatment. Cyclical oestrogen/progestogen therapy will usually establish withdrawal bleeding. If the amenorrhoea is due to mild pituitary failure menstruation may return after treatment with clomiphene. Clomiphene is a non-steroidal agent which competes for oestrogen receptors in the hypothalamus. The patients who are most likely to respond to clomiphene are those who have some evidence of endogenous oestrogen and gonadotrophin production.

MENORRHAGIA Excessive menstruation may be due to the same general conditions which produce amenorrhoea, the same diseases, such as glomerulonephritis or tuberculosis, causing stoppage or excess in different women. Thus, in some people an excessive loss is brought about by these conditions, and the effects of the general disease are much increased by the loss of blood. In heart disease, the womb may share in the general internal congestion, and the menses in consequence are increased. In some people, menstruation at its first appearance is excessive; whilst this is so often the case as to be almost the general rule at the time when the menstrual periods are about to stop, i.e. at the menopause, when they also tend to become irregular. But it is most often a local condition that produces menorrhagia: in this case, as a rule, not only is the periodic loss increased but there is bleeding at irregular times (metrorrhagia). Polypus, fibroid, and other tumours, displacements of the womb, and some inflammation consequent upon childbirth or miscarriage, are the most common causes of this type. In the treatment, rest and various internal remedies which check haemorrhage, together with careful attention to the general health between the periods, are essential. (See UTERUS, DISEASES OF.)

DYSMENORRHOEA may vary from mere discomfort to agonizing colic, accompanied by prostration and vomiting. Anaemia is sometimes a cause of painful menstruation as well as of stoppage of this function. Chills and exhaustion may produce pain for a single period in women whose periods are usually painless.

Inflammation of various internal organs, e.g. of the womb itself, the ovaries, or the Fallopian tubes, is one of the commonest causes of dysmenorrhoea which comes on for the first time late in life, especially when the trouble follows the birth of a child. In this case the pain exists more or less at all times, but is aggravated at the periods. It is relieved by various local means directed towards checking the inflammation present.

Many cases of dysmenorrhoea appear with the beginning of menstrual life, and accompany every period. It has been estimated that 5 to 10 per cent of girls in their late teens or early twenties are severely incapacitated by dysmenorrhoea for several hours each month. Various causes have been suggested for the pain, one being an excessive production of prostaglandins (q.v.). In not a few – indeed some would say the majority – there is a large psychological factor. This may be the sole cause, or it may be an ancillary cause exacerbating the pain, or discomfort, induced by some physical cause. Whatever the psychological factor – whether due to inadequate sex instruction, fear, mental, domestic, or work disharmony – the sooner it is discovered and dealt with, the more likely is the dysmenorrhoea to come under control. For the temporary relief of dysmenorrhoea, rest in bed, or, at all events, in the recumbent position, a hot water bottle to the lower part of the abdomen, and aspirin orally, are the remedies which prove most useful.

MENTAL HANDICAP is a generalized, though often not uniform, intellectual, developmental and social impairment, deriving from brain dysfunction, requiring additional support, supervision and attention to enable an affected person to live as normal a life as possible. (See LEARNING DISABILITY.)

MENTAL ILLNESS is not strictly a medical term but is used generally to refer to the more severe disorders treated by psychiatrists. Mental illness may be due to organic causes, such as brain tumours or disease of the arteries, and in these cases there is usually a disturbance of orientation and short-term memory. Alzheimer's disease and senile dementia are the result of deterioration in the cells of the brain. The remainder, called 'functional' mental illness, is characterized by disorders of mood, perception, cognition (q.v.), motivation and insight – knowledge of oneself.

Description *Mood* may be raised, and then the individual talks excessively and is overactive. He or she may plan overenthusiastically and be unduly optimistic about the future; inappropriate spending, inflated self-esteem and, possibly, grandiose delusions about power, wealth and personal standing are other abnormal facets of behaviour. The opposite may occur, with depression of mood in which the patient feels inferior and has a pessimistic view of the future; the future may even appear absent. Depressed patients feel apathetic, have no interest in things which previously excited them, get no pleasure from life (anhedonia), find everything an enormous effort, feel tense and anxious, cannot concentrate or make decisions, feel excessively guilty, even for things they are not responsible for, feel unloved and unlovable, and suffer a change in sleep and appetite. A depressed person may be preoccupied with ideas of suicide, and both attempted suicide and completed suicide are common and hard to predict.

Disorder of *perception* usually takes the form of auditory hallucinations in which the patient hears the voices of what appear to be real people talking to or about them. Command hallucinations may order the patient to do things such as to commit suicide, to refuse treatment, or to keep the existence of the voices a secret. A patient may have hallucinations of smell, attributed either to others or to his or her own body, or of touch as of sexual interference, and these may give rise to false accusations of sexual assault. Parts of the body may feel moved from outside (kinaesthetic hallucinations) and the patient may feel like a puppet. Hallucinations of taste may give the idea of being poisoned. Visual hallucinations may take human or animal form, and if they are seen as evil or dangerous, the images may be attacked. Visual hallucinations, however, are not usually a major feature of functional mental illness, but rather suggest an organic mental disorder, such as the delirium which occurs on withdrawal of anxiolytic/hypnotic substances such as alcohol and benzodiazepines.

Disorders of *cognition* include delusions and thought disorder. Delusions may be secondary to mood change, such as the grandiose delusions of elevated mood, and the delusions of poverty, guilt and disease which are common with depressed mood. They may also be secondary to auditory hallucinations. Primary delusions are of many sorts, but often take the form of ideas of persecution, evidence for which is seen in ordinary or coincidental happenings which the normal person overlooks. It is usually possible to distinguish delusional from real persecution by the way the patient argues for their reality. Delusions of jealousy may be very troublesome in marriage, as may other delusions about the spouse, such as that he or she has been replaced by an imposter. The resulting marital disharmony often responds to antipsychotic medication, but is resistant to marriage guidance. Thinking may be generally disordered in mental illness, giving the speech of the patient a peculiar quality which leaves the hearer bemused; there may be discursive, tangential or 'knight's move' thinking, and the patient may assume that the hearer shares the personal knowledge of the speaker. The sign language of deaf patients is similarly affected.

Loss of *motivation* occurs, even in the absence of depression, and is manifested in self-neglect and restricted life-style.

Loss of *insight* describes the fact that some patients with mental illness do not recognize that they are ill; indeed, they may believe that those around them require treatment. This lack of insight causes major difficulties in management and treatment which will be discussed later.

Classification Many attempts have been made to classify functional mental illness. The medical approach began with the publication of Pinel's *Traité médico-philosophique sur l'aliénation mentale ou la manie* in 1801. Later in the century, the German psychiatrist Griesinger held that the integrity of each patient's ego was like a tree, subjected to gales from the stress of outside events and of mood changes from within. Some egos were strong, some flexible, and these recovered after the successive storms; but in other cases there was a step-like deterioration in the mental faculties after each assault, until the tree bent or broke and permanent mental illness resulted. Then Kraepelin at the turn of the century described the strong and flexible trees as 'manic-depressive' and the damaged trees as 'dementia praecox'. This division of functional mental illness into two categories challenged the existing unitary system, and also the 'Linnaean' system popular in France and Scandinavia, which had hundreds of different syndromes, each giving immortality to the psychiatrist who described it. Then the Swiss psychiatrist Bleuler gave a detailed description of the features of dementia praecox which he relabelled schizophrenia. Subsequently psychiatrists juggled with a classification which was partly based on the course of the illness, and partly on the features presented in the mental state of the patient. Attempts to find scientific evidence for the existence of two discrete forms of mental illness have not been successful.

Mental illness usually refers to the psychoses, which may be distinguished from other forms of 'functional' psychological malfunction such as the neuroses, including obsessions, personality disorders and stress disorders.

Stigma The anti-psychiatry movement has objected to people being 'labelled' as mentally ill. In fact, there are both advantages and disadvantages in being so labelled. The mentally ill person has access to services, not only statutory, but also voluntary such as the National Schizophrenia Fellowship (see APPENDIX 2: ADDRESSES) and in many cases they are eligible for private health insurance. Many mentally ill patents in England receive a Disability Living Allowance. In the case of crimes committed under the influence of delusions or hallucinations, a diagnosis of mental illness may direct the perpetrator to treatment in hospital rather than to punishment in prison. Mental illness is one of the categories of mental disorder which allows patients to be detained in hospital and treated against their will, and this is an important civil right for those patients who are tormented by severe illness but due to lack of insight cannot apreciate that the torment is of mental origin. On the other hand, the label of mental illness may lower self-esteem, and it may cause difficulty in obtaining life insurance, driving licences and jobs.

In the United Kingdom the policy is to treat as many people with mental illness as possible in the community and to persuade those needing institutional treatment to do so voluntarily. When, however, people's conduct becomes a risk to their own health and safety, or that of others, they can be compulsorily admitted to a psychiatric unit under mental health legislation. Less than 10 per cent of psychiatric admissions in Britain are compulsory. Many people with socially maladjusted personalities

end up in prison, however, sometimes because of a shortage of appropriate treatment facilities.

Treatment, general principles The first aim of treatment is to protect the patient against harming self or others, and, in achieving this, intensive nursing is seen as preferable to mechanical or chemical restraint. Antipsychotic (neuroleptic) drugs – formerly called major tranquillizers to distinguish them from the benzodiazepines which were called minor tranquillizers – have an immediate sedative effect and an antipsychotic effect which takes a week or more to materialize. These drugs may be given daily by mouth or by intramuscular injection every few weeks. They are not popular with patients, probably because they remove a certain excitement or 'buzz' from subjective experience; also, because they act by inhibiting dopamine (q.v.) transmission in the brain, they may cause movement disorders by interfering with the dopamine-mediated neural pathways that control movement. These drugs have been shown in numerous controlled trials to reduce or abolish the manifestations of mental illness, and when taken for long periods they prevent relapse. Other physical treatments include electric convulsive therapy (ECT) and a type of brain surgery, stereotactic tractotomy, which are used for severe mood disorders but have provoked controversy. Psychosocial rehabilitation is very important and takes the form of family therapy, residential provision, day-hospital treatment and work training.

Treatment of individual disorders *Depression* is the commonest psychiatric disorder encountered both in general practice and in hospital medicine. A relatively mild depression responds to supportive psychotherapy, whilst a psychotic depression with delusions and hallucinations will require admission to hospital and possible electro-convulsive therapy. Depressive illness has a spontaneous remission rate of about 50 per cent within several months and, if anti-depressant drugs are given, the recovery rate increases to over 70 per cent. The advantage of drugs treatment is that recovery is made more rapidly and the patient's suffering is therefore curtailed and the risk of suicide reduced. Tricyclic antidepressant drugs act, apparently, by promoting the transmission of impulses between nerves by noradrenaline or serotonin. Depressed patients with agitation or anxiety respond best to a sedative tricyclic antidepressant such as amitriptyline or dothiepin. Retarded, apathetic patients are best treated with a less sedative antidepressant, such as imipramine. The side-effects of the tricyclic antidepressants (particularly amitriptyline) are due to atropine-like effects which lead to a dry mouth, constipation, pupillary dilatation and blurring of close vision. The monoamine oxidase inhibitors, such as isocarboxazide and phenelzine, are best reserved for those neurotic or atypical cases, where the depression is accompanied by a great deal of anxiety and phobic behaviour. The monoamine oxidase inhibitors are associated with severe side-effects if the patient eats cheese or any substance that contains tyramine or catecholamines. Among other anti-depressant drugs are selective serotonin-reuptake inhibitors (SSRIs) which are less sedative than the tricyclic drugs with few anti-muscarinic or cardiotoxic effects. They do, however, have other side-effects and require careful monitoring. Fluoxetine (q.v.) and paroxetine are examples of SSRIs. Electroconvulsive therapy may also facilitate the transmission of nerve impulses. It is now given under brief general anaesthetic with a muscle relaxant. It is an effective treatment in severe depressive illness and the response is at least as good and probably more rapid than the response to tricyclic antidepressants.

People with *hypomania* require admission to hospital. The most useful drugs are the phenothiazines, such as chlorpromazine and the butyrophenones such as haloperidol, which act by blocking central dopamine receptors. Lithium carbonate has anti-manic properties but as it has little effect for seven to ten days it is generally reserved for prophylaxis of recurrent manic depressive disorder.

In the treatment of anxiety states, patients must be given an opportunity to ventilate their worries and be counselled on stress management and relaxation. Since many patients with anxiety states are often concerned that the commonly associated physical symptoms indicate an underlying organic disorder, they should be reassured (see PSYCHOSOMATIC DISEASES). If an acute stress cannot be managed in this way, long-acting benzodiazepines may be indicated (see BENZODIAZEPINES). Short-acting benzodiazepines are more suitable for elderly patients or patients with renal or hepatic impairment. These drugs should in general be prescribed only for a few weeks at most, as patients often become tolerant to their effects and dependent on them. In patients who experience a rapid pulse or tremor, beta-blockers (see ADRENERGIC RECEPTORS) are useful and do not cause dependence.

The treatment of *schizophrenia* usually requires admission to a psychiatric unit for clarification of the diagnosis. The treatment is both pharmacological and psycho-social. The drugs most commonly used for the treatment of schizophrenia are neuroleptics including the phenothiazines, such as chlorpromazine, and the butyrophenones, such as haloperidol. The efficacy of neuroleptics in acute schizophrenia is demonstrated by the fact that 75 per cent of patients given phenothiazines are substantially better after four weeks compared to 25 per cent given a placebo. Psycho-social treatment is also important. During the acute phase the schizophrenic patient needs support, reassurance and simple counselling. Schizophrenic individuals are vulnerable to social pressures that most people can take in their stride. Despite the introduction of drug treatment, schizophrenic patients still occupy about one-sixth of all hospital beds in England and Wales. Drug treatment needs to be prolonged as 50 per cent of patients will relapse when drugs are discontinued. As a high proportion of psychiatric outpatients fail to comply with oral medication, long-acting depot-neuroleptics are commonly used, such as fluphenazine and flupenthixol. Patients may experience side-effects with the neuroleptics. These take the form of abnormal muscle movements or rigidity, as well as restlessness in the legs and increased salivation. Some of them can be controlled with other medication and recede with time.

After treatment has been established and florid symptoms are controlled, the patient is encouraged to resume activities by degrees. If living at home is not desirable, a hostel or group home may be indicated.

Like the 1959 Mental Health Act, the 1983 Act continues the principles (1) that as much treatment as possible, both in hospital and outside, should be given on a voluntary and informal basis; (2) that the care of people with mental illness should be shifted as far as possible from the institutions to care within the community. Psychiatric units attached to or in district general hospitals are now regarded as the norm and many large separate mental hospitals have been closed, a policy that is being continued.

The 1983 Act strengthened the checks and protected the civil liberties of the 10 per cent of in-patients who are admitted to psychiatric hospitals involuntarily.

Under the Act, mental disorder is defined as mental illness, arrested or incomplete development of mind, psychopathic disorder, or any other disability of mind.

Under Section 2 it provides for the compulsory admission of a patient to hospital for a maximum of 28 days on the grounds: (a) that he is suffering from mental disorder of a nature or degree which warrants his detention for assessment (or for assessment followed by medical treatment); and (b) that he ought to be so detained in the interests of his own health or safety or with a view to the protection of other persons.

Under Section 3 compulsory admission to hospital for treatment is for a maximum of six months, subject to renewal.

Patients detained in hospital must be informed of their rights and may apply to a Mental Health Tribunal to be released. Medical staff and hospital managers also have the power to discharge a patient from the compulsory provisions at any time.

Other sections of the Act permit involuntary detention for shorter periods of time under certain conditions and provide for guardianship in the community, although this last provision has been little used.

Persons coming before the courts who are mentally disordered may be detained in hospital or received into guardianship if the court considers it a suitable course. In certain circumstances higher courts may also make restriction orders, in which case the patient may not be discharged without the consent of the Home Secretary. Persons detained in prison or approved school who are found to be mentally disordered may be transferred to hospital by the Home Secretary.

Institutions, known as Special Hospitals, exist for mentally disordered people who, in the opinion of the minister, require treatment under conditions of special security on account of their dangerous, violent, or criminal tendencies. Secure units have also been established in some NHS district general hospitals, but the pressure on secure places is such that unsuitable patients have been discharged to community care – the responsibility of local-authority social service departments – where problems have occurred in looking after them.

The Mental Health Act Commission has been set up to provide special safeguards for detained patients. It gives second opinions in certain matters affecting the treatment of patients, will visit detained patients, investigate complaints, review the use of legal powers and advise staff on good practice. Some treatments are not permitted without the patient's consent and an independent second opinion; some may be given without consent but only if the second opinion agrees, whilst others can be given for up to three months without consent or a second opinion.

The checks on and safeguards of civil liberties of detained patients in the 1983 Act are detailed. Further information can be obtained from the Mental Health Act Commission, and from MIND, The National Association for Mental Health. MIND also acts as a campaigning and advice organization on all aspects of mental health. (See APPENDIX 2: ADDRESSES.)

MEPACRINE HYDROCHLORIDE is a synthetic acridine product used in the treatment of malaria. It came to the fore during the 1939–45 War, when supplies of quinine were short, and proved of great value both as a prophylactic and in the treatment of malaria. It is now used only to treat infestation with tapeworms. (See TAENIASIS.)

MEPROBAMATE is one of the tranquillizer drugs. It is mainly used for the relief of states of tension, mild anxiety states and persistent insomnia.

MERALGIA PARAESTHETICA is a condition characterized by pain and paraesthesia (q.v.) on the front and outer aspect of the thigh. It is more common in men than in women, and the victims are usually middle-aged, overweight and out of condition. It is due to compression of the lateral cutaneous nerve of the thigh. It is exacerbated by an uncomfortable driving position when motoring long distances. Reduction in weight, improvement in general fitness and correction of faulty posture usually bring relief. If these fail, surgical decompression of the nerve may bring relief.

MERCAPTOPURINE is one of the anti-metabolite group of drugs, which includes methotrexate, fluorouracil and thioguanine. These drugs are incorporated into new nuclear material in the cell or combine irreversibly with vital cellular enzymes, preventing normal cellular metabolism and division. Mercaptopurine is used mainly for the maintenance treatment of acute leukaemias, though it is increasingly proving valuable in the treatment of Crohn's disease (q.v.). As with all cytotoxic drugs (q.v.), dosage must be carefully controlled; in particular it must be reduced if used concurrently with allopurinol. Side-effects include gastrointestinal upsets, including ulceration, and bone-marrow depression.

MERCURY, also known as QUICKSILVER or HYDRARGYRUM, is a heavy fluid metal which, with its salts, has been used in medicine for many centuries.
Action The salts of mercury fall into two groups: the mercuric salts, which are very soluble and powerful in action; and the mercurous salts, which are less soluble and act more slowly and mildly. The mercuric salts are all highly poisonous both to man and to bacterial life, so that they are strongly antiseptic. In strong solutions, several act as caustics, and in weaker solutions they are irritants. Taken internally, the first effect of the mercuric, and to a less degree of the mercurous salts, is by their irritating action to set up copious purging. They are also credited with the power of increasing the flow of bile, and for this reason blue pill, which contains mercury, and mercurous chloride, i.e. calomel, were at one time much used as purgatives.
Uses Externally the mercuric salts are used as antiseptics, anti-parasitic agents and fungicides. Mercury is widely used in dental amalgams for filling teeth, though doubts have recently been raised whether the metal can be absorbed into the body tissue, with unwanted results.

MESCALINE is derived from the Mexican peyote cactus, *Anhalonium lewinii*. It is probably the most powerful of all the hallucinogens and has been used for many centuries by Indian tribes in Mexico as an intoxicant to produce ecstatic states for religious celebrations. (See DRUG ADDICTION.)

MESENCEPHALON is the mid-brain connecting the cerebral hemispheres with the pons and cerebellum.

MESENTERY is the double layer of peritoneal membrane which supports the small intestine. It is of a fan shape, and its shorter edge is attached to the back wall of the abdomen for a distance of about 15 cm (6 inches), while the small intestine lies within its longer edge, for a length of over 6 metres (20 feet). The terms mesocolon, mesorectum, etc., are applied to similar folds of peritoneum that support parts of the colon, rectum, etc.

MESMERISM (see HYPNOTISM).

MESOCOLON is the double fold of peritoneum by which the large intestine is suspended from the back wall of the abdomen.

MESOTHELIOMA A malignant tumour of the pleura, the membrane lining the chest cavity. The condition is commoner in people exposed to asbestos dust. It may be asymptomatic or cause pain, cough, and breathing troubles. Surgery or radiotherapy may be effective but often the disease has spread too far before it is discovered.

MESTEROLONE is a synthetic androgen (q.v.) which is being used in the treatment of hypogonadism (q.v.). (See ANDROGEN.)

METABOLISM means tissue change and includes all the physical and chemical processes by which the living body is maintained, and also those by which the energy is made available for various forms of work. The constructive, chemical and physical, processes by which food materials are adapted for the use of the body are collectively known as anabolism. The destructive processes by which energy is produced with the breaking down of tissues into waste products is known as catabolism. *Basal metabolism* is the term applied to the energy changes necessary for essential processes such as the beating of the heart, respiration, and maintenance of body warmth. This can be estimated, when a person is placed in a state of complete rest, by measuring the amounts of oxygen and carbon dioxide exchanged during breathing under certain standard conditions. (See CALORIE.)

METACARPAL bones are the five long bones which occupy the hand between the carpal bones at the wrist and the phalanges of the fingers. The large rounded 'knuckles' at the root of the fingers are formed by the heads of these bones. (See HAND.)

METAPHYSIS is the extremity of a long bone where it joins the epiphysis (q.v.).

METAPLASIA is the term applied to a change of one kind of tissue into another.

METASTASIS and METASTATIC are terms applied to the process by which malignant disease spreads to distant parts of the body, and also to the secondary tumours resulting from this process. For example, a cancer of the breast may produce metastatic growths in the glands of the armpit, cancer of the stomach may be followed by metastases in the liver.

METATARSAL bones are the five bones in the foot which correspond to the metacarpal bones in the hand, lying between the tarsal bones, at the ankle, and the toes. (See FOOT.)

METATARSALGIA is pain affecting the metatarsal region of the foot. It is common in adolescents associated with flat-foot (q.v.). In adults it may be a manifestation of rheumatoid arthritis. *Morton's metatarsalgia* is a form associated usually with the nerve to the second toe cleft often induced by the compression of tight shoes.

METATARSUS is the group name of the five metatarsal bones in the foot (q.v.). *Metatarsus varus* is the condition characterized by deviation of the forefoot towards the other foot. It is a common condition in new-born babes and almost always corrects itself spontaneously. Only in the rare cases in which it is due to some deformity of the bones or muscles of the foot is any treatment required.

METEORISM means the distension of the abdomen by gas produced in the intestines. (See FLATULENCE.)

METFORMIN is a biguanide (q.v.) which lowers the blood sugar. This it does by increasing cellular uptake of glucose. It is active when taken by mouth and is proving of value in the treatment of certain cases of diabetes mellitus.

METHADONE, or PHYSEPTONE, is a synthetic drug structurally and pharmacologically similar to morphine. It is, however, less sedating and has a longer half-life. Furthermore, it is more reliable when taken orally, and although vomiting is common, it is generally less severe than with morphine.

Methadone is used for two main reasons. It is valuable as a cough suppressant for non-productive cough, acting on the medullary 'cough centre' in the central nervous system. It is also helpful in weaning addicts off morphine and heroin, having a slower onset of dependence and a less severe withdrawal syndrome. When used for prolonged periods, methadone should not be given more often than twice daily, to avoid the risks of accumulation and opioid overdosage. (See DRUG ADDICTION.)

METHAEMOGLOBIN is a derivative of haemoglobin in which the iron has been oxidized from ferrous to ferric form. It does not combine with oxygen and therefore plays no part in oxygen transport. Normal concentration of methaemoglobin in red blood cells is less than one per cent of the total haemoglobin. When a large concentration of the haemoglobin is in the form of methaemoglobin the patient will suffer from hypoxia and will be cyanosed. Most cases of methaemoglobinaemia are due to chemical agents.

METHAEMOGLOBINAEMIA is a condition due to the presence in the blood of methaemoglobin (q.v.). It is characterized by cyanosis (q.v.) which turns the skin and lips a blue colour, shortness of breath, headache, fatigue and sickness. There are two main forms: a *hereditary* form and a *toxic* form. The latter is caused by certain drugs, including acetanilide, phenacetin, the sulphonamides and benzocaine. The treatment of the toxic form is the withdrawal of the causative drug. In the more severe cases the administration of methylene blue or ascorbic acid may also be needed, and these are the drugs used in the hereditary form.

In recent years attention has been drawn to a form known as *infantile methaemoglobinaemia* in bottle-fed babies under the age of 6 months. This is due to the presence of excess nitrate in the drinking water. Nitrate pollution of water has been increasing due to the purification of sewage effluent to a high standard before its discharge to water-courses, and to changes in agricultural policy leading to better drainage of land and increased use of artificial fertilizers. As a result, especially where rainfall is low and the land low-lying, as in eastern and south-east England, underground supplies of water contain more than 50 mg of nitrate per litre, which is the level recommended by the World Health Organization, and may even exceed the maximum acceptable level of 100 mg per litre. High nitrate concentrations may also occur in surface waters after heavy rain. The cause of the methaemoglobinaemia is nitrite into which the nitrate is converted either in the baby's bottle or in his gut. Few serious cases have been recorded in Britain, and most of those which have occurred have been due to water from private sources.

Arrangements are now in force whereby water authorities inform the appropriate health authority if water with a nitrate content of 50 mg per litre has to be supplied, and alternative low-nitrate water is made available, sometimes in the form of bottled water, by local authorities for infants below the age of 6 months. The EEC has recommended an even more stringent criterion: that water used for baby feeds should not contain more than 25 mg of nitrate per litre.

METHIONINE is an essential amino-acid (q.v.) that contains sulphur and is necessary for normal growth in infants and to maintain nitrogen balance in adults.

METHOHEXITONE is an ultra-short-acting barbiturate which is proving of value as a short-acting anaesthetic – particularly in dentistry.

METHOTREXATE is an antimetabolite (q.v.) which is proving of value in the treatment of choriocarcinoma (q.v.). (See CYTOTOXIC.)

METHYL is an organic radical whose chemical formula is CH_3, and which forms the centre of a wide group of substances known as the methyl group. For example, methyl alcohol is obtained as a by-product in the manufacture of beet-sugar, or by distillation of wood; methyl salicylate is the active constituent in oil of wintergreen; methyl hydride is better known as marsh gas.

Methyl alcohol, or wood spirit, is distilled from wood and is thus a cheap form of alcohol. It has actions similar to, but much more toxic than, those of ethyl alcohol. It has a specially pronounced action on the nervous system, and in large doses is apt to cause neuritis, especially of the optic nerves, leading to blindness, partial or complete.

METHYLCELLULOSE is a colloid (q.v.) which absorbs water to swell to about 25 times its original volume. It is used in the treatment of constipation and also in the management of obesity. The rationale for its use in obesity is that by swelling up in the stomach it reduces the appetite.

METHYLDOPA is one of the drugs introduced for the treatment of high blood-pressure. It is the drug most commonly used to control high blood-pressure in pregnancy.

METHYLENE BLUE, or methylthionin chloride, is valuable in a dose of 75–100 mg, as a 1-per-cent intravenous injection, in the treatment of methaemoglobinaemia, which may occur following high doses of local anaesthetics such as prilocaine.

METHYLPREDNISOLONE is a preparation with an action comparable to that of prednisolone (q.v.), but effective at a somewhat lower dose.

METHYLTESTOSTERONE is a derivative of the testicular hormone, testosterone (q.v.), which is active when taken by mouth. (See ANDROGEN.)

METHYSERGIDE is a drug that is being used in the prevention of attacks of migraine (q.v.). The drug requires hospital supervision as it has to be used with care because of the toxic effects it sometimes produces, such as nausea, drowsiness and retroperitoneal fibrosis.

METOCLOPRAMIDE is a drug that is proving of value in the treatment of vomiting. It is said to restore normal co-ordination and tone to the upper digestive tract. It is proving of value in the early treatment, and prevention, of migraine (q.v.).

METOLAZONE (see BENZOTHIADIAZINES).

METOPROLOL is a beta-adrenergic receptor blocking agent. (See ADRENERGIC RECEPTORS.)

METRE is the basic unit of length in the modern version of the metric system, known as the International System of Units (SI). (See APPENDIX 6: MEASUREMENTS IN MEDICINE.) It is equivalent to 39·37 inches.

METRITIS means inflammation of the womb.

METRONIDAZOLE is a drug, administered by mouth, which is proving of value in the treatment of various diseases including balantidiasis (q.v.), giardiasis (q.v.), amoebic dysentery (see DYSENTERY) and trichomonal vaginitis. (See TRICHOMONAS VAGINALIS.) It is also active against Gram-negative anaerobic micro-organisms.

METROPATHIA HAEMORRHAGICA, or ESSENTIAL UTERINE HAEMORRHAGE, is a diseased state characterized by haemorrhage from the uterus, cysts in the ovaries, and thickening of the uterine mucosa.

METRORRHAGIA means bleeding from the womb otherwise than at the proper period. It is usually due to a uterine lesion. (See MENSTRUATION.)

METYRAPONE is a drug that is used in the treatment of Cushing's syndrome (q.v.).

MEXENONE is a substance that has the property of absorbing ultra-violet light over a wide range, and is therefore used in the prevention of sunburn. It has the practical advantage of not being readily removed from the skin by washing or sweating, and thereby provides long protection.

MICONAZOLE is one of the imidazole group of antifungals which includes clotrimazole and ketoconazole. Active against a wide range of fungi and yeasts, their main indications are vaginal candidiasis and dermatophyte skin infections. Miconazole is used as a cream or ointment; it may also be given orally (for oral or gastrointestinal infections), or parenterally (for systemic infections such as aspergillosis or candidiasis). (See MYCOSIS.)

MICROANGIOPATHY means disease of the capillaries (q.v.).

MICROBE (see BACTERIA).

MICROBIOLOGY is the study of all aspects of micro-organisms (microbes) – that is, organisms which individually are generally too small to be visible other than by microscopy. Few ecological habitats are devoid of micro-organisms – even extreme environments such as salt pans and thermal springs support microbial life – and the range of habitats the microbes can colonize is reflected in their extraordinary diversity in terms of morphology and development; metabolic abilities; and behaviour in response to stimuli in their immediate environment, adverse conditions, and other organisms.

The term micro-organism is applicable to viruses (q.v.); bacteria (q.v.); and microscopic forms of fungi (q.v.), algae, and protozoa. Some micro-organisms have affinities with both plants and animals, and it is preferable to consider micro-organisms as belonging to a separate kingdom, the protista, rather than attempting to categorize them according to the conventional dichotomy of the plant and animal kingdoms.

Among the smallest and simplest micro-organisms are the viruses. First described as filterable agents, and ranging in size from 20–30 nm to 300 nm, they may be directly visualized only by electron microscopy. They consist of a core of deoxyribonucleic or ribonucleic acid (DNA or RNA) (qq.v.) within a protective protein coat, or capsid, whose subunits confer a geometric symmetry. Thus viruses are usually cubical (icosahedral) or helical; the larger viruses (pox-, herpes-, myxo-viruses) may also have an outer envelope. Their minimal structure dictates that viruses are all obligate parasites, relying on living cells to provide essential components for their replication. Apart from animal and plant cells, viruses may infect and replicate in bacteria (bacteriophages) or fungi (mycophages), which are damaged in the process.

Bacteria are larger (0·01–5000μm) and more complex. They are prokaryotes, with a subcellular organization which generally includes DNA and RNA, a cell membrane, organelles such as ribosomes, and a complex and chemically variable cell envelope. Rickettsiae, chlamydia, and mycoplasmas, once thought of as viruses because of their small size and absence of a cell wall (mycoplasma) or major wall component (chlamydia), are now acknowledged as bacteria. Rickettsiae and chlamydia are obligate intracellular parasites of medical importance. Bacteria may also possess additional surface structures, such as capsules and organs of locomotion (flagella) and attachment (fimbriae and stalks). Individual bacterial cells may be spheres (cocci); straight (bacilli), curved (vibrio), or flexuous (spirilla) rods; or oval cells (coccobacilli). On examination by light microscopy bacteria may be visible in characteristic configurations (as pairs of cocci (diplococci), or chains (streptococci), or clusters); actinomycete bacteria grow as filaments with externally produced spores. Bacteria grow essentially by increasing in cell size and dividing by fission, a process which in ideal laboratory conditions some bacteria may achieve about once every 20 minutes. Under natural conditions growth is usually much slower.

As a group bacteria have a wide repertoire of metabolic and physiological capabilities. Some can synthesize their complex organic cellular components and biochemical intermediates if provided with light or chemical energy; others require sources of existing organic molecules from other micro-organisms, plants, or animals.

Eukaryotic micro-organisms comprise fungi, algae, and protozoa. These organisms are larger, and they have in common a well-developed internal compartmentation into subcellular organelles. Algae additionally have chloroplasts, which contain photosynthetic pigments; fungi lack chloroplasts; and protozoa lack both a cell wall and choroplasts but may have a contractile vacuole to regulate water uptake and, in some, structures for capturing and ingesting food. Fungi grow either as discrete cells (yeasts), multiplying by budding, fission, or conjugation, or as thin filaments (hyphae) which bear spores, though some may show both morphological forms during their life cycle. Algae and protozoa generally grow as individual cells or colonies of individuals and multiply by fission.

Micro-organisms of medical importance include representatives of the five major microbial groups that obtain their essential nutrients at the expense of their hosts. Many bacteria and most fungi, however, are saprophytes (q.v.), being major contributors to the natural cycling of carbon in the environment and to biodeterioration; others are of ecological and economic importance because of the diseases they cause in agricultural or horticultural crops or because of their beneficial relationships with higher organisms. Additionally, they may be of industrial or biotechnological importance. Fungal diseases of humans tend to be most important in tropical environments and in immuno-compromised subjects.

For the micro-organism to be considered pathogenic and therefore capable of causing disease, it should fulfil a classic set of criteria termed Koch's postulates, which are designed to establish pathogenicity unequivocally. Some pathogens, for example, those that are not cultivable *in vitro* or in an alternative animal host, cannot fulfil all of the criteria and their status as true pathogens may have to rely on indirect methods.

Pathogenic micro-organisms display to a varying extent special characteristics, or virulence factors, that enable them to colonize their hosts and overcome or evade physical, biochemical, and immunological host defences. For bacteria, whose pathogenic properties have been intensively researched, the role of specific virulence factors and their relation to disease is better understood. Thus the presence of capsules, as in the bacteria that cause anthrax (*Bacillus anthracis*), one form of pneumonia (*Streptococcus preumoniae*), scarlet fever (*S. pyogenes*), bacterial meningitis (*Neisseria meningitidis, Haemophilus influenzae*) is directly related to the ability to cause disease because of their antiphagocytic properties. Fimbriae are related to virulence, enabling tissue attachment – for example, in gonorrhoea (*N. gonorrhoeae*) and cholera (*Vibrio cholerae*). Many bacteria excrete extracellular virulence factors; these include enzymes and other agents that impair the host's physiological and immunological functions. Some bacteria produce powerful toxins (excreted exotoxins or endogenous endotoxin), which may cause local tissue destruction and allow colonization by the pathogen or whose specific action may explain the disease mechanism. In *Staphylococcus aureus* exfoliative toxin produces the staphylococcal scalded-skin syndrome, TSS toxin-1 toxic-shock syndrome, and enterotoxin food poisoning. The pertussis exotoxin of *Bordetella pertussis*, the cause of whooping cough, blocks immunological defences and mediates attachment to tracheal cells, and the exotoxin produced by *Corynebacterium diphtheriae* causes local damage resulting in a pronounced exudate in the trachea.

Viruses cause disease by cellular destruction arising from their intracellular parasitic existence. Attachment to particular cells is often mediated by specific viral surface proteins; mechanisms for evading immunological defences include latency, change in viral antigenic structure, or incapacitation of the immune system – for example, destruction of CD 4 lymphocytes by the human immunodeficiency virus.

Mechanisms of pathogenicity are generally less well understood for fungi and protozoa; further discussion of these topics is to be found in major textbooks on medical micro-biology.

MICROCEPHALY is abnormal smallness of the head.

MICROCYTE means a small red blood corpuscle.

MICROFILARIA The mobile embryo of certain parasitic nematode worms which are found in the blood or lymph of patients infected with filarial worms. The microfilariae develop into larva in the body of a blood-sucking insect, for example, a mosquito.

MICROGRAM is the 1/1000th part of a milligram. The abreviation for it is μg. (See APPENDIX 6: MEASUREMENTS IN MEDICINE.)

MICROMETRE, or MICRON, is the 1/1000th part of a millimetre. The abbreviation for it is μm. (See APPENDIX 6: MEASUREMENTS IN MEDICINE.)

MICRO-ORGANISM (see BACTERIA).

MICROPSIA Condition in which objects appear smaller than normal. It can be due to disease of the macula.

MICROSCOPE An optical instrument comprising adjustable magnifying lenses that greatly enlarge a small object under study – for example, an insect, blood cells, or bacteria. Some microscopes use electron beams to magnify minute objects such as chromosomes, crystals, or even large molecules. Optical microscopes are also used for microsurgery when the area being operated on is otherwise inaccessible, for example, in eye and inner ear surgery, for the removal of tumours from the brain or spinal cord and for resuturing damaged blood vessels and nerves.

MICROSPORON is the genus of fungi which includes the fungi responsible for ringworm of the scalp. (See RINGWORM.)

MICROSURGERY is surgery performed with the use of an operating microscope. It is used routinely in certain operations on the eye, the ear and the larynx. In recent years it has been used, with increasing success, in attempts to reunite severed legs and arms. Under the operating microscope, surgical sutures invisible to the naked eye are used to reunite blood vessels 0·5 millimetre in diameter. The severed limb will survive for up to eight hours at room temperature, longer if cooled – as by ice in the ambulance taking the patient to hospital. Success depends primarily on restoration of the circulation to the limb. Once this has been achieved, attention is later turned to restoring the continuity of the nerves.

MICROWAVES are non-ionizing electro-magnetic radiations in the frequency range of 30–300,000 megahertz. They are emitted from electronic devices, such as heaters, some domestic ovens, television receivers, radar units and diathermy units. There is no scientific evidence to justify the claims that they are harmful to man or produce any harmful effect in the genes (q.v.). The only known necessary precaution is the protection of the eyes in those using them in industry, as there is some evidence that prolonged exposure to them in this may induce cataract. (See also DIATHERMY.)

MICTURITION means the act of passing water.

MIDDLE EAR That portion of the ear lying between the tympanic membrane and the inner ear (q.v.). It contains the ossicles, the three small bones that transmit sound. (See EAR.)

MIDGES (see BITES AND STINGS).

MIDWIFE A member of the profession which provides care and advice during pregnancy, supervises the mother's labour and delivery and looks after her and the baby after birth. Should a pregnancy or labour develop complications, the midwife will seek medical advice. Most midwives are registered general nurses who have also done an 18-month course in midwifery. Trained midwives are registered with the UK Central Council for Midwifery and work in hospitals or a domiciliary setting.

MIDWIFERY (see LABOUR; MIDWIFE).

MIGRAINE, or HEMICRANIA as it is sometimes known from the Greek word for half a skull, is a common condition characterized by recurring intense headaches. It is much commoner in women than men. There are said to be six million victims of it in Britain. It has been defined as 'episodic headache accompanied by visual or gastro-intestinal disturbances, or both, attacks lasting hours with total freedom between episodes'.

It usually begins at puberty and often tends to stop in middle age: e.g. in women attacks often cease after menopause. It often disappears during pregnancy. In susceptible individuals attacks may be provoked by a wide variety of causes including: anxiety, emotion, depression, shock, and excitement; physical and mental fatigue; prolonged focusing on television or cinema screen; noise, especially loud and high-pitched sounds; certain foods: e.g. chocolate, cheese, citrus fruits, pastry; alcohol; prolonged lack of food; irregular meals; menstruation and the pre-menstrual period.

Indeed, it has been said that anything that can provoke a headache in the ordinary individual can precipitate an attack in a migrainous subject. It seems as if there is an inherited predispostion that triggers a mechanism whereby in the migrainous subject the headache and the associated sickness persist for hours, a whole day or even longer.

The precise cause is not known, but the generally accepted view is that in susceptible individuals one or other of these causes produces spasm or constriction of the blood-vessels of the brain. This in turn is followed by dilatation of these blood-vessels which also become more permeable and so allow fluid to pass out into the surrounding tissues. This combination of dilatation and outpouring of fluid is held to be responsible for the headache.

The typical attack is very characteristic. It consists of an intense headache, usually situated over one or other eye. The headache is usually preceded by a feeling of sickness and blurring of sight. In 15 to 20 per cent of cases this disturbance of sight takes the form of bright lights: the so-called aura of migraine. The majority of attacks are accompanied by vomiting. The duration of the headache varies, but in the more severe cases the victim is usually confined to bed for twenty-four hours.

Treatment consists, in the first place, of trying to avoid any precipitating factor. Patients must find out which drug, or drugs, give them most relief, and they must always carry these about with them wherever they go. This is because it is a not uncommon experience to be aware of an attack coming on and to find that there is a critical quarter of an hour or so during which the tablets are effective. If not taken within this period, they may be ineffective and the unfortunate victim finds himself prostrate with headache and vomiting. In addition he should immediately lie down, and at this stage a few hours' rest may prevent the development of a full attack. When an attack is fully developed, rest in bed in a quiet, darkened room is essential; any loud noise or bright light intensifies the headache or sickness. The less food that is taken during an attack the better, provided the individual drinks as much fluid as he wants. Group therapy, in which groups of around ten migrainous subjects learn how to relax, is often of help in more severe cases, whilst in others the injection of a local anaesthetic into tender spots in the scalp reduces the number of attacks. Drug treatment is not very satisfactory. Analgesics such as paracetamol (q.v.), aspirin and codeine phosphate sometimes help. A combination of buclizine hydrochloride and analgesics, taken when the visual aura occurs, prevents or diminishes the severity of an attack in some people. Perhaps the most effective remedy for the condition is ergotamine tartrate which causes the dilated blood vessels to contract, but this must only be taken under medical supervision. In many cases metoclopramide, followed ten minutes later by three tablets of either aspirin or paracetamol, provides a most effective form of treatment if taken early in an attack. In milder attacks, aspirin, with or without codeine and paracetamol, may be of value. A recently introduced drug Sumatriptan (a 5-hydroxytryptamine (see SEROTIN) agonist) is showing promise as a treatment for acute attacks.

People with migraine and their relatives can obtain help and guidance from the British Migraine Association (see APPENDIX 2: ADDRESSES).

MILIA These are small keratin cysts appearing as white papules on the cheek and eyelids.

MILIARIA is the name applied to the group of diseases of the skin caused by disturbances of perspiration. The best known is MILIARIA RUBRA, or PRICKLY HEAT (q.v.).

MILIARY is a term, expressing size, applied to various disease products which are about the size of millet seeds: e.g. miliary aneurysms, miliary tuberculosis.

MILIUM is the term applied to a small, whitish nodule in the skin, especially of the face. (See ACNE.)

MILK is the natural food of all animals belonging to the class of mammalia for a considerable period following their birth. It is practically the only form of animal food in which protein, fat, carbohydrate, and salt are all represented in sufficient amount, and it therefore contains all the constituents of a standard diet. Milk is important in human nutrition because it contains first-class animal protein of high biological value, because it is exceptionally rich in calcium, and because it is a good source of

vitamin A, thiamine and riboflavine. It also contains a variable amount of ascorbic acid (vitamin C) and of vitamin D, the amount of the latter being higher during the summer months than during the winter months. Raw milk yields 67 Calories per 100 millilitres, in which are present (in grams) 87·6 of water, 3·3 of protein, 3·6 of fat, 4·7 of carbohydrate, and 0·12 of calcium. Heat has no effect on the vitamin A or D content of milk, or on the riboflavine content, but it causes a considerable reduction in the vitamin C and thiamine content.

The ready digestibility of milk, especially when mixed with lime water, or when 125 to 200 mg of citrate of soda have been added for 30 ml of milk in order to soften the curd, makes it a specially suitable food for children, invalids, and people suffering from fever. For a person confined to bed and restricted in the matter of food, 1·5 litres (3 pints) daily afford sufficient nourishment for two or three weeks.

Preparation of milk Milk may be prepared for food in various ways. *Boiling* destroys the bacteria, especially any *Mycobacteria tuberculosis* which the milk may contain. It also partly destroys vitamin C and thiamine, as does *pasteurization*. *Curdling* of milk is effected by adding rennet, which carries out the initial stage of digestion and thus renders milk more suitable for people who could not otherwise tolerate it. *Souring* of milk is practised in many countries before milk is considered suitable for food; it is carried out by adding certain organisms such as the lactic acid bacillus, the Bulgarian bacillus, and setting the milk in a warm place for several hours. (See LACTIC ACID BACILLI.) *Sterilization*, which prevents fermentation and decomposition, is usually carried out by raising the milk to boiling temperature (100 °C) for fifteen minutes and then hermetically sealing it. *Condensed, unsweetened milk* – usually known as *evaporated milk* – is concentrated *in vacuo* at low temperature; the milk is then placed in tins, which are sealed, and is sterilized by heat at a temperature of 105 °C. This destroys 60 per cent of the vitamin C and 30 to 50 per cent of the thiamine. *Sweetened condensed milk* is not exposed to such a high temperature. The sugar, which prevents the growth of micro-organisms, is added before the condensing, and finally reaches a concentration of about 40 per cent. *Dried milk* is prepared by evaporating all the fluid so that the milk is reduced to the form of powder. *Humanized milk* is cow's milk treated to render it closely similar to human milk.

Grades of milk In the United Kingdom the grades of milk that are now officially recognized are: untreated milk and heat-treated milk, which is divided into three categories: pasteurized, sterilized, and ultra heat-treated.

Pasteurized milk is milk that has been treated in one of two ways. One is the 'Holder Process', in which the milk is retained at a temperature of not less than 63 °C and not more than 65·5 °C for at least half an hour and then immediately cooled to a temperature of not more than

10 °C. The other is the 'High Temperature Short Time Process', in which the milk is retained at a temperature of not less than 71·7 °C for at least fifteen seconds and then immediately cooled to a temperature of not more than 10 °C. Pasteurization will not make satisfactory milk that was unsatisfactory in the first instance but, provided satisfactory milk is used in the first instance, it does provide a safe milk of good keeping qualities without affecting its nutritive value to any appreciable extent. *Sterilized milk* is milk that has been filtered or clarified, homogenized and then heated to, and maintained at, a temperature of at least 100 °C for such a period as to ensure that it complies with the turbidity test as described in the appropriate regulations. *Ultra heat-treated milk* is milk which has been retained at a temperature of at least 132 °C for not less than one second. It is required to satisfy the bacteriology colony count test as laid down in the appropriate regulations. It keeps much better than pasteurized milk: packed in sterile cartons it will keep for several weeks without refrigeration.

MILK TEETH are the temporary teeth of children. (For the time of their appearance, see TEETH.)

MILLILITRE is the 1000th part of 1 litre. It is practically the equivalent of a cubic centimetre (1 cm³ = 0·999973 ml); ml is the usual abbreviation.

MINERALCORTICOID (see CORTICO-STEROIDS).

MINIMALLY INVASIVE SURGERY (MIS) Popularly called keyhole surgery, MIS is surgical intervention, whether diagnostic or curative, that causes patients the least possible physical trauma. It is commonly carried out by means of an operating laparoscope (a type of endoscope (q.v.)) that is slipped through a small incision in the skin. Operations done in this manner include extracorporeal shock-wave lithotripsy (q.v.) for stones in the gall bladder and biliary ducts and in the urinary system and removal of the gall bladder. MIS is also used to remove cartilage or loose pieces of bone in the knee joint. This method of surgery usually means that patients can be treated on a day or overnight basis allowing them to resume normal activities more quickly than with conventional surgery. It is also more cost effective, allowing hospitals to treat more patients in a year.

MINOCYCLINE is a long-acting tetracycline (q.v.) which is proving of value in the treatment of carriers of meningococci, or *Neisseria meningitidis* (see MENINGITIS), and in some cases of chronic bronchitis.

MIOSIS Condition of constriction of the pupil.

MISCARRIAGE (see ABORTION).

MITHRAMYCIN or PLICAMYCIN was once used as a cytoxic drug but is now used in low dose for emergency treatment of hypercalaemia (q.v.) in malignant disease.

MITHRIDATISM is a term applied to immunity against the effects of poisons produced by administration of gradually increasing doses of the poison itself. The process is named after Mithridates, King of Pontus, who rendered himself immune against poisoning by this means.

MITOCHONDRIA are the rod-like bodies in the cells of the body which contain the enzymes (q.v.) necessary for the activity of the cell. They have been described as the 'power plant of the cell'. (See CELLS.)

MITOSIS is the process of cell division for somatic cells and for the ovum after fertilization. Each chromosome becomes doubled by splitting lengthwise and forming two chromatids which remain held together by the centromere. These chromatids are exact copies of the original chromosomes and contain duplicates of all the genes they bear. When cell division takes place the pull of the spindle splits the centromere and each double chromatid separates, one passing to one pole of the nucleus and the other to the opposite pole. The nucleus and the cell itself then also divide, forming two new daughter cells containing precisely the same 23 pairs of chromosomes and carrying exactly the same complement of genes as did the mother cell. (See CHROMOSOMES, FERTILIZATION, GENES, HEREDITY.)

MITRAL INCOMPETENCE A defect in the mitral valve (q.v.) or the heart (q.v.) allows blood to leak from the left ventricle into the left atrium (qq.v.). It is also known as mitral regurgitation; incompetence may occur along with mitral stenosis (q.v.). The left ventricle has to work harder to compensate for the faulty valve, so it enlarges, but eventually the ventricle cannot cope with the extra load and left-sided heart failure may develop. A common cause of mitral incompetence is rheumatic fever or damage following a heart attack. The condition is treated with drugs to help the heart but in severe cases heart surgery may be required.

MITRAL STENOSIS is the narrowing of the opening between the left atrium and left ventricle of the heart as a result of rigidity of, and adhesion between, the cusps of the mitral valve. It is due, almost invariably, to the infection of rheumatic fever.

MITRAL VALVE, so called from its resemblance to a bishop's mitre, is the valve which guards the opening between the atrium and ventricle on the left side of the heart. (See HEART.)

MRI (see NUCLEAR MAGNETIC RESONANCE).

MMR VACCINE A combined vaccine offering protection against measles, mumps, and rubella (German measles), it was introduced in the UK in 1988 and has now replaced the measles vaccine. The combined vaccine is offered to all infants in their second year, and the present rate of uptake is around 90 per cent. Health authorities have an obligation to ensure that all children have received the vaccine by school entry – it should be given with the preschool booster doses against diphtheria, tetanus, and polio, if not earlier – unless there is a valid contra-indication (such as partial immunosuppression), parental refusal, or evidence of previous infection. MMR vaccine may also be used in the control of measles outbreaks, if offered to susceptible children within three days of exposure to infection. The vaccine is effective and safe, though minor symptoms such as malaise, fever and rash may occur 5–10 days after immunization. The incidence of all three diseases has dropped substantially since MMR was introduced in the UK and USA (see IMMUNIZATION).

MOLAR TEETH are the last three teeth on each side of the jaw. (See TEETH.)

MOLE is a term used in two quite different senses. In the first place, a mole on the skin is a darkly pigmented spot, usually raised above the surrounding surface, rough, and covered with hair. These moles are of developmental origin, and malignant melanomas (q.v.) may develop from some of them. Secondly the term hydatidiform mole is applied to cases in which, following upon conception, a degenerate mass forms in the womb, the embryo dying in the process; whilst the term carneous mole is applied to an ovum that has died in the early months of pregnancy.

MOLLUSCUM CONTAGIOSUM A disease in which small papules, seldom larger than peas, develop on the surface of the skin. It is due to a virus and is highly contagious, being most commonly conveyed from individual to individual in swimming pools and sauna baths. They usually disappear spontaneously and need no treatment.

MONGOLIAN BLUE SPOTS are irregularly shaped areas of bluish-black pigmentation found occasionally on the buttocks, lower back or upper arms in new-born infants of African, Chinese and Japanese parentage and sometimes in the babies of black-haired Europeans.

They measure from one to several centimetres in diameter, and usually disappear in a few months. They are commonly mistaken for bruises.

MONGOLISM (see DOWN'S SYNDROME).

MONILIASIS is the infection caused by monilia, the genus of fungi now known as *Candida albicans*. The infection may occur in the mouth, where it is known as thrush (q.v.), lungs, intestine, vagina, skin, or nails.

MONKEYPOX is a smallpox-like disease, due to a virus which occurs in monkeys kept in captivity. Since 1970, when first reported, 48 human cases have been recorded. Most of these have been in Zaïre, and all have been in the equatorial rain-forest of West and Central Africa (Zaïre, Liberia, Sierra Leone, Nigeria, Ivory Coast and Cameroon). The case-fatality rate to date has been 17 per cent. It does not appear to be highly infectious and it is not at the moment considered to be a great risk to human beings.

MONOAMINE OXIDASE INHIBITORS are drugs that destroy, or prevent the action of, monoamine oxidase (MAO). Monoamines, which include noradrenaline (q.v.) and tyramine, play an important part in the metabolism of the brain, and there is some evidence that excitement is due to an accumulation of monoamines in the brain. MAO is a naturally occurring enzyme (q.v.) which is concerned in the breakdown of monoamines.

An excessive accumulation of monoamines can induce a dangerous reaction characterized by high blood-pressure, palpitations, sweating and a feeling of suffocation. Hence the care with which MAO inhibitor drugs are administered. What is equally important, however, is that in no circumstances should a patient receiving any MAO inhibitor drug eat cheese, yeast preparations such as Marmite, tinned fish, or high game. The reason for this ban is that all these foodstuffs contain large amounts of tyramine which increases the amount of certain monoamines such as noradrenaline in the body. (See MENTAL ILLNESS.)

There are also certain drugs, such as amphetamine and pethidine, which must not be taken by a patient who is receiving an MAO inhibitor drug.

MONOCLONAL ANTIBODIES An artificially prepared *antibody* (q.v.) obtained from cell clones – a genetically identical group of cells – and comprising a single type of immunoglobulin. It neutralizes only one specific antigen (q.v.). The antibodies are prepared by linking antibody-forming lymphocytes (q.v.) from the spleen of mice with myeloma cells (q.v.) from mice. Monoclonal antibodies are used in the development of new vaccines and in the study of human cells, hormones, and micro-organisms. Research is under way for their use in the treatment of some forms of cancer. (See IMMUNOLOGY.)

MONOCYTE A type of white blood cell which has a single kidney-shaped nucleus. Present in the tissues and lymphatic system as well as the circulation, it ingests foreign particles such as tissue debris and bacteria. Monocytes are about 20µm in diameter and 1 mm³ of blood contains around 7500 of them, many times fewer than the five million erythrocytes (red blood cells).

MONOMANIA is a form of partial insanity, in which the affected person has a delusion upon one subject, though he can converse rationally and is a responsible individual upon other matters.

MONONUCLEOSIS An acute viral infection in which the patient developes a sore throat, swollen lymph glands and fever. Also known as glandular fever, infectious mononucleosis is caused by members of the Herpes group of viruses – Epstein Barr and cytomegalovirus (qq.v.). The disease is more common among adolescents aged 15 to 17, an age when their immune defence machanisms are not fully developed. In the UK many thousands of teenagers catch the disease every year, and kissing is believed to be the method of transmission among many of them. The blood contains many atypical lymphocytes and the diagnosis is confirmed with the heterophil antibodies test. Patients normally recover within six weeks without treatment, but they may feel tired and depressed for several months afterwards.

MONOPLEGIA means paralysis of a single limb or part. (See PARALYSIS.)

MONOSACCHARIDE is a sugar having six carbon atoms in the molecule, such as glucose, galactose, and laevulose.

MONOZYGOTIC TWINS Twins who develop from a single ovum fertilized by a single spermatozoa. Also known as identical or uniovular twins (see MULTIPLE BIRTHS).

MORBIDITY The condition of being diseased. The morbidity rate is the number of cases of disease occurring within a particular number of the population.

MORBILLI is another name for measles.

MORBILLIVIRUSES are the group of viruses which include those responsible for measles, canine distemper and rinderpest.

MORBUS, the Latin word for disease, is used in such terms as morbus cordis (heart disease), morbus coxae (hip-joint disease).

MORIBUND In a state of dying.

MORON is the term applied to a feeble-minded person whose defect is relatively slight and whose mental age is somewhere between 8 and 12 years.

MORPHINE, or MORPHIA, is the name of the chief alkaloid upon which the action of opium depends. (See OPIUM; DRUG ADDICTION.)

MORPHOEA is a form of circumscribed scleroderma. (See SCLERODERMA.)

MORTALITY (see DEATH, CAUSES OF; DEATH RATE; INFANT MORTALITY).

MORTIFICATION is another name for gangrene. (See GANGRENE.)

MOSAICISM If non-dysjunction occurs after the formation of a zygote, that is during a mitotic cell division and not a meiotic cell division, some of the cells will have one chromosome constitution and others another. The term mosaicism describes a condition in which a substantial minority of cells differ from the majority in their chromosome content. How substantial this minority is will depend on how early during cleavage the zygote undergoes non-dysjunction.

MOSQUITOES. (See ANOPHELES; BITES AND STINGS.)

MOTILIN is a hormone (q.v.) formed in the duodenum (q.v.) and the jejunum (q.v.) which plays a part in controlling the movements of the stomach and the gut.

MOTION Waste products evacuated in a bowel movement, also called faeces or stool. (See MOTION SICKNESS.)

MOTION (TRAVEL) SICKNESS is a characteristic set of symptoms experienced by many people when subjected to the constant changes of position caused, for example, by the pitching and rolling motion of a vessel at sea. Depression, giddiness, nausea and vomiting are the most prominent.
Causes Although the vast majority of people appear to be liable to this ailment at sea, they do not all suffer alike. Many endure distress of a most acute and even alarming kind, whilst others are simply conscious of transient feelings of nausea and discomfort. A smaller proportion of people suffer from air and car sickness.

The symptoms are a result of overstimulation of the organs of balance in the inner ear by continuous changes in the body's position. The movements of the horizon worsen this situation.

Symptoms The symptoms generally show themselves soon after the journey has started, by the onset of giddiness and discomfort in the head, together with a sense of nausea and sinking at the stomach, which soon develops into intense sickness and vomiting. Most people recover quickly when the motion stops.

Treatment Innumerable preventives and remedies have been proposed, but the most effective drug is hyoscine (q.v.). Antihistamines (q.v.), which have fewer side-effects, are often helpful taken in advance of a journey. Avomine and dramamine are commonly used.

MOTOR NEURONE DISEASE (MND) is a disorder of unknown origin. Certain cells in the neurological system's motor nerves degenerate and die. Upper and lower motor neurones may be affected but sensory cells retain their normal functions. Three types of MND are identified: amyotrophic lateral sclerosis (50 per cent of patients); progressive muscular atrophy (25 per cent) in which the prognosis is better than for AML; bulbar palsy (25 per cent). Men are affected more than women and the disorder affects about seven people in every 100,000. Those affected usually die within three to five years and the average age of death is 60 years. There is no medical treatment: patients need physical and psychological support with aids to help them overcome disabilities.

MOUNTAIN SICKNESS (see ALTITUDE SICKNESS).

MOUTH is the start of the alimentary canal. It is bounded anteriorly by the lips and posteriorly by the fauces which is the narrow passage between the tonsils. Immediately behind the lips are the teeth, embedded in the jaw, and behind the lower teeth is the tongue. The upper part of the mouth is the palate. The anterior or hard palate is firm and immovable as it consists of bone covered by mucosa, while the posterior part is soft and mobile. The soft palate moves during swallowing and speech. The salivary glands discharge their saliva into the mouth through small ducts. Two of these ducts are large and can be easily seen; the parotid duct opens into the cheek opposite the upper second molar tooth and the submandibular gland duct can be seen under the tongue in the midline.

Food in the mouth is prepared for digestion by being broken up by the teeth and mixed with saliva prior to being projected into the stomach via the oesophagus.

MOUTH, DISEASES OF The mucous membrane of the mouth can indicate the health of the individual and internal organs, e.g. pallor or pigmentation may indicate anaemia, jaundice or Addison's disease. The musculature of the tongue can also act as a guide to the health of other muscles and of the nervous system in generalized disease.

CONDITIONS OF THE TONGUE At rest the tongue touches all the lower teeth and is slightly arched from side to side. It has a smooth surface with a groove in the middle and an even but definite edge. It is under voluntary control and the tip can be moved in all directions.

Ankyloglossia or tongue-tie is found when the frenum or band connecting the lower surface of the tongue to the floor of the mouth is so short or tight that the tongue cannot be protruded. This is said to interfere with speech but, if it does, it is only to a small degree. The restricted movement makes it difficult to remove food from round the teeth which may encourage decay.

Gross enlargement of the tongue can make speech indistinct or make swallowing and even breathing difficult. This is known as macroglossia and may be such that the tongue is constantly protruded from the mouth. The cause may be congenital as in severe cases of Down's Syndrome or it may occur as a result of acromegaly or be due to abnormal deposits as in amyloid disease.

In general debility the tongue may appear flabby, large and pale with the edge indented by the teeth.

A marked tremor of the tongue when protruded may be seen in various nervous diseases but is common in excessive indulgence in alcohol and cannot be concealed.

After a stroke involving the motor nerve centre the control of one side of the tongue musculature will be lost. This will result in the protruded tongue pointing to the side of the body which is paralysed. The sense of taste on one side of the tongue may also be lost in some diseases of the brain and facial nerve.

The presence of fur on the tongue may be obvious and distressing. This is due to thickening of the superficial layers of the tongue which may appear like hairs which trap food debris and become discoloured. Furring is common in the presence of fever, mouth breathing and smoking. Debility and loss of appetite will prevent the normal cleaning movements of the tongue and result in a build-up of debris between elongated papillae.

In some conditions the tongue may appear dry, red and raw. An inflamed *beefy tongue* is characteristic of pellagra, a disease caused by deficiency of nicotinic acid in the diet. A magenta-coloured tongue may be seen when there is a lack of riboflavin.

THRUSH is characterized by the presence of white patches on the mucous membrane which bleeds if the patch is gently removed. It is caused by the growth of a parasitic mould known as *Candida albicans*. Thrush is frequently found under the upper denture of elderly people who wear their dentures day and night and whose oral hygiene is poor. A more florid form is seen in feeble babies and in adults with a chronic severe illness. A less obvious form may be found in some patients after they have been taking antibiotics. Antifungal agents usually suppress the growth of Candida. Candidal infiltration of the mucosa is often found in cancerous lesions.

LEUKOPLAKIA literally means a white patch. In the mouth it is often due to an area of thickened cells from the horny layer of the epithelium. It appears as a white patch of varying density and is often grooved by dense fissures. There are many causes, most of them of minor importance. If, however, it is associated with spirits, smoking, syphilis, chronic sepsis or trauma from a sharp tooth, then cancer must be excluded.

A bright red bare area of tongue surrounded by a definite whitish yellow margin is known as *geographical tongue*. The areas may change position from week to week and there may be a slight burning sensation. Apart from an association with digestive disorders, it is of no great importance.

Ulcers of the tongue are similar to those elsewhere in the mouth. The most common are aphthous ulcers which are small red and painful and last for about ten days. They are associated with stress, mild trauma, and occasionally with folic acid and vitamin B_{12} deficiency. Ulcers of the tongue are sometimes found in patients with chronic bowel disease.

STOMATITIS (inflammation of the mouth) arises from the same causes as inflammation elsewhere, but among the main causes are the cutting of teeth in children, sharp or broken teeth, excess alcohol, tobacco smoking and general ill-health. The mucous membrane becomes red, swollen and tender and ulcers may appear. The avoidance of spicy foods and other irritants make the patient more comfortable until the condition resolves. Treatment consists mainly of preventing secondary infection supervening before the stomatitis has resolved. Antiseptic mouthwashes are usually sufficient.

Gingivitis (see TEETH, DISEASES OF) is inflammation of the gum where it touches the tooth. It is caused by poor oral hygiene and is often associated with the production of calculus or tartar on the teeth. If it is neglected it will proceed to periodontal disease.

ULCERS OF THE MOUTH These are usually small and arise from a variety of causes. *Aphthous ulcers* are the most common. They are round with a bright red margin and uncomfortable as they tend to occur near a sharp tooth or on a mobile part of the mucosa where they are easily stretched open or torn. They last about ten days and usually heal without scarring. They may be associated with stress or dyspepsia. There is no ideal treatment.

Herpetic ulcers are similar but usually there are many ulcers and the patient appears feverish and lethargic. It is more common in children and may arise from mothers who have cold sores on their lip.

Undernourished children may develop an ulcer in the cheek which causes pain, an increased flow of saliva and a foetid breath. This rarely progresses to a condition known as cancrum oris in which much of the cheek may be destroyed.

In whooping cough the underside of the tongue may be frequently forced against the lower teeth as it is protruded during the coughing bouts and this will cause an ulcer under the tongue. Larger ulcers may be tuberculous, syphilitic or cancerous in origin.

ALVEOLAR ABSCESS, DENTAL ABSCESS or GUMBOIL This is an abscess caused by an infected tooth. It may present as a large swelling or cause trismus (inability to open the mouth). Treatment is drainage of the pus, extraction of the tooth or antibiotics.

CALCULUS (*a*) *Salivary* A calculus or stone may develop in one of the major salivary gland ducts. This may result in a blockage which will cause the gland to swell and be painful. It usually swells before a meal and then slowly subsides. The stone may be passed but often has to be removed in a minor operation. If the gland behind the calculus becomes infected, then an abscess forms and, if this persists, the removal of the gland may be indicated. (*b*) *Dental*, also called TARTAR: This is a hard substance which adheres to the teeth. Some people produce more than others. It is a mixture of calcified material and bacteria and often starts as the soft debris found on teeth which have not been well cleaned and is called plaque. If not removed, it will gradually destroy the periodontal membrane and result in the loss of the tooth.

RANULA This is a cystlike swelling found in the floor of the mouth. It is often caused by mild trauma to the salivary glands with the result that saliva collects in the cyst instead of discharging into the mouth. Careful surgical removal is required as cysts can become quite large.

MUCOCOELE or MUCOUS CYST This is a collection of saliva in the lip following mild trauma. It is similar to a ranula but does not become so large. Treatment is surgical removal.

MUMPS is an acute infective disorder of the major salivary glands. It causes painful enlargement of the glands which lasts for about two weeks.

TUMOURS occur in all parts of the mouth. They may be benign or malignant. Benign tumours are common and may follow mild trauma or are an exaggerated response to irritation. Polyps are found in the cheeks and on the tongue and become a nuisance as they may be bitten frequently. They are easily excised.

A *mucocoele* (q.v.) is found mainly in the lower lip.

An *epulis* is a lump on the gum. One form is seen during pregnancy and may bleed easily but disappears spontaneously at the end of the gestation. Another form is more persistent and may recur after excision and removal of the associated teeth. An *exostosis* or bone outgrowth is often found in the mid-line of the palate and on the inside of the mandible. This only requires removal if it becomes unduly large or pointed and easily ulcerated.

Malignant tumours within the mouth are

often large before they are noticed, whereas those on the lips are usually seen early and are more easily treated. The cancer may arise from any of the tissues found in the mouth including epithelium, bone, salivary tissue and tooth-forming tissue remnants. In England and Wales in 1988 there were over 3,000 new cases of malignant disease in the mouth and major salivary glands. Nearly 670 of these were in the tongue.

Cancer of the mouth is less common below the age of 40 years and more common in men. It is often associated with chronic irritation from a broken tooth or ill-fitting denture. It is also more common in those who smoke and those who chew betel leaves. Leukoplakia (q.v.) may be a precursor of cancer. Spread of the cancer is by way of the lymph nodes in the neck. Early treatment by surgery or radiotherapy will often give a five-year cure, except for the posterior of the tongue where the prognosis is very poor. Although surgery may be extensive and potentially mutilating, recent advances in repairing defects and grafting tissues from elsewhere have made treatment more acceptable to the patient.

MRI or MAGNETIC RESONANCE IMAGING (see NUCLEAR MAGNETIC RESONANCE).

MUCILAGE is prepared from acacia or tragacanth gum, and is used as an ingredient of mixtures containing solid particles in order to keep the latter from settling, and also as a demulcent.

MUCOCOELE is an abnormally dilated cavity in the body due to the accumulation of mucus; such a 'cyst' may therefore form wherever there is mucous membrane.

MUCOCUTANEOUS LYMPH NODE SYNDROME is a disease that has been reported from Japan, Korea, Hawaii, Greece and the USA, but not yet from Britain. The cause is not known. It occurs in young children, usually under the age of 5 years. It is characterized by fever, a generalized rash which becomes bright red on the hands and feet, and enlargement of the glands in the neck. Recovery usually occurs in two to four weeks. Complications sometimes occur in the form of meningitis, arthritis, jaundice, or myocarditis. The mortality rate is 1 to 2 per cent. There is no specific treatment.

MUCOLYTIC is the term used to describe the property of destroying, or lessening the tenacity of, mucus. It is most commonly used to describe drugs which have this property and are therefore used in the treatment of bronchitis (q.v.). The inhalation of steam, for example, has a mucolytic action.

MUCOSA A term for mucous membrane.

MUCOUS MEMBRANE is the general name given to the membrane which lines many of the hollow organs of the body. These membranes vary widely in structure in different sites, but all have the common character of being lubricated by mucus, derived in some cases from isolated cells on the surface of the membrane, but more generally from definite glands placed beneath the membrane, and opening here and there through it by ducts. The air passages, the alimentary canal and the ducts of glands which open into it, and also the urinary passages, are all lined by mucous membrane.

In structure a mucous membrane consists of a basis of fibrous tissue resembling the true skin, though looser and lighter in texture, in which the blood-vessels, nerves, and mucous glands lie. This is covered on its surface by a layer of epithelium resembling the epithelium covering the skin, although the cells are in all cases of a more soft and succulent nature than those on the outer surface of the body.

It is in the character and properties of these cells that the various mucous membranes chiefly differ. In the air passages they are – almost everywhere except over the vocal cords – of a pillar-like shape and provided with thread-like processes, being known as ciliated cells. On the vocal cords the cells, which are exposed to constant friction, resemble those of the skin. In the alimentary system generally they are of a simple pillar-like or columnar type placed side by side, though in the mouth and gullet, where the food causes much friction, the surface, like that of the vocal cords, closely resembles the epidermis of the skin.

Lying close beneath the epithelium there is, in most mucous membranes, a thin layer of involuntary muscle fibres, and to this, coupled with the extremely loose attachment of mucous membranes to the organs which they line, is due the great pliability and elasticity of these membranes.

MUCOVISCIDOSIS (see CYSTIC FIBROSIS).

MUCUS is the general name for the slimy secretion derived from mucous membranes. It is mainly composed of a substance called mucin, which varies according to the particular mucous membrane from which it is derived, and it contains other substances, such as cells cast off from the surface of the membrane, ferments, and dust particles. From whatever source derived, mucin has the following characteristics: it is viscid, clear, and tenacious; when dissolved in water it can be precipitated by addition of acetic acid; and when not in solution already, it is dissolved by weak alkalis, such as lime-water.

Under normal conditions the surface of a mucous membrane is lubricated by only a small quantity of mucus; the appearance of large quantities is a sign of inflammation.

MULLERIAN DUCTS The Mullerian and the Wolffian ducts are separate sets of primordia that transiently co-exist in embryos of both sexes. In female embryos the Mullerian ducts grow and fuse in the midline producing the Fallopian tubes, the uterus and the upper third of the vagina whereas the Wolffian ducts regress. In the male the Wolffian ducts give rise to the vas deferens, the seminal vesicles and the epididymis and the Mullerian ducts disappear. This phase of development requires a functioning testis from which an inducer substance diffuses locally over the primordia to bring about the suppression of the Mullerian duct and the development of the Wolffian duct. In the absence of this substance development proceeds along female lines regardless of the genetic sex.

MULTIGRAVIDA is a pregnant woman who has had more than one pregnancy.

MULTIPARA is a woman who has borne several children.

MULTIPLE BIRTHS Twins occur about once in eighty pregnancies, triplets once in 6000, quadruplets about once in 500,000. Quintuplets are exceedingly rare. Such is the natural state of affairs. In recent years, however, the position has been altered by the introduction of the so-called fertility drugs, such as clomiphene (q.v.), and human menopausal gonadotrophin which, through the medium of the pituitary gland, stimulate the production of ova. Their wide use in the treatment of infertility has resulted in an increase in the number of multiple births, a recognized hazard of giving too large a dose. So far as fraternal, or binovular, twins are concerned, multiple pregnancy may be an inherited tendency; it certainly occurs more often in certain families, but this may be partly due to chance. A woman who has already given birth to twins is ten times more likely to have another multiple pregnancy than one who has not previously had twins. In 1974, a Swedish mother, who had not had any fertility drugs, gave birth to her third lot of twin girls. Both she and her husband were twins themselves. The statistical chance of a third pair of twins is 1 in 512,000. Identical twins do not run in families.

Twins may be binovular or uniovular. Binovular, or fraternal, twins are the result of the mother's releasing two ova within a few days of each other and both being fertilized by separate spermatozoa. They both develop separately in the mother's womb and are no more alike than is usual with members of the same family. They are three times as common as uniovular, or identical, twins, who are developed from a single ovum fertilized by a single spermatozoon, but which has split early in development. This is why they are usually so remarkably alike in looks and mental characteristics. Unlike binovular twins, who may be of the same or different sex, they are always of the same sex.

The relative proportion of twins of each type varies in different races. Identical twins have much the same frequency all over the world: around 3 per 1000 maternities. Fraternal twins are rare in Mongolian races: less than 3 per 1000 maternities. In Whites they occur two or three times as often as identical twins: between 7 (Spain and Portugal) and 10 (Czechoslovakia and Greece) per 1000 maternities. They are more common in Negroes, reaching 30 per 1000 maternities in certain West African populations. (See also SIAMESE TWINS.)

'False twins' are not uncommon, when 'twin' children have been fathered by different men.

Parents of twins, triplets or more can obtain advice and help from the Twins and Multiple Births Association (TAMBA) (see APPENDIX 2: ADDRESSES).

MULTIPLE PERSONALITY DISORDER
The individual with this psychiatric disorder has two or more different personalities, often contrasting. The dominant personality at the time determines the behaviour and attitude of the individual, who customarily seems not to know about the other personality – or personalities. The switch from one personality to another is abrupt and the mental condition of the differing personalities is usually normal. It is possible that child abuse is a factor in the disorder, which is treated by psychotherapy.

MULTIPLE SCLEROSIS is a disease of the brain and spinal cord, which, though slow in its onset, in time may produce marked symptoms, such as paralysis and tremors, and may ultimately render people suffering from it confirmed invalids. It consists of hardened patches, from the size of a pin-head to that of a pea or larger, scattered here and there irregularly through the brain and cord, each patch being made up of a mass of the connective tissue (neuroglia), which should be present only in sufficient amount to bind the nerve-cells and fibres together. In the earliest stage, the insulating sheaths of the nerve-fibres in the hardened patches break up, are absorbed, and leave the nerve-fibres bare, the connective tissue being later formed between these.

Cause Although this is one of the most common diseases of the central nervous system in Europe – there are around 50,000 affected individuals in Britain alone – the cause is still not known. The disease comes on in young people (onset being rare after the age of 40), apparently without previous illness. It is more common in first and second children than in those later in birth order, and in small rather than big families. There may be a hereditary factor, but this is by no means proven. If such exists it is of an obscure nature and linked more to a defect in the individual's reaction to infection than to any precise defect in the nervous system. The actual changes in the nervous system appear to be due to the action of some substance which dissolves or breaks up the fatty matter of the nerve-sheaths.

Symptoms These depend greatly upon the part of the brain and cord affected by the sclerotic patches. Temporary paralysis of a limb, or of an eye muscle, causing double vision, and tremors upon exertion, first in the affected parts, and later in all parts of the body, are early symptoms. Stiffness of the lower limbs causing the toes to catch on small irregularities in the ground and trip the person in walking, is often an annoying symptom and one of the first to be noticed. Great activity is shown in the reflex movements obtained by striking the tendons and by stroking the soles of the feet. The latter reflex shows a characteristic sign (Babinski sign) in which the great toe bends upwards and the other toes spread apart as the sole is stroked, instead of the toes collectively bending downwards as in the normal person. Tremor of the eye movements (nystagmus) is usually found. Trembling handwriting, interference with the functions of the bladder, giddiness, and a peculiar 'staccato' or 'scanning' speech are common symptoms at a later stage. Numbness and tingling in the extremities occur commonly, particularly in the early stages of the disease. As the disease progresses, the paralyses, which were transitory at first, now become confirmed, often with great rigidity in the limbs. Many cases progress very slowly and show little or no tendency to shortening of the duration of life.

People with multiple sclerosis, and their relatives, can obtain help and guidance from the Multiple Sclerosis Society of Great Britain and Northern Ireland. Another helpful organization is the Multiple Sclerosis Resource Centre. Those with sexual or marital problems arising out of the illness can obtain information from SPOD (Association to Aid the Sexual and Personal Relationships of People with a Disability). See APPENDIX 2: ADDRESSES.

Treatment is unsatisfactory, because the most that can be done is to lead a life as free from strain as possible, to check the progress of the disease. It is important to keep the nerves and muscles functioning, and therefore the patient should remain at work as long as he or she is capable of doing it, and in any case should regularly exercise the lower limbs by walking and the upper limbs by carrying out movements requiring co-ordination, such as knitting or embroidery. Corticosteriods seem to be as effective a means as any of slowing up the progress of the disease, but they should only be used under medical supervision.

MUMPS, also known as EPIDEMIC PAROTITIS, is an infectious disease characterized by inflammatory swelling of the parotid and other salivary glands, often occurring as an epidemic, and affecting mostly young people. Its name comes from the old verb, 'mump', meaning to mope or assume a disconsolate appearance – an apt description of the victim of the disease at its height.

Causes Mumps is due to infection with a virus and is highly infectious from person to person.

It is predominantly a disease of childhood and early adult life, but it can occur at any age. Epidemics usually occur in the winter and spring. It is infectious for two or three days before the swelling of the glands appears. A vaccine is now available that gives a high degree of protection against the disease, the incidence of which is falling sharply. The vaccine is combined with those for measles and rubella (MMR). (See IMMUNIZATION.)

Symptoms There is a long incubation period of two to three weeks after infection before the glands begin to swell. The first signs are fatigue, slight feverishness, and sore throat, which may precede the swelling by a day or two. The gland first affected is generally the parotid, situated in front of and below the ear. Along with the swelling there is often some face-ache and considerable rise of temperature to 38·3 or even 40 °C (101 or 104 °F). The swelling usually spreads to the submaxillary and sublingual glands lying beneath the jaw, and to the glands on the side opposite that first affected. There is hardly ever any redness or tendency to suppuration in the swollen parts, although interference with the acts of chewing and swallowing may occasion a good deal of trouble, and the swelling is tender to touch. After continuing four or five days, the swelling abates, the temperature having generally already fallen. In 15 to 30 per cent of males, inflammation of the testicles (orchitis) develops. This usually occurs during the second week of the illness, but may not occur until two or three weeks later. It may result in partial atrophy of the testicles, but practically never in infertility. In a much smaller proportion of females with mumps, inflammation of the ovaries or breasts may occur. Inflammation of the pancreas, accompanied by tenderness in the upper part of the abdomen and digestive disturbances, sometimes occurs. Meningitis is also an occasional complication. The various complications are found much more often when the disease affects adults than when it occurs in childhood.

Treatment The patient may require bed rest and should be kept in isolation for 14 days from the onset of the disease or 7 days from the subsidence of all swelling. Soft food, and the protection of the inflamed parts by a strip of flannel or by cotton-wool and a handkerchief are all the treatment usually required. If there is much face-ache, it is relieved by warm fomentations or aspirin.

MUNCHAUSEN'S SYNDROME, also known as 'hospital addiction' syndrome, is a condition in which patients may present repeatedly to hospitals with symptoms and signs (often simulated) suggestive of serious physical illness. More common among men than women, it differs from malingering in that no obvious reward results from the imagined or simulated symptoms. Patients may simulate signs and symptoms in a bizarre way, for instance, by swallowing blood or inserting needles into the chest. Abdominal symptoms are particularly common. They have a history of multiple hospital admissions and operations, and show extensive pathological lying and lack of personal rapport. Although the cause is unclear, it is thought to be a form of hysterical behaviour in a severely disordered personality. Patients are often masochistic, attention seeking, and constantly trying to obtain analgesic drugs. Occasionally there may be a degree of treatable depression, but on the whole management is very difficult, as patients often abscond from psychiatric treatment.

A variation of the syndrome – Munchausen by proxy – has recently been identified. The persons affected inflict damage on others, usually children, in their care – thus drawing attention to themselves.

MURMUR is the uneven, rustling sound heard by auscultation over the heart and various blood-vessels in abnormal conditons. For example, murmurs heard when the stethoscope is applied over the heart are highly characteristic of valvular disease of this organ.

MUSCAE VOLITANTES ('FLYING FLIES') Spots before the eyes due to small opacities in the vitreous humour casting shadows on the retina. In themselves vitreous floaters are harmless but anyone with 'spots before the eyes' of sudden onset should seek specialist advice.

MUSCARINE is the poisonous principle found in some toadstools. (See FUNGUS-POISONING.) It is a cholinergic substance with pharmacological properties resembling those of acetylcholine (q.v.), a chemical neurotransmitter released at the junctions (synapses) of parasympathetic nerves (q.v.) and at the junctions where nerves enter muscles.

MUSCLE, popularly known as FLESH, is the tissue by which, because of its power of contraction, movements are made in the higher animals. Muscular tissue is divided, according to its function, into two main groups, voluntary muscle and involuntary muscle, of which the former is under control of the will, whilst the latter discharges its functions independently. The term striped muscle is often given to voluntary muscle, because under the microscope all the voluntary muscles show a striped appearance, whilst involuntary muscle is, in the main, unstriped or plain. There are exceptions to the latter statement, for the heart muscle, which is involuntary, is partially striped, while certain muscles of the throat, and two small muscles inside the ear, not controllable by will-power, are also striped.

Structure of muscle VOLUNTARY MUSCLE is disposed in a regular method over the body, being mainly attached to the skeleton, and hence often called skeletal muscle. There are certain definite muscles, and these vary as to shape only slightly in different persons, although in one person particular muscles may be developed to a much greater bulk than in others. Each muscle is enclosed in a sheath of fibrous tissue, known as fascia or epimysium, and, from this, partitions of fibrous tissue, known as perimysium, run into the substance of the muscle, dividing it up into small bundles. Each of these bundles, if carefully examined, will be found to consist in turn of a collection of fibres, which form the units of the muscle. Each fibre is about 50 micrometres in thickness and ranges in length from a few millimetres to 300 millimetres. If the fibre is cut across and examined under a high-powered microscope, it is seen to be further divided into fibrils. Each fibre is enclosed in an elastic sheath of its own, which allows it to lengthen and shorten, and is known as the sarcolemma. Within the sarcolemma lie numerous nuclei belonging to the muscle fibre, which was originally developed from a simple cell. To the sarcolemma, at either end, is attached a minute bundle of connective-tissue fibres which unites the muscle fibre to its neighbours, or to one of the connective tissue partitions in the muscle, and by means of these connections the fibre produces its effect upon contracting. The sarcolemma is pierced by a nerve fibre, which breaks up upon the surface of the muscle fibre into a complicated end-plate, and by this means each muscle fibre is brought under the guidance of the central nervous system, and the discharge of energy which produces muscular contraction is controlled. When the muscle fibre within the sarcolemma is examined by a high magnifying power, it is found to show alternate light and dark transverse stripes, with a fine dotted line, called Dobie's line or Krause's membrane, across the middle of each light stripe. These appearances are due to the fact that the fibre is composed of segments made up partly of fibrous connective material, partly of semi-fluid contractile tissue, in which visible changes take place as the fibre contracts.

Between the muscle fibres, which have, on account of their relative length and width, a pillar-like shape, run many capillary blood-vessels. They are so placed that the contractions of the muscle fibres empty them at once of blood, and thus the active muscle is ensured a specially good blood supply. None of these vessels, however, pierces the sarcolemma surrounding the fibres, so that the blood does not come into direct contact with the muscular tissue, whose nourishment is carried on by the lymph that exudes from the blood-vessels. The lymph circulation is also automatically varied, as required, by the muscular contractions. Between the muscle fibres, and enveloped in a sheath of connective tissue, lie here and there special structures known as muscle-spindles. Each of these contains thin muscle fibres, numerous nuclei, and the endings of sensory nerves. They appear to be the sensory organs of the muscles. (See TOUCH.)

INVOLUNTARY MUSCLE includes, as already stated, the heart muscle and unstriped muscle. The heart muscle stands in structure between striped and unstriped muscle. Each fibre is short, has a nucleus in its centre, communicates with its neighbours by short branches, shows a faintly striped appearance near its exterior, and is devoid of sarcolemma.

Plain or unstriped muscle is found in the following positions: the inner and middle coats of the stomach and intestines; the ureters and urinary bladder; the windpipe and bronchial tubes; the ducts of glands; the gall-bladder; the uterus and fallopian tubes; the middle coat of the blood- and lymph-vessels; the iris and ciliary muscle of the eye; the dartos muscle of the scrotum; and in association with the various glands and hairs in the skin. The fibres are very much smaller than those of striped muscle, although they vary greatly in size. Each is pointed at the ends, has one or more oval nuclei in the centre, and a delicate sheath of sarcolemma enveloping it. The fibres are grouped in bundles, much as are the striped fibres, but they adhere to one another by cement material, not by the tendon bundles found in voluntary muscle.

Development of muscle All the muscles of the developing individual arise from the central layer (mesoderm) of the embryo, each fibre taking origin from a single cell. Later on in life, muscles have the power both of increasing in size, as the result of use, for example, in athletes, and also of healing, after parts of them have been destroyed by injury. This takes place partly by the growth and splitting of the original fibres to form new fibres, and partly from reserve cells, known as sarcoplasts, which lie in every muscle between the muscle fibres. An example of the great extent to which unstriped muscle can develop, to meet the demands made upon its power, is given by the womb, whose muscular wall develops so much during pregnancy that the organ increases from the weight of 30 to 40 g (1 to 1½ oz.) to a weight of around 1 kg (2 lb.), decreasing again to its former small size in the course of a month after child-birth.

Physiology of contraction A muscle is an elaborate chemico- physical system for producing heat and mechanical work. The total energy liberated by a contracting muscle can be exactly measured. From 25 to 30 per cent of the total energy expended is used in mechanical work. The heat of contracting muscle makes an important contribution to the maintenance of the heat of the body. (See also MYOGLOBIN.)

The energy of muscular contraction is derived from a complicated series of chemical reactions. Complex substances are broken down and built up again, supplying each other with energy for this purpose. The first reaction is the breakdown of adenyl-pyrophosphate into phosphoric acid and adenylic acid (derived from nucleic acid); this supplies the immediate energy for contraction. Next phosphocreatine breaks down into creatine and phosphoric acid, giving energy for the resynthesis of adenyl-pyrophosphate. Creatine is a normal nitrogenous constituent of muscle. Then glycogen through the intermediary stage of sugar bound to phosphate breaks down into lactic acid to

supply energy for the resynthesis of phosphocreatine. Finally part of the lactic acid is oxidized to supply energy for building up the rest of the lactic acid into glycogen again. If there is not enough oxygen, lactic acid accumulates and fatigue results.

There are some points to be noticed in this version of muscular activity. First, muscle contraction and relaxation take place in the absence of oxygen – the anaerobic phase. Secondly, oxygen comes into the picture in the phase of recovery, and by oxidizing some of the lactic acid winds up the contractile mechanism once more. Thirdly, the energy of contraction does not come directly from the breakdown of glycogen.

All of the chemical changes are mediated by the action of several enzymes.

Involuntary muscle has several peculiarities of contraction. In the heart *rhythmicality* is an important feature, one beat appearing to be, in a sense, the cause of the next beat. *Tonus* is a character of all muscle, but particularly of unstriped muscle in some localities, as in the walls of arteries. Muscles are not held either slack or taut, but in a slightly stretched condition, so that when occasion arises they are ready for instant action, while the arteries owe their elasticity and strength mainly to this fact. The involuntary muscle, forming the middle coat of the bowels, gland-ducts, and other tubes, contracts in the so-called *vermicular movement*, or peristalsis, which means that a ring of contraction passes slowly along the tube, at a rate of about 25 mm (1 inch) per second, the muscle relaxing as the ring of contraction passes on.

Fatigue of muscle comes on when a muscle is made to act for some time. It is due, not to wearing out of the muscle's power, but to the accumulation of waste products, especially sarcolactic acid, produced by the muscle's activity. These substances affect the end plates of the nerve controlling the muscle, and so prevent destructive over-action of the muscle. As they are rapidly swept away by the blood, the muscle, after a rest, particularly if the rest is accompanied by massage or by gentle contractions to quicken the circulation, recovers rapidly from the fatigue. After great muscular activity over the whole body, a more lasting fatigue is produced by the accumulation of these products, and by their action upon the central nervous system, this being recovered from after a prolonged rest, during which the waste substances are excreted by the lungs, kidneys, and other excretory organs.

Another factor that comes into play is the accumulation of fluid in the muscles on unaccustomed exercise. Active tissues swell because of the increased blood flow through them. This results in an increased amount outside the blood-vessels but within the tissues themselves. Normally the body can cope with this state of affairs but on occasion, as when an undertrained individual undertakes excessive exercise, the accumulation of fluid in the muscles may be so great that the body cannot absorb it quickly

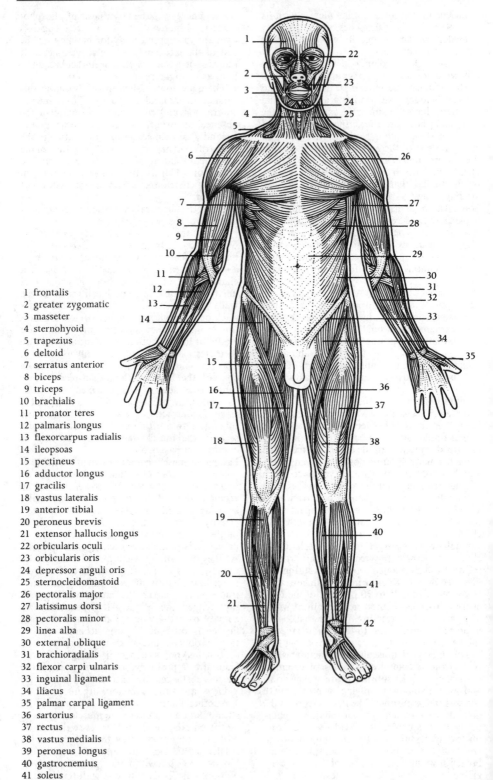

1 frontalis
2 greater zygomatic
3 masseter
4 sternohyoid
5 trapezius
6 deltoid
7 serratus anterior
8 biceps
9 triceps
10 brachialis
11 pronator teres
12 palmaris longus
13 flexorcarpus radialis
14 ileopsoas
15 pectineus
16 adductor longus
17 gracilis
18 vastus lateralis
19 anterior tibial
20 peroneus brevis
21 extensor hallucis longus
22 orbicularis oculi
23 orbicularis oris
24 depressor anguli oris
25 sternocleidomastoid
26 pectoralis major
27 latissimus dorsi
28 pectoralis minor
29 linea alba
30 external oblique
31 brachioradialis
32 flexor carpi ulnaris
33 inguinal ligament
34 iliacus
35 palmar carpal ligament
36 sartorius
37 rectus
38 vastus medialis
39 peroneus longus
40 gastrocnemius
41 soleus
42 superior extensor retinaculum

Muscles of the body: front view.

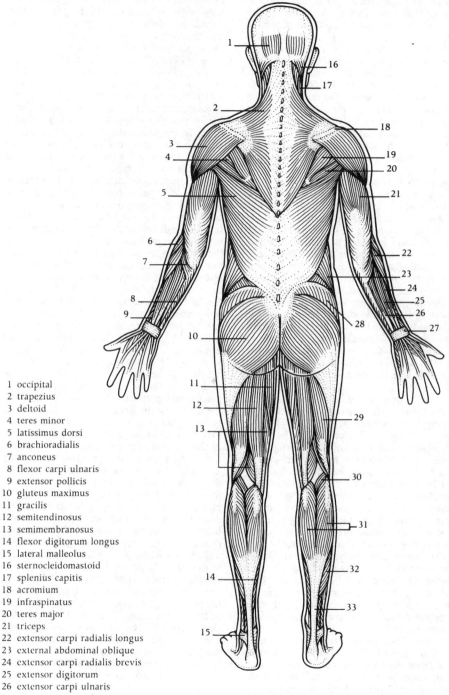

1 occipital
2 trapezius
3 deltoid
4 teres minor
5 latissimus dorsi
6 brachioradialis
7 anconeus
8 flexor carpi ulnaris
9 extensor pollicis
10 gluteus maximus
11 gracilis
12 semitendinosus
13 semimembranosus
14 flexor digitorum longus
15 lateral malleolus
16 sternocleidomastoid
17 splenius capitis
18 acromium
19 infraspinatus
20 teres major
21 triceps
22 extensor carpi radialis longus
23 external abdominal oblique
24 extensor carpi radialis brevis
25 extensor digitorum
26 extensor carpi ulnaris
27 extensor retinaculum
28 gluteus medius
29 vastus externus
30 plantaris
31 gastrocnemius
32 soleus
33 calcaneal tendon (Achilles)

Muscles of the body: back view.

enough, and the muscles swell and become tense and painful. This is the cause of the muscle stiffness which follows unaccustomed exercise. In those areas of the body where the space available for muscles is restricted, this increase of fluid may cause trouble and produce what is known as the compression syndrome. The classical example of this is the *anterior tibial syndrome*, in which the muscles on the front and outer aspect of the shin, lying within a tight fascial envelope, as they do, become tense and painful, and there may be actual damage to the muscles as a result of interference with their blood supply. (See MUSCLES, DISEASES OF.)

Rigor mortis is a condition which comes on in the muscles after death, and to which the general stiffening of the dead body is due. It consists in a state of permanent, wasteful contraction, beginning in the muscles of the neck and lower jaw at a period which varies from ten minutes to seven hours after death, and spreading gradually over the whole body. It comes on quickest after death from exhaustion, or from some weakening disease; and, occasionally, after violent injuries causing death, it comes on instantaneously, so that the posture of the body is fixed in the attitude in which death occurs. The rigidity lasts usually from sixteen to twenty-four hours, but its duration is extremely variable, being longer, as a rule, when its onset has been slow. (See DEATH, SIGNS OF.)

Muscular system, popularly known as 'the flesh', comprises all the voluntary muscles, and amounts in an average man of 70 kg (154 lb.) to about 35 kg (77 lb.), or half of the whole body weight. The total number of the voluntary muscles, each of which is named, amounts to around 620, including the muscles of both sides. Each muscle constitutes a separate organ, controlled by a special nerve or nerves, which connect it with the spinal cord and brain, where, however, actions and combined movements are represented rather than individual muscles. (See BRAIN.) The fleshy part of the muscle is known as its belly, and there is usually at either end a tendon, by which the muscle is inserted into bone or other structure, upon which it acts. One end is more fixed than the other, as a rule, the rigid end being known as the origin of the muscle, the more mobile end as its insertion.

UPPER LIMB *Between the trunk and limb* run the following muscles: the trapezius, latissimus dorsi, large and small rhomboids, and levator of the angle of the scapula, behind; and the large and small pectoral, the subclavius, and serratus anterior muscles in front. *In the shoulder region* lie the deltoid, supraspinatus, infraspinatus, large and small teres, and the subscapular muscles. *In the upper arm* the coracobrachialis, biceps, and brachialis occupy the front, while the triceps fills up the back of the arm. *In the forearm* the muscles in front that bend the wrist and fingers, or turn the hand palm downwards, are the pronator teres, the radial flexor of the wrist, the long palmar, the

ulnar flexor of the wrist, the superficial and deep flexors of the fingers, the long flexor of the thumb, and the pronator quadratus; while the muscles on the back of the forearm that extend the fingers and bend the wrist backwards, or turn the hand palm upwards, are the supinator, longer and shorter radial extensors of the wrist, extensor of the fingers, extensor of the little finger, ulnar extensor of the wrist, the extensors of the metacarpal bone, of the first joint, and of the second joint of the thumb, and the extensor of the forefinger. *In the palm of the hand* there are four lumbrical muscles, the short palmar muscle, three muscles each for the thumb and little finger, which respectively abduct, oppose, and flex these digits, an adductor of the thumb, and, in the spaces between the metacarpal bones, seven interosseous muscles.

LOWER LIMB *Muscles of the hip* are the iliacus in front, and, behind, the three gluteus muscles forming the prominence of the buttock, with the pyriform, external and internal obturator, two gemelli, and quadratus femoris muscles under cover of the largest gluteal muscle, while to the outer side lies the tensor of the sheath of the thigh. *On the back of the thigh* lie the biceps, semitendinosus, and semimembranosus muscles, whose tendons, standing out prominently behind the knee, are known collectively as the ham-strings. *In front of the thigh* are placed the sartorius, which is the longest, and the quadriceps extensor of the leg, which is the largest muscle of the body. *On the inner side of the thigh* lie the gracilis and pectineus muscles, with the long, the short, and the large adductors. *On the front of the leg* are placed the tibialis anterior, the long extensor of the great toe, the long extensor of the toes, and the peroneus tertius muscles. *On the outer side of the leg* are two muscles, the long and short peroneal muscles, whose tendons pass down behind the outer ankle to the foot. *On the back of the leg* are two groups of muscles. The superficial group of three muscles, consisting of the gastrocnemius, a doublebellied muscle, the soleus, which is flat and projects slightly beneath the gastrocnemius, and the small plantaris muscle, forms the calf of the leg, and ends in the tendo calcaneus, or Achilles tendon, behind the heel. The deep group lies close upon the bones, and consists of the popliteus, long flexor of the toes, long flexor of the great toe, and tibialis posterior muscles, the tendons of the last three passing down behind the inner ankle. *In the foot* there is one muscle, the short extensor of the toes, upon the 'dorsum' or upper surface; while in the sole of the foot are four layers of small muscles, comprising the short flexor of the toes, and abductors of the great and little toes; the accessory flexor of the toes, and four lumbrical muscles; the short flexor of the great toe, oblique and transverse adductors of the great toe, and short flexor of the little toe; and in the fourth layer seven interosseous muscles, as in the hand.

FACE AND HEAD Attached to the auricle of the ear are three weak muscles which raise, draw back, and flatten the auricle. The eyelids, nose, and lips are provided with numerous flattened muscles, which dilate and draw together these openings, and which form the means of varying facial expression.

The movements of the eye-ball are effected by six small muscles. (See EYE.) The movements of the lower jaw in chewing are controlled by four muscles on each side: the masseter muscle, which can be felt on the hinder part of the cheek as the jaws are closed; the temporal muscle, felt in the region of the temple; and the outer and inner pterygoid muscles, attached to the deep surface of the jaw-bone. Within the mouth the tongue consists of certain intrinsic muscle bundles, together with four muscles on each side, which connect it with the lower jaw, hyoid bone, and base of the skull. The floor of the mouth is formed by four muscles, which pass from the hyoid bone in front of the neck up to the lower jaw and base of the skull. The throat or pharynx, which is open in front to the nose, the mouth, and the larynx, one beneath the other, is closed behind by three broad, flat muscles, the superior, middle, and inferior constrictors of the pharynx, and is swung from the base of the skull by the stylopharyngeus muscle on either side. The soft palate, which separates the hinder part of the cavities of nose and mouth from one another, consists of five muscles on each side covered by mucous membrane. The larynx is controlled by eleven small muscles, which open or close its opening, and render the vocal cords more or less tense in the production of the voice.

FRONT OF NECK   The most prominent feature of the neck is the thick sternocleidomastoid muscle, which on each side runs from behind the ear downwards and forwards to the breast-bone and collar-bone. Partly under cover of these and protecting the front of the larynx are four small muscles on each side: the sternohyoid, sternothyroid, thyrohyoid, and omohyoid muscles. Deep in the neck, behind, and to either side of the windpipe, gullet, and large blood-vessels, lie the anterior, middle, and posterior scalene muscles, which pass from the spinal column to the upper two ribs. Lying close upon the spine are three rectus muscles on each side, which bend the head upon the spine, and the long muscle of the neck, which bends the spine in this region.

BACK OF THE NECK AND TRUNK   The muscles in this region form a very complicated system, most arising from the spine or transverse processes of several vertebrae or from a number of ribs, and running upwards to be attached to another series of vertebrae or ribs some distance above, whilst the upper muscles of the set are attached to the hinder portion of the skull. These muscles form a couple of strong columns running the whole length of the back from the loins to the head, with a groove between in which the line of vertebral spines can be felt. The upper and lower serrated muscles of the back are muscles of respiration passing from ribs to spine, and, together with the splenius muscle in the neck, form a superficial layer. Beneath them the erector spinae, the great

muscle which supports the back, runs the whole distance from the sacrum to the skull, obtaining at numerous points attachments to the spines and transverse processes of the vertebrae and to the neighbouring portions of the ribs. This muscle, along with those about to be mentioned, is of great power, having, even in moderately strong persons, a lifting power of 90 to 180 kg (200 to 400 lb.). Covered by the erector is the transversospinalis group of muscles, in which all the muscles ascend with an inward inclination; a series of short muscles connecting succeeding vertebrae with one another; and four small muscles passing from the uppermost two vertebrae to the skull. These last-named muscles incline and rotate the trunk and head from side to side.

CHEST   The diaphragm is the chief muscle of this part of the body. (See DIAPHRAGM.) Next in importance come the outer and inner intercostal muscles, which form a double layer of oblique fibres filling up the gaps between the ribs, the fibres of the two muscles running in different directions. There are also levators of the ribs, which pass each from a vertebra to the rib beneath it, and subcostal muscles which are of feeble development. All these muscles share in the act of inspiration.

ABDOMEN   The sides and front of the abdomen, unprotected by any bone beneath the level of the ribs, are enclosed by thick muscular layers strengthened by sheets of fibrous tissue. On the sides of the abdomen are three muscles: the external oblique, consisting of fibres which run downwards and forwards from the lower eight ribs; the internal oblique, under cover of the first, consisting of fibres which run upwards and forwards from the haunch-bone, and fibrous layers in its neighbourhood; and thirdly, the transversalis muscle, the fibres of which run horizontally forward from the lower six ribs, the lumbar vertebrae, and the haunch-bone. The fibres of all three muscles end along a curved line, the semilunar line, which is plainly visible upon the surface of the abdomen, running with a curve from its upper to its lower end, and distant, at the level of the navel, some 10 or 12·5 cm (4 or 5 inches) from the middle line. From the curved line a sheet of dense fibrous tissue runs inwards, those of the two sides meeting down the middle line of the body. Embedded in this fibrous sheet is a strong muscle upon each side, the rectus abdominis, which is 7·5 or 10 cm (3 or 4 inches) broad, almost 25 mm (1 inch) thick in muscular persons, and runs vertically from the front of the pelvis up to the lower part of the chest. It is a muscle of great strength, and is divided into four or five sections, by tendinous intervals, which run across the muscle, and which, in well-developed persons, form distinct transverse depressions on the front of the abdomen. The quadratus lumborum is still another muscle situated, behind, in the gap between the last rib and the haunch-bone. Other small muscles close the lower opening of the pelvis, and are associated with the functions of the bowel and genital organs.

MUSCLE CRAMP is a sudden painful involuntary maximal contraction of a muscle or muscle group. It may last up to 10 minutes and occurs in individuals with no neurological or muscle disease. Cramps usually occur in bed at night when the individual is at rest. Night cramps are especially common in the elderly, during pregnancy and in cases of diabetes or peripheral vascular disease. They can be caused by sodium loss from excessive sweating, vomiting or diarrhoea. It may also be due to hypokalaemia as a result of treatment with diuretics. Drugs such as the beta-adrenergic stimulants may be responsible. Sometimes an attack can be thwarted by actively contracting the opposing muscle. The most common cramp is in the calf or foot, so the foot should be dorsiflexed at the ankle and the leg straightened. When the cramp is in the calf muscles, getting out of bed and standing up will stretch the calf muscles and ease the attack. When attacks of cramp occur frequently at night, treatment with quinine bisulphate is beneficial.

MUSCLE RELAXANTS produce partial or complete paralysis of skeletal muscle. Drugs in clinical use are all reversible and are used to help insert a breathing tube into the trachea (endotracheal tube) during general anaesthesia and artificial ventilation. They may be broadly divided into depolarizing and non-depolarizing muscle relaxants. Depolarizing muscle relaxants act by binding to acetylcholine receptors at the motor end plate where nerves are attached to muscle cells and producing a more prolonged depolarization than acetylcholine which results in initial muscle fasciculation (overactivity) and then flaccid paralysis of the muscle. The only commonly used depolarizing drug is succinylcholine which has a rapid onset of action and lasts approximately three minutes. It is degraded by the plasma enzyme cholinesterase and its action is prolonged in congenital or acquired deficency of this enzyme. Non-depolarizing muscle relaxants bind to the acetylcholine receptors, preventing acetylcholine from gaining access to them. They have a slower onset time and longer duration than depolarizers, though this varies widely between different drugs. They are competitive antagonists (q.v.) and they may be reversed by increasing the concentration of acetylcholine at the motor end plate using an anticholinesterase agent such as neostigmine. These drugs are broken down in the liver and excreted through the kidney and their action will be prolonged in liver and renal failure. Other uses include the relief of skeletal muscle spasms in tetanus, Parkinson's disease and spastic disorders. Dantrolene and diazepam are used in these circumstances.

MUSCLES, DISEASES OF The muscles are singularly free from liability to diseases which commonly affect other tissues, this being the result, probably, of their activity, good blood supply, and the changes constantly taking place in them. Wasting of muscles sometimes occurs as a symptom of disease in other organs: for example, damage to the nervous system, as in poliomyelitis or in the disease known as progressive muscular atrophy. (See PARALYSIS.)

INFLAMMATION (MYOSITIS) of various types may occur. As the result of injury, an abscess may develop (see ABSCESS), although wounds affecting muscle generally heal well. Tuberculous inflammation in muscles is almost unknown. A growth due to syphilis, known as a gumma, sometimes forms a hard, almost painless swelling in a muscle. Rheumatism is a vague term traditionally used to define intermittent and often migratory discomfort, stiffness or pain in muscles and joints with no obvious cause. Sometimes used as a general term to cover any disorder with symptoms of pain in muscles or joints such as osteoarthritis, rheumatoid arthritis and gout. The most common form of myositis is the result of immunological damage as a result of auto-immune disease. Because it affects many muscles it is called polymyositis.

MYOSITIS OSSIFICANS, or deposition of bone in muscles, may be congenital or acquired. The congenital form, which is rare, first manifests itself as painful swellings in the muscles. These gradually harden and extend until the child is encased in a rigid sheet – the 'stone man' who used to be one of the unfortunate 'freaks' in circus side-shows. There are usually associated congenital abnormalities of the toes and fingers. The condition is fatal sooner or later. There is no effective treatment, though in some cases diphosphonates seem to delay the onset of calcification.

The acquired form arises as a sequel of a direct blow on muscle, most commonly on the front of the thigh. The condition should be suspected whenever there is severe pain and swelling following a direct blow over muscle. The diagnosis is confirmed by hardening of the swelling. Even when the condition is only suspected it is essential to avoid immobilization of the patient, and to avoid massage. Treatment consists of short-wave diathermy (see DIATHERMY) with gentle active movements. Recovery is usually complete, though slow surgical removal of residual calcified areas may be necessary.

RUPTURE of a muscle may occur, without any external wound, as the result of a spasmodic effort. It may tear the muscle right across, as sometimes happens to the feeble plantaris muscle in running and leaping, or part of the muscle may be driven through its fibrous envelope, forming a hernia of the muscle. The severe pain experienced in many cases of lumbago is due to tearing of one of the muscles in the back. These conditions give rise to considerable pain, but are relieved by rest and massage. Partial muscle tears, such as occur in sport, require more energetic treatment. In the early stages this consists of the application of cold (see COLD, USES OF), firm compression, elevation of the affected limb and rest. After forty-eight hours gradual mobilization is started, with active exercises and short-wave diathermy (see DIA-THERMY) or ultrasound (q.v.).

COMPRESSION SYNDROME is the tense painful state of muscles induced by excessive accumulation of interstitial fluid (q.v.) in them, following unusual exercise. It is particularly likely to occur in those parts of the body where the space available for muscles is restricted, as on the front and outer aspect of the shin, where the muscles lie within a tight fascial membrane. Here the syndrome is known as the *anterior tibial syndrome*. Prevention consists of always keeping fit and in training for the amount of exercise to be undertaken. Equally important is what is known in sporting circles as 'warming down': i.e., at the end of training or a game, exercise should be gradually tailed off. Treatment consists of elevation of the affected limb, compression of it by compression bandages, with ample exercise of the limb within the bandage, and massage. In more severe cases diuretics (q.v.) may be given. Occasionally surgical decompression may be necessary.

MYASTHENIA (see MYASTHENIA GRAVIS) is muscle weakness due to a defect of neuro-muscular conduction.

PAIN, quite apart from any inflammation or injury, may be experienced on exertion. This type of pain, known as myalgia, occurs especially in weakly persons, and is then relieved by rest and physiotherapy. It is also one of the common forms of rheumatism. In young children, pains of an aching character are often experienced in the muscles, especially of the legs and back, and are known as growing pains (q.v.). These come on especially after exertion and are relieved by resting.

PARASITES sometimes lodge in the muscles, the most common being *Trichinella spiralis*, producing the disease known as trichinosis (q.v.).

TUMOURS are occasionally met with, the most common being fibroid, fatty, and sarcomatous growths.

MYOPATHY is a term applied to an acquired or developmental defect in certain muscles. (See MYOPATHY.)

MUSCULAR DYSTROPHY (see MYOPATHY).

MUSHROOM POISONING (see FUNGUS-POISONING).

MUSHROOM-WORKER'S LUNG is a form of lung disease that occurs in mushroom workers as a result of their being hypersensitive to mushrooms. (See ALVEOLITIS.)

MUSTINE is the British Pharmacopoeia name for the bis form of nitrogen mustard. The nitrogen mustards have an action comparable to that of ionizing radiation and inhibit cell division. Mustine is used in the treatment of chronic leukaemia and Hodgkin's disease. (See CYTOTOXIC.)

MUTAGEN A chemical or physical agent that has the property of increasing the rate of mutation (q.v.) among cells. A mutagen does not usually increase the range of mutations. Chemicals, ionizing radiation, and viruses may act as mutagens.

MUTATION A change occurring in the genetic material (DNA) in the chromosomes of a cell. It is caused by a fault in the replication of a cell's genetic material when it divides to form two daughter cells. Mutations may occur in somatic cells which may result in a local growth of the new type of cells. These may be destroyed by the body's defence mechanism or they may develop into a tumour. If mutation occurs in a germ cell or gamete – the organism's sex cells – the outcome may be a changed inherited characteristic in succeeding generations. Mutations occur rarely but a small steady number are caused by background radiation in the environment. They are also caused by mutagens (q.v.). (See CHROMOSOME; GENETIC DISORDERS.)

MUTISM (see VOICE AND SPEECH).

MYALGIA means pain in a muscle. (See BORNHOLM DISEASE; LUMBAGO.)

MYALGIC ENCEPHALOMYELITIS (ME) A syndrome in which tiredness, muscle pain, lack of concentration, panic attacks, memory loss and depression occur. Its existence and causes have been the subject of controversy reflected in the variety of names given to the syndrome: post-viral fatigue syndrome, Royal Free disease, epidemic neuromyasthenia and Icelandic disease. ME often follows virus infections of the upper respiratory tract or gut. It may occur in epidemics or as individual cases. Physical examination shows no evidence of disease and there is no diagnostic test. The sufferer usually recovers in time, though sometimes recovery may take many months. There is no specific curative treatment, but symptomatic treatment such as resting in the early stages, may help. Sufferers may find it helpful to consult the ME Association (see APPENDIX 2: ADDRESSES).

MYASTHENIA GRAVIS is a serious disorder in which the chief symptoms are muscular weakness and a special tendency for fatigue to come on rapidly when efforts are made. The prevalence is around 1 in 30,000. Two-thirds of the patients are women, in whom it develops in early adult life. In men it tends to develop later in life.

It is a classical example of an auto-immune disease (see AUTO-IMMUNITY). The body develops antibodies which interfere with the working of the nerve endings in muscle that are acted on by acetylcholine (q.v.). It is acetylcholine that transmits the nerve impulses to muscles. If this transmission cannot be effected, as in myasthenia gravis, then the muscles are unable to contract. Not only the voluntary muscles, but those connected with the acts of swallowing, breathing, and the like, become progressively weaker, though there is no very marked wasting. Rest and avoidance of undue exertion, so as carefully to husband the strength, are necessary, and regular doses of neostigmine bromide, or pyridostigmine at intervals enable the muscles to be used and in some cases have a curative effect. These drugs act by inhibiting the action of cholinesterase. This is an enzyme (q.v.) produced in the body which destroys any excess of acetylcholine. In this way they increase the amount of available acetylcholine which compensates for the deleterious effect of antibodies on the nerve endings.

The dose of anticholinesterase that gives the maximum therapeutic response must be established. This may not restore muscle strength to normal and patients often have to live with some degree of disability. If the dose of drugs is increased above the maximum response level, in the forlorn hope of improving physical activity, the opposite effect will be produced, with progressive muscle weakness, possibly ending in what is called a cholinergic crisis. Anticholinergic drugs have no affect on the underlying disease, they merely increase the concentration of acetylcholine at receptor level.

The thymus gland plays the major part in the cause of myasthenia gravis, possibly by being the source of the original acetylcholine receptors to which the antibodies are being formed. At all events, thymectomy, or removal of the thymus, is increasingly important in the management of patients with myathenia gravis. The incidence of remission following thymectomy increases with the number of years after the operation. Complete remission or substantial improvement can be expected in 80 per cent of patients.

The other important aspect in the management of patients with myasthenia gravis is immunosuppression. Drugs are now available that suppress antibody production and so reduce the concentration of antibodies to the acetylcholine receptor. The problem is that they not only suppress abnormal antibody production, but also suppress normal antibody production. The main groups of immunosuppressive drugs used in myasthenia gravis are the corticosteroids and azathioprine. Improvement following steroids may take several weeks to become manifest and an initial deterioration is often found during the first week or ten days of treatment. Azathioprine is also effective in producing clinical improvement and reducing the antibodies to acetylcholine receptors. These affects occur more slowly than with steroids and the mean time for an azathioprine remission is nine months.

The Myasthenia Gravis Association has been established to relieve and comfort those who suffer from myasthenia gravis, to bring myasthenics together into a meaningful association where they may be offered help and understanding, and to provide the opportunity where myasthenics also help each other to overcome many of their common problems and disabilities. The association also encourages families and friends to accompany myasthenics in order that they too may learn more about the symptoms and effects of the disorder, and so offer the real help and understanding that is required. The Myasthenia Gravis Association was created and is supported by myasthenics, their families and friends (see APPENDIX 2: ADDRESSES).

MYCOBACTERIUM A Gram-positive rod-like genus of aerobic bacteria, some species of which are harmful to man and animals. For example, *M. tuberculosis* (Koch's bacillus) and *M. leprae* cause, respectively, tuberculosis and leprosy.

MYCOPLASMA is a genus of micro-organisms which differ from bacteria in that they lack a rigid cell wall. They are responsible for widespread epidemics in cattle and poultry. For a long time the only member of the genus known to cause disease in man was *Mycoplasma pneumoniae* which is responsible for the form of pneumonia known as primary atypical pneumonia (see PNEUMONIA). Another, *Mycoplasma genitalium*, has now been isolated which is responsible for certain cases of non-gonococcal urethritis. (See NON-SPECIFIC GENITAL INFECTION.)

MYCOSIS is the general term applied to diseases due to the growth of fungi in the body. Among some of the simplest and commonest mycoses are ringworm, favus, and thrush. The Madura foot of India, actinomycosis, and occasional cases of pneumonia and suppurative ear disease are also due to the growth of moulds in the bodily tissues. Other forms of mycosis include aspergillosis (q.v.), candidiasis (q.v.), cryptococcosis (q.v.) and histoplasmosis (q.v.).

MYCOSIS FUNGOIDES is a rare neoplastic condition of the reticulo-endothelial system, characterized in its later stages by multiple tumours of the skin. The course is prolonged and almost invariably ends fatally.

MYDRIASIS Condition of dilatation of the pupil.

MYELIN A substance made up of protein and phospholipid that forms the sheath surrounding the axons (q.v.) of some neurons (q.v.). These are described as myelinated or medullated nerve fibres (see NERVES), and electric impulses pass along them faster than along non-myelinated nerves. Myelin is produced by Schwann cells which occur at intervals along the nerve fibre.

MYELITIS is inflammation of the spinal cord.

MYELOCYTE is the name given to one of the cells of bone-marrow from which the granular white corpuscles of the blood are produced. They are found in the blood in certain forms of leukaemia.

MYELOGRAPHY is the injection of a radio-opaque substance into the central canal of the spinal cord in order to assist in the diagnosis of diseases of the spinal cord or spine.

MYELOID An adjective that relates to the granulocyte precursor cell in the bone marrow. For example, myeloid leukaemia, which arises from abnormal growth in the blood-forming tissue of the marrow.

MYELOMA (see MYELOMATOSIS).

MYELOMATOSIS, or MULTIPLE MYELOMA, is a malignant disorder of plasma cells, derived from B lymphocytes. In most patients the bone marrow is heavily infiltrated with atypical, monoclonal plasma cells, which gradually replace the normal cell lines, inducing anaemia, leucopenia, and thrombocytopenia. Bone absorption occurs, producing diffuse osteoporosis. In some cases only part of the immunoglobulin molecule is produced by the tumour cells, appearing in the urine as Bence Jones proteinuria. The disease is rare under the age of 30, frequency increasing with age to peak between 60 and 70 years. It is more common in men than women, and in black people than white. There may be a long pre-clinical phase, sometimes as long as 25 years. When symptoms do occur, they tend to reflect bone involvement, reduced immune function, renal failure, anaemia or hyperviscosity of the blood. Vertebral collapse is common, with nerve root pressure and reduced stature. The disease is usually fatal, infection being a common cause of death. Local skeletal problems should be treated with radiotherapy, and the general disease with chemotherapy, chiefly melphalan or cyclophosphamide. Red-blood-cell transfusion is usually required, together with plasmapheresis, and orthopaedic surgery may be necessary following fractures. With sensitive counselling to increase the patient's morale, the prognosis may be significantly improved.

MYOCARDIAL INFARCTION (see CORONARY THROMBOSIS).

MYOCARDITIS means inflammation of the muscular wall of the heart.

MYOCARDIUM is the muscular substance of the heart.

MYOCLONUS is a brief, twitching muscular contraction which may involve only a single muscle or many muscles. It may be too slight to cause movement of the affected limb, or so violent as to throw the victim to the floor. The cause is not known, but in some cases may be a form of epilepsy. A single myoclonic jerk in the upper limbs occasionally occurs in petit mal. (See EPILEPSY.) The myoclonic jerks which many people experience in falling asleep are a perfectly normal phenomenon.

MYOGLOBIN is the protein which gives muscle (q.v.) its red colour. It has the property of combining loosely and reversibly with oxygen. This means that it is the vehicle whereby muscle extracts oxygen from the haemoglobin in the blood circulating through it, and then releases the oxygen for use by the muscle.

MYOGLOBINURIA The occurrence of myoglobin in the urine. This is the oxygen-binding pigment in muscle and mild myoglobinuria may occur during exercise. Severe myoglobinuria will result from severe injuries, particularly crushing injuries, to muscles.

MYOMA is the term applied to a tumour, almost invariably of a simple nature, which consists mainly of muscle fibres. These muscle tumours often occur in the uterus.

MYOMECTOMY Removal by surgery of FIBROIDS from the muscular wall of the uterus (q.v.).

MYOMETRIUM is the muscular coat of the uterus (q.v.).

MYOPATHY is a generic term covering all primary muscle disease. It is not a neurological disease, and should be distinguished from neuropathic conditions (see NEUROPATHY) such as motor neurone disease, which tend to affect the distal limb muscles. The main subdivisions are genetically determined, congenital, metabolic, drug induced, and myopathy (often inflammatory) secondary to a distant carcinoma. Progressive muscular dystrophy is characterized by symmetrical wasting and weakness, the muscle fibres being largely replaced by fatty and fibrous tissue, with no sensory loss. Inheritance may take several forms, thus affecting the sex and age of victims.

The commonest type is Duchenne's muscular dystrophy which is inherited as a sex-linked disorder. It nearly always occurs in boys.

Symptoms There are three chief types of myopathy. The commonest, known as pseudo-hypertrophic muscular dystrophy, affects particularly the upper part of the lower limbs of children. The muscles of the buttocks, thighs and calves seem excessively well developed, but nevertheless the child is clumsy, weak on his legs, and has difficulty in picking himself up when he falls. In another form of the disease, which begins a little later, as a rule about the age of 14, the muscles of the upper arm are first affected, and those of the spine and lower limbs become weak later on. In a third type, which begins about this age, the muscles of the face, along with certain of the shoulder and upper arm muscles, show the first signs of wasting. All the forms have this in common: that the affected muscles grow weaker till their power to contract is quite lost. In the first form, the patients seldom reach the age of 20, falling victims to some disease which, to ordinary people, would not be serious. In the other forms the wasting, after progressing to a certain extent, often remains stationary for the rest of life. Myopathy may also be acquired when it is the result of disease such as thyrotoxicosis, osteomalacia or Cushing's disease, and the myopathy resolves when the primary disease is treated.

Treatment Some myopathies may be the result of inflammation or arise from an endocrine or metabolic abnormality. Treatment of these is the treatment of the cause with supportive physiotherapy and any necessary physical aids while the patient is recovering. Treatment for the hereditary myopathies is supportive since, at present, there is no cure, though developments in gene research raise the possibility of future treatment. Physiotherapy, physical aids, counselling and support groups may all be helpful in caring for these patients.

The education and management of these unfortunate children raise many difficulties. Much help in dealing with these problems can be obtained from the Muscular Dystrophy Group of Great Britain (see APPENDIX 2: ADDRESSES).

MYOPIA (see REFRACTION).

MYOSITIS means inflammation of a muscle. (See MUSCLES, DISEASES OF.)

MYOSITIS OSSIFICANS (see MUSCLE).

MYOTONIA is a condition in which the muscles, though possessed of normal power, contract only very slowly. The stiffness disappears as the muscles are used.

MYRINGOTOMY is the operation of cutting the drum of the ear in cases of acute inflammation of the middle ear.

MYRRH is a gum-resin obtained from *Commiphora molmol*, an Arabian myrtle tree. It stimulates the function of mucous membranes with which it is brought in contact or by which it is excreted. Tincture of myrrh is used for a gargle in sore throat, as a tooth-wash when the gums are inflamed, and as an ingredient of cough mixtures.

MYXOEDEMA is a disease due to underactivity of the thyroid gland. The thyroid gland secretes two hormones – thyroxine and triodothyronine – and these hormones are responsible for the metabolic activity of the body. Hypothyroidism may result from developmental abnormalities of the gland or a deficiency of the enzymes necessary for the synthesis of the hormones. It may be a feature of endemic goitre (q.v.) and cretinism, but the most common cause of hypothyroidism is the auto-immune destruction of the thyroid known as chronic thyroiditis. It may also occur as a result of radio-iodine treatment of thyroid overactivity and is occasionally secondary to pituitary disease in which inadequate TSH production occurs. It is a common disorder, occurring in fourteen per one thousand females and one per one thousand males. Most patients present between the age of thirty and sixty years. The term myxoedema was introduced in 1878 to describe the swelling of the skin and sub-cutaneous tissues that characterized severe forms of hypothyroidism.

Symptoms As thyroid hormones are responsible for the metabolic rate of the body hypothyroidism usually presents with a general slowing-up. This affects both physical and mental activities. The intellectual functions become slow, the speech deliberate and the formation of ideas and the answers to questions take longer than in healthy people. Physical energy is reduced and patients frequently complain of lethargy and generalized muscle aches and pains. Patients become intolerant of the cold and the skin becomes dry and swollen. The larynx also becomes swollen and gives rise to a hoarseness of the voice. Most patients gain weight and develop constipation. The skin becomes dry and yellow due to the presence of increased carotine. Hair becomes thinned and brittle and even baldness may develop. Swelling of the soft tissues may give rise to a carpal tunnel syndrome and middle-ear deafness. The diagnosis is confirmed by measuring the levels of thyroid hormones in the blood which are low and of the pituitary TSH which is raised in primary hypothyroidism.

Treatment consists of the administration of thyroxine. Although triodothyronine is the metabolically active hormone, thyroxine is converted to triodothyronine by the tissues of the body. Treatment should be started cautiously with a small dose of not more than 0·05 mg of thyroxine and this can be slowly increased to 0·2 mg daily, the equivalent of the maximum output of the thyroid gland. If too large a dose is given initially palpitations and tachycardia are likely to result and in the elderly heart failure may be precipitated.

MYXOMA is a tumour consisting of very imperfect connective tissue, and containing a peculiar mucus-like juice.

MYXOVIRUSES include the influenza viruses A, B and C; the para-influenza viruses, types 1 to 3. Respiratory syncytial virus, which is an important cause of respiratory disease in the early years of life, is caused by the related paramyxoviruses. Myxoviruses have an affinity for protein receptors in red blood cells.

N

NADOLOL (see ADRENERGIC RECEPTORS).

NAEVUS Vascular naevi, or cutaneous angiomata, develop in around one in three children within the first month or two of life, though they are not usually apparent at birth and most resolve spontaneously. Formed by a mass of superficial dilated blood-vessels, there are two main variants, though in many cases components of both are combined. Capillary naevi are characterized by increased numbers of capillaries, and present as macular areas of vascular dilatation – typically the port-wine stain on the face. They show little tendency to resolve spontaneously. Cosmetic cover was for many years the best available treatment, although cryosurgery and particularly lasers (q.v.) have revolutionized therapy in the past decade. Strawberry naevi, or cavernous angiomata, are raised, bright red, and sometimes very large and disfiguring. Ulceration and bleeding may occur, and is common when they occur in the napkin area. They tend to enlarge for the first year, then after a short static period they gradually resolve, generally leaving a fold of redundant skin (which may require surgical removal) by the age of 8 or 9. Treatment should be conservative until complete spontaneous resolution has occurred. Spider naevi are much smaller and commonly occur on the face, particularly in association with liver cirrhosis (see LIVER DISEASES).

NAIL-BITING is a common practice in schoolchildren, most of whom gradually give it up as they approach adolescence. Too much significance should therefore not be attached to it. In itself it does no harm, and punishment or restraining devices do nothing but harm. It is a manifestation of tension or insecurity, the cause of which should be removed.

NAILS (see SKIN).

NAILS, DISEASES OF The nails are subject to relatively few diseases. On the other hand, any interference with the natural appearance of the finger-nails is very unsightly, whilst the sensitive matrix of both finger- and toe-nails is extremely tender when diseased.
INFLAMMATION of the nails and of the bed in which they rest occurs in various skin diseases: e.g. psoriasis, eczema, fungus infections (see RINGWORM). The nails then become rough, thickened, irregular, discoloured, and split readily into layers. Most acute febrile diseases are accompanied by irregularities in growth of the nails, producing a transverse furrow in the nail, as it grows onwards, and these furrows on the nails serve to date a severe illness fairly accurately, the furrow gradually approaching the

free margin of the nail and disappearing in about six months' time.
Brittle nails tend to be troublesome in the elderly.
Spoon-shaped or concave nails (KOILONYCHIA) are often associated with iron deficiency, especially in middle-aged women, and become normal when this is treated.
ABSCESS may occur at the root of the nail (see WHITLOW) or underneath it near its edge. Antibiotic treatment or local surgery is effective, though the nail may be lost.
INJURY to the nail by a blow is often followed by an extravasation of blood beneath it, the nail first turning black, and then often being shed. In all these cases in which the nail is shed, a new nail generally appears quickly, and replaces the old one in six months, unless the matrix has been very seriously diseased or injured.
INGROWING NAIL is a troublesome condition affecting only the nails of the toes. It is due to a variety of causes, chief among which are the pressure of badly fitting shoes, cutting away of the corners in paring the nails, and want of attention to the nails. Proper attention to the nails is usually effective but, if the nail is troublesome, the patient should consult a chiropodist or doctor. Occasionally surgery is required to cure the condition.

NALIDIXIC ACID is a drug, active against Gram-negative micro-organisms, which is proving useful in the treatment of infections of the urinary tract.

NALORPHINE reduces or abolishes most of the actions of morphine and similarly acting narcotics, such as pethidine. It was used as an antidote in the treatment of over-dosage with these drugs but has now been superseded by naloxone (q.v.).

NALOXONE is the most efficient drug in the treatment of morphine poisoning. It blocks the effects of most opiates. Administration by mouth is unreliable but, when given intravenously, it acts within two or three minutes.

NANOMETRE is a millionth of a millimetre (q.v.). The approved abbreviation is nm.

NAPPY RASH is the eruption which tends to occur on the buttocks of infants, due to too infrequent changing of soiled nappies or inadequate laundering of nappies. There is some evidence that it is more common in bottle-fed, than in breast-fed, babies. It has become much less common since the advent of disposable nappies.
Prevention consists of the following measures. (i) When the baby is bathed, particular attention must be paid to the creases and folds of the skin which must be carefully washed, then equally carefully dried and sprinkled with a bland baby powder. (ii) Nappies must not be

washed in strong soaps or detergent solutions. After washing they must be carefully rinsed out in several changes of clean water. (iii) Soiled nappies must be changed frequently.

Should the skin become inflamed, washing it with a 1-per-cent solution of sodium sulphate, followed by the application of calamine lotion, is often useful. An alternative application is zinc and castor oil ointment.

NAPRAPATHY is a system of healing which attributes disease to disorder in the ligaments and connective tissues.

NAPROXEN (see NON-STEROIDAL ANTI-INFLAMMATORY DRUGS).

NARCISSISM is an abnormal mental state characterized by excessive admiration of self.

NARCOLEPSY is a condition in which uncontrollable episodes of sleep occur two or three times a day. It starts at any age and persists for life. The attacks, which usually last for 10 to 15 minutes, come on at times normally conducive to sleep, such as after a meal, or sitting in a bus, but they may occur when walking in the street. In due course, usually after some years, they are associated with cataplectic attacks when for a few seconds there is sudden muscular weakness affecting the whole body. The cataplectic attacks are controlled by imipramine or clomipramine.

Familial narcolepsy is well recognized and recently a near-100-per-cent association between narcolepsy and the histocompatability antigen HLA-DR2 has been discovered. This has given rise to the notion that narcolepsy is an immune-related disease. The Narcolepsy Association (UK) has been founded to help patients with this strange disorder. (See APPENDIX 2: ADDRESSES.)

NARCOSIS is a condition of profound insensibility, resembling sleep so far that the unconscious person can still be roused slightly by great efforts, or at all events is not entirely indifferent to sensory stimuli. It is most commonly produced by drugs, such as opium, but may also be due to poisons formed within the body, as in uraemia.

NARCOTICS (see HYPNOTICS).

NARES is the Latin word for the nostrils.

NASOGASTRIC TUBE A small-bore plastic or rubber tube passed into the stomach through the nose, pharynx and then the oesophagus. It is used either to aspirate gas and liquid from the stomach or to pass food or drugs into it.

NASOPHARYNX is the upper part of the throat, lying behind the nasal cavity. (See NOSE.)

NATAMYCIN is an antibiotic isolated from *Streptomyces natalensis* which is proving of value in the treatment of moniliasis (q.v.).

NATIONAL HEALTH SERVICE (NHS) The United Kingdom's National Health Service was created by Act of Parliament and inaugurated on 5 July 1948. Its original aim was to provide a comprehensive system of health care to everyone, free at the point of delivery. The service is funded by National Insurance contributions and from general taxation (approximately £31 billion, excluding patient charges, or 6 per cent of gross domestic product was spent on health in 1994–5). The system has been reformed several times. The latest occurred in 1991 when the 1990 National Health Service and Community Health Act came into force and further changes are being introduced. This aims to improve efficiency and accountability within all branches of the health service by introducing competition and 'market forces'. There has also been some separation between those branches of the service which 'provide' health care and those that 'purchase' it. Hospital groups and community health services were enabled to become NHS trusts, independent providers of services, and general practitioners (GPs) to hold funds with which to buy certain services from the 'providers'.

The Secretary of State for Health is responsible to Parliament for the provision of health services in England and Wales. Within the Department of Health the Policy Board (chaired by the Secretary of State) makes the strategic plans for the health service and the NHS Executive deals with implementation of strategy and operational management. Below the Department of Health in the management structure are the eight regional health authorities (RHAs), NHS trusts, special health authorities, district health authorities (DHAs) and family health service authorities (FHSAs). Many DHAs and FHSAs have amalgamated or will be doing so. Community health councils are outside the management structure but are statutory bodies at local level which represent the interests of their communities within the NHS.

RHAs develop services within the national guidelines, allocate resources to the DHAs, FHSAs and GP fund-holders and monitor their performances. In 1996 the government plans to replace RHAs with fewer, smaller regional boards accountable to the NHS Management Executive. The revenue of DHAs is decided on weighted capitation basis and they are responsible for purchasing hospital and community services for their residents (they are also responsible for managing units that are not yet NHS trusts). In England FHSAs (and in future amalgamated authorities) are responsible for managing the services provided by GPs, dentists, opticians and retail pharmacists (who are all independent practitioners under contract to the NHS). An increasing number of GPs are now fund-holders.

NHS trusts are hospitals and other units providing patient care which are self governing and are directly accountable to the Secretary of State. They are run by small directly appointed executive boards and their revenue is generated by 'winning' contracts from the various purchasers – including fundholding GPs – and they are free to control their own assets, management structure and the terms of employment of their staff. Special health authorities which provide highly specialized services, including psychiatric care for mentally ill patients who may be a public danger, are also directly responsible to the Secretary of State.

Scotland, Wales and Northern Ireland have broadly similar structures but there are no RHAs, responsibility being held by the Scottish, Welsh and Northern Ireland Offices. In Northern Ireland the health and social services are administratively integrated.

NATIONAL LISTENING LIBRARY is a charity which produces recorded books for handicapped people who cannot read, with the exception of the blind who have their own separate organization, the Royal National Institute for the Blind. (See APPENDIX 2: ADDRESSES.). (See also CALIBRE.)

NAUSEA means a feeling that vomiting is about to take place. (See VOMITING.)

NAVEL, or UMBILICUS, is the scar on the abdomen marking the point where the umbilical cord joined the body in embryonic life. (See PLACENTA.)

NEAR SIGHT (see REFRACTION).

NEBULA is the term applied to a slight opacity on the cornea producing a haze in the field of vision, and also to any oily preparation to be sprayed from a nebulizer, an apparatus for splitting up a fluid into fine droplets.

NEBULIZERS A nebulizer makes an aerosol by blowing air or oxygen through a solution of a drug. Many inhaled drugs such as salbutamol, ipratropium and beclomethasone can be given in this way. It has the advantage over a medihaler in that no special effort is required to co-ordinate breathing and a nebulizer allows a much greater concentration of the drug to be delivered compared with that of a medihaler. The use of higher doses of bronchodilator drugs made possible by the nebulizer means that the risk of unwanted side-effects is also increased.

NECATOR AMERICANUS is a hookworm, closely resembling but smaller than the *Ancylostoma duodenale*. (See ANCYLOSTOMIASIS.)

NECK is that portion of the body which extends from the upper limit of the chest to the base of the skull. Its main function is to support the head. Through its front part run the passages for the air and the food. The great bulk of the neck is composed of seven cervical vertebrae with the muscles attached thereto, in front and behind. (See MUSCLE.) Within the canal formed by the rings of these vertebrae lies the cervical part of the spinal cord, from which proceed the nerves that control the movements of the neck and arms.

In front of the spinal column lies the pharynx, or throat-cavity, extending from the base of the skull above down to the lower edge of the sixth vertebra, where the gullet continues it directly downwards, while the larynx opens out of it in front. The larynx is close to the surface of the front of the neck, and the thyroid cartilage can be readily seen and felt beneath the skin. (See LARYNX.) The larynx is continued downwards by the windpipe, and just beneath the larynx the isthmus of the thyroid gland can be felt crossing the windpipe and connecting the two lobes of the gland which lie one on either side of the larynx. The strong sternocleidomastoid muscle is prominent on each side of the neck, running from the mastoid process of the skull down to the breast-bone and inner end of the clavicle; under cover of it lies a fibrous sheath containing the carotid artery, internal jugular vein and vagus nerve. The sternocleidomastoid muscle divides each side of the neck into two triangular areas, in which lie important nerves and branches of these blood-vessels, as well as chains of lymphatic glands. Several large superficial veins run down the neck, and are of importance, because in wounds of the neck they may give rise to much bleeding. The chief of these are the external jugular vein, running straight downwards from the angle of the jaw, and the anterior jugular vein, running downwards from beneath the chin, not far from the middle line. At the root of the neck the apex of each lung projects a short distance from the chest into the neck.

NECROPSY is a post-mortem examination which produces almost no disfigurement. The brain is examined by an opening across the scalp, afterwards hidden by the hair, and the contents of chest and abdomen are inspected through an opening down the middle line in front. If necessary minute pieces of organs are removed for microscopic examination. It is a social duty of the deceased person's relatives to permit or request a post-mortem examination in cases in which the disease was a matter of uncertainty.

NECROSIS means death of a limited portion of tissue, the term being most commonly applied to bones when, as the result of disease or injury, a fragment dies and separates. (See BONE, DISEASES OF.)

NECROTIZING FASCIITIS or CELLULITIS is a potentially lethal infection caused by the Gram-positive bacterium *Streptococcus pyogenes* (q.v.) which has the property of producing dangerous exotoxins. The infection may spread very rapidly, destroying tissue as it spreads. Urgent antibiotic treatment may check the infection, and surgery is sometimes required, but even with treatment patients may die (see STREPTOCOCCUS).

NEEDLING is an operation performed in the treatment of cataracts (q.v.), in which the anterior lens capsule is torn open with a needle, allowing the aqueous fluid to dissolve the opaque soft lens matter, which is gradually washed away into the bloodstream. This 'extra-capsular extraction' may need to be repeated several times before all the opaque lens matter disperses. Although a relatively simple procedure, it is unsuitable for patients over the age of 35 (when the nucleus of the lens becomes increasingly hard), and cryosurgery (q.v.) and laser therapy (q.v.) have become the preferred methods of treatment.

Needling is also used for certain minor dermatological procedures, such as removal of small facial cysts and scabies mites.

NEGATIVISM means a morbid tendency in a person to do the opposite of what he is desired or directed to do. It is specially characteristic of schizophrenia, but is not uncommon in non-psychotic persons.

NEISSERIA is a group, or genus, of rounded bacteria that occur in pairs and are therefore known as diplococci (see MICROBIOLOGY). They are named after Albert Neisser, the German physician who discovered the gonococcus, the causative organism of gonorrhoea (q.v.), which is now known as *Neisseria gonorrhoea*. The group also includes the causative organism of cerebrospinal meningitis (see MENINGITIS): *Neisseria meningitidis*.

NEMATODE is a roundworm. (See ASCARIASIS.)

NEOMYCIN is an antibiotic derived from *Streptomyces fradiae*. It has a wide antibacterial spectrum, being effective against the majority of Gram-negative bacilli. Its use is limited by the fact that it is liable to cause deafness and kidney damage. For this reason it is never given by injections. Its main use is for application to the skin, either in solution or as an ointment, for the treatment of infection of the skin. It is also given by mouth for the treatment of certain forms of enteritis due to *E. coli*.

NEONATAL means pertaining to the first month of life.

NEONATAL MORTALITY is the mortality of infants under one month of age. In England and Wales this has fallen markedly in recent decades: from over 28 per 1000 related live births in 1939 to around 4 in 1992. This improvement can be attributed to various factors: better antenatal supervision of expectant mothers; care to ensure that expectant mothers receive adequate nourishing food; improvements in the management of the complications of pregnancy and of labour. Nearly three-quarters of neonatal deaths occur during the first week of life. For this reason, increasing emphasis is being laid on this initial period of life. Between 1960 and 1990, in England, the number of deaths in the first week fell from 9772 to 2174, representing a fall in the rate per 1000 live births from 13·2 to 3·3. The chief causes of deaths in this period are immaturity of the infant, birth injuries, congenital abnormalities and asphyxia. After the first week the commonest cause is infection.

NEOPLASM, which means literally a 'new formation', is another word for tumour.

NEPHRECTOMY is the operation for removal of the kidney. (See KIDNEYS, DISEASES OF.)

NEPHRITIS means inflammation of the kidneys. (See KIDNEYS, DISEASES OF: glomerulo-nephritis.)

NEPHROLITHIASIS is the term applied to a condition in which calculi are present in the kidney.

NEPHROLOGY The branch of medicine concerned with the study and management of kidney disease.

NEPHRON Each kidney comprises over a million of these microscopic units which regulate and control the formation of urine. A tuft of capillaries invaginates the Bowmans capsule which is the blind-ending tube (glomerulus) of each nephron. Plasma is filtered out of blood and through the Bowmans capsule into the renal tubule. As the filtrate passes along the tubule most of the water and electrolytes are reabsorbed. The composition is regulated with the retention or addition of certain molecules (e.g. urea, drugs, etc.). The tubules eventually empty the filtrate, which by now is urine, into the renal pelvis from where it flows down the ureters into the bladder. (See KIDNEYS.)

NEPHROPEXY is the fixation of a floating kidney in its original position.

NEPHROPTOSIS means the condition in which a kidney is movable or 'floating'.

NEPHRORRHAPHY is the operation by which a movable kidney is fastened by stitches in its proper place.

NEPHROSTOMY is the operation of making an opening into the kidney to drain it.

NEPHROTIC SYNDROME is one of proteinuria, hypo-albuminaemia and gross oedema. The primary cause is the leak of albumin through the glomerulus. When this exceeds the liver's ability to synthesise albumin the plasma level falls and oedema results. The nephrotic syndrome is commonly the result of primary renal glomerular disease (see KIDNEYS, DISEASES OF: glomerulonephritis). It may also be a result of metabolic diseases such as diabetic glomerular sclerosis and amyloidosis. It may be the result of systemic auto-immune diseases such as systemic lupus erythematosis and polyarteritis. It may complicate malignant diseases such as myelomatosis, Hodgkin's disease and lymphocytic leukaemia. It is sometimes caused by nephrotoxins such as gold or mercury and certain drugs, and it may be the result of certain infections such as malaria and Crohn's disease.

NEPHROTOMY means the operation of cutting into the kidney, in search of calculi or for other reasons.

NERVE BLOCK (see ANAESTHESIA, local anaesthetics).

NERVE INJURIES are produced by several causes. Continued or repeated severe pressure may be enough to damage a nerve seriously, as in the case of a badly made crutch pressing into the armpit and causing drop-wrist. Bruising due to a blow which drives a superficially placed nerve against a bone may inflict severe damage upon a nerve such as the radial nerve behind the upper arm. A wound may sever nerves, along with other structures; this accident is specially liable to occur to the ulnar nerve in front of the wrist, owing to falls upon broken glass, and to various nerves in the armpit when the humerus is fractured near its upper end.
Symptoms When a sensory nerve is injured, sensation is immediately more or less impaired in the part supplied by the nerve. When the nerve in question is a motor one the muscles governed through it are instantly paralysed. In the latter case, the portion of nerve beyond the injury degenerates and the muscles gradually waste, and lose their power of contraction in response to electrical applications. Finally, deformities result and the joints become fixed. This is particularly noticeable when the ulnar nerve is injured, the hand and fingers taking up a claw-like position. The skin may also become

cold, glossy and even ulcerate, owing to the loss of its nerve supply.
Treatment The nerve, if wounded, should be carefully stitched with the ends touching one another, and, if injured by other causes, should be carefully protected from a repetition of the injury. In some cases recovery takes place within a few days, but usually, if the nerve is completely severed or seriously injured, the muscles supplied by it do not regain their power for several weeks at least. The reason for this is that the part cut off from connection with the brain and cord degenerates rapidly, and the new nerve has to grow all the way down the sheath of the old one. (See NERVES.)

NERVES The nervous system consists in part of cells and in part of fibres, each of which is a long process extending from a nerve-cell. The brain and spinal cord are often spoken of together as the central nervous system; the nerves which proceed from them, forty-three on each side, are named the cerebrospinal, or peripheral nerves; whilst the third great division, situated in the neck, thorax and abdomen, and intimately connected with the cerebrospinal nerves (though in its action largely independent of the brain and cord) is known as the autonomic nervous system. The last-named consists of ganglia containing nerve-cells, which are profusely connected by plexuses of nerve-fibres.

The nerve-cells originate, or receive, impulses and impressions of various sorts, which are conveyed from them to muscles, blood-vessels, and elsewhere, by efferent nerves, or received by them through afferent nerves coming from the skin, organs of sense, joints, etc. The autonomic system is concerned mainly with the movements and other functions of the internal organs, secreting glands and blood-vessels, the activities of which proceed independently of the will.
Structure (1) NERVE-FIBRES: The nerves vary much in size. The sciatic nerve, deeply buried in the muscles on the back of the thigh, is the largest nerve in the body, being as thick as a pencil or more; other nerves reach about the size of goose-quills, and from these there are all gradations, down to the minute single fibres distributed to muscle-fibres or to skin. A nerve, such as the sciatic, possesses a strong, outer fibrous sheath, called the epineurium, within which lie bundles of nerve-fibres, divided from one another by partitions of fibrous tissue, in which run blood-vessels that nourish the nerve. Each of these bundles is surrounded by its own sheath, known as the perineurium, and within the bundle fine partitions of fibrous tissue, known as endoneurium, divide up the bundle into groups of fibres. The blood-vessels and lymphatics of the nerves divide into fine branches, which run in these sheaths and partitions of fibrous tissue. The finest subdivisions of the nerves are the fibres, and these are of two kinds: medullated and non-medullated fibres. The *medullated fibres* vary in thickness

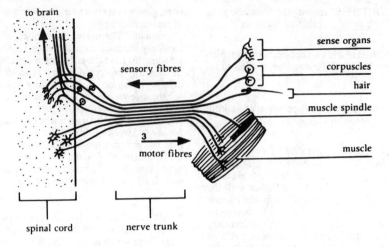

Diagram showing nervous connections between the central nervous system
and muscle and skin.

from 2 to 15 micrometres, some nerves containing a greater proportion of the small fibres than others. Under the microscope, all have the appearance of tubes, this being due to the fact that each has an outer membranous sheath, the neurilemma, within which is a clear white material, the medullary (or myelin) sheath, in the centre of which runs the axis-cylinder or nerve-fibre proper. The neurilemma is a strong but thin sheath with nuclei at regular intervals on its inner surface. The medullary sheath is composed of fatty material containing lecithin and cholesterin, and to it the white colour of the nerves is mainly due. It is divided at regular intervals by short gaps, situated about 1 mm apart, known as the nodes of Ranvier, but across these gaps the neurilemma and axis-cylinder are continuous. This medullary, or myelin, sheath is regarded as fulfilling a purpose similar to the insulating material upon electric wires and preventing nerve impulses from passing beyond the nerve-fibre by which they are conveyed. The axis-cylinder, or axon, is the conducting part of the nerve, for whilst the neurilemma is absent from the fibre in its course through the brain and spinal cord, and the medullary sheath is absent from non-medullated nerves, the axis-cylinder never fails. It has a striped appearance, seeming to consist of a number of fibrils which, however, cannot be separated from one another. The *non-medullated fibres* are very much thinner than the average of medullated fibres, from which they differ only in the fact of not possessing a medullary sheath, and of being therefore grey-ish in colour.

(2) NERVE-CELLS, from one of which springs each nerve-fibre, are found in the grey matter of the brain and spinal cord. In the brain alone it is calculated there are some 600,000,000 of these cells. They also exist in the ganglia of the sympathetic system, in connection with some of the nerves of special sense, and on the posterior roots of the spinal nerves. The shape of these nerve-cells varies. The most common appearance is that of a large clear cell, containing an oval nucleus, and running out at various points into long processes, which, as a rule, branch again and again, after the manner of a tree,

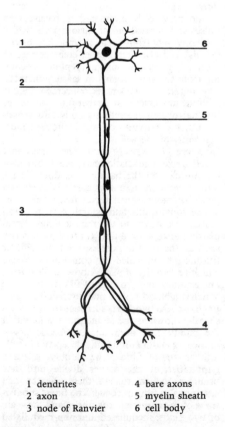

1 dendrites	4 bare axons
2 axon	5 myelin sheath
3 node of Ranvier	6 cell body

Diagram of a nerve.

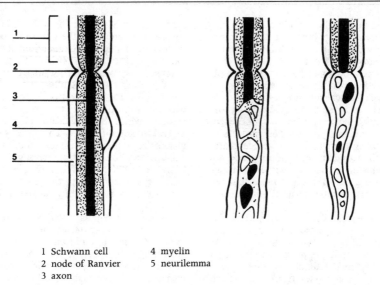

1 Schwann cell   4 myelin
2 node of Ranvier   5 neurilemma
3 axon

Diagram of (left) a healthy nerve, (centre) degenerating nerve cell after
two days, (right) and after a week.

these dendritic processes, as they are called,
meeting with similar processes from neighbouring cells. The ends of the branching processes
from one cell meet the ends of similar processes
from another cell, the points of apposition
being known as *synapses*. The state of closure
or openness of these synapses is believed to be
of great importance in quickening or blocking
nerve impulses. The body of the cell has a
mottled appearance, owing to its containing
many bodies, known as Nissl's granules, which
appear to be of the nature of food material,
destined to be used up when the cell is stimulated to work till reduced to a state of fatigue.

In the cerebrum, the cells are distinctly
pyramidal in shape, and one of the processes of
each cell is much longer than the rest, forming
indeed a nerve-fibre, which may run a long
distance down the spinal cord. Other cells are
bipolar, i.e. they possess just two processes, and
others are unipolar, i.e. they possess only one
process, which, a short distance from the cell,
divides in a T-shaped manner, as, for example,
the cells in the ganglia upon the posterior roots
of the spinal nerves. Other cells are found in the
grey matter of the brain, which are known as
neuroglia cells. These are provided with innumerable processes that form a supporting felt-
work for the nerve-cells and nerve-fibres, and
act merely as connective tissue cells.

(3) NERVE-ENDINGS Each nerve-fibre proceeds
from a nerve-cell to end in a definite organ, to
or from which it carries a special form of nerve
impulse. The manner in which the fibre ends in
the organ to which it proceeds varies in different cases. The simplest mode of ending is that
of the non-medullated fibres which proceed to
the involuntary muscle-fibres, as, for example,
those of the intestine. These fibres form a
complex network between the layers of muscle,

from which fine fibres pass between the muscle-
fibres. In the heart the nerves end in a similar
manner. In voluntary muscles the arrangement
is more complicated. Each nerve-fibre splits up
into numerous branches, which go to neighbouring muscle-fibres. Each branch pierces the
membrane surrounding its muscle-fibre, and
ends by spreading out into a plate composed of
granular material and numerous nuclei. The
endings of sensory nerves in the skin have a
special arrangement. Most of these end, not in
the epidermis, which is devoid of sensation, but
in the projections of the corium beneath it,
where each nerve-fibre enters a small rounded
bulb. Some of these bulbs found beneath the
skin of the fingers are known as Pacinian
corpuscles: around 2·5 mm long and half that
in width. These consist of a large number of
thin coats enclosing the swollen end of a nerve-
fibre. Other much smaller bodies, around 0·08
mm long, known as touch-corpuscles, are found
close beneath the epidermis all over the skin,
and consist of a framework of connective tissue
in which the nerve-fibre winds round and
round. Similar bodies are found on the front of
the eye. In other cases the nerves appear to end
abruptly in cells in the deepest layer of the
epidermis.

Development and repair The whole nervous
system is developed from the ectoderm or outer
layer of the embryo, the brain and spinal cord
arising from an infolding of the surface along
the back to form a tube, and all the nerves being
formed directly or indirectly as out-growths
from this tube, which increase in length till they
reach the muscle, skin or other structure for
which they are destined. Each nerve-fibre, as
already stated, is the process of a nerve-cell,
and, if a nerve is cut, that portion of its fibres
which is separated from the cells immediately

starts to degenerate, the medullary sheath and axis-cylinder, as a rule, breaking up. Within a few days or weeks, however, a bundle of small new fibres grows out from the cut end of each fibre in that portion which has not been cut off from connection with the nerve-cells, and these grow through the scar and down the sheath of the degenerated portion till they reach the organs to which the nerve originally proceeded. Thus the nerve is restored. This process is quickened when the cut ends have been carefully brought together, and indeed there are reasons for believing that, sometimes when this is done, no degeneration takes place, but the nerve heals and again transmits impulses at once.

Functions of nerves The greater part of the bodily activity originates in the nerve-cells, food material being used up in the process. As a result of this activity, impulses are sent down the nerves, which act simply as transmitters. The impulse which passes from a nerve-cell along a nerve-fibre to a muscle may be compared to the electric spark which explodes a mine, since the nerve impulse causes sudden chemical changes in the muscles as the latter contract. (See MUSCLES.) Similarly, the impulse which passes from a sensory ending in the skin along a nerve-fibre to affect nerve-cells in the spinal cord and brain, where it is perceived as a sensation, may be compared to the electric current which passes along a telephone cable to affect the receiver. Nevertheless, it must be understood that the impulse passing along a nerve is a form of motion quite different from electricity: travelling at the slow rate of about 30 metres (100 feet) per second, and probably more nearly resembling the motion of air-particles which produces sound. (See NERVOUS IMPULSE.)

The important fact that the anterior root of each spinal nerve is motor in function was discovered in 1811 by Sir Charles Bell. This was confirmed by Magendie in 1822, and the discovery also made that the posterior roots are sensory in function. They therefore concluded that the anterior roots consist of motor fibres to muscles, the posterior roots of sensory fibres from the skin. The terms, efferent and afferent, are applied to these roots more correctly, because, in addition to motor fibres, fibres through which blood-vessels are contracted and relaxed, and fibres which control secreting glands leave the cord in the anterior roots, while, in addition to sensory fibres, fibres which bring in impulses from muscles, joints and other organs, and inform the sense of locality as well as the sense of feeling, also enter the cord by the posterior roots.

Sensation is popularly supposed to be derived through five senses: smell, sight, hearing, taste and touch. In addition to these, impulses are brought by special nerve-fibres and converted in the brain into sensations which furnish a sense of movement and locality, a sense of pain, and a sense of heat and cold. (See TOUCH.)

The connection between the sensory and motor systems of nerves is important. The simplest form of nerve action is that known as *automatic action*. In this a part of the nervous system, controlling, for example, the lungs, goes on rhythmically, making discharges from its motor cells sufficient to keep the muscles of respiration in regular action, influenced only by occasional sensory impressions and chemical changes from various sources, which increase or diminish its activity according to the needs of the body.

In *reflex action* the parts engaged are a sensory ending, say in the skin; a sensory nerve leading from it to the spinal cord, where it ends by splitting up into processes near the nerve-cells; a nerve-cell which is stimulated by the sensory impulse, and which immediately sends a motor impulse down its nerve; and a muscle

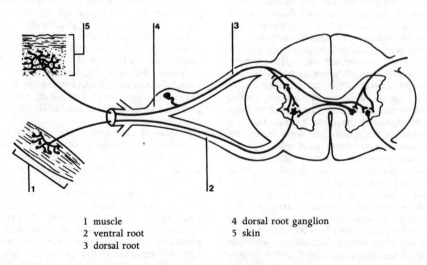

1 muscle
2 ventral root
3 dorsal root

4 dorsal root ganglion
5 skin

Diagram of a reflex arc.

which contracts as the result. A simple example of reflex action is given by the drawing away of the hand when it is pricked with a pin, before and independently of the conscious perception of pain.

Voluntary acts are more complicated than reflex ones. The same mechanism is involved, but, in addition, the controlling power of the brain is brought into play. This exerts first of all an inhibitory or blocking effect, which prevents immediate reflex action, and then the impulse, passing up to the cerebral hemispheres, sets up activity in a series of cells there, the complexity of these processes depending upon the intellectual processes involved. Finally, the inhibition is removed and an impulse passes down to motor cells in the spinal cord, and a muscle or set of muscles is brought into play through the motor nerves.

The *trophic function* of nerves is another most important part of their activity, for it appears as if the constant passage of nerve impulses down the nerves of any part were important for its nutrition. Thus, if sensory nerves are diseased or injured, ulceration of the skin, bed sores and other changes are liable to occur, while muscles waste and disappear if their motor nerves are permanently destroyed.

Nervous system   The brain and its twelve pairs of cranial nerves are treated under BRAIN; the spinal cord and the origin of its thirty-one pairs of nerves are treated under SPINAL CORD.

Each of these spinal nerves arises by two roots, the posterior root being larger than the anterior, and being furnished with a ganglion. Just before they emerge from the side of the spinal canal, the two roots unite to form a single nerve, their fibres mix, and then the nerve separates into two divisions.

One division immediately turns backwards to supply the skin and muscles of the back (posterior division), the other runs forwards (anterior division).

These anterior divisions supply the skin on the front and sides of the body and on the limbs, as well as all the muscles of the trunk and limbs, excepting those on the back. They do not run straight to these parts, but form a series of plexuses in which the nerve-fibres from different levels of the cord to the limbs are given off. The upper four cervical nerves unite to produce the *cervical plexus*. From this the muscles and skin of the neck are mainly supplied, and the phrenic nerve, which runs down through the lower part of the neck and the chest to innervate the diaphragm, is given off. The *brachial plexus* is formed by the union of the lower four cervical and first dorsal nerves, and, in addition to nerves which proceed to some of the muscles in the shoulder region, and others to the skin about the shoulder and inner side of the arm, it gives off the following large nerves that proceed down the arm: the musculocutaneous nerve, the median nerve, the ulnar nerve, and the radial nerve, each of which is about the size of a goose-quill. The musculocutaneous nerve supplies the large muscles in front of the upper arm, as well as the skin on the radial side of the

forearm as far as the wrist. The radial nerve winds round the back of the upper arm, where it supplies the triceps muscle, and then gives branches which innervate the skin on the outer side of the arm and forearm, the muscles behind the forearm, and finally the skin on the outer part of the back of the hand and fingers. The median nerve and the ulnar nerve run through the upper arm without giving off branches, and it is possible to feel the ulnar nerve as a cord running between the two marked bony prominences behind the elbow. The median nerve supplies most of the muscles in front of the forearm, a few of the small muscles in the hand and the skin of the palm and front of the thumb, index finger, middle finger and half of the ring finger. The ulnar nerve supplies two muscles in the forearm, most of the small muscles in the hand and the skin down the inner side of the forearm and palm and the skin in front of the little finger and half the ring finger.

The *thoracic* or *dorsal nerves*, with the exception of the first, do not form a plexus, but each runs round the chest along the lower margin of the rib to which it corresponds, whilst the lower six extend on to the abdomen. In this course they supply both the skin and muscle of the trunk.

The *lumbar plexus* is formed by the upper four lumbar nerves, and its branches are distributed to the lower part of the abdomen, and front and inner side of the thigh.

The *sacral plexus* is formed by parts of the fourth and fifth lumbar nerves, and the upper three and part of the fourth sacral nerves. It gives branches directly to the muscles and skin about the hip and fork, and supplies the skin down the back of the thigh, but the main bulk of the plexus is collected into the sciatic nerve. This, the largest nerve in the body, is buried in the muscles on the back of the thigh, which it supplies. It continues down to the back of the knee, and there divides into two branches, the internal popliteal (tibial) nerve and the external (common) popliteal nerve, which between them supply all the muscles below the knee and the greater part of the skin covering the leg and the foot.

The *sympathetic system* is joined by a pair of small branches given off from each spinal nerve, close to the spine. This system consists of two great parts. There is, first, a pair of cords running down on the side and front of the spine, and containing on each side three ganglia in the neck, and beneath this a ganglion opposite each vertebra. From these two ganglionated cords numerous branches are given off, and these unite in the second place to form plexuses connected with various internal organs, and provided with numerous large and irregularly placed ganglia. The chief of these plexuses are the cardiac plexus, the solar or epigastric plexus, the diaphragmatic, suprarenal, renal, spermatic, or ovarian, aortic, hypogastric and pelvic plexuses, the name in each case indicating the organ upon which, or the part of the abdomen within which, the plexus is placed.

NERVOUS DEBILITY (see NEURASTHENIA).

NERVOUS DISEASES This class of disease is one of the most difficult to diagnose. The brain and spinal cord being enclosed in the skull and spine, beyond the reach of direct examination, and the nerves being almost everywhere deeply buried in the tissues, the nature of nervous diseases must be made out from the disturbances of organs governed by the affected nerves.

The following conditions are discussed under their individual headings: APHASIA; BRAIN, DISEASES AND INJURIES OF; CATALEPSY; CHOREA; CRAMP; EPILEPSY; HYSTERIA; LEARNING DISABILITY; MEMORY; MENTAL ILLNESS; MULTIPLE SCLEROSIS; NERVE INJURIES; NEURALGIA; NEURITIS; PARALYSIS; PSYCHOSOMATIC DISEASES; SPINE AND SPINAL CORD, DISEASES AND INJURIES OF; STROKE; TABES.

NERVOUS IMPULSE The effects of nervous activity are now believed in all cases to be transmitted chemically, by the formation at nerve-endings of chemical substances. When, for example, a nerve to a muscle is stimulated, there appears at the neuromuscular junction (q.v.) the chemical substance, acetylcholine. Acetylcholine also appears at endings of the parasympathetic nerves and transmits the effect of the parasympathetic impulse. When an impulse passes down a sympathetic nerve, the effect of it is transmitted at the nerve-ending by the chemical liberated there: adrenaline or an adrenaline-like substance.

NETTLE-RASH (see URTICARIA).

NEURALGIA, literally 'nerve pain', is a term which is often employed both technically and popularly in a somewhat loose manner, to describe pains the origin of which is not clearly traceable. In its strict sense it means the existence of pain in some portion of, or throughout the whole of, the distribution of a sensory nerve, without any distinctly recognizable structural change in the nerve or nerve-centres. This strict definition, if adhered to, however, would not be applicable to a large number of cases of nerve pain; for in many instances the pain is connected with pressure on, or inflammation of, the nerve. Hence the word is generally used to indicate pain affecting a particular nerve or its branches, whatever be the cause.
Treatment With all forms of neuralgia it is of the first importance to ascertain, if possible, whether any constitutional condition is associated with the symptom.

Naturally also one looks for, and as speedily as possible removes, any local cause such as pressure on a nerve.

During the time an acute attack lasts, various local applications may give symptomatic relief e.g. warmth or massage. Analgesics applied locally or systemically may be necessary.

Some cases resist all forms of medicinal treatment, and for these surgical procedures are sometimes tried, such as division and removal of a portion of the nerve, or injection of absolute alcohol into the nerve.

NEURALGIA TRIGEMINAL affects the sensory nerve which supplies most of the face. Usually two out of the three main branches are involved. It is a severe pain often initiated by light pressure on the skin. It is generally diagnosed after excluding all other likely causes of facial pain. Treatment may be with the long-term use of the analgesic carbamazepine or partial or complete destruction of the appropriate branch of the nerve. The nerve may be destroyed by freezing, coagulating or injection of an alcohol round it. If untreated or suppressed the pain may be present for many months, then disappear, only to recur a year or so later.

NEURASTHENIA means a condition of nervous exhaustion in which, although the patient suffers from no definite disease, he becomes incapable of sustained exertion. It was never a very well-defined entity, and the term has now been largely given up. The condition which it represented is now recognized to be a form of neurosis (q.v.) or psychosomatic disease (q.v.).

NEURECTOMY is an operation in which part of a nerve is excised: for example, for the relief of neuralgia.

NEURILEMMA is the thin membranous covering which surrounds every nerve-fibre. (See NERVES.)

NEURITIS means inflammation affecting a nerve or nerves which may be localized to one part of the body, as, for instance, in sciatica, or which may be general, being then known as multiple neuritis, or polyneuritis. Owing to the fact that the most peripheral parts of the nerves are usually at fault in the latter condition, i.e. the fine subdivisions in the substance of the muscles, it is also known as peripheral neuritis.
Causes In cases of LOCALIZED NEURITIS the fibrous sheath of the nerve is usually at fault, the actual nerve-fibres being only secondarily affected. This condition may be due to inflammation spreading into the nerve from surrounding tissues, to cold or to long-continued irritation by pressure on the nerve, and the symptoms produced vary according to the function of the nerve, in the case of sensory nerves being usually neuralgic pain (see NEURALGIA), in the case of motor nerves more or less paralysis in the muscles to which the nerves pass.

In POLYNEURITIS, which is always due to some general or constitutional cause, the nerve-fibres themselves in the small nerves degenerate and break down. Hence the very protracted nature of this malady, since, if recovery takes place, it must be brought about by the growth of new nerve-fibres from the healthy part of the nerve, down the sheath of the nerve, to the muscle.

The cause of this degeneration may be said, in general terms, to be some poison either taken into or produced in the body, and circulating in the blood. By far the commonest of these poisons is alcohol. Next in importance comes lead, wrist-drop and other features of neuritis being among the most prominent symptoms of lead-poisoning. (See LEAD POISONING.) Arsenic is occasionally responsible for neuritis, particularly when the effect of arsenic is combined with over-indulgence in alcohol, as in an epidemic of neuritis, due to beer contaminated with arsenic, in the Midlands of England about the year 1900. Bisulphide of carbon, naphtha and other solvents of rubber are apt to produce the disease when inhaled in large quantity by the workmen in rubber factories. People with diabetes mellitus are prone to neuritis, the condition sometimes being the result of deficiency of thiamine in the diet. This deficiency probably also accounts for some cases of alcoholic neuritis. The disease known as beriberi (q.v.) is a form of neuritis which persists in certain localities of the world, in consequence of thiamine deficiency.

Symptoms The chief symptom of a LOCALIZED NEURITIS, whether pain or paralysis, varies according to the functions of the nerve.

POLYNEURITIS, as a rule, takes longer to show itself. In most cases it begins with vague pains and tingling in the limbs; weakness and wasting of the muscles in the feet and legs, in the hand and arms, or in other parts, following later. Wrist-drop, the peculiar steppage gait in which the person lifts his feet as if he were constantly stepping over small obstacles, squinting, loss of voice, difficulty of breathing, enfeeblement of the heart's action appear according to the muscles whose nerves are affected. The knee-jerks and other deep reflexes are generally lost in all forms of severe neuritis. A peculiar feature of alcoholic neuritis is the wandering delirium from which the patient often suffers, her imagination conjuring up the most vivid delusions as to journeys she is making, and the mind being quite confused, especially in matters regarding time and place.

The course of the disease is usually very slow, but if treated the mortality is low.

Treatment: For the treatment of LOCALIZED NEURITIS see under NEURALGIA.

The first essential in the treatment of POLYNEURITIS is to discover and remove the cause. This applies particularly to alcoholism, lead poisoning and neuritis due to manufacture of rubber. Physiotherapy helps to prevent wasting of muscles, and the deformities which arise through fixation of the joints in one position.

NEURODERMATOSES, sometimes grouped under the name of NEURODERMATITIS, are disorders of the skin in which stress is one of the important factors, if not the most important cause. In some conditions, such as pruritus (see ITCHING) and rosacea (q.v.) this is the principal cause. In others, such as atopic eczema (see ECZEMA) and *Lichen simplex* (see LICHEN), it is

a secondary, but none the less often important, factor, any mental or emotional stress or strain bringing on an exacerbation, or flaring up, of the skin condition. In others again, such as *Dermatitis artefacta* the emotional, or mental, instability may be the sole cause, the individual deliberately damaging his or her skin, without divulging the cause. The extreme form of this manifestation of mental illness is parasitophobia, in which the individual has a morbid terror of parasites and is quite convinced that he or she is infested with some parasite which is causing the itching which in turn has been scratched until the skin has broken down.

NEUROFIBROMATOSIS (see VON RECKLING-HAUSEN'S DISEASE).

NEUROGLIA is the name applied to a fine web of tissue and branching cells which supports the nerve fibres and cells of the nervous system. (See NERVES.)

NEUROLEPTICS Although many of these drugs have sedative properties they should not be regarded as tranquillizers. They are used to quieten disturbed patients, whether this is the result of brain damage, mania, delirium, agitated depression or an acute behavioural disturbance. They relieve the florid psychotic symptoms such as hallucinations and thought disorder in schizophrenia and prevent relapse of this disorder when it is in remission.

Most of these drugs are dopamine antagonists (see DOPAMINE) and act by blocking dopamine receptors. As a result they can give rise to the extra pyramidal effects of Parkinsonism (q.v.) and they may also cause hyperprolactinaemia. The extrapyramidal symptoms are the most troublesome side-effects and they can usually be controlled by anticholinergic drugs. The main anti-psychotic drugs are: (i) chlorpromazine, methotrimeprazine, and promazine. These drugs are characterized by pronounced sedative effects and a moderate anticholinergic and extrapyramidal effect. (ii) pericyazine, pipothiazine and thioridazine. These drugs have moderate sedative effects, marked anticholinergic effects but less extrapyramidal effects than the other groups. (iii) fluphenazine, perphenazine, prochlorperazine, sulpiride and trifluoperazine. These drugs have fewer sedative effects, fewer anticholinergic effects but more pronounced extrapyramidal effects.

NEUROLOGY is the branch of medical practice and science which deals with the nervous system and its diseases.

NEUROMA means a tumour connected with a nerve, such tumours being generally composed of fibrous tissue, and of a painful nature.

NEUROMUSCULAR BLOCKADE In clinical practice the transmission of impulses at the neuromuscular junction (q.v.) may be competitively blocked in order to paralyse reversibly a patient for a surgical procedure or to assist treatment on the intensive care unit. There are two main types of drug, both of which competitively block the acetylcholine receptors on the motor end plates: (1) Depolarizing neuromuscular blocking agents: these act by first producing stimulation at the receptor and then blocking it. There are characteristic muscle fasciculations before the rapid onset of paralysis which is of short duration (less than five minutes with the commonly used drug, suxamethonium). The drug is removed from the receptor by the enzyme plasma, cholinesterase. (2) Non-depolarizing neuromuscular blocking agents: these drugs occupy the receptor and prevent acetylcholine from becoming attached to it. However, in sufficiently high concentrations acetylcholine will compete with the drug and dislodge it from the receptor and the effect of these drugs is reversed by giving an anticholinesterase, which allows the amount of acetylcholine at the neuromuscular junction to build up. These drugs have varying durations of action but all are slower in onset and of longer duration than the depolarizers.

NEUROMUSCULAR JUNCTION The specialized area where a motor nerve ends in close proximity to the muscle membrane and is able to initiate muscle contraction. The motor nerve ending is separated from the motor end plate by the synaptic cleft which is only 50–70 nm wide. When a nerve impulse arrives at the motor nerve ending molecules of acetylcholine are released which cross the synaptic cleft and attach to receptors on the motor end plate. This initiates depolarization of the muscle which in turn initiates the process of contraction. Acetylcholinesterase (an enzyme) rapidly breaks down the molecules of acetylcholine, thus ending their action and freeing the receptor in preparation for the next impulse.

NEURON is a single unit of the nervous system, consisting of a nerve cell with its various processes and the nerve fibre or fibres to which it gives origin. As applied to the motor part of the nervous system, two neurons are specially recognized: the *upper neuron*, which includes a cell on the surface of the brain and a fibre extending down into the spinal cord; the *lower neuron*, which consists of a cell in the grey matter of the cord with a nerve fibre extending outwards to end in a fibre of the muscle with which it is connected. The former has a controlling influence over the latter, whilst the latter is more directly concerned with the changes that result in the contraction of the muscle fibre and with nutritional influences over it. (See NERVES.)

NEUROPATHIC BLADDER A bladder with complete or partial loss of sensation. As there is no sensation of fullness, the individual either develops complete retention of urine or the bladder empties reflexly. The condition predisposes affected individuals to urinary-tract infections and back pressure on the kidneys, leading to renal failure. It may be caused by spinal injury, spina bifida (q.v.) or any disorder which produces neuropathy (q.v.).

NEUROPATHY A disease affecting nerves. It may affect a single nerve (mononeuropathy) or be a generalized disorder (polyneuropathy). Symptoms will depend on whether motor, sensory, or autonomic nerves are affected. Trauma or entrapment is a common cause of mononeuropathy, pressure or stretching of a nerve occurring in various situations. Complete recovery in four to six weeks is usual. Common causes of polyneuropathy include diabetes (q.v.), B vitamin deficiency (often alcohol associated), some viral infections, and carcinomatous. Genetic and toxic neuropathies are also seen.

NEUROSIS is a general term applied to mental or emotional disturbance in which, as opposed to psychosis, there is no serious disturbance in the perception or understanding of external reality. However, the boundaries between neurosis and psychosis are not always clearly defined. Neuroses are usually classified into anxiety neuroses, depressive neuroses, phobias, hysteria and obsessional neuroses.
ANXIETY NEUROSIS, or ANXIETY STATE, constitutes the commonest form of neurosis. Fortunately it is also almost the most responsive to treatment. It is more likely in people of anxious personality. Once the neurosis develops, they are in a state of persistent anxiety and worry, 'tensed up', always feeling fatigue and unable to sleep at night. In addition, there are often physical complaints, e.g. palpitations or headache.
OBSESSIONAL NEUROSES are much less common and constitute only about 5 per cent of all neuroses. Like other neuroses, they usually develop in early adult life. (See MENTAL ILLNESS.)

NEUROSURGERY is surgery performed on some part of the nervous system, whether brain, spinal cord or nerves.

NEUROTIC is a general term of indefinite meaning applied to a person of nervous temperament, whose actions are largely determined by emotions or instincts rather than by reason.

NEUROTRANSMITTER is a substance which transmits the action of a nerve to a cell. It is now recognized that this is how nerves work. If there should be a lack or deficiency of the appropriate neurotransmitter, then the nerve cannot carry out its action. A classical example of this is dopamine (q.v.), lack of which is responsible for the condition known as Parkinsonism (q.v.). Other neurotransmitters include acetylcholine (q.v.) which is the neurotransmitter for the parasympathetic nervous system (q.v.) and noradrenaline which is the neurotransmitter for the sympathetic nervous system.

NEUTRON is one of the particles that enter into the structure of the atomic nucleus. (See ISOTOPES.)

NEUTROPENIA denotes a reduction in the number of neutrophil leucocytes per cubic millimetre of circulating blood to a figure below that found in health. There is still some disagreement over the precise limits of normality, but a count of less than 2500 per mm^3 would be generally accepted as constituting neutropenia. Several infective diseases are characterized by neutropenia, including typhoid fever, influenza and measles. It may also be induced by certain drugs, including chloramphenicol, phenylbutazone, the sulphonamides and chlorpromazine.

NEUTROPHIL   A type of leucocyte (q.v.) or white blood cell (see BLOOD).

NICLOSAMIDE is the drug of choice in the treatment of tapeworm infestation. It is also known as YOMESAN.

NICOTINAMIDE, the amide of nicotinic acid, is usually used instead of nicotinic acid (q.v.) in the treatment of vitamin B deficiency.

NICOTINE is the active principle in tobacco. (See TOBACCO.)

NICOTINIC ACID, or NIACIN, is a member of the vitamin B complex. It is essential for human nutrition, the normal daily requirement for an adult being about 15 to 20 mg. A deficiency of nicotinic acid is one of the factors in the etiology of pellagra (q.v.), and either nicotine acid or nicotinamide is used in the treatment of this condition. Nicotinic acid also reduces the concentration of blood lipids. (See HYPER-LIPIDAEMIA.)

NIDUS   A site of infection within the body from which it can spread to other tissues.

NIFEDIPINE is a drug that is being used in the treatment of angina pectoris (q.v.). It is said to reduce the requirements of the heart muscle for oxygen. It is also proving of value in the treatment of high blood-pressure. It is one of the calcium antagonists. (See CALCIUM-CHAN-NEL BLOCKERS.)

NIGHT BLINDNESS (see BLINDNESS).

NIGHTMARE (see SLEEP).

NIGHT SWEATS consist in copious perspiration occurring in bed at night and found in conditions such as tuberculosis, brucellosis and lymphomas.

NIKETHAMIDE is a drug which stimulates the respiratory centre.

NIPPLES, DISEASES OF (see BREASTS, DISEASES OF).

NIRIDAZOLE is a drug which is proving of value in the treatment of schistosomiasis (q.v.) and guinea-worm infections (see DRACUN-CULIASIS).

NITRAZEPAM is a tranquillizer introduced as a hypnotic. (See TRANQUILLIZERS, BENZO-DIAZEPINES.)

NITRIC ACID is one of the strongest of the mineral acids, and is a clear, heavy liquid, becoming brownish with age. It is kept in dark, stoppered bottles, and immediately the stopper is removed from the bottle, irritating white fumes are given off.
Action   In its pure state, nitric acid acts as a powerful caustic upon the tissues of the body, which it turns a bright yellow colour. In weaker solution it is, like all acids, an antiseptic, but is very irritating. Internally, in small doses it has a stimulating action upon the gastric mucous membrane.
Uses   Although a powerful antiseptic and caustic, nitric acid is rarely used now in Britain for the removal of warts (where it has been superseded by cryotherapy) or treatment of septic ulcers.

NITRIC OXIDE (NO)   An important naturally occurring chemical that performs a wide range of biological roles. It is involved in the laying down of memories in the brain, killing viruses, bacteria and cancer cells, and helping to control blood pressure. NO, comprising a nitrogen atom attached to an oxygen one, is one of the smallest of biologically active compounds as well as having such diverse functions. The chemical is a muscle relaxant and is important in maintaining the heart and circulation in good condition. NO is the toxic agent released by macrophages (q.v.) to kill invading germs and spreading cancer cells. It acts as an essential neurotransmitter and protects nerve cells against stress. Researchers are studying how it might be used to treat diseases.

NITRITES are salts which have a powerful effect in paralysing the action of involuntary muscle, and they therefore dilate the blood-vessels, and check spasm of all sorts. The most commonly used nitrites are nitrite of amyl, of ethyl, and of sodium. Erythrol tetranitrate and nitroglycerin have a similar action. (See GLYCERYL TRINITRATE.)

NITROFURANTOIN is a synthetic nitrofuran derivative which has a wide range of antibacterial activity and is effective against many Grampositive and Gram-negative micro-organisms. It is used mainly in the treatment of infections of the urinary tract.

NITROGEN MUSTARDS are nitrogen analogues of mustard gas. They are among the most important alkylating agents (q.v.) used in the treatment of various forms of malignant disease. They include mustine, trimustine, uramustine, busulphan, chlorambucil and melphalan.

NITROUS OXIDE GAS, also known as LAUGH-ING GAS, is, at ordinary pressures, a gas devoid of odour but of a slightly sweetish taste. Its use in medicine is to produce insensibility to pain, which it does very quickly, and with a great degree of safety, though the effect is of very short duration, not extending beyond two or three minutes. Its use is therefore applicable only for short operations, such as extraction of a tooth, unless it is repeatedly administered in association with oxygen. (See ANAESTHESIA.)

NOCICEPTORS Nerve endings which detect and respond to painful or unpleasant stimuli.

NOCTURIA denotes excess passing of urine during the night. Among its many causes are glomerulonephritis (see KIDNEY, DISEASES OF) and enlargement of the prostate. (See also URINE, EXCESS OF.)

NOCTURNAL ENURESIS is the involuntary passing of urine during sleep. It is a condition predominantly of childhood. In a small minority of cases it is due to some organic cause such as infection of the genito-urinary tract, but in the vast majority of cases it is due to inadequate or improper training of the child or psychological ill health. Traditionally it is said to be associated with threadworms, but there is little, if any, evidence to support this tradition.

Before deciding that a child is suffering from nocturnal enuresis, it is necessary to remember that the age at which a child achieves full control of bladder function varies considerably. Such control is usually achieved in the second year, but more commonly in the third year of life, and there are some children who do not normally achieve such control until the fourth, or even fifth, year.

It is a difficult condition to cure in the absence of an organic cause. If there should be an organic cause, treatment consists of its eradication. In the absence of such a cause, treatment consists essentially of reassurance and firm but kindly and understanding training. In quite a number of cases the use of a buzzer alarm which wakens the child should he start passing water is helpful provided that it is backed up by psychological support from the parents and the family doctor.

NODE The term node is widely used in medicine. For instance, the smaller lymphatic glands are often termed lymph nodes. It is also applied to a collection of nerve cells forming a subsidiary nerve centre found in various places in the sympathetic nervous system, such as the sinuatrial node and the atrio-ventricular node which control the beating of the heart.

NOISE (see DEAFNESS; OCCUPATIONAL DISEASES).

NOMA is another name for cancrum oris. (See CANCRUM ORIS.)

NOMIFENSINE (see ANTIDEPRESSANTS).

NON-SPECIFIC GENITAL INFECTION, or NON-SPECIFIC URETHRITIS, is an inflammatory condition of the urethra (q.v.) due to infection with certain types of micro-organism. The most common is *Chlamydia trachomatis* – over 35,000 cases were identified by laboratories in England and Wales in 1992. It produces pelvic inflammatory disease in women, which often results in sterility, the risk of ectopic pregnancy (see ECTOPIC), and recurrent pelvic pain. Most cases respond well to tetracycline (q.v.). Abstinence from sexual intercourse should be observed during treatment and until cure is complete. Children born to infected mothers may have their eyes infected during birth, producing the condition known as ophthalmia neonatorum. This is treated by the application to the eye of chlortetracycline eye ointment. The lungs of such a child may also be infected, resulting in pneumonia.

NON-STEROIDAL ANTI-INFLAMMATORY DRUGS act by inhibiting the formation of prostaglandins which are mediators of inflammation. They act both as analgesics to relieve pain and as inhibitors of inflammation. Aspirin is a classic example of such a compound. Newer compounds have been synthesized with the aim of producing fewer and less severe side-effects. They are sometimes preferred to aspirin for the treatment of conditions such as rheumatoid arthritis, osteoarthritis, sprains, strains and sports injuries. Their main side-effects are gastro-intestinal. Gastric ulcers and gastric haemorrhage may result. This is because prostaglandins are necessary for the production of the mucous protective coat in the stomach and, when the production of prostaglandin is inhibited, the protection of the stomach is compromised. They should therefore be used with caution in patients with dyspepsia and gastric ulceration. The various non-steroidal anti-inflammatory drugs differ little from each other in efficacy though there is considerable variation in patient response. Naproxen is one of the first choices in this group of drugs as it combines good efficacy with a low incidence of side-effects and administration is only required twice daily. Other drugs in this series include azapropazone, fenbufen, fenclofenac, fenoprofen, feprazone, flurbiprofen, ibuprofen, indomethacin, indoprofen, ketoprofen, piroxicam, sulindac, tiaprofenic acid and tolmetin.

NORADRENALINE is a precursor of adrenaline (q.v.) in the medulla of the suprarenal glands. It is also present in the brain. Its main function is to mediate the transmission of impulses in the sympathetic nervous system (q.v.). It also has a transmitter function in the brain.

NOREPINEPHRINE (see NORADRENALINE).

NORETHISTERONE is a synthetic preparation that has the action of progesterone (q.v.), but is active when given by mouth.

NORMAL is a term used in several different senses. Generally speaking, it is applied to anything which agrees with the regular and established type. In chemistry the term is applied to solutions of acids or bases of such strength that each litre contains the number of grams corresponding to the molecular weight of the substance in question. In physiology the term normal is applied to solutions of such strength that, when mixed with a body fluid, they are isotonic and cause no disturbance: e.g. normal saline solution. (See ISOTONIC.)

NORMOBLAST is the term applied to the precursor of a red blood corpuscle which still contains the remnant of a nucleus.

NORMOTENSIVE Having a blood pressure within the normal range for an individual's age and sex.

NORTRIPTYLINE is an antidepressant drug which is also a sedative. (See ANTIDEPRESSANTS.)

NOSE The nose has three main functions. It is the natural pathway whereby air enters the body in the course of respiration (q.v.). In the nose the incoming air is warmed, moistened and filtered before passing on into the lungs. It has also a protective function. Irritation of it by dust or the like induces sneezing (q.v.) which expels the irritant from the nose and so prevents it getting into the lungs. It is also the organ of smell (q.v.).

The *external nose* is formed partly of bone and partly of cartilage, covered by skin. In its upper part, the two nasal bones, one on each side, project downwards from the frontal bone for about 25 mm (1 inch) from, and, supported by a process of the upper jaw-bone, form the hard bridge of the nose between the eyes. The ending of the bony part can be seen or felt on most noses, and, beneath this, two cartilages on each side, the lateral cartilages and the cartilages of the aperture give shape, firmness, and pliability to the lower two-thirds of the nose. The gap between the cartilages of the aperture can be distinctly felt on the point of the nose. The spaces between the cartilages are filled up and the cartilages firmly bound to the bones and to one another by fibrous tissue. When the nose is injured, some of the cartilages are apt to be dislocated, thus altering the shape of this organ. However, most injuries resulting in deformity of the nose are due to injuries to the bones of the nose.

In its *interior*, the nose is completely divided into two narrow cavities, one on each side, by a septum or partition running from front to back. This septum is a thin plate composed partly of bone, partly of cartilage, consisting in about its hinder two-thirds of the central plate of the ethmoid bone and of the vomer bone, and in about its anterior third of a four-sided plate of cartilage, which along one edge touches the nasal bones, the lateral cartilages, and the cartilages of the aperture. On both surfaces this septum is covered by the general mucous membrane that lines the nose.

The cavities on either side of the septum, known as the *nasal fossae*, are extremely narrow, being at their widest point less than 6 mm (¼ inch) in breadth, though in height they correspond to the length of the nose, and run directly backwards about 5 cm (2 inches). At its upper end each cavity is separated from the interior of the skull by a thin plate of bone containing many minute apertures for the passage of the filaments of the olfactory nerve. The front part of each cavity consists of the space enclosed by the cartilages of the nose, is lined by skin, which is furnished with stiff hairs or vibrisae that grow downwards and protect the entrance, and is known as the vestibule. Further back the outer surface of each cavity is rendered very complicated, and the space in the cavity greatly filled up, by three projections known as the nasal conchae or turbinates. These bones form ridges which run from before backwards with an inclination downwards, and, in section, each ridge is curled over so that its edge looks downwards. There are therefore three passages (meatus) running from before backwards, each under cover of a corresponding nasal turbinate. As each of these bones, in common with the whole of the cavity, is covered with very vascular and thick mucous membrane, the air in its passage through the nose is by this arrangement brought in contact with a large surface of mucous membrane, and thus is considerably warmed before it enters the broncial tubes and lungs. In addition, this mucous membrane, which is covered with cilia (q.v.), secretes more that 500 millilitres of sticky mucus every 24 hours. This traps dust particles and the like, which are then moved on by the cilia and usually swallowed unnoticed. It is the excessive production of this mucus, in response to irritations or infection, that is known as

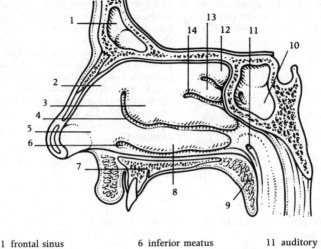

1 frontal sinus	6 inferior meatus	11 auditory tube
2 atrium of middle meatus	7 maxilla	12 sphenoethmoidal recess
3 middle nasal concha	8 inferior nasal concha	and higher nasal concha
4 middle meatus	9 soft palate	13 superior nasal concha
5 vestibule	10 sphenoidal sinus	14 superior meatus

The lateral wall of the right half of the nasal cavity.

nasal catarrh (q.v.). The front portion of the inferior and of the middle nasal concha can be seen as two red projections by looking up the nostril with a bright light, when the nostril is slightly opened by a speculum. The superior meatus beneath the superior nasal concha is a narrow passage, and, upon this bone and passage as well as upon the corresponding part of the septum, the nerves of smell end in the mucous membrane. The wider and longer middle meatus and inferior meatus are the passages through which the air mainly passes out and in during respiration.

Certain *sinuses* lie concealed in the bones of the skull, into which air enters freely by apertures connecting them with the nose. These cavities occupy spaces in the frontal bone over the eyebrow (frontal sinus), in the upper jawbone, filling in the angle between the eye and the nose (maxillary sinus or antrum of Highmore), in the sphenoid bone (sphenoidal sinus), and in the lateral part of the ethmoid bone (ethmoidal sinus). The function of the sinuses is, as yet, unknown. The most capacious is the maxillary sinus, which is a cubical cavity, often over 12 mm (½ inch) in measurement each way. The frontal sinus, maxillary sinus, and ethmoidal sinus open by small apertures about the centre of the middle meatus, the sphenoidal sinus above this. Into the front part of the inferior meatus opens the nasal duct, which carries the tears off from the eye. (See EYE.) The latter fact explains the frequent blowing of the nose which becomes necessary when a person is weeping. On a level with the inferior meatus, but situated in the part of the throat into which the nose opens, is placed the orifice of the Eustachian, or auditory, tube leading to the middle ear. (See EAR.)

NOSE, DISEASES OF The nose, so far as the skin-covering is concerned, is subject to the same diseases as the skin of other parts. Redness of the skin of this part may, on account of its disfiguring character, be very annoying. It may be due to poor circulation in cold weather, partaking of the nature of a chilblain (see CHILBLAIN); occasionally it is due to acne rosacea. Among the skin diseases, acne (q.v.), lupus (q.v.), and erysipelas (q.v.) are specially prone to affect this site.

ACUTE INFLAMMATION of the nose is generally a viral infection affecting the mucous membrane of the nose and paranasal sinuses and is commonly known as a cold in the head. (See CHILLS AND COLDS.) It may be due, though less commonly, to the inhalation of irritating gases. Boils occasionally develop just within the entrance to the nose, in connection with the hairs there, and in this locality give rise to great pain and considerable danger. (See BOILS.) Diphtheria used to be a form of severe rhinitis but this is now extremely rare. Hay fever is a distressing form of acute rhinitis. (See HAY FEVER.)

MALFORMATIONS OF THE NOSE are of various kinds. The external nose varies much in shape in different races, even in different families, and it is possible for persons who desire for aesthetic reasons to alter the character of their noses to undergo some form of surgery. This is known as rhinoplasty. As to the interior of the nose, the two cavities are practically never of equal size, the septum almost always bulging to one or other side, so that the passage of air is slightly freer on one side than on the other. When this bulging is so marked that the septum touches the nasal conchae on one side, or when, owing to injury or other cause, spurs and crests have developed on the septum, considerable irritation may arise, and this may form the starting-point for chronic inflammation of the nose, hay fever or asthma. These imperfections, though they often exist without the least ill-effect, and are only discovered accidentally, are readily removed by the specialist if necessary, such operations being attended by but little pain. A more common abnormality is that in which the nose becomes obstructed as the result of nasal polyps, adenoids and other causes and in consequence the person breathes through the mouth.

ADENOIDS means an overgrowth of the glandular tissue which is naturally found in small amount on the back of the upper part of the throat, into which the nose opens.

This glandular tissue is similar in structure to the tonsils and lymphatic glands, and in children may be large enough to obstruct the posterior openings of the nose into the naso-pharynx. This obstruction therefore leads to nasal obstruction and may also obstruct the Eustachian tubes.

The association between enlarged adenoids and Eustachian-tube dysfunction remains controversial, but a substantial number of children with enlarged adenoids do have secretory otitis media (glue ear). Children with a problem of enlarged adenoids and some or all of these symptoms should seek specialist opinion.

If symptoms are severe, operation is usually necessary.

POLYPI   Nasal polyps are growths of soft, jelly-like character, with more or less of a stalk, usually arising from the ethmoid and maxillary sinuses, but they may also grow from the middle nasal turbinate. They arise from chronic inflammation associated with allergic rhinitis, chronic sinusitis, asthma and aspirin abuse. This chronic inflammation leads to oedema or swelling of the mucous membrane of the nose and paranasal sinuses which becomes so extensive as to produce polypi.

When polyps become large they can cause erosion of the nasal bones and should therefore generally be removed.

BLEEDING FROM THE NOSE, or EPISTAXIS (see HAEMORRHAGE).

FOREIGN BODIES   At first the foreign body may set up no reaction and produce no symptoms but, in time, there will be obstruction of the affected nostril, with a foul-smelling discharge, which is often bloody from that side. The foreign body may remain in the nose for years until symptoms are noticed, but the presence of a unilateral foul-smelling bloody discharge should always alert one to the possible presence of a foreign body.

Foreign bodies require removal.

LOSS OF SENSE OF SMELL, or ANOSMIA may be temporary or permanent. Temporary anosmia is caused by conditions of the nose which are reversible, whereas permanent anosmia is caused by conditions which destroy the olefactory nerves. Temporary conditions are those such as the common cold, or other inflammatory conditions of the nasal mucosa or the presence of

nasal polyps. Permanent anosmia may follow and influenzal neuritis or it may also follow injuries to the brain and fractures of the skull involving the olfactory nerves.

SINUSITIS is of fairly frequent occurrence and most commonly follows an upper-respiratory-tract infection involving the nose and paranasal sinuses. The maxillary sinus is the sinus most commonly prone to sinus infection, followed by the ethmoid sinuses, then the frontal sinuses and, finally, the cells of the sphenoid sinus. Maxillary sinusitis may also arise from dental infection if the roots of the upper teeth penetrate into the floor of that sinus.

Sinusitis is generally treated by the administration of antibiotics and decongestants, preferably topical ones. In more severe cases, it may be necessary to drain the sinus through an opening made between the sinus and the nose.

NOSOLOGY is the term applied to scientific classification of diseases.

NOSTALGIA means a form of melancholy or aggravated home-sickness occurring in persons who have left their home.

NOTIFIABLE DISEASES are diseases, usually of an infectious nature, which are required by law to be made known to a health officer or local authority. (See INFECTION.) Certain occupational diseases (q.v.) are also notifiable.

Notifiable Diseases in the U.K. as at 1 October 1994

Acute encephalitis
Acute poliomyelitis
Anthrax
Cholera
Diphtheria
Dysentery (amoebic or bacillary)
Food poisoning
Lassa fever
Leprosy (reported to Chief Medical Officer at the Department of Health)
Leptospirosis
Malaria
Marburg disease
Measles
Meningitis
Meningococcal septicaemia (without meningitis)
Mumps
Ophthalmia neonatorum
Paratyphoid fever
Plague
Rabies
Relapsing fever
Rubella
Scarlet fever
Smallpox
Tetanus
Tuberculosis
Typhoid fever
Typhus
Viral haemorrhagic fever (including Lassa fever)
Viral hepatitis
Whooping cough
Yellow fever

Reporting AIDS is voluntary (and in confidence) to the Director, Communicable Diseases Surveillance Centre (PHLS) (see APPENDIX 2: ADDRESSES).

NOVOBIOCIN is an antibiotic derived from cultures of *Streptomyces spheroides* or *Streptomyces niveus*. It is particularly active against staphylococci, and has proved especially useful in the treatment of staphylococcal infections which have not responded to treatment with other antibiotics, or in which the causative micro-organism is resistant to such antibiotics.

NUCHA is the Latin name for the back of the neck.

NUCLEAR MAGNETIC RESONANCE or MAGNETIC RESONANCE IMAGING (MRI) A non-invasive method of imaging the body and its organs. It may also be used to study tissue metabolism. The body is placed in a magnetic field which causes certain atomic nuclei to align in the direction of the field. Pulses of radio-frequency radiation are then applied and interpretation of the frequencies absorbed and re-emitted allows an image in any body plane to be built up.

NUCLEAR MEDICINE is that branch of medicine that is concerned with the use of radioactive material in the diagnosis, investigation and treatment of disease.

NUCLEIC ACID is a substance constructed out of units known as nucleotides which consist of a purine or pyrimidine base linked to a pentose sugar which in turn is esterified with phosphoric acid. Two types of nucleic acid occur in nature: deoxyribonucleic acid (DNA) and ribonucleic acid (RNA). (See DNA; RNA.)

NUCLEUS means the central body in a cell, which controls the activities of the latter. (See CELLS.)

NUCLEUS PULPOSUS is the inner core of an intervertebral disc. (See SPINAL COLUMN.)

NULLIPARA is the term applied to a woman who has never borne a child.

NUMBNESS (see TOUCH).

NURSING as a profession requires an elaborate training, although people are often called upon to nurse relatives and friends without any previous experience of the subject. The functions and skills required in nursing range from nursing assistants, who provide basic 'bedside' services, through ward and outpatient nurses registered with the UKCC (see below) who are authorized to give (and sometimes prescribe) drugs and technical treatment to nurses working in operating theatres and intensive-care units. Nurses can also become managers, teach students or do research. The basic registration course is also required for those wanting to become midwives, health visitors or district nurses – all of which require extra training. Changes are taking place in the organization and training of nurses aiming for registration, with greater emphais on an academic and vocational approach in place of the traditional 'apprenticeship' type training. Registered nurses in the United Kingdom now have to complete a recognized three-year university-style course during which they spend time in hospitals. Full details about openings in nursing, details of training and of training schools can be obtained from the Royal College of Nursing (see APPENDIX 2: ADDRESSES). The Nurses, Midwives and Health Visitors Act 1979 led to the establishment of a United Kingdom Central Council and four National Boards for nursing, midwifery and health visiting. The Central Council, supported by the Boards, has responsibility for registration and the setting and maintaining of standards of education and of conduct of nurses, midwives and health visitors throughout the United Kingdom. Over 382,000 nurses and midwives were employed in the NHS in England in 1992.

NUTRITION The process by which the living organism physiologically absorbs and used food to ensure growth, energy production and repair of tissues. The science of nutrition includes the study of diets and deficiency diseases (see DIET).

NUX VOMICA is the seed of *Strychnos nux-vomica*, an East Indian tree. It has an intensely bitter taste. The medicinal properties of the plant are almost entirely due to two alkaloids, strychnine and brucine, which it contains. (See STRYCHNINE.)

NYSTAGMUS (see EYE DISEASES).

NYSTATIN is an antibiotic isolated from *Streptomyces noursei*. It was the first antibiotic to be isolated which was active against fungus diseases, and is proving particularly useful in the treatment of moniliasis (q.v.).

O

OAT CELL   A type of cell found in one highly malignant form of lung cancer. The cell is small and either oval or round. The nucleus stains darkly and the cytoplasm is sparse and difficult to identify. Oat-cell carcinoma of the bronchus is usually caused by smoking and comprises around 30 per cent of all bronchial cancers. It responds to radiotherapy and chemotherapy but, because the growth has usually spread widely by the time it is diagnosed, the prognosis is poor. Results of surgery are unsatisfactory.

OBESITY is a condition in which the energy stores of the body (mainly fat) are too large. It is a prevalent nutritional disorder in prosperous countries. The Quetelet Index or Body Mass Index (BMI), which relates weight in kilograms (W) to height^2 in metres (H^2), is a widely accepted way of classifying obesity in adults according to severity, e.g.

Grade of obesity	BMI (W/H^2)
III	>40
II	30–40
I	25–29·9
not obese	<25

There is no advantage in further classifying obesity according to frame size since this does not improve the accuracy with which levels of body fat are predicted. (See APPENDIX 6: section C.)

Causes   For obesity to occur, energy intake must exceed energy output over a sufficiently long period of time. All aetiological factors must ultimately act by reducing energy output or increasing energy intake or both.

Obesity tends to aggregate in families. This has led to the suggestion that some people inherit a 'thrifty' gene which predisposes them to obesity in later life by lowering their energy output. Indeed patients often attribute their obesity to such a metabolic defect. Total energy output is made up of the resting metabolic rate (RMR), which represents about 70 per cent of the total, the energy cost of physical activity and thermogenesis, i.e. the increase in energy output in response to food intake, cold exposure, some drugs and psychological influences. In general, obese people are consistently found to have a higher RMR and total energy output, per person and also when expressed against fat-free mass, than do their lean counterparts. Most obese people do not appear to have a reduced capacity for thermogenesis. Although a genetic component to obesity remains a possibility, it is unlikely to be great or to prevent weight loss from being possible in most patients by reducing energy intake. Environmental influences are believed to be more important in explaining the familial association in obesity.

An inactive lifestyle is thought to play a minor role in the development of obesity, but it remains unclear if people are obese because they are inactive or are inactive because they are obese.

For the majority of obese people a reduction in energy output does not appear to be the main aetiological factor. It follows then that the explanation must lie in an excessive energy intake. Unfortunately, it is difficult to demonstrate this directly since the methods used to assess habitual energy intake are unreliable. For most obese people it seems likely that the defect lies in their failure to regulate energy intake in response to a variety of cognitive factors (i.e. ease of fitting of clothes) in the long term.

Rarely, obesity has an endocrine basis and is caused by hypothyroidism, hypopituitarism, hypogonadism or Cushing's syndrome (qq.v.)

Symptoms   Obesity has adverse effects on morbidity and mortality which are greatest in young adults and increase with the severity of obesity. It is associated with an increased mortality and/or morbidity from cardiovascular disease, non-insulin-dependent diabetes mellitus, diseases of the gall bladder, osteoarthritis, hernia, gout and possibly certain cancers (i.e. colon, rectum and prostate in men, and breast, ovary, endometrium and cervix in women). Menstrual irregularities and ovulatory failure are often experienced by obese women. Obese people are also at greater risk when they undergo surgery. With the exception of gallstone formation, weight loss will reduce these health risks.

Treatment   Creation of an energy deficit is essential for weight loss to occur. An average deficit of 1000 kcal/day will produce a loss of 1 kg of fat/week and should be aimed for. Theoretically, this can be achieved by increasing energy expenditure or reducing energy intake. In practice, a low-energy diet is the usual form of treatment since attempts to increase energy expenditure, either by physical exercise or a thermogenic drug, are relatively ineffective.

Anorectic drugs, gastric stapling and jaw wiring are sometimes used to treat severe obesity. They are said to aid compliance with a low-energy diet by either reducing hunger (anorectic drugs) or limiting the amount of food the patient can eat. Unfortunately, the long-term effectiveness of gastric stapling is not known and it is debatable if the modest reduction in weight achieved by use of anorectic drugs is worthwhile. For some grossly obese patients jaw wiring can be helpful but a regain of weight once the wires are removed must be prevented. Fitting a waist cord as a means of alerting a person to an increase in weight may help to maintain weight loss.

OBSESSION in medicine means the sudden domination of the mind by an idea or emotion, leading to impulsive acts which are beyond the control of the will, the power of judgment being for a time lost. (See MENTAL ILLNESS.)

OBSTETRICS is the branch of medicine dealing with pregnancy and giving birth. Derived from the Latin word for midwifery, it is closely allied to gynaecology. It is concerned with the health of the woman and fetus, from early in pregnancy through to a successful labour (q.v.). Close monitoring of both is essential, and has been greatly facilitated by advances in ultrasound (q.v.), amnioscopy (q.v.), amnio- and cordocentesis (see PRENATAL DIAGNOSIS). Numerous problems may occur at all stages, and early detection, followed rapidly by sensitive and appropriate treatment, is vital. Doctors and nurses can specialize in obstetrics after suitable training.

OBSTIPATION Severe constipation.

OBSTRUCTION OF THE BOWELS (see INTESTINE, DISEASES OF).

OCCIPUT is the lower and hinder part of the head where it merges into the neck.

OCCLUSION The way that the teeth fit together when the jaws close. Also the closing or obstruction of a duct, hollow organ, or blood vessel.

OCCULT Describing something that is not easily seen. Occult blood in the faeces is present in very small amounts and can be identified only by a chemical test or under the microscope.

OCCUPATIONAL DISEASES Work has been the cause of human illness and injury for centuries. The earliest accounts concentrated on the rigours of underground mining where, in earliest times, the risks to health were severe enough to relegate such 'occupations' to slaves and criminals. Such activities are inherently dangerous but the advent of industrialization widened and broadened the range of health risks to which employed people could be exposed. Control of workplace exposures in modern industrialized society has limited the toll of disease and injury but cannot abolish it entirely.

In the country such as Britain with 30 million employable people, over 400 are killed and another 150,000 injured each year as a direct result of work. One in 4,500 develops an occupational disease annually. By contrast, the Scandinavian figures for occupational disease are ten time 'worse'. Such differences are more to do with reporting criteria than true differences in occupational health. Whilst compensation for such disease rests with government social-security departments, the control of workplace hazards is in the hands of labour inspectorates. In Britain, this responsibility lies in the Department of Employment with the Health and Safety Commission and its Executive. The Executive includes both inspectorates

and a medical division staffed by doctors and nurses who have responsibility for giving advise to employers and employees on workplace risk to health in relation to health and safety legislation. Increasingly the laws governing health and safety at work are moving into a European arena as the European Commission promulgates directives which are binding on member states. Although a new European list of compensatable occupational diseases is currently being drafted, member states have widely differing criteria. What follows are brief notes on the numerically more important compensatable occupational diseases in the United Kingdom.

Inhaled materials PNEUMOCONIOSIS covers a group of diseases which cause fibrotic lung disease following the inhalation of dust. Around 500 new cases receive benefit each year – mostly due to coal dust with or without silica contamination. Silicosis is the more severe disease. The contraction in the size of the coal-mining industry as well as improved dust suppression in the mines have diminished the importance of this disease, whereas *asbestos-related diseases* now exceed 1,000 per year. Asbestos fibres cause a restrictive lung disease but also are responsible for certain malignant conditions such as pleural and peritoneal mesothelioma and lung cancer. The lung-cancer risk is exacerbated by cigarette smoking.

OCCUPATIONAL ASTHMA is of increasing importance – not only because of the recognition of new allergic agents but also in the number of reported cases. Twenty-two specific agents are listed at present of which the most common offending agents are isocyanates, flour and other grain dusts, soldering flux, epoxy resins and wood dusts. Other notable allergens are platinum salts, proteolytic enzymes, arthropods and crustaceans, antibiotics and reactive dyes. The disease develops after a short symptomless period of exposure and symptoms are temporally related to work exposures and relieved by absences from work. Removal of the worker from exposure does not necessarily lead to complete cessation of symptoms. For many agents, there is no relationship with a previous history of atopy (q.v.). Occupational asthma now accounts for about 10 per cent of all asthma cases.

BYSSINOSIS is considered by many authorities to be a variant of occupational asthma. The condition is, however, broader and more complex than this. In susceptible individuals, exposure to the dusts of cotton, sisal, hemp, or flax can cause acute dyspnoea with cough and reversible airways obstruction. It is first noticed on the first day of the working week and then subsides. Later, with continued exposure, symptoms recur on subsequent days of the week until even weekends and holidays are not free of symptoms.

Other organic dusts can produce extrinsic allergic alveolitis with resultant lowering of respiratory gas transfer in the alveoli. Most of the agents causing this condition are fungal spores and the most common condition in

Cause	Occupation	Disease
Coal dust	Coal mining	Coal-workers' pneumoconiosis
Silica	Gold mining	Silicosis
	Iron and steel industries (metal casting)	
	Metal grinding	
	Stone dressing	
	Pottery	
Asbestos	Asbestos mining	Asbestosis
	Manufacturer of fireproof and insulating materials	
Iron oxide	Arc welding	Siderosis
Tin dioxide	Tin ore mining	Stannosis
Beryllium	Aircraft and atomic energy industries	Berylliosis
Cotton, flax or hemp dust	Textile industries	Byssinosis
Fungal spores from mouldy hay, straw or grain, bagasse, mushroom compost	Agriculture and related industries	Farmer's lung
		Metalworker's lung
		Bagassosis
		Mushroom worker's lung

Some occupational lung diseases. Davidson and Macleod.

Britain is FARMER'S LUNG (see ALVEOLITIS). These diseases frequently start as an influenza-like illness and, if exposure is continued, lead to subacute and chronic pulmonary fibrotic disease.

Dermatitis The risk of dermatitis caused by an allergic or irritant reaction to substances used or handled at work is present in a wide variety of jobs. This condition is the commonest of all the occupational diseases. Whilst changes in the compensation criteria over the last twenty years have reduced successful claims from 11,000 a year to a few hundred, general-practice-based surveys suggest that over 50,000 new cases are diagnosed each year. About three-quarters of these cases are irritant-contact dermatitis due to such agents as acids, alkalis and even soap and water. Allergic contact dermatitis is a more specific response by susceptible individuals to a range of allergens. The main occupational contact allergens include chromates, nickel, epoxy resins, rubber additives, germicidal agents, dyes, topical anaesthetics and antibiotics as well as certain plants and woods.

Musculo-skeletal disorders Apart from the commonest problems of injured backs from manual handling, there are two groups of disorders caused by repeated injury – the 'beat' conditions and work-related upper-limb disorders. The *beat conditions* such as beat knee and beat elbow are caused by repeated damage to a joint from kneeling or crawling – problems associated with mining and carpet-laying, for example. The *work-related upper-limb disorders* range from clear-cut occupationally induced repetitive movement conditions such as tendinitis, tenosynovitis (q.v.), carpal tunnel syndrome (q.v.) and epicondylitis to less well-defined disorders of prolonged or repetitive posture disturbances which may lead to shoulder or cervical spine discomfort. These disorders are common in the general population and

their occupational attribution is frequently controversial. Particular high-risk occupations include poultry processors, packers, electronic assembly workers, data processors, supermarket check-out operators and telephonists. These jobs often contain a number of the relevant exposures of dynamic load, static load, a full or excessive range of movements and awkward postures.

Physical agents A number of physical agents cause occupational ill health of which most important is *occupational deafness*. Workplace noise exposures in excess of 85 decibels for a working day are likely to cause damage to hearing which is initially restricted to the vital frequencies associated with speech – around 3–4 KHz. Protection from such noise is imperative as hearing aids do nothing to ameliorate the neural damage once it has occurred.

Hand–arm vibration syndrome is a disorder of the vascular and/or neural endings in the hands leading to episodic blanching and numbness which is exacerbated by low temperature. The condition, which is caused by vibrating tools such as chain saws and pneumatic hammers, is akin to Raynaud's disease (q.v.) and can be disabling.

Decompression sickness is caused by a rapid change in ambient pressure and is a disease associated with deep-sea divers, tunnel workers and high-flying aviators. Apart from the direct effects of pressure change such as ruptured tympanic membrane or sinus pain, the more serious damage is indirectly due to nitrogen bubbles appearing in the blood and blocking small vessels. Central and peripheral nervous-system damage and bone necrosis are the most dangerous sequelae.

Radiation *Non-ionizing radiation* from lasers or microwaves can cause severe localized heating leading to tissue damage of which cataracts are a particular variety. *Ionizing radiation* from radioactive sources can cause similar acute tissue damage to the eyes as well as cell damage to rapidly dividing cells in the gut and bone marrow. Longer-term effects include genetic

damage and various malignant disorders of which leukaemia and aplastic anaemia are notable. Particular radioactive isotopes may destroy or induce malignant change in target organs, for example, I^{131} (thyroid), Sr^{90} (bone).
Other occupational cancers Occupation is directly responsible for about 5 per cent of all cancers and contributes to a further 5 per cent. Apart from the cancers caused by asbestos and ionising radiation, a number of other occupational exposures can cause human cancer. The International Agency for Research on Cancer lists 50 agents or processes of which occupational agents or processes account for 31. The more important of these are polynuclear aromatic hydrocarbons such as mineral oils, soots, tars (skin and lung cancer), the aromatic amines in dyestuffs (bladder cancer), certain hexavalent chromates, arsenic and nickel refining (lung cancer), wood and leather dust (nasal sinus cancer), benzene (leukaemia) and vinyl chloride monomer (angiosarcoma of the liver). Elimination of all known occupational carcinogens, if possible, would lead to an annual saving of 5,000 premature deaths in Britain.
Infections Two broad categories of job carry an occupational risk. These are workers in contact with animals (farmers, veterinary surgeons and slaughtermen) and those in contact with human sources of infection (health care staff and sewage workers). Estimates of current annual incidences of work related cases are leptospirosis (q.v.) (40 cases), tuberculosis (q.v.) (30 cases), hepatitis B (q.v.) (25 cases), chlamydiosis (see CHLAMYDIA) (16 cases), Q fever (q.v.) (12 cases), brucellosis (q.v.) (10 cases). The less severe orf (q.v.) accounts for at least 50 cases but this is even more of an underestimate than the figures for the other diseases. Other compensatable infections are anthrax, glanders, ancylostomiasis (qq.v.), streptococcus suis, and hydatidosis.
Poisonings In earlier decades, chemical poisonings by lead, phosphorus, arsenic, mercury, cadmium and a number of organic solvents were much more common. Today, around 2,000 poisonings are reported annually with 20–30 fatalities. The commonest agents are now solvents, gases, acids, alkalis and irritant vapours. The lead regulations specify that persons with blood lead levels above 69μg/100 ml (above 39 for females of reproductive age) should be suspended from working with lead. In 1989–90, of 22,000 male lead workers, there were 534 suspensions. The success in diminishing morbidity is largely one of prevention.
Prevention There are certain principles of prevention which, if followed, can significantly diminish the risk of occupationally induced diseases. Indeed as these diseases cannot be eliminated from the world – in comparison with smallpox – prevention is the utmost importance. This is a hierachy of control measures. The ideal solution is elimination of the offending substance or process. Failing this, substitution by a less hazardous material or process could be undertaken and/or more effective enclosure or exhaust ventilation, thereby di-

minishing exposure of the worker. The least satisfactory method is personal protection for the worker.

OCCUPATIONAL THERAPY is the treatment of physical and psychiatric conditions through specific selected activities in order to help people reach their maximum level of function and independence in all aspects of daily life.
Occupational therapists work from hospital and community bases. They do much more than keep patients occupied with diverting hobbies. The arts and crafts still have a place in modern therapy techniques but these now also include household chores, industrial work, communication techniques, social activities, sports and educational programmes. An Occupational Therapy Department may have facilities for woodwork, metalwork, printing, gardening, cooking, art and drama. Occupational therapists will use any combination of activities to strengthen muscles, increase movement and restore co-ordination and balance. With mentally ill people similar activies are used. They help provide order, comfort and support and aim to build up self-confidence. Occupational therapists plan courses of treatment which are individually tailored to the needs of the patient. The aim is to help the patient practise all the activites involved in daily life. The therapists are part of a team including doctors, nurses, social workers, home helps, housing officers, physiotherapists, speech therapists and psychologists. Occupational therapists are mainly employed by the National Health Service and by Local Authority Social Services and they work in hospitals, special centres and in the handicapped person's own home. State Registration is essential for employment as an occupational therapists. There are 15 occupational therapy schools in the United Kingdom where the course leading to the diploma of the College of Occupational Therapists can be followed. The course lasts three academic years. (See REHABILITATION; REMPLOY.)

OCHRONOSIS is a rare condition in which the ligaments and cartilages of the body, and sometimes the conjunctiva, become stained by dark brown or black pigment. This may occur in chronic carbolic poisoning, or in a congenital disorder of metabolism in which the individual is unable to break down completely the tyrosine of the protein molecule, the intermediate product, homogentisic acid, appearing in the urine – this being known as alkaptonuria.

OEDEMA means an abnormal accumulation of fluid beneath the skin, or in one or more of the cavities of the body.
Causes Oedema is not a disease, although this is a popular idea, supported by the fact that at one time many deaths were recorded as due to 'dropsy' without a further statement of cause. Oedema may be due to one of three

conditions: (1) weakening of the walls of the capillary vessels, by injury of the part in which oedema occurs, by ill-health of the body generally, by poverty of the blood circulating through and nourishing the vessels, or by poisonous materials in the blood; (2) obstruction to the blood-flow through the veins; (3) a watery condition of the blood allowing fluid to escape through the capillary walls. Oedema may also result from obstruction to the flow of lymph in the lymph channels.

Heart disease, which produces increased pressure in the veins, and also an impaired circulation of the blood, in consequence of the defective pumping action of the heart, and *glomerulonephritis* in which the kidneys fail in their functions of excreting poisonous substances and a certain amount of water from the blood, are the main causes of general oedema. In heart disease the oedema is more marked after exertion; in kidney disease it is found chiefly after resting. Thus one of the chief characters of oedema due to glomerulonephritis is that it appears in the morning, affects loose tissues like the skin beneath the eyes, and passes off as the day advances. Oedema due to heart disease, on the other hand, tends to appear towards evening, affects dependent parts like the feet, and diminishes during the night.

In *hunger oedema* due to diminution of the amount of protein in the blood as a result of starvation, the oedema is generalized, but in the earlier stages is most marked in the feet and legs, especially after exertion. The swelling which sometimes follows snake bites, bee-stings or the eating of poisonous shell-fish, and constitutes an extreme and rapidly ensuing form of *nettle-rash*, is a special variety of oedema. *White-leg*, which may appear after some acute disease like typhoid fever or pneumonia, or after the birth of a child, due to a thrombosis or plugging of the main vein in the affected limb, is one of the localized forms of oedema. A similar condition may be caused by a *tumour* pressing upon a large vein of the arm or leg. Oedema in the legs may be due to varicose veins. *Cirrhosis*, tumours, and other diseases of the liver may, by interference with the circulation through it, cause oedema, first of the abdomen and later of the lower limbs.

Treatment There is no general treatment which will meet every case. The particular cause has, in each case, to be removed. Oedema due to heart or kidney disease yields as the disease producing it is alleviated. In cases of localized oedema, elevation of the oedematous part is of great importance, and the person should adopt the recumbent position. In the case of heart disease, digitalis, which improves the action of the heart, and benzothiadiazine diuretics form the chief means employed. In acute kidney disease the treatment of the oedema consists in the routine treatment of glomerulonephritis. In oedema due to liver conditions, occasional purges with blue-pill or calomel may help the condition. When the oedema will not yield to drugs, some of the fluid may have to be drawn off (see ASPIRATION); when this is done partially,

the kidneys are sometimes enabled to cope with the remainder of the fluid.

OEDEMA OF THE LUNGS results when the left ventricular myocardium is unable to handle the blood delivered to it. There is an abrupt increase in the venous and capillary pressure in the pulmonary vessels followed by flooding of fluid into the interstitial spaces and alveoli. The commonest cause of acute pulmonary oedema is myocardial infarction which reduces the ability of the left ventricular myocardial muscle to handle the blood delivered to it. Pulmonary oedema may result from other causes of left ventricular failure such as hypertension or valvular disease of the mitral and aortic valves. The initial symptoms are cough with breathlessness and occasionally with wheezing. The patient becomes extremely short of breath with a sensation of imminent death. In a severe attack the patient is pale, sweating and cyanosed and obviously gasping for breath. Frequently frothy sputum is produced which may be blood stained.

OEDIPUS COMPLEX A description used by psychoanalysts of the subconscious attraction of a child for its parent of the opposite sex. This is accompanied by a wish to get rid of the parent of the same sex. The origin of the phrase lies in the Greek story in which Oedipus kills his father without realizing who he is and then marries his mother.

OESOPHAGOSCOPE is an instrument constructed on the principle of the telescope, which is passed down the oesophagus and enables the observer to see the state of the oesophagus. (See ENDOSCOPE.)

OESOPHAGUS, or GULLET, is the tube passing from the throat into the stomach, down which passes swallowed food and drink. It consists of three coats: a strong outer coat of muscle fibres in two layers, the outer running lengthwise, the inner being circular; inside this a loose connective tissue coat containing bloodvessels, glands, and nerves; and finally a strong mucous membrane lined by epithelium, which closely re-sembles that of the mouth and skin.

OESOPHAGUS, DISEASES OF The oesophagus, or gullet, may be the seat of inflammatory conditions causing discomfort in swallowing, but the more important ailments are those which arise from local injuries, such as the swallowing of scalding or corrosive substances. This may cause ulceration followed by the formation of a scar which narrows the passage and produces the symptoms of *stricture* of the oesophagus: namely, pain and difficulty in swallowing, with regurgitation of the food. The severity of the case will necessarily depend upon the amount of narrowing and consequent mechanical obstruction, but in some instances this has occurred to such an extent as practically to close the canal. Cases of oesophageal stricture of this kind may sometimes be dilated by the use of suitable instruments or surgery may be necessary.

A still more serious and frequent cause of oesophageal stricture is that due to *cancer*, which may occur at any part, but is most common at the lower end, near the entrance into the stomach. The chief symptoms of this condition are increasing difficulty in swallowing, steady decline in strength, together with enlargement of the glands in the neck. The condition usually occurs in middle age or beyond. In 1989 2,957 men and 2,224 women developed cancer of the oesophagus in England and Wales. In many cases treatment can only be palliative, but recent advances in surgery are producing promising results. In some cases treatment with irradiation produces relief, if not cure. In those in whom neither operation nor radiation can be performed life may be prolonged and freedom from pain obtained by fluid food which is either swallowed or passed down a tube. The operation of gastrostomy, by which an opening is made through the front of the abdomen, allows food to be directly introduced into the stomach.

Strictures of the oesophagus may also be produced by the pressure of tumours or aneurysms within the cavity of the chest but external to the gullet.

An important cause of difficulty in swallowing is the condition known as *cardiospasm* or *achalasia of the cardia* is due to failure of the cardiac sphincter (the sphincter at the lower end of the oesophagus) to relax when food is swallowed. The cause is not known. The condition occurs usually in young adults. Treatment consists of passing special bougies down the oesophagus to dilate the sphincter.

Finally, difficulty in swallowing sometimes occurs in certain serious nervous diseases from paralysis affecting the nerves supplying the muscular coats of the pharynx, which thus loses its propulsive power (*bulbar paralysis*).

Foreign bodies which lodge in the respiratory part of the throat, i.e. at the entrance to, or in the cavity of, the larynx, set up immediate symptoms of choking. (See CHOKING.) Those which lodge in the gullet, on the contrary, do not usually set up any immediately serious symptoms, although their presence causes considerable discomfort. Medical attention is usually required.

OESTRADIOL is the name given to the oestrogenic hormone secreted by the ovarian follicle. Oestradiol is responsible for the development of the female sexual characteristics, of the breasts, and of part of the changes that take place in the uterus before menstruation.

OESTRADIOL VALERATE (see OESTROGEN).

OESTRIOL (see OESTROGEN).

OESTROGEN is the term applied to any substance that will induce oestrus or 'heat'. In human medicine it is applied to the substances, natural or synthetic, that induce the changes in the uterus that precede ovulation. They are also responsible for the development of the secondary sex characteristics in women: that is the physical changes that take place in a girl at puberty, such as enlargement of the breasts, appearance of pubic and axillary hair and the deposition of fat on the thighs and hips. They are used in the management of disturbances of the menopause, and also in the treatment of cancer of the prostate and certain cases of cancer of the breast.

The oestrogenic hormones of the ovary are oestradiol and oestrone and they are interconvertible. The natural oestrogens, like the hormones of the testis and the adrenal cortex, are steroids. They are rapidly metabolized in the body and excreted in the urine as inactive conjugates. The rapid degradation of natural oestrogens limits their use as therapeutic agents. Chemical substitution of the steroid molecule, as in ethinyl oestradiol, or the use of a non-steroidal synthetic oestrogen such as stilboestrol, greatly reduces the rate of degradation and enhances the therapeutic action. A further development has been the use of compounds which are not actually oestrogenic themselves, but which are slowly metabolized to oestrogenic substances, or substances such as chlorotrianisene, which are taken up in the body fat and then slowly released into the circulation. There is in fact little to choose between the various synthetic oestrogens. Preparations such as equine oestrogens or chlorotrianisene have little therapeutic advantage and are considerably more expensive. Ethinyl oestradiol is the most potent oral oestrogen, being twenty times more active than stilboestrol.

The following oestrogens are in therapeutic use: chlorotrianisene, cyclofenil, cyproterone, dinoestrol, equine oestrogens, ethinyl oestradiol, hexoestrol, methallenoestril, oestradiol valerate, oestriol, oestrone, piperazine oestrone sulphate, quinestradol, stilboestrol, stilboestrol diphosphate, quinestrol.

OESTRONE (see OESTROGEN).

OFFICE OF POPULATION CENSUSES AND SURVEYS A central government department in the United Kingdom that compiles and publishes statistics of local and national populations as well as the demography of births, marriages, and deaths. It also records the medical cause of deaths. Every ten years the OPCS conducts a national survey of the population on a particular night. The figures it provides are used by other government departments and local authorities for planning services for the public.

OINTMENTS are semi-solid mixtures of medicinal substances with lard, benzoated lard, paraffin or yellow soft paraffin, and wool- fat (lanolin), intended for external application. They are used for three main purposes: (i) as emollients, that is to soften the skin; (ii) as a protective preparation to be applied to the skin; (iii) as a means for the local application of medicaments to be absorbed through the skin.

Other substances occasionally used to form the body of an ointment are almond oil, beeswax, camphor, glycerin, oleic acid, spermaceti, and prepared suet.

Among the most useful ointments are the following: *Simple Ointment* BP, which contains 5 per cent each of wool fat, hard paraffin, and cetostearyl acid in white or yellow soft paraffin, and is used for application to chafed surfaces. *Cold Cream*, made of beeswax, spermaceti, almond oil, rose water, and attar of rose, is used for a similar purpose. *Zinc and Castor Oil Ointment* BP, which contains 7·5 per cent zinc oxide and 50 per cent w/w castor oil has a well-earned reputation for the prevention and treatment of napkin rash.

OLD AGE (see AGEING).

OLEANDOMYCIN is an antibiotic derived from *Streptomyces antibioticus*. It is active against many Gram-positive micro-organisms and some Gram-negative micro-organisms.

OLEIC ACID is the commonest of naturally occurring fatty acids, being present in most fats and oils in the form of triglyceride. It is used in the preparation of ointments, but not eye ointments.

OLFACTORY NERVE, the nerve of smell, is the first cranial nerve.

OLIGAEMIA means a diminution of the quantity of blood in the circulation.

OLIGOMENORRHOEA is infrequent menstruation.

OLIGURIA means an abnormally low excretion of urine, such as occurs in acute nephritis.

OLIVE OIL is the oil obtained by pressure from the fruit of *Olea europaea*. It is practically a pure fat.

OMENTUM is a long fold of peritoneal membrane, generally loaded with more or less fat, which hangs down within the abdominal cavity in front of the bowels. It is formed by the layers of peritoneum that cover the front and back surfaces of the stomach in their passage from the lower margin of this organ to cover the back and front surfaces of the large intestine. Instead of passing straight from one organ to the other, these layers dip down and form a sort of fourfold apron. It is to the increasing deposit of fat in this structure that the prominence of the abdomen is largely due in people of middle age who are large eaters. This omentum is known as the greater omentum, to distinguish it from two smaller peritoneal folds, one of which passes between the liver and stomach (the hepatogastric omentum), and the other between the liver and duodenum (the hepatoduodenal omentum). Together they are known as the lesser omentum.

OMPHALOCELE is another name for exomphalos – a hernia of abdominal organs through the umbilicus.

ONCHOCERCIASIS is infestation with the filarial worm, *Onchocerca volvulus*. It is found in many parts of tropical Africa south of the Sahara, in Central and South America, and in the Yemen and Saudi Arabia. It is estimated that there are more than 20 million victims of it. It is transmitted by gnats of the genus *Simulium*. After a period of nine to eighteen months, the young filarial worms, injected into the body by the bite of an infected *Simulium*, mature, mate and start producing young microfilariae. The females live for up to fifteen years and during this period each may produce several thousand microfilariae a day. It is these microfilariae, which have a life-span of up to two years, that produce the characteristic features of the disease: an itching rash of the skin and the appearance of nodules in different parts of the body. There may also be involvement of the eyes and the worm may invade the optic nerve and so cause blindness; hence the name of African river blindness. Treatment consists of diethylcarbamazine and suramin. An international campaign is now under way in an attempt to destroy *Simulium* in the affected zones. Meanwhile the only means of prevention is to avoid so far as possible being bitten by the gnat. One means of achieving this is by wearing long trousers, shoes and socks.

ONCOGENE is a gene (q.v.) found in mammalian cells and viruses that can cause cancer. It is believed to manufacture the proteins that control the division of cells. In certain circumstances this control malfunctions and a normal cell may be changed into one with malignant properties.

ONCOLOGY is that part of medical science which is concerned with the management of malignant disease such as cancer.

ONYCHIA means an inflammation affecting the nails. (See NAILS, DISEASES OF.)

ONYCHOGRYPHOSIS is a distortion of the nail in which it is much thickened, overgrown and twisted on itself. This usually affects a toenail and is the result of chronic irritation and inflammation.

ONYCHOLYSIS means separation of the nail from the nail-bed.

OÖCYTE An immature ovum (q.v.). When the cell undergoes meiosis in the ovary it becomes an ovum and is ready for fertilization by the spermatozoa. Only a small number of the many oöcytes produced survive until puberty (q.v.), and not all of them will become ova and be ejected into the fallopian tubes (q.v.).

OÖPHORECTOMY is a term applied to removal, by operation, of an ovary. When the ovary is removed for the presence of a cyst, the term ovariotomy is usually employed.

OÖPHORITIS is another name for ovaritis or inflammation of an ovary.

OÖPHORON is another name for the ovary.

OPHTHALMOLOGY The study of the structure and function of the eye and the diagnosis and treatment of the diseases that affect it.

OPHTHALMOPLEGIA means paralysis of the muscles of the eye. Internal ophthalmoplegia refers to paralysis of the iris and ciliary body, external ophthalmoplegia refers to paralysis of one or all of the muscles that move the eyes.

OPHTHALMOSCOPE An instrument for examining the interior of the eye. There are different types of ophthalmoscope, all have a light source to illuminate the inside of the eye and a magnifying lens to make examination easier.

OPIATE is a preparation of opium (q.v.).

OPIOID A substance with a pharmacological action that is like that of opium or its derivatives.

OPIPRAMOL is a drug with antidepressant properties.

OPISTHOTONOS is the name given to a position assumed by the body during one of the convulsive seizures of tetanus. The muscles of the back, by their spasmodic contraction, arch the body in such a way that the person for a time may rest upon the bed only by his heels and head.

OPIUM is the dried juice of the unripe seed-capsules of the white Indian poppy, *Papaver somniferum*. It is cultivated mainly in India, but it is also produced in Iran, China, and the Asiatic provinces of Turkey. Opium possesses its medicinal properties only when produced under favourable conditions of soil and climate, and the juice of other species of poppies grown in temperate climates is almost useless. The juice is obtained by scarifying the seed-capsules of the poppies before they are ripe, and next day collecting the gummy sap which has exuded from the cuts. This is dried with great care, kneaded, and carefully tested. Good opium should contain about 10 per cent of morphine, to which its action is chiefly due. It is a brown, resinous-looking substance, or brown powder, with characteristic smell and bitter taste. The action of opium depends upon the twenty to twenty-five alkaloids it contains. Of these, the chief is morphine, the amount of which varies from around 9 to 17 per cent. Other alkaloids include codeine, narcotine, thebaine, papaverine, and naceine, and as the action of these differs considerably, the effect of the opium naturally varies according to the proportion of each that it contains. Turkish opium, which is purest in morphine, is generally regarded as the best, the use of Indian opium, which contains a large proportion of narcotine, being more apt to cause sickness. Opium, which is exported from the country of its production in balls or cakes, is often adulterated with sugar, vegetable extracts, gum, molasses, and even stones concealed in the middle of the cakes, and it is therefore very carefully tested before sale.

The importation into Britain of opium is very carefully regulated under the *Dangerous Drugs Acts*. Similar regulations govern the sale and distribution of any preparation of morphine or diamorphine (heroin) stronger than 1 part in 500.

The alkaloids, morphine and codeine, are administered in various forms. Morphine hydrochloride and morphine sulphate are given in doses from 7·5 to 20 mg; codeine phosphate in doses from 10 to 60 mg. Morphine hydrochloride solution (containing 1 per cent of morphine) is used in doses from 0·5 to 2 ml.

Action The action of opium varies considerably, according to the source of the drug and the preparation used; it varies even more according to the age, race, and temperament of the individual. Children are profoundly affected by even the smallest doses, so that the drug is unsuited for use, except with great care, during childhood.

In small doses, opium produces a state of gentle excitement, the person finding his imagination more vivid, his thoughts more brilliant, and his power of expression greater than usual. This stage lasts for some hours, and is succeeded by languor. In larger, i.e. medicinal, doses this stage of excitement is short and is followed by deep sleep, from which the person can still be aroused as from natural sleep. When very large, i.e. poisonous, doses are taken, sleep comes on quickly, and passes into coma and death. The habitual use of opium produces great tolerance, so that opium users require to take large quantities daily before experiencing its pleasurable effects. The need for opium also confers tolerance, so that people suffering great pain may take, with apparently little effect beyond dulling the pain, quantities which at another time would be dangerous.

It checks all secretions, except the sweat, and slows the processes of tissue change, this action being sometimes useful, sometimes a hindrance to its employment. (See DRUG ADDICTION.)

OPIUM POISONING As a result of induced tolerance (see DRUG ADDICTION) and great individual variability, the amount of opium required to cause serious consequences varies enormously.

Symptoms When a poisonous dose of any of the preparations of the drug has been taken, sleep rapidly comes on, becomes deeper and deeper, and passes gradually into a state of complete insensibility. Increased sweating, contracted pupils and slow shallow breathing are characteristic. Opium paralyses the respiratory centre and death usually occurs up to 18 hours after a fatal dose has been taken.

Treatment An emetic should be given as soon as possible and full doses of naloxone, levallorphan or nalorphine should be given. Should none of these be immediately available, injections of caffeine sodium benzoate or nikethamide may be given.

It is important to keep the patient awake. Strong coffee, and other stimulants may be given internally. If, in spite of all these measures, he becomes unconscious and the breathing begins to fail, artificial respiration must be performed.

OPPORTUNISTIC A description usually applied to infection resulting from an organism that does not normally cause disease in a healthy individual. It is also used to describe widespread infection by an organism that usually causes local infection. The body's defence mechanism can usually combat these organisms but if it is impaired – as happens in AIDS – opportunistic infection, such as pneumonia, may develop. Some viral and fungal infections behave in this way. Antimicrobial treatment is often effective, even though the weakness in the body's defence mechanism cannot be rectified.

OPSONINS are substances present in the serum of the blood which act upon bacteria, so as to prepare them for destruction by the white corpuscles of the blood.

OPTIC ATROPHY A deterioration in the fibres of the optic nerve resulting in partial or complete loss of vision. It may be caused by damage to the nerve from inflammation or injury, or the atrophy may be secondary to disease in the eye.

OPTIC CHIASMA This is formed by a crossing over of the two optic nerves which run from the back of the eyeballs to meet in the midline beneath the brain. Nerve fibres from the nasal part of the retina cross to link up with fibres from the outer part of the retina of the opposite

eye. The linked nerves form two separate optic tracts which travel back to the occipital lobes of the brain.

OPTIC DISC Otherwise known as the blind spot of the eye, the disc is the beginning of the optic nerve, the point where nerve fibres from the retina's rods and cones – the light- and colour-sensitive cells – leave the eyeball.

OPTICIAN Someone who fits and sells glasses or contact lenses. An ophthalmic optician is trained to perform eye examinations to test for long and short sightedness but they do not treat disorders of the eye.

OPTIC NERVE (see EYE).

ORAL An adjective referring to the mouth or to substances taken by mouth.

ORAL CONTRACEPTIVES A contraceptive taken by mouth. It comprises one or more synthetic female hormones, usually an oestrogen, which blocks normal ovulation, and a progestogen which influences the pituitary gland and thus blocks normal control of the woman's menstrual cycle. Progestogens also make the uterus less congenial for the fertilization of an ovum by the sperm. (See CONTRACEPTION.)

ORANGE is an excellent source of vitamin C: 100 millilitres of orange juice contain 50 mg of ascorbic acid (ie. vitamin C). It is also used as a flavouring agent in the form of infusion, tincture and syrup of the peel. Fresh orange is also employed, often mixed with glucose, in feverish conditions for the action of the citric acid it contains. (See CITRIC ACID.)

ORBIT (see EYE).

ORCHIDECTOMY is the operation for the removal of the testicles (one or both).

ORCHIDOPEXY When testes do not descend into the scrotum normally in young children (cryptorchidism) an operation is necessary to bring the testes in to the scrotum. This is called surgical orchidopexy.

ORCHITIS means inflammation of the testicle. (See TESTICLE, DISEASES OF.)

ORF is a widespread viral infection of sheep and goats which is sometimes transmitted to man, in whom it manifests itself as a skin eruption, usually on the hands, fingers, forearms and face.

ORGAN A collection of different tissues that form a distinct structure in the body with a particular function or functions. The liver, for example, comprises a collection of different metabolic cells bound together with connective tissue and liberally supplied with blood vessels that performs vital functions in the breakdown of substances absorbed from the gastrointestinal tract. Other examples of organs are the kidneys, brain and heart.

ORGANIC DISEASE is a term used in contradistinction to the word functional, to indicate that some structural change is responsible for the faulty action of an organ or other part of the body.

ORGANIC SUBSTANCES are those which are obtained from animal or vegetable bodies, or which resemble in chemical composition those derived from this source. Organic chemistry has come to mean the chemistry of the carbon compounds.

ORGANO-PHOSPHORUS INSECTICIDES are a group of insecticides which act by inhibiting the action of cholinesterase. (See ACETYL-CHOLINE.) For this reason they are also toxic to man and must therefore be handled with great care. The most widely used are parathion (q.v.) and malathion (q.v.).

Some of them are of value in agriculture because, when applied to plants, they are absorbed, and distributed to all parts of the plant, where they may kill sucking insects such as aphids.

ORGASM The climax of sexual intercourse. In men this coincides with ejaculation of the semen when the muscles of the pelvis force the seminal fluid from the prostate into the urethra and out through the urethral orifice. In women orgasm is typified by irregular contractions of the muscular walls of the vagina followed by relaxation. The sensation is more diffuse in women than men and tends to last longer with successive orgasms sometimes occurring.

ORIENTAL SORE This term is a synonym for cutaneous leishmaniasis (see LEISHMANIASIS); others include: Cochin, Delhi, Kandahar, Lahore, Madagascar, Natal, Old World tropical, tropical sore, etc. As with many of the local names for this infection, it is now rarely used.

ORNITHOSIS is an infection of birds with the micro-organism known as *Chlamydia psittaci*, which is transmissible to man.

ORPHENADRINE is a drug used in the treatment of Parkinsonism (q.v.).

ORTHODONTICS is the branch of dentistry concerned with the prevention and treatment of dental irregularities and malocclusion.

ORTHOPAEDICS Originally the general measures, surgical and mechanical, which can be used for the correction or prevention of deformities in children. Now, that branch of medical science dealing with skeletal deformity, congenital or acquired.

ORTHOPNOEA is a form of difficulty in breathing so severe that the patient cannot bear to lie down, but must sit or stand up. As a rule, it occurs only in serious affections of the heart or lungs.

ORTHOPTIC TREATMENT involves the examination and treatment by exercises of squints and their sequelae.

OSGOOD-SCHLATTER'S DISEASE is the form of osteochondrosis (q.v.) involving the tibial tubercle – the growing point of the tibia (q.v.). It occurs around puberty, mainly in boys, and first manifests itself by a painful swelling over the tibial tubercle at the upper end of the tibia. The pain is worst during and after exercise. A limp with increasing limitation of movement of the knee joint develops. Treatment consists of immobilization of the knee joint in plaster of Paris for six to eight weeks, with gradual return to activity over the next few months.

OSMOLARITY The osmotic pressure of a particular concentration of an osmotic solute dissolved in water. It is defined by the number of active particles in a set volume.

OSMOSIS means the passage of fluids through a membrane, which separates them, so as to become mixed with one another. Osmotic pressure is a term applied to the strength of the tendency which a fluid shows to do this, and depends largely upon the amount of solid which it holds in solution.

OSSICLE A small bone, the term is usually applied to the three small bones of the middle ear – malleus, incus, and stapes – that conduct sound from the eardrum to the inner ear (q.v.). (See EAR.)

OSSIFICATION means the formation of bone. In early life, centres appear in the bones previously represented by cartilage or fibrous tissue, and from these the formation of true bone and deposit of lime salts proceed. When a fracture occurs, the bone mends by ossification of the clot which forms between the fragments. (See FRACTURES.) In old age an unnatural process of ossification often takes place in parts which should remain cartilaginous, e.g. in the cartilages of the larynx and of the ribs, making these parts unusually brittle.

OSTEITIS means inflammation in the substance of a bone. *Traumatic osteitis* is a condition particularly common in footballers, in which the victim complains of pain in the groin following exercise, particularly if this has involved much hip rotation. Examination reveals difficulty in spreading the legs and marked tenderness over the symphysis pubis. It responds well to rest and the administration of anti-inflammatory drugs such as indomethacin.

OSTEITIS DEFORMANS (see PAGET'S DISEASE OF BONE).

OSTEITIS FIBROSA CYSTICA is a pathological rather than a clinical entity. The term refers to the replacement of bone by a highly cellular and vascular connective tissue. It is the result of osteoclastic and osteoblastic activity and is due to excessive parathyroid activity. It is thus seen in a proportion of patients with primary hyperparathyroidism and in patients with uraemic osteodystrophy; that is, the secondary hyperparathyroidism that occurs in patients with chronic renal disease.

OSTEOARTHRITIS is a term used for joint problems where the primary problem is seen as a change in structure of cartilage and bone, rather than an inflammatory synovitis. Osteoarthritis usually implies a loss of the central load-bearing area of articular hyaline cartilage by a process of fibrillation, fissuring and fragmentation. This is usually associated with outgrowth of cartilage at the articular margin with subsequent ossification to form bony outgrowths known as osteophytes. Unfortunately there is confusion because the term is also used to cover joint pain that appears to have a mechanical basis in the absence of clinical or radiographic evidence of cartilage loss. Osteophytes form with increasing age, whether or not there is significant cartilage loss, and in the elderly osteophytes may lead to local frictional symptoms, and in the spine nerve compression. Despite major efforts, it has proved impossible to produce a single clear definition of osteoarthritis and this probably reflects the muddled nature of a concept which will need replacing.

The important problem of loss of central load-bearing articular cartilage occurs increasingly with age but is by no means inevitable. It has a wide range of causes, of which some, like dysplasia and trauma, are known and others have yet to be identified. The main clinical problems occur in the hip and knee. The cartilage loss in the hip usually occurs in the sixth or seventh decade. It may affect both hips in fairly rapid succession, or only one hip and such patients often have no problems in other joints. Cartilage loss in the knee occurs from the fifth decade onwards and is often associated with cartilage loss in small joints in the hand and elsewhere. Cartilage loss in the distal interphalangeal joints of the hand is associated with the formation of bony swellings known as Heberden's nodes.

Treatment Management is largely directed at maintaining activity, with physical and social support as necessary. Analgesics may be of some value, particularly in the management of night pain. Non-steroidal anti-inflammatory agents may help patients with early morning stiffness and may also reduce pain on movement and night pain. Their benefit, however, tends to be less marked than in rheumatoid arthritis and their long-term usage has considerable toxicity problems. Advanced cartilage loss is best treated by joint replacement. Hip and knee-joint replacements are now common surgical procedures which greatly improve the mobility of affected individuals.

People with arthritis and their relatives can obtain help and advice from Arthritis Care (see APPENDIX 2: ADDRESSES).

OSTEOCHONDRITIS is inflammation of both bone and cartilage. It is a not uncommon cause of backache in young people, particularly gymnasts.

OSTEOCHONDROSIS includes a group of diseases involving degeneration of the centre of ossification (see BONE) in the growing bones of children and adolescents. They include Kohler's disease, Osgood-Schlatter's disease (q.v.), and Perthes' disease (q.v.).

OSTEOCYTE A bone cell formed from an osteoblast or bone-forming cell that has stopped its activity. The cell is embedded in the matrix of the bone.

OSTEOGENESIS IMPERFECTA is a hereditary disease due to an inherited abnormality of collagen (q.v.). It is characterized by extreme fragility of the skeleton, resulting in fractures and deformities. It may be accompanied by blue sclera (the outermost, normally white coat of the eyeball), transparent teeth, hypermobility (excessive range of movement) of the joints, deafness, and dwarfism (shortness of stature). The cause is not known, though there is some evidence that it may be associated with collagen formation (see COLLAGEN). Parents of affected children can obtain help and advice from the Brittle Bone Society (see APPENDIX 2: ADDRESSES).

OSTEOMALACIA is the adult form of rickets. It is due to inadequate mineralization of osteoid tissue caused by a deficiency of vitamin D. This deficiency may arise because of inadequate intake or it may be due to impaired absorption such as occurs in intestinal malabsorption. It may also be due to renal disease as the kidney is responsible for the hydroxylation of cholecalciferol, which has virtually no metabolic action, to dihydroxy-cholecalciferol, the metabolically active form of the vitamin. (See VITAMIN D.)

OSTEOMYELITIS means inflammation in the marrow of a bone. (See BONE, DISEASES OF.)

OSTEOPATHY is the name applied to a system of healing in which diseases are treated by manipulating bones and other parts with the idea of thereby restoring functions in the bodily mechanism that have become deranged. Properly qualified osteopaths are included on the General Council and Register of Osteopaths (see APPENDIX 2: ADDRESSES).

OSTEOPHYTES are bony spurs or projections. They occur most commonly at the margins of points involved in osteoarthritis (q.v.).

OSTEOPOROSIS is a reduced mass of normal bone. It is due to excessive resorption of bone rather than decreased bone synthesis. The quality of the bone that is present is normal, it is just the quantity that is deficient. It is a feature of ageing so that osteoporosis is common in the elderly. After the menopause women lose one per cent of their bone each year so that post-menopausal osteoporosis is a common disorder unless hormone-replacement therapy is given. Osteoporosis is also a feature of Cushing's syndrome and of patients who have been on long-term treatment with corticosteroids. Information and advice about the disease can be obtained from the National Osteoporosis Society (see APPENDIX 2: ADDRESSES).

OSTEOSARCOMA or OSTEOGENIC SARCOMA is the most common, and most malignant, tumour of bone. It occurs predominantly in older children and young adults. The commonest site for it is at the ends of the long bones of the body: i.e. the femur, tibia and humerus. Treatment is by chemotherapy and surgical reconstruction or amputation of the affected limb. The 5-year survival rate is over 70 per cent.

OSTEOTOMY is the operation of cutting of a bone.

OS TRIGONUM is a small accessory bone behind the ankle joint which is present in about 7 per cent of the population. It may be damaged by energetic springing from the toes in ballet, jumping or fast bowling.

OTITIS means inflammation of the ear. (See EAR, DISEASES OF.)

OTOLOGY is that branch of medical science which is concerned with disorders and diseases of the organ of hearing, one practising this branch being called an OTOLOGIST.

OTORRHOEA means discharge from the ear. (See EAR, DISEASES OF.)

OTOSCLEROSIS is a condition in which abnormal bone is deposited around the footplate of the stapes resulting in fixation of that bone and causing a progressive conductive hearing loss due to immobility of the ossicular chain. There is an hereditary pattern to the disease and its onset is usually in the third decade. It tends to be slightly commoner in women and is often accelerated in pregnancy. Treatment involves supplying a hearing aid or performing an operation known as stapedectomy. Rarely the deposition of abnormal bone may affect the inner ear as well.

OTOSCOPE (see AURISCOPE).

OUABAIN, or Strophanthin-G, is a glycoside first obtained from the African tree, *Acokanthera ouabaio*: it was used as an arrow poison in West Africa. It is now obtained from the African tree *Strophanthus gratus*. It is a cardiac stimulant, having a similar action to that of digitalis.

OUTPATIENT A patient attending hospital on a day basis. He or she is not admitted to a bed. Most patients attend an outpatients' department after referral for a specialist opinion by their general practitioner. An increasing number of investigations and treatments, including surgery, are being done on an outpatient basis.

OVARIES are the glands in which are produced, in the female sex, the ova, capable, if fertilized, of developing into new individuals. They are situated, one on each side, in the cavity of the pelvis, corresponding on the surface of the body approximately to the centre of the groin. Each is shaped something like an almond, is about 3 cm long, 1·5 cm wide, and 1 cm in thickness, and is whitish in colour. It is attached to the broad ligament running from the womb to the side of the pelvis, by one edge along which blood-vessels and nerves enter. One end is connected to the expanded end of the Fallopian tube, as well as by a ligament to the side of the pelvis, and the other end to a ligament to the side of the womb. The ovary therefore lies to a considerable extent free in the pelvis. (See REPRODUCTIVE SYSTEM: diagram.)

The chief bulk of the ovary is made up of connective tissue, which differs from ordinary fibrous tissue in being composed of spindle-shaped cells. On the surface is a layer of columnar cells, and beneath this a dense connective tissue layer, the tunica albuginea. Beneath the tunica albuginea the structure appears to the naked eye to be of a granular character, this appearance being due to the presence of a layer of follicles, estimated at around 2,000,000 in number in each ovary at birth. By puberty they are reduced to around 40,000 in each ovary, a mere 400 of which will be shed at ovulation during the child-bearing period. Each follicle contains one (seldom more) ovum, each of these ova being capable of developing into a new individual. Every follicle consists essentially of a hollow ball of cells, embedded in which is a single large cell, the ovum. Each ovary contains follicles in all stages of maturity, from the rudimentary ones described above to several which are greatly increased in size to 35 micrometres in diameter through multiplication of the cells surrounding the ovum and the formation among them of a cavity distended with fluid. One at least of these follicles comes to maturity, when it is known as a Graafian follicle, about half-way between two menstrual periods, distends till it reaches the surface of the ovary, and finally bursts allowing the escape of the contained ovum, measuring 110 micrometres in diameter, which finds its way down the corresponding Fallopian tube into the womb. This process is know as ovulation. (See MENSTRUATION.)

For ovarian secretions, see Ovaries under ENDOCRINE GLANDS, and also OESTRADIOL; OESTROGEN; PROGESTERONE.

OVARIES, DISEASES OF Medical problems caused by the ovary arise as a result of a number of conditions, namely: infection, failure of ovulation, premature ovarian failure and the development of tumours.

Oöphoritis or infection of the ovaries rarely occurs alone, except in viral infections such as mumps. Usually it is involved with infection of the Fallopian tubes (salpingitis). It may occur as a complication of a miscarriage or a therapeutic abortion or the birth of a baby. Cases not associated with pregnancy are often the result of sexual activity. The most common organisms involved are *Chlamydia, Escherichia coli* and *Neisseria gonorrhoea*. Swabs should be taken from the cervical canal and sent for culture. The definitive treatment is with antibiotics. Pain should be relieved with analgesics. If the pain is severe or if the patient is vomiting, she should be admitted to hospital.

Failure of ovulation is the cause of infertility in about a third of couples seeking help with conception. It may also lead to menstrual problems. These may be in the form of an irregular menstrual cycle or menorrhagia. Treatment depends on the symptoms. Induction of ovulation will help those trying to conceive. Menstrual problems can be treated with the combined oral contraceptive pill or with cyclical progestogens. An uncommon cause of failure of ovulation is polycystic ovary syndrome often associated with acne (q.v.), hirsutism (q.v.) and obesity.

Early ovarian failure is the cause of a premature menopause (q.v.). Treatment is with hormone replacement therapy using a combination of oestrogen and progestogen.

Ovarian tumours may be physiological or pathological. Physiological cysts arise as a result of ovulation. Follicular cysts may cause pain when they rupture. The pain is transient and no specific treatment is required. Following ovulation the remains of the follicle forms a structure called the corpus luteum. Infrequently, this can form a cyst which ruptures and may bleed causing pain. The condition may be mistaken for an ecoptic pregnancy (q.v.). The diagnosis is made at laparoscopy (q.v.). Treatment consists of stopping the bleeding either by removing the cyst or by cauterizing or suturing the bleeding points.

Pathological tumours may be benign or malignant. They may cause pain as a result of a complication such as rupture, torsion, haemorrhage or infection. They may press on the bladder or rectum and cause symptoms that way. The commonest benign tumour in young women is a dermoid cyst (benign cystic teratoma). In the older women fibroma (see UTERUS, DISEASES OF) is more common. Benign tumours need to be removed surgically since malignancy can be excluded only after the specimen has been examined microscopically by a pathologist.

Malignant tumours may be primary or secondary, i.e. either they arise in the ovary or they are metastases (seedlings) from a cancer which has developed in another organ. The cancers which are most likely to metastasize to the ovaries are those from the bronchus, breast, stomach, colon, endometrium (q.v.) or lymphoma (q.v.). Treatment depends on the primary tumour.

Primary ovarian cancer causes more deaths each year than cervical and endometrial cancers combined. Most patients (85 per cent) present after the tumour has spread beyond the ovaries. Early tumours present with symptoms similar to benign tumours. Late ones present with abdominal distension and vague gastrointestinal symptoms. The disease should be totally removed if possible; if not possible, the tumour mass is reduced to the smallest possible amount. The benefit of such cytoreductive treatment needs to be evaluated. Nowadays, radiotherapy is only used for palliation. Chemotherapy is given to those patients with evidence of spread away from the ovaries or who have residual disease after surgery. The most active cytotoxic agents are cisplatin and its analogues. Recently paclitaxol (Taxol) has been shown to be extremely active, especially when combined with cisplatin. Ideally the surgery should be done by a gynaecological oncologist, a gynaecological surgeon specializing in the treatment of gynaecological tumours. The best results of treatment are obtained in specialist centres in which there is close co-operation between the gynaecological, medical and radiation oncologists.

OVARIOTOMY or OÖPHORECTOMY is the operation of removal of an ovary or an ovarian tumour.

OVULATION The development and release of an ovum (q.v.) (egg) from the ovary into the fallopian tube. Ovulation is initiated by the secretion of luteinizing hormone by the anterior pituitary gland and occurs half way through the menstrual cycle. If the ovum is not fertilized, it is lost during menstruation.

OVUM is the single cell derived from the female, out of which a future individual arises, after its union with the spermatozoon derived from the male. It is about 35 micrometres in diameter. (See FETUS; OVARIES.)

OXALIC ACID is not used in medicine, but it is of importance because it is an irritant poison, and has a domestic use for cleaning purposes. It is also found in many plants including rhubarb and sorrel. Oxalic acid, when swallowed, produces burning of the mouth and throat, vomiting of blood, breathlessness and circulatory collapse. Calcium salts, lime water or milk should be given by mouth. An injection of calcium gluconate is an antidote.

OXIMETRY The measurement by an oximeter of the proportion of oxygenated haemoglobin (q.v.) in the blood.

OXPRENOLOL (see ADRENERGIC RECEPTORS).

OXYCEPHALY, or STEEPLE HEAD, describes a deformity of the skull in which the forehead is high and the top of the head pointed. There is also poor vision and the eyes bulge.

OXYGEN is a colourless and odourless gas of molecular weight 32. It constitutes just less than 21 per cent of the Earth's atmosphere. Though not itself flammable, it supports combustion. It was first isolated by Priestley in 1772. Medical and industrial oxygen are manufactured by the fractional distillation of liquid air. In Britain it is supplied as a compressed gas at high pressure (13600 kilopascals (KPa)) in cylinders which are black with white shoulders. In hospitals oxygen is often stored as a liquid in insulated tanks and controlled evaporation allows the gas to be supplied via a pipeline at a much lower pressure.

Oxygen is essential for life. It is absorbed via the lungs and is transported by haemoglobin (q.v.) within the erythrocytes (q.v.) to the tissues. Within the individual cell it is involved in the production of adenosine triphosphate (ATP), a compound that stores chemical energy for muscle cells, by the oxidative metabolism of fats and carbohydrates. Hypoxia (q.v.) causes anaerobic metabolism with a resulting build-up in lactic acid, the result of muscle cell activity. If severe enough, the lack of ATP causes a breakdown in cellular function and the death of the individual.

When hypoxia occurs, it may be corrected by giving supplemental oxygen. This is usually given via a face mask or nasal prongs or in severe cases during artificial ventilation of the lungs. Some indications for oxygen therapy are high altitude, ventilatory failure, heart failure, anaemia (q.v.), pulmonary hypertension (q.v.),

carbon monoxide poisoning (q.v.), anaesthesia and post-operative recovery. In some conditions – e.g. severe infections with anaerobic bacteria (q.v.) and carbon monoxide poisoning – hyperbaric oxygen therapy has been used.

OXYGEN DEFICIT In a resting individual the potential oxygen supply to the tissues is greater than its consumption. During heavy exercise the energy required by the tissues is greater than can be supplied by aerobic cellular metabolism and the additional energy is supplied by a biochemical reaction called anaerobic metabolism. There is a build-up of lactate – a product of lactic acid – from anaerobic metabolism which is ultimately oxidized after conversion to citrate and metabolism via the citric acid cycle. The increased amount of oxygen above resting concentrations which needs to be consumed to perform this metabolism is known as the oxygen debt or deficit.

OXYGEN TOXICITY occurs when high concentrations of oxygen are breathed for long periods. It is thought that under hyperoxic conditions there is increased production of chemicals called free radicals by cellular metabolism which damages cells and organs. The most susceptible organs are the lungs, eyes (particularly in the neonate), central nervous system and gut. Oxygen toxicity in human lungs causes an acute oedema followed by fibrosis and pulmonary hypertension. In the neonate retrolental fibroplasia occurs and central-nervous-system damage may result in the infant having fits. Several factors are involved in toxicity and there is no absolute relationship to time or concentration, though inspired concentrations of under 50 per cent are probably safe for long periods.

OXYMETHOLONE is an anabolic steroid (q.v.) used to treat aplastic anaemia (q.v.).

OXYPERTINE is an anti-psychotic drug related to the phenothiazines.

OXYTETRACYCLINE is an antibiotic derived from a soil organism, Streptomyces rimosus. Its range of antibacterial activity is comparable to that of tetracycline (q.v.).

OXYTOCIC means hastening parturition or stimulating uterine contraction, or a drug or procedure that has this effect.

OXYTOCIN is the extract isolated from the pituitary posterior lobe which stimulates the uterine muscle to contract. It can also be synthesized. (See PITUITARY BODY.)

OXYURIS is another name for the threadworm.

OZAENA is a chronic disease of the nose of an inflammatory nature, combined with atrophy of the mucous membrane and the formation of extremely foul-smelling crusts in the interior of the nose. (See NOSE, DISEASES OF.)

OZONE is a specially active and poisonous form of oxygen in which three volumes of the gas are condensed into the space ordinarily occupied by two. It has a characteristic smell and is a strong oxidizing agent. Formed when an electrical charge is passed through oxygen or air, it is found at high altitudes in the atmosphere where it screens out much of the sun's ultraviolet radiation. The ozone layer, as it is called, is being damaged by pollutant gases from earth and, unless this damage is reversed, lethal quantities of ultraviolet radiation could penetrate to the earth's surface, with long-term damage to the environment.

P

PACEMAKER (see CARDIAC PACEMAKER).

PACHYDERMIA means hypertrophy or thickening of the skin. PACHYDERMIA LARYNGIS is a name applied to thickening of the vocal cords due to chronic inflammation or irritation.

PACHYMENINGITIS means inflammation of the dura mater of the brain and spinal cord. (See MENINGITIS.)

PACINIAN CORPUSCLES, or lamellated corpuscles, are minute bulbs at the ends of the nerves scattered through the skin and subcutaneous tissue, and forming one of the end-organs for sensation.

PACKED CELL VOLUME That fraction of the blood's total volume made up of red cells. The packed cell volume is established by centrifuging blood in a tube and measuring the depth of the column of red cells as a fraction of the whole column of blood. (See HAEMATOCRIT).

PAEDIATRICS means the branch of medicine dealing with diseases of children.

PAGET'S DISEASE OF BONE, or OSTEITIS DEFORMANS, is a chronic disease in which the bones – especially those of the skull, limbs, and spine – gradually become thick and also soft, causing them to bend. It is said to be the commonest bone disease in the world, and it is estimated that some 600,000 people in England may suffer from it. It seldom occurs under the age of 40. Pain is its most unpleasant manifestation. The cause is not known, and there is no known cure, but satisfactory results are being obtained from the use of calcitonin (q.v.) and a group of drugs known as diphosphonates (eg. etidronate). Those with the disease can obtain help and advice from the National Association for the Relief of Paget's Disease (see APPENDIX 2: ADDRESSES).

PAIN 'Pain is an unpleasant sensory and emotional experience associated with actual or potential tissue damage or described in terms of such damage' (International Association for the Study of Pain, 1979). Pain threshold is the least experience which the subject recognizes as pain. Pain tolerance is the greatest amount of pain which the subject is prepared to tolerate. The perception of a harmful or potentially harmful (*noxious*) stimulus by the nervous system in the conscious or unconscious state without the emotion of unpleasantness is not pain and should be called *nociception*.

In its usual and simplest form, pain is the result of a noxious external stimulus and the unpleasant nature of the experience causes the subject to react to the stimulus, thereby limiting the extent of the damage. The amount of pain that a person experiences is, in part, dependent on the strength of the stimulus, although it can be modified by association of thoughts and mood. It can be inhibited by distraction or anger or excitement and case histories abound of damage suffered and ignored in times of battle, sporting endeavour and passion. Conversely, pain can be increased by anticipation, fear, depression, fatigue or anxiety.

When tissues are damaged, the products of damage and the increased activity and secretions of the nerves cause increased sensitivity within the immediate area of damage (*primary hyperalgesia*) and over a larger area (*secondary hyperalgesia*). The pain perceived from further stimulation of this 'inflamed' area is dependent as much on the increase of sensitivity as on the strength of the stimulus.

Pain can be the result of damage, deterioration or functional changes within the nervous system itself (central pain). This typically gives rise to spontaneous pain, unrelated to any detectable stimulus, or to extreme hypersensitivity and pain in response to stimuli which are not normally painful such as light touch, gentle stroking or warmth (*allodynia*). Pain may be sensed when, or even because, other sensations are reduced, so that pain and numbness can occur at the same time in the same place (*anaesthesia dolorosa*). When pain is appreciated only after strong, prolonged or repeated stimuli but increases during and beyond the stimuli, this is termed *hyperpathia*.

Pain may also be due to changes in perception, or the interpretation of distress or misery, and be the presenting and primary symptom in depression, bereavement and, rarely, psychosis. More usually, the emotional components of pain such as annoyance, anger or frustration, fear of death and disability, guilt or embarrassment, accompany the sensation initiated by the noxious stimulus, especially when the pain is prolonged.

Pain also has associations with punishment – the word pain can be used to denote penalty ('on pain of death') – and pain is often used as a punishment in childhood, as a means of punishment by governments or persuasion in torture, or is considered as a form of divine retribution. Prolonged pain can lead to feelings of inadequacy and helplessness. Pain may persist in the absence of continuing damage but the association between 'hurt' and 'harm' leads to pain-avoidance, or pain-related behaviour, which can itself be harmful. For example, prolonged bed-rest for low back pain leads to wasting of the muscles of the spine and increased instability. 'Pain' reflexes are those automatic responses which occur in response to conscious pain or to nociception in the unconscious state (such as anaesthesia, sleep, or coma). These may include autonomic responses such as changes in pulse rate, blood pressure, pallor, sweating and pupil size, and muscular movements such as withdrawal, muscle spasm, vocalization or stridor.

LOCALIZATION   When pain is due to an external source and perceived by receptors of the nervous system on the body surface, the brain can localize the stimulus with considerable accuracy because of the relatively high density of receptors and the relative lack of branching of their neural pathways. When the stimulus arises from an internal organ such as the gut or heart, localization is poor. Sometimes the pain is felt to be not in the originating organ but in an external part of the body, the sensory nerves of which enter the same segment of the spinal cord. Thus pain arising in or just under the diaphragm may be perceived in the shoulder. This is called *referred pain*. Pain which is perceived in a part which has been amputated or denervated is called *phantom pain* and is caused by activity in a more proximal part of the nervous system.

CHARACTERISTICS OF PAIN SENSATION   Many words are used to describe the various kinds of pain. Some describe the timing or pattern of pain, some the character of sensation, some the emotion and others the intensity of the pain. Acute and chronic only describe pain of short or long duration, respectively. Colicky pain is one which increases and decreases rhythmically and usually reflects the waves of peristalsis in a hollow organ such as the gut or ureter (q.v.) with increased sensitivity and duration of contraction or reaction. Aching, burning, throbbing, sharp, shooting, stabbing, tender, all describe various sensations and can indicate the origin of the pain. Throbbing and tender are often associated with inflammation (e.g. toothache), whereas sharp, shooting, stabbing and aching, especially in combination, are more likely to be associated with compression, irritation or damage of nerve or muscle.

Treatment of pain should be directed primarily to the prevention or limitation of injury and the elimination of the cause of the pain. Diagnosis of the cause and mechanism of the pain is also necessary for the treatment of established pain. Much pain can be reduced or prevented by treatment of the patient's anxiety, by explanation and reassurance. Pain associated with trauma and inflammation is reduced by 'simple' analgesics such as paracetamol and non-steroidal anti-inflammatory drugs (NSAID) (q.v.) such as aspirin or diclofenac. Opioids (such as morphine) (q.v.) may be required for severe pain. Resistant, chronic and nerve-generated pain can sometimes be better treated by the tricyclic antidepressants (q.v.), anticonvulsants (q.v.) or agents that modify neural augmentation such as ketamine. Pain can also be treated by such stimulation techniques as acupuncture or transcutaneous nerve stimulation, or by relaxation, hypnotherapy, massage or cognitive-behavioural therapy. In recent years some hospitals have set up pain relief clinics to which doctors can refer patients whose pain is resistant to routine treatments. Patients with intractable pain may need surgery to cut the nerves transmitting the painful stimuli.

PAINTER'S COLIC (see COLIC; LEAD POISONING).

PALATE is the partition between the cavity of the mouth, below, and that of the nose, above. It consists of the *hard palate* towards the front, which is composed of a bony plate covered below by the mucous membrane of the mouth, above by that of the nose; and of the *soft palate* further back, in which a muscular layer, composed of nine small muscles, is similarly covered. The hard palate extends a little further back than the wisdom teeth, and is formed by the maxillary and palate bones. The soft palate is concave towards the mouth and convex towards the nose, and it ends behind in a free border, at the centre of which is the prolongation known as the uvula. When food or air is passing through the mouth, as in the acts of swallowing, coughing, or vomiting, the soft palate is drawn upwards so as to touch the back wall of the throat and shut off the cavity of the nose. Movements of the soft palate, by changing the shape of the mouth and nose cavities, are important in the production of speech.

PALATE, MALFORMATIONS OF   The palate is subject to certain alterations, as the result of defective development. The hard palate may be much more arched than usual: this is sometimes due to the failure to breathe through the nose, caused by the presence of adenoid vegetations in the throat. (See NOSE, DISEASES OF.)

In early embryonic life (see FETUS) there are certain clefts in the region of the throat and face, the nose being formed by the junction of one process which grows down from between the eyes (fronto-nasal process) and two which grow in, one from either side (maxillary processes). The fronto-nasal process produces the external nose, the septum of the nose, the central part of the upper lip, and that part of the upper jaw which carries the two front teeth. The maxillary processes form the remainder of the upper jaw and the palate on each side. These three should unite completely prior to birth, but if they fail to do so, a Y-shaped gap is left. This gap runs from the back of the palate forward to a point a little distance behind the front teeth, from which point a limb of the gap runs forwards to each nostril and through the upper lip. A complete state of *cleft palate* may occur; or there may be only a partial gap in the soft palate, the parts having closed in front; or again, there may be closure behind and only a notch be left in the lip or a single cleft in the edge of the upper jaw. The notch of the lip is known as *hare-lip*, from a fanciful resemblance to the hare, which has a notch in the centre of its lip.

The incidence of cleft lip (hare-lip) and cleft palate seems to be increasing and one child in approximately 700 normal births has some degree of cleft lip and palate. The increase is probably due to more of these babies surviving, as a result of improved surgical techniques, and getting married and having children. As a rough guide, it can be said that if a child is born with a cleft, and there is no family history as far back as the parents' grandparents, the chances of another malformed child is about the same as in the general population. When one parent is affected, the risk is around 1 in 80 but, when a mother with a cleft palate produces a daughter with a cleft palate, the risk to a second daughter is as high as 1 in 7.

Cleft-palate and hare-lip should, if possible, be rectified by operation, because both are a serious drawback to feeding in early life, while later, hare-lip is a great disfigurement, and cleft-palate gives to the voice a peculiar twang. When there is merely a slight degree of hare-lip, it is usual to operate a few weeks or even some days after birth, although, when the notch is very large, it may be necessary to wait till the

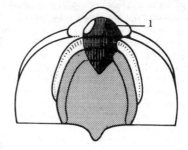

1 Unilateral cleft palate, involving lip and upper jaw

Cleft palate viewed from below.

child is several months old. The closure of a large cleft in the palate, which is a more formidable operation, is usually deferred till the child has gained some strength, and the most suitable time is generally held to be between eighteen months and two and a half years of age, because the fault must be remedied before the child has learned to speak. The operations performed vary greatly in details, but all consist in paring the edges of the gap and drawing the soft parts together across it.

Until a hare-lip has been remedied, it is often necessary to feed the child with a spoon, as he cannot suck. When a cleft palate is too wide for operation, its effects can be diminished in later life by wearing an artificial palate.

Parents of such children can obtain help and advice from the Cleft Lip and Palate Association, or the Dental and Maxillofacial Department, Hospital for Sick Children, Great Ormond Street (see APPENDIX 2: ADDRESSES).

PALINDROMIC An adjective describing symptoms or diseases that recur.

PALLIATIVE is a term applied to the treatment of incurable diseases, in which the aim is to mitigate the sufferings of the patient, not to effect a cure.

PALLOR Unusual paleness of the skin caused by a reduced flow of blood or a deficiency in normal pigments. Pallor may be a sign of shock, anaemia, or other diseases.

PALPATION means the method of examining the surface of the body and the size, shape, and movements of the internal organs, by laying the flat of the hand upon the skin.

PALPEBRAL Relating to the eyelid.

PALPITATION is a condition in which the heart beats forcibly or irregularly, and the person becomes conscious of its action.

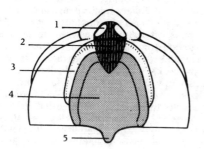

1 nostrils
2 primary palate
3 lips
4 palate
5 uvula

Normal palate viewed from below.

Causes As a rule we are quite unconscious of the beating of the heart, but when the nervous system is unduly excited its action may become unpleasantly palpable. A disorder of the rhythm of the heart (arrhythmia) may cause the heart to beat rapidly and give rise to palpitations. Sudden emotions, such as fright, and occasionally dyspepsia, may bring it on. A common cause consists in over-use of tobacco, tea, coffee, or alcohol. Sometimes it may appear in cases of organic heart disease.

Symptoms There may simply be a fluttering of the heart and a feeling of weakness, or the heart may be felt pounding and the arteries throbbing, causing great distress to the affected person. The subject may be conscious of the heart missing beats.

Treatment Although these symptoms can be unpleasant, they do not usually signify serious disease. Moderate exercise is a good thing. If the person is a smoker, he or she should stop. Tea, coffee, alcohol or other stimulants should be taken sparingly. A sensible diet is advisable. If symptoms persist or are severe, the individual should see a doctor and any underlying disorder should be investigated and treated. The beta adrenoreceptor antagonists are the most useful drugs in controlling the palpitations of anxiety and those due to some cardiac arrhythmias.

PALSY is another name for paralysis. (See PARALYSIS.)

PALUDRINE (see PROGUANIL HYDROCHLORIDE).

PAN- is a prefix meaning all or completely.

PANACEA is a term applied to a remedy for all diseases, or more usually to a remedy which benefits many different diseases.

PANCARDITIS means inflammation of the pericardium, myocardium, and endocardium at the same time.

PANCREAS, or SWEETBREAD, is a long secreting gland situated in the back of the abdomen, at the level of the first and second lumbar vertebrae. It lies behind the lower part of the stomach, an expanded portion, called the head of the pancreas, occupying the bend formed by the duodenum or first part of the small intestine, whilst a long portion known as the body extends to the left, ending in the tail, which rests against the spleen. A duct runs through the whole gland from left to right, joined by many small branches in its course, and, leaving the head of the gland, unites with the bile duct from the liver to open into the side of the small intestine about 7·5 to 10 cm (3 or 4 inches) below the outlet of the stomach.

Minute structure The gland resembles one of the salivary glands, being composed of tubes of columnar cells bound together by loose connective tissue. These cells are arranged with one end abutting on a central lumen into which the secretion of the cells passes, and each group of tubes ends in a small duct, which unites with other small ducts to join the main pancreatic duct running to the intestine. The cells present an outer, clear zone, and an inner zone filled with granules of the materials secreted by the activity of the cell. Blood-vessels and nerves in large numbers run in the connective tissue of the gland.

Scattered through the pancreas are collections of cells known as the islets of Langerhans, of which there are around a million in a normal individual. These do not communicate with the duct of the gland, and the internal secretion of the pancreas – insulin – is formed by these cells and absorbed directly into the blood.

Functions The most obvious function of the pancreas is the formation of the pancreatic juice, which is poured into the small intestine after the partially digested food has left the stomach. This is the most important of the digestive juices, is alkaline in reaction, and contains, in addition to various salts, four enzymes. These enzymes are: trypsin and chymotrypsin, which digest proteins; amylase, which converts starchy foods into the disaccharide maltose; lipase, which breaks up fats. For the action of these see DIGESTION.

Inadequate production of insulin by the islets of Langerhans leads to the condition known as diabetes mellitus (q.v.). In addition to insulin, another hormone is produced by the pancreas. This is glucagon which has the opposite effect to insulin and raises the blood sugar by promoting the breakdown of liver glycogen.

PANCREAS, DISEASES OF Abscesses, cysts, calculi, and tumours may occur in the pancreas as in other organs, but are not very common. The most important disease of the pancreas, though again, fortunately, not very common, is acute pancreatitis. This is an unpredictable disease which may start gradually or suddenly, accompanied by pain that can be very severe. Biliary-tract disease and alcohol account for 80 per cent of patients admitted to hospital with acute pancreatitis. Among other causes are drugs and infections such as mumps. The acute abdominal pain often radiates through to the back. Patients are acutely ill with tachycardia (q.v.), fever and low blood pressure. Many go into shock. Hospital admission is required, treatment is complicated and the prognosis is hard to forecast. Around 10 per cent of people with acute pancreatitis die. Of the rest some develop chronic pancreatitis, a much more indeterminate disease, commonly associated with disease of the gall-bladder, particularly gall-stones, and chronic alcoholism. Cancer of the pancreas is on the increase and around 7,000 cases are now diagnosed every year in the UK. There is an established association with heavy cigarette smoking, and it is twice as common in patients with diabetes mellitus as compared with the general population. Reference has already been made to the association between the islets of Langerhans (q.v.) and diabetes mellitus (q.v.).

PANCREATIN or PANCREATIC JUICE, contains the four powerful enzymes trypsin, chemotrypsin, lipase, and amylase, which continue the digestion of foods started in the stomach (see DIGESTION). It is given by mouth for the relief of pancreatic deficiency in conditions such as pancreatitis (see PANCREAS, DISEASES OF) and fibrocystic disease of the pancreas (see CYSTIC FIBROSIS). It is also used for the preparation of predigested, or so-called peptonized, foods, such as milk and some starchy foods.

PANCYTOPENIA A fall in the number of red and white blood cells as well as of platelets. The condition is found in aplastic anaemia, bone-marrow tumours, enlarged spleen, and other disorders.

PANDEMIC is an epidemic which affects a vast area, such as a country or a continent.

PANHYSTERECTOMY is an operation by which the uterus is completely removed.

PANNICULITIS means inflammation of the subcutaneous fat, and may occur anywhere on the body surface.

PANNUS Blood vessels growing into the cornea beneath its epithelium. Seen in trachoma and to a lesser extent in patients who are long-term soft-contact-lens wearers.

PANTOTHENIC ACID, which has now been prepared synthetically, is part of the vitamin B complex. It is known as the chick anti-dermatitis factor because if it is absent from the chick's diet the bird develops dermatitis, and degeneration of nerve-fibres in the spinal cord also occurs. In rats lack of pantothenic acid produces greying of the hair, but there is no evidence that in man greying is due to lack of this vitamin. Indeed, little is known about the significance of pantothenic acid in man, except that it is one of the essential constituents of the diet. The daily requirement is probably around 10 milligrams. It is widely distributed in foodstuffs, both animal and vegetable. Yeast, liver, and egg-yolk are particularly rich sources. (See APPENDIX 5: VITAMINS.)

PAPAIN, PAPYAOTIN, and PAPOID are names given to a ferment, or mixture of ferments, obtained from the juice of the pawpaw, the unripe fruit of *Carica papaya*, which has an action similar to that of the ferments of the gastric and pancreatic juices. It is accordingly sometimes used to peptonize foods for invalids,

as it does not give them the same bitter taste that pepsin gives. It is widely used as a meat tenderizer.

PAPANICOLAOU TEST (see CERVICAL SMEAR).

PAPAVERETUM consists of the hydro-chlorides of alkaloids of opium (q.v.). It has the pain-relieving and narcotic effects of morphine (q.v.), but fewer side-effects. It is largely used in association with anaesthesia.

PAPILLA means a small projection, such as those with which the corium of the skin is covered, and which project into the epidermis and make its union with the corium more intimate; or those covering the tongue and projecting from its surface.

PAPILLITIS is the term applied to inflammation of any papilla, but especially of the prominence formed by the end of the optic nerve in the retina, also known as optic neuritis.

PAPILLOEDEMA Swelling of the optic disc specifically due to raised intra-cranial pressure.

PAPILLOMA means a tumour composed of papillae growing from the surface of skin or mucous membrane. These tumours may be either simple or malignant in nature. Such a tumour is found occasionally in the bladder, and the chief symptom of its presence is the painless presence of blood in the urine.

PAPOVAVIRUS is a group of viruses, one of which is responsible for warts (q.v.).

PAPULE means a pimple.

PARA- is a prefix meaning near, aside from, or beyond.

PARA-AMINO SALICYLIC ACID was one of the early antituberculous antibiotics. It tended to cause a lot of dyspepsia and has been replaced by newer antituberculous drugs with fewer side-effects. The first-line drugs for tuberculosis are now rifampicin, isoniazid, and ethambutol.

PARACENTESIS is the puncture by hollow needle or trocar and cannula of any body cavity (e.g. abdominal, pleural, pericardial), for tapping or aspirating fluid pathologically accumulated. (See ASPIRATION.)

PARACETAMOL has antipyretic and analgesic actions similar to those of aspirin. The dose is 500 to 1000 milligrams.

PARACETAMOL POISONING Paracetamol is one of the safest of drugs when taken in correct dosage. When an overdose is taken, however, it is a very dangerous one because of the toxic effect on the liver. This is why cases of poisoning with it must be taken to hospital as quickly as possible. In the early stages there is only sickness and vomiting without any loss of consciousness. Once in hospital, treatment consists of washing out the stomach, and the administration of drugs, such as cysteamine and acetylcysteine, to protect the liver.

PARACUSIS means any perversion of the sense of hearing.

PARAESTHESIA is a term applied to unusual feelings, apart from mere increase, or loss, of sensation, experienced by a patient without any external cause: for example, hot flushes, numbness, tingling, itching. Various paraesthesiae form a common symptom in some nervous diseases.

PARAFFIN is the general name used to designate a series of saturated hydrocarbon bodies, discovered by Reichenbach in 1830 and first produced as a commercial product by Young in 1850. The higher members of the series, paraffin-waxes, are solid at ordinary temperatures, some being hard, others soft. Lower in the scale comes petroleum, which is liquid at ordinary temperatures. Naphtha, petroleum spirit, and hydramyl are lower members of the series which are very volatile, and lowest comes methane, better known as marsh-gas, which is a gaseous body.
Uses In the form of the *British Pharmacopoeia* preparation, liquid paraffin, it is used in the treatment of constipation.
Externally, the hard and soft paraffins are used in various consistencies, being very useful as ointments and lubricants as they are apparently harmless.

PARAFORMALDEHYDE is used as a source of formaldehyde. For disinfecting rooms it is prepared in the form of tablets which are vaporized on an electric hotplate. It is also used as lozenges. These should be allowed to dissolve slowly in the mouth. To keep catheters and other surgical instruments aseptic, it is enclosed with them in airtight containers.

PARAGANGLIOMA is the term used to describe two types of tumour. One known as a CHROMAFFINOMA or PHAEOCHROMOCYTOMA, is a tumour containing chromaffin cells (q.v.), most often found in the medulla of the suprarenal gland, where chromaffin cells are normal constituents. An important sign of these tumours is paroxysmal high blood-pressure. The other, also known as a CHEMODECTOMA, occurs in the carotid body (q.v.) and the comparable aortic

body. It is usually quite small and is more common in women than men.

PARAGONIMIASIS is the condition caused by *paragonimus*, a genus of trematode or fluke, the most common being *Paragonimus westermani*, which is most often found in the Far East, but is also found in India, South America and parts of Africa. The disease is also known as endemic haemoptysis, as the presenting feature is haemoptysis, or the coughing up of blood, due to the worm settling in the lungs. The infection is acquired by eating inadequately cooked crayfish or crab. Bithionol is the drug most commonly used in treatment. Chloroquine is also used.

PARAGRAPHIA is misplacement of words, or of letters in words, or wrong spelling, or use of wrong words in writing as a result of a lesion in the speech region of the brain.

PARAINFLUENZA VIRUSES are included in the paramyxovirus (see MYXOVIRUSES) and divided into four types, all of which cause infection of the respiratory system. Infection with type 3 begins in May, reaches a maximum in July or August and returns to baseline level in October. Types 1 and 2 are predominantly winter viruses. Children are commonly affected and the manifestations include croup (q.v.), fever, and a rash.

PARALDEHYDE is a clear, colourless liquid with a penetrating ethereal odour, and a burning taste followed by a cool sensation in the mouth. Although in small quantities it may cause excitement, in larger doses it is a soporific, with little depressing effect, and productive of quiet, refreshing sleep.
Uses It is given when a powerful hypnotic action is required, and is particularly useful in inducing sleep in mentally unstable patients. Its unpleasant taste restricts its use, but has the compensatory advantage that it usually prevents the patient receiving paraldehyde from becoming an addict.

PARALYSIS, or PALSY, means loss of muscular power due to interference with the nervous system. When muscular power is weakened as the result of some disorder of the nervous system, but not entirely lost in the parts concerned, the term *paresis* is often used instead of paralysis. Various terms are used to designate paralysis distributed in different ways. Thus *hemiplegia* is the term applied to paralysis affecting one side of the face, with the corresponding arm and leg, as the result of disease on one side of the brain; *diplegia* means a condition of more or less total paralysis, in which both sides are affected in this manner; *monoplegia* is the term applied to paralysis of a single limb; and *paraplegia* signifies paralysis of both sides of the body below a given level, usually from about the level of the waist; *quadriplegia* is paralysis of all four limbs.

Paralysis is a symptom of underlying disease and these paragraphs cover in general terms only the more common types.

(1) PARALYSIS DUE TO BRAIN DISEASE   Of this, by far the most common form is palsy affecting one side of the body, or *Hemiplegia*. It usually arises from disease of the hemisphere of the brain opposite to the side of the body affected, such disease being in the form of haemorrhage into the brain substance (*cerebral haemorrhage*), or the plugging up of blood-vessels by a locally formed clot (*cerebral thrombosis*) or by

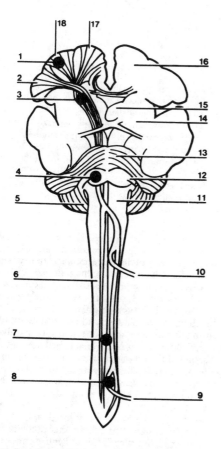

Brain and spinal cord, showing motor paths and positions of injuries causing various forms of paralysis. 1 position of haemorrhage causing paralysis of left arm; 2 face; 3 position of haemorrhage causing complete paralysis of left side; 4 position of haemorrhage followed by paralysis of left arm and leg with right side of face (crossed paralysis); 5 cerebellum; 6 spinal cord; 7 position of disorder causing paralysis of both lower limbs (paraplegia); 8 position of the disease responsible for poliomyelitis in the left leg; 9 to leg; 10 to arm; 11 medulla oblongata; 12 seventh nerve (facial); 13 pons; 14 lentiform nucleus; 15 thalamus; 16 cerebral hemisphere; 17 leg; 18 arm.

a clot dislodged from some other part of the body (*cerebral embolism*), and consequent arrest of blood supply to an area of the brain; or again, it may result from an injury, or be due to a tumour in the tissues of the brain. The character of the seizure and the amount of paralysis vary according to the situation of the disease or injury, its extent, and its sudden or gradual occurrence. The attack may come on as a stroke (see STROKE), in which the patient becomes suddenly unconscious, and loses completely the power of motion of one side of the body, or a like result may arise more gradually and without loss of consciousness. In either type of complete hemiplegia, the paralysis affects on one side the muscles of the face, tongue, body, and limbs. Speech is indistinct and thick, and the tongue, when protruded, points towards the paralysed side owing to the unopposed action of its muscles on the unaffected side. The muscles of the face implicated are chiefly those about the mouth. The paralysed side hangs loose, and the corner of the mouth is depressed, but the muscles closing the eye are, as a rule, unimpaired, because movements like that of shutting the eyes, which are performed usually on both sides together, are controlled from either side of the brain. As a result the eye on the paralysed side can be shut, unlike what occurs in another form of facial paralysis (Bell's palsy), in which the fault lies in the nerve. The muscles of respiration on the affected side are seldom more than slightly weakened for deep breathing, but those of the arm and leg are completely powerless. Sensation may at first be impaired (anaesthesia), but as a rule returns soon, unless the portion of the brain affected is connected with this function. Rigidity of the paralysed members is usually present as a later symptom. In many cases of even complete hemiplegia, improvement takes place after the lapse of weeks or months, and is in general indicated by a return of motor power, first in the face, next in the leg, while that of the arm follows after a longer or shorter interval, and is rarely complete. Such recovery of movement is, however, only partial in a large proportion of cases and the side remains weakened. Prolonged rehabilitative treatment is essential including the supply of physical aids to help minimize the effects of disability.

TREMBLING PALSY, PARALYSIS AGITANS; PARKINSONISM or SHAKING PARALYSIS (see PARKINSONISM). CEREBRAL PALSY (q.v.).

FUNCTIONAL PARALYSIS includes other forms of paralysis which, being of cerebral origin, should be mentioned here, although they are not connected with any discoverable disease of the brain. These forms of paralysis are amenable to psychological treatment, the cause of the paralysis often being traceable to some deepseated mental conflict having its origin in childhood. (See HYSTERIA.)

(2) PARALYSIS DUE TO DISEASE OF THE SPINAL CORD   Of paralysis from this cause, there are numerous varieties, depending on the nature, the site, and the extent of the disease. Frequently defects in muscular action, due to

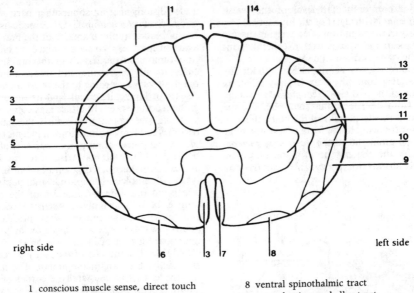

right side   left side

1 conscious muscle sense, direct touch   8 ventral spinothalmic tract
2 unconscious muscle sense   9 ventral spinocerebellar tract
3 voluntary control of striated muscle   10 lateral spinothalmic tract
4 involuntary control of striated muscle   11 rubrospinal tract (extrapyramidal
5 pain, heat and cold   12 lateral corticospinal tract (pyramidal)
6 crossed touch   13 dorsal spinocerebellar tract
7 ventral corticospinal tract (pyramidal)   14 posterior columns

Diagram of a cross-section of spinal cord. Nerve
tracts are shown on the right and their function
on the left.

disease in the spinal cord, are not of a paralytic nature, and these must be carefully distinguished.

PARAPLEGIA, paralysis of both lower extremities, including usually the lower portion of the trunk, and occasionally also the upper portion – indeed, all the parts below the seat of the disease in the spinal cord – is a form of paralysis which is a common result of injuries or disease of the vertebral column; also of inflammation affecting the spinal cord (myelitis), as well as of haemorrhage or tumours involving its substance. When it is due to disease, this is generally situated in the lower portion of the cord. The symptoms necessarily vary in relation to the locality and the extent of the disease in the cord. Thus, if in the affected area the posterior part of the cord, including the posterior nerve roots, suffer, the function of sensation in the parts below is impaired because the cord is unable to transmit the sensory impressions from the surface of the body to the brain, and the condition of ataxia affects the power of motion. If, on the other hand, the anterior portion of the cord and the anterior nerve roots be affected, the motor impulses from the brain cannot be conveyed to the muscles below the seat of the injury or disease, and consequently their power of movement is abolished. Whilst, if the lateral portions of the cord be affected, a condition of spastic paralysis is set up. In many

forms of this complaint, particularly in the case of injuries, the whole thickness of the cord is involved (transverse myelitis), and both sensory and motor functions are lost below the level at which the cord is affected. Further, the functions of the bladder and bowels are apt to suffer, and either spasm, or more often paralysis, of these organs is the result. Bed sores and wasting of the muscles are common. Occasionally, more especially in cases of injury, recovery takes place, but in general this is incomplete, the power of walking being more or less impaired. When the paralysis is due to pressure caused by a diseased or injured spine, an operation designed to relieve this pressure is often completely successful, and entire power is restored, even after the paralysis has lasted for several months. Advances in rehabilitative treatment and the provision of physical aids, some electronically controlled, have gone a long way towards ameliorating the lot of the paraplegic patient and allowing him or her to lead a reasonably active life at home and in the community. Patients and their relatives can obtain help and advice from the Spinal Injuries Association and Spinal Injuries Scotland (see APPENDIX 2: ADDRESSES).

INFANTILE PARALYSIS (see POLIOMYELITIS).

MOTOR NEURONE DISEASE is a disease usually occurring in middle life. Pathologically it is characterized by degeneration: (*a*) of the anterior horn cells of the grey matter of the spinal cord, with corresponding degeneration of the peripheral motor nerves and wasting of the muscles innervated by them; (b) of the nerve cells in the bulb of the brain from which the motor cranial nerves arise hypoglossal, facial, trigeminal, oculomotor, accessory, glossopharyngeal, vagus; (c) in some cases the large motor neurones of the cerebral cortex that give rise to the cortico-spinal tract. There is diffuse atrophy of the white matter of the spinal cord, excepting the posterior, sensory columns. The cause of the degeneration is not known. Approximately one person in 50,000 develops it each year, and it is estimated that there are around 5000 victims of it in the United Kingdom.

BULBAR PARALYSIS may occur as a form of motor neurone disease, or as a complication of other diseases, including rabies, diphtheria, and polyneuritis. The muscles of facial expression, of mastication, of articulation, and of swallowing suffer progressive loss of power.

Treatment All forms of motor neurone disease run an inexorable course to a fatal termination. There is no treatment in the strict sense of the term, but much can be done to make the lot of the victim more comfortable.

Much help can be obtained from the Motor Neurone Disease Association (see APPENDIX 2: ADDRESSES).

PROGRESSIVE MUSCULAR DYSTROPHY, MYOPATHY, or PSEUDOHYPERTROPHIC MUSCULAR DYSTROPHY, is one of the muscular dystrophies. (See MYOPATHY.)

(3) PERIPHERAL PARALYSIS, or local paralysis of individual nerves, is of frequent occurrrence. Only the most common and important examples of this condition will be briefly referred to.

FACIAL PARALYSIS and BELL'S PALSY are the terms applied to paralysis involving the muscles of expression supplied by the seventh cranial nerve. It is unilateral. The cause is not known, but it sometimes follows exposure of one side of the head to a draught of cold air, which sets up inflammation of the nerve. It may also be due to injury or disease either affecting the nerve near the surface or deeper in the bony canals through which it passes, or in the brain itself, involving the nerve at its origin. The paralysis is manifested by a marked change in the expression of the face, the patient being unable to move the muscles of one side in such acts as laughing, and whistling, or to close the eye on that side. Recovery usually takes place in about six weeks, the improvement being first shown in the power of closing the eye, which is soon followed by the disappearance of the other signs. Recovery may be speeded up by the administration of prednisolone (q.v.), especially if this is given at an early stage of the disease. It is more effective in younger patients (under the age of 45) than older ones. When the paralysis proceeds from damage to the nerve, disease of the temporal bone, or from tumours in the brain, it is more apt to be permanent.

A form of peripheral paralysis often results from chronic alcoholism. Other poisons also act similarly, as, for example, lead and arsenic. (See NEURITIS.) Injury to a nerve may cause paralysis in the muscles which it should supply, and this may follow on wounds, severe bruises, or even long-continued pressure, as in crutch-palsy. (See DROP-WRIST; NERVE INJURIES.)

Treatment Generally speaking, the treatment consists of measures which aim at supporting the patient's strength and maintaining his health while the nervous system is slowly restoring itself.

An important point in the treatment is that, since paralysed muscles tend to undergo degenerative changes, their action should be maintained as long as possible. With the view of improving the circulation in the muscles, and also in order to prevent stiffening of the joints, massage is very useful.

Patients with paraplegia need highly skilled nursing and rehabilitative support, since not only the patient's comfort but his life depends upon careful management, directed towards preventing bed sores (see BED SORES), and inflammation of the bladder (see CATHETERS).

PARAMEDICAL A generic title for the professions which work closely with or are reponsible to the medical profession in caring for patients. A paramedical worker has skills, experience and qualifications in certain spheres of health care. Examples are ambulance staff, primarily those trained to deal with emergencies, physiotherapists (q.v.), radiographers (q.v.) and dieticians (q.v.).

PARAMETER A measurement of a certain factor – for example, pulse rate, blood pressure, or haemoglobin concentration – that is relevant to a disorder under investigation.

PARAMNESIA is a derangement of the memory in which words are used without a comprehension of their meaning; it is also applied to illusions of memory in which a person in good faith imagines and describes experiences which never occurred to him.

PARANOIA is a form of mental illness characterized by fixed delusions, usually of persecution. Many sufferers are able to go about freely and carry out activities with which their delusions do not interfere. In loose English usage, 'paranoia' means 'subject to any sorts of feelings of persecution'. (See MENTAL ILLNESS).

PARAPHASIA is misplacement of words, or use of wrong words, in speech as a result of a lesion in the speech region of the brain.

PARAPHIMOSIS The constriction of the penis behind the glans by an abnormally tight foreskin that has been retracted. The condition causes swelling and severe pain. Sometimes the foreskin can be returned by manual manipulation after an ice pack has been applied to the glans. Sometimes an operation to cut the foreskin is required to release it.

PARAPHRENIA is a form of paranoia (q.v.). (See also MENTAL ILLNESS.)

PARAPLEGIA means paralysis of the lower limbs, accompanied generally by paralysis of bladder and rectum. (See PARALYSIS.)

PARAQUAT is a contact herbicide widely used in agriculture and horticulture. A mouthful is enough to kill. Its major misuse has resulted from its being decanted from the professional pack into soft-drink bottles and kept in the domestic kitchen. The resultant potential for accidental and probably fatal ingestion is obvious. It is involved in around 40 cases of suicide every year. The eyes and skin must be carefully protected so as not to come into contact with it. So widespread is its use that nineteen medical centres have been set up throughout the country to provide treatment in cases of poisoning with it. Details of these can be obtained from the National Poisons Information Service centres (see APPENDIX 2: ADDRESSES).

PARASITE An organism which lives in or on another organism, known as the host. A parasite derives all its nourishment from the host but provides no benefits in return. It may damage the host's bodily functions and in extreme cases cause the death of the host. Human parasites include worms, fungi, bacteria and viruses.

PARASITICIDE is a general term applied to agents or substances destructive to parasites.

PARASUICIDE is non-fatal self-poisoning or self-injury, or attempted suicide. It is most common in the 12–15 age-group. The intention is not as a rule to commit suicide, but a cry for help to resolve an acute domestic upset.

PARASYMPATHETIC NERVOUS SYSTEM is that part of the autonomic nervous system (q.v.) which is connected with the brain and spinal cord through certain nerve centres in the mid-brain, medulla, and lower end of the cord. The nerves from these centres are carried in the 3rd, 7th, 9th, and 10th cranial nerves and the 2nd, 3rd, and 4th sacral nerves. The action of the parasympathetic system is usually antagonistic to that of the sympathetic system. Thus it inhibits the action of the heart and augments the action of the intestine, whereas the sympathetic augments the action of the heart and inhibits that of the intestine. (See diagram of sympathetic and parasympathetic nervous systems under NERVES.)

PARATHION is one of the organo-phosphorus insecticides (q.v.). It is highly toxic to man and must therefore be handled with the utmost care.

PARATHYROID is the name applied to four small glands, about 5 mm in diameter, which lie to the side of and behind the thyroid gland. These glands regulate the metabolism of calcium and of phosphorus. If for any reason there is a deficiency of the secretion of the parathyroid glands, the amount of calcium in the blood falls too low and the amount of phosphorus increases. The result is the condition known as tetany (q.v.), in which there is great restlessness and spasm of muscles. The condition is checked by the injection of calcium gluconate – which causes an increase in the amount of calcium in the blood. The commonest cause of this condition, or hypoparathyroidism as it is known, is accidental injury to or removal of the glands during the operation of thyroidectomy for the treatment of Graves' disease (q.v.). This is one of the hazards of thyroidectomy in view of the very close relationship of the parathyroid glands to the thyroid gland. If there is over-production of the parathyroids there will be an increase of calcium in the blood. This extra calcium is drawn from the bones, in which, as a consequence, thin cysts form and greatly weaken the bones, these breaking easily as a result. This cystic disease of bone is known as OSTEITIS FIBROSA CYSTICA (q.v.). Tumours of the parathyroid glands result in this overactivity of the parathyroid hormone, and the resulting increase in the amount of calcium in the blood leads to the formation of stones in the kidneys. The only available treatment is surgical removal of the tumour. This state of increased activity of the parathyroid glands, or hyperparathyroidism, is always considered as a possible cause in dealing with a case of stones in the kidneys. (See KIDNEYS, DISEASES OF.)

PARATYPHOID FEVER (see ENTERIC FEVER).

PAREGORIC, or CAMPHORATED OPIUM TINCTURE, is a preparation of opium much used for cough mixtures. It contains 5 per cent of tincture of opium, together with oil of anise, benzoic acid and camphor. The dose is 2 to 10 ml. Scotch paregoric, or ammoniated opium tincture, contains 10 per cent of tincture of opium, together with dilute ammonia solution, oil of anise and benzoic acid. The dose is 2 to 4 ml.

PARENCHYMA is a term meaning originally all the soft tissues of internal organs except the muscular flesh, though now reserved for the secreting cells of the glandular organs.

PARENTERAL is the word applied to the administration of drugs by any route other than by the mouth or by the bowel.

PARENTERAL NUTRITION In severely ill patients, especially those who have had major surgery or with sepsis, burns, acute pancreatitis and renal failure, the body's reserves of protein become exhausted. This results in weight loss, reduction of muscle mass, a fall in the serum albumin and lymphocyte count and an impairment of cellular immunity. Severely ill patients are unable to take adequate food by mouth to repair the body protein loss so that enteral or parenteral nutrition is required. Enteral feeding is through the gastro-intestinal tract with the aid of a naso-gastric tube. Parenteral nutrition involves the provision of carbohydrate, fat and proteins by intravenous administration. Intitally the carbohydrate glucose was the sole energy substrate used, but it soon became appreciated that regimes supplying an equal proportion of carbohydrate and fat were preferable in the vast majority of cases. Over the last decade a multitude of nitrogen solutions have been developed for the purpose of intravenous nutrition. As with enteral nutrition there are few indications for the administrations of pure amino acids. All patients requiring intravenous nutrition will require, in addition, a supply of vitamins and essential minerals.

Methods of vascular access have improved remarkably over recent years. The preferred route for the infusion of hyperosmolar solutions is via a central venous catheter. If parenteral nutrition is required for more than two weeks it is advisable to use a long-term type catheter such as the Broviac, Hickman or extra corporeal type, which is made of silastic material and is inserted via a long subcutaneous tunnel, which not only helps to fix the catheter but minimizes the risk of ascending infection.

Dextrose is considered the best source of carbohydrate and may be used as a 20-per-cent or 50-per-cent solution. Amino acids should be in the laevo form and should contain the correct proportion of essential and non-essential amino acids. Preparations such as Vamin glucose 9, Synthamin 9 (low nitrogen solution), Synthamin 14 and 17 (high nitrogen solutions) are available with or without electrolytes. Intralipid is the safest fat emulsion and is used either as 10 per cent or 20 per cent solution.

The main hazards of intravenous feeding are blood-borne infections made possible by continued direct access to the circulation, and biochemical abnormalities related to the composition of the solutions infused. The continuous use of hypertonic solutions of glucose can cause hyperglycaemia and glycosuria and the resultant polyuria may lead to dehydration. Treatment with insulin is needed when hyperosmolality occurs, and in addition the water and sodium deficits will require to be corrected.

PARESIS means a state of partial paralysis. (See PARALYSIS.)

PARIETAL is the term applied to anything pertaining to the wall of a cavity: e.g. parietal pleura, the part of the pleural membrane which lines the wall of the chest.

PARIETAL LOBE A major section of each cerebral hemisphere (see BRAIN). The two lobes lie under the parietal bones and contain the sensory cortex.

PARKINSONISM, or PARKINSON'S DISEASE, so called after the London general practitioner who first described the condition in 1817, is also known as PARALYSIS AGITANS. It is a progressive disease of insidious onset which comes on in the second half of life, and is due to degenerative changes in the ganglia at the base of the cerebrum. This results in a deficiency of a neurotransmitter known as dopamine (q.v.), and it is this deficiency of dopamine which is responsible for most cases. In some, however, deficiency of neurotransmitters other than dopamine may be the cause. It is much commoner in men than in women. In some cases the disease is a sequel to encephalitis lethargica. The disease first manifests itself by increasing rigidity of the muscles. In the face this results in a loss of the natural play of expression and produces a mask-like expression. The voice is also affected by the rigidity of the muscles of the larynx, tongue and lips, loses its tone and inflexion and develops into a monotone. Later the limbs become rigid, and this is typified by the peculiar running gait. The patient always seems to be tottering and taking short steps as if running after himself. Later a coarse tremor develops in the muscles, best typified in the rolling movements of the fingers as if a cigarette were always being rolled. The tremor is exaggerated by excitement and self-consciousness and ceases during sleep. In the hands and arms it may interfere grossly with eating and dressing.

Treatment There is now an increasing number of drugs that keep the condition under control. None is curative, and the effort to find the most suitable one for any given individual is usually a matter of trial and error, the successful outcome of which depends largely upon understanding co-operation between family doctor and patient. Levodopa, a precursor of dopamine, is valuable. Its introduction has revolutionized the outlook in this disease. Unfortunately it has considerable side-effects, which means that it must only be administered under medical supervision. Levodopa produces spectacular improvement in one-fifth of patients, moderate improvement in two-fifths, modest improvement in one-fifth, and no improvement in one-fifth. A recently introduced drug proving of value in supplementing the benefit of levodopa is selegiline. A small number of other drugs are also available which may be of help to certain patients with the disorder.

Patients with the disease and their relatives, seeking advice and help, are recommended to get in touch with the Parkinson's Disease Society of the UK (see APPENDIX 2: ADDRESSES).

PARONYCHIA is the term applied to inflammation near the nail. In the *acute* form it is usually due to infection with *Staphylococcus aureus*, and is most often seen in nurses and others handling septic material. It usually starts at one corner of the nail-fold and then spreads to the other side and deeply under the base of the nail. There is local pain and tenderness, with swelling of the nail-fold. Treatment in mild cases consists of applying an adhesive dressing and giving penicillin. In more severe cases the swelling has to be opened. A new nail grows in two or three months, displacing the old one in front of it. *Chronic paronychia* occurs usually in women who have their hands much in water. In men it occurs in fishmongers and chefs. It may affect one or more fingers. Treatment consists of keeping the finger dry and giving a suitable antibiotic. (See WHITLOW.)

PAROSMIA means a perverted sense of smell; everything usually smells unpleasant to the affected individual. The most common cause is some septic condition of the nasal passages, but it may occasionally be due to a lesion in the brain involving the centre responsible for the sense of smell.

PAROTID GLAND is one of the salivary glands (q.v.). It is situated just in front of the ear, and its duct runs forwards across the cheek to open into the interior of the mouth on a little projection opposite the second last tooth of the upper row. The parotid gland is generally the first of the salivary glands to become enlarged in mumps.

PAROTITIS means inflammation of the parotid gland. Epidemic parotitis is another name for mumps (q.v.).

PAROXETINE is an antidepressant drug in the selective serotonin-reuptake inhibitors (SRRIs) group (q.v.). (See MENTAL ILLNESS.)

PAROXYSM A sudden temporary attack that may take the form of a convulsion or spasm. It may also occur when a patient with a disease suddenly deteriorates.

PARTHENOGENESIS is non-sexual reproduction. In other words, development of the ovum into an individual without fertilization by a spermatozoon. It has been produced in animals experimentally. There is, however, no certain record of the birth of a parthenogenetic animal. The most that has been achieved is that parthogenetic mice and rabbit embryos have developed normally to about halfway through pregnancy but have then died and been aborted.

PARTOGRAM is a method of recording the degree of dilatation, or opening, of the cervix (or neck) of the uterus in labour, which is of value in assessing how labour is progressing.

PARTURITION (see LABOUR).

PARVOVIRUSES (from *parvus*, Latin for small) is a group of viruses responsible for outbreaks of winter vomiting disease (q.v.).

P.A.S. is a commonly used abbreviation for para-aminosalicylic acid (q.v.).

PASSIVE MOVEMENT A movement induced by someone other than the patient. Physiotherapists manipulate joints by passive movement in order to retain and encourage function of a nerve or muscle that is not working normally because of injury or disease.

PASTEURELLA is a group of bacilli. They are essentially animal parasites that under certain conditions are transmitted to man. They include the micro-organism responsible for plague and tularaemia.

PASTEURIZATION is a method of sterilizing milk. In many parts of the world pasteurization has done away with milk-borne infections, of which the most serious is bovine tuberculosis, affecting the glands, bones, and joints of children. Other infections conveyed by milk are scarlet fever, diphtheria, enteric fever (typhoid and paratyphoid), undulant fever (brucellosis), and food poisoning (e.g. from salmonellae or the toxins of the staphylococcus). The case therefore is very clear for the compulsory pasteurization of all milk. Yet 10 per cent of all milk retailed in Scotland is neither pasteurized nor heat treated in any way. The comparable figure for England and Wales is 3 per cent.
HIGH-TEMPERATURE SHORT-TIME (HTST) PASTEURIZATION consists in heating the milk at a temperature not less than $71 \cdot 7$ °C (161 °F) for at least fifteen seconds, followed by immediate cooling to a temperature of not more than 10 °C (50 °F).
LOW-TEMPERATURE PASTEURIZATION, or 'HOLDER' PROCESS, consists in maintaining the milk for at least half-an-hour at a temperature between 63 to 65 °C (145 to 150 °F), followed by immediate cooling to a temperature of not more that 10 °C (50 °F). This has the effect of considerably reducing the number of bacteria contained in the milk and of preventing the diseases conveyed by milk referred to above. This procedure is sufficient for the sale of milk as 'pasteurized milk' in England. (See MILK.)

PATCH TEST This is used to identify possible substances that may be causing a patient's allergy. Small amounts of different substances are placed on the skin, usually the back or arm. If the patient is allergic a red flare and swelling will appear, usually within about 15 minutes.

Sometimes the reaction may take longer – up to three days – to develop.

PATELLA, also known as the knee-pan or knee-cap, is a flat bone shaped somewhat like an oyster-shell, lying in the tendon of the extensor muscle of the thigh, and protecting the knee-joint in front. (See BONE; KNEE; FRACTURES.)

PATELLAR REFLEX (see REFLEX ACTION).

PATENT DUCTUS ARTERIOSUS (see DUCTUS ARTERIOSUS).

PATHOGENIC means disease-producing, and is a term, for example, applied to bacteria, capable of causing disease.

PATHOGNOMONIC is a term applied to signs or symptoms which are specially characteristic of certain diseases, and on the presence or absence of which the diagnosis depends. Thus the discovery of the *Mycobacterium tuberculosis* in the expectoration is said to be pathognomonic of pulmonary tuberculosis.

PATHOLOGY is the science which deals with the causes of, and changes produced in the body by, disease.

PATIENT-CONTROLLED ANALGESIA A technique whereby a patient can deliver an analgesic substance in amounts related to the extent of the pain he is suffering. For example, to combat postoperative pain some hospitals use devices which allow patients to give themselves small intravenous amounts of opiates when they are needed. Pain is more effectively controlled if it is not allowed to reach a high level, a situation which tends to happen when patients receive analgesics only on ward drug rounds or when they ask the nursing staff for them.

PAUL-BUNNELL TEST is a test for mononucleosis (q.v.) which is based upon the fact that patients with this disease develop antibodies which agglutinate sheep red blood cells.

PECTIN is a polysaccharide substance allied to starch, contained in fruits and plants, and forming the basis of vegetable jelly. It has been used as a transfusion fluid in place of blood in cases of haemorrhage and shock.

PECTORAL means anything pertaining to the chest, or a remedy used in treating chest troubles.

PECTORILOQUY means the resonance of the voice, when spoken or whispered words can be clearly heard through the stethoscope. It is a sign of consolidation, or of a cavity, in the lung.

PEDICLE A narrow tube of tissue formed by folded skin which links a piece of tissue used for surgical grafting to its site of origin. A pedicle graft is used by the surgeon when the site under repair is unsuitable for an independent graft, usually because the blood supply at the recipient site is inadequate.

A pedicle is also found occurring between a tumour and its tissue of origin, and the term is used in anatomy to refer to any slim tubular process.

PEDICULOSIS is infestation with lice.

PEDICULI, or lice, are of three species, which vary in shape and size as well as in the area of the body they infest.

PEDICULUS HUMANUS var. CAPITIS (*Pediculus capitis*), or the head louse, is similar in practically all respects to the body louse, except that it occurs in the head and not on the trunk of the body. It is more common in girls and women than boys and men. The eggs, commonly known as nits and visible as little white specks, are usually laid in the hairs of the back of the head; behind the ears is also a favourite site. On infested heads the hairs are often matted together by the exudate which results from irritation and scratching. The glands behind the ears and in the back of the neck are often enlarged.

PEDICULUS HUMANUS var. CORPORIS (*Pediculus vestimenti*), or the body louse, is found on the underclothing on the trunk and upper arms, rather than on the skin. The female louse, which has a life of almost a month, lays seven to ten eggs a day. The eggs hatch out in 7 to 10 days and become mature in another week. Without food the adult dies in nine days and the newly hatched louse in two days. The eggs are viable for much longer (up to a month) and are usually found in the more inaccessible parts of the clothing: e.g. the seams.

PEDICULUS PUBIS, popularly known as the crab louse, is broader and shorter. It is found predominantly on the short hairs of the pubic region, to which it adheres very tenaciously. It may also infest the eye-lashes, beard, and leg and under-arm hairs. It causes intense itching. So far as is known, it does not carry any disease. It is most commonly transmitted from one person to another by sexual contact. Live lice have been found on lavatory seats, and the eggs may be spread from a lousy person by attachment of their infected hairs to towels and clothing.

(For further details, see INSECTS IN RELATION TO DISEASE.)

PEDUNCLE A stalk-like structure that usually acts as a support.

PELLAGRA is a nutritional disorder, showing a number of nervous, digestive, and skin symptoms.

Causes It occurs in those parts of the world where the inhabitants live on a diet of maize without adequate first-class protein in the form of milk and meat. It is due to deficiency of the nicotinic acid component of the vitamin B complex, in association with deficiency of protein. For long the puzzling feature was that it occurred predominantly in maize-eating areas of the world, yet maize has as much nicotinic acid as wheat but the disease did not occur in wheat-eating areas. The explanation is that the nicotinic acid in maize is in a bound form that the consumer cannot utilize. Further, maize is deficient in the amino-acid, tryptophan, from which the human body can make nicotinic acid.

Symptoms Pellagra is known as the disease of the three D's: dermatitis, diarrhoea and dementia. The course of pellagra lasts many years, with digestive disturbances including loss of appetite and diarrhoea or constipation, headache, and irritability of temper. The skin manifestations consist at first of redness resembling severe sunburn on the parts of the body exposed to the sun, such as the hands, forearms, chest, neck, and face. The irritation usually lasts about a fortnight, is followed by desquamation, and the skin remains rough, thickened, and permanently brownish in colour. This brownish and roughened appearance on the hands is the most prominent feature of the disease, and from this the disease takes its name. Tremors, sleepiness, and weakness of the legs also appear. For several years the disease may recur in this manner every spring, the attacks gradually becoming more severe, the patient slowly growing emaciated and in some cases completely paralytic or demented.

Treatment The disease is prevented or cured by adding to the diet foods such as fresh meat, eggs, milk, liver, and yeast extracts, and nicotinic acid, as well as by improvement of the general conditions of life.

PELVIC INFLAMMATORY DISEASE Acute or chronic infection of the ovaries, fallopian tube, or uterus. The condition is usually caused by infection spreading from the vagina or from a nearby infected organ – for example, the appendix. Blood-borne infection may also be the cause. Lower abdominal pain, sometimes severe, is characteristic of the condition. Treatment may be by antibiotics or sometimes surgery.

PELVIMETRY Measurement of the internal dimensions of the pelvis. The four diameters measured are: transverse, anterioposterior, and left and right oblique. These measurements help to establish whether a fetus can be delivered normally. If the outlet is abnormally small, the mother will have to be delivered by Caesarian section.

PELVIS The bony pelvis consists of the two hip bones, one on each side, with the sacrum and coccyx behind. It connects the legs with the spine. It connects the lower limbs with the spine. Each hip bone is composed of three originally separate bones, in the adult pelvis firmly fused together: the ilium; the ischium, with a rounded part below, the tuberosity, upon which the body rests in sitting; and the pubis in front. The expanded parts of the iliac bones incompletely surround the lower part of the abdomen, known as the false pelvis, and are separated by a distinct line, known as the brim or inlet, from the true pelvis beneath. The true pelvis, as its name implies, is basin-shaped; though in the dried state it has a wide outlet beneath, yet in the living body this is well closed and rounded off by ligaments and muscles so as to leave small openings only for the urinary and genital passages and for the rectum. This soft floor of the pelvis is composed mainly of two muscles, the levators of the anus, whilst the deep notch, between the haunch-bone and sacrum behind, is closed in by a pair of strong sacro-sciatic ligaments.

The pelvis varies considerably in the two sexes. In the female it is shallower and the ilia are more widely separated, giving great breadth to the hips of the woman; the inlet is more circular and the outlet larger; whilst the angle beneath the pubic bones (subpubic angle), which is an acute angle in the male, is obtuse in the female. All these points are of importance in connection with child-bearing.

The contents of the pelvis are the urinary bladder and rectum in both sexes; in addition the male has the seminal vesicles and the prostate gland surrounding the neck of the bladder, whilst the female has the womb, ovaries, and their appendages.

In addition to these sex differences, the pelvis differs between races. It tends to be wider from front to back and longer from top to bottom in black people than in white people: the so-called anthropoid pelvis.

PEMPHIGOID (see PEMPHIGUS).

PEMPHIGUS is an autoimmune skin condition characterized by the appearance of large blebs. *Pemphigus neonatorum* is really a form of impetigo in which bullae (or large blisters) occur. (The term pemphigus neonatorum is misleading and should be abandoned.) It is liable to occur in nurseries and maternity hospitals and is highly infectious. Strict isolation of cases is essential and the prognosis is satisfactory provided active treatment is started at an early stage. In addition to the local treatment recommended for impetigo in older children and adults, an antibiotic or sulphonamide should be given provided the staphylococcus responsible or the condition is sensitive to it. Unfortunately *Staphylococcus aureus*, especially that which occurs in hospital, is so often resistant to penicillin that this antibiotic is of no avail, and some other has to be used. *Pemphigus vulgaris*, which occurs in the middle-aged, particularly Jews, is a comparatively rare condition. The skin eruption is accompanied by marked constitutional disturbances and, until the introduction of the corticosteroids (q.v.) it was almost invariably fatal, though it still carries a mortality rate of 30–50 per cent. With large doses of corticosteroids, however, the condition can usually be kept under control. The local application of zinc cream or calamine lotion is soothing. *Pemphigus foliaceus*, in which practically the whole of the skin may be involved, is not marked by such constitutional disturbances. Treatment is as for pemphigus vulgaris. *Pemphigoid* is the form of the disease as it occurs in old age. It responds well to corticosteroids. It may occur as a complication of penicillamine or gold therapy and usually clears on withdrawal of the offending drug.

PENICILLAMINE is a metabolite of penicillin which is a chelating agent (q.v.). It is sometimes used in rheumatoid arthritis that has not responded to the first-line remedies and it is particularly useful when the disease is complicated by vasculitis. Penicillamine is also used as an antidote to poisoning by heavy metals, particularly copper and lead, as it is able to bind these metals and so remove their toxic effects. Because of its ability to bind copper it is also used in Wilson's disease where there is a deficiency in the copper-binding protein so that copper is able to become deposited in he brain and liver, damaging these tissues.

PENICILLIN is the name given by Sir Alexander Fleming, in 1929, to an antibacterial substance produced by the mould *Penicillium notatum*. This mould was first described in 1911 in Scandinavia, where it was discovered in decaying hyssop. The story of penicillin is one of the most dramatic in the history of medicine, and its introduction into medicine initiated a new era in therapeutics comparable only to the introduction of anaesthesia by Morton and Simpson and of antiseptics by Pasteur and Lister. The two names that will always be primarily associated with penicillin are those of Sir Alexander Fleming, of St Mary's Hospital, London, who discovered its anti-bacterial action, and Lord Florey, of Oxford, who did so much to develop its practical use during the 1939–45 War. The two great advantages of penicillin are that it is active against a large range of bacteria and that, even in large doses, it is non-toxic. Penicillin diffuses well into body tissues and fluids and is excreted in the urine, but it penetrates poorly into the cerebrospinal fluid. An important side-effect of penicillins is hypersensitivity which causes rashes and sometimes anaphylaxis (q.v.), which can be fatal. Among the organisms against which it is active are: staphylococcus, strepto-coccus, pneumococcus, meningococcus, gonococcus, and the organisms responsible for syphilis, and for gas gangrene.

Penicillin has been synthesized in the laboratory, and various forms of penicillin are now available. These include the following broad groups: benzylpenicillin and phenoxymethyl-penicillin; penicillinase-resistant penicillins; broad-spectrum penicillins; antipseudomonal penicillins; and mecillinams. Brief details of some of the commonly used penicillins follow. *Benzylpenicillin* is available as the sodium or potassium salt. It is given intramuscularly, and is the form that is used when a rapid action is required. It can also be given by mouth but, as the proportion absorbed varies greatly, it is unreliable in action when given in this way. *Procaine penicillin* is a relatively insoluble form of penicillin. A single daily intramuscular injection of 600,000 units will maintain a bacteriostatic level in the blood for twenty-four hours. *Phenoxymethylpenicillin* is given by mouth but is absorbed inconstantly.

Ampicillin is another of the penicillins derived by semi-synthesis from the penicillin nucleus. It, too, is active when taken by mouth, but its special feature is that it is active against Gram-negative micro-organisms such as *E. coli* and the salmonellae. *Cloxacillin* is yet another of the semi-synthesized penicillins. It has a relatively weak antibacterial action, but has the advantage of being active against penicillin-resistant staphylococci.

Methicillin is another penicillin derived from the penicillin nucleus. It is active against penicillin-resistant staphylococci but has to be given by injection as it is destroyed by the acid secretion of the stomach. *Carbenicillin*, a semi-synthetic penicillin, must be given by injection, which may be painful. Its main use is in dealing with infections due to *Pseudomonas pyocanea*. It is the only penicillin active against this micro-organism. *Piperacillin* and *Ticarcillin* are carboxypenicillins used to treat infections caused by *Pseudomonas aeruginosa* and *Proteus* spp. *Flucloxacillin*, also a semi-synthetic penicillin, is active against penicillin-resistant staphylococci and has the practical advantage of being active when taken by mouth. *Amoxycillin* is an oral semi-synthetic penicillin with the same range of action as ampicillin but less likely to cause side-effects. *Mecillinam* is yet another in this series, though of slightly different chemical origin. It is of value in the treatment of infections with salmonellae (see FOOD POISONING), including typhoid fever, and with *E. coli* (see ESCHERICHIA). It is given by injection. There is a derivative, *Pivmecillinam*, which can be taken by mouth.

PENIS is the organ down which, in the male, passes the urethra, the tube by which the contents of the urinary bladder and those of the seminal vesicles escape (see EJACULATION).

PENTAMIDINE is a drug that is used in the prevention and treatment of African trypanosomiasis, and in the treatment of leishmaniasis.

PENTAZOCINE is a pain-relieving drug with similar actions and uses to those of morphine, but much less likely to lead to addiction. It is given, usually by injection, for the relief of moderate to severe pain, especially postoperative pain, and to relieve the pain of myocardial infarction, or coronary thrombosis.

PEPPERMINT is the leaves and tops of *Mentha piperita*. It has an aromatic odour, due to the presence of an oil from which is obtained menthol, a camphor-like substance. Peppermint water is a useful remedy for flatulence and colic in infants. Oil of peppermint is used like the other volatile oils.

PEPSIN is an enzyme found in the gastric juice which digests proteins, converting them into peptides and amino acids. It is used in the preparation of predigested, or 'peptonized', foods (q.v.), or, more frequently, it is taken orally after meals. Available as a white powder or liquid, it is prepared from the mucous membrane of cow, sheep, or pig stomachs.

PEPTIC ULCER is the term commonly applied to ulcers in the stomach and duodenum. (See DUODENAL ULCER; STOMACH, DISEASES OF.)

PEPTIDE is a compound formed by the union of two or more amino-acids.

PEPTONIZED FOODS are foods which have been predigested by pancreatin (q.v.) and thereby rendered more digestible.

PERCUSSION is an aid to diagnosis practised by striking the body with the fingers, in such a way as to make it give out a note. It was introduced in 1761 by Leopold Auenbrugger (1722–1809) of Vienna, the son of an innkeeper, who derived the idea from the habit of his father tapping casks of wine to ascertain how much wine they contained. According to the degree of dullness or resonance of the note, an opinion can be formed as to the state of consolidation of air-containing organs, the presence of abnormal cavities in organs, and the dimensions of solid and air-containing organs, which happen to lie next to one another. Still more valuable evidence is given by auscultation (q.v.).

PERCUTANEOUS is a term applied to any method of administering remedies by passing them through the skin, as by rubbing in an ointment or carrying in drugs on the galvanic current.

PERFORATION The perforation of one of the hollow organs of the abdomen or major blood vessels may occur spontaneously in the case of an ulcer or an advanced tumour or may be secondary to trauma such as a knife wound or penetrating injury from a traffic or industrial accident. Whatever the cause, perforation is a surgical emergency. The intestinal contents, which contain large numbers of bacteria, pass freely out into the abdominal cavity and cause a severe chemical or bacterial peritonitis (q.v.). This is uaully accompanied by severe abdominal pain, collapse or even death. There may also be evidence of free fluid or gas within the abdominal cavity. Surgical intervention, to repair the leak and wash out the contamination, is often necessary. Perforation or rupture of major blood vessels, whether from disease or injury, is an acute emergency for which urgent surgical repair is usually necessary. Perforation of hollow structures elsewhere than in the abdomen – for example, the heart or oesophagus – may be caused by congenital weaknesses, disease or injury. Treatment is usually surgical but depends on the cause.

PERFUSION The transfer of fluid through a tissue. For example, when blood passes through the lung tissue, dissolved oxygen perfuses from the moist air in the alveoli to the blood. Fluid may also be deliberately introduced into a tissue by injecting it into the blood vessels supplying the tissue.

PERI- is a prefix meaning around.

PERIARTERITIS NODOSA (see POLYARTERITIS NODOSA).

PERICARDITIS means inflammation of the pericardium. (See HEART DISEASES.)

PERICARDIUM is the smooth membrane that surrounds the heart. (See HEART.)

PERICHONDRITIS Inflammation of cartilage (q.v.) and the tissue surrounding it, usually as a result of chronic infection.

PERICYAZINE (see NEUROLEPTICS).

PERIMETRITIS means a localized inflammation of the peritoneum surrounding the womb.

PERINATAL MORTALITY consists of deaths of the fetus after the 28th week of pregnancy and deaths of the new-born child during the first week of life. Today, more individuals die within a few hours of birth than during the following forty years. It is therefore not surprising that the perinatal mortality rate, which is the number of such deaths per 1000 total births, has come to be looked upon as a valuable indicator of the quality of care provided for the mother and her new-born baby. In 1992, the perinatal mortality rate was 7·6 in England, compared with 32·5 in 1960.

The causes of perinatal mortality include intrapartum anoxia (that is, difficulty in the birth of the baby, resulting in lack of oxygen), congenital abnormalities of the baby, antepartum anoxia (that is, conditions in the terminal stages of pregnancy preventing the fetus getting sufficient oxygen), and injuries to the brain of the baby during birth.

In 1992 perinatal deaths in England numbered 4,951 (which number includes still births). The deaths during the first weeks of life numbered 2,174. The commonest cause of perinatal death was some complication of placenta, cord or membranes. The next most common was congenital abnormality. Intra-uterine hypoxia and birth asphyxia comprised the third most common cause.

PERINEUM, or FORK, or CROTCH, is the region situated between the opening of the bowel behind and of the genital organs in front. In women it is apt to be lacerated in the act of childbirth.

PERIOD (see MENSTRUATION).

PERIODIC PARALYSIS is a condition characterized by the onset of weakness of the voluntary muscles. It usually occurs in young adults. As a rule the onset is in the morning on awakening. The weakness usually lasts for several hours. Attacks may also be brought on by a heavy meal or severe cold. It is a familial condition of obscure origin. There is one form, probably the most common, which is apparently due to a low level of potassium in the blood and is relieved by the taking of potassium chloride – 10 grams in water. There are other forms, however, in which the blood potassium may be raised or normal.

PERIODONTAL An adjective that relates to the tissues around the teeth.

PERIODONTAL MEMBRANE (see TEETH).

PERIOSTEUM is the membrane surrounding a bone. The periosteum carries blood-vessels and nerves for the nutrition and development of the bone. When it is irritated, an increased deposit of bone takes place beneath it; if it is destroyed, the bone may cease to grow and a portion may die and separate as a sequestrum. (See BONE.)

PERIOSTITIS means inflammation on the surface of a bone affecting the periosteum. (See BONE, DISEASES OF.)

PERIPHERAL NEURITIS means inflammation of the nerves in the outlying parts of the body. (See NEURITIS.)

PERISTALSIS is the worm-like movement by which the stomach and bowels propel their contents. It consists of alternate waves of relaxation and contraction in successive parts of the tube. When any obstruction to the movement of the contents exists, these contractions become more forcible and are liable to be accompanied by the severe form of pain known as colic.

PERITONEOSCOPY is viewing of the peritoneal cavity through a tube fitted with mirrors and light. The instrument (see ENDOSCOPE) is entered just below the umbilicus. The peritoneal cavity is then inflated with air. This simple operation may obviate a more drastic one: for example, if peritoneoscopy shows deposits of cancer in the peritoneum or the liver. Colour photographs of the liver have been taken through the peritoneoscope.

PERITONEUM is the membrane lining the abdominal cavity, and forming a covering for the organs contained in it. That part lining the walls of the abdomen is called the parietal peritoneum, and that part covering the viscera is known as the visceral peritoneum. The two are continuous with one another at the back of the abdomen, and form a closed sac. The folds of peritoneum passing from one organ to another are thus very complicated, and receive special names in various parts. (See MESENTERY; OMENTUM.)

Although the peritoneum is said to form a closed sac, there is an exception in the female, the Fallopian tube on each side having an opening into the cavity at its end large enough to admit a bristle. There is, however, no large outlet for drainage of fluid, so that a small amount is always present to lubricate the membrane, while a large amount collects in conditions that are associated with oedema.

In structure the peritoneum consists of a dense, though thin and elastic, fibrous membrane covered, on its inner side, by a smooth glistening layer of plate-like epithelial cells. Here and there between the cells are minute openings (stomas), each of which communicates with a lymphatic vessel, so that the fluid in the cavity is constantly draining off into the general lymphatic circulation.

PERITONITIS means inflammation of the peritoneum or membrane investing the abdominal and pelvic cavities and their contained viscera. It may exist in an acute or a chronic form, and may be either localized in one part or generally diffused. Inflammation of this membrane varies much as regards its causes, severity, and danger, according as it is acute or chronic.

ACUTE PERITONITIS **Causes** As a rule it arises because micro-organisms enter the peritoneal cavity, from wounds from the exterior or from the abdominal organs. The great danger which follows upon stabs and other penetrating wounds of the abdomen originates from the risk of peritonitis. Any conditions which lead to perforation of the stomach, bowels, bile-ducts, bladder, and other hollow organs may produce it. Thus gastric ulcer, typhoid fever, gall-stones, rupture of the bladder, strangulated hernia, and obstructions of the bowels may end in peritonitis; appendicitis, abscesses of the ovary and Fallopian tubes are other possible causes.

In some cases the peritonitis becomes *localized* by adhesions between neighbouring organs due to the deposit of fibrin upon their surface. This process takes place with great rapidity, and it makes a great deal of difference to the result of the disease whether it be thus shut in to one part of the abdomen or whether it spreads so rapidly as quickly to become *general*.

The bacteria causing peritonitis are numerous, but among the most common are the *Escherichia coli*, which is always present in the intestine; streptococci, which produce the most virulent form of inflammation; and the gonococcus.

Symptoms The symptoms usually begin by a rigor, together with vomiting and pain in the abdomen of a peculiarly severe and sickening character, accompanied with extreme tenderness, so that the slightest pressure causes intense aggravation of the pain. The patient lies on the back with the knees drawn up, breathing is rapid and shallow and performed by movements of the chest only, the abdominal muscles remaining rigid. The abdomen becomes swollen by flatulent distension of the intestines. There is usually constipation. The skin is hot, and the temperature rises to 40 to 40·5 °C (104 or 105 °F), although there may be no perspiration; the pulse is small in volume; the urine is scanty and dark coloured. These symptoms and signs may subside but, if they do not and the patient is untreated, he or she usually dies.

Treatment The patient should be admitted to hospital for investigation, diagnosis and treatment. Intravenous fluids, antibiotics and surgery for the causative condition form the usual course of action. Such treatment is usually successful. If hospital is not readily accessible, the patient should be given intravenous (or subcutaneous) fluids, strong analgesics such as pethidine by injection and antibiotics. Food should be withheld and the patient should not take fluids by mouth, although the mouth should be washed out regularly to keep it clean and moist. Every effort should be made to obtain skilled professional care.

PERITONSILLAR ABSCESS is the term applied to a collection of pus or an abscess which occurs complicating an attack of tonsillitis. The collection of pus forms between the tonsil and the superior constrictor muscle of the pharynx. This condition is also known as quinsy. The treatment of this condition involves drainage of the abscess and the administration of appropriate antibiotics.

PERNICIOUS ANAEMIA is an auto-immune disease in which the sensitized lymphocytes destroy the parietal cells of the stomach. These cells normally produce intrinsic factor which is the carrier protein for vitamin B_{12} that permits its absorption in the terminal ileum. Without intrinsic factor, vitamin B_{12} can not be absorbed

and this gives rise to a macrocytic anaemia. The skin and mucosa become pale and the tongue smooth and atrophic. A peripheral neuropathy is often present and this is commonly manifest by paraesthesiae and numbness, and even ataxia. The more severe neurological complication of sub-acute combined degeneration of the cord is fortunately more rare. The anaemia gets its name from the fact that before the discovery of vitamin B_{12} it was uniformly fatal. Now a monthly injection of vitamin B_{12} is all that is required to keep the patient healthy.

PERONEAL is the name given to structures, such as the muscles, and nerves, on the outer or fibular side of the leg.

PERPHENAZINE (see NEUROLEPTICS).

PERSEVERATION is the senseless repetition of words or deeds by a person with a disordered mind.

PERSISTENT VEGETATIVE STATE (PVS) may occur in patients with severe brain damage from hypoxia or injury. The victim lies helpless in a coma without feeling or contact with the outside world. Sleep alternates with apparent wakefulness, the patient's eyes may reflexly follow or respond to sound, his spastic limbs can withdraw from pain and his hands reflexly grope or grasp. Individuals in a PVS retain automatic breathing, heartbeat and circulation and their eyes may wander vaguely. Half such patients die within 2 to 6 months, but those alive at 3 months sometimes survive from 5 to 30 years with artificial feeding. The ethics of keeping patients alive with artificial support are controversial.

PVS must be distinguished from conditions which appear similar. These include the 'locked-in syndrome' (q.v.) which is the result of damage to the brain stem (see BRAIN). Patients with this syndrome are conscious but unable to speak or move except for certain eye movements and blinking. The psychiatric state of catatonia (q.v.) is another condition in which the patient retains consciousness and will usually recover.

PERSONALITY DISORDER Condition in which the sufferers fail to learn from experience or to adapt to changes. The outcome is impaired social functioning and personal distress. There are three broad overlapping groups. One group is characterized by eccentric behaviour with paranoid or schizoid overtones. The second group shows dramatic and emotional behaviour with self-centredness and antisocial behaviour as typical components of the disorder. In the third group anxiety and fear are the main characteristics, which are accompanied by dependency and compulsive behaviour. These disorders are not classed as illnesses but psychotherapy and behavioural therapy may help.

The individuals affected are notoriously resistant to any help that is offered, tending to blame other people, circumstances or bad luck for their persistent difficulties. (See MENTAL ILLNESS; MULTIPLE PERSONALITY DISORDER; MUNCHAUSEN'S SYNDROME.)

PERSPIRATION, or SWEAT, is an excretion from the skin, produced by microscopic sweat-glands, of which there are around 2·5 million, scattered over the surface. There are two different types of sweat-glands, known as eccrine and apocrine. Insensible perspiration takes place constantly by evaporation from the openings of the sweat-glands, well over a litre a day being produced. Sensible perspiration – to which the term sweat is usually confined – occurs with physical exertion and raised body temperature: up to three litres an hour may be produced for short periods.

Eccrine sweat is a faintly acid, watery fluid containing less than 2 per cent of solids, made up mainly of salts and to a slight extent of fatty material, and including 0·3 per cent of urea (about the same concentration as in the blood), the substance which the kidneys excrete in large amount. Patients with severe uraemia (q.v.) may produce deposits of urea crystals on their skin when sweat evaporates.

The *eccrine sweat-glands* in man are situated in greatest numbers on the soles of the feet and palms of the hands, and with a magnifying glass their minute openings or pores can be seen in rows occupying the summit of each ridge in the skin. Perspiration is most abundant in these regions, though it also occurs all over the body.

The chief object of perspiration is to maintain an even body temperature by regulating the heat lost from the body surface. Sweating is therefore increased by internally produced heat, such as muscular activity, or external heat. It is controlled by two types of nerves: vasomotor, which regulate the local blood flow, and secretory (part of the sympathetic nervous system) which directly influence secretion.

The *apocrine sweat-glands* are found in the armpits, the eyelids, around the anus in association with the external genitalia and in the areola and nipple of the breast. (The glands that produce wax in the ear are modified apocrine glands.) They are developed in close association with hairs and their ducts often open into hair follicles. They do not start functioning until puberty. The flow of apocrine sweat is evoked by emotional stimuli such as fear, anger, or sexual excitement.

Abnormalities of perspiration Decreased sweating may occur in the early stages of fever, in diabetes, and in some forms of glomerulonephritis. Some people are unable to sweat copiously, and are prone to heat-stroke (q.v.).

EXCESSIVE sweating, or HYPERIDROSIS, may take place in any feverish condition, and also in people with hyperthyroidism, obesity, diabetes mellitus, or an anxiety state. Offensive perspiration, or bromidrosis, commonly occurs on the feet or in the armpits, and is due to bacterial decomposition of skin secretions.

Treatment Decreased sweating may be treated with diaphoretic drugs or hot air baths. Excessive sweating in febrile diseases is reduced by treating the underlying fever. When the sweating is offensive, frequent baths with antiseptic soap, together with regular shaving of armpit hair may be helpful. The skin should be carefully dried, and shoes and clothes worn which encourage good air circulation. Numerous effective antiperspirants and deodorants are available; in cases of persistent and unresponsive armpit sweating, surgical removal of a small area of skin bearing the apocrine glands may be necessary.

PERTHES' DISEASE is an affection of the hip in children, due to fragmentation of the epiphysis (or spongy extremity) of the head of the femur. It occurs in the age-group, 4 to 10 years, with a peak between 6 and 8. It is ten times more common in boys than girls, and is bilateral in 10 per cent of cases. The initial manifestation is a lurching gait with a limp, accompanied by pain. Treatment consists of bed rest and traction of the affected limb so long as there is pain and spasm. The child is then allowed up and about with a walking calliper splint (q.v.) until the condition has healed. Spontaneous recovery occurs in about two years.

PERTUSSIS is another name for whooping-cough. (See WHOOPING-COUGH.)

PES CAVUS is the technical name for claw-foot (q.v.).

PES PLANUS is the technical name for flat-foot (q.v.).

PESSARIES are either instruments designed to support a displaced womb, or solid bodies suitably shaped for insertion into the vagina, which are made of oil of theobromine or a glycerin basis and are used for applying local treatment to the vagina.

PESTICIDES may be defined as any substance or mixture of substances intended for preventing or controlling any unwanted species of plants and animals, and includes any substances intended for use as plant growth regulators, defoliants or dessicants. The main groups of pesticides are: *herbicides* to control weeds; *insecticides* to control insects; *fungicides* to control or prevent fungal disease.

PET (see POSITRON EMISSION TOMOGRAPHY.)

PETECHIAE are small spots on the skin, of red or purple colour, resembling flea-bites. They are small haemorrhages in the skin, as in purpura.

PETHIDINE HYDROCHLORIDE is a synthetic analgesic and antispasmodic drug, which is used in the treatment of painful and spasmodic conditions in place of morphine and atropine. It was at first thought that the drug would have an advantage over morphine in not encouraging addiction, but this has not proved to be the case. Pethidine is a controlled drug (q.v.).

PETIT MAL means the lesser type of epileptic seizure. (See EPILEPSY.)

PETRI DISHES are shallow, circular glass dishes, usually 10 cm in diameter, which are used in bacteriology laboratories for the growth of micro-organisms.

PEYER'S PATCHES are conglomerations of lymphoid nodules in the ileum, or lower part of the small intestine. They play an important part in the defence of the body against bacterial invasion, as in typhoid fever.

PEYRONIES DISEASE Painful and deformed erection of the penis caused by the formation of fibrous tissue. The cause is unknown but it may be associated with Dupuytren's contracture (q.v.). The condition may be improved by surgery.

pH A measurement of the concentration of hydrogen ions in a solution that is calculated as a negative logarithm. A neutral solution has a pH of 7·0 and this figure falls for a solution with increasing acidity and rises if the alkalinity increases.

PHAEOCHROMOCYTOMA A disorder in which a vascular tumour of the adrenal medulla develops. The tumour may also affect the structurally similar tissues associated with the chain of sympathetic nerves. There is uncontrolled and irregular secretion of adrenaline and noradrenaline (qq.v.) with the result that the patient suffers from episodes of high blood pressure, raised heart rate, and headache. Surgery to remove the tumour may be possible; if not, drug treatment may help. (See HYPERTENSION.)

PHAGOCYTE Cells, including white blood cells and macrophages, that envelop and digest bacteria, cells, cell debris, and other small particles. These cells are a vital part of the body's defence system.

PHAGOCYTOSIS is a process by which the attacks of bacteria upon the living body are repelled and the bacteria destroyed through the activity of the white corpuscles of the blood.

PHALANX is the name given to any one of the small bones of the fingers and toes. The phalanges are fourteen in number in each hand and foot, the thumb and great toe possessing only two each, whilst each of the other fingers and toes has three.

PHALLUS An alternative name for the penis (q.v.), this word may also be used to describe a penis-like object. In embryology the phallus is the rudimentary penis before the urethral duct has completely developed.

PHANTASY, or FANTASY, is the term applied to an imaginary appearance or day dream.

PHANTOM LIMB Following the amputation of a limb it is usual for the patient to experience sensations as if the limb were still present. This condition is referred to as a phantom limb. In the vast majority of cases the sensation passes off in time.

PHARMACOKINETICS The way in which the body deals with a drug. This includes the drug's absorption, distribution in the tissues, metabolism, and excretion.

PHARMACOLOGY is the part of medical science dealing with knowledge of the action of drugs.

PHARMACOPOEIA is an official publication dealing with the recognized drugs and giving their doses, preparations, sources, and tests. Most countries have a pharmacopoeia of their own. That for Great Britain and Ireland is prepared by the British Pharmacopoeia Commission under the direction of the Medicines Commission. Many hospitals and medical schools have a small pharmacopoeia of their own, giving the prescriptions most commonly dispensed in that particular hospital or school. The *British National Formulary* (q.v.) is an authoritative pocket book for those concerned with the prescribing or dispensing of medicines.

PHARMACY is the term applied to the art of preparing and compounding medicines, or to a place where this is carried out.

PHARYNGITIS is an inflammatory condition affecting the wall of the pharynx or throat proper. It is most commonly due to a viral upper respiratory tract infection. It may be confined to the pharynx or may also involve the rest of the upper respiratory tract, i.e. the nose and the larynx. On examination the mucous membrane is red and glazed with enlarged lymph-follicles scattered over it. It produces considerable irritation, tickling in the throat and discomfort which may last longer if not treated. If a viral cause is suspected, then only symptomatic treatment is instituted, consisting of analgesia and various gargles. This may include the sucking of medicated pastilles or lozenges. If a bacterial cause is suspected, an antibiotic should be prescribed and in both conditions irritants, such as smoking and highly spiced foods should be avoided.

PHARYNX is another name for the throat. The term throat is popularly applied to the region about the front of the neck generally, but in its strict sense it means the irregular cavity into which the nose and mouth open above, from which the larynx and gullet open below, and in which the channel for the air and that for the food cross one another. It extends from the base of the skull down to the 6th cervical vertebra, separated from the upper six vertebrae only by some loose fibrous tissue, and is about 12·5 cm (5 inches) long.

It is completely closed behind by a layer of muscles, and by mucous membrane, but in front it opens into the nose, mouth, and larynx in succession from above down. In its upper part, the Eustachian tubes open one on either side, and between them on the back wall grows a mass of glandular tissue known as the third tonsil, which, if enlarged, produces the condition known as adenoids. (See NOSE, DISEASES OF.) The muscles which close in the sides and back of the pharynx are three in number on each side, and spring, one from the jawbone, the second from the hyoid bone, the third from the side of the larynx, each of these constrictors spreading out like a fan on the back of the pharynx. Two other small muscles run downwards on each side.

PHENACETIN is a white crystalline coal-tar product, at one time much used in fevers, influenza, headaches, and neuralgias of all kinds, on account of its power of reducing temperature and of deadening pain.

PHENAZOCINE is a powerful pain-reliever, or analgesic, which is said to be more potent, but less habit-forming, than morphine.

PHENCYCLIDINE (see DRUG ADDICTION).

PHENELZINE is one of the widely used antidepressant drugs which are classified as monoamine oxidase inhibitors (q.v.). (See ANTIDEPRESSANTS.)

PHENINDIONE is a synthetic anticoagulant (q.v.) which is effective by mouth, and is used for the same purpose as heparin. It is slower in action than heparin, the full anticoagulant effect not being obtained until 36 to 48 hours after the initial dose.

PHENOBARBITONE is the *British Pharmacopoeia* name for one of the most widely used of all the barbiturate group of drugs. It is given in doses of 30 to 125 mg to control epilepsy.

Phenobarbitone Sodium is a soluble preparation which can be given by injection.

PHENOL is another name for carbolic acid (q.v.).

PHENOLPHTHALEIN is a substance much used as an indicator of reaction in urine, and gastric juice, for example, being colourless in acid media, brilliant red with alkalis, and varying in tint according to the acid concentration. It is also given internally in 60 to 300 mg doses as an aperient.

PHENOTHIAZINES are the group of major antipsychotic or neuroleptic drugs, colloquially called 'tranquillizers', of value in the treatment of the psychoses (q.v.). They can be divided into three main groups. Chlorpromazine and methotrimeprazine are examples of group 1, usually characterized by their sedative effects and moderate antimuscarinic and extrapyramidal side-effects. Group 2 includes pericyazine and thioridazine, which have moderate sedative effects but significant antimuscarinic action and modest extrapyramidal side-effects. Fluphenazine, perphenazine, prochlorperazine and trifluoperazine comprise group 3. Their sedative effects are less than for the other groups and they have little antimuscarinic action; they have marked extrapyramidal side-effects.
Uses Phenothiazines should be prescribed and used with care. In the short term these therapeutically powerful drugs can be used to calm disturbed patients, whatever the underlying condition which might have a physical or psychiatric basis. They also alleviate acute anxiety and some have antidepressant properties, while others worsen depression.

PHENOTYPE An individual's characteristics as determined by the interaction between his genotype – his quota of genes – and the environment.

PHENOXYBENZAMINE is an alpha-adrenoceptor blocking drug (see ADRENERGIC RECEPTORS) used in the treatment of hypertension caused by phaeochromocytoma (q.v.).

PHENOXYMETHYLPENICILLIN Otherwise known as pencillin V, this drug, which can be taken orally, is used to treat tonsillitis (q.v.), otitis media (q.v.) and erysipelas (q.v.) and as a prophylactic for rheumatic fever (q.v.) and pneumococcal infection (q.v.). (See PENICILLIN.)

PHENYLALANINE A natural amino-acid essential for growth in infants and nitrogen metabolism in adults.

PHENYLKETONURIA is one of the less common, but very severe, forms of mental deficiency. The incidence in populations of European origin is around 1 in 15,000 births. It is due to the inability of the baby to metabolize the amino-acid, phenylalamine. Its outstanding interest lies in the fact that, if it is diagnosed soon after birth – and this can be done by a simple urine test or by a test carried out on a drop of blood – and the infant is then given a diet low in phenylalamine, the chances are that the infant will grow up mentally normal. Parents of children with phenylketonuria can obtain help and information from the National Society for Phenylketonuria (UK) Ltd. (See APPENDIX 2: ADDRESSES.)

PHENYTOIN SODIUM is one of the most effective drugs for the treatment of epilepsy. One of its advantages is that it does not make the patient feel particularly sleepy. Its use is not without risk and it must therefore be used only under medical supervision.

PHEROMONES are chemicals produced and emitted by an individual which produce changes in the social or sexual behaviour when perceived by other individuals of the same species. The precise role of these odours, for it is by their smell that they are recognized, in man is still not clear, but there is growing evidence of the part they play in the animal kingdom. Thus if a strange male rat is put into a group of female rats, this may cause death of the fetus in any pregnant rats, and this is attributed to the pheromones emitted by the male rat.

PHIMOSIS is a condition of great narrowing at the edge of the foreskin, for which the operation of circumcision (q.v.) may be necessary.

PHLEBITIS means inflammation of a vein. (See VEINS, DISEASES OF.)

PHLEBOGRAPHY is the study of the veins, particularly by means of X-rays after the veins have been injected with a radio-opaque substance.

PHLEBOLITH is the term applied to a small stone formed in a vein as a result of calcification of a thrombus.

PHLEBOTOMY is an old name for the operation of blood-letting by opening a vein. (See VENESECTION.)

PHLEGM is a popular name for mucus, particularly that secreted in the air passages. (See BRONCHITIS; EXPECTORANTS; MUCUS.)

PHLEGMASIA DOLENS is another name for white leg (q.v.).

PHLYCTENULE A hypersensitivity reaction of the conjunctiva. At the turn of the century the commonest cause was tuberculosis. Nowadays it is most commonly due to hypersensitivity to *staphylococci*.

PHOBIA is an irrational fear of particular objects or situations. A well-known American medical dictionary lists 206 'examples' of phobias, ranging, alphabetically, from air to writing. Included in the list are phobophobia (fear of phobias) and triskaidekaphobia (fear of thirteen at table). It is a form of obsession, and not uncommonly one of the features of the anxiety. (See MENTAL ILLNESS.) Those who suffer from what can be a most distressing condition can obtain help and advice from the Phobics Society (see APPENDIX 2: ADDRESSES).

PHOCOMELIA This is a great reduction in the size of the proximal parts of the limbs. In extreme cases the hands and feet may spring directly from the trunk.

PHOLCODINE is the 3-(2-morpholinoethyl) ester of morphine. As it resembles codeine in suppressing cough, it is used for the relief of unproductive coughs.

PHONOCARDIOGRAPH is an instrument for the graphic recording of heart sounds and murmurs.

PHOSPHATES are salts of phosphoric acid, and, as this substance is contained in many articles of food as well as in bone, the nuclei of cells, and the nervous system, phosphates are constantly excreted in the urine. The continued use of an excess of food containing alkalis, such as green vegetables, and still more the presence in the urine of bacteria which lead to its decomposition, produce the necessary change from the natural mild acidity to alkalinity, and lead to the deposit of phosphates and to their collection into stones.

PHOSPHATURIA means the presence in the urine of a large amount of phosphates.

PHOSPHORUS BURNS If particles of phosphorus settle on or become embedded in the skin, the resulting burn should be treated with a 2 per cent sodium bicarbonate solution, followed by application of a 1 per cent solution of copper sulphate. Fats and oils should not be employed.

PHOSPHORUS POISONING, now rare, is produced only by the yellow, soluble form of phosphorus found in certain rat poisons.
Signs and symptoms When swallowed, it acts first as an irritant, and on being absorbed, results in acute degeneration of the liver and

other abdominal organs. Exposure to phosphorus fumes in chemical works may lead to a chronic form of poisoning, with severe debility. Necrosis of the lower jaw bone (phossy jaw) occurs over months or years; this may be partly due to a secondary infection in the bone. Acute symptoms, most common in children after swallowing a large dose of poison, include pain, vomiting, colic, diarrhoea, and even convulsions. The breath often smells of garlic, and death may occur within a few hours. Partial recovery may occur, but jaundice and blood-stained urine develop after a few days, leading to death.

Treatment Phosphorus is slowly absorbed, so stomach wash-outs up to two hours after swallowing the poison may succeed, or emetics may be tried instead. If neither works, a large saline purge should be given. No oils, fats, or milk should be taken. If liver damage is threatened, then treatment with sodium bicarbonate, glucose, and insulin is indicated. Chronic poisoning in chemical works is prevented by good ventilation, cleanliness, and regular dental examination of the workers. (See POISONS and APPENDIX 2: ADDRESSES.)

PHOTOCOAGULATION Coagulation of the tissues of the retina by laser for treatment of diseases of the retina such as diabetic retinopathy (see RETINA, DISORDERS OF).

PHOTODERMATOSIS, or PHOTODERMATITIS, is the term applied to an eruption on areas of the skin exposed to sunlight, caused by sensitivity to sunlight. (See POLYMORPHIC LIGHT ERUPTION.) In some cases the sensitivity is caused by certain drugs, cosmetics or chemicals.

PHOTOPHOBIA Sensitivity to light. It can occur in disorders of the eye, or in meningitis.

PHOTOPSIA This is a description of the flashing lights which are a not uncommon aura preceding an attack of migraine.

PHOTOSENSITIVITY Abnormal reaction to sunlight. The condition usually occurs as a skin rash appearing in response to light falling on the skin, and it may be caused by substances that have been eaten or applied to the skin. These are called photosensitizers and may be dyes, chemicals in soaps, or drugs. Sometimes plants act as photosensitizers – for example, buttercups and mustard. The condition may occur in some illnesses such as lupus erythematosus (q.v.).

PHOTOSYNTHESIS is how green plants and some bacteria produce carbohydrates (q.v.) from water and carbon dioxide. They use energy absorbed from the sun's rays by a green pigment in the organism called chlorophyll. It is one of the earth's fundamental biological processes. As well as converting the carbon dioxide into the essential biological compound carbohydrate, the process removes the gas from the atmosphere where, if it builds to excess, the atmospheric temperature rises, thus contributing to global warming.

PHRENIC NERVE is the nerve which chiefly supplies the diaphragm. It springs from the 3rd, 4th, and 5th cervical spinal nerves, and has a long course down the neck, and through the chest to the diaphragm.

PHRENOLOGY is an old term applied to the study of the mind and character of individuals from the shape of the head. As the shape of the head has been shown to depend chiefly upon accidental characteristics, such as the size of the air spaces in the bones, and not upon development of special areas in the contained brain, this branch of science is now generally discredited.

PHTHISIS means wasting, and is the general term applied to that progressive enfeeblement and loss of weight that arise from tuberculous disease of all kinds, but especially from the disease as it affects the lungs.

PHYSICAL MEDICINE is a medical specialty founded in 1931 and recognized by the Royal College of Physicians of London in 1972. Physical-medicine specialists started by treating rheumatic diseases. Subsequently their work developed to include the diagnosis and rehabilitation of people with physical handicaps. The disabilities included those arising from asthma, poliomyelitis and injuries, especially those affecting limbs. Back injuries and backache were other disabling disorders treated by physical-medicine specialists. Their responsibilities overlap and are complementary to those specialists who practise rheumatology (q.v.).

PHYSIOLOGY is the branch of medical science that deals with the healthy functions of different organs, and the changes that the whole body undergoes in the course of its activities.

PHYSIOTHERAPY is the form of treatment involving the use of physical measures, such as exercise, heat, manipulation and remedial exercises in the treatment of disease. An alternative name is PHYSICAL MEDICINE. It is an essential part of the rehabilitation of convalescent or disabled patients. Those who practise physiotherapy – physiotherapists – have a recognized training and, on successful completion of this, they are placed on the profession's official register.

PHYSOSTIGMINE, or ESERINE, is an alkaloid obtained from Calabar bean, the seed of *Physostigma venenosum*, a climbing plant of

West Africa. Calabar bean is known also as the ordeal bean, because preparations derived from it were at one time used by the natives of West Africa to decide the guilt or innocence of accused persons, the guilty being supposed to succumb to its action, while the innocent escaped. Its action depends on the presence of two alkaloids, the one known as physostigmine or eserine, the other as calabarine, the former of these being much the more important.

Action Physostigmine produces the same effect as stimulation of the parasympathetic nervous system (q.v.): i.e. it constricts the pupil, stimulates the gut, increases the secretion of saliva, stimulates the bladder, and increases the irritability of voluntary muscle. In poisonous doses it brings on a general paralysis.

Uses It is used in medicine in the form of physostigmine salicylate. Its main use is to contract the pupil and thereby reduce the pressure inside the eyeball. For this purpose it is used as eye-drops or as lamellae. It is also given by subcutaneous injection to stimulate the gut when this is paralysed or atonic. It is the specific antidote (q.v.) to atropine and is therefore used in the treatment of atropine poisoning (q.v.).

PHYTOMENADIONE is the *British Pharmacopoeia* name for vitamin K. (See VITAMIN.)

PIA MATER is the membrane closely investing the brain and spinal cord, in which run blood-vessels for the nourishment of these organs. (See BRAIN; SPINAL CORD.)

PICA (Latin for magpie) is a term which means an abnormal craving for unusual foods. It is not uncommon in pregnancy. Among the unusual substances for which pregnant women have developed a craving are soap, clay pipes, bed linen, charcoal, ashes – and almost every imaginable foodstuff taken in excess. In primitive races it is taken to mean that it indicates the growing fetus requires such food. It is also not uncommon in children. (See APPETITE; LEAD POISONING.)

PICORNAVIRUSES derive their name from pico (small) and RNA (because they contain ribonuleic acid). They are a group of viruses which includes the enteroviruses (q.v.) and the rhinoviruses (q.v.).

PICRIC ACID, or TRINITROPHENOL, is used for preparing explosives, and so is employed in medicine only in solution. As it coagulates albumin, it produces a soothing pellicle over any raw surface with which it is brought into contact. It has antiseptic properties, but is rapidly going out of use because of its toxic effects.

PIGEON BREAST (see CHEST, DEFORMITIES OF).

PIGMENT is the term applied to the colouring matter of various secretions, blood, etc.; also to any medicinal preparation of thick consistence intended for painting on the skin or mucous membranes.

PILES, or HAEMORRHOIDS, consist of a varicose and often inflamed condition of the veins about the lower end of the bowel, known as the haemorrhoidal veins. They are very common affecting nearly half of the UK population at some time in their lives, with men having them more often and for a longer time.

Varieties Haemorrhoids are classified into first, second and third degree depending on how far they prolapse through the anal canal. First-degree ones do not protrude; second-degree piles protrude during defaecation; third-degree ones are trapped outside the anal margin, though they can be pushed back. Most haemorrhoids can be described as internal, since they are covered with glandular mucosa, but some large, long-term ones develop a covering of skin. Piles are usually found at the three, seven and eleven o'clock sites when viewed with the patient on his or her back.

Causes There is always a tendency for the veins in this situation to become distended, partly because they are unprovided with valves, partly because they form the lowest part of the portal system and are very apt to become overfilled when there is the least interference with the circulation through the portal vein, and partly because the muscular arrangements for keeping the rectum closed interfere with the circulation through the haemorrhoidal veins. An absence of fibre from Western diets is probably the most important cause. The result is that people strain to pass small hard stools, thus raising intra-abdominal pressure which slows the rate of venous return and engorges the network of veins in the anal mucosa. Pregnancy is a contributory factor in women developing haemorrhoids. In some people haemorrhoids are a symptom of disease higher up on the portal system, causing interference with the circulation. They are common in heart disease, liver complaints, such as cirrhosis or congestion, and any disease affecting the bowels.

Symptoms Piles cause itching, pain and often bleeding, which may occur whenever the patient defaecates or only sometimes. The piles may prolapse permanently or intermittently. The patient may complain of aching discomfort which, with the pain, may be worsened on opening the bowels.

Treatment Prevention is important and a high-fibre diet will help to do this and is also necessary after piles have developed. A bulking agent will help and patients should not spend a long time straining on the lavatory. Itching can be lessened if the perineum (q.v.) is properly washed, dried and powdered. Prolapsed piles can be replaced with the finger. Local anaesthetic and steroid ointments can help to relieve symptoms but do not remedy the underlying disorder. If conservative measures fail, then surgery may be required. Piles may be injected, stretched or excised according to the patient's particular circumstances.

Where haemorrhoids are secondary to another disorder such as cancer of the rectum or colon, the underlying condition must be treated, hence the importance of medical advice if piles persist.

PILLS are small round masses containing active drugs held together by syrup, gum, glycerin, or adhesive vegetable extracts. They are sometimes without coating, being merely rolled in French chalk, but often they are covered with sugar, gelatin, or gilt. Some pills, designed to act upon the bowels only, are coated with keratin, salol or other substances which are insoluble in the gastric juice.

PILOCARPINE is an alkaloid derived from the leaves of *Pilocarpus microphyllus* (jaborandi). It produces the same effects as stimulation of the parasympathetic nervous system: i.e. it has exactly the opposite effect to atropine (q.v.), but cannot be used in the treatment of atropine poisoning as it does not antagonize the action of poisonous doses of atropine on the brain. Its main use today is in the form of eye-drops to decrease the pressure inside the eyeball in glaucoma (q.v.).

PILONOIDAL SINUS A sinus (q.v.) that contains hairs, usually occurring in the cleft between the buttocks. It may get infected and cause considerable pain. Treatment is by antibiotics and, if necessary, surgical removal.

PIMPLES, technically known as papules, are small, raised, and inflamed areas on the skin. On the face the most common cause is acne (q.v.). Boils (q.v.) start as hard pimples. The eruption of smallpox and that of chicken-pox begin also with pimples. (See also SKIN DISEASES.)

PINEAL BODY is a small reddish structure, 10 mm in length and shaped somewhat like a pine cone (hence its name), situated on the upper part of the mid-brain. Many theories have been expounded as to its function, but there is increasing evidence that, in some animals at least, it is affected by light and plays a part in hibernation and in controlling sexual activity and the colour of the skin. This it seems to do by means of a substance it produces known as melatonin. There is also growing evidence that it may play a part in controlling the circadian rhythms of the body – the natural variations in physiological activities throughout the 24-hour day.

PINNA The part of the ear, formed of cartilage and skin, that is external to the head. In animals it is an important element in detecting the direction of sound.

PINS AND NEEDLES is a form of paraesthesia (q.v.), or disturbed sensation, such as may occur, for example, in neuritis (q.v.) or poly-neuritis (q.v.).

PINT is a measure of quantity containing 16 fluid ounces (wine measure) or 20 fluid ounces (Imperial measure). The metric equivalent is 568 millilitres. (See APPENDIX 6: MEASUREMENTS IN MEDICINE.)

PINWORM (see ENTEROBIASIS).

PIPERACILLIN (see ANTIBIOTIC).

PIPERAZINE is a drug used for the treatment of threadworms and ascariasis. (See ASCARIASIS; ENTEROBIASIS.)

PIPOTHIAZINE is an antipsychotic drug for maintenance treatment of schizophrenia. It is given as a depot injection that lasts four weeks. (See NEUROLEPTICS.)

PIROXICAM is used to treat pain and inflammation in rheumatic disease, other musculoskeletal disorders and acute gout. (See NON-STEROIDAL ANTI-INFLAMMATORY DRUGS.)

PITHIATISM is a group of disorders in which the patient is subject to cure by persuasion or suggestion, the term being used as an equivalent for hysteria. (See HYSTERIA.)

PITUITARY BODY, also known as the PITUITARY GLAND and the HYPOPHYSIS, is an ovoid structure, weighing around 0·5 gram in the adult, attached to the base of the brain, and lying in the depression in the base of the skull known as the sella turcica on account of its resemblance to a Turkish saddle. It consists of an anterior and a posterior section divided by a clear line of cleavage. For long these two parts were known, respectively, as the anterior and the posterior lobes of the pituitary body, and the part of the gland that connected it to the brain was known as the stalk or infundibulum. This, however, was too simple a classification to be accurate, as was realized once information concerning the multifarious functions of the gland began to accumulate. It was therefore decided to divide it up according to its origin. The reason for this is that the pituitary has a double origin. The anterior part is derived in the embryo from the ectoderm (see FETUS) of the primitive mouth, and this part of the gland is now known as the adenohypophysis. The posterior part is derived from the brain and is now known as the neurohypophysis. The gland is connected to the hypothalamus (q.v.) of the brain by a stalk known as the hypophyseal or pituitary stalk. The confusing thing about this new 'classification' of the pituitary is that it involves a certain amount of overlapping with the old classification. Thus, the adenohypophysis is made up of the anterior lobe which, in turn, is subdivided into a pars distalis and a pars tuberalis, and the pars intermedia of the posterior lobe. The neurohypophysis is also made up of three parts: the infundibular process (or neural lobe) of the posterior lobe, the nervous part of the stalk known as the infundibular or neural stalk, and the median eminence of the tuber cinereum.

The pars distalis, which accounts for the greater part of the gland, is composed of masses of cells which fall into three main groups: (1) chromophobe cells which do not stain and constitute about 50 per cent of the total; (2) acidophil cells which stain with acid dyes and constitute about 35 per cent of the total; and (3) basophil cells which stain with basic stains and constitute about 15 per cent of the total. The pars intermedia consists only of a few cells, whilst the pars tuberalis contains non-granular cells. The neurohypophysis is composed of nerve fibres and brown granular cells known as pituicytes.

The pituitary gland is the most important ductless, or endocrine, gland in the body. (See ENDOCRINE GLANDS.) It has been described as the master gland of the endocrine system, or the conductor of the endocrine orchestra. This over-all control it exerts through the media of a series of hormones which it produces. The adenohypophysis is the major producer of these, and those it produces will be dealt with first. Those which function through the media of other endocrine glands are known as trophic hormones and have therefore been given names ending with 'trophic' or 'trophin'. The thyrotrophic hormone, or thyroid-stimulating hormone (abbreviated to TSH) as it is also known, exerts a powerful influence over the activity of the thyroid gland. The adrenocorticotrophic hormone, also known as corticotrophin (ACTH), stimulates the cortex of the adrenal glands. The growth, or somatotrophic, hormone, also known as somatotrophin (SMH), controls the growth of the body. There are also two gonadotrophic hormones which play a vital part in the control of the gonads: these are the follicle-stimulating hormone (FSH), and the luteinizing hormone (LH) which is also known as the interstitial-cell-stimulating hormone (ICSH). (See GONADOTROPHINS.) The lactogenic hormone, also known as prolactin, mammotrophin and luteotrophin, induces lactation. The neurohypophysis produces two hormones. One is oxytocin which is widely used because of its stimulating effect on contraction of the uterus. The other is vasopressin, or the antidiuretic hormone (ADH), which acts on the renal tubules and the collecting tubules (see KIDNEYS) to increase the amount of water that they normally absorb.

Gigantism is the result of the over-activity of, or tumour formation of, the acidophil cells in the adenohypophysis which produce the growth hormone. If this over-activity occurs after growth has ceased a condition known as acromegaly (q.v.) arises, in which there is gross over-growth of the ears, nose, jaws, and hands and feet. Dwarfism may be due to lack of the growth hormone. Diabetes insipidus (q.v.), a condition characterized by the passing of a large volume of urine every day, is due to lack of the antidiuretic hormone. Enhanced production of ACTH by the basophil cells of the pituitary leads to Cushing's syndrome (q.v.). Excessive production of prolactin by micro or macro adenomas leads to hyperprolactinaemia and consequent amenorrhoea and galactorrhoea. Some chromophobe adenomas do not produce any hormone but cause effects by damaging the pituitary cells and inhibiting their hormone production. The most sensitive cells to extrinsic pressure are the gonadotrophin-producing cells and the growth-hormone producing cells, so that if the tumour occurs in childhood growth-hormone will be suppressed and growth will cease. Gonadotrophin hormone suppression will prevent the development of puberty and if the tumour occurs after puberty will result in amenorrhoea in the female and lack of libido in both sexes. The thyroid-stimulating hormone cells are the next to suffer and the pressure effects on these cells will result in hypothyroidism. Fortunately the ACTH-producing cells are the most resistant to extrinsic pressure and this is teleologically sound as ACTH is the one pituitary hormone that is essential to life. However, these cells do suffer damage from intracellular tumours, and adrenocortical insufficiency is not uncommon.

PITYRIASIS ALBA is a form of chronic eczema which occurs mainly in children. It is characterized by rounded, scaly, white patches, usually on the face, but also sometimes on the upper arms and back. It is a self-limiting condition, but may drag on for several years. A bland cream controls the scaling if this is troublesome.

PITYRIASIS ROSEA is a skin eruption of unknown origin that occurs in young people. It starts characteristically with an oval, slightly red and scaly area – known as the herald patch – between the shoulder blades or on the lower abdomen. Three or four days later the eruption spreads all over the trunk. It consists of pink papules (q.v.) and oval brownish macules (q.v.), which tend to itch considerably. It usually lasts about six weeks, and does not usually recur. No specific treatment is called for. Hot baths should be avoided as they tend to accentuate the itching. If this itching is unpleasant, it can be relieved with calamine lotion or antihistamine tablets.

PIVAMPICILLIN is a broad-spectrum oral penicillin active against some Gram-negative and Gram-positive organisms. (See ANTIBIOTIC.)

PIVMECILLINAM is a derivative of the antibiotic, mecillinam. It differs from the latter in being active when taken by mouth. (See PENI-CILLIN, ANTIBIOTIC.)

PLACEBO No treatments of specific value are found in all the pages of Hippocrates. Nevertheless the placebo response occurred with sufficient frequency to enable the physician to command respect. The therapeutic opportunities are now very different. However, man himself has not changed. He still wants and expects to take medicine when he is ill and is still just as subject to persuasion and suggestion. Despite the scientific advances of this century the physician is still the most important therapeutic agent.

Placebo is the Latin for 'I will please'. Traditionally, placebos were used to pacify without actually benefiting the patient. They were inactive substances formerly given to please or gratify the patient but now only used in controlled studies to determine the efficacy of drugs. We now realise that pharmacologically inert compounds can relieve symptoms and we call this the placebo effect. The reassurance that is associated with placebo administration is accompanied by measurable changes in body function which are affected through autonomic pathways and humoral mechanisms. Alterations in blood pressure and pulse frequency are especially common. Placebos have the ability to relieve a variety of symptoms in a consistent proportion of the population. On average, one third of patients with symptoms such as pain or cough will respond to placebo medications and an even higher proportion of patients with psychological symptoms such as anxiety or insomnia is relieved. Current scientific jargon defines the placebo as any therapy or component of therapy that is deliberately or unknowingly used for its non-specific psychological or psycho-biological effect and that is without specific activity for the condition being treated.

PLACENTA is the name of the thick, spongy disc-like cake of tissue which connects the embryo with the inner surface of the womb, the embryo otherwise lying free in the amniotic fluid. (See AMNION.) The placenta is mainly a new structure growing with the embryo, but, when it separates, a portion of the inner surface of the womb, called the maternal placenta, comes away with it. It is mainly composed of loops of veins belonging to the embryo, lying in blood-sinuses, in which circulates maternal blood. Thus, though no mixing of the blood of embryo and mother takes place, there is ample opportunity for the exchange of fluids, gases, and the nutriment brough by the mother's blood. The width of the full-sized placenta is about 20 cm (8 inches), its thickness 2·5 cm (1 inch). One surface is rough and studded with villi, which consist of the loops of foetal veins; the other is smooth, and has implanted in its centre the umbilical cord, or navel string, which is about as thick as a finger and 50 cm (20 inches) long. It contains two arteries and a vein, enters the foetus at the navel, and forms the sole connection between the bodies of mother and foetus. The name 'afterbirth' is given to the structure because it is expelled from the womb in the third stage of labour (see LABOUR).

PLACENTA PRAEVIA Implantation of the placenta in the bottom part of the uterus adjacent to or over the cervix. The condition may cause few problems during pregnancy or labour; it may, however, cause vaginal bleeding late in pregnancy and this requires medical attention.

PLACENTOGRAPHY is the procedure of rendering the placenta (q.v.), or afterbirth, visible by means of X-rays. This can be done either by using what is known as soft-tissue radiography, or by injecting a radio-opaque substance into the blood-stream or into the amniotic cavity. (See AMNION.) The procedure is not without danger to both mother and fetus, and must therefore only be carried out under expert supervision but it is sometimes of value in assessing the cause of antepartum haemorrhage. The placenta and fetus can now be visualized by the non-invasive and safe method of ultrasound (q.v.).

PLAGUE, or BUBONIC PLAGUE This infection is caused by the bacterium *Yersinis pestis* (identified by Yersin in Hong Kong in 1894). It has yielded vast amounts of morbidity and mortality in numerous epidemics and pandemics over many centuries. Originating in Asia, it probably caused the Plague of Athens (430 BC), and that of Justinian in AD 542. In the Middle Ages the 'Black Death' (1348) swept through Europe reducing the human population by one third to one half; it had a major impact on the educated classes in Britain. The Great Plague of London (1665) killed some 70,000 people in the capital, out of a total population of approximately 460,000. Small outbreaks have since occurred in Europe, the last in Britain being in Suffolk in the 1920s. Plague remains a major infection in many tropical countries; WHO statistics indicate significant annual mortality from this bacterial infection.

The reservoir for the bacillus in urban infection lies in the black (*Rattus rattus*), and less importantly the brown (sewer) rat (*Rattus norvegicus*). It is conveyed to man by the rat flea, usually *Xenopsylla cheopis*: *Y. pestis* multiplies in the gastrointestinal tract of the flea, which may remain infectious for up to 6 weeks. In the pneumonic form (see below), human-to-human transmission can occur by droplet infection. Many lower mammals (apart from the rat) can also act as a reservoir in sylvatic transmission which remains a major problem in the USA (mostly in the south-western States); ground-squirrels, rock-squirrels, prairie dogs, bobcats, chipmunks, etc., can be affected.

Clinically, symptoms usually begin 2–8 days

after infection; disease begins with fever, headache, lassitude, and aching limbs. In over two-thirds of patients, enlarged glands (buboes) appear – usually in the groins, but also in the axillae and cervical neck; this constitutes *bubonic* plague. Haemorrhages may be present beneath the skin causing gangrenous patches and occasionally ulcers; these lesions led to the epithet 'Black Death'. In a favourable case, fever abates after about a week, and the buboes discharge foul-smelling pus. In a rapidly fatal form (*septicaemic* plague), haematogenous transmission produces mortality in a high percentage of cases. *Pneumonic* plague is associated with pneumonic consolidation (person-to-person transmission) and death often ensues on the fourth or fifth day. (The nursery rhyme 'Ring-o-ring o' roses, a pocketful o' posies, atishoo! atishoo!, we all fall down' is considered to have originated in the 17th century and refers to this form of the disease.) In addition, *meningitic* and *pharyngeal* forms of the disease can occur; these are unusual. Diagnosis consists of demonstration of the causative organism.

Treatment was revolutionized by the introduction of sulphonamides, followed by streptomycin in 1948. Tetracycline or doxycycline is now frequently used and a range of other antibiotics has been shown to be efficacious. There is no indication of development of antibiotic-resistance in *Y. pestis*, which is a highly sensitive organism. Plague remains (together with cholera and yellow fever) a quarantinable disease. Prevention is dominated by vector control. Contacts should be disinfected with insecticide powder; clothes, skins, soft merchandise, etc., which have been in contact with the infection can remain infectious for several months; suspect items should be destroyed or disinfected with an insecticide. Ships must be carefully checked for presence of rats; the rationale of anchoring a distance from the quay prevents access of vermin. Vaccination is not widely available, although research is in progress.

PLANTAR Describing anything related to the sole of the foot.

PLANTAR DERMATOSIS is a condition usually affecting children, characterized by cracks, or fissures, in the skin of the soles of the feet. The skin also assumes a glazed appearance. It is usually relieved by the regular rubbing in of paraffin ointment BPC, or one of its proprietary equivalents.

PLANTAR FASCIITIS (See FASCIITIS.)

PLAQUE is a coating of the teeth which forms as a result of neglect. It consists of food debris and bacteria and later calcium salts will be deposited in it to form calculus. It is therefore associated with both caries and periodontal disease.

PLASMA is the name applied to the fluid portion of the blood composed of serum and fibrinogen, the material which produces clotting. When the plasma is clotted, the thinner fluid separating from the clot is the serum.

PLASMA EXCHANGE involves the removal of the circulating plasma (q.v.) from the patient. It is done by removing blood from a patient and returning the red cells with a plasma expander. The plasma exchange is carried out through an in-dwelling cannula in the femoral vein and the red cells and plasma are separated by a hemonetics separator. Usually a sequence of three or four sessions is undertaken, at each of which two to three litres of plasma are removed. The lost plasma can either be replaced by human serum albumin or a plasma expander.

In auto-immune disorders the disease is due to damage wrought by circulating antibodies or sensitized lymphocytes. If the disease is due to circulating humoral antibodies, removal of these antibodies from the body should theoretically relieve the disorder. This is the principle on which plasma exchange was used in the management of auto-immune diseases due to circulating antibodies. Such disorders include Goodpasture's syndrome, systemic lupus erythematosis and myasthenis gravis. One of the problems in the use of plasma exchange in the treatment of such diseases is that the body responds to the removal of antibody from the circulation by enhanced production of that antibody by the immune system. It is therefore necessary to suppress this homeostatic response with cytotoxic drugs such as azathioprine. Nevertheless remissions can be achieved in auto-immune diseases due to circulating antibodies by the process of plasma exchange.

PLASMAPHERISIS A way of removing plasma (q.v.) from the blood. Blood is taken from a donor and allowed to settle in a vessel after which the separated plasma is extracted. The blood cells are transfused back into a vein. The process may be repeated and is used to treat some auto diseases caused by antibodies circulating in the patient's plasma. (See AUTO-IMMUNITY.)

PLASMA TRANSFUSION is sometimes used instead of blood transfusion. Plasma, the fluid part of blood from which the cells have been separated, may be dried and in powder form kept almost indefinitely; when wanted it is reconstituted by adding sterile distilled water. In powder form it can be transported easily and over long distances. Transfusion of plasma is especially useful in the treatment of shock. One advantage of plasma transfusion is that it is not necessary to carry out testing of blood groups before using it. (See TRANSFUSION OF BLOOD.)

PLASMIDS A generic description of any discrete agents in cells that have genetic functions. They include plasmagenes (self-reproducing copies of a nuclear gene existing outside the cell nucleus) and viruses.

PLASMINOGEN A precursor of plasmin, an enzyme that digests the protein fibrin, the main constituent of blood clots. When tissue is damaged, activators are released which provoke the conversion of plasminogen into plasmin.

PLASMODIUM is the general term applied to minute protoplasmic cells, and particularly to those which cause malaria and allied diseases. (See MALARIA.)

PLASTER OF PARIS is a form of calcium sulphate, which, after soaking in water, sets firmly. For this reason it is widely used as a form of splinting in the treatment of fractures. It is used for this purpose in the form of bandages which consist of bleached cotton cloth impregnated with the plaster and suitably adhesive. Its great advantage, compared with an ordinary splint, is that it can be moulded to the shape of the limb. This technique was originally introduced by a Dutchman in 1852. A predecessor of it, which seemed to serve its purpose well, was a bandage stiffened by soaking in egg white and flour – a method still in use in parts of Africa.

PLASTIC SURGERY is that branch of surgery which is concerned with the reformation and restoration of parts of the body which are damaged, lost, or deformed. Skin grafting is widely used, especially in the treatment of burns or where large areas of skin have been lost because of injury or surgery for cancer. Cosmetic surgery on faces, noses, breasts and the abdomen is also carried out by plastic surgeons.

PLATELETS Blood platelets, or thrombocytes, are small spherical bodies in the blood, which play an important part in the process of blood coagulation (q.v.). Normally, there are around 300,000 per cubic millimetre of blood.

PLATING is a term used in connection with bacteriological investigation to mean the cultivation of bacteria on flat plates containing nutrient material. The term is also applied in surgery to the method of securing union of fractured bones by screwing to the sides of the fragments narrow metal plates, which hold them firmly together while union is taking place.

PLETHORA means a condition of fullness of the blood-vessels in a particular part or in the whole body. The term is applied to a condition in which the volume of the blood is increased above normal; there may or may not be an increase in the total number of red blood corpuscles.

PLETHYSMOGRAPH is an apparatus for estimating changes in the size of any part placed in the apparatus; in this way changes in the volume of blood in a part can be measured.

PLEURA, or PLEURAL MEMBRANE, is the name of the membrane which, on either side of the chest, forms a covering for one lung. The two pleurae are distinct, though they touch one another for a short distance behind the breastbone. (See LUNGS.)

PLEURAL CAVITY The normally restricted space between the parietal and visceral pleura (q.v.), which slide over one another as the individual breathes in and out. If gas or fluid are introduced as a result of injury or infection, the pleural surfaces are separated and the pleural space increases in volume. This usually causes breathing difficulties.

PLEURISY, or PLEURITIS, means inflammation of the pleura or serous membrane investing the lung and lining the inner surface of the ribs. It is a common condition, and may be either acute or chronic, the latter being usually tuberculous in origin.

Many cases of pleurisy are associated with only a little effusion, the inflammation consisting chiefly in exudation of fibrin. To this form the term *dry pleurisy* is applied. Further, pleurisy may be limited to a very small area, or, on the contrary, may affect, throughout a greater or less extent, the pleural surfaces of both lungs.

Causes Pleurisy is often associated with other forms of inflammatory disease within the chest, more particularly pneumonia, bronchiectasis, and tuberculosis, and also occasionally accompanies pericarditis. It may also be due to carcinoma of the lung, or be secondary to abdominal infections such as subphrenic abscess. Further, wounds or injuries of the thoracic walls are apt to set up pleurisy.

Symptoms The symptoms of pleurisy vary, being generally well marked, but sometimes obscure.

DRY PLEURISY In the case of dry pleurisy, which is, on the whole, the milder form, the chief symptom is a sharp pain in the side, felt especially on breathing. Fever may or may not be present. There is a slight, dry cough, and breathing is quicker than normal and shallow. PLEURISY WITH EFFUSION is usually more severe than dry pleurisy, and, although it may in some cases develop insidiously, it is in general ushered in sharply by shivering and fever, like other acute inflammatory diseases. Pain is felt in the side or breast, of a severe cutting or stabbing character. A dry cough is almost always present. The breathing is painful and difficult.

Treatment The treatment varies greatly with the form and severity of the attack. Bed rest, antibiotics, analgesics and antipyretics are advisable. A large pleural effusion may need to be drained via an aspiration needle.

PLEURODYNIA means a painful condition of the chest-wall. It may be due to rheumatism of the intercostal muscles or to neuralgia of the intercostal nerves, or, when of the sharp nature popularly known as a 'stitch in the side', to cramp.

PLEXUS is a network of nerves or vessels: e.g. the brachial and sacral plexuses of nerves and the choroid plexus of veins within the brain.

PLICAMYCIN (see MITHRAMYCIN).

PLUMBISM is another name for lead poisoning. (See LEAD POISONING.)

PLUMMER-VINSON SYNDROME is a syndrome associated with certain cases of hypochromic anaemia. It consists of hyochromic anaemia, and difficulty in swallowing due to an oesophageal web. It is found practically only in women. (See ANAEMIA.)

PNEUMOCOCCUS A type of streptococcal bacterium which is associated with pneumonia and other infections of the respiratory tract.

PNEUMOCONIOSIS is the general name applied to a chronic form of inflammation of the lungs which is liable to affect workmen who constantly inhale irritating particles at work. It has been defined by the Industrial Injuries Advisory Council as: 'Permanent alteration of lung structure due to the inhalation of mineral dust and the tissue reactions of the lung to its presence but does not include bronchitis and emphysema'. Some of the trades liable to suffer are those of stone-masons, potters, steel-grinders, ganister workers, colour-grinders, coalminers, millers, and workers in cotton, flax, or wool mills. Annually about 400 workers are diagnosed as having coalminer's pneumoconiosis; 120 other workers have asbestosis and under 100 silicosis. (See OCCUPATIONAL DISEASES; TUBERCULOSIS.)

PNEUMONECTOMY is the operation of removing an entire lung in such diseases as bronchiectasis, tuberculosis, and cancer of the lung.

PNEUMONIA Inflammation of the lung may be caused by allergic reactions, when the term *alveolitis* is used, or by chemical or physical agents, when the term *pneumonitis* is used. The classicial division of pneumonia into lobar and bronchial pneumonia is no longer relevant. The aetiology and management of pneumonia depends on whether it occurs in a healthy person or in a person who has some underlying chronic disease that has lowered his local bronchial defences or his general resistance to infection. Conditions predisposing to the lowering of local or general resistance are chronic bronchitis, diabetes mellitus, malnutrition, alcoholism, and in those patients in whom the immune mechanism is suppressed either by a disease such as leukaemia or by the treatment with immunosuppressive drugs which is always necessary after an organ transplant.

When pneumonia arises in a previously healthy person the three most common organisms are the *Streptococcus pneumoniae*, a virus or mycoplasma pneumoniae. *Staphlylococcus aureus* is an important cause of pneumonia following an attack of influenza. Rarer causes of pneumonia in a previously healthy person include psittacosis, which is caused by a chlamydia, Q fever caused by a rickettsia, and legionnaire's disease which is caused by a bacterium. Organisms responsible for pneumonia in patients with pre-existing disease include *Streptococcus pneumoniae*, *Staphlylococcus aureus*, *Haemophilus influenziae*, *Streptococcus pyogenes*, Klebsiella and Gram-negative bacilli such as *Pseudomomas aeruginosa*, *Escherichia coli* and Proteus.

Immunosuppressive drugs predispose to what are called opportunist infections of the lung, which are infections by organisms that rarely cause pneumonia in ordinary circumstances. These include bacteria such as nocardia, cytomegalovirus, fungi and protozoa (*Pneumocystic carinii*).

Symptoms The common symptoms with which pneumonia presents are cough, fever, especially when accompanied by rigors, pleuritic pain, dyspnoea or cyanosis. The elderly or infirm may have no fever. The sputum is usually purulent in patients with chronic bronchitis and watery and rusty in those with an overwhelming infection. In other cases sputum may be difficult to obtain during the early stages of the disease and this is partly because coughing is suppressed by pleuritic pain. It is however important to obtain a specimen of sputum so that the nature of the pneumonia can be ascertained by culturing the organism responsible.

Certain physical signs are usually present. Diminished movement of the affected side is noticeable, the healthy side of the chest performing most of the respiratory function. On percussion over the affected area a dull note is obtained which becomes particularly marked if fluid has collected in the pleural cavity. On auscultation over the affected area the breathing is usually harsh and high-pitched (bronchial breathing) but it sometimes shows no deviation from normal, especially in cases in which the deeper parts of the lung only are affected. Accompanying the breathing in the early stages of the disease crackling sounds may be heard.

It is advisable to obtain a specimen of

sputum and to do a blood culture before antibiotics are given.

Treatment The treatment of pneumonia requires eradication of the infection, correcting hypoxia, relieving cough and pleuritic pain, and dealing with any complications that may arise. If the patient is drowsy, cyanosed or confused, hospital admission is indicated. Treatment of the infection with antibiotics should start at the earliest possible moment. The choice of antibiotic is based on the clinical judgement of the type of pneumonia with any microbiological support that is available. Microscopic examination of the sputum with the relevant stains will provide a clue to the nature of the prevailing organism but the results of culture may take 24 to 48 hours. Pus cells in the sputum and a leucocytosis suggest that the infection is bacterial rather than viral in origin. Pneumonia in a previously healthy person, particularly if there are rigors and herpes labialis and if there are pus cells and diplococci in the sputum, means that pneumonia is almost certainly due to *Strep. pneumoniae* and the antibiotic of choice is benzylpenicillin. If the clinical symptoms and signs suggest that the pneumonia is due to a virus, mycoplasma or other non-bacterial infection, then a broad spectrum antibiotic such as erythromycin or tetracycline or ampicillin is indicated. Pneumonia complicating chronic bronchitis should be treated with a broad spectrum antibiotic such as ampicillin or co-trimoxazole. Acute fulminating pneumonia accompanied by signs of respiratory or circulatory failure is probably staphylococcal in origin and this requires urgent intravenous treatment with flucloxacillin and either gentamicin or tobramicin. The optimum duration of antibiotic treatment depends on the response of the patient and the nature of the infection. Good nursing is also important. Pain and difficulty in breathing may be relieved by the application of hot-water bottles and by the administration of analgesics. Cough may be relieved by expectorants. Excessive fever may be controlled by sponging with tepid water. As regards feeding, the digestive powers are much reduced in such an acute infection and the patient should be fed with milk, soups and other light forms of nourishment. Oxygen is important for the hypoxic patient. However if the patient has chronic obstructive airways disease oxygen is the drive to respiration and if oxygen is given in too great a concentration respiration will be suppressed and the patient will die of hypercapnia and acidosis. Oxygen is therefore administered in a concentration of 28 per cent usually through a Venturi mask.

PNEUMONITIS is an inflammation of the lung due to chemical or physical agents. When the inflammation of the lung is due to infections it is called pneumonia and when it is caused by allergic reactions it is known as alveolitis.

PNEUMOPERITONEUM means a collection of air in the peritoneal cavity. Air introduced into the peritoneal cavity collects under the diaphragm which is thus raised and collapses the lungs. This procedure was sometimes carried out in the treatment of pulmonary tuberculosis in the pre-antibiotic days as an alternative to artificial pneumothorax.

PNEUMOTHORAX means a collection of air in the pleural cavity, into which it has gained entrance by a lesion in the lung or a wound in the chest wall. When air enters the chest the lung immediately collapses towards the centre of the chest, but, air being absorbed from the pleural cavity, the lung expands again in a short time. (See LUNGS, DISEASES OF.)

Artificial pneumothorax was an operation often performed in the pre-antibiotic days by which in a case of pulmonary tuberculosis air was run into the pleural cavity to cause collapse of one lung, which rests it and allows cavities in it to heal.

PODAGRA is another name for gout affecting the foot. (See GOUT.)

PODOPHYLLIN is a resin derived from the root of *Podophyllum peltatum*, a plant of the United States and Canada, or from *Podophyllum emodi*, a plant which grows in the Himalayas. It has a purgative action but is seldom used for this purpose now. It is also used as a local application in the treatment of venereal warts.

POIKILOCYTOSIS This is a term used to describe the variation seen in the shape of red blood cells in some bone marrow disorders.

POISONS A poison is any substance which, if absorbed by, introduced into or applied to a living organism may cause morbidity or mortality. The term toxin is often used to refer to a poison of biological origin. Toxins are therefore a subgroup of poisons, but often little distinction is made between the terms. The study of the effects of poisons is toxicology and the effects of toxins is toxinology.

The concept of the dose-response is important for understanding the risk of exposure to a particular substance. This is embodied in a statement by Paracelsus (*c.*1493–1541): 'All substances are poisons; there is none which is not a poison. The right dose differentiates a poison and a remedy.'

Poisoning may occur in a variety of ways: deliberate – suicide, substance abuse or murder; accidental – including accidental overdose of medicines; occupational; environmental – including exposure during fire.

Ingestion is the most common route of exposure but poisoning may also occur through inhalation, absorption through the skin, by injection and through bites and stings of venomous animals. Poisoning may be described as acute, where a single exposure produces clinical effects with a relatively rapid onset, or chronic, where prolonged or repeated exposures may produce clinical effects which may be insidious in onset, cumulative and in some cases permanent.

Diagnosis of poisoning is usually by circumstantial evidence or elimination of other causes of the clinical condition of the patient. Some substances (e.g. opioids (q.v.)), anticholinergic agents (q.v.) produce a characteristic clinical picture in overdose that can help with diagnosis. In some cases laboratory analysis may be useful to determine or confirm the agent taken. Routine assays are not necessary. For a very small number of poisons, such as paracetamol, aspirin, iron and lead, the management of the patient may depend on measuring the amount of poison in the bloodstream.

Accurate statistics on the incidence of poisoning in the UK are lacking. Mortality figures are more reliable than morbidity statistics. In 1987 about 120,000 cases of poisoning were admitted to hospital. In the same year about 35,000 children under 4 years of age attended (but were not necessarily admitted to) hospital because of accidental poisoning in the home. The total figure for all ages was 40,000. The annual number of deaths from poisoning is relatively small, about 300. In most cases patients die before reaching hospital. Currently carbon monoxide is by far the commonest cause of death due to poisoning. The most common agents involved in intentional or accidental poisoning are drugs, particularly analgesics, antidepressants and sedatives. Alcohol is also commonly taken by adults, usually in combination with drugs. Children frequently swallow household cleaners, white spirit, plant material, aftershave and perfume as well as drugs. The use of child-resistant containers has reduced the number of admissions of children to hospital for treatment. Bixtrex® is an intensely bitter-tasting agent which is often added to products to discourage ingestion; however not everybody is able to taste it nor has any beneficial effect been proved.

Treatment of poisoning usually begins with decontamination procedures. For ingested substances this may involve making the patient sick or washing the stomach out. This is usually only worthwhile if performed soon after ingestion. It should be emphasized that salt (sodium chloride) water must never be given to induce vomiting since this procedure is dangerous and has caused death. For substances spilt on the skin the affected area should immediately be thoroughly washed and all contaminated clothing removed. When the eye has been exposed to a poison it should be thoroughly irrigated with saline or water. Treatment is then generally symptomatic and supportive with maintenance of the respiratory, neurological and cardiovascular systems, and where appropriate, monitoring of fluid and electrolyte balance and hepatic and renal function. Some substances have specific antidotes: the most important of these are paracetamol (q.v.), iron, cyanide (q.v.), opioids, digoxin, anticoagulant agents, organophosphorus insecticides and some heavy metals.

When a patient presents with an illness thought to be caused by exposure to substances at work, further exposure should be limited or prevented and investigations undertaken to determine the source and extent of the problem. Acutely poisoned workers will usually go to hospital, but those suffering from chronic exposure may attend their GP with non-specific symptoms.

In recent years the UK has approved legislation to improve safety in the workplace and to ensure that data on the hazardous constituents and effects of chemicals are most readily available. These official controls include the Control of Substances Hazardous to Health (COSHH) and the Chemicals (Hazard Information and Packaging) Regulations (CHIP) and introduced in response to European Union directives.

The National Poisons Information Service is a 24-hour emergency telephone service available to the medical profession which provides information on the likely effects of numerous agents and advice on the management of the poisoned patient (see APPENDIX 2: ADDRESSES). In the UK this is not a public access service. People who believe they, or their relatives, have been poisoned should seek medical advice from their GPs or attend their local hospital or, if the incident is acute, call the emergency services. Factories and other potentially hazardous work places should have appropriate first aid or emergency procedures available, with the staff informed about what steps to take.

POLIOMYELITIS, or INFANTILE PARALYSIS, is a viral infection involving the brain and spinal cord. After the first recorded epidemic in Sweden in 1881, the disease became increasingly important, but has become relatively rare since the successful introduction of oral polio vaccination. The disease has been notifiable in Great Britain since 1912; the annual number of cases is in single figures, with none being reported in some years. Although sporadic cases may occur at any time, there is a definite seasonal incidence, with epidemics tending to occur in the late summer and early autumn in the northern hemisphere. In the tropics infection continues throughout the year.

Pathology There are three types of virus, infection spreading by the stools – contaminated hands – mouth route. Children are most susceptible, but an increasing tendency to severe paralytic cases among young adults has been reported recently. Children vaccinated with Sabin live attenuated oral poliomyelitis vaccine (OPV) can pass the infection to unvaccinated adults who are caring for them for up to 6 weeks after vaccination.

One attack usually produces permanent immunity, and second attacks are rare. The virus typically affects the anterior horn cells, especially those in the lumbar section of the spinal cord, and the grey matter of the brain stem and cortex may also be damaged.

Symptoms The incubation period is around 7 to 14 days, the onset being marked by a mild fever and headache which improves after a few days. In many cases there is no further progression, but in some – after approximately one week – the symptoms recur, together with neck stiffness and signs of meningeal irritation. Weakness of individual muscle groups is common, and may progress – to a variable extent, depending on the distribution of the virus – to widespread paralysis. Involvement of the diaphragm and intercostal muscles may lead to respiratory failure and rapid death unless artificial respiration is provided. Involvement of the cranial nerves and brain may lead to nystagmus (q.v.), hoarseness, and difficulty in swallowing, and convulsions may occur in young children. The cerebrospinal fluid shows an early increase in lymphocytes, followed by a rise in protein concentration.

Treatment Oral vaccine given in childhood has practically banished the disease in many countries, but a booster dose should be given to adults when travelling outside Europe and the USA. When cases of polio occur, there may be great variation in the proportion of abortive and non-paralytic cases, and in mortality rate. Paralysis is greatest at the end of the first week of the major illness. Gradual recovery may then take place for several months, but any muscle showing no sign of recovery after a month is unlikely to regain any useful function. Treatment involves early bed rest, followed by physiotherapy and orthopaedic measures as required. At the onset of respiratory difficulties a tracheostomy (q.v.) and artificial ventilation should be started. In cases of severe paralysis with persistent wasting of the limbs, surgery may be necessary to minimize the resulting disability.

POLIOSIS means premature greying of the hair. It is also the term applied to whitening of the hair in segments, such as a forelock.

POLLEN consists of microspores formed in flowering plants and conifers. Between 4 and 7 million tons of it are said to be shed annually throughout the world. From ancient days it has had the reputation of being a specific against old age, and recent reports from Russia claim that bee-keepers live longer because they eat pollen. It contains protein, vitamins A, B, C, D and K, small amounts of minerals including calcium, copper, iron, magnesium, manganese, phosphorus, potassium, and sulphur, as well as several enzymes. It has a bitter taste, which is traditionally disguised by honey – the ambrosia of the Bible, the Koran and the Talmud. Sufferers from hay fever should not eat it during the hay-fever season as it may induce allergic reactions.

POLLEX is a Latin term for thumb.

POLYARTERITIS NODOSA, or PERIARTERITIS NODOSA as it is sometimes known, is a disease of unknown origin, in which prolonged fever and obscure symptoms referable to any system of the body are associated with local areas of inflammation along the arteries, giving rise to nodules in their walls. Recovery occurs in about 50 per cent of cases.

POLYCHROMASIA and **POLYCHROMATOPHILIA** are terms applied to an abnormal reaction of the red blood corpuscles in severe anaemia, whereby they have a bluish tinge instead of the normal red colour in a blood film stained by the usual method. It is a sign that the cell is not fully developed.

POLYCYSTIC DISEASE OF KIDNEY An inherited disease in which the kidneys contain many cysts. These grow in size until normal kidney tissue is largely destroyed. Cysts may also occur in other organs such as the liver. In adults the disease will cause hypertension and kidney failure. There is also a juvenile form. There is no effective treatment, though symptoms can be alleviated by dialysis and sometimes kidney transplant.

POLYCYSTIC OVARY SYNDROME In 1935 Stein and Leventhan described seven hirsute and infertile women with amenorrhoea or oligomenorrhoea in whom bilateral cystic ovarian enlargement was found at laparotomy and thereby gave their names to a polycystic ovarian disorder. Since then, however, the protean manner of clinical presentation and the variability of biochemical changes in patients with this condition have lead some people to doubt the existence of a disease entity. Enlarged cystic ovaries may occur in the absence of the classical clinical characteristics originally described. Polycystic ovaries may be found in those who have conceived and are not hirsute, and they may be seen in infertile women who menstruate regularly and even in some patients with menorrhagia. On the other hand, the clinical features of oligomenorrhoea, hirsutism and infertility may occur in the absence of bilateral ovarian enlargement and cystic change may be found in normal sized or small ovaries.

Polycystic ovaries may have several causes. Whether large or small ovaries result may be determined by the duration and severity of the particular cause. Sclerocystic ovarian change would therefore be a better description, but the term polycystic is now firmly established by common usage. The choice of treatment is determined by the clinical presentation and the main complaint. If hirsutism is the main problem and there is evidence of androgen suppression after dexamethasone, then corticosteroid treatment should be tried. The anti-androgen, cyproterone acetate, has recently been introduced and is probably more effective. If, however, fertility is the prime consideration then clomiphene should be given and wedge ressection of the ovaries considered if pregnancy does not result after three courses of the drug.

POLYCYTHAEMIA is an excess in the number of red corpuscles in the blood.

POLYCYTHEMIA RUBRA VERA A disorder in which the red blood cells increase in number along with an increase in the number of white blood cells and platelets. The cause is unknown. Severe cases may require treatment with cytotoxic drugs or radiotherapy.

POLYDACTYLY means the presence of extra, or supernumerary, fingers or toes.

POLYDIPSIA means excessive thirst, which is a symptom of diabetes mellitus and some other diseases.

POLYMER FUME FEVER occurs in people who work with polytetrafluoroethylene (PTFE, Teflon). The fever is caused by degradation products, including hydrofluoric acid, which are produced at temperatures of 170 °C and upwards. The likeliest source of these injurious products is cigarette smoking. Even the tiniest particles of PTFE on a burning cigarette will yield sufficient of these degradation products to cause fume fever.

The illness consists of an influenza-like illness, which lasts for a few hours.

POLYMORPH is a name applied to certain white corpuscles of the blood which have a nucleus of irregular and varied shape. These form between 70 and 75 per cent of all the white corpuscles. (See BLOOD.)

POLYMORPHIC LIGHT ERUPTION is a photodermatosis (q.v.) which occurs predominantly in females, appearing first as a rule in adolescence or early adult life. The eruption, which consists of a mixture of erythema (q.v.), papules (q.v.) and vesicles (q.v.), occurs on those parts of the body exposed to the sun, mainly the back of the hands, the forearms, the front of the neck, the cheeks and the nose. There are usually several attacks a year, depending on the amount of sunlight. The attacks start in the spring and continue until the winter. Apart from the fact that the rash is provoked by sunlight, the precise cause is not known. Treatment consists of avoiding sunlight, wearing protective clothing, and using sunscreening preparations. (See SUNBURN.)

POLYMYALGIA RHEUMATICA is a form of rheumatism characterized by gross early morning stiffness, which tends to ease off during the day, and pain in the shoulders and sometimes round the hips. It affects women more than men, and is rare under the age of 60. The cause is still obscure. It responds well to prednisolone, but treatment may need to be ng continued. On the other hand the condi- n is not progressive and does not lead to pling.

POLYMYOSITIS A disease of the muscles throughout the body. The disorder may be acute or chronic but it usually affects the muscles of the shoulders or hip areas. The muscles weaken and are tender to the touch. Diffuse inflammatory changes occur and symptomatic relief may be obtained with corticosteroid drugs (q.v.).

POLYMYXIN is the name applied to the group of antibiotics derived from various species of *Bacillus polymyxa*. One variety, colistin, is used to sterilize the bowels before surgery. Polymyxin B is the antibiotic of choice in the treatment of infections of the skin, eye and ear.

POLYNEURITIS means an inflammatory condition of nerves in various parts of the body. (See NEURITIS.)

POLYPEPTIDE A molecule in which several amino-acids (q.v.) are joined together by peptide bonds. Protein (q.v.) molecules are polypeptides.

POLYPHARMACY is a term applied to the administration of too many drugs to one person. Sometimes combinations of drugs are an effective means of treatment, reducing the risk of drug resistance. Polypharmacy, however, worsens the risk of drug interactions and of adverse effects, especially in the elderly.

POLYPOSIS means the presence of a crop, or large number, of polypi. The most important form of polyposis is that known as *familial polyposis coli*. This is a hereditary disease characterized by the presence of large numbers of polypoid tumours in the large bowel. Every child born to an affected parent stands a fifty-fifty chance of developing the disease. Its importance is that sooner or later one or more of these tumours undergoes cancerous change. If the affected gut is removed surgically before this occurs, and preferably before the age of 20, the results are excellent.

POLYPUS or POLYP is a general name applied to tumours which are attached by a stalk to the surface from which they spring. The term refers only to the shape of the growth and has nothing to do with its structure or nature. Most polypi are of a simple nature, though malignant polypi are also found. The usual structure of a polypus is that of a fine fibrous core covered with epithelium resembling that of the surrounding surface. The sites in which polypi are most usually found are the interior of the nose, the outer meatus of the ear, and the interior of the womb, bladder, or bowels (see POLYPOSIS).

Their removal is generally easy, as they are simply twisted off, or cut off, by some form of snare or ligature. Those which are situated in the interior of the bladder or bowels, and whose presence is usually recognized by the presence of blood in the urine or stools, require a more serious operation to reach the organ into which they project.

POLYSACCHARIDE A carbohydrate comprising several monosaccharides linked in long chains. Polysaccharides store energy – as starch in plants and glycogen in animals – and they also form the structural parts of plants (as cellulose) and animals (as mucopolysaccharides).

POLYTHELIA is the condition in which extra or supernumerary nipples appear along a line between the armpit and the groin.

POLYTHIAZIDE is a moderately potent diuretic (q.v.) drug of the thiazide group.

POLYURIA means the passage of an amount of urine considerably in excess of the 1500 ml or thereabout which is the usual daily quantity. It is a symptom of diabetes mellitus, diabetes insipidus, chronic renal failure and psychogenic polydipsia.

POMPHOLYX is a form of eczema characterized by the appearance of deeply set vesicles (q.v.) on the palms and soles, fingers and toes. When it occurs on the fingers and hands it is known as CHEIROPOMPHOLYX. On the toes and feet it is known as PODOPOMPHOLYX.

PONS VAROLII is the bridge of the brain, mainly composed of strands of white nerve-fibres which unite various parts of the brain. (See BRAIN.)

POPLITEAL SPACE, or HAM, is the name given to the region behind the knee. The muscles attached to the bones immediately above and below the knee bound a diamond-shaped space through which pass the main artery and vein of the limb (known in this part of their course as the popliteal artery and vein), the tibial and common peroneal nerves (which continue the sciatic nerve from the thigh down to the leg), the external saphenous vein, as well as several small nerves and lymphatic vessels. The muscles, which bound the upper angle of the space and which are attached to the leg bones by strong prominent tendons, are known as the hamstrings. The lower angle of the space lies between the two heads of the gastrocnemius muscle, which makes up the main bulk of the calf of the leg.

POPPY as used in medicine is of two species: *Papaver somniferum*, the white opium-poppy (see OPIUM), and *Papaver rhoeas*, the red corn-poppy. The corn-poppy is chiefly used as a colouring agent, the syrup made from it having a brilliant crimson colour.

PORE A small opening. The word is usually used to describe an opening in the skin that releases sweat or sebum, a waxy material secreted by the sebaceous glands in the skin.

PORPHYRIA is a condition, or rather a series of conditions, characterized by an excessive production and excretion of porphyrins. Porphyrins are constituents of various blood and respiratory pigments found throughout the animal kingdom, including human beings. They are also found in plants and micro-organisms.

In porphyria there is some disturbance of their metabolism and this results in a variegated picture which includes discoloration of the urine due to excessive excretion of porphyrins, skin rashes due to sensitization of the skin to light, various forms of indigestion and mental disturbances.

PORPHYRINS Complex organic compounds which are sensitive to light and form the basis of respiratory pigments, for example, haemoglobin and myoglobin. Porphyrins are crucial to many metabolic oxidation/reduction reactions in animals, plants, and micro-organisms.

PORT-A-CATH The Port-a-cath system consists of a silicon catheter connected to a stainless steel chamber in which there is a silicon injection port. The catheter is inserted into a central vein and connected by a sub-cutaneous tunnel to the portal which is implanted subcutaneously on the chest wall. Its purpose is to provide a central venous access while avoiding repeated cannulation with its inevitable risk of sepsis.

PORTAL HYPERTENSION Raised blood pressure in the portal vein. This results in increased pressure in the veins of the oesophagus and upper stomach and these grow in size to form varices – dilated tortuous veins. Sometimes these varices rupture causing bleeding into the oesophagus. The raised pressure also causes fluid to collect in the abdomen and form ascites. The commonest reason for portal hypertension is cirrhosis (see LIVER DISEASES) (fibrosis) of the liver. Thrombosis in the portal vein may also be a cause. Treatment requires the cause to be tackled, but bleeding from ruptured vessels may be stopped by injecting a sclerosant or hardening solution into and around the veins. Sometimes a surgical shunt may be done to divert blood from the portal vein to another blood vessel.

PORTAL SYSTEM A vein or collection of veins which finish at both ends in a bed of capillary blood vessels. An important example is the hepatic portal system, comprising the portal vein and its tributaries. Blood from the stomach, pancreas, spleen and intestines drains into the veins that join up to comprise the portal vein into the liver, where it branches into sinusoids.

PORTAL VEIN is the vein which carries to the liver blood that has been circulating in many of the abdominal organs. It is peculiar among the veins of the body in that it ends by breaking up into a capillary network instead of carrying the blood directly to the heart, a peculiarity which it shares only with certain small vessels in the kidneys. The portal system begins below in the haemorrhoidal plexus of veins round the lower end of the rectum, and from this point, along the whole length of the intestines, the blood is collected into an inferior mesenteric vein upon the left, and a superior mesenteric vein upon the right side. The inferior mesenteric vein empties into the splenic vein, and the latter, uniting with the superior mesenteric vein immediately above the pancreas, forms the portal vein. The portal vein is joined by veins from the stomach and gall-bladder, and finally divides into two branches which sink into the right and left lobes of the liver. (For their further course, see LIVER.)

The organs from which the portal vein collects the blood are the large and small intestines, the stomach, spleen, pancreas, and gall-bladder.

POSITRON-EMISSION TOMOGRAPHY (PET) A method for assessing the metabolic activity of tissues in the brain. The operator measures emissions of radiation from specially radiated deoxyglucose. The brain cells accept this substance in the same way as they do glucose. Metabolic activity is slowed down in injured brain tissues, which can therefore be identified. This type of tomography is used to diagnose and treat patients with cerebral palsy and similar brain damage.

POSSETTING is the technical term used to describe the quite common habit of healthy babies to regurgitate, or bring up, small amounts of the meal they have just taken.

POST- is a prefix signifying after or behind.

POST-COITAL CONTRACEPTION Action taken to prevent conception after intercourse. The hormonal (Yuzpe) method is suitable for occasional use, being taken up to three days after unprotected intercourse (see CONTRACEPTION).

POST-COITAL TEST A test for infertility. A specimen of cervical mucus, taken up to 24 hours after coitus (during the post-ovulatory phase of the menstrual cycle), is examined microscopically to assess the motility of the sperms. If motility is above a certain level then sperms and mucus are not interacting abnormally, thus eliminating one cause of sterility.

POST-MORTEM EXAMINATION (see NECROPSY).

POST-OPERATIVE Relating to the period after an operation, to the patient's condition after operation or to any investigations or treatment during this time.

POST-PARTUM is the term applied to anything happening immediately after child-birth: for example, post-partum haemorrhage.

POST-TRAUMATIC STRESS DISORDER (PTSD) An individual who has suffered great personal stress arising from an alarming event may develop this severe anxiety disorder. The event may be an injury, exposure to disaster resulting in casualties, participation in warfare as combatant or refugee, an assault or a rape or witnessing an assault or rape. Any reaction may be when the event occurs or months or even years later. Someone with PTSD has regular recurrences of memories or images of the stressful event. Insomnia, nightmares, feelings of guilt and isolation, an inability to concentrate and irritability may develop. The affected individual often becomes very depressed. Support from friends and family and skilled counselling help to resolve the condition, which usually – but not always – settles with time.

POST-VIRAL FATIGUE SYNDROME (see MYALGIC ENCEPHALOMYELITIS).

POSTURAL DRAINAGE is the process whereby the drainage of secretions from dilated bronchi of the lungs is facilitated. The patient lies on an inclined plane head downwards and is encouraged to cough up as much secretion from the lungs as possible. The precise position depends on which part of the lungs is affected. It may need to be carried out for up to three hours daily in divided periods. It is of particular value in bronchiectasis (q.v.) and lung abscess.

POTASH, or POTASSA, is the popular name for potassium carbonate. Hydrated oxide of potassium is usually known as caustic potash, and its solution as potash solution.

POTASSIUM is a metal which, on account of its great affinity for other substances, is not found in a pure state in nature. Its salts are used to a great extent in medicine but, as their action depends in general not on their metallic radicle but upon the acid with which it is combined, their uses vary greatly and are described elsewhere. All salts of potassium have a depressing effect on the heart's action by virtue of the potassium ion.

POTASSIUM ASCORBATE EYE-DROPS were originally introduced for the treatment of glaucoma. They are now largely used in helping to prevent ulceration and perforation of the cornea (see EYE DISEASES) following acid and alkali burns of the eye.

POTASSIUM CHLORATE, in addition to the general actions exerted by potassium salts, has a soothing action upon inflamed mucous membranes, and is used for a gargle in sore throat of every description.

POTT'S DISEASE is a name often applied to the angular curvature of the spine which results from tuberculous disease. (See SPINE AND SPINAL CORD, DISEASES AND INJURIES OF.) The disease is named after Percivall Pott, an English surgeon (1714–88), who first described the condition.

POTT'S FRACTURE is a term applied to a variety of fractures around the ankle, accompanied by a varying degree of dislocation of the ankle. In all cases the fibula is fractured. Named after Percivall Pott, who suffered from this fracture and was the first to describe it (see FRACTURES), it is often mistaken for a simple sprain of the ankle.

POULTICES (see also FOMENTATION) are soft moist applications to the surface of the body, generally used hot to soothe pain due to inflammation and promote resolution.

POUPART'S LIGAMENT, also known as the inguinal ligament, is the strong ligament lying in the boundary between the anterior abdominal wall and the front of the thigh.

POWDERS form a method in which drugs are prescribed, powerful drugs being made up with inert substances like sugar, gum, or ginger in order to give them sufficient bulk. The best known powders were Dover's powder (ipecacuanha and opium powder), containing opium; Gregory's powder (compound rhubarb powder); and Seidlitz powder (compound effervescent powder). Powders have largely been replaced by tablets.

PRAZIQUANTEL is a drug that is proving of value in the treatment of schistosomiasis (q.v.).

PRE- is a prefix meaning before.

PRECIPITIN An antibody that combines with an antigen and forms the immune complex as a precipitate. The reaction is used in some diagnostic serological tests to indentify antigens in the serum.

PRECORDIAL REGION is the area on the centre and towards the left side of the chest, lying in front of the heart.

PREDNISOLONE is a derivative of cortisone, which is five or six times as active as cortisone and has less of the salt- and water-retaining properties of cortisone. It is given by mouth.

PREDNISONE is the official name for deltadehydrocortisone, and has the same action as prednisolone.

PRE-ECLAMPSIA is a complication of pregnancy, of unknown cause, which in severe cases may proceed to eclampsia (q.v.). It is characterized by hypertension, renal impairment, oedema, often with proteinuria and disseminated intravascular coagulation. It usually occurs in the second half of pregnancy, mild cases (without proteinuria) occurring in about 10 per cent of pregnancies, severe cases in about 2 per cent. Predisposing factors include a first pregnancy, or pregnancy by a new partner; a family history of pre-eclampsia, hypertension, or other cardiovascular disorders; and pre-existing hypertension or diabetes mellitus. Increased incidence with lower socio-economic class may be linked to diet or to failure to attend for antenatal care. Although less common in smokers, fetal outlook is worse. Multiple prenancy and hydatiform mole (q.v.), together with hydrops fetalis (q.v.), predispose to early and severe pre-eclampsia
Treatment Severe pre-eclampsia is an emergency. Urgent admission to hospital should be arranged and, if available, the obstetric flying squad called. Treatment should be given to control the hypertension, the fetal heart rate carefully monitored, and in very severe cases urgent Caesarean section may be necessary.

PREGNANCY The time during which a woman carries a developing fetus in the uterus. (Occasional ectopic pregnancy (q.v.) occurs outside the uterus.)

Pregnancy lasts about 280 days from the first day of the last menstrual period. In exceptional cases there may be considerable variation. For the purpose of calculating the probable date of confinement, it is usual to take the first day of the last period that occurred, to allow seven days for the duration of this and then to add 273 days for the duration of gestation, making in all 280 days from the beginning of the last menstruation.

Signs of pregnancy (a) The sudden stoppage of the menstrual flow is the first sign. This symptom may, however, be due to many other causes (see MENSTRUATION). (b) Swelling of the breasts may start as soon as the second or third month of pregnancy. A thin fluid, known as colostrum, can, even at this early stage, be pressed from the nipples. The veins on the breasts become enlarged and visible, and the pigmented ring round the nipple (areola) becomes much darker than before, as well as showing small nodules (Montgomery's tubercles) round its edge. (c) Morning sickness is also a common sign, occurring in about two-thirds of all women. (d) Quickening, or the fluttering sensation felt by the mother in consequence of the child's rapid movements, is an important sign usually occurring during the fifth month of pregnancy or even later. (*e*) Enlargement of the abdomen, though for the first three months the enlargement is not apparent. (*f*) One certain sign of pregnancy is the beating of the fetal heart which can be heard by auscultation over the lower part of the abdomen from the middle of the fifth month onwards. (*g*) Other minor signs which are sometimes present include varicose veins, mucous discharge from the vagina, changes in the neck of the womb.

Pregnancy is a normal state and most women have few major problems and are delivered normally. All women should, however, attend regular antenatal clinics and be supervised by a doctor and/or a midwife. This ensures that any complications can be diagnosed early and dealt with appropriately.

PREGNANCY TESTS   There are several tests for pregnancy in its early stages, and these can be done on blood or urine; some of the urine tests may be carried out at home. Most tests are based on the detection of human chorionic gonadotrophin (HCG) (q.v.) in the woman's urine. They are nearly 100-per-cent accurate and may show positive as early as 30 days after the first day of the last normal period.
The Hogben test   This test is based upon the observation that the injection of pregnancy urine promotes ovulation in the female South African clawed toad (*Xenopus laevis*). It gives a result within twenty-four hours.
The Haemagglutination Inhibition test   This, and the subsequent tests to be mentioned, are known as immunological tests, as opposed to that already mentioned which is known as a biological test. They are based upon the effect of the urine from a pregnant woman upon the interaction of red-blood cells, which have been sensitized to human gonadotrophin (q.v.), and anti-gonadotrophin serum. They have the great practical advantage of being performed in a test-tube or even on a slide, and therefore not requiring animals. Because of their ease and speed of performance (a result can be obtained in two hours), these tests are being used on an increased scale. The *Latex test* and the *Gravindex test* are modifications of the haemagglutination test. (See also PRENATAL DIAGNOSIS.)

PREGNANDIOL is the excretion product of the hormone, PROGESTERONE (q.v.), manufactured by the corpus luteum of the ovary. Pregnandiol is excreted in the urine during the second half of the menstrual period, and its excretion rises steadily throughout pregnancy.

PREMATURE BEAT (see ECTOPIC BEAT).

PREMATURE BIRTH (see ABORTION; FETUS) is one that takes place before the end of the normal period of gestation, usually before 37 weeks. In practice, however, it is defined as a birth that takes place when the baby weighs less than 2·5 kilograms (5½ pounds). Between 5 and 10 per cent of babies are born prematurely and in around 40 per cent of premature births the cause is unknown. Pre-eclampsia is the commonest known cause; others include hypertension, chronic kidney disease, heart disease and diabetes mellitus. Multiple pregnancy is another cause. In the vast majority of cases the aim of management is to prolong the pregnancy and so improve the outlook for the unborn child. This consists essentially of rest in bed and sedation, but there are now several drugs, such as ritodrine (q.v.), that may be used to suppress the activity of the uterus and so help to delay premature labour. Prematurity was once a prime cause of infant mortality but modern medical care has greatly improved survival rates in development countries.

PREMATURE EJACULATION   A disorder in which ejaculation occurs before or immediately after the penis penetrates the vagina. The commonest sexual problem in men, persistent premature ejaculation, may have psychological causes, although many adolescents and some adults experience it occasionally. Sexual counselling may help to alleviate the condition.

PREMEDICATION   A drug or drugs given to a patient to produce sedation before an operation. A narcotic analgesic drug is usually used as this relieves pain as well as anxiety. An antisecretory drug is often added to reduce the secretions in the airways and thus lessen the risk of general anaesthesia. Premedication reduces the amount of anaesthetic needed to make the patient unconscious.

PREMENSTRUAL SYNDROME has been defined as 'any combination of emotional or physical features which occur cyclically in a woman before menstruation and which regress or disappear during menstruation'. It is characterized by mood changes, discomfort, swelling and tenderness in the breasts, swelling of the legs, a bloated feeling in the abdomen, headache, fatigue and constipation. The mood changes range from irritability and mild depression to outbursts of violence. It may last for three up to 14 days. How common it is is not known, as only the more severe cases are seen by doctors, but it has been estimated that 1 in 10 of all menstruating women suffer from it severely enough to require treatment. The cause is not known, but it is probably due to some upset of the hormonal balance of the body. In view of the multiplicity of causes that have been put forward, it is not surprising that there is an equal multiplicity of treatments. Among these one of the most widely used is progesterone (q.v.). Others include pyridoxine (q.v.), danazol (q.v.), and gamma linolenic acid available in the form of oil of evening primrose. Whatever drug may be prescribed, psychological treatment is equally essential and, in many cases, is all that is required.

PREMOLAR The two teeth on each side of the jaw positioned between the canines and the molars in the adult. The teeth are used with the molars for holding and grinding food.

PRENATAL DIAGNOSIS or SCREENING of fetal abnormalities may be the result of screening tests carried out on most or all pregnant women or as the result of specific diagnostic tests performed to detect specific conditions. Prenatal diagnosis is important as it will identify babies who might need medical or surgical treatment before or soon after birth. In addition it might also detect severe abnormalities for which parents might decide to have a therapeutic abortion (see ABORTION).

Ultrasound scanning (q.v.) is probably the most widely used diagnostic tool in obstetric practice. It can detect structural abnormalities such as spina bifida (q.v.) and cleft lip (q.v.) and even cardiac and renal problems. A series of scans can assess whether the baby is growing at a normal rate and it may also be used to assist with other diagnostic tests (e.g. amniocentesis (q.v.)).

Tests on the mother's blood can also diagnose fetal abnormalities. Alphafetoprotein (AFP) is produced by babies and 'leaks' into the amniotic fluid (q.v.) and is absorbed by the mother. In spina bifida (q.v.) and other neural tube defects there is increased leakage of AFP and a blood test at 16 weeks' gestation can detect a raised level which suggests the presence of these abnormalities.

The triple test, also performed at 16 weeks, measures AFP, and two hormones – human chorionic gonadotrophin and unconjugated oestradiol – and is used in diagnosing Down's syndrome (q.v.).

Amniocentesis involves inserting a needle through the mother's abdominal wall into the uterus to remove a sample of amniotic fluid at 16–18 weeks. Examination of the fluid and cells it contains is used in the diagnosis of Down's syndrome and other inherited disorders. The test carries a small risk of miscarriage.

Chorionic villus sampling may be used to diagnose various inherited conditions. A small amount of tissue from the developing placenta is removed for analysis and this test has the advantages of having a lower incidence of miscarriage than amniocentesis and is carried out at an earlier stage (9–13 weeks).

Analysis of a blood sample removed from the umbilical cord (cordocentesis) may diagnose infections in the uterus, blood disorders or inherited conditions.

Direct observation of the fetus via a viewing instrument called a fetoscope is also used diagnostically and will detect structural abnormalities.

Most tests have a recognized incidence of false positive and negative results and are therefore usually cross-checked with another test. Counselling of the parents about prenatal tests is important. This allows them to make an informed choice which may not necessarily involve terminating the pregnancy if an abnormality is found.

PREPUCE is the free fold of skin that overlaps the glans penis and retracts when the penis becomes erect. It is the part that is removed at circumcision (q.v.).

PRESBYACUSIS is the deafness that comes on with increasing years. It is caused by increasing loss of elasticity in the hearing mechanism, combined with the slowing down of the mental processes that accompanies old age. It is characterized by particular difficulty in hearing high notes such as the telephone and the voices of women and children. Hearing in a background of noise, is also early affected. Modern, miniaturized, transistor 'within-the-ear' hearing aids are now available that are proving helpful in making life more bearable for the elderly in this respect. (See also DEAFNESS; HEARING AIDS.)

PRESBYOPIA (see ACCOMMODATION; REFRACTION).

PRESCRIPTION is the written direction for drugs for medicinal use, given by the doctor to the patient, for dispensation by the pharmacist. Drugs should only be prescribed when essential for treatment, and when any possible risks involved to the patient (and fetus in cases of pregnancy) are outweighed by the potential benefits of giving the drug. When possible, non-proprietary, or generic, titles should be prescribed; by allowing the pharmacist to dispense any equivalent drug this avoids delay for the patient, as well as reducing the cost to the Health Service. Dosage is generally stated in metric units, and both the amount and frequency should be carefully explained to the patient by the doctor, and clearly written when the drug is dispensed (see also DOSAGE; DRUGS). Strict adherence to the Misuse of Drugs Act 1973 is necessary to restrict the inappropriate prescription and abuse of drugs, particularly controlled drugs (q.v.). Full details of drugs available on NHS prescription are given in the *British National Formulary*, which is published twice a year. Careful monitoring of prescribing in the UK is carried out by a government-appointed agency.

PRESENILE Describing the condition of premature ageing. The mental and physical faculties are adversely affected in presenility to an extent that does not usually occur until old age (see DEMENTIA).

PRESENTATION means the appearance in labour of some particular part of the child's body at the mouth of the womb. This is a head presentation in 96 per cent of cases, but in a certain number the breech (or buttocks) may present, or the face, or foot, or even a part of the trunk in cases of cross-birth.

PRESSOR is the term applied to anything that increases the activity of a function: for example, a pressor nerve or pressor drug.

PRESSURE SORES (see BED SORES).

PREVALENCE An epidemiological term describing the proportion of a defined group in the population having a condition at one point in time. It is an appropriate measure only in relatively stable conditions for example, chronic bronchitis – and is not suitable for measuring acute illnesses.

PREVENTIVE MEDICINE The branch of medicine concerned with the prevention of disease. Prevention is achieved by public health measures such as health education, health-screening programmes, immunization procedures against infectious diseases, the provision of clean water and the maintenance of a clean environment (see PUBLIC HEALTH).

PRIAPISM A persisting painful erection of the penis (q.v.) occurring without sexual stimulation. It is a rare but acute condition that requires immediate treatment. The cause is the failure of blood to drain from the spongy corpus caversonum tissues of the penis, thus maintaining an erection. This may happen because of infection, damage to the nerves controlling the blood vessels, or a clotting defect in the blood.

PRICKLY HEAT, or MILIARA RUBRA This common skin condition most often affects Europeans in a tropical climate. The outlet of sweat or sebaceous glands in the skin is obstructed; as a result, numerous minute vesicles appear which cause intolerable itching. Areas covered by clothing and subject to friction are usually involved. It is aggravated by any factor giving rise to perspiration – hot drinks, hot soup, close rooms, or warm clothing. A serious consequence is anhidrotic heat exhaustion. Secondary infection (with bacteria or fungi) is an important complication. Insomnia may result from intense irritation. Management consists of avoiding, as far as possible, all causes of excessive perspiration, reduction of salt intake, and maintenance of an adequate fluid intake. Following a bath, an astringent, antiseptic dusting powder – one composed of boric acid, zinc oxide, and starch in equal parts – should be applied; emollient creams or bath oil are also of value. Temporary relief can be obtained by the use of calamine lotion (either alone, or incorporating menthol crystals). Any associated heat illness must be treated promptly (see HEAT STROKE). Removal to a cool climate may be necessary.

PRIMIDONE is a drug used for the treatment of epilepsy.

PRIMIGRAVIDA A woman who is undergoing her first pregnancy.

PRIMIPARA is the term applied to a woman who has given birth, or is giving birth, to her first child.

PRO- is a prefix meaning forwards.

PROBE is a slender, flexible instrument usually made of metal designed for introduction into a wound or cavity either to explore its depth and direction, to discover the presence of foreign bodies, or to introduce medicinal substances.

PROBENECID is a benzoic acid derivative. It interferes with the excretion by the kidney of certain compounds, including penicillin and para-aminosalicylic acid, and was originally introduced into medicine for this reason, as a means of increasing and maintaining the concentration of penicillin in the body. It has also proved of value in the treatment of chronic gout.

PROBUCOL is a cholesterol-reducing drug. (See HYPERLIPIDAEMIA.)

PROCAINAMIDE is a derivative of procaine, which has been introduced for the treatment of certain cardiac arrythmias.

PROCAINE, or PROCAINE HYDROCHLORIDE, is a synthetic substance having a similar action to the natural alkaloid, cocaine. It is a powerful local anaesthetic with transitory effect. Procaine possesses the anaesthetic properties of cocaine, but has an advantage over the latter in being very much less poisonous, so that it can be administered in larger doses, and also in producing no tendency to contract a habit for its use.

PROCAINE PENICILLIN is an intramuscular preparation which is the preferred choice for the treatment of syphilis (see PENICILLIN).

PROCARBAZINE is a drug that is proving useful in the treatment of various forms of tumour, especially Hodgkin's disease (q.v.). It acts by interfering with the process of mitosis (q.v.), whereby the cells of the body, or tumours, reproduce themselves.

PROCHLORPERAZINE is an anti-psychotic drug. It is also an effective drug for the prevention or treatment of vomiting, and has therefore been used in the treatment of Menière's disease (q.v.). (See NEUROLEPTICS.)

PROCIDENTIA is another term for prolapse (q.v.).

PROCTALGIA is neuralgic pain in the anus or rectum. The term is usually reserved for rectal pain without local disease in the rectum to account for it.

Proctalgia fugax is a condition characterized by cramp-like pains in the rectum which may be excruciatingly painful. They are more common in men than women. They occur during the night, last up to fifteen minutes and may be accompanied by a feeling of faintness. The cause is not known. The taking of food or drink may bring relief, as may pressure on the perineum (e.g. by sitting astride the edge of the bath). A finger in the rectum may also bring relief. The sucking of a 1 mg tablet of glyceryl trinitrate is said by some to bring prompt relief. The attacks usually stop after the age of 50.

PROCTITIS means inflammation situated about the rectum or anus.

PRODROMATA is a term applied to the earliest symptoms of a disease, or those which give warning of its presence.

PROFLAVINE is a valuable antiseptic. It is an acridine derivative. Like all the acridine derivatives it is effective against both Gram-positive and Gram-negative bacteria and is not inactivated by body fluids or pus. It is also non-toxic and non-irritating.

PROGERIA is premature old age.

PROGESTERONE is the hormone of the corpus luteum (q.v.). After the escape of the ovum from the ruptured follicle, the corpus luteum secretes progesterone, which stimulates the growth and secretion of the endometrial glands of the uterus during the fourteen days before menstruation. In the event of pregnancy, the secretion of progesterone continues until parturition. (See also ETHISTERONE; NORETHISTERONE; PREGNANDIOL; CONTRACEPTION; MENSTRUATION.)

PROGESTOGEN is a preparation with an action like that of progesterone (q.v.).

PROGLOTTIS is a segment of a tapeworm.

PROGNATHISM Abnormal protusion of the lower jaw or sometimes of both jaws. The condition may make biting and chewing difficult, in which case corrective surgery is necessary.

PROGNOSIS is the term applied to a forecast as to the probable result of an illness or disease, particularly with regard to the prospect of recovery.

PROGRESSIVE MUSCULAR ATROPHY (see PARALYSIS).

PROGUANIL HYDROCHLORIDE is a synthetic antimalarial drug which has proved of value both in the treatment and the prevention of malaria, particularly the form known as malignant tertian malaria.

PROLACTIN is the pituitary hormone which initiates lactation. The development of the breasts during pregnancy is ascribed to the action of oestrogens (q.v.). Prolactin starts them secreting. If lactation does not occur or fails, it may be started by injection of prolactin.

The secretion of prolactin is normally kept under tonic inhibition by the secretion of a prolactin inhibitory hormone. This is formed in the hypothalamus and secreted into the portal capillaries of the pituitary stalk to reach the anterior pituitary cells. The prolactin inhibitory hormone has now been identified as the catecholamine dopamine. Drugs that deplete the brain stores of dopamine or antagonize dopamine at receptor level will cause hyperprolactinaemia and hence the secretion of milk from the breast and amenorrhoea. Methyldopa and reserpine deplete brain stores of dopamine and the phenothiazines act as dopamine antagonists at receptor level. Other causes of excess secretion of prolactin are pituitary tumours, which may be minute and are then called microadenomas, or may actually enlarge the pituitary fossa and are then called macroadenomas. The commonest cause of hyperprolactinaemia is a pituitary tumour. The patient may present with infertility, because patients with hyperprolactinaemia do not ovulate, or the patient may present with amenorrhea and even galactorrhoea.

Bromocriptine is a dopamine agonist. Treatment with bromocriptine will therefore control hyperprolactinaemia and restore normal menstruation and ovulation and suppress galactorrhoea. If the cause of hyperprolactinaemia is a macroadenoma, surgical treatment should be considered.

PROLAPSE means slipping down of some organ or structure. The term is applied chiefly to downward displacements of the rectum and womb. When the lower end of the bowel prolapses each time the bowels move – as may occur in children – it should be carefully sponged with cold water, replaced, and, if necessary, retained in place by a soft pad and bandage attached to a waist- belt, or by strapping the buttocks together with plaster. The condition tends to pass off as the child grows older. Prolapse which affects the womb may, in the earlier stages, cause protrusion of a fold of the bowel or bladder through the vagina, and in the later stages the womb itself may protrude to the exterior. The condition, which affects elderly women, is mainly due to injuries caused by childbirth. It may often be remedied by wearing a suitably shaped pessary, or by an operation designed to unite the torn parts.

PROLAPSED INTERVERTEBRAL DISC

The spinal column (q.v.) is built up of a series of bones, known as vertebrae, placed one upon the other. Between these vertebrae lies a series of thick discs of fibro-cartilage known as intervertebral discs. Each disc consists of an outer portion known as the anulus fibrosus, and an inner core known as the nucleus pulposus. The function of these discs is to give flexibility and resiliency to the spinal column and to act as buffers against undue jarring. In other words, they are most efficient shock absorbers. They may, however, prolapse, or protrude, between the two adjacent vertebrae. If this should happen they press on the neighbouring spinal nerve and cause pain. As the most common sites of protrusion, or prolapse, are between the last two lumbar vertebrae and between the last lumbar vertebra and the sacrum, this means that the pain occurs in the back, causing lumbago (q.v.) or down the course of the sciatic nerve causing sciatica (q.v.). The prolapse is most likely to occur in middle age, which suggests that it may be associated with degeneration of the disc involved, but it can occur in early adult life as well. It usually occurs when the individual is performing some form of exercise which involves bending, as in gardening. The onset of pain may be acute and sudden, or gradual and more chronic in intensity. (See INTERVERTEBRAL DISC.)

Treatment varies, depending, amongst other things, on the severity of the condition. In the acute phase rest in bed is essential. Later, exercise and physiotherapy are helpful, and in some cases manipulation of the spine brings relief by allowing the herniated, or prolapsed, disc to slip back into position. The injection of a local anaesthetic into the spine (epidural anaesthesia) is yet another measure that often helps the more chronic cases. The ultimate form of treatment is an operation to remove the prolapsed disc, but this is a procedure that is not now performed nearly as often as it once was. An alternative form of treatment is the injection into the disc of chymopapain, an enzyme (q.v.) obtained from the paw-paw, which dissolves the disc.

PROMAZINE is an antipsychotic drug used to tranquilize disturbed patients (see NEUROLEPTICS).

PROMETHAZINE HYDROCHLORIDE is a widely used antihistamine drug with a prolonged action and a pronounced sedative effect. (See ANTIHISTAMINE DRUGS.)

PROMETHAZINE THEOCLATE, or AVOMINE, is a drug that is widely used in the alleviation or prevention of sea-sickness.

PRONATION is the movement whereby the bones of the forearm are crossed and the palm of the hand faces downwards.

PRONE Lying with the face down, or positioning the arm and hand so that the palm faces downwards.

PROPANTHELINE, or PROPANTHELINE BROMIDE, is a substance with an anti-cholinergic, or atropine-like action, which is used in the treatment of conditions such as duodenal ulcer and spastic colon.

PROPHYLAXIS means treatment or action adopted with the view of warding off disease.

PROPRANOLOL is a drug that is used in the treatment of angina pectoris, myocardial infarction, certain abnormal rhythms of the heart, and high blood-pressure. It is also proving of value in preventing attacks of migraine, and in certain anxiety states, particularly those associated with unpleasant bodily sensations, such as palpitations. It is a beta-adrenoceptor-blocking drug. (See ADRENERGIC RECEPTORS.)

PROPRIETARY NAME The trade name of a drug registered by the pharmaceutical company which has developed and patented it. This protects the name, ingredients and manufacturing technique for a set period of time. Doctors may prescribe a drug by its trade name or by its official, approved name, though the NHS encourages the latter.

PROPRIOCEPTORS Sensory nerve endings in the muscles, tendons and joints which signal to the brain their position relative to the outside world and the state of contraction of the muscle. During movement of a regular flow of information to the brain from the proprioceptors, the eyes and ears ensure that actions are co-ordinated and the body's balance maintained.

PROPTOSIS A condition in which the eye protrudes from the orbit. Some causes include thyroid disorders, tumours within the orbit, inflammation or infection of the orbit. Proptosis due to endocrine abnormality, e.g. thyroid problems, is known as *exophthalmos*.

PROSTACYCLIN is a prostaglandin (q.v.) produced by the endothelial lining of the blood vessels. It inhibits the aggregation of platelets (q.v.), and thereby reduces the likelihood of the blood clotting. It is also a strong vasodilator.

PROSTAGLANDINS, so called because they were first discovered in the semen and thought to arise in the prostate gland, are a group of recently discovered substances with a wide range of activity. The richest known source is semen, but they are also present in many other parts of the body. Their precise mode of action is not yet clear, but they are potent stimulators of muscle contraction and they are also potent vasodilators (q.v.). They cause contraction of the womb and have been used to induce labour. They are also being used as a means of inducing therapeutic abortions. They play an important part in the production of pain, and it is now known that aspirin relieves pain by virtue of the fact that it prevents, or antagonizes, the formation of certain prostaglandins. In addition, they play some, though as yet incompletely defined, part in producing inflammatory changes. (See INFLAMMATION, NON-STEROIDAL ANTI-INFLAMMATORY DRUGS.)

Thus prostaglandins have potent biological effects but their instability and rapid metabolism make them short acting. They are produced but not stored by most living cells and act locally. The two most important prostaglandins are prostacycline and thromboxane. Prostacycline is a vaso-dilator and an inhibitor of platelet aggregation and may cause relaxation of the myometrium. Thromboxanes have the opposite effects and cause vaso-constriction and platelet aggregation. The non-steroidal anti-inflammatory drugs act by blocking an enzyme called cyclo-oxygenase which converts arachidonic acid to the precursors of the various prostaglandins. Despite their potent pharmacological properties, the role of prostaglandins in current therapeutics is limited and controversial. They have been used most successfully as an inhibitor of platelet aggregation in extra-corporeal haemoperfusion systems. The problems with the prostacyclines is that they have to be given intravenously as they are inactive by mouth, and continuous infusion is required because the drug is rapidly eliminated with a half-life of minutes. Side-effects tend to be severe because the drug is usually given at the highest dose the patient can tolerate. The hope for the future lies in the exploitation of the novel compound to generate stable orally active prostacycline analogues which will inhibit platelet aggregation and hence thrombotic events, and yet have minimal effects on the heart and blood vessels.

PROSTATE, DISEASES OF   Disease of the prostate can affect the flow of urine so that patients present with urological symptoms.
PROSTATITIS   This can be either acute or chronic. Acute prostatitis is caused by a bacterial infection, while chronic prostatitis may follow on from an acute attack, arise insidiously, or be non-bacterial in origin.
Symptoms   Typically the patient has pain in the perineum (q.v.), groins, or supra pubic region, and pain on ejaculation. He may also have urinary frequency, and urgency.
Treatment   Acute and chronic prostatitis are treated with a prolonged course of antibiotics. Patients with chronic prostatitis may also re-

quire anti-inflammatory drugs, and anti-depressants.
PROSTATIC ENLARGEMENT   This is the result of benign prostatic hyperplasia (BPH), causing enlargement of the prostate. The exact cause of this enlargement is unknown, but affects 50 per cent of men between 40 and 59 years and 95 per cent of men over 70 years.
Symptoms   These are urinary hesitancy, poor urinary stream, terminal dribbling, frequency and urgency of urination and the need to pass urine at night (nocturia). The diagnosis is made from the history, a digital examination of the prostate gland via the rectum to assess enlargement, and analysis of the urinary flow rate.
Treatment   This can be with tablets, which either shrink the prostate – an anti-androgen drug such as finasteride – or relax the urinary sphincter muscle during micturition. For more severe symptoms the prostate can be removed surgically, by trans-urethral resection of prostate (TURP), using either electrocautery or laser energy. An experimental treatment is the use of microwaves to heat up and shrink the enlarged gland.
CANCER   Cancer of the prostate is the fourth commonest cause of death from cancer in UK males: in 1988 over 12,500 cases of prostatic cancer were registered. Little is known about the cause, but the majority of prostate cancers require the male hormones, androgens, to grow.
Symptoms   These are similar to those resulting from benign prostatic hypertrophy. Spread of the cancer to bones can cause pain. The use of a blood test measuring the amount of an antigen (q.v.), prostatic specific antigen (PSA), can be helpful in making the diagnosis, as can an ultrasound scan of the prostate.
Treatment   This could be surgical, with removal of the prostate, either via an abdominal incision, total prostatectomy, or trans-urethrally, or could be by radiotherapy. In more advanced cancers treatment with anti-androgen drugs, such as cyprotexone acetate or certain oestrogens, is used to inhibit the growth of the cancer.

PROSTATE GLAND   This is an accessory sex gland in males which is wrapped round the urethra as this tube leaves the bladder. Opening into the urethra, the gland secretes an alkaline fluid during ejaculation and is a constituent of semen (q.v.). The gland grows during adolescence and is sensitive to the concentrations of sex hormones.

PROSTATISM is the condition induced by benign enlargement of the prostate gland (q.v.).

PROSTHESES   A prosthesis is an artificial replacement, such as an artificial limb or eye, or a denture. It is often necessary, for aesthetic or practical reasons, to replace part of the body, lost by injury or disease, with copies of the original, or PROSTHESES as they are now known. From ancient times this has been the case:

Herodotus speaks of a man with a wooden foot; the Romans carried the manufacture of limbs to a high degree of efficiency, as witnesssed by a leg, the oldest known artificial limb in existence, neatly formed of thin bronze plates, leather and iron, found in a tomb at Capua and dating from around 300 BC; the Etruscans fashioned gold teeth five centuries before the Christian era; Goetz von Berlichingen (1480–1562), to supply his lost right hand, had one made of iron and thus became known as Goetz of the Iron Hand; and Ambroise Paré, who wrote on surgery in the sixteenth century, has a chapter upon artificial limbs. From then there was little advance until 1800 when James Potts, of London, patented an artificial leg made of two hollow wooden cones with a steel knee joint and a wooden ankle joint. It became known as the Anglesey leg after its owner, the Marquis of Anglesey and, with few modifications, remained the basis of British designs until the 1914–18 War. Since the 1939–45 War there have been striking advances, particularly in artificial hands, as the result of the introduction of electronics and myoelectric means of control.

Arms Owing to the very delicate movements which the upper limb has to carry out, it is never amputated if there is any possibility of its being of any use. When amputation is decided upon, as little as possible of the arm is removed. Great strides have been made in the provision of artificial arms and hands, and it is now found that 50 per cent efficiency can be obtained when the amputation has been above the elbow, and 75 per cent efficiency when it is below the elbow. Appliances are now available which allow an individual who has lost an arm to engage, for example, in carpentry, many branches of engineering, and the electrical trades. Such an individual can also write, shoot, play golf and cricket, and even fly-fish.

Legs An artificial substitute can come much nearer to the usefulness of the original in the lower than in the upper limb. As result of experience gained in the two World Wars artificial lower limbs are now so efficient that the individual often suffers little disability. This applies particularly to amputations below the knee, but even in the case of amputations high in the thigh many individuals can often resume their old occupations. In addition, they can often ride a bicycle or a horse, or drive a car, whilst tennis and golf are quite normal pastimes. One of the great secrets of success in the fitting of artificial limbs is to restore the patient's morale and to stimulate his sense of independence. A considerable time must elapse after amputation, to allow for shrinkage of the stump, before a permanent prosthesis can be fitted. To overcome the practical disadvantages of this delay, a pneumatic post-amputation mobility aid is now available. This fits over the bandaged stump, and is inflated to 40 mm Hg to support a rigid frame. It can be fitted by nurses and paramendical staff without any special training in prosthetics. Using this device patients can now start learning to walk again

within a week of their amputation. It is suitable for amputation below, above and through the knee.

Eyes Artificial eyes are worn both for appearance and to protect the socket from dust, though, of course, vision is impossible. They are made of glass or plastic, and are thin shells of a boat-shape. representing the front half of the eye which has been removed. The stump which is left has still the eye-muscles in it, and so the artificial eye still has the power of moving with the other, though to a less extent, and it is often difficult for this reason to tell at a short distance that a person has a false eye. A glass eye has to be replaced by a new one every year. Plastic eyes have the advantage of being more comfortable to wear, and more durable and of being unbreakable.

Dental prosthesis is any artificial replacement of a tooth. There are three main types, a crown, a bridge and a denture. A crown is the replacement of the part of a tooth which sticks through the gum. It is fixed to the remaining part of the tooth and may be made of metal, porcelain, plastic or a combination of these. A bridge is the replacement of two or three missing teeth and is usually fixed in place. The replacement teeth are held in position by being joined to one or more crowns on the adjacent teeth. A denture is a removable prosthesis used to replace some or all the teeth. The teeth are made of plastic or porcelain and the base may be of plastic or metal. All these prostheses are individually made by skilled technicians and are matched to the patient's own teeth for size, shape and colour. Removable teeth may be held more firmly by means of implants.

Nose The making of a new nose is the oldest known operation in plastic surgery, Hindu records of such operations dating back to 1000 BC. Loss of a nose may be due to eroding disease, war wounds, gun-shot wounds or dog bites. In essence the operation is the same as that practised a thousand years before Christ: namely the use of a skin graft, brought down from the forehead. Alternative sources of the skin graft today are skin from the arm, chest or abdomen. As a means of support the new nose is built round a graft of bone or of cartilage from the ear.

PROTEIN is the term applied to members of a group of non- crystallizable nitrogenous substances widely distributed in the animal and vegetable kingdoms and forming the characteristic materials of their tissues and fluids. They are essentially combinations of amino-acids. They mostly dissolve in water and are coagulated by heat and various chemical substances. Typical examples of protein substances are white of egg and gelatin.

Proteins constitute an essential part of the diet as a source of energy and for the replacement of protein lost in the wear and tear of daily life. Their essential constituent from this point of view is the nitrogen they contain. To be absorbed, or digested, proteins have to be broken down into their constituent amino-acids. The adult human body can maintain nitrogenous equilibrium on a mixture of eight amino-acids, which are therefore known as the essential amino-acids. They are isoleucine, leucine, lysine, methionine, phenylalanine, threonine, tryptophan and valine. In addition, infants require histidine.

PROTEINURIA means a condition in which proteins, principally albumin, are present in the urine. It is of immense importance because it is often a symptom of serious heart or kidney disease, although some normal people have mild and transient proteinuria after exercise.

Causes (1) *Kidney disease* is the most important cause of proteinuria, and in some cases the discovery of proteinuria may be the first evidence of such disease. This is why an examination of the urine for the presence of albumin constitutes an essential part of every medical examination. Almost any form of kidney disease will cause proteinuria, but the most frequent form to do this is glomerulonephritis. In the subacute (or nephrotic) stage of glomerulonephritis the most marked proteinuria of all may be found. Proteinuria is also found in infections of the kidney (pyelitis) as well as in infections of the bladder (cystitis) and of the urethra (urethritis). The development of proteinuria in pregnancy requires investigation, as it may be the first sign of one of the most dangerous complications of pregnancy: toxaemia of pregnancy, glomerulonephritis, or eclampsia (q.v.). Proteinuria may also result from the contamination of urine with vaginal secretions. (2) *Cardiovascular disorders* are commonly accompanied by proteinuria, particularly when the right side of the heart is failing. In severe cases of failure, accompanied by oedema, the proteinuria may be marked. (3) *Fever* often causes proteinuria, even though there is no actual kidney disease. The proteinuria disappears soon after the temperature becomes normal. (4) *Drugs and poisons* These include arsenic, lead, mercury, gold, copaiba, salicylic acid and quinine. (5) *Anaemia* A trace of albumin may be found in the urine in severe anaemia. (6) *Postural or orthostatic albuminuria* This type is important because, if its true cause is unrecognized, it may be taken as a sign of kidney disease. The significance of postural proteinuria is unclear: it is more common among young people and is absent when the person is recumbent, hence the importance of testing a urine sample that is taken before rising in the morning.

Treatment The treatment is that of the underlying disease. (See KIDNEYS, DISEASES OF.)

PROTHROMBIN An inactive substance in the blood plasma that is the precursor of the enzyme thrombin, which clots the blood. The conversion occurs when a blood vessel is damaged and the process of blood coagulation occurs (see COAGULATION).

PROTOPLASM is the viscid, translucent, glue-like material containing fine granules and composed mainly of proteins, which makes up the essential material of plant and animal cells and has the properties of life.

PROTOZOA A simple, primitive animal comprising a single cell. Protozoa are microscopic in size but are much larger than bacteria. Most protozoa live freely but around 30 are parasitic in humans causing disease such as amoebiasis and giardiasis (intestinal infections), malaria, kala-azar and sleeping sickness. Some protozoa are able to excrete, respire, and absorb food particles and they may move around like a mobile jelly or by means of flagellae.

PROTRIPTYLINE is a tricyclic antidepressant drug. (See ANTIDEPRESSANTS.)

PROXIMAL is a term of comparison applied to structures which are nearer the centre of the body or the median line as opposed to more distal, or distant, structures.

PROZAC (see FLUOXETINE).

PRURIGO is the name of a chronic skin disease in which small papules (q.v.) develop in the skin, accompanied by intense itching. The condition may either be permanent or may come and go.

PRURITUS is another name for itching (q.v.).

PRUSSIC ACID POISONING (see CYANIDE POISONING).

PSEUDOCYESIS means spurious or false pregnancy, a condition characterized by enlargement of the abdomen, and even enlargement of the breasts and early morning sickness, the unfortunate woman being quite convinced that she is pregnant.

PSEUDOHYPERTROPHIC MUSCULAR DYSTROPHY, or PSEUDOHYPERTROPHIC PARALYSIS, is a condition in which certain muscles enlarge owing to a fatty and fibrous degeneration, giving a false appearance of increased strength.

PSEUDOXANTHOMA ELASTICUM This is a hereditary disorder of elastic tissue. Degenerating elastic tissue in the skin produces lesions in the skin which look like soft yellow papules. Elastic tissue in the eye and blood vessels is also involved, giving rise to visual impairment, raised blood pressure and haemorrhages.

PSITTACOSIS is an infectious disease of parrots and other exotic birds which may be transmitted to man and is caused by the micro-organism *Chlamydia psittaci*. It presents as pneumonia (q.v.) or a systemic illness in which the patient has an enlarged spleen and liver and pneumonitis (q.v.). Tetracycline is an effective treatment but relapses may occur. In the United Kingdom several hundred cases occur annually.

PSOAS is a powerful muscle which arises from the front of the vertebral column in the lumbar region, and passes down, round the pelvis and through the groin, to be attached to the inner side of the thigh-bone not far from its upper end. The act of sitting up from a recumbent posture, or that of bending the thigh on the abdomen, is mainly accomplished by the contraction of this muscle. Disease of the spine in the lumbar region is apt to produce an abscess which lies within the sheath of this muscle and makes its way down to the front of the thigh, where it threatens to burst. Such an abscess is known as a psoas abscess. (See ABSCESS, CHRONIC.)

PSORALENS are a family of chemical compounds that occur in many plants. They can be activated by ultraviolet light type A (UVA) to produce inflammation and pigmentation of the skin. One compound, 8-methoxypsoralen, is used with UVA as photochemotherapy (PUVA) in the treatment of psoriasis.

PSORIASIS is a chronic, relapsing inflammatory skin condition which may cause significant social embarrassment. There is currently no cure for this condition but the symptoms may be alleviated by regular use of topical or systemic therapies (see below). Psoriasis affects approximately 2 per cent of the British population and there is a strong genetic component; a child with one affected parent has a 25-per-cent chance of developing the disease. This risk increases to 60 per cent if both parents are affected. Psoriasis occurs equally in males and females, frequently appearing for the first time in young adulthood.

Different types of psoriasis are recognized, each with a distinct clinical appearance and prognosis, but all are thought to be part of the same disease process. Any type of psoriasis may be associated with nail changes (pitting), scalp involvement or arthritis (including gout). The commonest, PLAQUE-TYPE PSORIASIS, presents as well-demarcated salmon-pink, or red, patches of skin with adherent silvery scale, typically on the elbows, shins and buttocks. GUTTATE PSORIASIS is a variant which typically occurs in young children, often following a streptococcal (bacterial) throat infection; this type of psoriasis frequently responds well to ultraviolet-light therapy. Children with guttate psoriasis do not necessarily go on to develop plaque-type psoriasis as adults. ERYTHRODERMIC OR PUSTULAR PSORIASIS is a severe, often life-threatening condition associated with constitutional symptoms of fever, malaise and, occasionally, prostration.

Secondary infection and renal failure are serious complications; this condition requires very close monitoring, usually in hospital.

Treatments for psoriasis include bed-rest and topical application of corticosteroid, tar or dithranol products, often in association with ultraviolet light (UVB or psoralen and UVA therapy). Systemic immunosuppressive drugs, including methotrexate and cyclosporin, but not prednisolone, may be helpful in severe or recalcitrant psoriasis but need careful monitoring.

Patient information may be obtained through the Psoriasis Association (see APPENDIX 2: ADDRESSES).

PSYCHEDELIC DRUGS are drugs, such as lysergic acid diethylamide (LSD), that expand consciousness and perception. (See DRUG ADDICTION.)

PSYCHIATRY is that branch of medical science which treats mental disorder and disease and also helps with the management of people with learning disabilities (q.v.).

PSYCHO-ANALYSIS is the term applied to the theories and practice of the school of psychology originating with Freud. It depends upon the theory that states of disordered mental health have been produced by a repression of painful memories or of conflicting instincts. By such repression these hurtful memories or instincts are kept constantly in a subconscious condition. As a result, the individual's mental power is needlessly occupied and diverted from the proper objects with which it should be concerned and he finds difficulty in concentrating his attention upon and adapting himself to the practical realities of everyday life.

Psycho-analysis aims at discovering these repressed memories which are responsible for the diversion of mental power and of which the affected person usually is only dimly aware or quite unaware. The fundamental method of psycho-analytical treatment is the free expression of thoughts, ideas and fantasies on the part of the patient. To facilitate this, in classical analysis, he or she lies on a couch to relax mind and body, and the analyst may sit so as to observe the patient but not to be observed by him. The analyst's task is to adopt a neutral attitude to the patient, to encourage the free association of ideas and to explain where explanation is necessary for the continuance of free association. The analyst will receive by way of transference good and bad fantasies of the patient and represent for him or her from time to time objects of love and hate, especially members of the patient's family. In the course of analysis the patient will re-explore his early emotional attitudes and tensions.

There is much that is speculative in the theories of psycho-analysis by the standards of orthodox experimental science but, at the same time, its fundamental conceptions have been widely adopted and developed by other schools of psychology to their enrichment. The new approaches to the study of the mind in health and disease opened up by the concepts of Freud have changed the attitude of the lay and the medical public to the problems of the neurotic, the morbidly anxious, the fearful and to the mental and emotional development of the child.

PSYCHOLOGY is the branch of science that deals with the mind and its methods of working.

PSYCHONEUROSIS is a general term applied to various functional disorders of the nervous system. (See NEUROSIS.)

PSYCHOPATHIC Psychopathic disorder is defined by the Mental Health Act 1983 as a persistent disorder or disability of mind (whether or not including significant impairment of intelligence) which results in abnormally aggressive or seriously irresponsible conduct. The cardinal features are as follows: (1) Absence of normal feelings for other people such as love, affection, sympathy and condolence. (2) A tendency to anti-social impulsive acts with no forethought of the consequences. (3) A failure to learn by experience and to be deterred from crime by punishment. (4) Absence of any other form of mental disorder that would explain the unusual behaviour. The corresponding American terminology is 'anti-social personality disorder'.

PSYCHOSIS is a term applied to serious disorder of the mind, amounting to insanity.

PSYCHOSOMATIC DISEASES are illnesses resulting from the effects of excessive or repressed emotions upon bodily function or structure. They affect vast numbers of patients who are not out of their minds and yet do not have any organic disease to account for their illness. Functional symptoms must not be regarded as invented or imagined or as a mysterious state affecting an inferior personality. In psychosomatic disease the will may be strong and the mind normal, yet the emotions require treatment. Disorders precipitated by emotional factors may be psychotic, psychoneurotic or psychosomatic. In psychotic and psychoneurotic illnesses the symptoms are predoninantly psychological, whilst in psychosomatic disorders the symptoms may be entirely somatic. The concept of emotional disturbances contributing to bodily disease is not new. It was over 2400 years ago that Socrates stressed that 'as you ought not to attempt to cure the eyes without the head, or the head without the body, so you should not treat body without mind'. The rapid advances of scientific medicine have encouraged a preoccupation with the measurable and a neglect of the intangible. It has been estimated that one third of medical outpatients have psychiatric illness. In another third symptoms are largely dependent on an emotional factor even though organic disease is present. In gynaecological clinics emotional tensions are even more commonly encountered and exceed physical disease as a cause of illness. Over one quarter of all absence from work due to sickness is a result of an illness having an emotional basis.

The three major problems that lead to psychosomatic disorder are marital relationships; occupation, which includes the frustrations, disappointments and feelings of unfulfilment provoked by the patient's work; and finally, social relationships – the feelings which prevail between friends, neighbours and relations.

The many somatic symptoms due to anxiety result from enhanced activity of the sympathetic nervous system. Pain may be a manifestation of psychosomatic disease. Psychogenic factors may produce muscle tension and and cause a pain that is organic. The tension headache is due to the increased tone of the muscles of the neck and scalp.

The visceral reactions of emotional stimuli are of two types:

(1) *Sympathetic.* This is the part of the autonomic nervous system concerned with emergency situations in the external environment, the so-called preparation for fight or flight. The sympathetic nervous system which adjusts the body to such stresses inhibits the metabolic processes of the body and increases the heart rate and blood pressure, and mobilizes carbohydrate reserves. Its effects are mediated through the hormones adrenaline and noradrenaline.

(2) *Parasympathetic.* This is concerned with the conservation and anabolic processes of the body. Hence there is stimulation of gastrointestinal and bronchial secretions, a storing of sugar in the liver, and protective reflexes such as contraction of the pupil and spasm of the bronchiolar muscles as a protection against irritant substances. Parasympathetic effects are mediated through the secretion of acetylcholine. As a result of excess acetylcholine there is a feeling of warmth and flushing due to vasodilatation, and sweating due to cholinergic stimulation of the sweat glands. This is associated with nausea, vomiting and abdominal colic due to increased peristalsis and contraction of the intestines and the stomach. Thus, when emotional impulses are repressed, two possibilities arise. The patient may be in a constant state of preparedness for action and if this is never executed the sympathetic overactivity persists with a chronic increase in muscle tension, tachycardia and raised blood pressure, and these may give rise to symptoms. An alternative reaction is emotional withdrawal from action into a dependent state of para-sympathetic overactivity. This would include diarrhoea, gastric acid hypersecretion, oesophageal spasm and other parasympathetic effects on the gastro-intestinal tract. Since the autonomic nervous system innovates practically every portion of the body, a somatic

manifestation of emotional tension may be related to any area.

Autonomic nervous overactivity may be manifest in the various systems as follows:

(1) *Central nervous system.* Headache. Often described as a pressure on the head. Dizziness, feelings of faintness, nervousness, tremors, sleeplessness and physical exhaustion.

(2) *Cardiovascular system.* Tachycardia, arrhythmia and precordial pains.

(3) *Respiratory symptoms.* Sighing respirations and a feeling of an inability to breathe deeply. Vasomotor rhinitis, chronic sore throat and asthma.

(4) *Gastro-intestinal system.* Anorexia, nausea, vomiting, indigestion, wind, heartburn, diarrhoea, constipation and sensations of a lump in the throat.

(5) *Skin.* Itching, sweating, parasthesiae and neuro-dermatitis.

Direct observations on the human colon through fistulae and colostomy openings and on the gastric mucosa through gastrostomy have shown that fear, anxiety and pain can cause an increase in peristalsis with reddening and swelling of the mucous membrane, whilst depression causes reduced motility and pallor of the mucosa. Psychosomatic symptoms may be the result of disorders of secretory functions, such as salivation, dry mouth, hyperchlorhydria, functional hyperinsulinism and mucous colitis, or alternatively they may be due to disorders of motor function such as oesophageal spasm, gastric hypermotility, spastic colon, constipation and diarrhoea. The skin plays an important part in the regulation of body temperature by sweating and its functions are controlled by the autonomic nervous system.

Vasoconstriction, vasodilatation, pilomotor activity and sweating are the four common physiological processes of the skin and are all largely controlled by the autonomic nervous system. Emotional sweating is most evident on the palms and soles and in the axilla. The influence of emotion on respiratory function is well recognized by the everyday expression, 'it took my breath away'. The autonomic innervation of the respiratory tract, which includes the nasal mucosa, consists of sympathetic and para-sympathetic nerves. Parasympathetic nerves exert a constrictor effect on the smooth muscle of the respiratory tract and the sympathetic nerves have a relaxing influence. If para-sympathetic stimulation is excessive, mucous cells oversecrete and vasodilatation of blood vessels occurs. This produces swelling of the bronchial mucosa and congestion of airways.

Functional illness has its own characteristics and the diagnosis is not established by the mere exclusion of organic disease. It is suggested by the existence of emotional disturbance as a precipitating factor, by the presence of certain characteristic symptoms, by a family history of a similar disorder and by a phasic course characterized by remissions and relapses. It must always be remembered that organic disease may cause anxiety and may provide the stressful factor needed to precipitate psychosomatic disease.

PSYCHOSURGERY was introduced in 1936 by Egas Moniz, Professor of Medicine in Lisbon University, for the surgical treatment of certain psychoses. For his work in this field he shared the Nobel prize in 1949. The original operation, known as leucotomy, consisted of cutting white fibres in the frontal lobe of the brain. It was accompanied by certain hazards such as persistent epilepsy and undesirable changes in personality. Pre-frontal leucotomy is now regarded as obsolete. Modern stereotactic surgery may be indicated in certain intractable psychiatric illnesses in which the patient is chronically incapacitated, especially where there is a high suicide risk. Patients are only considered for psychosurgery when they have failed to respond to routine therapies. One contra-indication is marked histrionic or anti-social personality. The conditions in which a favourable response has been obtained are intractable and chronic obsessional neuroses, anxiety states and severe chronic depression.

Psychosurgery is now rare in Britain. The Mental Health Act 1983 requires not only consent by the patient, confirmed by an independent doctor, and two other representatives of the Mental Health Act Commission, but that the Commission's appointed medical representative must also advise on the likelihood of the treatment's alleviating or preventing a deterioration in the patient's condition.

PSYCHOTHERAPY is the term applied to any form of treatment which operates through the mind. Almost every type of disease or injury has a mental aspect, even if this relates only to the pain or discomfort that it causes. In some diseases and with some temperaments, the mental factor is much more pronounced than in others; for such cases psychotherapy is particularly important. The chief methods employed are the following:

Suggestion is a commonly employed method, used in almost every department of medicine. It may consist, in its simplest form, merely of emphasizing that the patient's health is better, so that this idea becomes fixed in the patient's mind. A suggestion of efficacy may be conveyed by the physical properties of a medicine or by the appearance of some apparatus used in treatment. Again, suggestion may be conveyed emotionally, as in religious healing. In occasional cases a therapeutic suggestion may be made to the patient in a hypnotic state.

Persuasion is a method of treatment in which appeal is made to a patient's reasoning faculties.

Analysis consists in the elucidation of the half-conscious or subconscious repressed memories or instincts that are responsible for some cases of mental disorder or personal conflicts.

Group therapy is a method whereby patients are treated in small groups and encouraged to participate actively in the discussion which ensues amongst themselves and the participating therapists. A modification of group therapy is *drama* therapy. Large group therapy also exists.

Education and employment may be important factors in rehabilitative psychotherapy.

Supportive therapy consists of sympathetically reviewing the patient's situation with him or her and encouraging the patient to identify and solve problems.

Short-term supportive psychotherapy is aimed at stabilizing and strengthening the psychological defence mechanisms of those patients who are confronted by a crisis which threatens to overwhelm their ability to cope, or who are struggling with the aftermath of major life events.

Long-term supportive psychotherapy is needed for patients with personality disorders or recurrent psychotic states, where the aim of treatment is to prevent deterioration and help the patient to achieve an optimal adaptation, making the most of his psychological assets. Such patients may find more profound and unstructured forms of therapy distressing.

Behavioural therapy and *cognitive therapy*, often carried out by psychologists, attempt to clarify with the patient specific features of behaviour or mental outlook respectively and identify step-by-step methods the patient can use for controlling the disorder. Behaviour therapy is commonly used for agoraphobia and other phobias, and cognitive therapy has been used for depression and anxiety.

PSYCHOTROPIC Affecting the mind. Psychotropic drugs include hallucinogens (q.v.), sleeping drugs, sedatives, tranquillisers (q.v.) and neuroleptic (q.v.) drugs.

PTERYGIUM A degenerative disorder of the conjunctiva which grows over the cornea medially and laterally. The overgrowths look like wings. They are commonly seen in people who live in areas of bright sunlight, particularly when reflected from deserts or snowfields. Treatment involves excision of the overgrowth. (See EYE DISEASES.)

PTOSIS (see EYE DISEASES).

PTYALIN is the name of the enzyme contained in the saliva, by which starchy materials are changed into sugar, and so prepared for absorption. It is identical with the amylase of pancreatic juice. (See DIGESTION; PANCREAS.)

PUBERTY means the change that takes place when childhood passes into manhood or womanhood. This change is generally a very definite one, taking place at about the age of fourteen years, although it is modified by race, climate, and bodily health, so that it may appear a year or two earlier or several years later. At this time the sexual functions attain their full development, the contour of the body changes from a childish to a more rounded womanly, or sturdy manly form, and great changes take place in the mode of thought and feeling. In girls it is marked by the onset of menstruation and development of the breasts. Development of the breasts is usually the first sign of puberty to appear, and may occur from 9 years onwards. Most girls show signs of breast development by the age of 13. The time from the beginning of breast development to the onset of menstruation is usually around two years but may range from six months to five years. The first sign of puberty in boys is an increase in testicular size between the age of 10 and 14. The larynx enlarges in boys, so that the voice after going through a period of 'breaking', finally assumes the deep manly pitch. Hair appears on the pubis and later in the armpits in both boys and girls, whilst in the former it also begins to grow on the upper lip, and skin eruptions are not uncommon on the face. (See ACNE.)

The period is one of transition from a physical and mental point of view. Puberty is not to be regarded as a physiological 'coming of age', for full development is not attained till between twenty and thirty years of age. (See also MENARCHE; MENSTRUATION.)

PUBIS is the bone that forms the front part of the pelvis. The pubic bones of opposite sides meet in the symphysis and protect the bladder from the front.

PUBLIC HEALTH Disease and health status can be studied and altered in populations as well as individuals. This understanding is central to the concept of public health. The term refers to a broad spectrum of activity organized at all levels of society. This activity, either directly or indirectly, aims to improve the health of the population by preventing disease, prolonging life or promoting health. The determinants of the health of the population are numerous. They range from personal habits such as smoking to environmental conditions such as housing and social factors such as unemployment. Public health activity can thus include the work of diverse professions: civil engineers improving sewer systems, veterinary scientists controlling animal-feed practices, government ministers changing alcohol taxation and health workers planning community services.

The term 'public health' can be used more specifically to refer to a public health system. This is a publicly funded service, the primary aim of which is to improve health by the use of population-based measures. The structure of these systems varies from country to country, reflecting differing social composition and political priorities. There are, however, some general elements that can be extracted. (1) Surveillance: the collection, collation and analysis of data to produce useful information about the distribution and determinants of health and disease in populations. These activities form the basis of epidemiology, which is often considered the backbone of public-health practice. (2) Intervention: the design and implementation of policies to improve health. This may be through the provision of preventive medical care, environmental measures, influencing the behaviour of individuals or the provision of appropriate services to limit disability and handicap. (3) Evaluation: assessment of the first two steps in order to determine their impact. This enables further action to be taken as required.

The practice of public health The situation in the United Kingdom will be described as, even though public health systems vary, it will give the reader a general impression of the type of work that is covered.

HISTORY Initially public health practice related to the environment and the control of infectious disease. Early examples include quarantine for plague and leprosy during the Middle Ages and the development of vaccination in the 18th century. However it was during the 19th century, in response to the health problems of rapid urban growth, that the foundations of a public health system were created. The concept of the 'sanitary idea' was fundamental to these developments. This suggested that overcrowding in insanitary conditions was the root of disease epidemics. Consequently sanitation measures such as improved sewerage systems and water supplies would prevent disease outbreaks. Although not based on the later, more accurate, knowledge relating the causes of disease to bacteriology, this idea led to the public health legislation of the 1870s. This gave local authorities the responsibility for sanitation and created the post of medical officer of health. These were the first official public-health doctors.

The role of the medical officer of health increased in importance in the first half of this century. It eventually encompassed not only sanitation but also food hygiene, maternal and child health, clinics for tuberculosis and sexually transmitted diseases and hospital administration. The medical officer of health was employed by local authorities but, in the reorganization of local government and the NHS in the 1970s, the post was abolished and the medical specialty of community medicine was formed and moved across to the health service. This drew together the existing medical officers of health and the academic discipline of social medicine. These changes altered the nature of the work the new public health doctors carried out. The organization of the discipline has been further changed as part of the management reforms that took place in the NHS during the 1980s and 1990s.

CURRENT PRACTICE There are a number of key personnel and structures that make up today's public-health system.

Public health doctors The medical specialty of community medicine changed its name to public health medicine in 1990. These doctors are usually attached to local public health departments within the health service, but can be employed in national units within government or in research establishments.

Public health departments employ public health doctors, statisticians, social scientists, health economists and other relevant information and research specialists. One of the primary roles of these departments is to assess the health needs of the population and to plan and evaluate services designed to meet those needs. For instance, they may advise health authorities how many hip replacements they need to provide. This would involve assessing the criteria for hip replacement and estimating how many of a given population fit these criteria. In addition the cost of providing the service may be calculated and competing priorities considered.

Disease prevention and health promotion are addressed through advice, co-ordination or evaluation of activities such as cancer-screening programmes, immunization schemes and health-education campaigns.

The spread of HIV infection and AIDS and the increased incidence of food and water-borne disease has emphasized the continued importance of the role of public health workers in infectious-disease control. Certain public health doctors have a statutory responsibility for this control.

National Departments such as the Department of Health, the Office of Population Censuses and Surveys (OPCS) and the Communicable Disease Surveillance Centre (CDSC) have a variety of roles. The one they share in common is surveillance and the co-ordinated production of statistics for the public-health system.

Environmental health officers are based in local authorities. These authorities have a statutory role in enforcing many aspects of public health legislation. These laws relate primarily to sanitation and environmental aspects of public health. These officers thus deal with food hygiene, pollution and environmental nuisance such as insanitary housing, pest and noise control. They also help with investigating outbreaks of infectious disease, for example food poisoning and legionnaire's disease.

PUERPERAL FEVER, now rare in developed countries, is characterized by a temperature above 38 °C within two weeks of delivery or miscarriage, particularly the first three days. (A slight fever is not uncommon on the first day.)

Causes The mother is specially liable during this period to pick up any infection to which she may be exposed. She is weakened by the strain of labour (q.v.), often with considerable blood loss, and her body's immunological defence system may be suppressed. Raw surfaces around the genital tract, and around the nipples (due to breast-feeding) allow easy access to micro-organisms, most commonly involved of which is the *Streptococcus haemolyticus* (q.v.).

Symptoms In its mildest form, the infection may develop as a localized inflammation (often of the urinary or genital tracts or breasts), with generalized discomfort and fever. Less commonly, the infection may spread to the surrounding lymph ducts and veins, leading to abscesses (q.v.), peritonitis (q.v.), and occasionally deep-vein thrombosis (see THROMBOSIS), often with considerable fever and pain. In the most severe cases septicaemia (q.v.) may result, usually accompanied by high fever and delirium.

Treatment The condition may be avoided by scrupulous attention to cleanliness and careful nursing during labour and in the post-natal period. Blood transfusion is indicated if the haemoglobin falls below 6g/dl. At the onset of even mild fever, full clinical investigation should be carried out, including the breasts and legs. Genital swabs should be taken, together with blood and sputum cultures. Penicillin or the appropriate antibiotic should be started as soon as possible.

PUERPERIUM is the period which elapses after the birth of a child until the mother is again restored to her ordinary health. It is generally regarded as lasting for a month. One of the main changes that occur is the enormous decrease in size that takes place in the muscular wall of the womb. (See MUSCLE.) There are often afterpains during the first day in women who have borne several children, less often after a first child. (See AFTERPAINS.) The discharge is blood-stained for the first two or three days, then clearer till the end of the first week, after which it becomes thicker and less in quantity, finally disappearing altogether, if the case goes well, at the end of two or three weeks. The breasts, which have already enlarged before the birth of the child, secrete milk more copiously, and there should be a plentiful supply on the third day of the puerperium.

Management It is now realized that prolonged rest in bed is not necessary for the mother after a normal birth. Indeed, it may be harmful. The mother should start practising exercises to help to ensure that the stretched abdominal muscles regain their normal tone. There is no need for any restriction of diet, but care must be taken to ensure an adequate intake of fluid, including at least 580 ml (a pint) of milk a day. The bowels are generally sluggish and it is usual to take an aperient on the second or third day.

Milk, as already stated, appears copiously on the third day, but this is preceded by a secretion from the breast, known as colostrum, which is of value to the new-born child. The child should therefore be put to the breasts within six to eight hours of being born, in order to obtain the small amount of fluid they are secreting, and also because suckling stimulates both the breasts and the natural changes taking place during this period. Suckling is beneficial for both child and mother.

PULMONARY DISEASES (see LUNGS, DISEASES OF).

PULMONARY EMBOLISM is the condition in which an embolus (see EMBOLISM), or clot, is lodged in the lungs. The source of the clot is usually the veins of the lower abdomen or legs in which clot formation has occurred as a result of the occurrence of thrombophlebitis. (See VEINS, DISEASES OF.) Thrombophlebitis, with or without pulmonary embolism, is a not uncommon complication of surgical operations, especially in older patients. This is one reason why nowadays such patients are got up out of bed as quickly as possible, or, alternatively, are encouraged to move and exercise their legs regularly in bed. The severity of a pulmonary embolism, which is characterized by the sudden onset of pain in the chest, with or without the coughing up of blood, and a varying degree of shock, depends upon the size of the clot. If large enough it may prove immediately fatal. In other cases immediate operation may be needed to remove the clot, whilst in less severe cases anticoagulant treatment, in the form of heparin (q.v.), is given to prevent extension of the clot.

PULMONARY HYPERTENSION In this condition increased resistance to the blood flow through the lungs occurs. This is usually the result of lung disease and the consequence is an increase in pulmonary artery pressure and in the pressure in the right side of the heart and in the veins bringing blood to the heart. Chronic bronchitis or emphysema (qq.v.) commonly constrict the small arteries in the lungs, thus causing pulmonary hypertension.

PULMONARY OEDEMA is a type of waterlogging in the lungs caused by left ventricular failure or mitral stenosis (q.v.).

PULMONARY STENOSIS A disorder of the heart in which obstruction of the outflow of blood from the right ventricle (see HEART) occurs. Narrowing of the pulmonary valve at the exit of the right ventricle and narrowing of the pulmonary artery may cause obstruction. The condition is usually congenital though it may be caused by rheumatic fever. In the congenital condition pulmonary stenosis may occur with other heart defects and is then known as Fallot's tetralogy. Breathlessness and enlargement of the heart and eventual heart failure may be the consequence of pulmonary stenosis. Surgery is usually necessary to remove the obstruction.

PULP (see TEETH).

PULSATION, or throbbing, is an appearance seen or felt naturally below the fourth and fifth ribs on the left side, where the heart lies, and also at every point where an artery lies close beneath the surface. In other situations, it may be a sign of aneurysm. In nervous people, particularly if thin, great pulsation can often be seen and felt in the upper part of the abdomen, due to the throbbing of the normal abdominal aorta.

PULSE If the tip of one finger is laid gently on the front of the forearm, about 2·5 cm (one inch) above the furrows that mark the wrist, and about 1 cm (half an inch) from the outer edge, the pulsations of the radial artery can be felt. This is known as *the pulse*, but a pulse can be felt wherever an artery of large or medium size lies near the surface.

The cause of the pulsation lies in the fact that, at each heart-beat, 80 to 90 millilitres of blood are driven into the aorta, and a fluid wave, distending the vessels as it passes, is in consequence transmitted along the arteries all over the body. This pulsation gets less and less marked as the arteries grow smaller, and is finally lost in the minute capillaries, where a steady pressure is maintained. For this reason, the blood in the veins flows steadily on without any pulsation. Immediately after the wave has passed, the artery, by virtue of its great elasticity, regains its former size. The nature of this wave enables the doctor to assess the state of the artery and the action of the heart.

The pulse rate is usually about 70 per minute, but it may vary in health from 50 to 100, and is quicker in childhood and slower in old age than in middle life; it increases in all feverish states.

In childhood and youth the vessel wall is so thin that, when sufficient pressure is made to expel the blood from it, the artery can no longer be felt. In old age, however, and in some degenerative diseases, the vessel wall becomes so thick that it may be felt like a piece of whipcord rolling beneath the finger.

Different types of heart disease have special features of the pulse associated with them. In atrial fibrillation the great character is irregularity. In patients with an incompetent aortic valve the pulse is characterized by a sharp rise and sudden collapse.

An instrument known as the sphygmograph registers the arterial waves and a polygraph enables tracings to be taken from the pulse at the wrist and from the veins in the neck and simultaneous events in the two compared.

The pressure of the blood in various arteries is estimated by a sphygmomanometer. (See BLOOD-PRESSURE.)

PULSES are the seeds of the *Leguminosa* family. They include peas, beans and lentils and constitute a valuable source of food. Most contain around 20 grams of protein per 100 grams of dry weight but the biological value of this protein requires supplementation to ensure an adequate intake of first class, or essential, amino- acids (q.v.). They have been described as 'the poor man's protein', and a combination of pulse and cereal proteins may have a nutritive value comparable to that of animal protein. They are a good source of the B group of vitamins with the exception of riboflavine. (See also DIET.)

PUNCTATE BASOPHILIA (see BASOPHILIA.)

PUNCTUM (see EYE).

PUPIL (see EYE).

PURGATIVES are drugs or other substances which promote evacuation of the bowels. The term is used synonymously with laxative, cathartic, aperient, and evacuant. They are classified according to their manner of action, the three main groups being bulk, stimulant, and faecal softeners. The time a purgative takes to act may vary, and determines whether it should be taken in the morning or evening.

Classification Bulk purgatives include bran and most high-fibre foods such as fruit, vegetables, and wholemeal foods. These leave a large indigestible residue upon which the intestine can contract, and by holding water in the gut promote a large, soft stool. If taken repeatedly with inadequate fluid they may cause intestinal obstruction, particularly if the normal bowel contractions (peristalsis) are weak. Inorganic salts (saline purges) used include magnesium sulphate (Epsom salt), sodium sulphate (Glauber's salt), and sodium potassium tartrate (Rochelle salt). These act in a similar way to the bulk purgatives, producing a fluid stool, but if taken in large doses may lead to dehydration. Stimulant purgatives include bisacodyl, phenolphthalein, cascara, senna, rhubarb and aloes. These substances stimulate peristalsis, though the action may be accompanied by griping pains. Rather more powerful is castor oil, which is sometimes used as a 'once for all' purgative, for example, after a dietetic indiscretion. Most patients find it objectionable to take, however, and it is little used. There are two groups of faecal softeners (emollients). Surface-active agents such as dioctyl sodium and sulphosuccinate retain water in the stools, and are often combined with a stimulant purgative. Liquid paraffin is chemically inert and is said to act by lubrication, though it probably also increases the rate of passage by retaining water in the bowel. Some paraffin is absorbed from the intestine, and large doses may leak out of the anus. Long-term use is associated with a slightly increased risk of gastro-intestinal cancer, and for these reasons it is generally used only for short periods, when straining at stool may be painful, as after anal surgery.

Uses Purgatives are most commonly used as a treatment for constipation (q.v.), though they may also be used in cases of diarrhoea or poisoning, with the object of getting rid of the offending substance. They are sometimes indicated before X-ray examinations of the bowel. Physical and psychological dependence may easily occur and is best prevented by eating a generally high-fibre diet, and stopping any necessary purgatives as soon as their purpose has been accomplished. The risk of water and electrolyte depletion should always be borne in mind.

PURPURA is a disease characterized by the occurrence of purple spots upon the surface of the body, due to extravasations of blood in the skin, associated occasionally with haemorrhages from mucous membranes.

Causes The condition is due either to an increased permeability of the smallest blood-vessels (ie. the capillaries) which allows blood to pass through their walls, or to a shortage of blood platelets which normally play an important part in sealing off any damage which may occur to the walls of the capillaries. The damage to the capillary wall may arise as a result of an infection, e.g. septicaemia; a toxic factor, e.g. certain drugs; or in scurvy.

A common cause of a lack of platelets is their auto-immune destruction in idiopathic thrombocytopenic purpura. Capillary damage is commonly due to anaphylactoid purpura which is an allergic condition, the increased permeability of the capillary wall being due to the individual's coming in contact with, inhaling, or ingesting, some substance to which he is sensitized. Two special forms of anaphylactoid purpura are recognized. One is *Henoch's purpura*, in which the purpuric haemorrhages occur in the wall of the intestine, causing symptoms resembling an acute abdominal emergency. This form occurs in children and young adults. The other is *Schönlein's purpura*, in which the purpura occurs around the joints causing them to be painful and tender. This form principally affects young adults.

Symptoms The complaint usually starts with lassitude and feverishness. This is soon followed by the appearance on the body of the characteristic spots in the form of small red points scattered over the skin of the limbs and trunk. Their colour soon becomes deep purple or nearly black; but after a few days they undergo the changes observed in an ordinary bruise. When of minute size they are termed petechiae, when in patches of considerable size ecchymoses. They may come out in fresh crops over a lengthened period.

Treatment The treatment of *secondary purpura* consists of that of the underlying cause: e.g. scurvy. The treatment of *primary thrombocytopenic purpura* consists of the administration of one of the cortisone-like drugs: e.g. prednisolone. In cases which do not respond to such therapy, removal of the spleen is often helpful, especially in children. In severe cases, with heavy loss of blood, blood transfusion may be necessary. The treatment of *anaphylactoid purpura* consists of the administration of antihistamine drugs. If these fail, then it is worth trying the effect of prednisolone. If, as is often the case, there is any anaemia, this must be treated by the administration of full doses of iron: e.g. ferrous sulphate.

PUS, or MATTER, is a thick, white, yellow, or greenish fluid, which is found in abscesses, on ulcers, and on inflamed and discharging surfaces generally. Its colour and consistency are due to the presence, in great numbers, of pus corpuscles. These are derived mostly from the white corpuscles of the blood, and consist also of the superficial cells of granulation tissue or of a mucous membrane which die and are shed off in consequence of the inflammatory process. (See ABSCESS; PHAGOCYTOSIS.)

PUSTULE means a small collection of pus. (See ABSCESS.) Malignant pustule is one of the forms taken by woolsorters' disease. (See ANTHRAX.)

PUTREFACTION is the change that takes place in the bodies of plants and animals after death, whereby they are ultimately reduced to carbonic acid gas, ammonia, and other simple substances. The change is almost entirely due to the action of bacteria, and, in the course of the process, various offensive and poisonous intermediate substances are formed. In the case of the human body, putrescine, cadaverine, and other alkaloids are among these intermediate products.

PUTRID FEVER is an old name for typhus fever.

PUVA is a method of treating severe cases of psoriasis (q.v.) which do not respond to other forms of treatment. This consists of giving the patient a tablet of a psoralen preparation (q.v.) which sensitizes the skin cells to sunlight and then exposing him in a special cubicle to high-intensity long-wave ultraviolet radiation (UVA). Hence the name PUVA: a combination of P for psoralen and UVA. Initially this treatment is given twice a week. Although not curative, it has proved highly effective, but can only be carried out in specially equipped hospital departments.

PYAEMIA means a form of blood-poisoning in which abscesses appear in various parts of the body. (See BLOOD-POISONING.)

PYELITIS means inflammation of that part of the kidney known as the pelvis, which is connected with the ureter. It is now realized, however, that the infection is seldom restricted to the pelvis, but involves the kidney tissue as well. In other words the correct diagnosis is pyelonephritis.

The inflammation may spread upwards from the bladder or may follow on febrile diseases in which bacteria leave the body by the urine. One of the commonest organisms productive of this condition is the *Escherichia coli*, which produces a highly acid state of the urine accompanied by the presence of pus. Pyelitis sometimes occurs as a complication of pregnancy. There are generally symptoms of feverishness, general malaise, loss of weight, discomfort in the region of the loins, and frequency in passing water. Examination reveals the presence of the infecting organism and of pus in the urine.

Treatment In some cases the administration of alkalis and the drinking of ample bland fluids are all that is required. As a rule, however, more active treatment with an antibiotic is required. As pyelitis may be due to some other condition of the kidney, such as a stone, a full investigation is necessary, as such cases will not clear up unless the underlying cause is removed.

PYELOGRAPHY is the term applied to the process whereby the kidneys are rendered radio-opaque, and therefore visible on an X-ray film. It constitutes a most important part of the examination of a patient with kidney disease. (See SODIUM DIATRIZOATE.)

PYELONEPHRITIS (see PYELITIS).

PYLEPHLEBITIS means inflammation of the portal vein. A rare but serious disorder, it usually results from the spread of infection within the abdomen – for example, appendicitis. The patient may develop liver abscesses and ascites (q.v.). Treatment is by antibiotics and surgery.

PYLORIC STENOSIS: Narrowing of the pylorus (q.v.), the muscular exit from the stomach. It is usually the result of a pyloric ulcer or cancer near the exit of the stomach. The result is that food is delayed when passing from the stomach to the duodenum and vomiting occurs. The stomach may become distended and peristalsis (muscular movement) may be seen through the abdominal wall. Unless surgically treated the patient will steadily deteriorate, losing weight, becoming dehydrated and developing alkalosis. Congenital pyloric stenosis occurs in babies (commonly boys) about 3 to 5 weeks old, and surgery produces a complete cure.

PYLOROSPASM means spasm of the pyloric portion of the stomach. This interferes with the passage of food in a normal, gentle fashion into the intestine and causes the pain that comes on from half an hour to three hours after meals and is associated with severe disorders of digestion. It is often produced by an ulcer of the stomach or duodenum.

PYLORUS is the lower opening of the stomach, through which the softened and partially digested food passes into the small intestine.

PYO- is a prefix attached to the name of various diseases to indicate cases in which pus is formed, such as pyonephrosis.

PYODERMIA GANGRENOSUM This is a disorder in which large ulcerating lesions appear suddenly and dramatically in the skin. It is the result of underlying vasculitis. It is usually the result of inflammatory bowel disease such as ulcerative colitis or Crohn's disease but can be associated with rheumatoid arthritis.

PYOGENIC is a term applied to those bacteria which cause the formation of pus and so lead to the formation of abscesses. Although many bacteria have this property, the most common cause of abscess is one of the rounded forms of bacterium (e.g. streptococcus).

PYORRHOEA is the name given to any copious discharge of pus. For *Pyorrhoea alveolaris* see under TEETH, DISEASES OF.

PYREXIA means fever. (See FEVER.)

PYRIDOXINE, or vitamin B₆, plays an important part in the metabolism of a number of amino-acids. Deficiency leads to atrophy of the epidermis, the hair follicles, and the sebaceous glands, and peripheral neuritis may also occur. Young infants are more susceptible to pyridoxine deficiency than adults: they begin to lose weight and develop a hypochromic anaemia; irritability and convulsions may also occur. Liver, yeast, and cereals are relatively rich sources of it. Fish is a moderately rich source, but vegetables and milk contain little. The minimal daily requirement in the diet is probably about 2 mg. (See APPENDIX 5: VITAMINS.)

PYRIMETHAMINE is an antimalarial drug which is particularly valuable as a prophylactic.

PYROSIS (see WATERBRASH).

PYURIA means the presence of pus in the urine, in consequence of inflammation situated in the kidney, bladder, or other part of the urinary tract. (See URINE.)

Q

A **QALY** is an outcome measure of health care devised by some health economists in the 1980s. It has proved controversial but nevertheless is an indication of the likely effectiveness of a particular treatment and can contribute to the assessment of treatment and care a patient should have. The initials stand for Quality Adjusted Life Year. It takes a year of healthy life expectancy to be worth 1 and a year of unhealthy life expectancy to be worth less than 1. The worse the forecast of an unhealthy person's quality of life, the lower will be his or her rating. If someone is expected to live five years in a healthy state, the grading will be 5; ten years of life estimated to be only 25-per-cent healthy will rate as 2·5 QALYs.

Q FEVER is a disease of worldwide distribution due to the organism *Coxiella burneti*. It is characterized by fever, severe headache and often pneumonia. It was first described in 1937 amongst abattoir workers in Brisbane. The disease was given the name 'Q' fever, the Q (?) referring to the unknown cause of the disease. The aetiology of the infection was later established by Burnet who cultured a micro-organism from the blood of an infected patient. This rickettsia-like organism was originally called *Rickettsia burneti* but was later renamed *Coxiella burneti* when Cox found that it had certain features which differentiated it from the true rickettsia.

The principal reservoir of human infection in Britain is probably cattle and sheep in which the infection is usually sub-clinical. The diagnosis is confirmed by the detection of serum antibodies to *Coxiella burneti*. The organism is sensitive to tetracycline.

QUADRANTANOPIA Inability to see in one quarter of the visual field. Homonymous quadrantanopia is loss of vision in the same quarter of the field in each eye.

QUADRICEPS is the large four-headed muscle occupying the front and sides of the thigh, which straightens the leg at the knee-joint and maintains the body in an upright position.

QUADRIPLEGIA means paralysis of the four limbs of the body.

QUADRUPLETS (see MULTIPLE BIRTHS).

QUARANTINE is the principle of preventing the spread of infectious disease by which people, baggage, merchandise, and so forth likely to be infected or coming from an infected locality are isolated at frontiers or ports till their harmlessness has been proved to the satisfaction of the authorities. (See INFECTION.)

Originally quarantine, as its name implies, involved detention for forty days; but, as this proved intolerable for people engaged in business, the time of detention is now calculated so as simply to cover the incubation period of the disease, the presence of which is suspected.

Numerous international conferences upon the subject have been held with the view of arriving at a uniform practice as regards quarantine in different countries. The diseases to which quarantine applies are cholera, yellow fever, plague, smallpox, typhus and relapsing fever.

The general practice with regard to quarantine is that when a serious disease breaks out in any country, the government of that country notifies surrounding governments as to the ports and other places that have become centres of infection. Any people travelling from these centres and attempting to enter another country, are subject to measures prescribed in the appropriate Regulations. These measures vary with the disease involved; as often as not, today they merely involve keeping under the surveillance of the local medical officer through the incubation period of the disease in question.

QUARTAN FEVER Description of intermittent fever with paroxysms developing every fourth day. Usually applied to malaria (q.v.).

QUASSIA is the wood of *Picrasma excelsa*, a large West Indian tree. Its virtues depend upon the presence of an active principle, quassin, which is excessively bitter and also irritating. The various preparations of the wood are mainly used as a bitter tonic. Quassia cups were for long to be found in many households. Made of quassia wood, they were filled with hot

Disease	Patients	Contacts
Chickenpox	6 days from the date of the appearance of the rash.	None.
Diphtheria	Until 3 consecutive throat and nose swabs are negative.	Until nose and throat swabs are bacteriologically clear.
German measles	5 days from the appearance of the rash.	None.
Measles	7 days after the appearance of the rash if the child appears well.	Infants who have not had the disease should be excluded for 14 days from the date of appearance of the rash in the last case in the house. Other contacts can attend school. Any contact suffering from a cold, chill or red eyes should be immediately excluded.
Mumps	9 days from the onset of the disease or 7 days from the subsidence of all swelling.	None.
Whooping-cough	21 days from the beginning of the characteristic cough.	Infants who have not had the disease should be excluded for 21 days from the date of onset of the disease in the last case in the house.

Quarantine periods for the commoner infectious diseases.

water. This resulted in a bitter water which was drunk as a 'bitter' to stimulate the appetite. These quassia cups could be used over and over again for several years, retaining their ability to produce a bitter extract.

QUICKENING (see PREGNANCY).

QUINIDINE is an alkaloid obtained from cinchona bark and closely related in chemical composition and in action to quinine. It is commonly used in the form of quinidine sulphate in doses of 200 to 600 mg. It is used in the treatment of the cardiac irregularity known as atrial fibrillation, being particularly useful in cases of recent onset.

QUININE is an alkaloid obtained from the bark of various species of cinchona trees. This bark is mainly derived from Peru and neighbouring parts of South America and the East Indies. Other alkaloids and acid substances are also derived from cinchona bark, such as quinidine and cinchonine.

Quinine is generally used in the form of one of its salts, such as the sulphate of quinine, or dihydrochloride of quinine. All are sparingly soluble in water, much more so when taken along with an acid.
Action Quinine is a powerful antiseptic. Its best-known action is in checking the recurrence of attacks of malaria, and this action it exerts by virtue of its destructive power against the malarial parasite in the blood. In fevers it acts as an antipyretic (q.v.).

Among its side-effects are ringing in the ears, temporary impairment of vision, and sometimes irritation of the kidneys: all these pass off when the drug is discontinued.
Uses The most important use of quinine is its original one in malaria, attacks of which it quickly cuts short or prevents altogether. After many years it was largely replaced by the more effective and less toxic anti-malarial drugs that were available. (See MALARIA.) Development of malarial parasites resistant to newer drugs has prompted a revival in the use of quinine. For intravenous injection, when this is necessary in cases of malaria, a soluble form of quinine, the dihydrochloride, is used in doses of 300 to 600 mg. Quinine can also be given in combination with other anti-malarial drugs on medical advice. The drug is sometimes used in the treatment of cramps.

QUINSY is a corruption of *cynanche*, and is an old name for a peritonsillar abscess (q.v.).

QUINTUPLETS (see MULTIPLE BIRTHS).

R

RABIES is an acute and fatal disease which affects animals, particularly carnivora, and may be communicated from them to man. Infection from man to man is very rare, but those in attendance on a case should take precautions to avoid being bitten or allowing themselves to be contaminated by the patient's saliva as this contains the causative virus.
Cause The disease is in existence constantly among dogs and wolves in some countries, and from these it spreads widely now and then in epidemics. It also occurs in foxes, coyotes and skunks, as well as vampire bats. Thanks to quarantine measures, it has been rare in Great Britain since 1897. Britain still retains strict measures to prevent the entry of infected animals including a six months' quarantine period and vaccination.

It is highly infectious from the bite of an animal already affected, but the chance of infection from different animals varies. Thus only about one person in every four bitten by rabid dogs contracts rabies, whilst the bites of rabid wolves and cats almost invariably produce the disease. The disease is due to a virus which has a special affinity for attacking the nervous system.
Symptoms In animals there are two types of the disease: mad rabies and dumb rabies. In the former, the dog runs about, snapping at objects and other animals, unable to rest; in the latter, which is also the final stage of the mad type, the limbs become paralysed, and the dog crawls about or lies still.

In man the incubation period is usually six to eight weeks, but may be as short as ten days or as long as two years. The disease begins by mental symptoms, the person becoming irritable, restless, and melancholy. At the same time, feverishness and difficulty of swallowing gradually come on. After a couple of days or so, the irritability passes into a state of wildness or terror, and there is great difficulty in swallowing either food or drink.
Treatment The best treatment is, of course, preventive. Local treatment consists of immediate, thorough, and careful cleansing of the wound surfaces and surrounding skin. This is followed by a course of rabies vaccine therapy. Only people bitten or in certain circumstances licked, either by a rabid animal or by one thought to be infected with rabies need treatment with rabies vaccine and antiserum and immunoglobulin (q.v.). A person previously vaccinated against rabies who is subsequently bitten by a rabid animal should be given three to four doses of the vaccine. The vaccine is also used to give protection to those liable to infection, such as kennel workers and veterinary surgeons.

RADIAL ARTERY This artery arises from the brachial artery at the level of the neck of the radius. It passes down the forearm to the wrist where it is easily palpated laterally. It then winds around the wrist to the palm of the hand to supply the fingers.

RADIAL NERVE This nerve arises from the brachial plexus in the axilla. At first descending posteriorly and then anteriorly it ends just above the elbow by dividing into the superficial radial and interosseous nerves. It supplies motor function to the muscles which extend the arm, wrist, and some fingers and supplies sensation to parts of the posterior and lateral aspects of the arm, forearm, and hand.

RADIATION Energy in the form of waves or particles. Radiation is mainly electromagnetic and includes, among others, X-rays, gamma rays, infra-red, ultraviolet, and the visible spectrum.

RADIATION SICKNESS is the term applied to the nausea, vomiting, and loss of appetite which may follow the use of radiotherapy in the treatment of cancer and other diseases. The phenothiazine group of tranquillizers, such as chlorpromazine (q.v.), as well as the antihistamine drugs (q.v.), are of value in its prevention and treatment. Radiotherapy may also be accompanied by irritation and itching of the skin. To prevent this, or at least to reduce its incidence, the skin should be protected from all unnecessary irritation by avoiding, for example, tight collars, hot baths, brisk towelling, wet shaving and cosmetics. Should itching occur, this may be relieved by a weak solution of sodium bicarbonate (1 teaspoonful in a cup of warm water) applied to the skin and dabbed dry with cotton-wool. The application of a bland dusting powder, such as a baby powder, also helps.

RADIOACTIVE ISOTOPES (see ISOTOPES).

RADIOGRAPHY (see X-RAYS).

RADIO-IMMUNO ASSAY is a technique introduced in 1960 which enables the minute quantities of circulating hormones to be measured. A radio-immuno assay depends on the ability of an unlabelled hormone to inhibit, by simple competition, the binding of isotopically labelled hormone by specific antibodies. The requirements for a radio-immuno assay include adequate amounts of the hormone; a method for labelling the hormone with a radio active isotope; the production of satisfactory antibodies; and a technique for separating antibody-bound from free hormone. Radio-immuno assay is more sensitive than the best bio-assay for a given hormone and most sensitive radio-immuno assays permit the detection of picogram (pg = 10^{-12}g) and femtogram (fg = 10^{-15}g) amounts of material.

RADIOLOGY (see X-RAYS).

RADIONUCLIDE is another word for a radioactive isotope. (See ISOTOPES.)

RADIO-OPAQUE Substances which absorb X-rays, rather than transmitting them, appear white on X-rays and are known as radio-opaque. This is true of bones, teeth, certain types of gallstones, renal stones and contrast media used to enhance the accuracy of radiographic imaging. (See X-RAYS.)

RADIOTHERAPY is treatment by radium or other radioactive matter, including X-rays. For long, radium and X-rays were the only sources available. Developments in our knowledge of atomic energy, however, have changed the picture entirely, and we have now at our disposal radioactive isotopes (see ISOTOPES) and X-ray machines which have largely replaced radium, except in the case of certain tumours.

Supervoltage X-ray machines are now available capable of producing X-rays generated at up to 22 million electron volts (22 MeV). These include linear accelerators which produce X-rays at four or more million electron volts, and betatrons which produce X-rays at 22 million electron volts. The advantage of these supervoltage machines is that it is predominantly gamma-rays they produce, which are penetrating rays and can therefore be used to treat deep-seated tumours.

Almost equally high concentrations of gamma-rays can now be obtained from the use of certain radioactive isotopes, particularly cobalt and caesium. Thus a telecobalt machine is now in use which contains 2000 curies or more of radioactive cobalt (Co^{60}), an amount equivalent to 3000 grams of radium (an unheard-of amount in the pre-1939 days when the ordinary radium beam units contained only 10 grams of radium). Not only does this machine give a high concentration of gamma-rays (equivalent to that from a 3 million-volt X-ray machine), it is absolutely safe for both patient and operators, and allows the beam to be directed accurately on the tumour.

Other forms of radiant energy are now coming into use in radiotherapy. One of these is electron-beam therapy. The usual source of electrons, one of the particles in the atomic nucleus, is the betatron, which can produce either electrons or X-rays at energies ranging from 18 to 42 MeV. Whilst the effect of electrons in the tissues of the body is the same as that of X-rays, their great practical advantage is that their effect can be concentrated on the part being treated, without any adverse effect on the surrounding normal tissue. The other form of radiant energy now being used is neutron therapy. Neutrons of 6 MeV energy are obtained from a cyclotron. One of the advantages of neutron therapy is that even if a cell is only partially damaged by neutrons it never recovers, but inevitably dies.

RADIUM The radiations of radium consist of: (1) alpha-rays, which are positively charged helium nuclei; (2) beta-rays, negatively charged electrons; (3) gamma-rays, similar to X-rays but of shorter wave-length.

At the present day the use of radium is largely restricted to the treatment of carcinoma of the neck of the womb, the tongue, and the lips.

Neither X-rays nor radium supersede active surgical measures when these are available for the complete removal of a tumour.

RADIUS is the outer of the two bones in the forearm. (See BONE.)

RÂLE (see CREPITATIONS).

RANITIDINE is a drug used in the treatment of duodenal ulcer (q.v.) by reducing the hyperacidity of the gastric juice. It is a histamine antagonist to the type-2 receptor. Maintenance treatment usually prevents relapse but does not stop the disorder which may return if the drug is discontinued. The drug is best given to patients with frequent severe recurrences.

RANULA is a swelling which occasionally appears beneath the tongue, caused by a collection of saliva in the distended duct of a salivary gland. (See MOUTH, DISEASES OF.)

RAPHE means a ridge or furrow between the halves of an organ.

RAREFACTION is the term applied to the diminution in the density of a bone as a result of withdrawal of calcium salts from it.

RASH (see ERUPTION).

RAT-BITE FEVER is an infectious disease following the bite of a rat. There are two causative organisms – *Spirillum minus* and *Actinobacillus muris* – and the incubation period depends upon which is involved. In the case of the former it is 5 to 30 days; in the case of the latter it is 2 to 10 days. The disease is characterized by fever, a characteristic skin rash and often muscular or joint pains. It responds well to penicillin.

RAUWOLFIA is a drug that has been used in the treatment of high blood-pressure, and as a tranquillizer. It is a peripheral acting adrenergic antagonist. It is derived from the root of *Rauwolfia serpentina*, a plant which grows widely in India, Ceylon, Burma, and Malaya. The active medicinal properties, which reside mainly in the root of the plant, have been recognized for centuries in India, where extracts of the root were used for the treatment of fevers, insomnia, and nervousness.

The drug and its alkaloid derivatives have been largely superseded by more effective antihypertensive agents with fewer side-effects.

RAYNAUD'S DISEASE, so called after Maurice Raynaud (1834–81), the Paris physician who published a thesis on the subject in 1862, is a condition in which the circulation becomes suddenly obstructed in outlying parts of the body. It is supposed to be due to spasm of the smaller arteries in the affected part, as the result of nervous influences, and its effects are increased both by cold and by various diseases involving the blood-vessels. It is predominantly a disease of women, the majority of cases occurring before the age of 40.

Symptoms The condition is most commonly confined to the occurrence of dead fingers, the fingers or the toes, ears, or nose becoming white, numb, and waxy looking. This condition may last for some minutes, or may not pass off for several hours, or even for a day or two.

Treatment People who are subject to these attacks should be careful in winter to protect the feet and hands from cold, and should always use warm water when washing the hands. In addition, the whole body should be kept warm, as spasm of the arterioles in the feet and hands may be induced by chilling of the body. Victims of this disease should be advised to give up smoking. Vasodilator drugs are helpful, especially the calcium antagonists (q.v.). In all cases which do not respond to such medical treatment, surgery should be considered in the form of sympathectomy: i.e. cutting of the sympathetic nerves to the affected part. This results in dilatation of the arterioles and hence an improved blood supply. This operation is more successful in the case of the feet than in the case of the hands.

REACTIVE ARTHRITIS is an aseptic arthritis secondary to an episode of infection elsewhere in the body. It often occurs in association with enteritis caused by Salmonella and certain Shigella strains and in both yersinea and campylobacter enteritis. Non-gonococcal urethritis, usually due to clamydia, is another cause of reactive arthritis and Reiter's syndrome is a particularly florid form with mucocutaneous and ocular lesions. The synovitis usually starts acutely and is frequently asymmetrical with the knees and ankles most commonly affected. Often there are inflammatory lesions of tendon sheaths and entheses such as plantar faschitis. The severity and duration of the acute episode are extremely variable. Individuals with the histocompactibility antigen HLA-B27 are particularly prone to severe attacks.

READ CODES These form an agreed UK thesaurus of health-care terminology named after the general practitioner who devised them initially in the 1970s. The coding system, now in its third version, provides a basis for computerized clinical records that can be shared across professional and administrative boundaries. Such records have essential safeguards for security and confidentiality. The codes accommodate the different views of specialists but use simple terms without any loss of the fine detail necessary in specialist terminology.

RECEPTOR (1) Organs, which may consist of one cell or a small group of cells, which respond to different forms of external or internal stimuli by conveying impulses down nerves to the central nervous system, alerting it to changes in the internal or external environment.
(2) A small, discrete area on the cell membrane or within the cell with which molecules or molecular complexes (e.g. hormones, drugs, and other chemical messengers) interact. When this interaction takes place it initiates a change in the working of the cell.

RECESSIVE Tending to recede. In genetic terms a recessive gene is one whose expression remains dormant if paired with an unlike allele. The trait will only be manifest in an individual homozygous for the recessive gene. (See GENES.)

RECOMBINANT DNA DNA (q.v.) or deoxyribonucleic acid containing genes from various sources that have been combined by genetic engineering (q.v.). (See GENES.)

RECRUDESCENCE The reappearance of a disease after a period without signs or symptoms of its presence.

RECTUM is the last part of the large intestine. It pursues a more or less straight course downwards through the cavity of the pelvis, lying against the sacrum at the back of this cavity. This section of the intestine is about 23 cm (9 inches) long. Its first part is freely movable and corresponds to the upper three pieces of the sacrum, the second part corresponds to the lower two pieces of the sacrum and the coccyx, whilst the third part, known also as the anal canal, is about 25 mm (1 inch) long, runs downwards and backwards, and is kept tightly closed by the internal and external sphincter muscles which surround it. The opening to the exterior is known as the anus. The structure of the rectum is similar to that of the rest of the intestine. (See INTESTINE.)

RECTUM, DISEASES OF Owing to the fact that this part of the intestine is more exposed to external influences than the rest of the bowels, and that it forms the place of lodgment of the stools prior to the evacuation of the bowels, and is therefore often subject to considerable irritation, the rectum is specially liable to various diseases.
Peculiarities of the motions are treated under STOOLS, while PILES and FISTULA are described

under these headings. DIARRHOEA and CONSTIPATION are also treated separately.
IMPERFORATE ANUS, or absence of the anus, may occur in newly born children, and, unless the condition is relieved by operation within a few days, the child dies.
ITCHING at the anal opening, or PRURITUS ANI, is often very troublesome. It may be due to slight abrasions, piles, the presence of threadworms, and anal sex. The anal area should be bathed once or twice a day. Clothing should be loose and smooth – preferably cotton or linen next to the skin. Calamine lotion, containing 1 per cent phenol, or 0·1 to 0·5 per cent camphor, is soothing – applied as a compress on gauze at night and dabbed on during the day. The local application of Eurax or hydrocortisone ointment is often effective.
PAIN of an acute cutting character, at stool, is often due to the presence of a small ulcer or 'fissure'. Pain of an aching nature is not uncommonly caused by the presence of piles. (See also PROCTALGIA.)
ABSCESS in the cellular tissue at the side of the rectum, known from its position as an ischiorectal abscess, is fairly common and may produce a fistula. (See FISTULA.)
PROLAPSE or protrusion of the rectum is sometimes found in children, usually between the ages of 6 months and 2 years. In slight cases, where a ring of bright red mucous membrane 12 or 25 mm (½ or 1 inch) in width protrudes as the result of straining at stool, the condition is generally easily curable. Any irritable condition of the bowels due to diarrhoea, constipation or worms, must be removed and the evacuations regulated by diet and laxatives, so as to avoid all straining. Each time the bowels move, the protruded portion must be returned by steady pressure with a cloth or sponge wrung out of cold water. When the protruded part is very large and the condition does not yield to simple treatment it can be remedied by operation but this is not usually necessary, as the prolapse ceases to occur as the child grows older.
TUMOURS of small size situated on the skin near the opening of the bowel, and consisting of nodules, tags of skin, or cauliflower-like excrescences, are common, and may give rise to pain, itching, and watery discharges. These are easily removed if necessary. Polypi occasionally develop within the rectum, and may give rise to no pain, though they may cause frequent discharges of blood. Like polypi elsewhere, they may often be removed by a minor operation. (See POLYPOSIS.)
CANCER of the rectum is fairly common. In 1989, in England and Wales there were over 10,000 registrations of new cases of cancer of the rectum and anus, and in 1990 nearly 6,000 people died of anorectal cancer. It is a disease of later life, seldom affecting young people, and its appearance is generally insidious. The tumour begins commonly in the mucous membrane, its structure resembling that of the glands with which the membrane is furnished, and it quickly infiltrates the other coats of the intestine and

then invades neighbouring organs. Secondary growths in most cases occur soon in the lymphatic glands within the abdomen and in the liver. The symptoms appear gradually and consist of diarrhoea, alternating with attacks of constipation, and, later on, discharges of blood or of thin blood-stained fluid from the bowels, together with increasing loss of weight and weakness, and pains about the lower part of the back and down the thighs. Upon examination, the tumour can be felt projecting from one side or in a ring-form into the interior of the bowel. These cases are usually far advanced before they give rise to much disturbance, but a lot can now be done to help them by surgical operation. In the majority of cases this consists of removal of the whole of the rectum and the distal two-thirds of the sigmoid colon, and the establishment of a colostomy (q.v.). Depending on the extent of the tumour approximately 50 per cent of the patients who have this operation are alive and well after five years. In some cases in which the growth occurs in the upper part of the rectum it is now possible to remove the growth and preserve the anus so that the patient is saved the discomfort of having a colostomy. Radiotheraphy and chemotherapy may also be of value.

RECURRENT LARYNGEAL NERVE is a branch of the vagus nerve which leaves the latter low down in its course, and, hooking round the right subclavian artery on the right side and round the arch of the aorta on the left, runs up again into the neck, where it enters the larynx and supplies branches to the muscles which control the vocal cords. The importance of this nerve is the fact that it is apt in its long course either to be injured by surgical procedures to the neck, by trauma to the neck, or to be pressed upon by enlarged lymph glands in the neck, by aneurysms of the aorta or right subclavian artery, resulting in defects of vocalization. These defects may therefore arise within the larynx itself or may arise from disease in the chest, which affects the left recurrent laryngeal nerve. If both recurrent laryngeal nerves are involved in the disease process or are injured, the vocal cords come to lie in the midline, causing embarrassment of the airway and this may necessitate some form of airway intervention, usually in the form of a tracheostomy.

RED BLOOD CELL (see ERYTHROCYTE and BLOOD).

REDUCTION The manipulation of part of the body from an abnormal position to the correct one (e.g. fractures, dislocations or hernias).

REFERRED PAIN Pain felt in one part of the body which is actually arising from a distant site (e.g. pain from the diaphragm is felt at the shoulder tip). This occurs because both sites develop from similar embryological tissue and therefore have common pain pathways in the central nervous system. (See PAIN.)

REFLEX ACTION is one of the simplest forms of activity of the nervous system. (For the mechanism upon which it depends, see NERVES.) Reflex acts are divided usually into three classes. *Superficial reflexes* comprise the sudden movements which result when the skin is brushed or pricked, such as the movement of the toes that results from stroking the sole of the foot. *Deep reflexes* depend upon the state of mild contraction in which muscles are constantly maintained when at rest, and are obtained, as in the case of the knee-jerks, by sharply tapping the tendon of the muscle in question. *Visceral reflexes* are those connected with various organs, such as the narrowing of the pupil when a bright light is directed upon the eye, and the contraction of the bladder when distended by urine.

Faults in these reflexes, both in the direction of excess and of diminution, give valuable evidence as to the presence of nervous diseases and the part of the nervous system in which such disease is situated. Thus, absence of the knee-jerk, when the patellar tendon is tapped, means some interference with the sensory nerve, nerve-cells, or motor nerve upon which the act depends, as, for example, in poliomyelitis, or peripheral neuritis; whilst an excessive jerk implies that the controlling influence exerted by the brain upon this reflex mechanism has been cut off, as, for example, by a tumour high up in the spinal cord, or in the disease known as multiple sclerosis (q.v.).

The condition of the plantar reflex (obtained by stroking the skin of the sole of the foot) is an important point in diagnosing organic disease of the nervous system. The normal reflex consists in bending downwards of the toes towards the sole. In organic disease of the higher parts of the nervous system the great toe tends to bend upwards with spreading out of the other toes (extensor plantar response).

The reflex of the pupil to light is also of great diagnostic importance. The pupil quickly contracts when light falls upon the eye or when the eyes are directed suddenly to a near object. In certain serious diseases of the nervous system, especially in general paralysis and tabes dorsalis the contraction on looking at a near object remains, while the effect of light is lost (Argyll-Robertson pupil).

REFLUX Fluid flowing in the opposite direction to normal (e.g. backflow). Often refers to regurgitation of stomach contents into the oesophagus.

REFRACTION The deviation of rays of light on passing from one transparent medium into another of different density. The refractive surfaces of the eye are the anterior surface of the cornea (which accounts for approximately two-thirds of the focusing or refractive power of the eye) and the lens (one-third of the focusing power of the eye). The refractive power of the lens can change, whereas that of the cornea is fixed. *Errors of refraction* (Ametropia) will occur when the focusing power of the lens and cornea do not match the length of the eye, so that rays of light parallel to the visual axis are not focused at the fovea centralis (see EYE). There are three types of refractive error: (i) *Hypermetropia* or long sightedness: the refractive power of the eye is too weak, or the eye is too short so that rays of light are brought to a focus at a point behind the retina. Long-sighted people can see well in the distance but generally require glasses with convex lenses for reading. Uncorrected long sight can lead to headaches and intermittent blurring of vision following prolonged close work, i.e. *eye strain*. As a result of ageing the eye becomes gradually long sighted, resulting in many people's needing reading glasses in later life. This normal process is known as *presbyopia*. A particular form of long sightedness occurs after cataract extraction. (ii) *Myopia* (short sight or near sight): rays of light are brought to a focus in front of the retina because the refractive power of the eye is too great or the eye is too short. Short-sighted people can see close to but need spectacles with concave lenses in order to see in the distance. (iii) *Astigmatism*: the refractive power of the eye is not the same in each meridian. Some rays of light may be focused in front of the retina while others are focused on or behind the retina. Astigmatism can accompany hypermetropia or myopia. It may be corrected by cylindrical lenses (these consist of a slice from the side of a cylinder, i.e. curved in one meridian and flat in the meridian at right angles to it).

REFRACTORY Unresponsive or resistant to treatment.

REGIMEN A course of treatment, possibly combining drugs, exercise, diet, etc., designed to bring about an improvement in health.

REGIONAL ANAESTHESIA (see ANAESTHESIA, Local).

REGIONAL ILEITIS (see under ILEITIS).

REGISTRAR (1) A grade of British junior hospital doctor between senior house officer and senior registrar. Under recent government recommendations registrar numbers should be regulated to ensure a balance with the National Health Service's need for consultants, the senior grade for career doctors in hospitals. (2) A public official responsible for registering births, deaths, and marriages.

REGURGITATION is a term used in various connections in medicine. For instance, in diseases of the heart it is used to indicate a condition in which, as the result of valvular disease, the blood does not entirely pass on from the atria of the heart to the ventricles, or from the ventricles into the arteries. The defective valve is said to be incompetent, and a certain amount of blood leaks past it, or regurgitates back, into the cavity from which it has been driven. (See HEART DISEASES.)

The term is also applied to the return to the mouth of food already swallowed and present in the gullet or stomach.

REHABILITATION is the restoration to health and working capacity of a person incapacitated by disease, mental or physical, or by injury. It is a word that came into prominent use during the 1939–45 War, reflecting the growing awareness of the medical profession that the treatment of a sick or injured person does not end at the moment of recovery from the immediate effects of illness or injury. For example, a man with a fractured limb or spine has to recover full use not only of the injured part but of his whole body; and he has to recover confidence in his ability to work and enjoy life. (See DISABLED PERSONS; REMPLOY.)

REITER'S SYNDROME For some 40 years the concurrence of polyarthritis, non-gonococcal urethritis and ocular inflammation has been called Reiter's Syndrome. The syndrome has over the years been associated with promiscuous sexual contact because urethritis is a common feature. The evidence for this is, however, circumstantial. It is now well recognized that urethritis can occur unrelated to sexual contact as a result of gastro-intestinal infection with *Yersinia enterocolitica*. Possession of the HLA antigen B27 affects the severity of the disease and the prognosis, but the syndrome is not confined to patients with this antigen. (See REACTIVE ARTHRITIS.)

REJECTION A term used in transplant medicine to describe the body's immunological response to foreign tissue. Various drugs, such as cyclosporin A, can be used to dampen the host's response to a graft and reduce the risk of rejection.

RELAPSE means the return of a disease during the period of convalescence.

RELAPSING FEVER, so-called because of the characteristic temperature chart showing recurring bouts of fever, is an infectious disease caused by spirochaetes. There are two main forms of the disease.

LOUSE-BORNE RELAPSING FEVER is an epidemic disease, usually associated with wars and famines, which has occurred in practically every country in the world. For long confused with typhus and typhoid, it was not until the 1870's that the causal organism was described by Obermeier. It is now known as the *Borrelia recurrentis*, a motile spiral organism 10 to 20

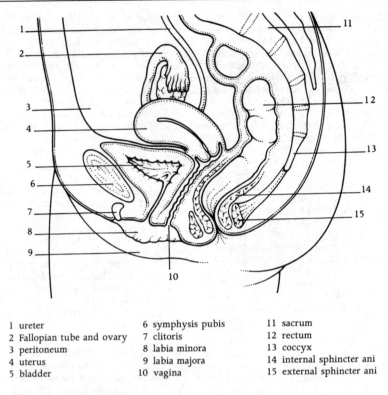

1 ureter	6 symphysis pubis	11 sacrum
2 Fallopian tube and ovary	7 clitoris	12 rectum
3 peritoneum	8 labia minora	13 coccyx
4 uterus	9 labia majora	14 internal sphincter ani
5 bladder	10 vagina	15 external sphincter ani

Vertical section of female pelvis viewed from left.

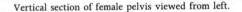

micrometres in length. The organism is transmitted from man to man by the louse, *Pediculus humanus*.

Symptoms The incubation period is up to 12 days, usually 7 days. The onset is sudden, with high temperature, generalized aches and pains, and nose-bleeding. In about half the cases a rash appears at an early stage, beginning in the neck and spreading down over the trunk and arms. Jaundice may occur; and both the liver and the spleen are enlarged. The temperature subsides after five or six days, to rise again in about a week. There may be up to four such relapses (see the introductory paragraph above).

Treatment Preventive measures are the same as those for typhus (q.v.). Rest in bed is essential, as are good nursing and a light, nourishing diet. There is usually a quick response to penicillin. The tetracyclines and chloramphenicol are also effective. Following such treatment the incidence of relapse is about 15 per cent. The mortality rate is low, except in a starved population.

TICK-BORNE RELAPSING FEVER is an endemic disease which occurs in most tropical and subtropical countries. The causative organism is *Borrelia duttoni*, which is transmitted by a tick, *Ornithodorus moubata*. David Livingstone suggested that it was a tick-borne disease, but it was not until 1905 that Dutton and Todd produced the definite evidence.

Symptoms The main differences from the louse-borne disease are: (*a*) the incubation period is usually shorter, 3 to 6 days, but may be as short as 2 days or as long as 12; (*b*) the febrile period is usually shorter and the afebrile periods are more variable in duration, sometimes only lasting for a day or two; (*c*) relapses are much more numerous.

Treatment Preventive measures are more difficult to carry out than in the case of the louse-borne infection. Protective clothing should always be worn in 'tick country'. Old, heavily infected houses should be destroyed. Curative treatment is the same as for the louse-borne infection.

RELATE MARRIAGE GUIDANCE The idea of a marriage guidance council came from a group of doctors, clergy and social workers who were concerned for the welfare of marriage. It is based upon two major concepts: that marriage provides the best possible way for a man and woman to live and love together and rear their children, and that the counsellors share a basic respect for the unique personality of the individual and his (or her) right to make his (or her) own decisions. The organization consists of between 120 and 130 Marriage Guidance Councils throughout the country, comprising about 1250 counsellors. These

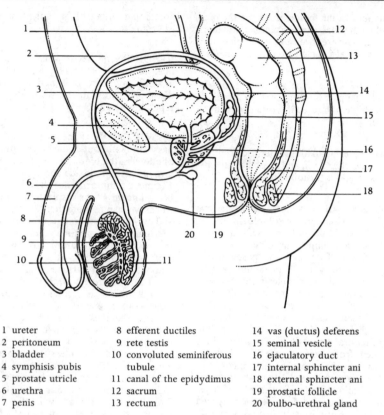

1 ureter	8 efferent ductiles	14 vas (ductus) deferens
2 peritoneum	9 rete testis	15 seminal vesicle
3 bladder	10 convoluted seminiferous	16 ejaculatory duct
4 symphisis pubis	tubule	17 internal sphincter ani
5 prostate utricle	11 canal of the epidydimus	18 external sphincter ani
6 urethra	12 sacrum	19 prostatic follicle
7 penis	13 rectum	20 bulbo-urethral gland

Vertical section of male pelvis viewed from left.

Councils are affiliated to Relate National Marriage Guidance, which is responsible for the selection, training and continued supervision of all counsellors. Anyone seeking help can telephone or write for an appointment. No fees are charged, but those receiving help are encouraged to donate what they can. (See APPENDIX 2: ADDRESSES.)

REMITTENT FEVER is the term applied to the form of fever in which, during remissions, the temperature falls, but not to normal.

REMPLOY is Britain's largest employer of severely disabled people, set up under the provisions of the 1944 Disabled Persons (Employment) Act. (See APPENDIX 2: ADDRESSES.)

REMISSION A period when a disease has responded to treatment and there are no signs or symptoms present.

REM SLEEP Rapid-eye-movement sleep – a stage during sleep in which the eyes are seen to move rapidly beneath the lids and during which dreaming occurs. It occurs for several minutes at a time approximately every 100 minutes. (See SLEEP.)

RENAL Related to the kidney.

RENAL DISEASES (see KIDNEYS, DISEASES OF).

RENIN is a protein-like substance extracted from the kidney which, when injected into animals, causes a rise of blood-pressure. This it does, apparently, by reacting with a substance normally present in the blood plasma to produce angiotensin. Angiotensin has been obtained in crystalline form, and it is angiotensin which causes the rise in blood-pressure. This work may have an important bearing on the problem of high blood-pressure in man.

RENNET, a substance obtained from the stomach of the calf, clots and partially digests milk, and is used in the preparation of cream cheese. Its activity depends on the enzyme rennin.

REPAIR of tissues after injury is described generally under WOUNDS, and the repair of special tissues which present various peculiarities is described under BONE; MUSCLE; NERVES, etc.

REPETITIVE STRAIN INJURY (see TENDINITIS).

REPRODUCTIVE SYSTEM A collective term for all the organs involved in sexual reproduction. In the female these are the ovaries, Fallopian tubes, uterus, vagina and vulva. In the male these are the testes, vasa deferentia, prostate, seminal vesicles, urethra and penis.

RESECTION is the name given to an operation in which a part of some organ is removed, as, for example, the resection of a fragment of dead bone.

RESERPINE is an alkaloid obtained from the root of Rauwolfia (q.v.), and is used as an antihypertensive and a tranquillizing agent.

RESINS are solid or semi-solid exudations from plants, which are insoluble in water, mostly soluble in alcohol or ether, soften or melt at moderate temperatures, and burn with a smoky flame. They are transparent when pure, but opaque when they contain water. They are non-conductors of electricity. Some of them are acids and combine with alkalis to form soaps. A *natural resin* is one that occurs as an exudation, such as mastic. A *prepared resin* is made from a drug, such as podophyllin, or from a natural oleoresin such as rosin which is obtained from various species of *Pinus. Oleoresins* may be either natural oleoresins, which are mixtures of volatile oils and resins generally obtained by incising trunks of trees, such as turpentine and copaiba; or prepared oleoresins which are concentrated liquid preparations made from drugs containing both volatile oil and resin, such as capsicum. *Gum resins* are natural mixtures of gums and resins, usually obtained as exudations from plants, such as myrrh and asafoetida. (See also ION EXCHANGE RESINS.)

RESOLUTION is a term applied to infective processes, to indicate a natural subsidence of the inflammation without the formation of pus. Thus a pneumonic lung is said to resolve when the material exuded into it is absorbed into the blood and lymph, so that recovery takes place naturally; an inflamed area is said to resolve when the inflammation fades away and no abscess forms; a glandular enlargement is said to resolve when it decreases in size without suppuration. Resolvents was an old term applied to procedures capable of assisting this process. (See BLISTERS; INFLAMMATION.)

RESONANCE means the lengthening and intensification of sound produced by striking the body over an air-containing structure. Decrease of resonance is called dullness and increase of resonance is called hyper-resonance. The process of striking the chest or other part of the body to discover its degree of resonance is called percussion, and according to the note obtained, an opinion can be formed as to the state of consolidation of air-containing organs, the presence of abnormal cavities, and the dimensions and relations of solid and air-

containing organs lying together. (See also AUSCULTATION.)

RESORCIN, or RESORCINOL, is a white, crystalline, antiseptic substance soluble in water, alcohol, and oils. It is mainly used in skin diseases which require a stimulating and antiseptic application.

RESPIRATION is the process in which air passes into and out of the lungs with the object of allowing the blood to absorb oxygen and to give off carbon dioxide and water. This occurs 18 times a minute in a healthy adult at rest, this being known as the respiratory rate. In other words we inspire more than 25,000 times a day and during this time inhale around 16 kg of air. **Mechanism of respiration** For the structure of the respiratory apparatus see AIR PASSAGES; CHEST; LUNGS. The air passes rhythmically into and out of the air passages, and mixes with the air already in the lungs, these two movements being known as inspiration and expiration. INSPIRATION is due to a muscular effort which enlarges the chest in all three dimensions, so that the lungs have to expand in order to fill up the vacuum that would otherwise be left, and the air accordingly enters these organs by the air passages. There is no direct pull upon the lungs, each of which is simply suspended within the corresponding pleural cavity by its root, and made to fill this cavity in all conditions of the chest by the pressure of the outer air exerted through the nose, mouth, and air passages. The increase of the chest in size from above downwards is mainly due to the diaphragm, the muscular fibres of which, by their contraction, reduce its domed shape and cause it to descend, pushing down the abdominal organs beneath it. The increase from before back is mainly due to a tilting forwards of the lower end of the breastbone, and of the lower rib cartilages. The increase from side to side can best be understood by examining a skeleton, noting the very oblique position of the lower ribs, and observing how greatly the capacity of the chest is increased when each is raised, in the manner of a bucket-handle, taking its fixed points at the spine and breast-bone. (See RIBS.)

The muscles which chiefly bring about these changes in ordinary quiet inspiration are the diaphragm, intercostal muscles, and levators of the ribs, whilst in forced or extraordinary inspiration, when a specially deep breath is taken, the sternocleidomastoid, serratus magnus, trapezius, and pectoral muscles are also brought powerfully into play. Many other muscles take part to a slight extent, steadying the spine and the upper and lower ribs, while even the muscles of the face and of the larynx are thrown rhythmically into activity, dilating the nostrils and the entrance to the larynx at each breath. EXPIRATION is in ordinary circumstances simply an elastic recoil, the diaphragm rising and the ribs sinking into the position that they naturally occupy, when muscular contraction is finished. Expiration occupies a slightly longer period than inspiration. In forced expiration many powerful muscles of the abdomen and thorax are brought into play, and the act may be made a very forcible one, as, for example, in coughing.

Nervous control Respiration is usually either an automatic or a reflex act, each expiration sending up afferent, sensory impulses to the central nervous system, from which efferent impulses are sent down various other nerves to the muscles that produce inspiration. It appears that there are several centres which govern the rate and force of the breathing, although all are presided over by a chief respiratory centre in the medulla oblongata, which is sometimes spoken of as the vital knot (*noeud vital*). Although this centre appears to be absolutely essential to life, it in turn is under the control of the higher centres in the cerebral hemispheres, through which the will acts, so that breathing can be voluntarily stopped, quickened, or otherwise changed at will. It would be impossible, however, to cause death by voluntarily holding the breath, because, as the blood becomes more venous, the vital centre in the medulla again assumes control and breathing starts again. Apart from changes due to willpower, the respirations follow one another rhythmically at the rate of about 18 per minute, being in general one for every four heart-beats.

Quantity of air The lungs do not by any means completely empty themselves at each expiration and refill at each inspiration. An amount equivalent, in quiet respiration, to less than one-tenth of the total air in the lungs passes out and is replaced by the same quantity of fresh air, which mixes with the stale air in the lungs. This renewal, which in quiet breathing amounts to about 500 millilitres, is known as the *tidal air*. By a special inspiratory effort, one can, however, draw in about 3000 millilitres, this amount being known as *complemental air*. By a special expiratory effort, too, after an ordinary breath one can expel much more than the tidal air from the lungs, this extra amount being known as the *supplemental* or *reserve air*, and amounting to about 1300 millilitres. If one takes as deep an inspiration as possible and then makes a forced expiration, one breathes out the sum of these three, which is known as the *vital capacity*, and amounts to about 4000 millilitres in a healthy adult male of average size. These figures all apply to a man of average height. Figures for women are about 25 per cent lower. The vital capacity varies with size, sex, age and ethnic origin. The formulae in the table, incorporating age, height and sex, give an approximate guide to the vital capacity:

Men:
vital capacity (*in millilitres*)
$$= [27 \cdot 63 - (0 \cdot 112 \times age)] \times height$$
(in centimetres)

Women:
vital capacity (*in millilitres*)
$$= [21 \cdot 78 - (0 \cdot 101 \times age)] \times height$$
(in centimetres)

Over and above the vital capacity, the lungs contain air which cannot be expelled by the strongest possible expiration. This *residual air*, as it is known, which remains in the lungs even after death, amounts to another 1500 millilitres.

Tests of respiratory efficiency are being increasingly used to assess lung function in health and disease. The most widely used one is based on an analysis of a single forced expiration after a maximal inspiration. The volume expelled in the first second of expiration (known as FEV_1) correlates well with the respiratory efficiency. Normal values for FEV_1 vary with age, sex and, to a lesser extent, with the size of the body but, by and large, healthy persons can breathe out 15 per cent or more of vital capacity within the first second.

Abnormal forms of respiration Apart from mere changes in rate and force, respiration is modified in several important ways, either involuntarily or voluntarily. *Sighing* is a long-drawn inspiration following a pause when breathing has been checked by mental preoccupation. This form of breathing also characterizes some conditions of extreme weakness of the nervous system, such as shock and diabetic coma. *Sobbing* is a series of convulsive inspirations, at each of which the larynx is partially closed; it follows grief or great exertion. *Snoring* (q.v.), or stertorous breathing, is due to a flaccid state of the soft palate causing it to vibrate as the air passes into the throat, or simply to sleeping with the mouth open, which has a similar effect. *Coughing* (q.v.) is a series of violent expirations, at each of which the larynx is suddenly opened after the pressure of air in the lungs has risen considerably; its object is to expel some irritating substance from the air passages. *Sneezing* (q.v.) is a single sudden expiration, which differs from coughing in that the sudden rush of air is directed by the soft palate up into the nose in order to expel some source of irritation from this narrow passage. *Cheyne-Stokes breathing* (q.v.) is a type of breathing found in persons suffering from apoplexy, heart disease, and some other conditions, in which death is impending; it consists in an alternate dying away and gradual strengthening of the inspirations. Other disorders of breathing are found in CROUP and in ASTHMA (qq.v.).

RESPIRATORY DISTRESS SYNDROME may occur in adults as adult respiratory distress syndrome or in new-born children, when it is also known as hyaline membrane disease (q.v.). The adult syndrome consists of pulmonary oedema of non-cardiac origin. It is a complication of shock, systemic sepsis and viral respiratory infections. It was first described in 1967 and despite advances with assisted ventilation it remains a serious disease with a mortality of more than 50 per cent. The maintenance of adequate circulating blood volume, peripheral perfusion, acid base balance and arterial oxygenation is important and assisted ventilation should be instituted early. The aetiology is not understood though the process begins when tissue damage stimulates the autonomic nervous system, releases vaso-active substances, precipitates complement activation and produces abnormalities of the clotting cascade – the serial process that leads to clotting of the blood. The activation of complement causes white cells to lodge in the pulmonary capillaries where they release substances which damage the pulmonary endothelium.

RESPIRATORY SYNCYTIAL VIRUS, or RS VIRUS as it is usually known, is one of the myxoviruses (q.v.). It is the major cause of bronchiolitis and pneumonia in infants under the age of 6 months and its incidence has been increasing, possibly due to atmospheric pollution.

RESTLESS LEGS SYNDROME: A condition in which the patient experiences unpleasant sensations, and occasionally involuntary movements, in the legs when at rest, especially at night. No pathological changes have been identified. It is sometimes indicative of iron-deficiency anaemia, but in many cases the cause remains a mystery and the variety of cures offered are a testimony to this. Some anti-epileptic drugs are said to help.

RESUSCITATION (see APPENDIX 2: BASIC FIRST AID).

RETARDATION Slowing down; developmental delay.

RETCHING is an ineffectual form of vomiting. (See VOMITING.)

RETENTION OF URINE (see URINE, RETENTION OF).

RETICULOCYTES are newly formed red blood corpuscles, in which a fine network can be demonstrated by special staining methods.

RETICULO-ENDOTHELIAL SYSTEM consists of highly specialized cells scattered throughout the body, but found mainly in the spleen, bone marrow, liver, and lymph glands. Their main function is the ingestion of red blood cells and the conversion of haemoglobin to bilirubin. They are also able to ingest bacteria and foreign colloidal particles.

RETICULOSES is the term used to describe a group of conditions characterized by progressive widespread proliferation of the cells of the reticulo-endothelial system. The two most important members of this group are Hodgkin's disease (q.v.) and lymphosarcoma (q.v.).

RETINA (see EYE).

RETINA, DISORDERS OF The retina can be damaged by disease that affects the retina alone, or by diseases affecting the whole body. *Retinopathy* is a term used to denote an abnormality of the retina without specifying a cause. Some retinal disorders are discussed below.

DIABETIC RETINOPATHY Retinal disease occurring in patients with diabetes mellitus. It is the commonest cause of blind registration in Great Britain of people between 20 and 65 years of age. Diabetic retinopathy can be divided into several types. The two main causes of blindness are those that follow, first, development of new blood vessels from the retina, with resultant complications and, second, those following 'water logging' (oedema) of the macula. Treatment is by maintaining rigid control of blood-sugar levels combined with laser treatment for certain forms of the disease – in particular to get rid of new blood vessels.

HYPERTENSIVE RETINOPATHY Retinal disease secondary to the development of high blood pressure. Treatment involves control of the blood pressure.

SICKLE CELL RETINOPATHY People with sickle cell disease can develop a number of retinal problems including new blood vessels from the retina.

RETROLENTAL FIBROPLASIA A disorder affecting low-birth-weight premature babies exposed to high oxygen pressures. Essentially new blood vessels develop which cause extensive traction on the retina with resultant retinal detachment and poor vision.

RETINAL ARTERY OCCLUSION, RETINAL VEIN OCCLUSION These result in damage to those areas of retina supplied by the affected blood vessel. The blood vessels become blocked. If the peripheral retina is damaged the patient may be completely symptom free, although areas of blindness may be detected on examination of field of vision. If the macula is involved, visual loss may be sudden, profound and permanent. There is no effective treatment once visual loss has occurred.

SENILE MACULAR DEGENERATION ('senile' indicates age of onset and has no bearing on mental state) is the leading cause of blindness in the elderly in the western world. The average age of onset is 65 years. Patients initially notice a disturbance of their vision which gradually progresses over months or years. They lose the ability to recognize fine detail, e.g. they cannot read fine print, cannot sew or recognize people's faces. They always retain the ability to recognize large objects such as doors and chairs. They are therefore able to get around and about reasonably well. There is no effective treatment in the majority of cases.

RETINITIS PIGMENTOSA A group of rare, inherited diseases characterized by the development of night blindness and tunnel vision. Symptoms start in childhood and are progressive. Many patients retain good visual acuity, although their peripheral vision is limited. One of the characteristic findings on examination is collections of pigment in the retina which have a characteristic shape and are therefore known as 'bone spicules'. There is no effective treatment. RETINAL DETACHMENT usually occurs because of development of a hole in the retina. Holes can occur because of degeneration of the retina, because of traction on the retina by the vitreous, or due to injury. Fluid from the vitreous passes through the hole causing a split within the retina. The inner part of the retina becomes detached from the outer part, the latter remains in contact with the choroid. Detached retina loses its ability to detect light with consequent impairment of vision. Retinal detachments are more common in the short sighted, in the elderly or following cataract extraction. Symptoms include spots before the eyes (*floaters*), flashing lights and a shadow over the eye with progressive loss of vision. Treatment by laser is very effective if caught early, at the stage when a hole has developed in the retina but the retina has not become detached. The edges of the hole can be 'spot welded' to the underlying choroid. Once a detachment has occurred, laser therapy cannot be used, the retina has to be repositioned. This is usually done by indenting the wall of the eye from the outside to meet the retina, then making the retina stick to the wall of the eye by inducing inflammation in the wall. This is done by freezing the wall. The outcome of surgery depends largely on the extent of the detachment and its duration. Complicated forms of detachment can occur due to diabetic eye disease, injury or tumour. Each requires a specialized form of treatment. (See EYE DISEASES.)

RETINOIC ACID is a synthetic vitamin A derivative. (See APPENDIX 5: VITAMINS.)

RETINOL is the official chemical name of vitamin A. (See APPPENDIX 5: VITAMINS.)

RETINOPATHY (see RETINA, DISEASES OF).

RETRACTOR An instrument for pulling apart the edges of an incision to allow better surgical access to the organs and tissues being operated on.

RETRO- is a prefix signifying behind or turned backward.

RETROBULBAR NEURITIS Inflammation of the optic nerve behind (rather than within) the eye. It usually occurs in young adults and presents with a rapid deterioration in vision over a few hours. Colour vision is also impaired. Usually vision recovers over a few weeks, but colour vision may be permanently lost. It can be associated with certain viral illnesses and with multiple sclerosis.

RETROFLEXION means bending of an organ so that its top is thrust backwards. Retroversion is a similar displacement in which the whole organ is turned backwards. These terms are particularly applied to the uterus.

RETROGRADE Movement in a contrary or backward direction from normal (e.g. a retrograde pyelogram introduces dye into the pelvis of the kidney by passing it up the ureters).

RETROPHARYNGEAL ABSCESS is an abscess occurring in the cellular tissue behind the throat. It is the result in general of disease in the upper part of the spinal column.

RETROVERSION An abnormal position of the uterus, occurring in about 20 per cent of women, in which its long axis is pivoted backwards in relation to the cervix and vagina instead of forwards.

REYE'S SYNDROME is a condition which occurs predominantly in young children following a virus infection of the upper respiratory tract or a viral infection such as chickenpox or influenza. The cause is not known, but there is some evidence that aspirin may play a part in its causation. It is of worldwide distribution, but relatively rare in Western Europe. The initial feature is severe, persistent vomiting and fever. This is followed by outbursts of wild behaviour, delirium and convulsions terminating in coma and death. The mortality rate is around 23 per cent, and 50 per cent of the survivors may have persistent mental or neurological disturbances. The younger the patient the higher the death rate and the more common the permanent residual effects.

RHABDOVIRUSES is a group of viruses which includes the rabies virus.

RHATANY, or KRAMERIA, is the root of *Krameria triandra*, a South American plant, which contains an astringent principle. It is mainly used in diarrhoea in the form of a tincture or extract, and to make lozenges for use in cases of relaxed throat.

RHESUS FACTOR (see BLOOD GROUPS).

RHEUMATIC FEVER describes an acute febrile illness, usually seen in children which may include arthralgia, arthritis, chorea (qq.v.), carditis and rash. The illness has been shown to follow a streptococcal infection and a streptococcal cause is now implicit in the term.

Rheumatic fever has become extremely uncommon in developed countries, but remains common in developing areas. It is rare before the age of 3, occurring most commonly in mid-childhood and adolescence. If chorea is excluded (commoner in girls), the disease is equally common in the two sexes. Recurrences of the acute illness may occur over a period of years. Long-term consequences include damage to heart valves and less commonly a non-erosive deforming arthritis or persistent neurological problems.

The streptococci responsible are the beta haemolytic type. Their presence may be confirmed by a positive throat swab or a rising anti-streptolysin antibody titre in serum.

Clinical features Fever is marked with attacks of shivering or rigor. Joint pain and swelling affect the knee, ankle, wrist or shoulder and may migrate from one joint to another. Tachycardia may be out of proportion to other constitutional features and indicate cardiac involvement. Subcutaneous nodules may occur, particularly over the back of the wrist or over the elbow or knee. Erythema marginatum is a red rash characteristic of the condition.

Cardiac involvement includes pericarditis, endocarditis, and myocarditis (qq.v.). The main long-term complication is damage to the mitral and aortic valves (qq.v.).

The chief neurological problem is chorea (St Vitus's dance) which may develop after the acute symptoms have subsided.

Treatment Eradication of streptococcal infection is essential. Other features are treated symptomatically. Paracetamol may be preferred to aspirin as an antipyretic in young children. A non-steroidal anti-inflammatory drug (q.v.) may benefit the joint symptoms. Corticosteroids (q.v.) may be indicated for more serious complications.

Patients who have developed cardiac valve abnormalities require antibiotic prophylaxis during dental treatment and other procedures where bacteria may enter the bloodstream. Secondary cardiac problems may occur several decades later and require replacement of affected heart valves.

RHEUMATISM is an obsolete medical term which no longer has a defined meaning. It remains a lay term covering any painful condition of the arms, legs or spine.

RHEUMATOID ARTHRITIS is the term used to describe a chronic inflammation of the synovial lining of several joints, tendon sheaths or bursae which is not due to sepsis or a reaction to crystals. Most cases show a typical symmetrical pattern, suggesting a single aetiology. However, several atypical patterns occur. It is likely that the problem is of multifactorial origin, and that there is some variation in the genetic and environmental factors involved in individual cases. Rheumatoid arthritis is distinguished from other patterns of inflammatory arthritis by the symmetrical involvement of a large number of peripheral joints, by the common association with serum rheumatoid factor antibody, by the presence of bony erosions around joints and, in a minority, the presence of subcutaneous nodules with necrobiotic (decaying) centres.

Causes There is a major immunogenetic predisposition to rheumatoid arthritis in people carrying the HLA-DR4 antigen. Other minor immunogenetic factors have also been implicated. In addition, there is a degree of familial clustering which suggests other unidentified genetic factors. Genetic factors cannot alone explain aetiology, and environmental and chance factors must be important, but these have yet to be identified. Rheumatoid arthritis appears to be more common in developed countries and in rural populations that have moved to an urban lifestyle. No convincing effect of diet has been demonstrated.

Epidemiology Rheumatoid arthritis most commonly occurs in women from the age of 30 onwards, the sex ratio being approximately 4 to 1. Typical rheumatoid arthritis may occur in adolescence, but in childhood chronic synovitis (q.v.) usually take one of a number of different patterns, classified under juvenile chronic arthritis.

Pathology The primary lesion is an inflammation of the synovial lining, with an accumulation of macrophages on the lining surface and an infiltration of the deeper tissue with lymphocytes, plasma cells, macrophages, and small numbers of neutrophil polymorphs. The synovial fluid becomes diluted with inflammatory exudate, containing a mixture of leukocytes. If inflammation persists for several months, there is often progressive destruction of articular cartilage and bone. Cartilage is replaced by inflammatory tissue known as pannus. A similar tissue invades bone to form erosions. Synovitis also affects tendon sheaths, and may lead to adhesion fibrosis or attrition and rupture of tendons. Subcutaneous and other bursae may be involved. Necrobiotic nodules also occur at sites outside synovium, including the subcutaneous tissues, the lungs, the pericardium and the pleura.

Clinical features Rheumatoid arthritis varies from the very mild to the severely disabling. Many mild cases probably go undiagnosed. At least 50 per cent of known cases continue to lead a reasonably normal life, about 25 per cent are significantly disabled in terms of work and leisure activities and a minority become markedly disabled and are limited in their independence. There is often an early acute phase, followed by substantial remission, but in other patients gradual stepwise deterioration may occur, with progressive involvement of an increasing number of joints.

The diagnosis of rheumatoid arthritis is largely based on clinical symptoms and signs. Approximately 70 per cent of patients have rheumatoid factor antibodies in the serum but, because of the large number of false positives and false negatives, this test cannot be considered diagnostic and has very little value in clinical practice. It may be a useful pointer to a worse prognosis in early cases if the titre is high. The erythrocyte sedimentation rate (see ESR) and plasma viscosity (stickiness) are usually raised during periods when the patient has clinical symptoms. They may remain abnormal during periods of clinical remission. Their value in long-term management is arguable. Joint radiographs will show progressive loss of the cartilage joint space and the development of body erosions in many cases. Radiographs may assist in diagnosis in early cases and are particularly helpful when considering surgery or possible complications such as pathological fracture. Patients commonly develop anaemia, which may be partly due to gastrointestinal blood loss from anti-inflammatory drug treatment. Treatment involves physical, pharmacological, and surgical measures, together with psychological and social support tailored to the individual patient's needs. Regular activity should be maintained. Resting of certain joints such as the wrist with splints may be helpful at night or to assist prolonged manual activities. Sound footwear is important. Drug treatment includes simple analgesics, non-steroidal anti-inflammatory agents and slow-acting antirheumatics including gold, penicillamine, sulphasalazine and azathioprine. The non-steroidal agents are largely effective in reducing pain, and early morning stiffness, and have no effect on the chronic inflammatory process. The slow-acting drugs take approximately three months to act but have a more global effect on chronic inflammation with a greater reduction in swelling and an associated fall in erythrocyte sedimentation rate and rise in the level of haemoglobin. Local corticosteroids are useful, given into individual joints. Systemic corticosteroids carry serious problems if continued long term, but may be useful under special circumstances.

RHEUMATOLOGY   The medical speciality concerned with the study and management of diseases of the joints and connective tissues.

RH FACTOR (see BLOOD GROUPS).

RHINITIS means inflammation of the mucous membrane of the nose. (See NOSE, DISEASES OF.)

RHINOPHYMA is the condition characterized by enlargement of the nose due to enormous enlargement of the sebaceous glands which may develop in the later stages of rosacea (q.v.).

RHINOPLASTY means the repair of the nose or modification of its shape by operation. This operation is performed by plastic and ENT surgeons alike. It may involve alteration of the bony skeleton of the nose and/or alteration of the septum (septorhinoplasty). It is mostly performed for cosmetic reasons. However, any disease process or injury which has caused defect in the nose may be repaired as well. The latter problem would usually involve the utilization of some form of skin flap, whereas this would not be required for cosmetic surgical purposes.

RHINOVIRUSES are a large group of viruses; to date around 80 distinct rhinoviruses have been identified. Their practical importance is that some of them are responsible for around one- quarter of the cases of the common cold.

RHIZOTOMY is the surgical operation of cutting a nerve root, as, for example, to relieve the pain of trigeminal neuralgia.

RHONCHI denotes the harsh cooing, hissing, or whistling sounds (wheezing) heard by auscultation over the bronchial tubes when they are the seat of infection. (See BRONCHITIS.)

RHYTHM METHOD   A method of contraception which attempts to prevent conception by avoiding intercourse during the fertile part of the menstrual cycle. (See CONTRACEPTION; SAFE PERIOD.)

RIBOFLAVINE is the *British Pharmacopoeia* name for what used to be known as vitamin B_2. Riboflavine belongs to a group of animal and plant pigments which give a greenish fluorescence on exposure to ultra-violet rays. It is present especially in milk, and is not destroyed during pasteurization. Other rich sources are eggs, liver, yeast and the green leaves of broccoli and spinach. It is also present in beer. Deficiency of riboflavine in the diet is thought to cause inflammation of the substance of the cornea, sores on the lips, especially at the angles of the mouth (cheilosis (q.v.)), and dermatitis.
   The minimal daily requirement for an adult is 1·5 to 3 mg, but is greater during pregnancy and lactation. (See APPENDIX 5: VITAMINS.)

RIBONUCLEIC ACID (see RNA).

RIBOSOME   Granules either found free within the cell or attached to a reticular network within the cell's endoplasm. Consisting of approximately 65 per cent RNA and 35 per cent protein, they are the sites where protein is made.

RIBS are the bones, twelve on each side, which enclose the cavity of the chest. The upper seven are joined to the breast-bone by their costal cartilages and are therefore known as true ribs. The lower five do not reach the breast-bone, and are therefore known as false ribs. Of the latter, the 8th, 9th and 10th are joined by their costal cartilages, each one to the rib immediately above it, while the 11th and 12th are free from any such connection, and are therefore known as floating ribs. Each rib has a head, by which it is joined to the upper part of the body of the vertebra with which it corresponds, as well as to the vertebra immediately above. Next comes a narrow part known as the neck, and then a tubercle, by which the rib is joined to the transverse process of the corresponding vertebra. Finally, the greater part of the bone is made up of the shaft, which runs at first

he sees. His descriptions and ideas about the blots are noted and an elaborate system of scoring is said to afford indications of the kind of personality and psychological make-up of the person investigated. Much work has been done on the test and it is thought highly of by experienced psychiatrists.

ROSACEA, or ACNE ROSACEA as it is sometimes known, is a condition in which there is chronic congestion of the flush areas of the face and forehead, leading to the formation of red papules. In the earlier stages the erythema, or redness of the skin, tends to wax and wane, being more marked after a meal or excessive drinking of alcohol or exposure to sunlight. Ultimately, however, the erythema becomes permanent, and may be accompanied by gross enlargement of the sebaceous glands (see SKIN), leading to the gross enlargement of the nose known as rhinophyma (q.v.) or grog blossoms.
Symptoms In the milder forms there is simple redness, burning, and tingling of the nose, the redness lasting at first only for a few hours every day, but later tending to become permanent, and also to appear upon the cheeks, forehead and chin. In the severer form the nose becomes very red and the skin thick and lumpy, while the openings of the sebaceous glands are seen as quite wide pits. In exceptional cases, more commonly in men than in women, there may be enormous enlargement of the sebaceous glands of the nose, the condition known as rhinophyma (q.v.).
Treatment Tetracycline is the treatment of choice and most patients respond to 250 mg twice daily for a period of 3 to 6 months.

ROSEOLA is a term applied to any rose-coloured rash.

ROSE-WAALER TEST is a blood test which is proving of value in the diagnosis of rheumatoid arthritis. It is positive in over 70 per cent of patients with this disease, compared with only 4 per cent of people not suffering from rheumatoid arthritis.

ROSE-WATER is prepared by soaking rose-petals in water and distilling over part of the fluid. It is used as an ingredient of cold-cream, etc. Rose oil, or attar of rose, is prepared by distilling the fresh flowers of *Rosa damascena*. It is largely used in perfumery, and in lozenges, dentifrices and ointments.

ROTAVIRUSES are a group of viruses (so-called from their wheel-like structure: *rota* is Latin for wheel) which are a common cause of gastroenteritis in infants (see DIARRHOEA). They are rarely found in children over 6 years of age. They cause from 25 to 80 per cent of childhood diarrhoea in different parts of the world. In the United Kingdom they are responsible for 60 to 65 per cent of cases. They infect only the cells

lining the small intestine. In the United Kingdom death from rotavirus is rare.

ROUGHAGE, or dietary fibre, has long been known to affect bowel function. How it does this is still not quite clear but the probability is that it achieves this through its capacity to hold water in a gel-like form. But fibre is not an inert substance as was long thought to be the case. It is digested and metabolized in the colon by the micro-organisms there. It plays a role in the prevention of constipation, diverticular disease (see DIVERTICULOSIS) and the irritable bowel syndrome (q.v.). There is also some evidence that it may reduce the incidence of cancer of the colon. Though bran is not the panacea it is made out to be by some, modern western diets do not contain as much roughage, such as wholemeal flour, as they should.

ROULEAUX is the term applied to the heaps into which red blood corpuscles collect as seen under the microscope.

ROUNDWORMS (see ASCARIASIS).

ROUS SARCOMA is a malignant tumour of fowls which is caused by a virus. This tumour has been the subject of much experimental work bearing upon the nature of cancer.

RUBBING (see MASSAGE; LINIMENTS).

RUBELLA is another name for GERMAN MEASLES (q.v.).

RUPTURE is a popular name for hernia. (See HERNIA.)

RYLE'S TUBE (see NASOGASTRIC TUBE).

S

SABIN VACCINE Introduced in 1962, the attenuated live oral vaccine (Sabin) against poliomyelitis (q.v.) replaced the previous inactivated vaccine (SALK) introduced in 1956. Since the introduction of vaccine, notifications of paralytic poliomyelitis have dropped substantially in the UK, with occasional outbursts of infection with wild virus among unimmunized people, thus showing the importance of maintaining a high level of uptake of the vaccine in the community (see SALK VACCINE).

SACCHARIN is a soluble coal-tar product of white crystalline appearance. It has an extremely sweet taste, being prepared in various strengths so as to equal in sweetness from 300 to 500 times its own weight of cane-sugar. It escapes from the body unchanged, having practically no effect upon the tissues beyond its influence upon the sensation of taste. Accordingly it is used by diabetics, fat people and others to whom sugar is harmful. It tends to give a bitter flavour to drinks to which it is added.

SACCHAROMYCES is another name for yeast.

SACRAL NERVES The five pairs of spinal nerves that leave the spinal column in the sacral area. They carry motor and sensory fibres from the anal and genital regions and from both legs.

SACRAL VERTEBRAE The five fused vertebrae that link the thoracic spine and the coccyx and form the sacrum.

SACROILEITIS Inflammation of one or both of the sacroiliac joints, which lie between the sacrum and the iliac bones. The condition may be the result of rheumatoid arthritis, ankylosing spondylitis, Reiter's syndrome (qq.v.), or the arthritis that occurs with psoriasis (q.v.) or infection. Sacroileitis causes pain in the lower back, buttocks, thighs, and groin. Stiffness may occur with ankylosing spondylitis. Non-steroidal anti-inflammatory drugs relieve the symptoms and if the cause is infection antibiotics should be used.

SACRUM is the portion of the spinal column near its lower end. The sacrum consists of five vertebrae fused together to form a broad triangular bone which lies between the two haunch-bones and forms the back wall of the pelvis.

SADISM (Marquis de Sade) is the term applied to a form of sexual perversion, in which satisfaction is derived from the infliction of cruelty upon another person.

SAFE PERIOD is that period during the menstrual cycle when fertilization of the ovum is unlikely to occur. Ovulation usually occurs about 15 days before the onset of the menstrual period. A woman is commonly believed to be fertile for about 11 days in each menstrual cycle: i.e. on the day of ovulation and for 5 days before and 5 days after this. This would be the eighth to the eighteenth day of the usual 28-day menstrual cycle. Outside this fertile period is the SAFE PERIOD: the first week and the last ten days of the menstrual cycle. On the other hand, there is increasing evidence that the safest period is the last few days before menstruation. In the case of irregular menstruation it is not possible to calculate the safe period. In any event the safety is not absolute.

SAFETY OF DRUGS The Medicines Act of 1968, which came into force in 1971, is a comprehensive measure replacing most of the previous legislation on the control of medicines for human and veterinary use. It is administered by the Health and Agriculture Ministers of the United Kingdom. It decreed the setting up of a Medicines Commission – reorganized in 1993 as the Medicines Control Agency – by the Ministers to give them advice generally relating to the execution of the provisions of the Act. On the advice of the Medicines Commission a series of expert advisory committees was set up. These are Standing Committees of independent experts, and consist of the Committee on Safety of Medicines, the Committee on the Review of Medicines, the Committee on Dental and Surgical Materials, the British Pharmacopoeia Commission which is responsible for the production of the *British Pharmacopoeia*, and the Veterinary Products Committee.

The Committee on Safety of Medicines (CSM) has the function of scrutinizing the efficacy, quality and safety of new drugs before clinical trial and before marketing, as well as the surveillance of each drug after marketing so that adverse reactions are monitored and documented, and warnings issued as required. Early clinical trial for a drug can only be carried out after a clinical trial certificate has been issued by the licensing authority: i.e. all Ministers specified in the Act. In the case of human medicines the Minister acts through the Medicines Control Agency.

The major defect in this carefully worked out system is the difficulty in obtaining reports of adverse reaction. The present evidence suggests that at most about 10 per cent of such reactions are reported. One method of trying to obtain this information is the yellow card system. It is so called because it is based on the distribution of yellow cards to all doctors and dentists, on which they are asked to report any adverse reaction they may encounter to a drug even though initially the evidence may not be 100 per cent certain. Alternatively the CSM has a Freephone line and on-line computer facilities (ADROIT) for practitioners to use. Even though the annual number of adverse reactions reported in this way has risen from around 5,000 in 1975 to over 20,000 in 1993, this is only a fraction of the adverse reactions that actually occur.

Two further committees in this safety screen are the Joint Committee on Vaccination and Immunization and the Adverse Reactions to Vaccines and Immunological Substances Committee. The function of the Committee on Review of Medicines is to review all medicinal products on the British market.

SAGITTAL is the term applied to a structure or section running from front to back in the body.

ST VITUS'S DANCE is an out moded name for CHOREA (q.v.).

SALBUTAMOL is a drug that is proving of value, and safe, for the relief of spasm of the bronchi in asthma.

SALICYLIC ACID is a white substance in fine crystals, of sweetish taste, and sparingly soluble in water.

Action Salicylic acid is an antiseptic. Externally it is used in ointments to check various skin affections due to bacteria, and, since it has in addition a softening action on the surface of the skin, salicylic acid plasters are used to remove corns and various other superficial overgrowths.

SALINE in the form of normal saline is a solution containing 0·9 per cent of sodium chloride (common salt). Saline is used clinically to dilute drugs given by injection and is also given as an intravenous infusion to restore blood volume if blood loss from accident or operation is not too serious or to tide a patient over until plasma (q.v.) or blood for transfusion becomes available.

Saline is also given orally to severely dehydrated children or adults suffering from diarrhoea and, in particular, cholera (q.v.).

SALIVA is the fluid which is always present to some extent in the mouth, and is secreted in specially copious amount during a meal, or when the salivary glands are stimulated, as for example by an acid substance placed in the mouth. Saliva contains much mucus and an enzyme known as ptyalin, which changes starch into dextrose and maltose (see DIGESTION); also many cells of different types. About 750 millilitres are produced daily.

The principal function of saliva is to aid in the initial processes of digestion. When food is taken into the mouth, an increased output of saliva is evoked. This saliva is essential for the process of mastication (q.v.), whereby food is reduced to a homogeneous mass before being swallowed. In addition, the ptyalin in the saliva initiates the digestion of starch in the food.

An excessive flow of saliva known as *salivation* occurs as the result of taking certain drugs over a considerable period. Salivation also occurs as the result of irritation in the mouth, as for instance, in the teething child, and from dyspepsia. Dribbling of saliva is a common symptom of bulbar paralysis. The converse state of lack, or deficiency, of saliva is known as xerostomia (q.v.).

SALIVARY GLANDS are the glands situated near, and opening into, the cavity of the mouth, by which the saliva is manufactured. They include the *parotid gland*, placed in the deep space that lies between the ear and the angle of the jaw; the *submandibular gland*, lying beneath the horizontal part of the jaw-bone; and the *sublingual gland*, which lies beneath the tongue.

Each gland is made up of branching tubes closely packed together, and supported by strong connective tissue. These tubes are lined by large cells that secrete the saliva, and from their interior lead ducts that unite with one another to form ultimately the large main ducts that open into the mouth. The appearance and character of the secreting cells vary in different glands. In the parotid gland they secrete a clear fluid containing the enzyme, ptyalin; in the sublingual gland they mainly produce mucus, whilst the submandibular gland contains cells of both types.

SALK VACCINE Treating the poliomyelitis virus with formalin stops it causing the disease but still allows the virus to stimulate the production of antibodies. Salk vaccine is given by injection and protects the recipient against the disease. The orally given Sabin vaccine is used in the United Kingdom.

SALMONELLA INFECTIONS, or SALMONELLOSIS (see FOOD POISONING, ENTERIC FEVER and DYSENTERY).

SALMON PATCHES are small pink patches found in some new-born infants – on the eyelids, on the forehead between the eyes, and on the nape of the neck. Those on the first two of these three sites have usually faded by the baby's first birthday, but those on the nape of the neck may be more persistent. (See also BIRTH-MARKS.)

SALPINGITIS is inflammation situated in the Fallopian tubes.

SALPINGO- is a prefix indicating a connection with either the Fallopian (or uterine) tubes or the Eustachian (or auditory) tubes.

SALT is the substance produced by the replacement of the acidic hydrogen of an acid by a metal or basic radical. It is also a synonym for common salt or sodium chloride.

SAL VOLATILE is another name for aromatic solution of ammonia, a liquid of burning taste and great stimulating powers. Its action depends upon various volatile oils, ammonia, and bicarbonate of ammonia which it contains. It is used as a stimulating expectorant in cough mixtures, and is valuable as a stimulant in faints. The dose is from half to one teaspoonful (1 to 5 millilitres) in a wineglassful of water. (See AMMONIA.)

SANDFLY FEVER, also known as PHLEBOTOMUS FEVER, THREE-DAY FEVER, and PAPATACI FEVER, is a short, sharp fever occurring in many parts of the tropics and subtropics, including most of the Mediterranean littoral, due to a virus, called phlebovirus, conveyed by the bite of a small hairy midge or sandfly (*Phlebotomus* *papatasi*). The incubation period is three to seven days.

Symptoms There are headache, feverishness, general sensations like those of influenza, flushed face and bloodshot eyes, but no signs of catarrh. The fever passes off in three days, but the patient may take some time to convalesce. **Treatment** As there is no specific remedy, prophylaxis is important. This consists of the spraying of rooms with an insecticide such as Gammexane (q.v.); the application of insect repellents such as dimethyl phthalate to the exposed parts of the body (e.g. ankles, wrists and face), particularly at sunset; and the use of sandfly nets at night. Once the infection is acquired, treatment consists of rest in bed, light diet and aspirin and codeine.

SANGUINEOUS means containing blood.

SAPHENOUS is the name given to the two large superficial veins of the leg. The small saphenous vein which runs up the outside and back of the leg joins the deep veins at the bend of the knee; the great saphenous vein, the longest vein in the body, which has a long course from the inner ankle to the groin, is specially subject, with its branches, to become the site of varicose veins.

SAPROPHYTE is the term applied to organisms which live usually upon decaying and dead matter and produce its decomposition.

SARCO- is a prefix signifying flesh or fleshy.

SARCOIDOSIS is a chronic disease of unknown origin. It involves the skin, lymph nodes, eyes, salivary glands, lungs, heart and bones of the hands and feet. The Kveim Test is used to confirm the diagnosis. The disease is usually self limiting but occasionally treatment with corticosteroids is required.

SARCOMA (see CANCER).

SARCOPTES SCABIEI is the mite which causes scabies (q.v.).

SAUNA is a hot-air, steam or smoke bath, combined with ice-cold water bathing or douching. An old Finnish practice, practically every house or block of flats there has its sauna. The precise therapeutic value of saunas may not be clear, though the Finns claim that they are a well-proven means of maintaining health. There is some evidence that they may be good for the skin, the upper air passages, weight reduction, and for the relief of rheumatic pains.

SCAB is the crust which forms on superficial injured areas. It is composed of fibrin, which is exuded from the raw surface, together with blood corpuscles and epithelial cells entangled in its meshes. Healing takes place naturally under this protection, and the scab dries up and falls off when healing is complete. Scabs appearing on the face without any previous abrasion are often of infectious nature. (See IMPETIGO.)

SCABIES is a skin disease caused by the *Sarcoptes scabiei* which resembles the cheese mite in appearance. It is a minute oval-shaped mite possessing four pairs of legs. It is just visible to the naked eye, the female measuring about 250 to 350 micrometres in length; the male is smaller. The female burrows in the skin, particularly that on the front of the wrist, the web and sides of the fingers, the buttocks, the genitals, and the feet, forming small tunnels in which she lays her eggs (25 to 30). The sides and legs may also be affected in the same way, though rarely the upper parts of the body. The eggs hatch in the burrows in four to five days, and it is the movement of the larvae which causes the intense itching which gives scabies its popular name of itch. The scratching caused by this itching is responsible for much of the eruption of scabies. The larvae ultimately leave the burrows and develop in the skin, a female becoming mature in about two weeks.

Scabies is rife among the population of Great Britain. Personal contact is the most important factor in keeping this infestation going. This is why it is so important that all members of a household in which a case occurs should be carefully examined, and treated if found to be infected. Less stress is now laid on dissemination of the mite by infested clothes and blankets.

Symptoms The person complains of great itchiness and heat, felt particularly soon after he goes to bed, and preventing sleep in the early part of the night. The spaces between the fingers, the backs of the hands, and the front of the wrists are red and scabbed as the result of scratching, or the surface in these localities may even be much inflamed.

Treatment The patient is scrubbed with soft soap in a hot bath, to open up the burrows. Immediately after drying, the official *British Pharmacopoeia* 25 per cent preparation of benzyl benzoate, known as Benzyl Benzoate Application BP, is applied to the whole surface of the body below the chin. A second and a third application is made at twelve-hourly intervals. The patient then has a bath, puts on clean underclothes, and has his bed clothes changed. In infants and young children, in whom benzyl benzoate may cause unpleasant stinging, monosulfiram or 1 per cent gamma benzene hexachloride may be used as an alternative.

SCALDS (see BURNS AND SCALDS).

SCALP is the soft covering of the skull on the top of the head. It consists of five layers, which from the surface inwards are as follows: the skin, thickly furnished with hair; next a subcutaneous layer of fat, rendered tough and stringy by many bands of fibrous tissue passing through it to bind the skin and the third layer together; thirdly, a tough membrane composed of fibrous tissue, known as the epicranium; fourthly, a loose layer of connective tissue attaching the epicranium to the deepest layer, and permitting the free movements of which the scalp is capable; and, finally, another fibrous layer clinging closely to the skull, and known as the pericranium.

SCALPEL is a small, straight, surgical knife.

SCANNING SPEECH A speech disorder in which articulated syllables are wrongly spaced and each is given the same vocal emphasis. The condition occurs as a result of disease in the cerebellum or its connecting nerves.

SCAPHOID BONE The outside bone on the thumb side of the hand in the row of carpal (wrist) bones nearest to forearm. Fracture of the scaphoid is a common wrist injury that usually occurs when someone falls on to their outstretched hand. The fracture may be missed in which case pain in and permanent damage to the wrist can occur.

SCAPULA is the technical name for the shoulder-blade. (See SHOULDER-BLADE.)

SCAR is the name applied to a healed wound, ulcer or breach of tissue. A scar consists essentially of fibrous tissue, covered by an imperfect formation of epidermis in the case of scars on the surface of the skin. The fibrous tissue is produced by the connective tissue corpuscles that wander into the wound in the course of its repair (see WOUNDS), and is at first delicate in texture and richly provided with blood-vessels. Accordingly a scar at first is soft, and has a redder tint than the surrounding skin. Gradually this fibrous tissue contracts, becomes more dense, and loses its blood-vessels, so that an old scar is hard and white. (See KELOID.)

SCARLET FEVER is caused by the erythrogenic toxin of the streptococcus (q.v.). The symptoms of pyrexia, headache, vomiting and a punctate erythematous rash follow a streptococcal infection of the throat or even a wound. The rash is symmetrical and does not itch. The skin subsequently peels. In the latter half of the 19th century it was the commonest cause of death in children over the age of one year. The mortality was already decreasing by the year 1900 and had virtually ceased by 1965.

Symptoms The period of incubation (i.e. the time elapsing between the reception of infection and the development of symptoms) varies somewhat. In most cases it lasts only two to three days, but in occasional cases the patient may take a week to develop his first symptoms. The invasion of fever is usually short and sharp, with rapid rise of temperature to 40 °C (104 °F) or thereabouts in the first few hours. There also occur shivering, vomiting, headache, sore throat and marked increase in the rate of the pulse. In young children convulsions or delirium may also usher in the fever. The rash usually appears within 24 hours of the onset of fever. Sometimes the redness is accompanied by small vesicles containing fluid. The rash is at its height in about two days and then begins to fade, being gone at the end of a week from its first appearance.

Complications The most common and serious of these is *glomerulonephritis*, which may arise during any period in the course of the fever, but is specially apt to appear in convalescence, while desquama-tion is in progress. Occasionally this condition does not wholly pass off, and consequently lays the foundation for chronic glomerulonephritis. (See KIDNEYS, DISEASES OF.) Another complication is *infection of the ears*, due to the extension of the inflamatory process from the throat along the Eustachian tube into the middle ear. (See EAR DISEASES.) Other disorders affecting the heart and lungs occasionally arise in connection with scarlet fever, the chief of these being *endocarditis*, which may lay the foundation of valvular disease of the heart later in life. Arthritis or *scarlatinal rheumatism* is another complication of the disease, producing swelling and pain in the smaller rather than in the larger joints. This complication usually occurs in the second week of illness. As scarlet fever is predominantly a strepto-coccal infection, penicillin should be given.

SCHISTOSOMIASIS, also known as BIL-HARZIASIS Infection results from one of the human *Schistosoma* spp. (identified by Theodore Bilharz in Egypt in 1851). It is common in Africa, South America, the Far East, Middle East, and, to a limited extent, the Caribbean. The life-cycle is dependent on fresh-water snails which act as the intermediate host for the fluke; the cercarial stage enters via intact human skin and matures in the portal circulation. Clinically, 'swimmers' itch' may occur at the site of cercarial skin penetration. Acute schistosomiasis (Katayama fever) can result in fever, an urticarial rash, and enlargement of liver and spleen. The adult male is about 12 mm and the female 24 mm in length. *S. haematobium* causes cystitis and haematuria – passage of blood in the urine; bladder cancer and ureteric obstruction, giving rise to hydronephrosis and kidney failure, are long-term sequelae in a severe case. *S. mansoni* can cause colonic symptoms and in a severe case, polyposis of the colon; diarrhoea, which may be bloody, can be a presenting feature. In a heavy infection, eggs surrounded by granulomas are deposited in the liver, giving rise to extensive damage (pipe-stem fibrosis) associated with portal hypertension, oesophageal varices, etc; however, unlike cirrhosis, hepatocellular function is preserved until late in the disease. *S. japonicum* (which is confined to the Far East, especially Indonesia) behaves similarly to *S. mansoni* infection; liver involvement is often more severe.

Diagnosis can be made by microscopic examination of urine or faeces. The characteristic eggs (*S. haematobium* which causes the urinary form has a terminal spine; *S. mansoni*, which causes colonic and liver disease, has a lateral spine; and *S. japonicum* is smooth and oval) are usually detectable. Alternatively, rectal or liver biopsy are of value. Serological tests, including an ELISA, have now largely replaced invasive procedures used in making a parasitological diagnosis. Chemotherapy has been revolutionized by the introduction of praziquantel (administered orally); this compound has no serious side-effects, although its cost may limit its use in developing countries. Oxamniquine is cheaper and effective in *S. mansoni* infection, although evidence of resistance has been recorded in several countries. Metriphonate is also relatively cheap and is of value in *S. haematobium* infection. Compounds formerly used – which included antimonial preparations and niridazole – are now rarely used. Prevention is by complete avoidance of exposure to contaminated water; all travellers to infected areas should know about this disease. It is increasing in frequency as new expanses of fresh water appear as a result of irrigation schemes and dam projects. Mollusciciding can be employed for snail-control.

SCHIZO- is a prefix signifying splitting.

SCHIZOGONY is an asexual phase in the life cycle of a sporozoan (q.v.) that occurs in red blood cells or liver cells.

SCHIZOPHRENIA (See MENTAL ILLNESS.)

SCHWANN CELL The cells that produce the myelin (q.v.) sheath of the axon (q.v.) of a medullated nerve. They are wrapped around a segment of the axon, forming concentric layers.

SCIATICA means pain in the distribution of the sciatic nerve. It is often accompanied by pain in the back, or lumbago. It may be due to a number of causes, such as a tumour in the spine or spinal column, tuberculosis of the spine, ankylosing spondylitis (see SPINE AND SPINAL CORD, DISEASES AND INJURIES OF) or a tumour in one of the organs in the pelvis such as the uterus. In the majority of cases, however, it is due to a prolapsed intervertebral disc (q.v.) pressing on one or more of the nerve roots issuing from the lower part of the spinal cord that make up the sciatic nerve. The precise distribution of the pain will thus depend on which of the nerve roots are affected. As a rule, the pain is felt in the buttock, the back of the thigh and the outside and front of the leg,

sometimes extending on to the top of the foot, the back of the thigh and the calf, and then along the outer border of the foot towards the little toe. What probably happens is that degenerative changes take place in the annulus fibrosus. (See SPINAL COLUMN.) Ultimately this ruptures, either as a result of some special strain such as is induced by heavy lifting, or spontaneously. The cushioning disc between the two neighbouring vertebral bodies slips through the rent in the annulus fibrosus, and presses on the neighbouring roots, thus causing the pain.

The condition usually occurs in adults under the age of 60. The pain may come on suddenly when the person is lifting, and may be so severe that he may be locked in one position. More commonly it comes on gradually and keeps on recurring over long periods of time.
Treatment consists essentially of rest in bed in the early stages until the acute phase is over. Analgesics, such as aspirin and codeine, are given to relieve the pain. Expert opinion varies as to the desirability of wearing a plaster of Paris jacket or a specially made corset. Opinion also differs as to the desirability of manipulation of the spine and operation. Surgeons are now very selective about which patients might benefit from a laminectomy (q.v.).

SCIRRHUS is a hard form of cancer in which much fibrous tissue develops.

SCLERA (see EYE).

SCLERITIS (see EYE DISEASES).

SCLERODERMA is a condition in which the skin becomes hard – like leather – causing stiffening of the joints, and leading to gradual wasting of the muscles.

SCLEROSIS means literally hardening, and is a term applied to conditions in which portions of organs become hard and useless as the result of an excessive production of connective tissue. The term is especially applied to a change of this type taking place in the nervous system. (See MULTIPLE SCLEROSIS.) When a change of this nature takes place in other organs it is generally known as cirrhosis or fibrosis. (See CIRRHOSIS.) These conditions are generally attributed to some form of chronic inflammation.

SCLEROTHERAPY A treatment that involves injecting varicose veins (see VEINS, DISEASES OF) with a sclerosing fluid. This causes fibrosis of the lining of the vein and its eventual obliteration. Sclerotherapy is also used to treat varicose veins in the legs, anus (haemorrhoids) and at the junction of the oesophagus (q.v.) with the stomach.

SCOLIOSIS is the name applied to curvature of the spine consisting partly of a bend to one side, partly of a rotary twist. It may result from disease of the spine, but in weakly children it may arise from so slight a cause as a bad habit in standing or in leaning one arm on the table at lessons. It also arises from disease affecting one side of the chest, such as chronic pleurisy or tuberculosis. (See SPINE AND SPINAL CORD, DISEASES OF.)

SCORBUTIC signs are those characteristic of scurvy (q.v.); typically swollen, spongy gums that bleed easily, and spontaneous haemorrhages and bruising anywhere in the body.

SCOTOMA   An area of blindness in the field of vision.

SCREENING TEST   The screening of apparently healthy people to identify those who may have treatable diseases. Cervical smears are done when screening women to detect if they have cancer or precancer of the neck of the womb (cervix). Factors to be assessed when planning screening procedures include the severity, frequency, and distribution of the disease and the availability and effectiveness of treatment. Convenience, safety, sensitivity and cost should also be assessed. In the United Kingdom the government has supported the extension of screening procedures for breast cancer, cervical cancer, hypertension and diabetes.

SCRIVENER'S PALSY is another name for writer's cramp. (See CRAMP.)

SCROFULA, or STRUMA, is tuberculosis of the glands in the neck. It was formerly known in England as 'king's evil', from the belief that the touch of the sovereign could effect a cure. This superstition can be traced back to the time of Edward the Confessor in England, and to a much earlier period in France. Samuel Johnson was touched by Queen Anne in 1712, and the same supposed prerogative of royalty was exercised by Prince Charles Edward in 1745. The disease, which is treated with antituberculous drugs, is now rare and usually affects young children.

SCROMBOTOXIN POISONING occurs from eating poorly preserved scromboid fish such as tuna, mackerel and other members of the mackerel family. In such fish, a toxic histamine-like substance is produced by the action of bacteria or histidine, a normal component of fish flesh. This toxin produces nausea, vomiting, headache, upper abdominal pain, difficulty in swallowing, thirst, itching (q.v.) and sometimes urticaria (q.v.). The condition settles as a rule in 12 hours. Antihistamine drugs (q.v.) are sometimes of value in ameliorating the condition.

SCROTUM is the pouch of integument within which the testicles are suspended. It consists of a purse-like fold of skin, within which each testicle has a separate investment of muscle fibres, several layers of fibrous tissue, and a serous membrane known as the tunica vaginalis.

SCRUM-POX, or PROP-POX, is a popular name for a contagious affection of the face affecting Rugby football players. It is most likely to occur in forwards as a result of face-to-face contact with cases in the opposing side of the scrum. In one investigation, 47 of 48 cases were forwards. Other possible sources of infection are changing rooms and communal baths. The condition may take the form of impetigo (q.v.) or herpes simplex (q.v.).

SCURF, or DANDRUFF, is a popular name for the scaly condition that is often found on the scalp, and often precedes baldness. (See SEBORRHOEA.)

SCURVY, or SCORBUTUS, is a disease caused by a deficiency of vitamin C, or ascorbic acid (q.v.), in the diet and characterized by spontaneous bleeding into body tissues. (See APPENDIX 5: VITAMINS.)

Causes   In former times this disease was extremely common among sailors, and was responsible for a high mortality rate. It is now of rare occurrence at sea. Lack of vitamin C, which is soluble in water and is found chiefly in citrus fruits, potatoes, green vegetables and black currants, is the essential deficient factor. A reduction in the total amount of food, poor cooking methods, and increased trauma or anxiety, all contribute to the development of the disease.

Symptoms   The symptoms of scurvy come on gradually, and its onset is not marked by any special indications beyond a certain failure of strength. Breathlessness and exhaustion are thus easily induced, along with mental depression; the gums are tender and the breath offensive almost from the onset. Later the gums are livid, spongy, ulcerating and bleeding; the teeth are loosened and drop out. Extravasations of blood occur in the skin and joints. Anaemia also occurs with profound exhaustion and various complications, such as diarrhoea and lung or kidney troubles, any of which may bring about a fatal result.

Treatment consists of the administration of vitamin C in adequate amounts, either in the form of tablets of ascorbic acid or foodstuffs rich in this vitamin such as potatoes, cabbages, tomatoes, swede turnips, many fresh fruits, especially black currants, oranges, grapefruit and lemons. Orange-juice or lemon-juice is often employed, either fresh or canned. The use of fresh lime-juice in the British Navy, which has been practised since 1795, had the effect of virtually extinguishing scurvy in the Service.

SEA-SICKNESS (see MOTION SICKNESS).

SEASONAL AFFECTIVE DISORDER SYNDROME Known colloquially as SADS, this is a disorder in which an affected individual's mood changes with the seasons. He or she is commonly depressed in winter, picking up again in the spring. The diagnosis is controversial and its prevalence is not known. The mood change is probably related to light, with melatonin (q.v.) playing a key role.

SEBACEOUS CYST is the term applied to a cyst in the skin formed as a result of blockage of the duct of a sebaceous gland.

SEBACEOUS GLANDS are the minute glands situated alongside of hairs and opening into the follicles of the latter a short distance below the point at which the hairs emerge on the surface . These glands secrete an oily material, and are especially large upon the nose, where their openings form pits that are easily visible. Some varieties of eczema, as well as acne, result from disorders of these glands. (See SKIN.)

SEBORRHOEA is a group of diseases of the skin in which the sebaceous or oil-forming glands are at fault. It manifests itself either by accumulation of dry scurf, or by the formation of an excessive oily deposit on an otherwise healthy skin.

SEBUM is the secretion of the sebaceous glands (q.v.). It acts as a natural lubricant of the hair and skin and protects the skin from the effects of moisture or excessive dryness. It may also have antibacterial action.

SECONDARY PREVENTION The early detection of disease that reduces or prevents its serious outcome. Routine regular examination of particular age groups – for example, children or the elderly – and screening tests are examples of secondary prevention.

SECONDARY SEXUAL CHARACTERISTICS The physical characteristics that develop during puberty as the body matures sexually. Girl's breasts and genitals increase in size and like boys they grow pubic hair. Boys also grow facial hair, their voice breaks and their genitals grow to adult size.

SECRETIN is a hormone secreted by the mucous membrane of the duodenum, the first part of the small intestine, when food comes in contact with it. On being carried by the blood to the pancreas, it stimulates the secretion of pancreatic juice.

SECRETION is the term applied to the material formed by a gland as the result of its activity. For example, saliva is the secretion of the salivary glands, gastric juice that of the glands in the stomach wall, bile that of the liver.

(See GLANDS.) Some secretions consist apparently of waste material which is of no further use in the chemistry of the body. These secretions are often spoken of as excretions: for example, the urine and the sweat. (For further details, see SALIVA; URINE; ENDOCRINE GLANDS, and also under the headings of the various organs.)

SECTION (1) A thin slice of a tissue specimen taken for examination under a microscope. (2) The act of cutting in surgery; for example, an abdominal section is done to explore the abdomen. (3) The issuing of an order under the United Kingdom's Mental Health Act to admit someone compulsorily to a psychiatric hospital.

SECUNDINES is another name for the afterbirth, consisting of the placenta and membranes expelled in the final stage of labour.

SECUNDUM ARTEM is a Latin expression meaning in a skilful professional manner.

SEDATIVES are drugs and other measures which have a calming effect, reducing tension and anxiety. They are hypnotics (q.v.) given in smaller doses than is needed to induce sleep.

SEDIMENTATION RATE (see ESR).

SELECTIVE SEROTONIN-REUPTAKE INHIBITORS (SSRIs) are a group of antidepressant drugs which are less sedative than tricyclic (q.v.) antidepressants, with few antimuscarinic effects and little effect on the heart. Examples are fluoxetine (q.v.) and paroxetine (q.v.).

SELENIUM SULPHIDE is used as a shampoo in the treatment of dandruff and seborrhoeic dermatitis of the scalp. In view of its potential toxicity it should only be used under medical supervision. It must never be applied to inflamed areas of the scalp, and it must not be allowed to get into the eyes, as it may cause conjunctivitis or keratitis. It is also used in the treatment of tinea versicolor. (See RINGWORM.)

SELF-POISONING has increased over the past 40 years and is a common cause of acute admission to hospital. Drugs are usually taken in overdosage on impulse because of a crisis in coping with social or personal difficulties and most patients have previously been prescribed psychotrophic drugs. It is predominantly a disease of young people, the mean age being in the 30s with a peak incidence in the 20s. There is a higher incidence of female patients. Fortunately about 98 per cent of patients admitted with drug overdosage will recover. There have been changes in the types of drugs used in deliberate self-poisoning. In 1962 barbiturates were used in 55 per cent of episodes whereas the benzodiazapines are now the most common drug used. The incidence of salicylate poisoning has declined but overdosage with paracetamol has become more common.

Admission to hospital for self-poisoning reached its peak in 1977 and the figures have been falling since then. This is also true of the number of fatal suicidal poisonings. There may be more than one explanation for this decrease but the most likely cause is that since 1976 the annual number of prescriptions for hypnotics and tranquillizers has also fallen steadily. The tranquillizers which are so popular for overdoses are prescribed for the very patients who are most likely to wish to poison themselves. There was, in fact, a parallel decrease in the rate of carbon monoxide poisoning when carbon monoxide was removed from domestic gas.

Treatment Emptying the stomach by gastric lavage is sometimes necessary but the risks of this procedure must be balanced against the toxicity of the ingested poison. Emptying the stomach by gastric lavage is of doubtful value more than four hours after ingestion of a poison. There are, however, two exceptions, namely salicylates and tricyclic antidepressants. Salicylates may be recovered up to 24 hours and tricyclic antidepressants up to 8 hours after ingestion. Gastric lavage is seldom practical or desirable before the patient reaches hospital.

The more common poisons seen today include the amphetamine-related drugs, aspirin and other salicylates, tranquillizers, iron salts, lithium salts, morphine, paracetamol, phenothiazines, tricyclic antidepressants, carbon monoxide, paraquat and organophosphorus insecticides.

SELLA TURCICA is the deep hollow on the upper surface of the sphenoid bone in which the pituitary gland (q.v.) is enclosed.

SEMEN is the richly albuminous fluid in which spermatozoa are suspended.

SEMILUNAR CARTILAGES are two crescentic layers of fibro- cartilage on the outer and inner edges of the knee-joint, which form hollows on the upper surface of the tibia in which the condyles at the lower end of the femur rest. The inner cartilage is especially liable to be displaced by a sudden and violent movement at the knee. (See KNEE.)

SEMINAL VESICLE is one of the small paired sacs lying on either side of the male urethra (q.v.), which collect and store spermatozoa. (See TESTICLE.)

SENILE DEMENTIA Dementia has traditionally been divided into presenile and senile types. This is increasingly recognized as an arbitrary division of a condition in which there is a general and often slow decline in mental capabilities. Around 10 per cent of people over 65 years of age and 20 per cent over 75 are affected by dementing illness, but people under 65 may also be affected. Treatable causes such as brain tumour, head injury, encephalitis and alcoholism are commoner in younger people. Other causes such as cerebrovascular disease, which is a major factor, especially among older people, or Alzheimer's disease are not readily treatable, although antihypertensive treatment for the former disorder may help and symptomatic treatment for both is possible. Individuals with dementia suffer a gradual deterioration of memory and of the ability to grasp what is happening around them. They often cover up their early failings and the condition may first become apparent as a result of emotional outbursts or uncharacteristic behaviour in public. Eventually personal habits and speech deteriorate and they become thoroughly confused and difficult to look after. Treatment is primarily a matter of ameliorating the symptoms, coupled with a sympathetic handling of the sufferer and the relatives. Admission to hospital or nursing home may be necessary if relatives are unable to look after the patient at home.

SENILITY (see AGEING).

SENNA is the leaves of various species of *Cassia senna*, being known as Tinnerelly senna and Alexandrian senna, according to its source. It is one of the most active of the simple laxative drugs, producing considerable griping if used alone. Senna is excreted in the urine, giving it a dark red or yellow colour. In the case of nursing mothers, some of the drug is excreted in the milk and may have a purgative effect upon the nursling. A standardized preparation of senna, Senokot, is now available which has none of the disadvantages of senna itself and is widely used for the management of constipation in old people.

SENSATION (see PAIN; TOUCH).

SENSITIVITY The extent to which a screening test (q.v.) detects the proportion of true cases of the disease being screened.

SENSITIZATION (see ALLERGY; ANAPHYLAXIS).

SEPSIS means poisoning by the products of the growth of micro- organisms in the body, and the general symptoms which accompany it are those of inflammation. (See INFLAMMATION.) It is prevented by the various procedures mentioned under ASEPSIS, and is neutralized, when it has occurred, by various substances. (See ANTISEPTICS.)

SEPTAL DEFECT A congenital abnormality of the heart affecting about 260 babies in every 100,000 in which there is a hole in the septum – the dividing wall – between the left and right sides of the heart. The effects of the defect depend on its size and position. A defect in the wall between the atria (upper chambers of the heart) is called an atrial septal defect and that between the ventricles a ventricular septal defect, the commonest form (25 per cent of all defects). Both defects allow blood to circulate from the left side of the heart, where pressures are highest, to the right. This abnormal flow of blood is described as a shunt and the result is that too much blood flows into the lungs. Pulmonary hypertension occurs and, if the shunt is large, heart failure may develop. A small septal defect may not need treatment but a large one will need to be repaired surgically.

SEPTICAEMIA is a serious condition caused by the presence of micro-organisms in the blood stream. A very high temperature may be the only sign, but there is often associated shivering (rigor), profuse sweating and pains in the joints and muscles.

The introduction of aseptic surgery by Lister immensely reduced the frequency of blood-poisonig, and the problem was further improved by the introduction of antibiotics.

SEPTIC SHOCK A dangerous disorder characterized by a severe fall in blood pressure and damage to the body tissues as a result of septicaemia (q.v.). The toxins from the septicaemia cause widespread damage to tissue, provoke clotting in small blood vessels and seriously disturb the circulation. The kidneys, lungs, and heart are particularly affected. The condition occurs most commonly in people who already have a chronic disease such as cancer, cirrhosis of the liver or diabetes mellitus. Septic shock may also develop in patients with immunodeficiency illnesses such as AIDS. The symptoms are those of septicaemia, coupled with those of shock, cold, cyanotic limbs, fast thready pulse and a lowered blood pressure. Septic shock requires urgent treatment with antibiotics, intravenous fluids, and oxygen.

SEPTUM A dividing wall within a structure in the body. Examples are the divisions between the chambers of the heart and the layer of bone and cartilage that separates the two nostrils of the nose.

SEQUELAE is the term applied to symptoms or effects which are liable to follow certain diseases. For example, bronchitis and other chest complaints may be sequelae of measles; heart disease is often a sequel of rheumatic fever; paralysis may follow diphtheria.

SEQUESTRUM is the name given to a fragment of dead bone cast off from the living bone in the process of necrosis. (See BONE, DISEASES OF.) A sequestrum often remains in contact with, and partly enveloped by, newly formed bone, so that a sinus is produced, and a constant discharge goes on, till the dead bone is removed.

SEROCONVERSION The production of specific antibodies to antigens present in the body. This may happen as a result of infection by a virus or immunization with a vaccine.

SEROTONIN A substance widely distributed in the body tissue, but especially in the platelets in the blood, the lining of the gastrointestinal tract and the brain. Serotonin is believed to have a similar function to that of histamine in inflammation. In the gut it inhibits gastric secretion and stimulates smooth (involuntary) muscle in the walls of the intestine. Serotonin participates in the transmission of nerve impulses and may have a function in controlling mood and states of consciousness. (See SELECTIVE SEROTONIN-REUPTAKE INHIBITORS.)

SEROTYPE A classification of a substance according to its serological activity. This is done in the context of the antigens (q.v.) it contains or the antibodies (q.v.) it may provoke. Micro-organisms of the same species may be classified according to the different antigens that they produce.

SEROUS Relating to, containing or resembling serum.

SEROUS MEMBRANES are smooth, transparent membranes that line certain large cavities of the body. The chief serous membranes are the peritoneum, lining the cavity of the abdomen; the pleurae, one of which lines each side of the chest, surrounding the corresponding lung; the pericardium, in which the heart lies; and the tunica vaginalis on each side, enclosing a testicle. The name of these membranes is derived from the fact that the surface is moistened by thin fluid derived from the serum of blood or lymph. Every serous membrane consists of a visceral portion, which closely envelops the organs concerned, and a parietal portion, which adheres to the wall of the cavity. These two portions are continuous with one another so as to form a closed sac, and the opposing surfaces are close together, separated only by a little fluid. This arrangement enables the organs in question to move freely within the cavities containing them. For further details see under PERITONEUM.

SERPIGINOUS is a term used in connection with ulcers or eruptions that spread in a creeping manner.

SERUM is the fluid which separates from blood, lymph (q.v.), and other body fluids when clotting occurs (see HAEMORRHAGE). Plasma (q.v.) is the fluid of the blood, including fibrin (q.v.), which carries the circulating blood cells and platelets (q.v.).

Serum is a clear, yellowish fluid containing around 7 per cent proteins and globulins, small quantities of salts, fat, sugar, urea, and uric acid, and even smaller quantities of immunoglobulins, essential in the prevention of disease (see IMMUNITY; IMMUNOLOGY). The serum given in the commonly used vaccines (q.v.) is generally derived from horses' blood, after they have been subjected to a long course of treatment.

SERUM SICKNESS is a hypersensitivity reaction due to circulating antigen antibody complexes. It got its name because it was a not uncommon reaction to the administration of foreign serum which used to be given as a form of passive immunity before the days of antibiotics. By definition it is a manifestation of sensitivity to serum but the same clinical and pathological picture can occur one to three weeks after the administration of drugs such as penicillin, streptomycin and sulphonamides. It is characterized by fever, arthralgia and lymphadenopathy and is usually self-limiting as it resolves when the supply of antigen is used up.

SERUM THERAPY (see IMMUNOLOGY).

SESAMOID BONES are rounded nodules of bone usually embedded in tendon. They are usually a few millimetres in diameter, but some are larger, such as the patella (q.v.), or knee-cap.

SESSILE A growth or tumour that has no stalk.

SEX CHROMOSOMES In the human being there are 23 pairs of chromosomes. Male and female differ in respect of one pair. In the nucleus of the female somatic cell the two members of the pair are identical and are called X-chromosomes. In the male nucleus there is one X-chromosome and another, unequal, dissimilar chromosome called the Y-chromosome. In the sex cells, after reduction division, all cells in the female will contain X-chromosomes. In the male, half will contain X-chromosomes and half Y-chromosomes. If, then, a sperm with an X-chromosome fertilizes an ovum (with, of course, an X-chromosome) the offspring will be female. If a sperm with a Y-chromosome fertilizes the ovum the offspring will be male. It is the sex chromosomes which determine the sex of an individual.

Sometimes during cell division chromosomes may be lost or duplicated, or abnormalities in the structure of individual chromosomes may occur. The surprising fact is the infrequency of such errors. About one in two hundred live-born babies has an abnormality of development caused by a chromosome and two-thirds of these involve the sex chromosomes. There is little doubt that the frequency of these abnormalities in the early embryo is much higher but because of the serious nature of the defect early spontaneous abortion occurs.

Chromosome studies on such early abortions show that half have chromosome abnormalities with errors of autosomes being three times as common as sex chromosome anomalies. Two of the most common abnormalities in such fetuses are triploidy with 69 chromosomes and trisomy of chromosome 16. These two anomalies almost always cause spontaneous abortion. Abnormalities of chromosome structure may arise because of:

(1) *Deletion*: where a segment of a chromosome is lost.

(2) *Inversion*: where a segment of a chromosome becomes detached and re-attached the other way around. Genes will then appear in the wrong order and thus will not correspond with their opposite numbers on homologous chromosomes.

(3) *Duplication*: where a segment of a chromosome is included twice over. One chromosome will have too little nuclear material and one too much. The individual inheriting too little may be non-viable and the one with too much may be abnormal.

(4) *Translocation*: where chromosomes of different pairs exchange segments.

(5) *Errors in division of centromere*: sometimes the centromere divides transversely instead of longitudinally. If the centromere is not central, one of the daughter chromosomes will arise from the two short arms of the parent chromosome and the other from the two long arms. These abnormal daughter chromosomes are called isochromosomes.

These changes have important bearings on heredity as the effect of a gene depends not only on its nature but on its position on the chromosome with reference to other genes. Genes do not act in isolation but against the background of other genes. Each gene normally has its own position on the chromosome and this corresponds precisely with the positon of its allene on the homologous chromosome of the pair. Each member of a pair of chromosomes will normally carry precisely the same number of genes in exactly the same order. Characteristic clinical syndromes, due to abnormalities of chromosome structure, are less constant than those due to loss or gain of a complete chromosome. This is because the degree of deletion, inversion and duplication is inconstant. However, translocation between chromosomes 15 and 21 of the parent is associated with a familial form of mongolism in the offspring and deletion of part of an X chromosome may result in Turner's syndrome.

NON-DISJUNCTION: Whilst alterations in the structure of chromosomes arise as a result of deletion or translocation, alterations in the number of chromosomes usually arise as a result of non-disjunction occurring during maturation of the parental gametes. The two chromosomes of each pair (homologous chromosomes) may fail to come together at the beginning of meiosis and continue to lie free. If one chromosome then passes to each pole of the spindle, normal gametes may result but if both chromosomes pass to one pole and neither to the other, two kinds of abnormal gametes will be produced. One kind of gamete will contain both chromosomes of the pair and the other gamete will contain neither. Whilst this results in serious disease when the autosomes are involved, the loss or gain of sex chromosomes seems to be well tolerated. The loss of an autosome is incompatible with life and the malformation produced by a gain of an autosome is proportional to the size of the extra chromosome carried.

Only a few instances of a gain of an autosome are known. An additional chromosome 21 (one of the smallest autosomes) results in mongolism and trisomy of chromosome 13 and 18 are associated with severe mental, skeletal and congenital cardiac defects. Diseases resulting from a gain of a sex chromosome are not as severe. A normal ovum contains 22 autosomes and an X sex chromosome. A normal sperm contains 22 autosomes and either an X or a Y sex chromosome. Thus as a result of non-disjunction of the X chromosome at the first meiotic division during the formation of female gametes the ovum may contain two X chromosomes or none at all, whilst in the male the sperm may contain both X and Y chromosomes (XY) or none at all. (See aso CHROMOSOMES, GENES.)

SEX HORMONES   These hormones control the development of primary and secondary sexual characteristics. They also regulate sex-related functions – for example, menstruation and the production of sperm and eggs. The three main types of sex hormone are androgens (q.v.), or male sex hormones; oestrogens (q.v.), or female sex hormones; and progesterones (q.v.), which are involved in pregnancy.

SEX-LINKED INHERITANCE   The way in which a characteristic or an illness determined by the sex chromosomes in an individual's cells is passed on to the succeeding generation. Men have one X and one Y sex chromosome and women have two X chromosomes. Disorders that result from an abnormal number of sex chromosomes include Klinefelter's syndrome, which affects only men, and Turner's syndrome, which affects mainly women (qq.v.). Recessive genes on the X chromosome cause most other sex-linked characteristics and in women these may well be masked because one of their two X chromosomes carries a normal (dominant) gene. In men, who have but one X chromosome, no such masking occurs, so more men than women are affected by X-linked characteristics or diseases.

SEXUAL ABUSE   (see CHILD ABUSE).

SEXUAL DEVIATION   Any type of pleasurable sexual practice which society regards as abnormal. Deviation may be related to the activity such as exhibitionism or sadomasochistic sex, or to the sexual object, for example, women's shoes or clothes (fetishism). Different cultures have different values, and treatment is probably not required unless the deviation is harmful to the participant(s). Aversion therapy or conditioning a person's behaviour may help if treatment is thought necessary.

SEXUAL DYSFUNCTION   Inadequate sexual response may be due to a lack of sexual desire or to an inadequate performance, or it may be that there is a lack of satisfaction or orgasm. The lack of sexual desire may be due to any generalized illness or endocrine disorder or to the taking of drugs that antagonize endocrine function. Disorders of performance in men can occur during arousal, penetration and ejaculation. In the female dyspareunia and vaginismus are the main disorders of performance. Diabetes mellitus (q.v.) can cause a neuropathy which results in loss of erection. Impotence can follow nerve damage from operations on the prostate and lower bowel and can be the result of neurological diseases affecting the autonomic system. Disorders of satisfaction include, in men, emission without forceful ejaculation and pleasureless ejaculation. In women such dis-orders range from the absence of the congestive genital response to absence of orgasm.

Sexual dysfunction may be due to physical or psychiatric disease, or it may be the result of the administration of drugs. The main group of drugs likely to cause sexual problems are the anti-convulsants, psychotrophic drugs, the anti-hypertensive drugs and drugs such as metoclopramide that induce hyperprolactinaemia. The benzodiazepine tranquillizers can reduce libido and cause failure of erection. Tricyclic antidepressives may cause failure of erection and clomipramine may delay or abolish ejaculation by blockade of alpha-adrenergic receptors. The mono-amine oxidase inhibitors often inhibit ejaculation. The phenothiazides reduce sexual desire and arousal and may cause difficulty in maintaining an erection. Methyldopa causes impotence in over 20 per cent of patients on large doses. The beta-blockers and the diuretics can also cause impotence. The main psychiatric causes of sexual dysfunction include stress, depression and guilt.

SEXUALLY TRANSMITTED DISEASES (STDs) are infections transmitted by sexual intercourse. In the United Kingdom they are treated in genito-urinary medicine (GUM) clinics. Although wart-virus infections (84,600), non-specific infection or urethritis (q.v.) (64,930), chlamydia (q.v.) (35,400) and gonorrhoea (q.v.) (14,280) were by far the commonest STDs registered in England in 1992, HIV/AIDS (see AIDS/HIV) maintained the highest public profile. In 1993, 1,473 cases of AIDS were reported in

England, bringing the cumulative total since 1982 to 7,890, of whom 5,203 are known to have died. On average, it is estimated that people newly diagnosed with AIDS were infected with HIV 10 years previously. Projected figures suggest 2,440 new cases in 1997 with 2,375 deaths and 4,205 people needing care for the infection.

Despite regular health-education campaigns and the ready availability of preventive measures, the incidence of STDs, especially among young people, fell only slightly between 1991 and 1992 when nearly 363,000 new cases were diagnosed at GUM clinics in England.

SHAKING PALSY is another name for Parkinsonism (q.v.).

SHELLFISH POISONING in the United Kingdom occurs in two main forms. Shellfish may be the cause of typhoid fever (see ENTERIC FEVER) as a result of their contamination by sewage containing the causative organism. They may also be responsible for what is known as paralytic shellfish poisoning. This is caused by a toxin, or poison, known as saxotoxin, which is present in certain planktons which, under unusual conditions, multiply rapidly, giving rise to what are known as 'red tides'. In these circumstances this toxin accumulates in mussels, cockles and scallops which feed by filtering plankton. The manifestations of such poisoning are loss of feeling in the hands, tingling of the tongue, weakness of the arms and legs, and difficulty in breathing. There is also growing evidence that shellfish poisoning may be due to a virus infection. (See FOOD POISONING.)

SHELL-SHOCK was a post-traumatic stress disorder which presented one of the major medical problems in the 1914–18 War.

SHELTERED HOUSING Accommodation that has been adapted to cater for the special requirements of those elderly people who can largely look after themselves but benefit from some discreet supervision. The accommodation is usually a small flat and a warden will supervise a group of flats. Meals and other services may be provided, and the payment system varies depending on whether the accommodation is privately owned or run by a local social-services department.

SHIGELLA is the name given to a group of rod-shaped, Gram-negative bacteria that are the cause of bacillary dysentery. (See DYSENTERY.)

SHINGLES is a popular name for herpes zoster, which forms more or less of a belt round the body. (See HERPES ZOSTER.)

SHIN SPLINTS (see MEDIAL TIBIAL SYNDROME).

SHOCK is a state of acute circulatory failure in which the cardiac output is inadequate to provide normal perfusion of the major organs. It represents a failure of blood flow rather than a failure of blood pressure. While shock is accompanied by a fall in arterial blood pressure, a fall in blood pressure is not necessarily indicative of shock. Shock can arise from a variety of causes and produce variable clinical signs according to the state of deterioration of the underlying disease. Direct bedside measurements of blood flow are not available so that physicians must usually rely on indirect evidence of inadequate perfusion. Shock is therefore a clinical syndrome and is characterized by systemic arterial hypotension (arterial blood pressure less than 80 mm of mercury) sweating and signs of vasoconstriction. These signs include pallor, cyanosis, a cold clammy skin and a low-volume pulse. These may be associated with clinical evidence of poor tissue perfusion, such as mental apathy, confusion or restlessness and oliguria. In haemodynamic terms shock is a state of circulatory failure associated with a low cardiac output and high peripheral resistance.

Shock results from many situations which give rise to inadequate perfusion of tissues and organs. It may occur because of increased resistance to blood flow, pooling or loss of blood or because of cardiac insufficiency, but the end result of impaired tissue perfusion is the same. As perfusion depends on blood flow and not blood pressure the sphygmomanometer reading is a poor indicator of circulatory failure.

The blood volume is approximately 5 litres. The heart puts out this volume each minute, a stroke volume of 70 ml being ejected 70 times per minute in the resting subject. Only 15 per cent of the blood volume lies in the arterial bed so that variations in arterial calibre have little effect on the vascular capacity. The arterioles are extremely muscular vessels and the tone of the arteriolar muscle varies the blood flow enormously. Because the greatest decline in pressure occurs at this level the arterioles are called resistance vessels. Over two-thirds of the circulating blood volume lies on the venous side of the circulation, particularly in the venules. Hence the venous system is called the capacitance system. The veins are less muscular than the arterioles but are also under autonomic nervous control. The pressure in veins is only about 7 mm of mercury. They have a relatively large diameter and correspondingly low resistance. The tension of venous musculature, although not great, has a critical influence on venous return and on venous pressure. Passive assumption of the erect posture will reduce the cardiac output by 25 per cent. Nervous adjustment through the sympathetic nervous system is intended to prevent pooling in the capacitance system. Failure of venous tone with pooling of blood in venules and capillaries is associated with a large fall in cardiac output and failure of the peripheral circulation. Failure of arteriolar tone, on the other hand, with consequent arteriolar dilatation is associated with hypotension but blood flow remains normal and there is only a transient decrease in the venous return to the heart. The normal regulatory mechanisms for the circulation, that is the Baro receptors and the autonomic innervation of the arterioles and venules, are geared to cope with the adjustments necessary in postural alterations, physical exercise and acute trauma. The adrenergic system regulates blood pressure, the distribution of blood, the capacity of the venous system and the force and rate of cardiac contraction. The autonomic nervous system can adequately compensate for 10 per cent alterations in blood volume, moderate systemic infections and a good deal of myocardial damage, by shunting away blood from visceral organs into cerebral, coronary and skeletal muscle beds. The haemodynamic response to shock inevitably produces inadequate perfusion of viscera in order to preserve circulation to the brain and coronary vessels. If this is prolonged the effects are disastrous. The ischaemic intestine permits the transfer of toxic bacterial products and proteins across its wall into the blood. Renal ischaemia prevents the maintenance of a normal electrolyte and acid base balance.

Shock may result from loss of blood or plasma volume. This may occur as a result of haemorrhage or severe diarrhoea and vomiting. It may also result because of peripheral pooling of blood due to such causes as toxaemia or anaphylaxis. The toxaemia is commonly the result of a septicaemia. Another form of shock is called cardogenic shock which is due to failure of the heart as a pump. It is most commonly seen as a result of myocardial infarction. The treatment of shock is dependent on its cause. If it is the result of haemorrhage or diarrhoea or vomiting, replacement of blood and lost electrolytes is of prime importance. If it is due to septicaemia the treatment of the infection is of paramount importance and in addition intravenous fluids and vasopressor drugs will be required.

SHOCK LUNG (see ADULT RESPIRATORY DISTRESS SYNDROME).

SHORT-SIGHT is a condition in which objects near at hand are seen clearly, while objects at a distance are blurred. The condition is technically known as myopia. (See REFRACTION; SPECTACLES; VISION.)

SHOULDER is the joint formed by the upper end of the humerus and the shoulder-blade or scapula. The acromion process of the scapula and the outer end of the collar-bone form a protective bony arch above the joint, and from this arch the wide and thick deltoid muscle passes downwards, protecting the outer surface of the joint, and giving to the shoulder its rounded character. The joint itself is of the ball-and-socket variety, the rounded head of the humerus being received into the hollow glenoid cavity of the scapula, which is further deepened by a rim of cartilage. One tendon of the biceps muscle passes through the joint, grooving the humerus deeply, and being attached to the upper edge of the glenoid cavity. The joint is surrounded by a loose fibrous capsule, strengthened at certain places by ligamentous bands. The main strength of the joint comes from the powerful muscles that unite the upper arm with the scapula, clavicle and ribs.

SHOULDER-BLADE, or SCAPULA, is a flat bone, about as large as the flat hand and fingers, placed on the upper and back part of the thorax. Many of the large muscles that move the arm are attached to it. It is not in contact with the ribs, and its only attachment to the trunk of the body is through a joint between its acromion process and the clavicle on the tip of the shoulder and by the powerful muscles which suspend it from the backbone and ribs. With the arm hanging by the side the scapula extends from the second to the seventh rib, but, as the arm is raised and lowered, it slides freely over the back of the chest. From the hinder surface of the bone springs a strong process, the spine of the scapula, which arches upwards and forwards into the acromion process. The latter forms the bony prominence on the top of the shoulder, where it unites in a joint with the outer end of the clavicle.

SHUNT   Passage of blood through a channel that is not its normal one. This may occur as a result of a congenital deformity (see SEPTAL DEFECT) or of surgery – for example, a portocaval shunt in which the main portal vein is joined up to the inferior vena cava.

SIALAGOGUES are substances which produce a copious flow of saliva.

SIAMESE TWINS, or CONJOINED TWINS, is the term applied to twins who are united bodily but are possessed of separate personalities. Their frequency is not known, but it has been estimated that throughout the world six or more conjoined twins are born every year who are capable of separation. The earliest case on record is that of the 'Biddendon Maids' who were born in England in 1100. The 'Scottish Brothers' lived for 28 years at the court of James III of Scotland. Perhaps the most famous, however, were Chang and Eng, who were born of Chinese parents in Siam in 1811. It was they who were responsible for the introduction of the term, 'Siamese twins', which still remains the popular name for 'conjoined twins'. They were joined together at the lower end of the chest bone, and achieved fame by being shown in Barnum's circus in the United States. They subsequently married English sisters and settled as farmers in North Carolina. They died in 1874.

The earliest attempt at surgical separation is

said to have been made by Dr Farius of Basle in 1689. The first successful separation in Great Britain was in 1912. Both twins survived the operation and one survived well into adult life. This is said to be the first occasion in which both twins survived the operation. The success of the operation is largely dependent upon the degree of union between the twins. Thus, if this is only skin, subcutaneous tissue and cartilage, the prospects of survival for both twins are good, but if some vital organ such as the liver is shared the operation is much more hazardous.

SIBLING is a brother or sister.

SICKLE-CELL ANAEMIA is a form of anaemia characteristically found in black people, so-called because of the sickle shape of the red blood cells. It is caused by the presence of the abnormal haemoglobin (q.v.), haemoglobin S, due to amino-acid (q.v.) substitutions in their polypeptide chains, reflecting a genetic mutation. Deoxygenation of haemoglobin S leads to sickling, which increases the blood viscosity and tends to obstruct flow, thereby increasing the sickling of other cells. Thrombosis (q.v.) and areas of tissue infarction (q.v.) may follow, causing severe pain, swelling, and tenderness. The resulting sickle cells are more fragile than normal red blood cells, and have a shorter life span, hence the anaemia. Advice is obtainable from the Sickle Cell Society (see APPENDIX 2: ADDRESSES).

SICKNESS (see VOMITING; MOTION-SICKNESS).

SIDE-EFFECT A consequence of or reaction to treatment that is extra to the effect the doctor wants. The term is usually applied to harmful or unwanted consequences and generally refers to drug treatment. A side-effect may also be a stronger action of the drug than expected or it may be quite unrelated to the intention of the treatment – for example, the drowsiness that occurs from antihistamine drugs given to combat an allergy. Sometimes the side-effects may be potentially lethal as happens when a person develops anaphylactic shock after the administration of, say, antitetanus vaccine. Doctors are expected to report side-effects of drugs to the manufacturers and the committee on safety of medicines (see SAFETY OF DRUGS).

SIDEROSIS is the name given to chronic fibrosis (q.v.) of the lungs occurring in iron-workers and due to the inhalation of fine iron particles. The term is also applied to the condition in which there is an excessive deposit of iron in the tissues of the body.

SIDS (see SUDDEN INFANT DEATH SYNDROME).

SIGHT (see VISION).

SIGMOIDOSCOPY Examination of the rectum and sigmoid colon with a viewing device called a sigmoidoscope. The procedure is done to investigate rectal bleeding or presistent diarrhoea with the aim of detecting or excluding cancer of the rectum and colitis. Sigmoidoscopy, which nowadays is performed with a flexible instrument, can usually be performed in the outpatients department. (See ENDOSCOPE.)

SILICA is a major constituent of the earth's crust. Its main danger to health arises from free silica, present mainly as quartz and flint and as an important constituent of granite, sandstone and slate. (See SILICOSIS.)

SILICONES are organic compounds of silicon, with a structure of alternate atoms of silicon and oxygen with organic groups, such as methyl and phenyl attached to the silicone atoms. As they produce a flexible and stable water-repellent film on the skin, they are used as barrier creams (q.v.).

SILICOSIS constitutes the most important industrial hazard in those industries in which silica is encountered: i.e. the pottery industry, the sandstone industry, sand-blasting, metal grinding, the tin-mining industry, anthracite coal mines. It is a specific form of pneumoconiosis (q.v.) caused by the inhalation of free silica. Among pottery workers the condition has for long been known as potter's asthma, whilst in the cutlery industry it was known as grinder's rot. For the production of silicosis the particles of silica must measure 0·5 to 5 micrometres in diameter and they must be inhaled into the alveoli of the lungs, where they produce fibrosis. This diminishes the efficiency of the lungs, which manifests itself by slowly progressive shortness of breath. The main danger of silicosis, however, is that it is liable to be complicated by tuberculosis. The incidence of silicosis is steadily being reduced by various measures which diminish the risk of inhaling silica dust. These include adequate ventilation to draw off the dust; the suppression of dust by the use of water; the wearing of respirators where the risk is particularly great and it is not possible to reduce the amount of dust: e.g. in sand-blasting; periodic medical examination of workpeople exposed to risk. In 1976, there were 171 notified cases.

SIMMONDS' DISEASE, or PITUITARY CACHEXIA, is a rare condition in which wasting of the skin and the bones, impotence, and loss of hair occur as a result of destruction of the pituitary gland.

SINGER'S NODULE is a small excrescence on the vocal cords which causes hoarseness. This tends to develop in people who abuse their voices, e.g. singers, people who shout excessively.

SINOATRIAL NODE This is the natural pacemaker of the heart and comprises a collection of specialized muscle cells in the wall of the upper chamber (atrium) of the heart. The cells initiate electrical impulses at a rate of up to 100 a minute. These impulses stimulate the muscles of the heart to contract. The rate is altered by the effects of certain hormones and various impulses from the nervous system. Damage or disease of the node affects the regular beating of the heart.

SINUS is a term applied to narrow cavities of various kinds, occurring naturally in the body, or resulting from disease. Thus it is applied to the air-containing cavities which are found in the frontal, ethmoidal, sphenoidal and maxillary bones, and which communicate with the nose. The function of these paranasal sinuses, as they are known, is doubtful, but they do lighten the skull and add resonance to the voice. They enlarge considerably around puberty and in this way are a factor in the alteration of the size and shape of the face. The term is also used in connection with the wide spaces through which the blood circulates in the membranes of the brain. Cavities which are produced when an abscess has burst but remain unhealed, are also known as sinuses. (See ABSCESS; FISTULA.)

SINUSITIS is inflammation of a sinus. It is usually applied to inflammation of the sinuses in the face. (See NOSE, DISEASES OF.)

SINUSOID A small blood vessel like an enlarged capillary occurring, for example, in the liver, which contains a large number of them. The sinusoids in the liver are drained by the hepatic veins.

SI UNITS The international system of measurement units used throughout the sciences. SI Units, which derive from metres, kilograms, and seconds, comprise seven basic units and two supplementary ones. Among the other base units are ampere (electric current) and mole (amount of a substance). Derived SI units include joule (energy), pascal (pressure), becquerel (activity), and newton (force). (See APPENDIX 6: MEASUREMENTS IN MEDICINE).

SJOGREN'S SYNDROME Sjogren described the association of dryness of the mouth (xerostomia) and dryness of the eye (kerato conjunctivitis sieca) with rheumatoid arthritis. It occurs in approximately 10 per cent of patients with rheumatoid arthritis but it can occur, and frequently does so, independently of rheumatoid disease. The lack of tears gives rise to symptoms of dryness and grittiness of the eyes. The dry mouth can occasionally be so severe as to cause a dysphagia. The disease is due to the auto-immune destruction of the salivary glands and the lacrimal glands. The disorder is usually associated with specific HLA antigen. The treatment is unsatisfactory and is limited to oral and ocular hygiene as well as the provision of artificial tears in the form of cellulose eye drops.

SKELETAL MUSCLE Muscle under a person's voluntary control. (See MUSCLE and VOLUNTARY MUSCLE).

SKELETON is the comprehensive term applied to the hard structures that support or protect the softer tissues of the body. Many animals are possessed of an exoskeleton, consisting of superficial plates of bone, horn, or the like; but in man the skeleton is entirely an endoskeleton, covered everywhere by soft parts, and consisting mainly of bones, but in places also of cartilage. The chief positions in which cartilage is found in place of bone are the larynx and the front of the chest. (For the details of the skeleton, see BONE.)

SKIN is the membrane which envelops the outer surface of the body, meeting, at the various orifices of the body, with the mucous membrane which lines the internal cavities. The skin consists of two distinct layers which differ entirely in structure and in origin. These are (a) *the epidermis*, also known as *scarf-skin*, *cuticle*, or *epithelium*, which is a cellular covering formed from the outer layer of the embryo; and (b) *the corium*, also known as the *cutis vera*, *true skin*, or *dermis*, which is a fibrous covering developed from the middle embryonic layer.

(a) **The epidermis** is the cellular layer which covers the outer surface of the body, varying in thickness from 1 mm on the palms and soles to 0·1 mm on the face. It is composed of four layers, which, from the surface inwards, are as follows:

(1) THE HORNY LAYER, or STRATUM CORNEUM, made up of several thicknesses of flat cells, forming an impervious covering pierced only by the openings of the sweat-glands and by the hairs. The flat cells are rubbed off the surface constantly as minute white scales, being replaced by growth from below.

(2) THE CLEAR LAYER, or STRATUM LUCIDUM, in which the cells are firmly fixed together into a kind of membrane.

(3) THE GRANULAR LAYER, or STRATUM GRANULOSUM, in which the cells are undergoing a change in form and substance from those of the fourth layer to those of the two on the surface.

(4) THE MALPIGHIAN LAYER, or GERMINATIVE ZONE, as it is sometimes known, which is made up of the STRATUM SPINOSUM (or PRICKLY CELL LAYER) and the STRATUM BASALE, which comprises living cells that divide continually; as they multiply they are pushed upwards to supply the constant wear and tear on the surface of the horny layer. There are no blood-vessels in the epidermis, but fine sensory nerves terminate between the cells of the Malpighian layer. The cells in the stratum basale include the

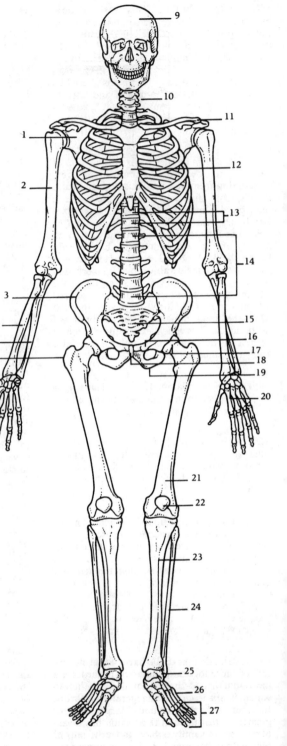

1 scapula (shoulder blade)
2 humerus
3 ilium (hip bone)
4 radius
5 ulna
6 greater trochanter
7 metacarpals (palm facing forward)
8 phalanges (palm facing forward)
9 skull (for details see diagram: SKULL)
10 cervical vertebrae
11 clavicle (collar bone)
12 sternum (breastbone)
13 eleventh and twelfth thoracic vertebrae
14 lumbar vertebrae
15 sacrum
16 pubis
17 hip joint
18 symphisis pubis
19 ischium
20 carpus (palm facing backwards)
21 femur (thigh bone)
22 patella (knee cap)
23 tibia
24 fibula
25 tarsus
26 metatarsals
27 phalanges

Diagram of human skeleton.

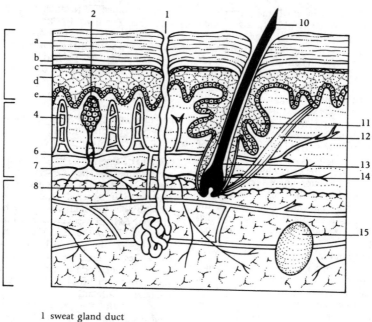

1 sweat gland duct
2 tactile corpuscle in corium
3 epidermis {
    (a) stratum corneum
    (b) stratum lucidum
    (c) stratum granulosum
    (d) stratum spinosum
    (e) stratum basale
}
4 fascicular papilla in corium
5 corium
6 blood vessel
7 nerve
8 bulb of hair
9 subcutaneous fat
10 hair
11 sebaceous gland
12 arrector pili muscle
13 medulla of hair
14 papilla of hair
15 pacinian corpuscle
16 body of sweat gland

Vertical section through the skin including hair and sweat gland.

melanocytes which are responsible for the production of melanin, the pigment responsible for suntan. (See MELANIN; SUNBURN.)

NAILS are analogous to the horny layer, but the cells of which they are composed are harder and more adherent. Beneath the nail is the nail bed, which is made up of the germinative zone together with the corium. Underneath the greater part of the nail the corium has a very liberal blood supply, which gives the nail its pink colour. All growth of the nail occurs at its root. Finger nails grow at an average rate of 0·5 mm a week.

(b) **The corium** is the fibrous layer which forms the chief part of the bodily covering. It varies greatly in thickness from about 0·5 to 3 mm, being coarser on the back than on the front of the body, and thicker in men than in women. It contains many nerves, which play an important part in affording sensations of touch, pain and temperature, and blood-vessels which, in addition to nourishing the skin, are largely concerned in regulating the temperature of the body. The corium bears also the hairs which pierce the epidermis, and the sweat-glands, whose ducts also penetrate the epidermis to reach the surface. Beneath the corium lies a loose fibrous layer of subcutaneous tissue which joins the skin to deeper parts and contains more or less fat, according to the stoutness of the person.

The fibrous tissue of the corium is composed of interlacing bundles of white fibrous tissue and elastic fibres that form a dense feltwork.

The corium is crossed everywhere by numerous folds, which are specially plentiful over joints and on the palms of the hands, and which are followed closely by the epidermis. The palms and soles are faced with continuous ridges with intervening grooves. These ridges remain permanent throughout life, and provide unique fingerprinting identification.

The endings of the sensory nerves in the skin are described under NERVES.

HAIRS grow from the true skin, each having a root and a stem or shaft. The varying tint of hair is due to pigment scattered in varying amount throughout the hair, while a white hair is produced by the formation of very numerous air-spaces throughout the cells composing it. The root of the hair ends in a knob in the corium, and is set upon a fibrous papilla, from which the hair obtains its principal nutriment.

GLANDS are found in immense numbers in the skin, and are of two kinds: *sebaceous glands*, which secrete a fatty substance, and *sweat glands*, which secrete a clear, watery fluid.

The *sebaceous glands* lie in the true skin, and open into the follicles of the hairs a little way from the surface. Each consists of a bunch of small sacs, within which fatty material is produced. The secretion reaches the surface by the hair-follicle, and serves to lubricate the hair and give pliability to the surface of the skin.

Sweat glands, or sudoriparous glands, are very numerous (there are around 3 million of them), are found all over the surface of the body at a slightly deeper level than the sebaceous glands, and have no connection with the hairs. In the fibrous tissue between the coils of the glands run many small blood-vessels, and from the blood in these the materials that form the sweat are extracted.

Functions of the skin The main use of the skin is a *protective* one. It covers the underlying muscles, both protecting them from injury and helping to maintain an even body temperature. The epidermis forms a highly impenetrable surface.

Secretion is an important function of the skin, the two secretions being sebaceous material and perspiration. Of these, the former is a lubricant for the hair and skin, the latter is treated of under PERSPIRATION.

Heat regulation is one of the most important functions of the skin. When cold air or water come into contact with the surface, the skin blanches, the numerous blood-vessels of the true skin contracting and thus preventing much blood from circulating through the skin, and being thereby unduly cooled. On the other hand, when the surface is exposed to a temperature approaching that of the body, say one of 26·7 or 32·2 °C (80 or 90 °F), or when an excessive amount of heat is produced by great muscular efforts, or when the environment is hot, the blood-vessels of the surface dilate and there is a copious secretion of perspiration, which produces great cooling as it evaporates from the surface. These actions of narrowing and dilatation of vessels, and of sweat secre-

tion, are controlled through reflex nerve influence. (See also HEAT STROKE.)

Respiration is a function of the skin in some animals but is of little relevance in humans.

Social function The skin also provides a major pathway for social communication, by virtue of its vascular responses associated with signalling of emotional states, muscular responses of expression, creating a complex sign language, and by the equally subtle possibilities of tactile communication.

SKIN DISEASES These form a large and important class. They are very extensive, owing to the varied forms of change which the skin texture may undergo, and to the different structures in the skin which may be specially affected. Skin diseases are of great importance, not only from the fact that they have an influence on the general health, but also because these diseases are often the expression of constitutional conditions, inherited or acquired, the recognition of which is essential to their effectual treatment.

CANCER of the skin occurs in various forms. *Rodent ulcer* (q.v.), or basal cell epithelioma responds well to treatment. Cure is obtained in 98 per cent of cases if treated early. Anyone over the age of 50 with a persistent superficial crusted ulcer on the cheek or the side of the nose which has not healed over a period of months should seek medical advice in case it is a rodent ulcer. *Squamous cell carcinoma* which usually starts as a hard nodule, is usually the result of long excessive exposure to sunlight. *Malignant melanoma* (see MELANOMA) develops in a pigmented spot. Cancer of the skin may also be induced by exposure to tar, pitch, bitumen, the mineral oils, and X-rays.

(See also ACNE; BOILS; BROMIDROSIS; DERMATITIS; ECTHYMA; ECZEMA; ERYSIPELAS; ERYTHEMA; ERYTHRASMA; HERPES SIMPLEX; HERPES ZOSTER; HYPERIDROSIS; ICHTHYOSIS; IMPETIGO; ITCHING; KERATOSIS; LEUCODERMA; LICHEN; LUPUS; MOLLUSCUM CONTAGIOSUM; NAPPY RASH; NEURODERMATOSES; PEMPHIGUS; PITYRIASIS ROSEA; POMPHOLYX; PRURIGO; PRURITUS; PSORIASIS; RINGWORM; ROSACEA; SEBORRHOEA; URTICARIA.)

SKIN-GRAFTING is an operation in which large breaches of surface due to wounding or ulceration are closed by transplantation of skin from other parts. There are three methods by which this is done. Most frequently the epidermis only is transplanted, according to a method introduced by Reverdin and by Thiersch, and known by their names. For this purpose, a broad strip of epidermis is shaved off the thigh or upper arm, after the part has been carefully purified, and is transferred bodily to the raw or ulcerated surface, or is cut into smaller strips and laid upon it. By a second method, small pieces of the skin in its whole thickness are removed from the arm and thigh, or even from other people, and are implanted and bound upon the raw surface. This method has the disadvantage that the true skin must contract at

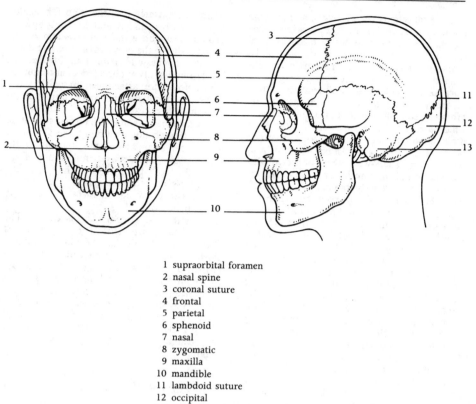

1 supraorbital foramen
2 nasal spine
3 coronal suture
4 frontal
5 parietal
6 sphenoid
7 nasal
8 zygomatic
9 maxilla
10 mandible
11 lambdoid suture
12 occipital
13 temporal

Frontal (left) and left lateral (right) views of the skull.

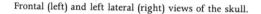

the spot from which the graft is taken, leaving an unsightly scar. When very large areas require to be covered, a third method is sometimes adopted, as follows. A large flap of skin, amply sufficient to cover the gap, is raised from a neighbouring or distant part of the body, in such a way that it remains attached along one margin, so that blood-vessels can still enter and nourish it. It is then turned so as to cover the gap; or, if it be situated on a distant part, the two parts are brought together and fixed in this position till the flap grows firmly to its new bed. The old connection of the flap is then severed, leaving it growing in its new place.

SKULL is the collection of 22 flat and irregularly shaped bones which protect the brain and form the face. The names of the individual bones composing the skull are given under BONE.

Arrangement of the bones In early life the brain and organs of special sense are enclosed in a case which is formed partly of cartilage, partly of fibrous membrane. At various parts of this investment, ossification begins early in life, and the bone gradually spreads outwards from each of these centres. Certain of the bones so formed fuse together in early childhood, thus constituting the twenty-two bones of the adult skull, which maintain their independence throughout the greater part of life. In old age, however, the bones fuse so completely that the cranium comes to be a solid bony case. Even before this happens, the bones are fastened to one another by sutures so tightly that their separation without breaking is very difficult. The sutures are joints in which each edge is locked with the edges of neighbouring bones by exactly fitting projections and depressions, resembling a complicated mortise-work. Occasionally small bones develop in the sutures between the ordinary, named ones, these extra bones being known as sutural bones.

The growth of the bones spreads outwards, as already stated, from certain centres, and at the time of birth the growth of several bones has not been quite completed, so that an infant's head presents six soft spots or fontanelles where the brain is covered only by skin and membranes, and at some of which the pulsations of its blood-vessels can be seen. One of these spots, the anterior fontanelle, situated on the top of the head, does not completely close till the child is 2½ years old. Another change takes place as age advances, consisting in the development of an outer and inner hard table in each of the cranial bones, the tables being separated by a layer of cancellous bone (*diplöe*), and in some positions by spaces containing air, which communicate with the respiratory passages. (See SINUS.) This change begins at the age of 10 years, and leads to great thickening and increased strength in the skull.

Parts of the skull The skull consists of two distinct parts: the cranium, which encloses the brain and consists of eight bones; and the face, which forms a bony framework for the eyes, nose, and mouth, and is composed of fourteen bones. These two parts can be detached from one another. The lower jaw is connected with the base of the cranium by a movable joint on each side, and when the bones are bare of soft parts there is no union between them. The ear, which lies just behind and above this joint, is enclosed in the substance of the temporal bone, lying beneath the brain and separated from it in places only by a very thin shell of bone. The interior of the cranium is moulded so as to form a support for the brain. Its base is divided by bony ridges into three fossae, which from before back support the frontal lobes, the temporosphenoidal lobes, and the cerebellum. Further, the inner surface of the bone shows grooves and hollows corresponding to the convolutions and blood-vessels of the brain. The bones, especially on the base of the skull, are pierced by many small canals (*foramina*) which transmit nerves, blood-vessels and the like. Of these, the largest is the foramen magnum, through which the medulla oblongata and the spinal cord are continuous with one another.

Shape of the skull In the lower animals, the cranium is placed in the back part of the head, and the face looks upwards to a great extent as well as forwards. In man, as a consequence of the great development of the cerebral hemispheres of the brain, in connection with his mental activity, the cranium extends above, as well as behind, the face, which therefore looks straight forwards. One method of classification is obtained by taking what is known as the cephalic index: i.e. the percentage that the skull's breadth forms of its length. Long-headed peoples, like the Australian aborigines, are known as *dolichocephalic*; peoples with rounded heads, like most European races, are called *mesocephalic*; while races with broad heads, like some American Indians, are said to be *brachycephalic*.

Age makes considerable changes in the skull. The persistence of soft spots in the skull during the first two years of life, as well as the gradual obliteration of the sutures in later life, have been already mentioned. In children the size of the cranium is large compared with that of the face, which measures only one-eighth of the whole head, but increases till in adult life cranium and face are of almost equal proportions. In old age the face once more decreases, owing largely to loss of the teeth and consequent absorption of their bony sockets, which allows the cheeks to sink inwards and gives the appearance known as nut-cracker jaws. A similar result is produced earlier in life by premature extraction of the teeth. The child's head is gently rounded, and does not show the prominences above the eyebrows and behind the ears, due to the presence of air-cells at these localities in the full-grown skull. Further, the skull is thinner in childhood, does not show the heavy ridges for attachment of muscles displayed in later life, and is more vertical on the front and sides.

Sex also makes some differences, so that, as a rule, though not invariably, the skull of a woman can be told from that of a man. In the woman the characters resemble those of the child, the skull being lighter, smoother, and having less marked prominences. The woman's skull has on an average nine-tenths the capacity of the male skull.

Deformities result from various causes. The head is rarely symmetrical, one side almost always bulging more than the other. Premature closure of one of the sutures leads to increased growth at other sutures. Thus if the suture running from before backwards on the vertex of the head (sagittal suture) close too early, the result is a very long boat-shaped head. Some races, as, for example, the flat-head Indians of North America, show striking deformities of the head produced by applying boards and bandages in infant life.

SLAPPED CHEEK DISEASE (see ERYTHEMA).

SLEEP is a state which alternates with wakefulness and in which awareness and responsiveness to the environment are reduced. It is not, however, uniform and can be divided into two main states which are differentiated according to electrical recordings of brain activity (EEG), of the muscles (EMG), and of the eye movements (EOG).

NON-RAPID-EYE MOVEMENT (NREM) SLEEP This is subdivided into four stages of which stage 1 is the lightest and stage 4 is the deepest. The activity of the cerebral cortex is diminished and the body's functions are mainly regulated by brain-stem activity. The metabolic rate is reduced and in keeping with this the temperature falls, respiration is reduced, cardiac output, heart rate, and blood pressure fall, and activity of the sympathetic nervous system is reduced. NREM sleep normally occurs at the onset of sleep except in neonates. During adult life the duration, particularly of stages 3 and 4, of NREM sleep becomes less and very little of this deep sleep occurs after the age of 60 years.

NREM sleep has been thought to have several functions such as energy conservation and growth. Growth hormone is produced in bursts during stages 3 and 4 NREM sleep and more cell division occurs during this type of sleep than during wakefulness. It has also been proposed that processing of information which has been acquired during wakefulness occurs during NREM sleep.

RAPID-EYE-MOVEMENT (REM) SLEEP This is characterized by the presence of rapid eye movements and a reduction in muscle tone. Cerebral cortical activity is prominent and its blood flow is increased. This activity is, however, different to wakefulness and may cause irregular movements of the body as well as of the eyes. Most dreams occur in REM sleep. These may represent a process of reorganizing mental associations after the period of wakefulness. The analysis of the content of dreams has been subject to a variety of interpretations but no consensus view has evolved.

Physiological changes, such as a fall in temperature and blood pressure, take place just before sleep and continue during the early stages of NREM sleep. There is an intrinsic rhythm of sleep which in most subjects has a periodicity of around 25 hours. This can be modified by external factors to bring it into line with the 24-hour day. Two peaks of a tendency to sleep have been identified and these usually occur between around 1400 hrs and 1800 hrs and 02.00 and 06.00 hours. There are, however, differences according to age, in that, for instance, infants sleep for most of the 24 hours and during adolescence there is also an increase in the duration of sleep. Sleep requirements fall later in life but there are wide genetic differences in the amount of sleep that people require and also the time at which they fall asleep most readily.

The internal clock can be disturbed by a variety of external factors which include irregular sleeping habits due, for instance, to shift work or jet lag. Sleep is also more likely to occur after physical exertion, reading and social activity. The duration and intensity of exposure to light can also modify sleep profoundly. Light promotes wakefulness and is the main factor that adjusts the 25-hour internal rhythm to the 24-hour daily cycle. Neural connections from the retina act on an area in the brain called the supra-chiasmatic nucleus which stimulates the pineal gland (q.v.) which produces melatonin (q.v.). This is thought to trigger the range of neurological and metabolic processes that characterize sleep.

SLEEP, DISORDERS OF There are three main groups of sleep disorders:

PARASOMNIAS These include medical disorders such as asthma (q.v.), angina (q.v.) or epilepsy (q.v.) which are exacerbated by sleep and the range of behavioural alterations which are usually related to a specific sleep stage or to a change from one state of sleep to another. Sleep walking, night terrors, and nightmares are examples.

INSOMNIA Insomnia is defined as a difficulty in initiating or maintaining sleep. It affects around 15 per cent of the population at any one time. It is often due to a poor pre-sleep routine (e.g. taking excessive stimulants such as caffeine), unsatisfactory sleep due to poor environments such as an uncomfortable bed or a cold or noisy bedroom, anxiety, depression or occasionally due to a physical problem, for example, pain or a medical disorder associated with sleep such as

obstructive sleep apnoeas or periodic limb movements.

EXCESSIVE DAYTIME SLEEPINESS This is usually due to sleep deprivation caused either by inadequate duration of sleep or by poor quality sleep. The individual's lifestyle is often a cause and modification of this may relieve the problem. Other common causes of excessive daytime sleepiness are depression, obstructive sleep apnoeas, periodic limb movements, excessive alcohol intake, and, less commonly, narcolepsy (q.v.).

SLEEP APNOEAS A sleep apnoea is conventionally defined as the cessation of breathing for ten seconds or more. Apnoeas may occur as frequently as 400 times per night. They can be due to a failure of the drive to breathe (central sleep apnoeas) but much more often are due to a transient obstruction of the airway between the level of the soft palate and the larynx (obstructive sleep apnoeas) when the airway dilator muscles overrelax. Any factor such as alcohol or sedative drugs that accentuates this, or that makes the airway narrower, such as obesity or large tonsils, will tend to cause sleep apnoeas.

Vigorous respiratory movements are made to overcome the obstruction during each apnoea. These are associated with snoring and snorting noises. The apnoea ends with a mini-arousal from sleep. As a result sleep becomes fragmented and sleep deprivation, manifested as sleepiness during the day, is common. This may result in accidents, for instance, at work or while driving, and sleep apnoea is also linked with an increased risk of strokes, heart attacks and hypertension.

Initial treatment is directed at correcting the cause, e.g., weight loss, but if the apnoeas persist or are severe a nasal mask and pump which introduces air under slight pressure into the upper airway (continuous positive airway pressure, CPAP) is almost invariably effective.

SLEEPING SICKNESS Also termed African trypanosomiasis, this infection is endemic in west, east, central and South Africa between latitudes 14° N and 25° S. Pioneering work was carried out by David Bruce in Zululand and Uganda in 1894 and 1903, respectively. There are two major forms of the disease: *Trypanosoma brucei gambiense* is confined to west and central Africa, and *T.b. rhodesiense* to central, east, and south-east Africa; there is a significant overlap, and it is probable that the two strains form part of a continuous spectrum. The infection is caused by the bite of tsetse fly (*Glossina* spp.). Clinically, a trypanosomal chancre may develop at the site of the tsetse-fly bite. After introduction into the bloodstream, the protozoan parasite develops in blood and lymphatic glands. After the blood stage, it enters the central nervous system, causing characteristic neurological sequelae (see below). Infection may be followed by a generalized macular papular reaction. In *T.b. gambiense* infection, enlarged glands in the neck (Winterbottom's sign) may be striking. Onset of disease is accompanied by fever, progressive anaemia, and enlarged glands; these signs and symptoms are followed by increasing lethargy, slowing of mentality, and physical weakness, and give way to headache and an increasing tendency to sleep. These symptoms are caused by proliferation of parasites in the patient's cerebral blood vessels; this is accompanied by inflammatory changes and disorganization of nervous tissue. Patients become emaciated and develop bed sores. Death finally takes place either as a result of gross emaciation or an intercurrent infection.

Diagnosis is by detection of trypanosomes in a blood specimen or, alternatively, a sample of cerebrospinal fluid. Recently introduced serological tests are of great value in diagnosis.

Treatment is with suramine or pentamidine; when cerebral involvement has ensued, melarsoprol – which penetrates the blood-brain barrier – is of value. In *T.b. gambiense* infection, eflornithine has recently given encouraging results; however, this form of chemotherapy is not effective in a *T.b. rhodesiense* infection. From the point of view of prevention, control of the tsetse-fly population is crucial; even so, only a very small percentage of these vectors is infected with *Trypanosoma* spp.

SLING means a hanging bandage for the support of injured or diseased parts. Slings are generally applied for support of the upper limb, in which case the limb is suspended from the neck. The lower limb may also be supported in a sling from an iron cage placed upon the bed on which the patient lies, the object usually being to aid the circulation, and so quicken the healing of ulcers on the leg.

SLIPPED DISC is the popular name for a prolapsed intervertebral disc (q.v.). (See SPINAL COLUMN; SCIATICA.)

SLOUGH means a dead part separated by natural processes from the living body. The term is applied to hard external parts which the lower animals cast off naturally in the course of growth, like the skin of snakes or the shell of crabs. In man, however, the process is generally associated with disease, and is then known as gangrene. (See GANGRENE.) Sloughs may be of very small size, as in the case of the core of a boil, or they may include a whole limb, but in general a slough involves a limited area of skin or of the underlying tissues. The process of separation of a slough is described under gangrene.

SLOW VIRUSES A group of viruses whose effects take a long time to show after their initial infection of the nervous system. The diseases may take years to develop during which time gradual but widespread damage of the nerve tissue occurs. The outcome is a loss of brain function and eventually death. Slow-virus disease was many years ago recognized as causing scrapie in sheep, and more recently bovine spongiform encephalopathy (BSE) has been identified in cows, the disease being spread through feedstuffs contaminated with nervous tissue from sheep and cattle. In humans the Creutzfeldt-Jakob syndrome (a type of dementia) (q.v.), kuru (laughing sickness) (q.v.) and a type of meningitis are among several diseases thought to be caused by a slow virus.

SMALLPOX, so called to distinguish it from syphilis, the great pox (pox being the plural of pock, the Old English term for a pustule (q.v.)), is also known as VARIOLA (from *varus*, the Latin for pimple). It is an acute, highly infectious disease due to a virus.

Until recent times it was one of the major killing diseases. In the 1960s the World Health Organization undertook an eradication scheme by means of mass vaccination. As a result, the last naturally occurring case was recorded in October 1977, and on 8 May 1980, the World Health Assembly solemnly agreed a Resolution confirming that smallpox has finally been eradicated from the world. This was indeed a historic occasion; the first occasion on which man has attempted to eradicate a disease and has succeeded in so doing. The public lack of interest in it is explained by the fact that so few of those living today have had any experience of it – even doctors.

Since 1960, there have been only 141 reported cases, with 28 deaths, in England and Wales, and not a single naturally occurring case since 1973. (See VACCINATION.)

SMEGMA is a thick, cheesy secretion formed by the sebaceous glands of the glans penis. A bacillus, closely resembling the tubercle bacillus morphologically, develops readily in this secretion.

SMELL The sense of smell is picked up in what is known as the olfactory areas of the nose. Each of these is about 3 square centimetres in area and contains 50 million olfactory, or smelling, cells. They lie, one on either side, at the highest part of each nasal cavity. This is why we have to sniff if we want to smell anything carefully, as in ordinary quiet breathing only a few eddies of the air we breathe in reaches an olfactory area. From these olfactory cells the olfactory nerves (one on each side) run up to the olfactory bulbs underneath the frontal lobe of the brain (q.v.), and here the impulse is translated into what we describe as smell.

SMELLING SALTS (see AMMONIA).

SMOKE INHALATION Smoke is made up of small particles of carbon in hot air and gases. The particles are covered with organic chemicals and smoke may also contain carbon monoxide and acids. When smoke is inhaled the effects on breathing may be immediate or delayed depending on the density of smoke and its composition. Laryngeal stridor (obstruction of the larynx), lack of oxygen and pulmonary oedema are life-threatening symptoms that require urgent treatment. Immediate removal of the victim from the smoke is imperative, as is the administration of oxygen. The victim may require admission to an intensive-care unit.

SMOKING (see TOBACCO).

SMOOTH MUSCLE   Muscle that is under the 'involuntary' control of the central nervous system (see MUSCLE).

SNAKE-BITE (see BITES AND STINGS).

SNEEZING means a sudden expulsion of air through the nose, designed to expel irritating materials from the upper air passages. In sneezing, a powerful expiratory effort is made, the vocal cords are kept shut till the pressure in the chest has risen high, and air is then suddenly allowed to escape upward, being directed into the back of the nose by the soft palate. One sneeze projects 10,000 to 100,000 droplets a distance of up to 10 metres at a rate of over 60 kilometres an hour. As such droplets may contain micro-organisms, it is clear what an important part sneezing plays in transmitting infections such as the common cold. Though usually transitory, sneezing may persist for days on end – up to 204 days have been recorded.

Sneezing may be caused by the presence of irritating particles in the nose, such as snuff, the pollen of grasses and flowers. It is also an early symptom of colds, influenza, measles, and hay-fever, being then accompanied or followed by running at the nose.

SNELLEN CHART   The most commonly used chart for testing the acuity of distant vision. The chart comprises rows of capital letters with the letters in each row being smaller than the one above. The top line of large letters can be seen by a normally sighted person standing 60 metres away. The subject under test sits six metres from the screen and, if he can read the six metre line of letters, his visual acuity is normal at 6/6 (see VISION).

SNORING is usually attributed to vibrations of the soft palate, but there is evidence that the main fault lies in the edge of the posterior pillars of the fauces (q.v.) which vibrate noisily. Mouth breathing is necessary for snoring, but not all mouth-breathers snore. The principal cause is blockage of the nose, such as occurs during the course of the common cold or chronic nasal catarrh. Such blockage also occurs in some cases of deviation of the nasal septum or nasal polypi. (See NOSE, DISEASES OF.) In children,

mouth-breathing, with resulting snoring, is often due to enlarged tonsils and adenoids. A further cause of snoring is loss of tone in the soft palate and surrounding tissues due to smoking, overwork, fatigue, obesity, and general poor health. One in eight people are said to snore regularly. The intensity, or loudness, of snoring is in the range, 40 to 69 decibels. (Pneumatic drills register between 70 and 90 decibels.)

Treatment therefore consists of the removal of any of these causes of mouth-breathing that may be present. Should these not succeed in preventing snoring, then measures should be taken to prevent the victim from sleeping lying on his back, as this is a habit which strongly conduces to snoring. Simple measures include sleeping with several pillows so that the head is raised quite considerably when asleep. Alternatively, a small pillow may be put under the nape of the neck. If all these measures fail, there is much to be said for the old traditional method of sewing a hair-brush, or some other hard object such as a stone, into the back of the snorer's pyjamas. This means that if he does turn on to his back while asleep, he is quickly awakened and therefore able to turn on his side again. (See also STERTOR.)

SNOW BLINDNESS   Damage caused to the cornea of an unprotected eye by the reflection of the sun's rays from snow. Ultraviolet light is the damaging agent and people going out in snow and sunlight should wear protective goggles. The condition is painful but resolves if the eyes are covered with pads for a day or two. Prolonged exposure may seriously damage the cornea and impair vision.

SNUFFLES is the name applied to noisy breathing in children due to the constant presence of nasal discharge. (For treatment, see NOSE, DISEASES OF.)

SOAP is a substance made by boiling a fat or oil with an alkali. The most commonly used oil is olive oil, and the most frequent alkali is caustic soda. In the process of manufacture the fatty acids of the oil unite with the alkali, glycerin separating out. In soft soap or green soap, caustic potash is used in place of soda; marine soap is made with coconut oil; curd soap has tallow for its fat: while many toilet soaps have palm oil or almond oil. Barilla soap is made from soda got by burning plants; in superfatted soaps care is taken that the fatty part is in excess, so that no crude alkali is left to irritate the skin; whilst glycerin soaps have a specially emollient action. Medicated soaps of various kinds are prepared, the chief drugs added to soap being of an antiseptic nature, such as carbolic acid, coal-tar, formalin, hexachlorophane, terebene.

Uses   The chief use of soap is, mixed with water, as a cleansing agent. Internally, hard soap is often used to make up the bulk of pills containing very active ingredients. As a purgative enema, soap is used made up into a strong solution in warm water. Soap liniment, better known as 'opodeldoc', is used as a popular remedy for stiffness or sprains.

SOCIAL CLASSES As factors such as the cause of death and the incidence of diseases vary in different social strata, the Registrar-General evolved the following social classification, which has now been in official use for many years:
Class I Professional occupations, such as lawyers, clergymen, and commissioned officers in the Armed Forces.
Class II Intermediate occupations, such as teachers, managers and nurses.
Class III N Non-manual – for example, clerical workers.
Class III M Skilled manual occupations such as miners and bricklayers.
Class IV Partly skilled occupations, such as agricultural workers.
Class V Unskilled occupations, such as building and dock labourers.

SODIUM is a metal, the salts of which are white, crystalline, and very soluble. The fluids of the body contain naturally a considerable quantity of sodium chloride.
SODIUM CARBONATE, commonly known as SODA or WASHING SODA, has a powerful softening action upon the tissues.
SODIUM BICARBONATE, or BAKING SODA, is used as an antacid in relieving indigestion associated with increased acidity of the gastric secretion. It is taken in doses of 600 or 1,200 mg, as a rule. The citrate and the acetate of sodium are used as diuretics and in the treatment of inflammatory conditions of the kidneys and bladder, though the corresponding potassium salts are more often used.

SODIUM CHLORIDE is the chemical name for common salt.

SODIUM CROMOGLYCATE is the main drug used in the prophylaxis of asthma. It is administered by inhalation and can reduce the incidence of asthmatic attacks but is of no value in the treatment of an acute attack. It acts by preventing the release of pharmacological mediators of bronchospasm, particularly histamine, by stabilizing mastcell membranes. It is thus of particular use in patients whose asthma has an allergic basis. The dose frequency is adjusted to the patient's response but is usually administered by inhalation four times daily.

SODIUM DIATRIZOATE is an organic iodine salt that is radio-opaque and is therefore used as a contrast medium to outline various organs in the body in X-ray films. It is given intravenously. Its main use is in pyelography (q.v.), that is in rendering the kidneys radio-opaque, but it is also used to outline the blood-vessels (angiography) and the gall-bladder and bile ducts (cholangiography).

SODIUM HYPOCHLORITE is a disinfectant by virtue of the fact that it gives off chlorine. For domestic use, as, for example, for sterilizing baby feeding bottles, it is available in a variety of proprietary preparations. (See also CHLORINATED LIME.)

SODIUM VALPROATE is a drug that is proving of value in the treatment of some cases of epilepsy which will not respond to any of the other drugs used for the treatment of this condition. It must be used with care as it may cause liver damage.

SODOMY Sexual intercourse in which the penis penetrates the anus and rectum. Sodomy may occur between men, between a man and a woman or between a man and an animal (bestiality).

SOLARIUM is a room enclosed by glass in which sun baths are taken while protection is afforded from the weather.

SOLAR PLEXUS A large network of sympathetic nerves and ganglia situated in the abdomen behind the stomach, where it surrounds the coeliac artery. Branches of the vagus nerve, the most important part of the parasympathetic system, lead into the solar plexus, which in turn distributes branches to the stomach, intestines and several other abdominal organs. A severe blow in the solar plexus may cause temporary unconsciousness.

SOLUTION or LIQUOR as it used to be known, is a liquid preparation containing one or more soluble drugs, usually dissolved in water.

SOLVENT ABUSE Also known as volatile-substance abuse, this is the deliberate inhalation of intoxicating fumes given off by some volatile liquids. Glue sniffing was the most common type of solvent abuse, but inhalation of fuel gases such as butane, especially in the form of lighter refills, is now the major problem in the United Kingdom. The problem has become common among children, particularly teenagers. Solvents or volatile substances are applied to a piece of cloth or put into a plastic bag and inhaled, sometimes until the person loses consciousness. He or she may become acutely intoxicated; chronic abusers may suffer from ulcers and rashes over the face as well as damage to peripheral nerves. Death can occur, probably as a result of an abnormal rhythm of the heart. Tolerance to the volatile substances may develop over months, but acute intoxication may lead to aggressive and impulsive behaviour. Treatment of addiction is difficult and requires professional counselling. Victims with acute symptoms require urgent medical attention. In 1990 about 130 deaths in the United Kingdom were associated with volatile substance abuse, mostly in young people under 20 years of age; 80 per cent of the deaths were in males. This compares with 82 deaths in 1983. (See ADDICTION; DRUG ADDITION.)

SOMATIC means relating to the body, as opposed to the mind.

SOMNAMBULISM means sleep-walking. (See SLEEP.)

SOPORIFICS are measures which induce sleep. (See HYPNOTICS.)

SORE is a popular term for ulcer (q.v.).

SOTALOL (see ADRENERGIC RECEPTORS).

SOUND is a rod with a curve at one end used mainly for passing into the bladder to determine whether a stone is present or not. (See URINARY BLADDER, DISEASES OF.)

SOUTHEY'S TUBES are long, fine tubes for drawing off fluid slowly from the tissues (usually from the legs) in patients with oedema. The procedure is rarely used now. (See ASPIRATION.)

SOYA BEAN is the bean of *Glycine soja*, a leguminous plant related to peas and beans. The outstanding characteristic of the soya bean is its high protein and fat content. There is an almost complete absence of starch, but a large amount of mineral matter. Soya flour contains 40 per cent of protein and 20 per cent of fat. It yields 470 Calories per 100 grams as compared with 370 Calories for white wheat flour. Soya flour contains 0·2 per cent of calcium (about ten times as much as in white flour). It also contains a variable but large amount of iron: 6·7 to 30 mg per 100 grams of soya flour compared with 1 mg in white flour and 3 mg in 100 grams of wholemeal flour. It is a good source of thiamine and riboflavine, and of vitamin A in the form of carotene.

SPANISH FLY is a popular term for cantharides, which is used as a blistering agent. (See CANTHARIDES.)

SPASM means an involuntary, and, in severe cases, painful contraction of a muscle or of a hollow organ with a muscular wall. Spasm may be due to affections in the muscle where the spasm takes place, or it may originate in some disturbance of that part of the nervous system which controls the spasmodically acting muscles. Spasms of a general nature are usually spoken of as convulsions; spasms of a painful nature are known as cramp when they affect the muscles of the limbs, and as colic when they are situated in the stomach, bowels, or other organs of the abdomen. Spasm of the heart receives the name of breast-pang or angina pectoris, and is both a serious and an agonizing condition. When the spasm is a prolonged firm contraction, it is spoken of as tonic spasm; when it consists of a series of twitches or quick alternate contractions and relaxations, it is known as clonic spasm. Spasm is a symptom of many diseases.

SPASMODIC TORTICOLLIS is the term applied to a chronic condition in which the neck is rotated or deviated laterally, forwards, or backwards, often with additional jerking or tremor. It is a form of focal dystonia, and should not be confused with the far commoner transient condition of acute painful wry-neck. (See DYSTONIA.)

SPASMOLYTICS are remedies which diminish spasm. They may achieve this in one of three ways: (*a*) by interfering with the transmission of the nerve impulses that are causing the spasm; (*b*) by a direct action on the affected muscle; (*c*) by depressing the central nervous system.
Varieties: In the past many of the favourites in this field, such as oil of cinnamon, oil of cloves, oil of peppermint, and valerian, achieved their reputation by virtue of their depressing effect on the sensitivity of the nerve endings. Others, such as lobelia and stramonium, often in the form of cigarettes to be inhaled, achieved a wide reputation as asthma cures.

Today, a more scientific approach is maintained, though there is still much to be said for the use of preparations, such as oil of cinnamon or of peppermint for the relief of mild spasm of the gut, and not a few asthmatics have implicit faith in the relieving power of lobelia or stramonium. The most widely used spasmolytics today are atropine and its derivatives, or its many synthetic substitutes. These act by paralysing the action of the parasympathetic nerve fibres that induce contraction of smooth muscle. They are most widely used in relieving spasm in the alimentary and renal tracts. For the relief of the spasm of asthma adrenaline and ephedrine are still great standbys, though isoprenaline and other similarly acting drugs are being used to an increasing extent. All these act through the sympathetic nervous system.

Of the spasmolytics acting directly on muscle, the best known group is the nitrites – amyl nitrite and glyceryl trinitrate – which are the great standby for the relief of the spasm that induces angina pectoris. Other drugs that act in this way are theophylline and aminophylline. If the spasm is really severe, and therefore painful enough, general depression of the brain may be necessary by means of general anaesthetics. In less severe cases, the lesser degrees of depression of the brain induced by hypnotics may have a spasmolytic action, and, though it should seldom be used for this purpose because of its habit-forming propensities, even alcohol could rank as a spasmolytic.

SPASTIC is a term applied to any condition showing increased muscle tone: e.g. spastic gait. This is specially associated with some disease affecting the upper part of the nervous system connected with movement (upper neuron), so that its controlling influence is lost and the muscles are in a state of over-excitability.

SPASTIC COLON (see IRRITABLE BOWEL SYNDROME).

SPATULA is a flat, knife-like instrument used for spreading plasters and ointments, and also for depressing the tongue when the throat is being examined.

SPECIFICITY An epidemiological term describing the extent to which a screening test (q.v.) throws up false positives. A specific test has few false positives.

SPECTACLES can be worn for a variety of reasons including correction of a refractive error, correction of a squint, for protection (from foreign bodies or, with tinted lenses, from bright light), or occasionally to hold a prosthesis.

SPECULUM is an instrument designed to aid the examination of the various openings on the surface of the body. Many specula are provided with small electric lamps so placed as to light up the cavity brilliantly.

SPEECH DISORDERS may be of physical or psychological origin – or a combination of both. Difficulties may arise at various stages of development: due to problems during pregnancy, at birth, childhood illnesses, or delayed development. Congenital defects such as cleft palate or lip (q.v.) may make speech unintelligible until major surgery is performed, thus discouraging talking and delaying development. Recurrent ear infections may make hearing difficult; the child's experience of speech is thus limited, with similar results. Childhood dysphasia (q.v.) occurs if the language development area of the brain develops abnormally; specialist education and speech therapy (q.v.) may then be required.

Dumbness is the inability to pronounce the sounds that make up words. Deafness is the most important cause, being due to a congenital brain defect, or acquired brain disease, such as tertiary syphilis. When hearing is normal or only mildly impaired, dumbness may be due to a structural defect such as tongue-tie or enlarged tonsils and adenoids, or to inefficient voice control, resulting in lisping or lalling. Increased tension is a common cause of stammering (q.v.); speech disorders may occasionally be a hysterical manifestation.

Normal speech may be lost in adulthood (see DYSPHASIA) as a result of a stroke (q.v.) or head injury. Excessive use of the voice may be an occupational hazard; and throat cancer may require a laryngectomy (q.v.), with subsequent help in communication. Severe psychiatric disturbance may be accompanied by impaired social and communication skills (see VOICE AND SPEECH).

Treatment The underlying cause of the problem should be diagnosed as early as possible; psychological and other specialist investigations should be carried out as required, and any physical defect should be repaired. Deaf-mutes should start training in lip-reading as soon as possible, and special educational methods aimed at acquiring a modulated voice should similarly be started in early childhood, provided by the local authority, and continued as required. Various types of speech therapy or psychotherapy may be appropriate, alone or in conjunction with other treatments, and often the final result may be highly satisfying, with a good command of language and speech being obtained.

Help and advice may be obtained from AFASIC (Overcoming Speech Impairment) (see APPENDIX 2: ADDRESSES).

SPEECH THERAPY is a small independent graduate profession. Speech therapists assist, diagnose and treat the whole spectrum of acquired or developmental communication disorders. They work in medical and education establishments often in an advisory or consultative capacity. The medical conditions in which speech therapy is employed include: dysgraphia, dyslexia, dysathria, dysphasia, dysphonia, dyspraxia, autism, Bell's palsy, cerebral palsy, deafness, disordered language, delayed speech, disordered speech, Down's syndrome, laryngectomy, macroglossia, mental subnormality, motor neurone disease, malformations of the palate, Parkinsonism, psychiatric disorders, stammering, stroke and disorders of voice production.

It is a caring profession; most speech therapists work for the National Health Service in community clinics and hospitals. They may also work in schools or in units for the handicapped, paediatric assessment centres, language units attached to primary schools, adult training centres and day centres for the elderly.

A speech therapist undergoes a four-year degree course which covers the study of disorders of communication in children and adults, phonetics and linguistics, anatomy and physiology, psychology and many other related subjects. Further information on training can be obtained from the College of Speech Therapists (see APPENDIX 2: ADDRESSES).

If the parents of a child are concerned about their child's speech, they may approach a speech therapist for assessment and guidance. Their general practitioner will be able to give them local addresses or they should contact the district speech therapist. Adults are usually referred by hospital consultants.

The College of Speech Therapists keeps a register of all those who have passed a recognized degree or equivalent qualification in speech therapy. It will be able to direct you to your nearest NHS or private speech therapist.

SPERMATIC is the name applied to the blood-vessels and other structures associated with the testicle.

SPERMATORRHOEA is the passage of semen without erection of the penis or orgasm.

SPERMATOZOON (plural: SPERMATOZOA) is the male sex or germ cell which unites with the ovum to form the embryo or fetus. It is a highly mobile cell approximately 4 micrometres in length, much smaller than an ovum, which is about 35 micrometres in diameter. Each millilitre of semen (q.v.) contains on average about 100 million spermatozoa, and the average volume of semen discharged during ejaculation in sexual intercourse is between 2 and 4 ml. Once ejaculated during intercourse it travels at a rate of 1·5 to 3 millimetres a minute and remains mobile for several days after insemination, but quickly loses its potency for fertilization. As it takes only about 70 minutes to reach the ovarian end of the uterine tube, it is assumed that there must be factors other than its own mobility, such as contraction of the muscle of the womb and uterine tube, that speed it on its way. (See also FETUS.)

SPHAGNUM MOSS, or peat or bog moss, has been used as a wound dressing from time immemorial. A skeleton from the Bronze Age in Scotland showed a large pad of sphagnum moss applied to what had been a chest wound. It was used on a large scale as a wound dressing in the 1914–18 War. It is widely distributed in Scotland, Ireland and Western England. Its main value lies in its great absorptive powers: it can absorb up to seven times its weight of water. It is deodorizing and does not allow discharges from wounds to pass through it as does cotton wool.

SPERMICIDE Contraceptive preparations that kill sperm. They may be in the form of gels, pessaries, cream, or foam and should be used with a barrier contraceptive such as a diaphragm or a condom.

SPHENOID is a bone lying in the centre of the base of the skull, and supporting the others like a wedge or keystone. (See SKULL.)

SPHINCTER means a circular muscle which surrounds the opening from an organ, and, by maintaining a constant state of moderate contraction, prevents the escape of the contents of the organ. Sphincters close the outlet from the bladder and rectum, and in certain nervous diseases their action is interfered with, so that the power to relax or to keep moderately contracted is lost, and retention or incontinence of the evacuation results.

SPHYGMOGRAPH is an instrument for recording the pulse. (See PULSE.)

SPHYGMOMANOMETER is the name of an instrument for measuring blood-pressure (q.v.) in the arteries. It usually consists of a pneumatic armlet, the interior of which communicates by a rubber tube with an air-pressure pump and a gauge. The armlet is bound about the upper arm and pumped up sufficiently to obliterate the pulse as felt at the wrist or as heard in the artery at the bend of the elbow. The pressure – measured in mm of mercury – registered on the gauge at this point is regarded as the pressure of the blood at each heart-beat (systolic pressure). The pressure at which the sound heard in the artery suddenly changes its character marks the diastolic pressure.

SPINA BIFIDA is one of the commonest of the congenital malformations. It is one of the three types of neural tube anomaly, the other two being anencephaly and cranium bifidum. It takes two main forms, spina bifida occulta – said to affect about one in ten individuals – being much the commoner. There is a deficit in the posterior part of the spinal wall, usually in the lumbar region, and it is generally asymptomatic, unless the underlying spinal cord is affected. Occasionally it is associated with a hairy patch or birth mark on the back, and a few children develop a mild spastic gait or bladder problems.

Much more serious is spina bifida cystica, in which the spinal wall defect is accompanied by a protrusion of the spinal cord. This may take two forms: a meningocele, in which the meninges (q.v.), containing cerebrospinal fluid, protrude through the defect; and a meningomyelocele, in which the protrusion contains spinal cord and nerves. Meningocele is less common and has a good prognosis. Hydrocephalus (q.v.) and neurological problems affecting the legs are rare, though the bladder may be affected. Treatment consists of surgery in the first few days of life; long-term follow-up is necessary to pick up any neurological problems that may develop during subsequent growth of the spine. Meningomyelocele is much more serious and more common, accounting for 90 per cent of all cases. Usually affecting the lumbo-sacral region, the range of severity may vary considerably and, while early surgery with careful attention in a minor case may achieve good mobility, normal bladder function and intellect, a more extensive protrusion may cause complete anaesthesia of the skin, with increased risk of trauma, extensive paralysis of the trunk and limbs, with severe deformities, and paralysis and insensitivity of the bladder and bowel. Involuntary movements may be present, and hydrocephalus occurs in 80 per cent of cases.

The decision to operate can only be made after a full examination of the infant to determine the extent of the defect and any co-existent congenital abnormalities. The child's potential can then be estimated, and appropriate treatment discussed with the parents. Carefully selected patients should receive long-term treatment in a special centre, where full attention can be paid to all their various problems.

There is growing evidence of the value of vitamin supplements before and during pregnancy in reducing the incidence of spina bifida. Parents of affected infants may obtain help, advice, and encouragement from the Association for Spina Bifida and Hydrocephalus which has branches throughout the country, or the Scottish Spina Bifida Association (see APPENDIX 2: ADDRESSES).

SPINAL ANAESTHESIA A method of anaesthesia that involves injecting an anaesthetic drug into the cerebrospinal fluid, which surrounds the spinal cord. This suppresses sensation in a part of the body, the area affected being dependent on the level at which the anaesthetic is injected and the strength of drug used. Two types are used for surgery. In one, epidural, the anaesthetic is injected into the outer lining of the cord. In the other, subarachnoid, the drug is injected into the lumbar region of the vertebral column, the needle being inserted between the vertebrae.

The technique is valuable in patients who cannot take a general anaesthetic because, for example, they have heart or chest disease. Spinal anaesthesia is also useful in obstetrics or in circumstances in which a skilled general anaesthestist is unavailable. It is more often used in the United States and Scandinavia than in the United Kingdom.

Spinal anaesthesia also describes the loss of sensation in an area of the body as a result of disease or injury to the spinal cord, the extent of anaesthesia depending on the location of the disease or injury. (See ANAESTHESIA.)

SPINAL COLUMN, also known as the SPINE, CHINE, BACKBONE, and VERTEBRAL COLUMN, forms an important part of the skeleton, acting both as the rigid pillar which supports the upper parts of the body and as a protection to the spinal cord and nerves arising from it. The spinal column is built up of a number of bones placed one upon another, which, in consequence of having a slight degree of turning-movement, are known as the vertebrae. The possession of a spinal cord supported by a vertebral column distinguishes the higher animals from the lower types, and gains for them the general name of vertebrates. Of the vertebrates, man alone stands absolutely erect, and this erect carriage of the body gives to the skull

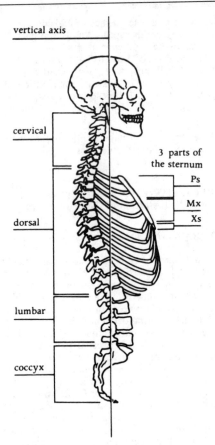

The spinal column.

and vertebral column certain distinctive characters.

The human backbone is about 70 cm (28 inches) in length, and varies little in full-grown people; differences in height depend mainly upon the length of the lower limbs. The number of vertebrae is 33 in children, although in adult life 5 of these fuse together to form the sacrum, and the lowest 4 unite in the coccyx, so that the number of separate bones is reduced to 26. Of these there are 7 in the neck, known therefore as *cervical vertebrae*; 12 with ribs attached, in the region of the thorax, and known as *thoracic* or *dorsal vertebrae*; 5 in the loins, called *lumbar vertebrae*; 5 fused to form the *sacrum*; and 4 joined in the *coccyx*. These numbers are expressed in a formula thus: C7, D12, L5, S5, Coc4 = 33. Although the vertebrae in each of these regions have distinguishing features, all the vertebrae are constructed on the same general plan. Each has a thick, rounded, bony part in front, known as the body, and these bodies form the main thickness of the column. Behind the body of each is a ring of bone, the neural ring, these rings placed one above another forming the bony canal which lodges the spinal cord. From each side of the ring a short

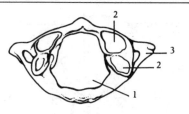

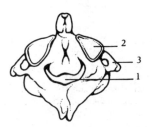

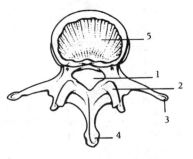

1 neural ring
2 articular process
3 transverse process
4 spinous process
5 body of vertebra

The atlas (1st cervical vertebra) and axis (2nd
cervical vertebra) vertebrae and a lumbar
vertebra seen from above.

process of bone known as the transverse process stands out, and from the back of the ring a larger process, the spinous process, projects. These processes give attachment to the strong ligaments and muscles which unite, support, and bend the column. The spines can be seen or felt beneath the skin of the back lying in the centre of a groove between the muscular masses of the two sides, and they give to the column its name of the spinal column. One of these spines, that of the 7th cervical vertebra, is especially large and forms a distinct bony prominence, where the neck joins the back. Between the bodies of the vertebrae lies a series of thick discs of fibro-cartilage known as intervertebral discs. Each disc consists of an outer portion, known as the annulus fibrosus, and an inner core, known as the nucleus pulposus. To these 23 discs the upper part of the spine owes much of

its pliability, as well as a great deal of its resiliency and power of diminishing the effect of jars and blows communicated through the feet or head. There is also a small joint at each side upon the ring of the vertebra so that each vertebra comes in contact with the one above and the one beneath in three places.

The first and second cervical vertebrae are modified in a very special manner. The first vertebra, known as the atlas, is devoid of a body, but has a specially large and strong ring with two hollows upon which the skull rests, thus permitting of nodding movements. The second vertebra, known as the axis, has a pivot upon its body which fits into the first vertebra and thus permits of free rotation of the head from side to side.

An important feature of the spinal column, and one especially marked in human beings, is the presence of four curves from behind forwards. Thus the cervical vertebrae are arranged with a curve whose hollow looks backwards, the dorsal vertebrae have a marked curve with the hollow forwards; in the lumbar region the hollow is directed backwards, while the sacrum and coccyx form a marked hollow to the front. The effect of the dorsal and sacral curves is greatly to increase the size of the cavities of chest and pelvis, while the compensating curves of the neck and loins serve to keep the general axis of the spinal column in a vertical line. The curves have also an action very similar to that of the springs of a vehicle, in minimizing jolting and jarring of the internal organs. There is usually a very slight curve to one side in the upper dorsal region, resulting from the greater development and use of one arm.

The neural rings placed one above another form a canal, which is wide in the neck, smaller and almost round in the dorsal region, and wide again in the lumbar vertebrae. This canal lodges the spinal cord, and the nerves that issue from the cord pass out from the canal by openings between the vertebrae which are produced by notches on the upper and lower margins of each ring. The intervertebral foramina formed by these notches are so large in comparison with the nerves passing through them that there is no chance of pressure upon the latter, except in very serious injuries which dislocate and fracture the spine.

SPINAL CORD is the lower portion of the central nervous system which is situated within the spinal column. Above, it forms the direct continuation of the medulla oblongata, this part of the brain changing its name to spinal cord at the *foramen magnum*, the large opening in the base of the skull through which it passes into the spinal canal. Below, the spinal cord extends to about the upper border of the second lumbar vertebra, where it tapers off into a fine thread, known as the filum terminale, that is attached to the coccyx at the lower end of the spine. The spinal cord is thus considerably shorter than the spinal column, being only 37 to 45 cm (15 to 18 inches) in length, and weighing around 30 grams. In its course from the base of the skull to the lumbar region the cord gives off thirty-one nerves on each side, each of which arises by an anterior and a posterior root that join before the nerve emerges from the spinal canal. The openings for the nerves formed by notches on the ring of each vertebra have been mentioned under SPINAL COLUMN. To reach these openings the upper nerves pass almost directly outwards, whilst lower in the series their obliquity increases, until below the point where the cord terminates there is a sheaf of nerves, known as the cauda equina, running downwards to leave the spinal canal at their appropriate openings. In shape the cord is a cylinder, about the thickness of the little finger, and slightly flattened from before backwards. It has two slightly enlarged portions, one in the lower part of the neck, the other at the last dorsal vertebra, and from these thickenings arise the nerves that pass to the upper and lower limbs. (See NERVES.) The spinal cord, like the brain, is surrounded by three membranes, the dura mater, arachnoid mater, and pia mater, from without inwards. The arrangement of the dura and arachnoid is much looser in the case of the cord than their application to the brain. The dura especially forms a wide tube which is separated from the cord by fluid and from the vertebral canal by blood-vessels and fat, this arrangement protecting the cord from pressure in any ordinary movements of the spine.

IN SECTION, the spinal cord consists partly of grey, but mainly of white, matter. It differs from the upper parts of the brain in that the white matter in the cord is arranged on the

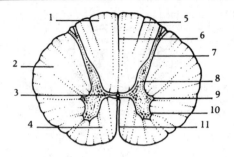

1 posterior white column
2 lateral white column
3 central canal
4 anterior white column
5 posterior lateral sulcus
6 posterior median septum
7 posterior horn of grey column
8 thoracic nucleus
9 lateral horn
10 anterior horn
11 anterior median fissure

Cross-section of spinal cord at level of 5th thoracic vertebra.

surface, surrounding a mass of grey matter, while in the brain the grey matter is superficial. The arrangement of grey matter, as seen in a section across the cord, resembles the letter H, each half of the cord possessing an anterior and a posterior horn, and the masses of the two sides being joined by a wide posterior grey commissure. In the middle of this commissure lies the central canal of the cord, a small tube which is the continuation of the ventricles in the brain. The horns of grey matter reach almost to the surface of the cord, and from their ends arise the roots of the nerves that leave the cord, but elsewhere the grey matter is completely surrounded by white matter. The white matter is divided almost completely into two halves by a posterior septum and anterior fissure that project inwards from the back and front surfaces, the posterior septum reaching down to the grey commissure, but the anterior fissure being separated from it by a small anterior white commissure that joins the white matter of the two sides together. The white matter is further divided into three columns, on each side, by the horns of grey matter and the nerve roots passing from them to the surface; these are known as the anterior, lateral, and posterior columns.

Functions The cord is, in part, a receiver and originator of nerve impulses, and in part merely a conductor of such impulses along fibres which pass to it and from the brain. The presence of centres in the cord, capable of receiving sensory impressions and originating motor impulses, is proved by several facts. Thus, it has been calculated that the number of nerve-fibres entering or leaving the cord by the spinal nerves is twice as great as the number of

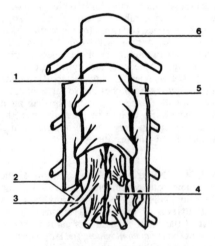

1 arachnoid
2 spinal ganglion
3 ventral nerve root
4 ligamentum denticulatum
5 dura mater, cut and turned backwards
6 dura mater

The membranes of the spinal cord.

fibres contained in the upper end of the cord, where it is continued into the brain. Again, if the cord is severed in the dorsal region, as by a fracture of the spine, the centres which govern the evacuation of the bladder and bowel do not lose their power of controlling these organs immediately upon being severed from the brain. Many of these centres are known to exist in the cord, such as centres for regulating the size of the blood-vessels, for altering the size of the pupil of the eye, for sweating, for breathing. Over most, if not all, of these centres, however, the brain exerts a controlling influence, and before any incoming sensation can produce an effect upon consciousness, it is in all probability necessary that it should obtain a clear passage up to the brain.

Many of these centres act in a rhythmical or *automatic* way. Other cells of the cord are capable of originating movements in response to impulses brought direct to them through sensory nerves, such activity being known as *reflex* action. (For a fuller description of the activities of the spinal cord, see NERVES.)

By observing the process of degeneration that takes place when nerve-fibres are cut off by disease or injury from the cells to which they belong, and by observing also the manner in which the fibres in different portions of the cord develop, it has been found possible to divide the three white columns of the cord into tracts, in each of which the fibres have a special function. Thus the posterior column consists of the *fasciculus gracilis* and the *fasciculus cuneatus* both conveying sensory impressions upwards. The lateral column contains the ventral and the dorsal spino-cerebellar tracts passing to the cerebellum, the crossed pyramidal tract of motor fibres carrying outgoing impulses downwards together with the rubro-spinal, the spino-thalamic, the spino-tectal, and the postero-lateral tracts. And, finally, the anterior column contains the direct pyramidal tract of motor fibres and an anterior mixed zone. The pyramidal tracts have the best-known course. Starting from cells near the central sulcus on the brain (see BRAIN), the motor nerve-fibres run down through the internal capsule, pons, and medulla, in the lower part of which many of those coming from the right side of the brain cross to the left side of the spinal cord, and vice versa. Thence the fibres run down in the crossed pyramidal tract to end beside nerve-cells in the anterior horn of the cord. From these nerve-cells other fibres pass outwards to form the nerves that go direct to the muscles. Thus the motor nerve path from brain to muscle is divided into two sections of neurons, of which the upper exerts a controlling influence upon the lower, while the lower is concerned in maintaining the muscle in a state of health and good nutrition, and in directly calling it into action.

SPINE AND SPINAL CORD, DISEASES AND INJURIES OF

SCOLIOSIS is a condition where the spine is curved to one side. The spine is normally straight when seen from behind. The deformity may be mobile and reversible or fixed. If fixed, it is accompanied by vertebral rotation and does not disappear with changes in posture. Fixed scoliosis is idiopathic (q.v.) in 65–80 per cent of cases. There are three main types. The infantile type occurs in boys under three and in 90 per cent of cases resolves spontaneously. The juvenile type affects 4-to-9-year-olds and tends to be progressive. The commonest is adolescent idiopathic scoliosis. Girls are affected in 90 per cent of cases and the incidence is 4 per cent. Treatment may be conservative with a Milwaukee or Boston brace, or surgical fusion may be needed if the curve is greater than 45 degrees. Scoliosis can occur as a congenital condition and in nuromuscular diseases where there is muscle imbalance such as Friedreich's ataxia.

KYPHOSIS is a backward curvature of the spine causing a hump back. It may be postural and reversible in obese people and tall adolescent girls who stoop but it may be fixed. Scheuermann's disease is the term applied to adolescent kyphosis. It is more common in girls. Senile kyphosis occurs in elderly people who probably have osteoporosis (bone weakening) (q.v.) and vertebral collapse.

DISC DEGENERATION is a normal consequence of ageing. The disc loses its resiliance and becomes unable to withstand pressure. Rupture (prolapse) of the disc may occur with physical stress. The disc between the fourth and fifth lumbar vertebrae is most commonly involved. The jelly-like central nucleus pulposus is usually pushed out backwards, forcing the annulus fibrosus to put pressure on the nerves as they leave the spinal canal.

Pain is felt in the back and in the distribution of the compressed nerve. If the disc prolapses forwards into the centre of the spinal canal, it may compress the cauda equina.

Treatment is bed rest with traction and pain relief. Rarely removal of the disc is needed. Compression of the cauda equina is a surgical emergency.

ANKYLOSING SPONDYLITIS is a rheumatic disease of young adults, mostly men. It is a familial condition which starts with lumbar pain and stiffness which progresses to involve the whole spine. The discs and ligaments are replaced by fibrous tissue making the spine rigid. Treatment is physiotherapy and anti-inflammatory drugs to try to keep the spine supple for as long as possible.

A National Association for Ankylosing Spondylitis has been formed which is open to those with the disease, their families, friends and doctors. (See APPENDIX 2: ADDRESSES.)

SPONDYLOSIS is a term which covers disc degeneration and joint degeneration in the back. Osteoarthritis is usually implicated. Pain is commonly felt in the neck and lumbar regions and in these areas the joints may become unstable. This may put pressure on the nerves leaving the spinal canal and in the lumbar region pain is generally felt in the distribution of the sciatic nerve – down the back of the leg.

In the neck the pain may be felt down the arm. Treatment is physiotherapy; often a neck collar or lumbar support helps. Rarely surgery is needed to remove the pressure from the nerves.

SPONDYLOLISTHESIS means that the spine is shifted forward. This is nearly always in the lower lumbar region and may be familial, or due to degeneration in the joints. Pressure may be put on the cauda equina. The usual complaint is of pain after exercise. Treatment is bed rest in a bad attack with surgery indicated only if there are worrying signs of cord compression.

SPINAL STENOSIS is due to a narrowing of the spinal canal which means that the nerves become squashed together. This causes numbness with pins and needles (paraesthia) in the legs. Computed tomography and nuclear magnetic resonance imaging scans can show the amount of cord compression. If improving posture does not help, surgical decompression may be needed.

WHIPLASH INJURIES occur to the neck usually as the result of a car accident when the head and neck are thrown backwards and then forwards rapidly. This causes pain and stiffness in the neck and the arm and shoulder may feel numb. Often a support collar relieves the pain but recovery commonly takes between 18 months to three years.

TRANSECTION OF THE CORD occurs usually as a result of trauma when the vertebral column protecting the spinal cord is fractured and becomes unstable. The cord may be concussed or it may have become sheared by the trauma and not recover (transected). Spinal concussion usually recovers after 12 hours. If the cord is transected the patient remains paralysed.

SPINNER'S FINGER is a cricket injury. Bowlers are liable to develop callosities (q.v.) of the fingers of the bowling hand. These tend to crack, and this is the condition known as spinner's finger.

SPIRAMYCIN is an antibiotic isolated from *Streptomyces ambofaciens*, which is useful in the treatment of certain cases of staphylococcal infection.

SPIRILLUM is a form of micro-organism of wavy or spiral shape. (See MICROBIOLOGY.)

SPIRIT is a strong solution of alcohol in water. (See ALCOHOL.) Proof spirit is one containing 57 per cent of alcohol by volume or 49 per cent by weight, and is so named because it can stand the proof of just catching fire. Rectified spirit contains 90 per cent of alcohol by volume or over 85 per cent by weight. Proof spirit is generally used in the preparation of tinctures. Spirits of various drugs contain a solution of any given drug in rectified spirit, examples include aromatic spirit of ammonia (sal volatile), and spirit of ether. Methylated spirit (also known as wood naphtha or wood spirit) is distilled from wood. When taken internally, it is a dangerous poison producing neuritis, especially neuritis of the optic nerves which may result in blindness. Methylated spirit is used to harden the skin for the prevention of bed sores and foot soreness.

SPIRITS consist of medicinal substances or flavouring agents dissolved in alcohol.

SPIROCHAETE is an order of bacteria which has a spiral form.

SPIROMETER A test of how the lung is working used to assess the effects of lung disease or the progress of treatment. The spirometer records the total volume of air breathed out – the forced vital capacity. The machine also records the volume of air breathed out in one second – the forced expiratory volume. In diseases such as asthma, in which the airways are obstructed, the ratio of the forced expiratory volume to the forced vital capacity is reduced.

SPIRONOLACTONE belongs to the group of substances known as spirolactones. These are steroids similar to aldosterone (q.v.) in structure which competitively act as inhibitors of it. They can thus antagonize the action of aldosterone in the renal tubules. As there is evidence that there is an increased output of aldosterone in oedematous conditions, such as congestive heart failure, which accentuates the oedema, spironolactone is used, along with other diuretics, in resistant cases of oedema – to antagonize the fluid-retaining action of aldosterone. (See DIURETICS.)

SPLANCHNIC means anything belonging to the internal organs of the body as distinguished from its framework.

SPLEEN is an organ deeply placed in the abdomen and is a major constituent of the reticulo-endothelial system (q.v.).

Position and size The spleen lies behind the stomach, high up on the left side of the abdomen, and corresponds to the position of the 9th, 10th, and 11th ribs, from which it is separated by the diaphragm. It is a soft, highly vascular, plum-coloured organ, and has a smooth surface, being almost completely covered by peritoneum. There are two wide peritoneal ligaments that support the spleen, the one attaching it to the stomach, the other to the kidney. Through the latter ligament the large vessels that supply the spleen with blood make their way. The size of the spleen varies widely. It is usually about 12·5 to 15 cm (5 to 6 inches) in length, and weighs about 170 grams or more. In diseased conditions the organ may reach a weight of 8 to 9 kg.

Structure The spleen is enveloped by peritoneal membrane beneath which is a strong elastic tunic, composed partly of fibrous tissue containing many elastic fibres, and partly of

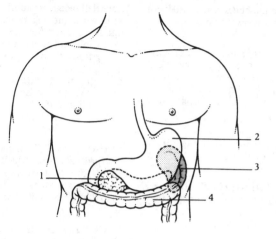

1 pancreas
2 stomach
3 spleen
4 transverse colon

Position of spleen in relation to other abdominal organs.

unstriped muscle. This elastic coat allows of the free expansion and contraction of the organ according to the varying amount of blood present in it. From the inner surface of the membrane fibrous partitions known as trabeculae run down into the substance and

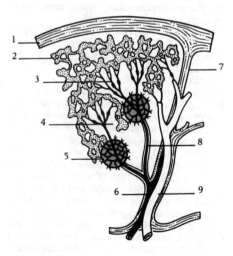

1 capsule
2 venous sinuses
3 arterial capillaries ending in sinuses
4 small arteries
5 Malphigi corpuscles
6 artery
7 trabecula of capsule
8 central artery of Malphigi corpuscle
9 vein

Cross-section of cone of tissue from spleen.

form a network in which the dark spleen pulp is contained. The pulp consists of delicate connective tissue fibres passing between the various trabeculae and of white and red blood corpuscles lying in this meshwork. The spleen is very vascular and venous blood leaves by the splenic vein and then enters the portal vein from the liver. There are also numerous lymphatics in the organ, which run in the trabeculae or surround the veins.

Functions The organ produces lymphocytes and acts as a reservoir of red blood cells for use in emergencies. It is also one of the sites for the manufacture of red blood cells in the fetus, but not after birth. Useless or worn-out red and white blood corpuscles and blood platelets are broken up by this organ. This results in the production of bilirubin (q.v.), which is conveyed to the liver, and of iron, which is used in the bone marrow for the production of new red blood cells.

SPLEEN, DISEASES OF In certain diseases associated with marked changes in the blood, such as leukaemia, and malaria, the spleen becomes chronically enlarged. In some of the acute infectious diseases, it becomes congested and acutely enlarged: for example, in typhoid fever, anthrax, and infectious mononucleosis. Rupture of the spleen may occur, like rupture of the other internal organs, in consequence of extreme violence, but in malarious countries, where many people have the spleen greatly enlarged and softened as the result of malaria, rupture of this organ occurs now and then as the result of some quite trivial blow upon the left side. The spleen, in consequence of its structure, bleeds excessively when torn, so that this accident is generally followed by collapse, signs of internal haemorrhage – and death if not dealt with promptly by operation.

SPLENECTOMY means removal of the spleen. This operation may be necessary if the spleen has been severely injured or in the treatment of the severe form of acholuric jaundice or auto-immune thrombocytopenic purpura. (See PURPURA.)

SPLENOMEGALY means enlargement of the spleen beyond its normal size.

SPLINTER HAEMORRHAGES are linear bleeds under the finger nails. Although they may result from injury they are a useful physical sign of infective endocarditis.

SPLINTS are supports for an injured or wounded part. They are most commonly employed in cases in which a bone is fractured, and consist then of some rigid substance designed to take the place of the broken bone in maintaining the shape of the limb, as well as to keep the broken ends at rest and in contact, and thus to ensure their union. Splints are most commonly made of wood either shaped to the limb or consisting merely of strips of wood about the width of the injured limb, and carefully padded with wool or similar soft material. Splints are also made of metal, poroplastic felt, leather, and cotton stiffened with plaster of Paris, as well as other materials. Splints may be improvized for first-aid out of walking-sticks, rifles, broom-handles, branches, folded-up newspapers, and in fact anything of suitable length and rigidity. (See FRACTURES.)

SPONDYLITIS is another name for arthritis of the spine. (See SPINE AND SPINAL CORD, DISEASES AND INJURIES OF.)

SPONDYLOLISTHESIS (see SPINE AND SPINAL CORD, DISEASES AND INJURIES OF).

SPONDYLOSIS (see SPINE AND SPINAL CORD, DISEASES AND INJURIES OF.)

SPONGIFORM ENCEPHALOPATHY A disease of the neurological system caused by slow virus (q.v.) Spongy degeneration of the brain with progresive dementia occurs. Known examples of the disorder in humans are Creutzfeldt-Jakob disease and kuru. Among animals scrapie in sheep and bovine spongiform encephalopathy (BSE) (q.v.) are caused by slow viruses. They are believed not be be transferable to humans, but research on this aspect is continuing.

SPORADIC is the term applied to cases of disease occurring here and there, as opposed to epidemic outbreaks.

SPORE Part of the life cycle of certain bacteria when the vegetative cell is encapsulated and metabolism falls to a low level. The spore is resistant to changes in the environment and, when these are unfavourable, the spore remains dormant; when they improve, it starts to grow. Certain dangerous bacteria, such as clostridium (q.v.), produce resistant ubiquitous spores so sterilization procedures need to be very effective.

SPOROZOA The name of a group of parasitic protozoa (q.v.) which includes the parasitic Plasmodium that causes malaria (q.v.). The life cycles of sporozoa are complex, often with sexual and asexual stages.

SPOROZOITES is one cell type of the many that are formed during the life cycle of sporozoans. In the case of malaria (q.v.) sporozoites pass into the salivary glands of the mosquito and and are the infecting agent of the human host when the insect next feeds on human blood.

SPORTS INJURIES, PREVENTION OF There are four basic rules for the prevention of sports injuries. (1) Be fit for the sport or game. (2) Obey the rules, written and unwritten. (3) Wear the right clothes and shoes. (4) Use common sense. The first of these is obvious. In amplification of the others, Dr John Williams, Medical Director of the Regional Sports Injuries Centre, Farnham Park Rehabilitation Centre, Slough, makes some cogent comments in his book, *Injury in Sport.*

'Obedience to the rules of the game (the spirit as well as the letter) is an essential component of injury prevention.' 'Reckless play is a not uncommon cause of injury.' 'It is the self-discipline of each individual player that finally determines whether sport will be safe or not. Since self-discipline is an essential component of sport, he who cannot discipline himself must be regarded as a menace on the sports field and if necessary permanently banned.'

Emphasis is laid on the importance of correct clothing and footwear. Clothing is often made of unsuitable material. Worn-out shoes and laces, jagged trouser buckles and sweat-rotted collars can all cause serious injury. The design of shoes may be faulty (e.g. the wrong siting of studs on football boots), or inappropriate (e.g. the same pair of shoes would not be suitable for running both on tartan track and asphalt road). A warning is given against advertisements that claim sports gear is in some way medically tested. Natural materials are better than man-made for clothes and footwear because of their absorbent and sweat evaporation qualities. When man-made fibres are worn, open weave is recommended.

All participants in sports should be immunized against tetanus (q.v.), and maintain this immunity by receiving regular booster injections every three years.

SPOTS BEFORE THE EYES can arise from a variety of causes including inflammation and bleeding in the eye, or preceding a retina detachment. They may also occur for a variety of totally harmless reasons.

SPOTTED FEVER (see MENINGITIS; EPIDEMIC; TYPHUS FEVER).

SPRAINS are injuries in the neighbourhood of joints, consisting usually in tearing of a ligament with effusion of blood. (See JOINTS, DISEASES OF.)

SPRUE, or PSILOSIS, is a disease occurring most commonly in patients in or from the tropics, and characterized by diarrhoea with large, fatty stools, anaemia, sore tongue, and weight loss. Its manifestations resemble those of non-tropical sprue, or gluten enteropathy, and coeliac disease (q.v.).

Causes Tropical sprue is thought to be due to an inborn error of metabolism, characterized primarily by an inability to absorb fats from the intestines. Its epidemiological pattern suggests that an infection such as dysentery may be the precipitating factor. Subsequently there is interference with the absorption of carbohydrates, vitamins, and minerals, leading to anaemia and hypocalcaemia.

Symptoms Of gradual or rapid onset, there is initial weakness, soreness of the tongue, difficulty swallowing, indigestion, and diarrhoea with pale frothy stools and poor appetite. Anaemia is typically macrocytic, and mild hypoglycaemia may occur. Untreated, the patient steadily loses weight and, unless appropriate treatment is started early, death may be expected because of exhaustion and some intercurrent infection.

Treatment This consists of bed rest, a high protein diet (initially skimmed milk), and treatment of the anaemia and any other deficiencies present. Minimum fat should be given to sufferers, who should also take folic acid and cyanocobalamin for the anaemia; large vitamin-B-complex supplements (such as Marmite®) are helpful. Vitamins A and D, together with calcium supplements, help to raise the concentration of calcium in the blood. A long convalescence is often required, which may lead to marked depression, and patients should be sent home to a temperate climate.

Non-tropical sprue is the result of gluten (q.v.) hypersensitivty and is treated with a gluten-free diet.

SPUTUM means material spat out of the mouth. It may consist of saliva from the mouth, of mucous secretions from the throat or back of the nose, but is generally expectorated by coughing from the lower air passages. (See EXPECTORATION.)

SQUINT or STRABISMUS A condition in which the visual axes of each eye are not directed simultaneously at the same fixation point (i.e. each eye is not pointing at the same object at the same time). Squints may be: (a) Paralytic, where one or more of the muscles, or their nerve supply is damaged; this type usually results in double vision. (b) Non-paralytic, where the muscles and nerves are normal. It is usually found in children. This type of squint can either result in poor vision, or occasionally may result from poor vision. Squints may be convergent (where one eye 'turns in') or divergent (one eye 'turns out'). Vertical squints can also occur but are less common. All squints should be seen by an eye specialist as soon as possible. Some squints can be corrected by exercises or spectacles; others require surgery.

STABS (see WOUNDS).

STAGHORN CALCULUS A branched renal stone formed in the image of the collecting system of the kidney. It fills the calyces and pelvis and is commonly associated with an infection of the urine, particularly *Proteus vulgaris*. The calculus may lead to pyonephrosis and an abscess of the kidney.

STAMMERING is a disruption of the forward flow of speech. The individual knows what he wants to say but he temporarily loses his ability to execute linguistically formulated speech. Stammering is characterized by a silent or audible involuntary repetition/prolongation of an utterance, be it a sound, syllable or word. Sometimes it is accompanied by accessory behaviours, or speech-related struggle. Usually there are indications or the report of an accompanying emotional state, involving excitement, tension, fear or embarrassment.

Idiopathic stammering begins sometime between the onset of speech and puberty, mostly between 2 and 5 years of age. Acquired stammering at a later age due to brain damage is rare. The prevalence of stammering (the percentage of the population actually stammering at any point in time) is approximately 0·9 per cent. Three times as many boys as girls stammer. About 70 per cent of stammering children recover with little or no therapy. Stammerers have not been shown to demonstrate differences in personality from non-stammerers. There are, however, indications that at least some stammerers show minimal differences from fluent speakers in cerebral processing of verbal material.

There is a genetic predisposition towards stammering. The risk of stammering among first-degree relatives of stammerers is more than three times the population risk. In 77 per cent of identical twins either both stammer or both are fluent. Only 33 per cent of non-identical twins agree in this way. As there are identical twins who differ for stammering, environmental factors must be important for some stammerers. There are relatively large numbers of stammerers in highly competitive societies, where status and prestige are important and high standards of speech competence are valued.

Different treatments have been demonstrated to produce considerable benefit, their basic outline being similar. A long period of time is spent in training stammerers to speak in a different way (fluency-shaping techniques). This may include slowing down the rate of speech, gentle onset of utterance, continuous flow with correct juncturing, etc. When the targets have been achieved within the clinic a series of planned speech assignments outside the clinic is undertaken. In these assignments, and initially in everyday situations, the fluency-enchancing techniques have to be used conscientiously. Gradually speech is shaped towards normality requiring less and less effort. Therapy may also include some work on attitude change (i.e. helping the client to see himself as a fluent speaker) and possibly general communicative skills training.

For information about organizations concerned with stammering, see APPENDIX 2: ADDRESSES.

STANNOSIS is the form of pneumoconiosis (q.v.) caused by the inhalation of stannous (tin) oxide, which occurs in tin ore mining.

STANOZOLOL (see ANABOLIC STEROIDS).

STAPES The innermost of the small trio of bones in the middle ear. It is stirrup shaped and articulates with the incus and is linked to the oval window of the inner ear. (See EAR.)

STAPHYLOCOCCUS is a genus of Gram-positive bacterium which under the microscope appears in small masses like bunches of grapes. It is one of the commonest infectious micro-organisms and is found, for example, in the pus discharged from boils (see MICROBIOLOGY).

STARCH is a substance belonging to that group of carbohydrates known as the amyloses. It is the form in which utilizable carbohydrate is stored in granules within the seeds and roots of many plants. It is converted into sugar when treated with heat in presence of a dilute acid. It is changed largely into dextrin when exposed to a considerable degree of dry heat, as in toasting bread; and a similar change into dextrin and malt-sugar takes place under the action of various ferments such as the ptyalin of the saliva. Starch forms a chief constituent of the carbohydrate foods (see DIET), and in the process of digestion the above-mentioned change takes place to prepare it for absorption. It is also slowly broken down in the process of cooking.

Starch is used externally to form a poultice for softening the skin in skin diseases. (See POULTICES.) It is also used as a constituent of dusting powders for application to chafed or irritable areas of the skin. (See CHAFING OF THE SKIN.) Starch enema is administered in inflammatory conditions of the bowel. (See ENEMA.)

STARVATION Partial starvation, as a method of treatment, is used in certain diseases associated with previous excess of food, particularly obesity. (See OBESITY.) When a person is completely deprived of food for a time, not only is there great loss of weight but the chemical processes of the body are altered, and a poisoning effect is produced by the formation of acetone and other ketone bodies. In cases of slow starvation, the vitality of the tissues is reduced and they become more liable to tuberculosis and other diseases. (See also FASTING.)

STASIS is a term applied to stoppage of the flow of blood in the vessels or of the food materials down the intestinal canal. (For Blood Stasis, see CIRCULATION, DISORDERS OF.)

STATUS ASTHMATICUS Repeated attacks of asthma, with no respite between the spasms, usually lasting for more than 24 hours. The patient is seriously distressed and, untreated, the condition may lead to death from respiratory failure and exhaustion. Corticosteroid treatment and other skilled medical care are urgently required.

STATUS EPILEPTICUS Repeated epileptic fits with no return to consciousness between them. Breathing stops between each fit and the body is deprived of oxygen which causes damage to the brain. Urgent medical attention is required to control the condition or the patient may die.

STEATOMA is a fatty, cystic tumour.

STEATORRHOEA is any condition characterized by the passing of stools containing an excess of fat. (See MALABSORPTION SYNDROME.)

STENOSIS is a term applied to a condition of unnatural narrowing in any passage or orifice of the body. The word is specially used in connection with the four openings of the heart at which the valves are situated. (See HEART DISEASES.)

STENT A surgical device used to assist the healing of an operative anastamosis – a joining up of two structures. A splint is left inside the lumen of a duct and this drains the contents.

STEREOGNOSIS means the faculty of recognizing the solidity of objects, and thus their nature, by handling them.

STEREOTAXIS is the procedure whereby precise localization in space is achieved. It is applied to that branch of surgery known as *stereotactic neurosurgery*, in which the surgeon is able to localize precisely those areas of the brain on which he wishes to operate.

STERILIZATION means either (1) the process of rendering various objects, such as those which come in contact with wounds, and various foods, free from microbes, or (2) the process of rendering a person incapable of producing children.

The manner of sterilizing bedding, furniture, and the like, after contact with a case of infectious disease, is given under DISINFECTION, whilst the sterilization of instruments, dressings, and skin surfaces, necessary before surgical procedures, is mentioned in the same article and also under ANTISEPTICS, ASEPSIS, and WOUNDS. For general purposes, one of the cheapest and most effective agents is boiling water or steam.

Use of sterilization Milk is the chief article of food that calls for special sterilization. With regard to other foods, ordinary cooking has this for one of its chief objects.

Method of sterilization One of the most effective modes is simply to boil the milk for a prolonged period in a covered pan; but this changes its taste considerably, and is therefore unsuitable for children and invalids, who tend to drink large amounts of milk.

Another method is to place the milk in a flask or bottle of which the neck is closed by a plug of cotton-wool, and set it in a pot of water, from the bottom of which it is separated by a triangle of wire or other means. The pot is placed on the stove and the water boiled for three-quarters of an hour, by which time the milk is sufficiently sterilized without appreciably affecting its taste. Many forms of sterilizer are on the market, but all depend upon this principle of having an inner vessel or set of bottles suspended within an outer pot containing water, which is boiled for three-quarters of an hour to one hour. Care must be taken that the milk is not uncovered, after being sterilized, until just before it is to be used.

Pasteurization is a slightly different method of treatment, which is sufficient to destroy the microbes that cause gastroenteritis, as well as those of many other diseases such as tuberculosis and typhoid fever, while preserving the natural state of the milk. (See PASTEURIZATION.)

Koch's method of sterilization is used in bacteriological investigation, where even the spores of bacteria must be destroyed. It is carried out by steaming the objects to be sterilized on three successive days. (See BACTERIOLOGY.)

BACTERIOLOGICAL STERILIZATION may be effected in many ways, and different methods are used in different cases, for it is evident that processes applicable to clothing or to a room may be quite unsuited for the sterilization of food.

SEXUAL STERILIZATION is being used to an increasing extent. In women it is performed by ligating, or cutting, and then tying the Fallopian tubes (q.v.), the tubes that carry the ovum from the ovary to the uterus. Alternatively the tubes may be sealed off by means of plastic and silicone clips or rings. It is usually performed through a small incision, or cut, in the lower abdominal wall. It has no effect on sexual or menstrual function, and, unlike the comparable operation in men, it is immediately effective. The sterilization is almost always permanent, but occasionally, for some unknown reason, the two cut ends of the Fallopian tubes reunite, and pregnancy is then again possible. Removal of the uterus and/or the ovaries also causes sterilization, but such procedures are only used when there is some special reason, such as the presence of a tumour.

The operation for sterilizing men is known as vasectomy (q.v.).

STERNUM is another name for the breastbone.

STEROID is the group name for compounds that resemble cholesterol chemically. The group includes the sex hormones, the hormones of the adrenal cortex, and bile acids.

STERTOR is a form of noisy breathing, similar to snoring (q.v.), and is usually due to flapping of the soft palate. Whereas ordinary snoring results from sleeping with the mouth open, stertor is the result of paralysis of the soft palate, which may be the result of a stroke, suffocation, concussion, drunkenness, or poisoning by opium (q.v.) or chloroform. In severe cases of paralysis, the tongue may loll back against the back of the throat, resulting in a very loud sound. In such cases breathing may be rapidly relieved by pulling the lower jaw forward, pulling the tongue out of the mouth, or turning the person on to one side.

Stertor should not be confused with sniffing or puffing breathing, though all three result from paralysis of different muscles. Stridor, or crowing breathing, due to spasmodic laryngeal narrowing, and wheezy, asthmatic breathing, due to narrowing of the bronchial tubes, should also be distinguished.

STETHOSCOPE is an instrument used for listening to the sounds produced by the action of the lungs, heart, and other internal organs. (See AUSCULTATION.)

STEVENS-JOHNSON SYNDROME This is a form of erythema multiforme which is characterized by annular lesions which can develop into blisters. In addition to the skin lesions in this syndrome there is severe involvement of the eyes and the mucosa, giving rise to ulceration. It is commonly a hypersensitivity reaction to drugs particularly the sulphonamide group of antibiotics.

STIFFNESS is a condition which may be due to a change in the joints, ligaments, tendons, or muscles, or to the influence of the nervous system over the muscles of the part affected. Stiffness is associated with various forms of rheumatism. Stiffness of the neck muscles resulting in bending backward the head, and of the hamstring muscles, causing difficulty in straightening the lower limbs, is a sign of meningitis. Stiffness or spasticity also occurs in certain diseases of the central nervous system.

STIGMA means any spot or impression upon the skin. The term, stigmas of degeneration, is applied to physical defects that are found in mentally handicapped persons. (See LEARNING DISABILITY.)

STILBOESTROL is a synthetic oestrogen. Its physiological actions are closely similar to those of the natural ovarian hormone, and it has the great merit of being active when taken by mouth. The drug may help patients suffering from cancer of the prostate, inducing in some cases regression of the primary tumour and of secondary deposits in bone. (See OESTROGEN.)

STILBOESTROL DIPHOSPHATE (see OESTROGEN).

STILET, or STILETTE, means the delicate probe or the wire used to clear a catheter or hollow needle.

STILLBIRTH A stillborn child is 'any child which has issued forth from its mother after the twenty-eighth week of pregnancy and which did not at any time after being completely expelled from its mother, breathe or show any other sign of life'. In England, in 1992, the number of stillbirths was 2,981. (See PERINATAL MORTALITY.)

STILL'S DISEASE, or JUVENILE RHEUMATOID ARTHRITIS, is a disease of childhood first described by Sir Frederic Still (1868–1941). The characteristic of the disease is that the arthritis is usually symmetrical. It tends to start in the fingers, which become spindle-shaped due to the swelling of the affected joints. It then spreads to involve other joints, practically always in a symmetrical manner, including the wrists, elbows, knees and ankles. Occasionally, only one joint, such as the knee, may be involved initially. The onset may be abrupt, with high temperature, or gradual. The cervical spine is often involved, leading to stiffness of the neck, and some of these cases go on to ankylosing spondylitis (see SPINE AND SPINAL CORD, DISEASES AND INJURIES OF). As a result of the child's not moving the affected joints because of the pain this causes, there is marked wasting of the muscles. The heart is seldom involved, but there is often a characteristic rash. The age of onset is usually between 2 and 5 years, and the disease is marked by repeated recurrences. The disease is usally self-limiting,

but tends to relapse and may persist for several years. Treatment is as for rheumatoid arthritis (q.v.) in the adult.

STIMULANTS are drugs and other agents employed to call forth special powers of the body or of individual organs in order to effect some special purpose or to offer resistance to some acute attack of disease. The use of stimulants presupposes a certain amount of reserve power on the part of the body or of the organ stimulated, which is lying dormant and requires an appropriate stimulus before it can be brought into action. In its broadest sense, the term stimulant includes all remedies which are not simply foods destined to supply the wear and tear of the body and to provide it with a store of energy-producing material. It also excludes remedies which have a sedative action upon the nervous system or other organs, and remedies which act directly upon the causes of disease without any reference to the body, such as antiseptics.

(For drugs which stimulate the intestines, see PURGATIVES; for those that stimulate the liver, see CHOLAGOGUES; for those that stimulate the kidneys, see DIURETICS.) Many substances, such as aromatics, spices, and bitters, stimulate the function of the stomach.

STINGS (see BITES AND STINGS).

STITCH is a popular name for a sharp pain in the side. It is generally due to cramp following unusually hard exertion (see CRAMP), but care must be taken that this trivial condition is not taken for pleurisy or for a fractured rib.

STOKES-ADAMS SYNDROME is a term applied to a condition in which slowness of the pulse is associated with attacks of unconsciousness, and which is due to a state of heart-block.

STOMA A stoma refers to an opening constructed when the bowel has to be brought to the skin surface to convey gastrointestinal contents to the exterior. It is derived from the Greek word meaning mouth. In the United Kingdom there are about 100,000 patients with a colostomy, 10,000 with an ileostomy and some 2,000 with a urostomy in which the ureters are brought to the skin surface. They may be undertaken because of malignancy of the colon or rectum or as a result of inflammatory bowel diseases such as Crohn's disease. Urostomies usually take the form of an isolated loop of ilium into which the ureters have been implanted and which in its turn is brought to the skin's surface. This is undertaken because of bladder cancer or because of neurological diseases of the bladder. The stomas drain into appliances such as disposable plastic bags. Most of the modern appliances collect the effluent of the stoma without any leak or odour.

Patients with stomas often find explanatory booklets helpful. *Living with your Colostomy* and *Understanding Colostomy* are examples. They are published by the British Colostomy Association (see APPENDIX 2: ADDRESSES).

STOMACH The stomach is a hollow dilation of the alimentary tract, shaped like a leather wine bottle, situated in the left upper abdomen and separated from the left lung and heart by the diaphragm. The stomach is divided into two distinct structural and functional parts – the corpus (body), which is the main part, and the antrum, which is the part furthest from the mouth. The oesophagus enters the right upper part of the corpus at an acute angle, which preserves the function of the lower oesophageal sphincter (and so prevents reflux of gastric contents into the oesophagus). The junction of the oesophagus and stomach is called the 'cardia'. At the far end of the stomach the gastric antrum ends in the pylorus, a thick circumferential muscular sphincter that separates the stomach from the duodenum.

The different functions of the corpus and the antrum of the stomach are reflected by differences in the structure of their mucosae linings. The mucosa of the corpus consists of oxyntic (acid-secreting) tubular glands which end in small pits in the mucosa. The cells lining the pits and necks of glands are columnar and produce mucus which covers the surface of the mucosa with a protective layer. Deeper within the glands lie parietal cells, which secrete hydrochloric acid and intrinsic factor (necessary for the absorption of vitamin B_{12} in the ileum (q.v.)), and also cells which secrete pepsinogen. The latter enzyme is converted into the digestive enzyme pepsin by hydrochloric acid.

Nerve plexuses, with parasympathetic (vagal) and sympathetic (q.v.) input occur especially between the longitudinal and circular muscle layers of the gastric wall. The vagal nerves (cranial nerve X) are important components of the parasympathetic nervous system (q.v.) and are connected to the nerves that supply the secreting cells as well as the stomach-wall muscles. Surgical section of the vagus nerves (vagotomy) reduces the stomach's ability to secrete gastric juice and also interferes with gastric motor function.

The mucosa of the antrum differs from corpus mucosa because the pyloric glands secrete mucus and a little sodium bicarbonate. More importantly, situated deep to the glands, are functionally significant endocrine cells, the most numerous of which are the G cells which secrete a hormone – gastrin – into the circulation. Its main function is to stimulate the parietal cells to secrete acid. The other important antral endocrine cells are the D cells, which secrete somatostatin, an important factor in the body's feedback control of gastric secretion.

Functions of the stomach The stomach has several functions. The corpus, including the fundus, acts as a distensible reservoir for food

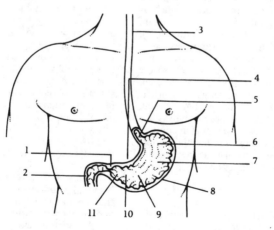

1 pyloric sphincter
2 duodenum
3 oesophagus
4 lesser curvature
5 cardiac orifice
6 fundus
7 cardia of stomach
8 greater curvature
9 pyloric part of stomach
10 pyloric canal
11 pylorus

Interior of stomach.

as it is processed and slowly propelled into the duodenum and small intestine for digestion.

The gastric juice in the stomach sterilizes swallowed food and saliva by killing contaminating bacteria. Patients with poor acid secretion suffer from colonization and overgrowth of oral and faecal bacteria in the stomach and intestine, as well as from increased susceptibility to infection with enteric pathogenic bacteria such as Salmonella (see FOOD POISONING) and Shigella (see DYSENTERY) organisms. These bacteria may cause chemical reactions that produce nitrogen compounds which are powerful carcinogens.

Pepsin is a protease enzyme active under acid conditions which starts the digestion of proteins in the stomach. The partly digested proteins then trigger the release of gastrin and other hormones from the small intestine. Pancreatic digestive enzymes are stimulated and the gall bladder discharges bile into the duodenum. Gastric acid stimulates the release of hormones from the duodenal lining, so stimulating further digestion.

Gastric juice also promotes the absorption of micronutrients – small amounts of essential ingredients. The most important is vitamin B_{12} (q.v.) which can only be absorbed in the presence of intrinsic factor, secreted by the stomach. Gastric juice also promotes the absorption of metal salts, especially iron and calcium. Malabsorption of both of these elements occurs, for example, after gastrectomy and results in anaemia and bone disease, such as osteomalacia (q.v.).

The antral part of the stomach has a motor function to grind and mix food (which is disturbed after surgical removal of the antrum, causing patients to develop severe indigestion). The antral mucosa releases hormones such as gastrin which stimulate gastric secretion and influence the function of organs such as the pancreas and colon. When excessive secretion of gastrin occurs, this results in general gastric hypersecretion, causing duodenal ulceration, severe oeosophagitis, and occasionally diarrhoea and steatorrhoea. The stomach controls body weight by adjusting an individual's appetite through complex control measures. Disruption of all of these functions occurs after gastrectomy.

STOMACH, DISEASES OF Gastritis is the description for several unrelated diseases of the gastric mucosa. Four principal aspects are important. First, infiltration of the mucosal surface cells and of the submucosa by neutrophil granulocytes (q.v.) indicates the presence of 'acute gastritis'. Infiltration with mononuclear cells, lymphocytes and plasma cells reflects 'chronic gastritis'. When the cellular infiltrate affects the superficial part of the mucosa, the term 'superficial' or 'mild' is added to the type of gastritis.

In addition, the glands of the gastric mucosa may atrophy; this 'atrophic gastritis' is a disorder of proliferation of unknown cause. While atrophic gastritis is usually patchy, a more complete and uniform type of atrophy, called 'gastric atrophy' characterizes a familial disease called pernicious anaemia (q.v.). The cause of the latter disease is not known but it may be an autoimmune disorder (q.v.).

ACUTE GASTRITIS is an inflammatory reaction of the gastric mucosa to various precipitating factors, ranging from physical and chemical injury to infections. Acute gastrits (especially of the antral mucosas) may well represent a reaction to infection by a bacterium called *Heliobacter pylori* (q.v.). The inflammatory changes usually go after appropriate antibiotic treatment for the *H. pylori* infection.

Acute and chronic inflammation occurs in response to chemical damage of the gastric mucosa. For example, reflux of duodenal contents may predispose to inflammatory acute and chronic gastritis. Similarly, multiple small erosions or single or multiple ulcers have resulted from consumption of chemicals, especialy aspirin and antirheumatic nonsteroidal anti-inflammatory drugs (NSAIDs) (q.v.).

Acute gastritis may cause anorexia, nausea, upper abdominal pain and, if erosive, haemorrhage. Treatment involves removal of the offending cause.

CHRONIC GASTRITIS Accumulation of cells called round cells in the gastric mucosal characterizes chronic gastritis. Most patients with chronic gastritis have no symptoms, and treatment of *H. pylori* infection usually cures the condition.

ATROPHIC GASTRITIS A few patients with chronic gastritis may develop atrophic gastritis. With or without inflammatory change, this disorder is common in Western countries. The incidence increases with age, and over 50 per cent of people over 50 may have it.

Functional changes and disease implications Since atrophy of the corpus mucosa results in loss of acid- and pepsin-secreting cells, gastric secretion is reduced or absent. Patients with pernicious anaemia or severe atrophic gastritis of the corpus mucosa may secrete too little intrinsic factor for absorption of vitamin B_{12} and so can develop severe neurological disease (subacute combined degeneration of the spinal cord).

Patients with atrophic gastritis often have bacterial colonization of the upper alimentary tract, with increased concentration of nitrite and carcinogenic N-nitroso compounds. These, coupled with excess growth of mucosal cells, probably result in cancer. In chronic corpus gastritis, the risk of gastric cancer is about 3–4 times that of the general population.

POSTGASTRECTOMY MUCOSA The mucosa of the gastric remnant after surgical removal of the distal part of the stomach is usually inflamed and atrophic and is also premalignant, with the risk of gastric cancer being very much greater than for patients with duodenal ulcer who have not had surgery.

STRESS GASTRITIS Acute stress gastritis develops, sometimes within hours, in individuals who have undergone massive physical trauma, burns (Curling ulcers), severe sepsis or major diseases such as heart attacks, strokes, intracranial trauma or operations (Cushing's ulcers). The disorder presents with multiple superficial erosions or ulcers of the gastric mucosa, with haematemesis (q.v.) and melaena (q.v.) and sometimes with perforation when the acute ulcers erode through the stomach wall. Treatment involves inhibition of gastric secretion with intravenous infusion of an H_2-receptor-antagonist drug such as ranitidine (q.v.) or famotidine (q.v.), so that the gastric contents remain at a near neutral pH. Despite treatment a few patients continue to bleed and may then require radical gastric surgery.

GASTRIC ULCER   Gastric ulcers were common in young women during the 19th century, markedly fell in frequency in many Western countries during the first half of the 20th century, but remained common in coastal northern Norway, Japan, in young Australian women, and in some Andean populations. During the latter half of this century, gastric ulcers have again become more frequent in the West, with a peak incidence between 55 and 65 years.

The cause is not known. The two factors most strongly associated with the development of duodenal ulcers – gastric acid production and gastric infection with *H. pylori* bacteria – are not nearly as strongly associated with gastric ulcers. The latter occur with increased frequency in individuals who take aspirin or NSAIDs. In healthy individuals who take NSAIDs, as many as 6 per cent develop a gastric ulcer during the first week of treatment, while in patients with rheumatoid arthritis who are being treated long term with drugs, gastric ulcers occur in 20–40 per cent. The cause is inhibition of the enzyme cyclo-oxygenase which in turn inhibits the production of repair-promoting prostaglandins (q.v.).

Gastric ulcers occur especially on the lesser curve of the stomach. The ulcers may erode through the whole thickness of the gastric wall, perforating into the peritoneal cavity or penetrating into liver, pancreas or colon.

Gastric ulcers usually present with a history of epigastric pain of less than one year. The pain tends to be associated with anorexia and may be aggravated by food, although patients with 'prepyloric' ulcers may obtain relief from eating or taking antacid preparations. Patients with gastric ulcers also complain of nausea and vomiting, and lose weight.

The principal complications of gastric ulcer are haemorrhage from arterial erosion or perforation into the peritoneal cavity resulting in peritonitis (q.v.), abscess or fistula.

Aproximately one in two gastric ulcers heal 'spontaneously' in 2–3 months. However, up to 80 per cent of the patients relapse within 12 months. Repeated recurrence and rehealing results in scar tissue around the ulcer, ultimately causing a circumferential narrowing, a condition called 'hour-glass stomach'.

The diagnosis of gastric ulcer is confirmed by endoscopy. All patients with gastric ulcers should have multiple biopsies to exclude the presence of malignant cells. Even after healing, gastric ulcers should be endoscopically monitored for a year.

Treatment of gastric ulcers is relatively simple. A course of an H_2 receptor antagonist (q.v.) heals gastric ulcers in 3 months. In patients who relapse, long-term indefinite treatment with an H_2 receptor antagonist such as ranitidine may be necessary since the ulcers tend to recur. Recently it has been claimed that gastric ulcers can be healed with a combination of a bismuth salt or a gastric secretory inhibitor, together with two antibiotics such as amoxycillin (q.v.) and metronidazole (q.v.). The long-term outcome of such treatment is not known.

CANCER OF THE STOMACH   Cancer of the stomach is common and dangerous and, world wide, accounts for approximately 1 in 6 of all deaths from cancer. There are marked geographical differences in frequency, with a very high incidence in Japan and low incidence in the USA. Studies have shown that environmental factors, rather than hereditary ones, are mainly responsible for the development of gastric cancer. Diet, including highly salted, pickled and smoked foods, and high concentrations of nitrate in food and drinking water, may well be responsible for the environmental effects.

Most gastric ulcers arise in abnormal gastric mucosa. The three mucosal disorders which especially predispose to gastric cancer include pernicious anaemia, postgastrectomy mucosa, and atrophic gastritis. Around 90 per cent of gastric cancers have the microscopic appearance of abnormal mucosal cells (and are called 'adenocarcinomas'). Most of the remainder look like endocrine cells of lymphoid tissue, although tumours with mixed microscopic appearance are common.

Early gastric cancer may be symptomless and, in countries like Japan with a high frequency of the disease, is often diagnosed during routine screening of the population. In more advanced cancers, upper abdominal pain, loss of appetite and loss of weight occur. Many present with obstructive symptoms, such as vomiting (when the pylorus is obstructed) or difficulty with swallowing. The diagnosis is made by endoscopic examination of the stomach and biopsy of abnormal-looking areas of mucosa. Treatment is surgical, often with additional chemotherapy.

STOMACH TUBE is a soft rubber or plastic tube with rounded end, and usually about 75 cm (30 inches) in length, which is used for washing out the stomach when it contains some poisonous material, or when it is dilated and filled with fermenting food. (See WASHING OUT STOMACH.) A narrower tube, 90 cm (36 inches) in length, is used for the purpose of obtaining a sample of gastric juice for examination. (See also TEST MEAL.) Such a tube can also be allowed to pass out of the stomach into the duodenum so that the contents of the upper part of the small intestine are similarly obtained for analysis.

STOMATITIS means inflammation of the mouth. (See MOUTH, DISEASES OF.)

-STOMY is a suffix signifying formation of an opening in an organ by operation: e.g. colostomy (q.v.).

STONE (see URINARY BLADDER, DISEASES OF; GALL-BLADDER, DISEASES OF).

STOOLS, or FAECES, consist of the remainder of the food after it has passed through the alimentary canal and been subjected to the action of the digestive juices, and after the nutritious parts have been absorbed by the intestinal mucous membrane. The stools also contain various other matters, such as pigment, derived from the bile, and large quantities of bacteria which are the main component of human stools. The stools are passed once daily by most people, but infants have several evacuations of the bowels in twenty-four hours and many adults may defaecate only two or three times weekly. Sudden changes in bowel habit, persistent diarrhoea or a change from the normal dark brown (caused by the bile pigment stercobilin) to very pale or very dark stools are reasons for seeking medical advice. Blood in the stools may be due to haemorrhoids (q.v.) or something more serious, and anyone with such symptoms should see a doctor.

Incontinence of the bowels, or inability to retain the stools, is found in certain diseases in which the sphincter muscles, that naturally keep the bowel closed, relax. It is also a symptom of disease in, or injury to, the spinal cord.

Pain at stool is a characteristic symptom of a fissure at the anus or of inflamed piles, and is usually sharp. Pain of a duller character associated with the movements of the bowels may be caused by inflammation in the other pelvic organs.

CONSTIPATION and DIARRHOEA are considered under separate headings.

STRABISMUS (see SQUINT).

STRANGULATION The constriction of a passage or tube in the body that blocks the blood flow and disturbs the working of the affected organ. It is usually caused by compression or twisting. Strangulation customarily occurs when part of the intestine (q.v.) herniates either inside the abdomen or outside as in an inguinal HERNIA (q.v.). If a section of the intestine twists this may strangulate and is known as a volvulus.

Strangulation of a person's neck either with a ligature or the hands obstructs the jugular veins in the neck preventing the normal outflow of blood from the brain and head. The trachea is also compressed, cutting off the supply of air to the lungs. The combination of these effects leads to hypoxia and damage to the brain. If not quickly relieved, unconsciousness and death follow. Strangulation may be deliberate or accidental – the latter being a particular hazard for children, for example, when playing with a rope. Removal of the constriction, artificial respiration, and medical attention are urgently necessary.

STRANGURY is a condition in which there is constant desire to pass water, accompanied by a straining sensation, though only a few drops can be voided. It is a symptom of inflammation situated in the kidneys, bladder or urinary passages.

STRAPPING means the application of strips of adhesive plaster, one overlapping the other, so as to cover a part and make pressure upon it. This method of treatment is used in cases of injury or disease when it is desired to keep a part at rest: for example, strapping may be applied to the chest in cases of pleurisy and fracture of the ribs. Also, it is often used to prevent the movement of joints which are sprained or otherwise injured.

STREPTOCOCCUS is a variety of Gram-positive bacterium which under the microscope has much the appearance of a string of beads. Most species are saprophytic (q.v.). A few are pathogenic (q.v.) and these include haemolytic types which can destroy red blood cells in a culture of blood agar. This offers a method of classifying the varying streptococcal strains. Alpha-haeomolytic streptococci are usually associated with bacterial endocarditis. Scarlet fever is caused by a β-haeomolytic streptococcus called *S. pyogenes*. *S. pneumonia*, also called pneumococcus, causes respiratory-tract infections, including pneumonia. *S. pyogenes* may on its own, or with other bacteria, cause severe necrotizing fasciitis or cellulitis in which oedema and death of subcutaneous tissues occur. The infection can spread very rapidly and, unless urgently treated with antibiotics and sometimes surgery, death may quickly result. This spread is related to the ability of *S. pyogenes* to produce toxic substances called exotoxins. Although drug-resistant forms are occurring, streptococcal infections usually respond to antibiotic treatment.

STREPTOKINASE is an enzyme produced by certain streptococci. It acts as a plasminogen (q.v.) activator, and hence enhances fibrinolysis (q.v.). It may be given as an infusion to treat severe thrombosis (q.v.) or embolism (q.v.), particularly when they occur in a limb, and in deep venous thrombosis. Being antigenic and very expensive it is rarely used for more than two days, and is followed by anticoagulation therapy. The chief risk is haemorrhage, so an antifibrinolytic such as aminocaproic acid should always be available.

STREPTOMYCIN is an anti-bacterial substance obtained from the soil mould, *Streptomyces griseus*. It was first isolated in 1944 by Dr Waksman in the United States of America. It was the first antibiotic to be effective against the tubercle bacillus.

Streptomycin has two disadvantages. The most important of these is the tendency of organisms to become resistant to it. This means that the administration of this antibiotic must be carefully supervized to ensure that correct dosage is being used. The other disadvantage is that streptomycin produces toxic effects, especially disturbance of the vestibular and hearing apparatus. This may result in deafness, giddiness, and tinnitus (q.v.). Whilst in many cases these toxic manifestations disappear when the antibiotic is withdrawn, they may be permanent. For this reason therefore streptomycin must always be used with special care.

STRESS FRACTURES are comparatively common in sportsmen. They tend to occur when an undue amount of exercise is taken: an amount of exercise which an individual is not capable of coping with in his (or her) state of training. The main initial feature is pain over the affected bone. This is usually insidious in onset, and worse at night and during and after exercise. It is accompanied by tenderness, and a lump may be felt over the affected site. X-ray evidence of them only appears after several weeks. Treatment consists of rest, some form of external support, and in the initial stage analgesics (q.v.) to deaden or kill the pain.

STRIAE ATROPHICAE is the term applied to atrophied strips of skin where this has been excessively stretched, as, for example, in pregnancy, when the greyish atrophied strips are known as STRIAE GRAVIDARUM.

STRICTURE means a narrowing in any of the natural passages of the body, such as the gullet, the bowel, or the urethra. It may be due to the development of some growth in the wall of the passage affected, or to pressure upon it by such a growth in some neighbouring organ, but in the majority of cases a stricture is the result of previous ulceration on the inner surface of the passage, followed by contraction of the scar. (See INTESTINE, DISEASES OF; URETHRA, DISEASES OF.)

STRIDOR is a noise associated with inspiration due to narrowing of the upper airway, in particular the larynx.

STROKE Stroke or cerebrovascular accident (CVA) is sudden damage to brain tissue caused either by a lack of blood supply or rupture of a blood vessel. The affected brain cells die and the parts of the body they control or receive sensory messages from cease to function.

Causes Blood supply to the brain may be interrupted by arteries furring up with atherosclerosis (q.v.) (which is accelerated by hypertension and diabetes, both of which are associated with a higher incidence of strokes) or being occluded by blood clots arising from distant organs such as infected heart valves or larger clots in the heart. Hearts with an irregular rhythm are especially prone to develop clots. Patients with thick or viscous blood, clotting disorders or those with inflamed arteries, e.g. in systemic lupus erythematosis, are particularly in danger of having strokes. Bleeding into the brain arises from areas of weakened blood vessels, many of which may be congenital.

Symptoms Minor episodes due to temporary lack of blood supply and oxygen (called transient ischaemic attacks or episodes (q.v.)) are manifested by short-lived weakness or numbness in an arm or leg and may precede a major stroke. Strokes cause sudden weakness or complete paralysis of the muscles controlled by the part of the brain affected as well as sensory changes, e.g., numbness or tingling. In the worst cases these symptoms and signs may be accompanied by loss of consciousness. If the stroke affects the area of the brain controlling the larynx and throat, the patient may suffer slurring or loss of speech with difficulty in initiating swallowing. When the face is involved the mouth may droop and the patient dribble. Strokes caused by haemorrhage may be preceded by headaches. Rarely, CVAs are complicated by epileptic fits. If, on the other hand, numerous small clots develop in the brain rather than one major event, this may manifest itself as a gradual deterioration in the patient's mental function, leading to dementia.

Investigations Tests on the heart or computed tomography or ultrasonic scans on arteries in the neck may indicate the original sites of distantly arising clots. Blood tests may show increased thickness or tendency to clotting and the diagnosis of general medical conditions can explain the presence of inflamed arteries which are prone to block. Special brain X-rays, e.g., computed tomography, show the position and size of the damaged brain tissue and can usually distinguish between a clot or infarct and a rupture of and haemorrhage from a blood vessel in the brain.

Management It is better to prevent a stroke than try to cure it. The control of a person's diabetes or high blood pressure will reduce the risk of a stroke. Anticoagulation treatment prevents the formation of clots and regular small doses of aspirin stop platelets clumping together to form plugs in blood vessels and both treatments reduce the likelihood of minor transient ischaemic episodes proceeding to a major stroke. Once the latter has occurred, there is no effective treatment to reduce the damage to brain tissue. Function will return to the affected part of the body only if and when the brain recovers and messages are again sent down the appropriate nerves. Simple movements are more likely to recover than delicate ones and sophisticated functions have the worst outlook. Thus, movement of the thigh may improve more easily than fine movements of fingers, and any speech impairment is more likely to be permanent. A rehabilitation team can help to compensate for any disabilities the subject may have. Physiotherapists maintain muscle tone and joint flexibility, whilst waiting for power to return; occupational therapists advise about functional problems and supply equipment to help patients overcome their disabilities; and speech therapists help with difficulties in swallowing, improve the clarity of remaining speech or offer alternative methods of communication. District nurses or home helps can provide support to those caring for victims of stroke at home. Advice about strokes may be obtained from the Stroke Association (see APPENDIX 2: ADDRESSES).

STROMA is the name applied to the tissue which forms the framework and covering of an organ.

STRONGYLOIDIASIS This infection is caused by nematode worms of the genus *Strongyloides* spp. – the great majority being from *S. stercoralis*. This helminth is present throughout most tropical and subtropical countries; a single case report has been made in England – about an individual who had not been exposed to such an environment. Larvae usually penetrate intact skin, especially the feet (as with hookworm infection). Unlike hookworm infection, eggs mature and hatch in the lower gastrointestinal tract; thus larvae can immediately re-enter the circulation in the colorectum or perianal region, setting up an auto-infection cycle. Therefore, infection can continue for the remaining lifespan of the individual. Severe malnutrition may be a predisposing factor to infection, as was the case in prisoners of war in south-east Asia during World War II (1939–45). Whilst an infected patient is frequently asymptomatic, heavy infection can cause jejunal mucosal abnormalities, and an absorptive defect, with weight loss. During the migratory phase an itchy linear rash (larva currens) may be present on the lower abdomen, buttocks, and groins; this gives rise to recurrent transient itching. In an immunosuppressed individual, the 'hyperinfection syndrome' may ensue; migratory larvae invade all organs and tissues, including the lungs and brain. Associated with this widespread infection, the patient may develop an *Enterobacteriacae* spp. septicaemia; this, together with *S. stercoralis* larvae, produces a meningoencephalitis. There is no evidence that this syndrome is more common in patients with HIV infection.

Diagnosis consists of visualization of *S. stercoralis* (larvae or adults) in a jejunal biopsy-section or aspirate. Larvae may also be demonstrable in a faecal sample, especially following culture. Eosinophilia may be present in peripheral blood, during the invasive stage of infection. Chemotherapy consists of albendazole. The formerly used benzimidazole compound, thiabendazole, is now rarely prescribed in an uncomplicated infection due to unpleasant side-effects. Even so, in the 'hyperinfection syndrome' it probably remains the more effective of the two compounds.

STRYCHNINE is an alkaloid derived from *Strychnos nux-vomca*, the seeds of an East Indian tree, as well as from the seeds of several other closely allied trees and shrubs. It is a white crystalline body possessed of an intensely bitter taste, more bitter perhaps than that of any other substance, and it is not very soluble in water. It stimulates all parts of the nervous system, and was at one time widely used for this purpose. Strychnine poisoning is fortunately rare. It shows itself in convulsions, which come on very speedily after the person has taken the poison. The mental faculties remain unaffected, and the symptoms end in death or recovery within a few hours.
Treatment The patient should be kept quiet. Artificial respiration may be necessary. At the earliest moment a benzodiazepine is injected intravenously in a large enough dose to stop the convulsions and put the patient to sleep. (See POISONS and APPENDIX 2: ADDRESSES.)

STUPOR (see UNCONSCIOUSNESS).

STUTTERING (see STAMMERING).

STYE (see EYE DISEASES).

STYPTICS are applications which check bleeding, either by making the blood-vessels contract more firmly or by causing rapid clotting in the blood. Some possess both modes of action.
Varieties Many substances have this action on account of their chemical or physical properties. Among them may be mentioned ice; hot water at 49 °C if brought directly in contact with the bleeding surface; perchloride of iron; acetate of lead and Goulard's water; nitrate of silver; sulphate of copper; sulphate of zinc; alum; tannin; hazeline; ergot; adrenaline; and Russell-viper venom.
Uses The use of styptics is described under HAEMORRHAGE.

SUB- is a prefix signifying under, near, or moderately.

SUBACUTE The description applied to a disease the duration of which lies between *acute* and *chronic*. An example is subacute endocarditis, a disorder that may not be diagnosed for several weeks or months, during which time it can severely damage valves in the heart.

SUBACUTE COMBINED DEGENERATION OF THE CORD is a degenerative condition of the spinal cord which most commonly occurs as a complication of pernicious anaemia. The motor and sensory nerves in the cord are damaged, causing spasticity of the limbs and an unsteady gait. Treatment is with vitamin B_{12} (see APPENDIX 5: VITAMINS; ANAEMIA).

SUBACUTE SCLEROSING PANENCEPHA-LITIS is a rare complication of measles due to infection of the brain with the measles virus. It develops two to eighteen years after the onset of the measles, and is characterized by mental deterioration leading on to convulsions, coma and death. The annual incidence in Britain is about 1 per million of the childhood population. The risk of its developing is five to twenty times greater after measles than after measles vaccination.

SUBARACHNOID HAEMORRHAGE is a haemorrhage into the subarachnoid space. It is usually the result of rupture of an aneurysm on the circle of Willis (q.v.).

SUBARACHNOID SPACE is the space between the arachnoid and the pia mater, two of the membranes covering the brain (q.v.).

SUBCLAVIAN is the name applied to a large artery and vein which pass to the upper arm between the collar bone and the first rib.

SUBCLINICAL A description of a disease that is suspected but which has not developed sufficiently or is too mild in form to produce clear signs and symptoms in an individual. Even so, damage may be caused to tissues and organs.

SUBCONSCIOUS is a state of being partially conscious, or the condition in which mental processes occur and outside objects and events are perceived with the mind nearly or quite unconscious of them. Such subconscious impressions or events may be forgotten at the time but may nevertheless exert a continued influence over the conscious mind, or may at a subsequent time come fully into consciousness. Much importance is attached to the influence of painful or unpleasant experiences which, though forgotten, continue to influence the mind, and these are held to be largely responsible for neurasthenic and similar states. This injurious influence is removed when the subconscious impressions come fully into consciousness and are then remembered and clearly seen in their relative importance.

SUBCUTANEOUS means anything pertaining to the loose cellular tissue beneath the skin: e.g. a subcutaneous injection. (See HYPODERMIC.)

SUBDURAL Relating to the space between the strong outer layer of the meninges, the membrane which cover the brain, and the arachnoid, which is the middle layer of the meninges. A subdural haemorrhage occurs when bleeding takes place into this space. The trapped blood forms a large blood clot or haematoma within the skull and this causes pressure on the underlying brain. Bleeding may occur slowly as the result of disease or suddenly as the result of injury. Headaches, confusion, and drowsiness result, sometimes with paralysis. Medical attention is required urgently if a serious haematoma occurs soon after injury. (See BRAIN.)

SUBINVOLUTION is a term used to indicate that the womb has failed to undergo the usual involution, or decrease in size, which naturally takes place within one month after a child is born.

SUBJECTIVE is a term applied to symptoms, and sensations, perceived only by the affected individual. For example, numbness is a purely subjective sensation, whilst the jerk given by the leg on tapping the tendon of the knee is an objective sign.

SUBLIMATION is the conversion of a solid substance into a vapour and its recondensation. The term is also used in a mental sense for the process of converting instinctive sexual desires to new aims and objects devoid of sexual significance.

SUBLUXATION means a partial dislocation, and is a term sometimes applied to a sprain.

SUBMUCOSA The layer of connective tissue that occurs under a mucous membrane – for example, in the intestinal wall.

SUBPHRENIC ABSCESS An abcess that develops under the diaphragm, usually on the right side of the abdomen between the liver and the diaphragm. The cause may be an organ that has perforated – for instance, a peptic ulcer in the stomach or intestine. An abscess may also occur after an abdominal operation, usually when the bowel or stomach has been operated on. Antibiotics and sometimes surgery are the method of treatment.

SUCCUSSION is a method of examination by shaking the body of a patient in order to elicit splashing sounds, with a view to determining the presence of gas and fluid in a cavity such as the interior of the stomach or the pleural cavity.

SUCKLING (see INFANT FEEDING; BREASTS, DISEASES OF).

SUCRALFATE is a drug that is proving of value in the treatment of peptic ulcer (q.v.).

SUCROSE, or CANE SUGAR (see SUGAR).

SUCTION The use of a reduction in pressure to clear away fluids or other material through a tube. Suction is used to remove blood from the site of a surgical operation. Suction is commonly necessary to remove secretions from the airways of newly born babies to help them breathe.

SUDDEN INFANT DEATH SYNDROME (SIDS), or cot death, refers to the unexpected death, usually during sleep, of an apparently healthy baby. Well over 1,500 such cases are thought to have occurred in the United Kingdom each year until 1992 when government advice was issued about laying babies on their backs. The figure is now below 500 and falling. Boys are affected more than girls, and over half these deaths occur between 2 and 6 months. More common in lower social classes, the incidence is highest in the winter, and most of the infants have been bottle fed.

Causes Unknown, possible multiple aetiology. Prematurity and low birth weight may play a role. The sleeping position of a baby and an over-warm environment may be major factors, since deaths have fallen sharply since mothers were officially advised to place babies on their backs and not to overheat them. Some deaths are probably the result of respiratory infections, usually viral, which may stop breathing in at-risk infants, while others may result from the infant's smothering in a soft pillow. Milk allergy is a possible factor, as may be a sudden disturbance of fluid balance resulting from bottle feeding. Other possible factors include vitamin E deficiency, or smoking, drug addiction or anaemia in the mother. Help and advice may be obtained from the Foundation for the Study of Infant Deaths (see APPENDIX 2: ADDRESSES).

SUDEK'S ATROPHY Osteoporosis (q.v.) in the hand or foot which develops quickly as a result of injury, infection or malignant growth.

SUDORIFICS are drugs and other agents which produce copious perspiration.

SUFFOCATION (see ASPHYXIA; CHOKING).

SUGAR is a substance containing carbon, hydrogen, and oxygen, and belonging therefore to the chemical group of carbohydrates. This group includes three subdivisions:

(1) Monosaccharides ($C_6H_{12}O_6$)
   e.g. Glucose, or dextrose, or grape sugar.
        Fructose, or laevulose, or fruit sugar.
        Galactose.
(2) Disaccharides ($C_{12}H_{22}O_{11}$)
   e.g. Sucrose, or cane sugar, or beet sugar.
        Lactose or milk sugar.
        Maltose or malt sugar.
(3) Polysaccharides ($C_6H_{10}O_5$)
   e.g. Starch.
        Glycogen or animal starch.

Glucose, also known as grape sugar because it is found in various kinds of fruit, including grapes, is the form of sugar produced by the tissues and excreted in large amount by the kidneys in diabetes mellitus.

Sucrose is widely distributed through the vegetable kingdom, though it is specially plentiful in the juice of the sugar-cane, beetroot, and maple. When taken as a food, it is converted by the digestive juices into glucose before it is absorbed, this process being known as inversion. It is a valuable food, being utilized in the production of heat and energy, although it is also to a certain extent a tissue-builder so far as fat is concerned. It is to be avoided by people who tend to get fat as well as by diabetics.

Lactose is found in milk, and it is to the fermentation of this sugar and consequent production of lactic acid by certain bacteria that the souring of milk is due. The extent to which it is present in the milk of different animals is mentioned under INFANT FEEDING. It has little sweetening power compared with cane sugar, but it is used sometimes as a laxative.

Maltose is produced by the action of the enzyme, diastase, upon the starch contained in barley, and also by the ferments of the saliva and pancreatic juice, and is still further changed by the intestinal ferments into glucose before it is absorbed.

Invert sugar is a natural mixture of dextrose and laevulose resulting from a chemical decomposition of cane sugar or of starch.

Starch is mentioned under a separate heading, and its use as a food under DIET and CEREAL.

The energy-producing value of sugars generally is taken as being, on the average, 4 Calories for each gram of sugar.

SUICIDE (see under MENTAL ILLNESS).

SULCUS is the term applied to any groove or furrow, but especially to a fissure of the brain.

SULFADOXINE is a long-acting sulphonamide (q.v.) which along with pyrimethamine is used in the prevention of malaria (see FANSIDAR), although in many areas in which it is endemic the malaria parasite is resistant to the combination.

SULINDAC is a drug of value in the treatment of rheumatic conditions. (See NON-STEROIDAL ANTI INFLAMMATORY DRUGS.)

SULPHADIAZINE is one of the sulphonamides. It is a highly active drug and in moderate dosage produces a high and persistent blood concentration. It is relatively non-toxic and is particularly useful in the treatment of meningitis and in preventing the recurrence of rheumatic fever (q.v.).

SULPHADIMIDINE is comparable in activity to sulphadiazine, and has the advantage of being even more non-toxic and of producing higher blood concentrations. Used for treating urinary infections and meningococcal meningitis.

SULPHAEMOGLOBIN is an abnormal pigment sometimes found in the blood as a result of the interaction of certain drugs derived from aniline, such as phenacetin and acetanilide.

SULPHAMETHOXAZOLE is one of the long-acting sulphonamides. It is related to sulphafurazole, has a duration of action of 12 hours, and is effective against streptococci. Combined with trimethoprim (as co-trimoxazole) there is a synergistic effect. Increasing bacterial resistance to sulphonamides and the incidence of side-effects are reducing the value of these drugs.

SULPHANILAMIDE, or p-aminobenzene-sulphonamide, is a drug the discovery of which is one of the most important in medicine in the twentieth century. It was the first of the sulphonamide drugs. In 1935 the German chemist, Gerhard Domagk, announced the discovery of the effect of prontosil on streptococci. It was later found that this action was due to conversion in the body of prontosil into sulphanilamide, which acts by inhibiting the growth of various bacteria, especially the ubiquitous and dangerous *Streptococcus haemolyticus.* Its use has been overtaken by other sulphonamides and by antibiotic drugs. (See also SULPHONAMIDE.)

SULPHASALAZINE is a sulphonamide which is of value in the treatment of ulcerative colitis and rheumatoid arthritis.

SULPHINPYRAZONE is a derivative of phenylbutazone which is of value in the treatment of gout.

SULPHONAMIDE A drug having the sulphonamide grouping – SO_2NH_2. In 1935, Gerhard Domagk, a German chemist, announced the discovery of the effect of prontosil on streptococci. Subsequent work showed that this action was due to the conversion in the body of prontosil to sulphanilamide. The action of the sulphonamides is bacteriostatic and not bactericidal: i.e. they do not directly kill the bacteria but so interfere with their growth that they are unable to multiply. This action of the sulphonamides is now believed to be due to the similarity of their chemical structure to that of p-aminobenzoic acid. This latter substance is essential for the growth of many bacteria. If the bacteria are surrounded by a sulphonamide in greater concentration than p-aminobenzoic acid, then the bacteria take up the sulphonamide. This interferes with their development and they therefore never mature; nor are they able to reproduce themselves. Although the sulphonamides have been largely replaced by other antibiotics in the treatment of infections, they still have a useful role in antibacterial therapy.

SULPHONES are a group of drugs allied to the sulphonamides. They are used in the treatment of leprosy. The members of this group include dapsone (q.v.).

SULPHONYLUREAS are sulphonamide derivatives which lower the blood sugar when they are given by mouth by enhancing the production of insulin. They are effective only when some residual pancreatic beta cell function is present. All may lead to a hypoglycaemia if given in overdose and this is particularly common when long-acting sulphonylureas are given to elderly patients. Tolbutamide (q.v.) was the first of the sulphonlyurea drugs. It has a short duration of action and is usually given twice daily. Chlorpropamide (q.v.) has a more prolonged action and only needs to be given once daily. Other oral hypoglycaemic agents of this family include glibenclamide, which has a duration of action intermediate between tolbutamide and chlorpropamide. Other sulphonlyureas include acetohexamide, glibornuride, gliclazide, glipizide, gliquidone and tolazamide. Glymidine is a related compound with a similar action to the sulphonylureas. It is particularly useful in patients who are hypersensitive to sulpho-nylureas.

Sulphonylureas are best avoided in patients who are overweight as they tend to stimulate the appetite and aggravate obesity. They should be used with caution in patients with hepatic or renal disease. Side-effects are infrequent and usually not severe, the most common being epigastric discomfort with occasional nausea, vomiting and anorexia. In about 10 per cent of patients chlorpropamide and tolbutamide may cause facial flushing after drinking alcohol (see DIABETES MELLITUS). Some patients are hypersensitive to oral hypoglycaemic agents and develop rashes which may progress to erythema multiforme and exfoliative dermatitis. These reactions usually appear in the first 6 to 8 weeks of treatment.

SULPHUR, in chemical combinations (sulphides and sulphates), has disinfectant and antiparastitic powers, and is used in low concentrations as a topical treatment for various skin diseases. It is available in several commercial preparations for acne (q.v.), the aim being to produce a keratolytic (peeling) and bacteriostatic effect. Although topical treatment is of doubtful value in rosacea (q.v.), weak sulphur creams are occasionally prescribed for nocturnal use. In the treatment of scabies (q.v.), 2·5 per cent sulphur ointment is often recommended for infants. Other applications of sulphur are not generally recommended.

SULPHURIC ACID, or OIL OF VITRIOL, is, in its undiluted state, one of the most powerful of the mineral acids. It is a heavy, colourless liquid of oily consistence and is largely used in various manufacturing operations, so that poisoning by sulphuric acid is not uncommon. It chars any organic substance with which it is brought in contact, and acts as a violent corrosive poison. The treatment of sulphuric acid poisoning is that for corrosive poisons generally: e.g. to administer weak alkalis such as baking soda, milk, egg white or water followed by gastric lavage (see APPENDIX 1: BASIC FIRST AID).

SULPHUROUS ACID is a saturated solution of sulphur dioxide. It has an extremely pungent odour and strong disinfectant power.

SUMMER DIARRHOEA (see DIARRHOEA; INFANT FEEDING).

SUNBURN This term includes various sequelae resulting from skin exposure to the sun's rays – the most important of which is ultraviolet (UV) light (q.v.). Effects are far more common in fair-skinned individuals than in those with brown and black skins; relative protection is afforded by the pigment melanin (q.v.). UV light causes thickening of the superficial layer of the skin. Physiological production of melanin is preceded by skin reddening, due to dilatation of the blood vessels (erythema); this begins several hours after initial exposure. Two to three days later, it is gradually replaced by tanning or darkening – the depth of which depends on length of exposure and intensity of sunlight. Overexposure to UV light produces itching and tingling; the superficial layer of skin becomes swollen, and is followed by blister-formation and peeling (desquamation). In a severely affected person, systemic symptoms – including headache – may supervene; these are accompanied by fever. Prolonged exposure, especially in the light-skinned individual, can predispose to skin cancer (melanoma (q.v.)). Someone who has been sunburned should avoid further exposure to the sun's rays; itching and tingling may be alleviated by the application of calamine lotion. Prevention depends on avoiding excessive exposure to the sun's rays – especially by those who are light-skinned. In areas where sunlight intensity is high, an individual should increase his or her exposure slowly, bearing in mind that those areas of the body not normally exposed to UV light are most susceptible. A range of proprietary protective suncreams is available; these are graded to the degree of protection required, but they do not necessarily offer complete protection. Sunscreen products must be applied regularly and those exposed to the sun should still take sensible precautions including the use of protective head gear.

SUPER- is a prefix signifying above or implying excess.

SUPINATION means the turning of the forearm and hand so that the palm faces upwards.

SUPINE Lying on the back, face upwards. or the position of the forearm where the hand lies face upwards.

SUPPOSITORY is a small conical mass made of oil of theobroma, to which white beeswax is sometimes added, or glycerin-jelly, and containing drugs intended for introduction into the rectum. This method of using drugs, which is more popular on the Continent than in the United Kingdom, may be chosen for various reasons. For example, the suppository, as in the case of soap or glycerin suppositories, may be used to produce an aperient action. Other suppositories, such as those of morphine, are used to quiet pain and check the action of the bowels. Others are used for the sake of their influence on neighbouring organs.
Method of use The suppository is placed with its pointed end against the anus and with a firm but gentle screwing movement is pushed upwards. With the point of the forefinger, it must be pushed onwards for about 25 mm (1 inch), past the sphincter muscle, otherwise it will not be retained. It must be quickly introduced, as the material of which it is composed rapidly softens when brought into contact with the body. It may be retained in position by crossing the legs or lying on the side. To facilitate insertion it may be lubricated with a small amount of olive oil before insertion.

SUPPRESSION (1) The stopping of any physiological activity. (2) A psychological defence mechanism by which an individual intentionally refuses to acknowledge an idea or memory that he finds distasteful or unpleasant. (3) A treatment that stops the visible signs of an illness or holds back its usual progress.

SUPPURATION means the process of pus formation. When pus forms on a raw surface the process is called ulceration, whilst a deep-seated collection of pus is known as an abscess. (For more detailed information, see ABSCESS; INFLAMMATION; PHAGOCYTOSIS; ULCER; WOUNDS.)

SUPRA- is a prefix signifying above or upon.

SUPRAPUBIC operation is one in which the abdomen is opened in its lower part, immediately above the pubic bones. (See LITHOTOMY.)

SUPRARENAL GLANDS, (see ADRENAL GLANDS).

SURAMIN is the *British Pharmacopoeia* name for a drug which has been much used, and with success, in the treatment of sleeping sickness (q.v.).

SURFACTANT is a surface-active agent lining the alveoli of the lungs, which plays an essential part in respiration (q.v.) by preventing the alveoli collapsing at the end of expiration. Absence, or lack, of surfactant is one of the factors responsible for hyaline membrane disease (q.v.), and it is now being used in the treatment of this condition by means of instillation into the trachea.

SURROGATE is a term applied in medicine to a substance used as a substitute for another.

SUSCEPTIBILITY A reduced ability to combat an illness, usually an infection. The patient may be in poor general health or immunization or disease may have affected his defence mechanisms. For example, a person with AIDS (q.v.) is particularly susceptible to infection.

SUTURE is the name given either to the close union between two neighbouring bones of the skull, or to the series of stitches by which a wound is closed. (See WOUNDS.)

SWAB is a term applied to a small piece of gauze, lint, or similar material used for wiping out the mouth of a helpless patient or for drying out a wound. The term is also applied to a tuft of sterilized cotton-wool wrapped round a wire and enclosed in a sterile glass tube used for obtaining matter or membrane from the throat, from wounds, or the like, in order that this may be subjected to bacteriological examination.

SWAN-GANZ CATHETER is a flexible tube with a double lumen and a small balloon at its distal end. It is introduced into a vein in the arm and advanced until the end of the catheter is in the right atrium. The balloon is then inflated with air through one lumen and this enables the blood stream to propel the catheter through the right ventricle to the pulmonary artery. The balloon is deflated and the catheter can then record the pulmonary artery pressure. When the balloon is inflated the tip is isolated from the pulmonary artery and measures the left atrial pressure. These measurements are important in the management of patients with circulatory failure as under these circumstances the central venous pressure or the right atrial pressure is an unreliable guide to fluid replacement.

SWEAT (see PERSPIRATION).

SWEAT GLANDS (see SKIN).

SWEETBREAD is a popular term applied to several glands used for food, including the thymus gland of young animals (neck sweetbread), the pancreas (stomach sweetbread), and the testis.

SYCOSIS is a skin disease in which the hair follicles, especially of the chin, are inflamed, forming pustules round the hairs, surrounded by a swollen and reddened area of skin. The disease is directly due to infection of the hair follicles with staphylococcus or ringworm. The infection is generally attributed to a barber's utensils, and the condition is sometimes known as barber's itch, foul shave, or ringworm of the beard. (For treatment, see IMPETIGO; RINGWORM.)

SYDENHAM'S CHOREA Also called St Vitus dance, this type of chorea (q.v.) is a disease of the central nervous system that occurs after rheumatic fever (q.v.) – up to six months later – and is probably an inflammatory complication of a β-haemolytic streptococcal (q.v.) infection. The patient presents with jerky, purposeless, involuntary movements of a limb and tongue, similar to the symptoms of cerebral palsy. Chorea is best treated as a transitory reversible form of cerebral palsy. The disorder usually lasts six to eight months and residual symptoms are rare.

SYMPATHETIC is a term applied to certain diseases or symptoms which arise in one part of the body in consequence of disease in some distant part. Inflammation may arise in one eye, in consequence of injury to the other, by the spread of organisms along the lymphatic channels connecting the two, and is then known as sympathetic inflammation. Pain also may be of a sympathetic nature. (See PAIN.)

SYMPATHETIC SYSTEM is part of the autonomic nervous system (q.v.). It consists of scattered collections of grey matter known as ganglia, united by an irregular network of nerve-fibres, those portions where the ganglia are placed most closely and the network of fibres is specially dense being known as plexuses. The chief part of the sympathetic system consists of two ganglionated cords that run through the neck, chest, and abdomen, lying close in front of the spine. (For further details, see NERVES.)

SYMPATHOMIMETIC DRUGS are those producing an effect comparable to those produced by stimulation of the sympathetic nervous system: e.g. adrenaline (q.v.).

SYMPHYSIS An anatomical description of a joint in which two bones are connected by strong fibrous cartilage. One example is the joint between the two pubic bones in the front of the pelvis.

SYMPTOM is a term applied to any evidence of disease. The term, physical sign, is generally applied to evidence of disease of which the patient does not complain but which is elicited upon examination. For the symptoms indicative of the various diseases see under the headings of each disease.

SYN- is a prefix signifying union.

SYNAPSE is the term applied to the anatomical relation of one nerve-cell with another which is effected at various points by contact of their branching processes. The state of shrinkage or relaxation at these points (synapses) is supposed in some cases to determine the readiness with which a nervous impulse is transmitted from one part of the nervous system to another. Many drugs act upon the nervous system through their effect in closing or widening these junctions.

SYNCOPE, or fainting, is a loss of consciousness due to a fall in blood pressure. This may result because the cardiac output has become reduced or because the peripheral resistance provided by the arterioles has decreased. The simple faint or vaso-vagal attack is a result of a failure to maintain an adequate venous return of blood to the heart. This is likely to occur after prolonged periods of standing, particularly if one is standing still or if the climatic conditions are hot. It can also result from an unpleasant or painful experience. Pallor, sweating and a slow pulse are characteristic. Recovery is immediate when the venous return is restored by lying flat. Syncope can also result when the venous return to the heart is impaired as a result of a rise in intra-thoracic pressure. This may happen after prolonged vigorous coughing, the so-called cough syncope, or when elderly men with prostatic hypertrophy strain to empty their bladder. This is known as micturition syncope. Syncope is particularly likely to occur when the arterial blood pressure is unusually low. This may result from overtreatment of hypertension with drugs or it may be the result of diseases, such as Addison's disease, which are associated with low blood pressures. It is important that syncope is distinguished from epilepsy.

SYNDACTYLY is the condition which a child is born with, in which two or more fingers or toes are fused together to a varying extent. The condition is popularly known as webbed fingers or toes (q.v.).

SYNDROME is a term applied to a group of symptoms occurring together regularly and thus constituting a disease to which some particular name is given: e.g. *Cushing's Syndrome* comprising obesity, hypertension, purple striae and osteoporosis; *Korsakoff's Syndrome*, of loss of appreciation of time and place combined with talkativeness, forming signs of alcoholic delirium.

SYNECHIAE Adhesions between the iris and adjacent structures, e.g. cornea, lens. They usually arise as a result of inflammation of the iris.

SYNERGIST (1) A muscle that works in concert with an agonist muscle to perform a certain movement. (2) An agent, for example a drug, that acts with another to produce a result that is greater than adding together the separate effects of the two agents. Synergism in drug treatment may be beneficial as in the case of combined levodopa and selegiline, a selective monoamine oxidase inhibitor (q.v.), in the treatment of Parkinson's disease (q.v.). It may be potentially dangerous, however, as when monoamine oxidase inhibitors boost the effects of barbiturates (q.v.).

SYNOSTOSIS is the term applied to a union by bony material of adjacent bones normally separate.

SYNOVIAL MEMBRANE forms the lining of the soft parts that enclose the cavity of a joint. (See JOINTS.)

SYNOVITIS means inflammation of the membrane lining a joint. It is usually painful and accompanied by effusion of fluid within the synovial sac of the joint. It is found in acute rheumatism, various injuries and inflammations of joints, and in the chronic form in tuberculosis. (See JOINTS, DISEASES OF.)

SYNTHETIC is a term applied to substances produced by chemical processes in the laboratory or by artificial building up.

SYPHILIS is a contagious disease of slow development, which, at its start, shows a characteristic sore at the site of infection, later brings on constitutional effects resembling those of other infectious diseases, and at a still later period produces certain changes in the central nervous system, the arteries and elsewhere. Because, in the majority of cases the disease is acquired as a result of sexual intercourse with an infected individual, it is classed as one of the *venereal* diseases, or sexually transmitted diseases as they are now known. Syphilis affects only human beings, though it has been experimentally produced in anthropoid apes.

The disease seems to have first attracted public attention about or soon after the year 1494 in consequence of a severe and widespread outbreak among the French soldiers then occupied in the siege of Naples. An association with martial activity has persisted ever since. Thus it has been estimated that during the 1914–18 War a quarter of the armies in Europe were incapacitated by syphilis and gonorrhoea. For long it was known as the Neapolitan disease, French Pox, or Great Pox; and, in consequence probably of the licentiousness and the want of cleanliness that then prevailed, it spread in epidemic form. Later, it came to be called syphilis, the name being derived from that of the chief character in a Latin poem published by Fracastoro in 1530. It has been suggested that the disease existed in ancient times among the natives of America, and that the infection was brought to Europe by the followers of Columbus, but there are also grounds for supposing that the disease occurred among the Eastern races in ancient times, although it was most likely often confused with leprosy and tuberculosis. Today, according to the World Health Organization, around 40 million new cases are notified annually in the world, and, according to many, this is an underestimate.

Causes The causative organism is the *Treponema pallidum*, a long, thread-like wavy organism with pointed tapering ends. It is found in large numbers in the sores in the primary stage of the disease and in the skin lesions in the secondary stage.

The number of cases of infectious syphilis reported in England in the year ending 30 June 1992, was around 338, while the total number of people with the disease was 1,312.

Syphilis may be *acquired* from people already suffering from the disease, or it may be *congenital*. The acquired form is usually got by sexual intercourse, but it may also result from kissing or from contact with a sore upon another person through some wound or abrasion. The epithelium covering the general surface of the skin seems to be an efficient protection, but the infective material apparently has the power of penetrating mucous membranes. The acquired form of the disease is infectious from contact with sores, both in its primary and secondary stages; whilst infants suffering from the congenital form are also highly infectious. Accordingly any one frequently handling such an infant runs great risk of infection, although the mother may handle the babe with impunity (Colles' Law).

Symptoms The *acquired form* of the disease is commonly divided into three stages – PRIMARY, SECONDARY, and TERTIARY, although in many cases the tertiary stage is wanting, whilst in others there is no dividing line between the secondary and tertiary symptoms. The disease presents great variations of intensity, being occasionally of a 'malignant' type, in which widespread ulceration speedily comes on and even causes death; and in other cases showing little more than a slight skin eruption. There are several laboratory tests for confirming the diagnosis.

The incubation period ranges from 10 to 90 days, though most frequently it occupies about four weeks. Then a small ulcer appears at the site of infection, which is accompanied by a typical cartilaginous hardness of the tissues immediately round and beneath it, and characterized by its resistance to all healing treatment. This, which is known as the PRIMARY SORE (or *chancre*), may be very much inflamed, or it may be so small and occasion so little trouble as to pass almost or quite unnoticed. A few days after this sore has appeared, the lymphatic glands in its neighbourhood, and later those all over the body, become swollen and hard. This condition lasts for several weeks as a rule, and then the sore slowly heals and the glands subside. After a variable period, usually about two months from the date of infection, the SECONDARY SYMPTOMS appear and resemble the symptoms of an ordinary fever in so far as they include rise of temperature and feverishness, loss of appetite, vague pains through the body, and a faint red rash seen best upon the front of the chest. The duration of this stage is largely dependent upon the efficiency with which it is treated.

In untreated or inadequately treated cases manifestations of the TERTIARY STAGE develop after the lapse of some months or years. These consist in the growth, here and there throughout the body, of masses of granulation tissue known as *gummas*. These gummas may appear as hard nodules in the skin, or form tumour-like masses in the muscles, or cause great thickening of bones, or they may develop in the brain and spinal cord, where their presence causes very serious symptoms. Gummas yield readily, as a rule, to appropriate treatment, and generally disappear speedily.

Still later effects are apt to follow, such as disease of the arteries, leading to aneurysm (see ARTERIES, DISEASES OF; ANEURYSM), to stroke, and to early mental failure (see MENTAL ILLNESS); also certain nervous diseases, of which tabes dorsalis and general paralysis are the chief.

The *congenital form* of syphilis, now rare, may affect the child before birth, leading then as a rule to miscarriage, or to a stillbirth if born at full time. Or he (or she) may show the first symptoms a few weeks after birth, the appearances then corresponding to the secondary manifestations of the acquired form.

Treatment Any person who suffers from this disease forms a source of infection, and should take precautions not to spread it. Penicillin is the drug of choice in the treatment of syphilis in all its stages. Treatment must be instituted as soon as possible after infection is acquired; (1) a full course of treatment is essential in every case, no matter how mild the disease may appear to be; (2) periodic blood examinations must be carried out on every patient for at least two years after he or she has been apparently cured.

SYRINGE is an instrument for injecting liquids into the body. Syringes vary considerably in shape and size according to the purpose for which they are used. (For the method of using a hypodermic syringe, see HYPODERMIC.)

SYRINGOMYELIA is a rare disease affecting the spinal cord, in which are found irregular cavities surrounded by an excessive amount of the connective tissue of the central nervous system. These cavities encroach upon the nerve tracts in the cord, producing especially loss of the sense of pain or of that for heat and cold in parts of the limbs, although the sensation of touch is retained. Another symptom sometimes present is wasting of certain muscles in the limbs. Changes affecting outlying parts like the fingers are also found. On account of their insensitiveness to pain, the fingers, for example, are often burnt or wounded, and troublesome ulcers, or loss of parts of the fingers, result. The condition of the spinal cord is probably present at birth, though the symptoms do not usually appear till young adulthood is reached. The disease is slowly progressive, though sudden exacerbations may occur after a cough, a sneeze, or sudden straining. Treatment consists simply in the maintenance of general good health.

SYRUP, formed of a mixture of sugar and water, is a fluid often used for the administration of drugs. It is employed partly on account of its pleasant taste, and largely also because it retards changes in drugs which deteriorate on exposure to the air.

SYSTEMIC   A description of something, for example, a drug, that affects the whole body and not just part of it.

SYSTEMIC LUPUS ERYTHEMATOSUS (SLE) is an autoimmune disease occurring predominantly in women (see LUPUS) that causes chronic inflammation of the connective tissue which affects the skin and various internal organs. The skin is red and scaly, joints develop inflammatory arthritis, and the kidneys may be damaged. The brain, heart and lungs may also be affected, with inflamed tissue ultimately becoming scarred. Treatment is with corticosteroids or immunosuppressive drugs.

SYSTOLE means the contraction of the heart, and alternates with the resting phase, known as diastole. The two occupy, respectively, about one-third and two-thirds of the cycle of heart action.

SYSTOLIC PRESSURE (see BLOOD PRESSURE).

T

TABES means, literally, a wasting disease, and is an old name applied to various diseases, such as tabes dorsalis and tuberculosis accompanied by enlargement of glands. At present the name *tabes dorsalis* is used for locomotor ataxia and *tabes mesenterica* is used for tuberculosis affecting the glands in the abdomen: two diseases totally different in their nature and cause.

TABLET is the name given to a solid disc-like preparation made by compression and containing drugs mixed usually with sugar and other indifferent material. Tablets are widely used because of their convenience and accurate dosage. The word, 'tabloid', indicates a proprietary preparation.

TACHYCARDIA means a rapid pulse rate. (See HEART DISEASE.)

TACHYPHYLAXIS is rapidly developing tolerance to a drug (see TOLERANCE.)

TACHYPNOEA means unusual quickness of breathing.

TACTILE   Perceptible to, pertaining to or related to the sense of touch.

TAENIASIS is the disease caused by taeniae, or tapeworms. Their shape is modified to present as large an absorbing surface as possible to the digested food passing down the intestine, so that they are flat, white and long (up to 12 metres [40 feet] in length), like a piece of tape, as their name implies. Each consists of a head, the size of a small pin's head, provided with suckers, and sometimes with hooklets, for adhesion to the bowel wall, and from this head segments are produced that gradually increase in size and develop ova the further they recede from the head. The mature segments at the extremity of the worm are crammed full of ova, and are constantly splitting off to be discharged in the stools. When these mature segments, or proglottides, are discharged, they fall upon the ground, and the ova they contain are afterwards conveyed either by food or drink into the stomach of an intermediate host, which may be a pig, ox or cattle, in the case of different parasites. The geographical distribution of different tapeworm infestation depends largely upon the eating habits of the inhabitants. Thus *Taenia saginata*, or the beef tapeworm, is found in beef-eating areas, especially in Europe and Mohammedan countries. *Taenia solium*, the pork tapeworm, is found most commonly in Germany and the Slav countries. *Echinococcus granulosus* is found where dogs are widely used, as in Iceland or sheep-rearing countries such as Australia, New Zealand and Argentina. When the ova reach the stomach of the intermediate host their capsule is dissolved, the embryos escape and find their way through the wall of stomach or intestine into the blood-vessels, by which they are carried to distant parts of the body. In the case of TAENIA SOLIUM the intermediate host is the pig, in the case of TAENIA SAGINATA it is cattle. In the muscles of these animals the embryos of the worm become encysted and remain so till they die, or till the animal's flesh happens to be eaten by the proper host, when they develop again into a new tapeworm in his intestine. The flesh of a pig thus infected shows plainly the encysted embryo (known as *Cysticercus cellulosae*), and is called measly pork. DIPHYLLOBOTHRIUM LATUM is seldom met with, except in the north of Europe and Asia, and the intermediate hosts are several varieties of fish. In the case of the tapeworm known as *Echinococcus granulosus*, relations are reversed, and man plays the rôle of intermediate host, the host of the mature tapeworm being the dog, from which the human being derives the embryo worm by allowing the dog to lick his hands and face, or to contaminate his food. Although the worm in the dog is very small (having only three segments, as a rule), the encysted form in man, known as a hydatid cyst, may reach a large size, situated in the liver, lungs, kidney or brain.

In the case of infestation with *Taenia saginata* there may be no symptoms or signs at all, and the 'host' only becomes aware that he is infested, when he sees the tapeworm, or rather part of it, in the stools. In the case of *Taenia solium*, the outlook is more serious because the eggs, when swallowed, are liable to migrate into the tissues of the body, as they do in the pig, and cause cysts. If these occur in the muscles they may cause little trouble but, if they occur in the brain, they can prove very serious.

Hydatid cysts often grow to a great size, budding off in their interior smaller cysts, which may have still smaller ones within them, the final contents of the smallest cysts being a salt, watery fluid and numerous heads of echinococci, each provided with a circle of hooks, and each capable, under proper conditions, of forming a new worm. The symptoms produced by a hydatid cyst depend mainly upon the effects of its size and consequent pressure. Very small cysts in the brain may produce serious results, like those of a tumour, whilst in the liver a cyst may grow to the size of a man's head before causing much trouble.

Treatment of tapeworm infestation consists of the administration of mepacrine, niclosamide or dichlorophen, followed by a purgative. Castor oil must not be used for this purpose. During treatment the stools must be carefully examined for the head of the tapeworm. Unless the head is passed in the stools, the worm will grow again. The treatment of hydatid cyst is surgical: i.e. the cyst must be removed by operation.

TALC is a soft mineral consisting of magnesium silicate. It is much used as an ingredient of dusting powders.

TALIPES is the technical name for club-foot (q.v.).

TALUS is the somewhat square-shaped bone which forms the lower part of the ankle-joint and unites the leg bones to the foot.

TAMOXIFEN is a hormonal drug of value in the treatment of some cases of cancer of the breast. It is used for treating postmenopausal women in whom the breast cancer has spread, as well as a first-line treatment for premenopausal women with breast cancer. Tamoxifen acts by combining with hormone receptors in the tumour to inhibit the effect of oestrogen.

TAMPON A plug or compressed gauze or cotton wool inserted into a wound or orifice to arrest haemorrhage. Also inserted into the vagina to absorb the flow of blood during menstruation. Infected tampons may cause toxic shock (q.v.), a potentially dangerous but fortunately uncommon reaction.

TAMPONADE The insertion of a tampon. It also may be used to describe the potentially life-threatening compression of the heart by the accumulation of fluid in the pericardial sac. This is characterized by tachycardia, pulsus paradoxus, low blood pressure, raised pressure in the jugular vein and abnormally quiet heart sounds.
Treatment consists of draining the fluid (which may be blood or an effusion) and treating the underlying cause.

TANNIN, or TANNIC ACID, is an uncrystallizable white or yellowish-white powder, which is soluble in water or glycerin. It is extracted from oak galls in large amount, but it is also present in almost all vegetable infusions. Tannic acid, acts as an astringent and also leads to rapid clotting of blood with which it is brought in contact.

TAPEWORM (see TAENIASIS).

TAPPING is the popular name for the withdrawal of oedema fluid from the cavities or the subcutaneous tissues of the body. (See ASPIRATION.)

TAR, or PIX LIQUIDA, is a thick, dark, oily substance obtained by the destructive distillation of several species of pine-tree. It is slightly soluble in water, more readily so in alcohol, oils, and strong alkaline solutions. Other tars of similar physical and medicinal properties are obtained from other woods, as well as from coal, shale, and peat. Tar is a substance of complex chemical composition, varying not only according to the source from which it is derived, but still more with the temperature at which it has been distilled. Generally speaking, wood-tar contains resin, creosote, and turpentine in considerable quantities, also benzol, carbolic acid, acetic acid, wood-spirit or methyl alcohol, methyl acetate, acetone, and wood-naphtha. The aniline dyes, many antipyretic bodies, saccharin, and various other medicinal substances and disinfectants are obtained indirectly from coal-tar.
Action In consequence of the numerous medicinally active bodies it contains, tar exerts

many marked effects upon the body. By reason of the creosote, carbolic acid, and methyl alcohol that it contains, it possesses an antiseptic and preservative power. Certain of its ingredients are of an irritating nature, and tar therefore stimulates the action of any skin surface with which it is brought in contact, as well as the respiratory and other mucous membranes by which it is excreted after being taken internally.

Uses Externally, tar is one of the most efficient preservatives of animal and vegetable tissues that we possess. For its germicidal action and stimulating properties it is used in chronic skin diseases, particularly psoriasis and dry eczema.

TARGET CELL Erythrocytes (q.v.) which are large and 'floppy' and have a ringed appearance, similar to that of a target, when stained and viewed under the microscope. This may occur with iron-deficiency anaemia, liver disease, a small spleen, haemoglobinopathies (disorders of haemoglobin) and thalassaemias (q.v.).

TARSAL Of or pertaining to the tarsus (q.v.) of the foot and ankle – this comprises talus, calcaneus navicular, cuboid and three cuneiform bones – or eyelid.

TARSUS is the region of the instep with its seven bones, the chief of which are the talus supporting the leg-bones and the calcaneus or heel-bone, the others being the navicular, cuboid, and three cuneiform bones.

TARTAR is a concretion that forms on the teeth near the margin of the gum, consisting chiefly of phosphate of lime deposited from the saliva. Mixed with this are food particles, and in it flourish numberless bacteria. It is important that it should be prevented from forming by regular brushing of the teeth, or removal after it has formed by regular visits to the dentist, because it gives rise to wasting of the gums and loosening of the teeth.

TASTE (see TONGUE).

TATTOOING has been a cult, or fashion, since the earliest days of history. Apart from the mixed motives for its use, it has a definite therapeutic indication in matching the colour of skin grafts. It is performed by implanting particles of colour pigment into the deeper layer of the skin known as the corium (see SKIN). This is done by means of a needle or needles. The pigments commonly used are carbon for black, cinnabar (red mercuric sulphide) or cadmium salts for red, chrome salts for greens and yellows, cobalt for blue, ferric (iron) salts for browns, pinks and yellows, and titanium for white. The main medical hazard of tattooing is infection, particularly hepatitis (q.v.), which

may be fatal. The tattooed person may also become allergic to one of the pigments used, particularly cinnabar. Removal, which should be done by a plastic surgeon, always leaves a residual scar, and often needs to be followed by a skin graft. Removal is not allowed under the National Health Service unless there is some medical reason: for example, allergic reactions to it. Other methods of removal are by cryosurgery (q.v.), dermabrasion (q.v.) and salabrasion. These, too, must only be carried out under skilled medical supervision. Promising results are also being obtained from the use of laser (q.v.), a method that appears to produce less scarring than other methods, if it is carried out under expert medical supervision.

In order to reduce the health hazards, tattooists, along with acupuncturists, cosmetic skinpiercers and hair electrolysers, are required, under the Local Government (Miscellaneous Provisions) Act 1982, to register their premises with health and local authorities before starting business. The practitioners have to satisfy the authorities that adequate precautions have been taken to prevent the transmission of infections, such as hepatitis.

TAXIS is the method of pushing back, into the abdominal cavity, a loop of bowel which has passed through the wall in consequence of a rupture.

TEARS (see EYE).

TECHNETIUM-99 An isotope of the artificial element technetium. It emits gamma rays and is used as a tracer in building up a scintigraphic radioactive image of organs such as the brain.

TEETH are hard organs developed from the mucous membranes of the mouth and embedded in the jawbones. They are used to bite and grind food and to aid clarity of speech. In some animals the teeth may be modified in shape to enable them to be used as weapons.

Structure Each tooth is composed of enamel, dentine, cement, pulp and periodontal membrane.

ENAMEL is the almost translucent material which covers the crown of a tooth. It is the most highly calcified material in the body, 96–97 per cent being composed of calcified salts. It is arranged from millions of long six-sided prisms set on end on the dentine. It is thickest over the biting surface of the tooth. With increasing age or the ingestion of abrasive foods the teeth may be worn away on the surface so that the dentine becomes visible. The outer sides of some teeth may be worn away by bad tooth-brushing technique.

DENTINE is a dense yellowish-white material from which the bulk and the basic shape of a tooth are formed. It is like ivory and it is harder than bone but softer than enamel. The crown of the tooth is covered by the hard protective

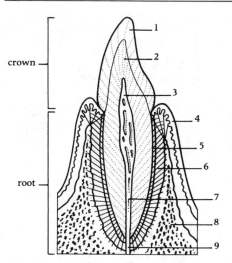

1 enamel
2 dentine
3 pulp (contains blood vessels and nerves)
4 gingiva (gum)
5 cementum
6 periodontal membrane
7 pulp canal
8 bone
9 apical foramen

Vertical section through incisor tooth.

enamel and the root is covered by a bonelike substance called cement. Dentine is formed from cells which produce cylinders of calcified material in the centre of which are tubules which contain protoplasmic processes which are extensions of the cells. These processes can transfer pain from the enamel to the sensitive pulp in the centre of the tooth. Dentine is formed from inorganic and organic matter. The composition is approximately 75 per cent inorganic salts and 25 per cent organic matter and water. Decay can erode dentine faster than enamel.

CEMENT or CEMENTUM is a thin bonelike material which covers the roots of teeth and helps hold the teeth in the bone. Fibres of the periodontal membrane are embedded in the cement and the bone. When the gums recede, part of the cement may be exposed and the cells die. Once this has happened, the periodontal membrane can no longer be attached to the tooth and, if sufficient cement is destroyed, the tooth support will be so weakened that the tooth will become loose.

PULP This is the inner core of the tooth and is composed of a highly vascular, delicate fibrous tissue with many fine nerve fibres. The outer layer is formed by the odontoblasts which formed the dentine and are now dormant unless required to lay down a further thickness of dentine in response to a destructive stimulus at the outer edge of the dentine. The pulp is the

tissue remaining after the tooth has been formed and may have helped in its eruption. The pulp is very sensitive to temperature variation and touch. If the pulp becomes exposed it will become infected and usually cannot overcome this. Root-canal treatment or extraction of the tooth may be necessary.

PERIODONTAL MEMBRANE This is a layer of fibrous tissue arranged in groups of fibres which surround and support the root of a tooth in a bone socket. The fibres are interspersed with blood-vessels and nerves. Loss of the membrane leads to loss of the tooth. The membrane can release and re-attach the fibres to allow the tooth to move when it erupts or is being moved by orthodontic springs.

Arrangement and form Teeth are present in most mammals and nearly all have two sets: a temporary or milk set followed by a permanent or adult set. In some animals, like the toothed whale, all the teeth are similar, but in man there are four different shapes: incisors, canines (eye-teeth), premolars (bicuspids), and molars. The incisors are chisel shaped and the canine is pointed. Premolars have two cusps on the crown (one medial to the other) and molars have at least four cusps. They are arranged together in an arch in each jaw and the cusps of opposing teeth interdigitate. Some herbivores have no upper anterior teeth but use a pad of

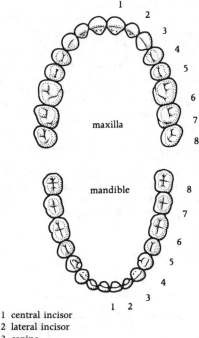

1 central incisor
2 lateral incisor
3 canine
4 1st premolar
5 2nd premolar
6 1st molar
7 2nd molar
8 3rd molar

The permanent teeth of the upper (top) and lower (bottom) jaws.

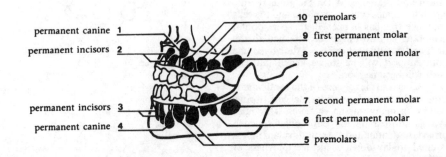

maxilla

mandible

8   7   6   5   4   3   2   1

1 central incisor
2 lateral incisor
3 canine
4 1st premolar
5 2nd premolar
6 1st molar
7 2nd molar
8 3rd molar

The permanent teeth of the left side of upper and lower jaws.

gum instead. As each arch is symmetrical, the teeth in an upper and lower quadrant can be used to identify the animal. In man the quadrants are the same, i.e. in the child there are two incisors, one canine and two molars (total teeth 20). In the adult there are two incisors, one canine, two premolars and three molars (total 32). This mixture of tooth form suggests that man is omnivorous. Anatomically the crown of the tooth has mesial and distal surfaces which touch the tooth next to it. The mesial surface is the one nearer to the centre line and the distal is the further away. The biting surface is called the incisal edge for the anterior teeth and the occlusal surface for the posteriors.

Development The first stage in the formation of the teeth is the appearance of a downgrowth of epithelium into the underlying mesoderm. This is the dental lamina, and from it ten smaller swellings in each jaw appear. These become bell shaped and enclose a part of the

mesoderm, the cells of which become specialized and are called the dental papillae. The epithelial cells produce enamel and the dental papilla forms the dentine, cement and pulp. At a fixed time the teeth start to erupt and a root is formed. Before the deciduous teeth erupt, the permanent teeth form, medial to them. In due course the deciduous roots resorb and the permanent teeth are then able to push the crowns out and erupt themselves. If this process is disturbed, the permanent teeth may be displaced and appear in an abnormal position or be impacted.

Eruption of teeth is in a definite order and at a fixed time, although there may be a few months leeway in either direction which is of no significance. Excessive delay is found in some congenital disorders such as cretinism. It may also be associated with local abnormalities of the jaws such as cysts, malformed teeth and supernumerary teeth.

permanent canine 1
permanent incisors 2

permanent incisors 3
permanent canine 4

10 premolars
9 first permanent molar
8 second permanent molar

7 second permanent molar
6 first permanent molar
5 premolars

Teeth of a six-year-old child. The permanent teeth are coloured black.

The usual order of eruption of deciduous teeth is:

Middle incisors	6–8 months
Lateral incisors	8–10 ,,
First molars	12–16 ,,
Canines (eye-teeth)	16–20 ,,
Second molars	20–30 ,,

The usual order of eruption of permanent teeth is:

First molars	6–7 years
Middle incisors	6–8 ,,
Lateral incisors	7–9 ,,
Canines	9–12 ,,
First and second premolars	10–12 ,,
Second molars	11–13 ,,
Third molars (wisdom teeth)	17–21 ,,

TEETH, DISEASES OF Teeth are important for appearance and speech and in the proper preparation of the food for its onward journey into the stomach. With modern foods biting and chewing are less important. Damage to the teeth can be painful.

TEETHING, or the process of eruption of the teeth, may be accompanied by symptoms which are particularly distressing in the child. There may be irritability, salivation, loss of sleep and a failure to feed. The child will tend to rub or touch the painful area. To a lesser extent this may also occur in the adult as the third molars try to erupt. Relief may be obtained in the child by allowing it to chew on a hard object such as a toy or rusk. If this is not sufficient, then various tinctures and pastes can be applied to the reddened area of gum. These remedies may contain salicilates or local anaesthetics.

TOOTHACHE is the pain felt when there is inflammation of the pulp or periodontal membrane of a tooth. It can vary in intensity and may be recurring. The commonest cause is caries when the cavity is close to the pulp. Once the pulp has become infected, this is likely to spread from the apex of the tooth into the bone to form an abscess (gumboil). A lesser but more long-lasting pain is felt when the dentine is unprotected. This can occur when the enamel is lost due to decay or trauma or because the gums have receded. This pain is often associated with temperature change or sweet foods. General debility makes a person more aware of minor discomforts. Expert dental advice should be sought early before the decay is extensive, even though the pain has disappeared temporarily. If a large cavity is accessible, temporary relief may be obtained by inserting a small piece of cotton wool soaked in one of the essential oils such as oil of cloves. A paste made from oil of cloves and zinc oxide powder is longer lasting but may make the pain more severe if the pulp is exposed and infected. Such a tooth requires root-canal therapy or extraction.

CARIES OF THE TEETH or dental decay is very common in the more affluent countries and is commonest in children and young adults. Increasing awareness of the causes has resulted in a considerable improvement in dental health, particularly in the last ten years. This has coincided with a rise in general health. Now 50 per cent of five-year-old children are caries free and of the others 10 per cent have half of the remaining carious cavities. Since the start of the National Health Service the emphasis has been on saving teeth. In south-east England, which has a high ratio of dentists for the population, less than 5 per cent of the people under 45 years have dentures. Now edentulous patients are mainly found among the elderly who had their teeth removed before 1948.

The precise cause of caries is still uncertain but the acidic theory is most widely held. Acid is produced by oral bacteria from dietary carbohydrates, particularly refined sugar, and this dissolves part of the enamel. The dentine is eroded more quickly as it is softer and the first time the person is aware of trouble is when the now hollow tooth collapses. Decay usually starts in a part of the tooth where cleaning is difficult, i.e. in the pits and fissures of the crown and between two teeth. The exposed smooth surfaces are usually protected as they are easily cleaned during normal eating and by brushing. Irregular and overcrowded teeth are more at risk from decay as they are difficult to clean. Primitive people who chew coarse foods rarely get caries. Fluoride in the drinking water at the rate of about 1 part per million is associated with a reduction in the caries rate. Prolonged severe disease in infancy is associated with poor calcification of the teeth, making them more vulnerable to decay. As the teeth are formed and partly calcified by the time of birth, the diet and health of the mother are also important to the teeth of the child. Pregnant mothers and children should have a good balanced diet with sufficient calcium and vitamin D. A fibrous diet will also aid cleansing of the teeth and stimulate the circulation in the teeth and jaws. The caries rate can be reduced by regular brushing with a fluoride toothpaste two or three times per day and certainly before going to sleep. This can be carried out with a brush and a tooth powder or paste. Powders tend to be more abrasive and, if used too often and with too much force, can wear the teeth away. Confectionery should be avoided between meals. The provision of sweet or sugary juices in a pacifier or bottle to help an infant sleep will rapidly lead to the loss of the upper front teeth.

The dental health of children has improved greatly in the past fifteen years in most industrial countries. This appears to be due to a number of factors. Public awareness of the need to brush and clean the teeth has greatly increased. Toothpastes now contain additives which reduce the formation of plaque and fluoride will strengthen the enamel up to 50 per cent. Fluoride in the water, whether it occurs naturally or is added, is associated with a lower caries rate. Fluoride is also available in tablet form for children but probably the most common source of the ion is in toothpaste.

IRREGULARITY OF THE PERMANENT TEETH may be due to an abnormality in the growth of the jaws or to the early or late loss of the deciduous set.

Most frequently it is due to an imbalance in the size of the teeth and the length of the jaws. Some improvement may take place with age but many will require the help of an orthodontist (specialist dentist) who can correct many mal-occlusions by removing a few teeth to allow him to move the others into a good position by means of springs and elastics on various appliances which are worn in the mouth.

LOOSENING OF THE TEETH may be due to an accident or inflammation of the gum. Teeth loosened by trauma may be replaced in the socket, even if knocked right out. If they are then splinted to the neighbouring teeth for a few weeks they may re-attach themselves to the bone. If the loosening is due to periodontal disease the prognosis is less favourable. The removal of any calculus and the use of some antiseptic mouthwashes will help.

DISCOLORATION of the teeth may be intrinsic or extrinsic, i.e. the stain may be in the calcified structure or stuck on to it. Intrinsic staining may be due to jaundice or the antibiotic tetracycline. Dark teeth are due to blood-breakdown products entering the dentinal tubules as a result of some trauma that has damaged the pulp. It may be possible to bleach such teeth but it usually needs to be repeated frequently. Extrinsic stain may be due to tea, coffee, tobacco, pan (a mixture of chuna and betel nuts wrapped in a leaf), iron-containing medicines or excess fluoride. Some of these can be removed by brushing with an abrasive paste but where the stain is within the tooth or the surface of the tooth is damaged, an artificial crown or veneer may be required.

GINGIVITIS or inflammation of the gums may occur as an acute or chronic condition. In the acute form it is often part of a general infection of the mouth and principally occurs in children or young adults and resolves after ten to fourteen days. The chronic form occurs later in life and tends to be progressive. There is moderate pain but the gums appear congested, bleed easily and may be ulcerated. Later calculus appears on the teeth. Eating may be difficult if the ulceration is extensive. Various micro-organisms may be found on the lesions including anaerobes. Treatment is initially supportive but the mouth should be kept as clean and moist as possible. Antiseptic mouthwashes may help and once the painful stage is past, the gums should be thoroughly cleaned and any calculus removed. In severe conditions an antibiotic may be required.

PERIODONTAL DISEASE is the spread of gingivitis to involve the periodontal membrane of the tooth and in its florid form used to be called pyorrhoea. In this, the membrane becomes damaged by the inflammatory process and a space or pocket is formed into which a probe can be easily passed. As the pocket becomes more extensive the tooth loosens. Although neglect hastens the process, the cause is still largely unknown. The production of calculus from plaque increases the trauma on the gingival margins and the injection of micro-organisms.

The loss of the periodontal membrane also leads to the loss of supporting bone. Chronic inflammation soon occurs and is difficult to eradicate. The effect of chewing on mobile teeth is debatable but some shedding of bacteria into the bloodstream occurs and this may affect damaged organs such as heart valves after rheumatic fever. Acute flare-ups of the disease may occur when the patient is unwell and also during pregnancy. Pain is not a feature of the disease but there is often an unpleasant odour (halitosis). The gums bleed easily and there may be dyspepsia. Treatment is largely aimed at stabilizing the condition rather than curing it. This is done by meticulous care of the mouth and teeth and the removal of calculus. Where there is excess tissue, the edge of the gums can be reshaped by surgical means, but attempts at replacing bone have only been partially successful.

DENTAL ABSCESS or ALVEOLAR ABSCESS is an infection that arises in or round a tooth and spreads to involve the bone. It may occur many years after a blow has killed the pulp of the tooth or more quickly after caries has reached the pulp. At first the pain may be mild and intermittent but eventually it will become severe and a swelling will develop in the gum over the apex of the tooth. The tooth may be sensitive to hot and cold at first, then will not respond but will feel extruded from the socket and be tender when touched. The swelling will enlarge until it feels like a bag of fluid, then may burst to discharge pus and will be more comfortable for a time. The discharge may become chronic. A radiograph of the tooth will show a round clear area at the apex of the tooth. Treatment may be by painting the gum with a mild counter-irritant such as a tincture of aconite and iodine in the early stages but later root-canal therapy or apicectomy may be required. If a swelling is present, it may need to be drained and antibiotics given. Where the tooth is beyond repair or of little use, then extraction may be preferable.

INJURIES TO TEETH are common. The more minor injuries include crazing and the loss of small chips of enamel, and the major ones include a broken root and avulsion of the entire tooth. A specialist dental opinion should be sought as soon as possible. The exposure of dentine will be painful for some weeks but can be easily treated by covering the tooth with a substance that does not easily conduct heat. Nail varnish or chewing gum will help for a few hours at least. When the pulp is exposed, it will almost certainly have to be removed before it becomes infected. A tooth that has been knocked out can be re-implanted if it is clean and replaced within a few hours. It will then require splinting in place for 4–6 weeks. Tinfoil can be used as a temporary splint. If the tooth was on the ground, then prevention of infection, including tetanus, will be necessary.

PREVENTION OF DENTAL DISEASE As with other matters, prevention is better than cure. Children should be taught at an early age to keep their teeth and gums clean and to avoid refined sugars between meals. It is better to finish a meal with a drink of water rather than a sweetened drink. Sweetened drinks are particularly harmful just before going to sleep. Fluoride in some of its forms is useful in the reduction of dental caries and a vaccine now being developed may be useful. Overcrowding of the teeth, obvious maldevelopment of the jaw and persistent thumbsucking into the teens are all indications for seeking the advice of an orthodontist. Generally adults have less trouble with decay but more with periodontal disease and, as its onset is insidious, regular dental inspections are desirable. Dentures are also not without problem and should be checked at least every five years. If worn day and night, there is a risk of developing thrush under the denture and damaging the gum and mucous membrane.

TEETH GRINDING, or BRUXISM as it is technically known, is quite common in children during sleep, when it is of no significance unless really persistent. During the day it may be an attention-seeking device. There is no treatment for it and if ignored it will stop. It is more common and persistent in mentally retarded children.

In adults it is usually associated with stress or anxiety, but may be due to some local condition in the mouth such as an unsatisfactory filling. It may also be caused by certain drugs, including fenfluramine and levodopa. More rarely it may be due to brain disease. If not controlled, it produces excessive wear of the enamel covering of the teeth. Treatment consists of alleviation of any condition in the mouth and any anxiety and stress. It may be useful to wear a splint covering the teeth of one jaw at night.

TEETHING (see TEETH, DISEASES OF).

TEICHOPSIA This refers to zigzag lines that patients with migraine often experience as an aura preceding an attack.

TELANGIECTASIS means an abnormal dilatation of arterioles and capillaries, forming sometimes a tumour or TELANGIOMA.

TEMAZEPAM is a relatively quick-acting hypnotic of short duration so that there is little or no 'hangover' the next morning. It is a derivative of diazepam. (See BENZODIAZEPINES.)

TEMPERAMENT is a term that includes those vague general peculiarities of mind and body that render some people more liable than others to be affected by particular diseases.

TEMPERATURE of the body is the result of a balance of heat-generating forces, chiefly metabolism (q.v.) and muscular activity, and heat-loss, mainly from blood circulation through and evaporation from the skin and lungs. The physiological process of homeostasis – a neurological and hormonal feedback mechanism – maintains the healthy person's body at the correct temperature. Disturbance of temperature, as in disease, may be caused by impairment of any of these bodily functions, or by malfunction of the controlling centre in the brain.

Animals are divided into two groups: cold-blooded animals, including reptiles, amphibians, fish, and invertebrates generally, whose temperature varies considerably with that of the environment; and warm-blooded animals, and mammals and birds, whose temperature remains almost constant. In man the 'normal' temperature is around 37 °C (98·4 °F). It may rise as high as 43 °C or fall to 32 °C in various conditions, but the risk to life is only serious above 41 °C or below 35 °C.

Fall in temperature may accompany major loss of blood, starvation, and the state of collapse (q.v.) which may occur in severe fever and other acute conditions. Certain chronic diseases, notably myxoedema (q.v.), are generally accompanied by a subnormal temperature. Increased temperature is a characteristic of many acute diseases, particularly infections. Indeed, many diseases have a characteristic pattern, such that a study of the patient's temperature chart in the early stages may be sufficient to make a confident diagnosis, or to detect any complications. In most cases the temperature gradually abates as the patient recovers, but in others, such as pneumonia and typhus fever, the disease ends rapidly by a crisis in which the temperature falls, perspiration breaks out, the pulse rate falls, and breathing becomes quieter. This crisis is often preceded by an increase in symptoms, including an epicritical rise in temperature.

Temperature in man is usually measured on the Celsius scale, on a thermometer reading from 35 °C to 43·3 °C. Measurement may be taken in the mouth (under the tongue), in the armpit, or (occasionally in infants) in the rectum. In each case the thermometer must be carefully washed and dried before use, and the mercury shaken down to below 35·5 °C. It must be left in place for at least three minutes, or five minutes in the armpit, for a representative reading.
Treatment Abnormally low temperatures may be treated by application of external heat, or reduction of heat loss from the body surface. High temperature may be treated in various ways, apart from the primary treatment of the underlying condition (see ANTIPYRETICS; COLD, USES OF; FEVER).

TEMPLE is the side of the head above the line between the eye and ear. The term, temporal, is applied to the muscles, nerves, and artery of this region. The hair usually begins to turn grey first at the temples.

TEMPORAL Referring or relating to the temporal region.

TEMPORAL ARTERITIS Inflammation of the temporal artery. Also known as giant cell arteritis, it often affects other arteries too, mainly in the head. It predominantly affects the elderly. The artery becomes tender with reddening of the overlying skin. Headache and blindness may also occur. The diagnosis is confirmed by temporal artery biopsy, and treatment is with steroids.

TEMPORAL LOBE EPILEPSY Epilepsy in which the abnormal cerebral activity originates in the temporal lobe of the brain. It is characterized by hallucinations of smell and sometimes of taste, hearing, or sight. There may be disturbances of memory, including déjà vu phenomena. Automatism (q.v.) may occur, but consciousness is seldom lost.

TENDERNESS is the term usually applied in medical nomenclature to pain experienced when a diseased part is handled, the term, pain, being reserved for unpleasant sensations felt apart from any manipulation.

TENDINITIS Inflammation of a tendon. Usually caused by unusual or excessive physical activity, it may also be infective in origin or secondary to a connective tissue disorder. The pain and inflammation may be treated with non-steroidal anti-inflammatory drugs (q.v.), immobilization splinting and steroid injections. Repetitive strain injury, caused by constant use of a keyboard (typewriter, word processor or computer) is tendinitis occurring in the hands and arms.

TENDON, SINEW, or LEADER, is the cord that attaches the end of a muscle to the bone or other structure upon which the muscle acts when it contracts. Tendons are composed of bundles of white fibrous tissue arranged in a very dense manner, and are of great strength. Some are rounded, some flattened bands, whilst others are very short, the muscle-fibres being attached almost directly to the bone. Most tendons are surrounded by sheaths lined with membrane similar to the synovial membrane lining joint-cavities. In this sheath the tendon glides smoothly over surrounding parts. The fibres of a tendon pass into the substance of the bone and blend with the fibres composing it. One of the largest tendons in the body is the tendo Achilles, or tendo calcaneus as it is now known, which attaches the muscle of the calf to the calcaneus or heel-bone.
TENDON INJURIES are one of the hazards of sports. They usually result from indirect violence, or overuse, rather than direct violence. *Rupture* usually results from the sudden application of an unbalanced load. Thus complete rupture of the Achilles tendon is common in taking an awkward step backwards playing squash. There is sudden pain, the victim is often under the impression that he received a blow. This is accompanied by loss of function, and a gap may be felt in the tendon. *Partial rupture* is also accompanied by pain, but there is no breach of continuity or complete loss of function. Treatment of a complete rupture usually means surgical repair followed by immobilization of the tendon in plaster of Paris for six weeks. Partial rupture usually responds to physiotherapy and immobilization, but healing is slow.

TENDOVAGINITIS means inflammation of a tendon and of the sheath enveloping it.

TENESMUS is a term applied to a symptom of disease affecting the lower part of the large intestine, such as dysentery, piles, or tumour. It consists of a constant sense of weight about the lower bowel and desire to go to stool, coupled with straining at stool and the passage of little but mucus and perhaps some blood.

TENNIS ELBOW (see ELBOW).

TENO- is a prefix denoting some relation to a tendon.

TENOSYNOVITIS, or TENOSITIS, means inflammation of a tendon.

TENOTOMY means an operation in which one or more tendons are divided, usually with the object of remedying some deformity.

TENTORIUM is a wide process of dura mater forming a partition between the cerebrum and cerebellum and supporting the former.

TERATOGENESIS is the production of physical defects in the fetus. It is understandable that a drug may interfere with a mechanism that is essential for growth and result in arrested or distorted development of the fetus and yet cause no disturbance in adults, in whom these growth processes have ceased to be relevant. Thus the effect of a drug upon a fetus may differ qualitively as well as quantitively from its effect on the mother. The susceptibility of the embryo will depend on the stage of development it has reached when the drug is given. The age of early differentiation, that is from the beginning of the third week to the end of the tenth week of pregnancy is the time of greatest susceptibility. After this time the likelihood of congenital malformation resulting from drug treatment is less, although the death of the fetus can occur at any time as a result of drugs crossing the placenta or as a result of their effect on the placental circulation. The term teratogenesis has come into common usage since the thalidomide disaster.
Thalidomide was an effective non-barbiturate hypnotic which had passed stringent tests before being released for general use. In spite of this it produced a number of congenital defects,

especially of the limbs, in children born to mothers who had taken the drug while pregnant. As soon as this was discovered the drug was withdrawn from use. Subsequently the government set up a Committee of Drug Safety to try and ensure that there was no recurrence of such a distressing episode with subsequent drugs. Even the most stringent precautions, however, cannot ensure the complete elimination of this risk. Fortunately the risk is a remote one, but it is now realised that no drug should be given to a pregnant woman, particularly during the first few months of pregnancy, unless it is absolutely essential for her health or that of her unborn child. There is no satisfactory test on animals that will clear a drug of the possibility of producing congenital malformation in man. Indeed drugs such as aspirin, caffein, insulin and thyroxine cause fetal abnormalities in some animal species but there is no evidence that they do so in man. Furthermore, the problem must be kept in perspective and it should be appreciated that only 1 per cent of congenital malformations are the results of environmental factors, which include not only drugs but infections such as German measles and irradiation. The risk that any random pregnancy will end in some serious malformation is about 1 in 40. Of drugs in current use there is circumstantial evidence that the alkylating agents and antimetabolites used in the treatment of reticulosis and leukaemia are teratogenic. There is some evidence that oral hypoglycaemic agents and antihistamine agents may also be responsible for a few congenital malformations.

TERATOMA is a tumour that consists of partially developed embryonic tissues. The most common sites of this tumour are the ovary and the testicle.

TERBUTALINE is a drug that is proving of value in the treatment of asthma. It is given by injection under the skin or by inhalation. It is a beta adrenoreceptor agonist.

TERTIAN FEVER is the name applied to that type of malaria in which the fever reappears every other day. (See MALARIA.)

TESTICLE The testes, or testicles, are the two male sexual glands. Each is developed in the corresponding loin, but before birth they descend through openings in the lower part of the front of the abdomen into a fold or pouch of skin known as the scrotum. This fold is strengthened by a layer of muscle fibres and fibrous tissues, and within it each testicle possesses a separate covering known as the tunica vaginalis. This tunic is a double layer of serous membrane similar in structure to the peritoneum or pleura, and it is derived from the peritoneum while the testicle is still within the abdomen. Occasionally, as the result of defective development, a more or less open channel

of communication is left between the peritoneum and tunica vaginalis, and down this channel a hernia is liable to form in childhood or later. Throughout life, the openings in the abdominal wall remain, but each inguinal canal should be just large enough to allow the passage of one of the two spermatic cords, each of which is composed of the vas (or ductus) deferens, together with the blood-vessels, nerves, and lymphatics proceeding to the gland. Within the tunica vaginalis lies a dense fibrous coat known as the tunica albuginea, which affords protection to the gland. On microscopic examination, each testicle is found to consist of a series of minute tubes, from eight hundred to one thousand in number, supported by fibrous tissue in which the nerves and blood-vessels run, and lined by cells from which the spermatozoa are formed. Around 4·5 million spermatozoa are produced per gram of testicle per day. These tubes communicate with one another near the centre of the testicle, and are connected by a much convoluted tube, the epididymis, with the ductus, or vas deferens, which enters the abdomen, and passes on to the base of the bladder. This duct, after joining a reservoir known as the seminal vesicle, opens, close to the duct from the other side of the body, into that part of the urethra which is surrounded by the prostate gland. Owing to the convulutions of these ducts leading from the testicles to the urethra, and their indirect route, the passage from testicle to urethra is over 6 metres (20 feet) in length. In addition to producing spermotozoa, the testicle also forms an internal secretion which is responsible for the development of male characteristics. This hormone has been isolated and is known as testosterone.

TESTICLE, DISEASES OF The pouch of skin, or scrotum, in which the testicles lie is liable to various general skin diseases, but particularly to eczema, which in many cases is often difficult to cure. Cancer of the skin in this region is specially common among chimney-sweeps, shale workers and cotton spinners, the result of chronic irritation by a carcinogenic agent in soot and paraffin products. Hernia, which in some cases passes into the scrotum, is treated under a special heading. (See HERNIA.) Sometimes, owing to defective development, the testicles are retained within the abdomen. HYDROCOELE is a local dropsy affecting one tunica vaginalis, and distending that side of the scrotum with fluid. (See HYDROCOELE.) VARICOCOELE is a condition in which the veins of the spermatic cord, especially on the left side, become unusually numerous and distended, the causes being much the same as those of varicose veins in other parts. The chief symptom is a dragging sensation in the testicle, which in some cases becomes at times very painful. This symptom is specially marked in warm weather and after exertion, the mass of veins at such a time becoming very distinct and resembling a 'bag of worms', though they empty quickly when the person lies down. Cold sponging of the part, careful regulation of the bowels, and the support of a suspensory net bandage afford all the treatment that is necessary in many cases; but an operation may sometimes be advisable.

INFLAMMATION of an acute type (orchitis) may arise in people suffering from cystitis, stone in the bladder, and various forms of inflammation in the urinary organs, the most common cause of all being gonorrhoea. It may follow also upon some cases of mumps. The symptoms are intense pain and swelling with redness of the skin over the affected testicle; and the usual treatment consists of rest in bed, support of the scrotum with a suspensory bandage or wads of cotton-wool, the administration of analgesics (in some cases the pain may be so severe that morphine is necessary), and the administration of antibiotics if there is some definite causative micro-organism. In some cases the condition goes on to the formation of an abscess which bursts through the skin with immediate relief of pain. The condition is then treated as an abscess elsewhere.

TORSION, or twisting or rotation, of the testes, or, strictly speaking, of the spermatic cord, is a relatively common occurrence in adolescent and young adult males. It can occur during sleep, at rest, while playing games or doing hard physical work. About half the cases occur in the early hours of the morning during sleep. It is more liable to happen more often in the colder, than the warmer, months of the year. It makes itself felt by pain of varying severity – from slight to excruciating – either in the lower part of the abdomen or in the scrotum. In time the pain diminishes or disappears. The testes become hard and swollen. Treatment consists of immediate undoing of the torsion. If this is done within a few hours no harm ensues as a rule, but it should be followed within six hours by surgical operation to ensure that the torsion has been successfully undone and to fix the testes so that there should be no recurrence.

TUBERCULOSIS occurs in the testicle occasionally, especially when some other organ, such as the bladder, is already the seat of the disease. It causes practically no pain, and is therefore often far advanced before it attracts attention. It responds well to chemotherapy with streptomycin, paraaminosaliylic acid and/or isoniazid.

TUMOURS of the testes occur in around 600 males annually in Britain. They represent the second commonest form of malignant growth in young males. There are two types: seminomas and teratomas (q.v.). When adequately treated the survival rate for seminomas is 95 per cent, whilst that for teratomas is 50 per cent.

INJURIES of the testicles are relatively rare. A severe blow may lead to shock and symptoms of severe collapse for a time, and may cause an effusion of blood into the tunica vaginalis. These symptoms are usually relieved by rest in bed.

TEST MEAL or gastric function test is a term originally applied to a meal given for the purpose of testing digestive function. The original gruel meal has been replaced by the injection of histamine (q.v.), which is a powerful stimulator of gastric juice, or pentagastin. After the stimulant has been injected, the digestive juices are withdrawn through a stomach tube (inserted through the nose and throat) and their volume and chemistry measured. A similar test is used to assess the working of the pancreas gland (q.v.).

TESTIS (see TESTICLE).

TESTOSTERONE is the name given to the male sex hormone secreted by the testes. It has also been prepared synthetically and has the formula $C_{19}H_{28}O_2$. In true eunuchoid conditions it has the power of restoring male sexual characteristics. (See ANDROGEN.)

TESTOSTERONE ENANTHATE (see ANDROGEN).

TESTOSTERONE PROPIONATE (see ANDROGEN).

TESTOSTERONE UNDECANOATE (see ANDROGEN).

TEST-TUBE is a tube of thin glass closed at one end, which is used for observing chemical reactions or for bacterial culture.

'TEST-TUBE BABY' (see EMBRYO TRANSFER).

TETANUS, or LOCKJAW, is a disorder of the nervous system. Increased excitability of the spinal cord results in painful and prolonged spasms of the voluntary muscles throughout the body, rapidly leading to death unless treated. **Causes** The disease is caused by the bacillus *Clostridium tetani*, found generally in earth and dust, especially in places where animal manure is collected. Infection usually follows a wound, especially a deeply punctured or gunshot wound, and is favoured by the presence of some foreign body. It is therefore particularly common in conditions of war, and may also be a hazard among farmers, gardeners and those in the construction industry. The bacillus develops a poison in the wound, which is absorbed through the motor nerves into the spinal cord. Here it leads to excessive sensitivity, such that the nerves react to quite mild stimuli

Symptoms Most commonly appearing within four to five days of the primary wound, the patient's symptoms may be delayed for several weeks – by which time the wound may have healed. Although generally the longer the delay, the better the outlook, a long delay with an acute onset may occasionally be dangerous, if it suggests that a dormant strain of the organism has suddenly started to produce large amounts of poison. Initially appearing as muscle stiffness around the wound, this symptom is followed by stiffness around the jaw, leading to lockjaw, or trismus. This extends to the muscles of the neck, back, chest, abdomen, and limbs, leading to strange, often changing, contorted postures, accompanied by frequent seizures – often provoked by quite minor stimuli. The patient's breathing may be seriously affected, in severe cases leading to asphyxia (q.v.); the temperature may rise substantially, often with copious sweating; and severe pain is a common feature. Mental clarity is a characteristic feature of the disease, adding to the patient's anxiety. In severe infections death may rapidly ensue from asphyxia, pneumonia, or general exhaustion. More commonly, the disease takes a more chronic course, leading to a gradual recovery. Outcome depends on several factors, chiefly the patient's immune status and age, and early administration of appropriate treatment.

Tetanus may occur in newborn babies, particularly when birth takes place in an unhygienic environment. It is particularly common in the tropics and Third-World countries, with a very high mortality rate. Local tetanus is a rare manifestation, in which only muscles around the wound are affected, though stiffness may last for several months. Strychnine poisoning and rabies, although similar in some respects to tetanus, may be easily distinguished by taking a good history.

Prevention and treatment The incidence of tetanus in the United Kingdom has been substantially reduced by the introduction of the vaccine (q.v.). Children are routinely immunized, and boosters are given later in life to at-risk workers, or those travelling to tropical parts.

Treatment should be started as soon as possible after sustaining a potentially dangerous wound. An intravenous injection of antitoxin should be given immediately, and the wound thoroughly cleaned. Benzylpenicillin should be given six hourly. Expert nursing is most important, and the patient should lie in a quiet, darkened room. Spasms may be minimized by reducing unexpected stimuli, and diazepam (q.v.) is often valuable. Good nutrition is vital, and intravenous feeding should be started immediately if the patient cannot swallow. Aspiration of bronchial secretions and antibiotic treatment of pneumonia may be necessary.

TETANY is a condition characterized by spasm of muscle usually caused by a fall in the ionic calcium of the blood. This fall in ionic calcium results in hyperexcitability of the muscles, which are thus liable to go into spasm on the slightest stimulus. This is well demonstrated in two of the classical signs of the disease: *Chvostek's sign*, in which the muscles of the face contract when the cheek is tapped over the facial nerve as it emerges on the cheek; *Erb's sign*, in which muscles go into spasm in response to an electrical stimulus which normally causes only a contraction of the muscle. Tetany is most common in infants, in whom it may arise as a result of rickets, excessive vomiting, or certain forms of nephritis. It may also be due to lack of the active principle of the parathyroid glands. Overbreathing may also cause it. Treatment consists of the administration of calcium salts, and in severe cases this is done by giving calcium gluconate intravenously or intramuscularly. High doses of vitamin D are also required: calcitriol is the most active preparation.

TETRACYCLINES are a group of broad-spectrum antibiotics which include chlortetracycline, oxytetracycline, tetracycline, doxycline, lymecycline, minocycline, and demeclocycline. Chlortetracycline, which is derived from *Streptomyces aureofaciens*, was the first to be discovered, followed by oxytetracycline which is derived from *Streptomyces rimosus*. Subsequently it was discovered that the active constituent of both these antibiotics was tetracycline, which can be prepared on a large scale by the catalytic hydrogenation of chlortetracycline.

From the point of view of antibacterial activity, all the preparations are virtually identical, being active against both Gram-negative and Gram-positive bacteria. Their value has, however, lessened owing to increasing resistance to the group among bacteria. They remain the treatment of choice for brucellosis (q.v.), mycoplasma (q.v.), Lyme disease (q.v.) as well as certain rickettsiae (q.v.) and chlamydia including those causing Q fever, trachoma, psittacosis, salpingitis, urethritis and lymphogranuloma inguinale.

It is this wide range of activity, which has given them the name of broad-spectrum antibiotics, combined with the fact that they are given by mouth, that has made them such a useful contribution to the treatment of infective diseases. They must be used with discrimination in young children as they are liable to produce permanent discoloration of the teeth.

TETRALOGY OF FALLOT is the most common form of cyanotic congenital heart disease. The tetralogy consists of: (*a*) stenosis of the pulmonary valve; (*b*) a defect in the septum separating the two ventricles; (*c*) the aorta overrides both ventricles; (*d*) marked hypertrophy of the right ventricle.

THALAMUS is one of two masses of grey matter lying on either side of the third ventricle of the brain. It is an important relay and co-ordinating station for sensory impulses such as those for sight. (Plural: Thalami.)

THALASSAEMIA, also known as Cooley's anaemia, is a condition characterized by severe anaemia, due to the individual's having an abnormal form of haemoglobin in his blood. It is a genetically inherited disease which is widely spread across the Mediterranean through the Middle East and into the Far East. It has a particularly high incidence in Greece and in Italy.

THALIDOMIDE A sedative and hypnotic drug now withdrawn from the market because it causes teratogenesis (q.v.). If taken during the first trimester of pregnancy it may cause an unusual limb deformity in the fetus known as phocomelia ('seal' of 'flipper' extremities).

THALLIUM An element that is toxic to nerve and liver tissues. The radio-isotope thallium-201 is used as a tracer during special imaging studies of blood flow through the heart muscle in the diagnosis of myocardial ischaemia.

THECA A sheathlike structure enclosing an organ or part.

THENAR EMINENCE is the projecting mass at the base of the thumb: what is popularly known as the ball of the thumb.

THEOPHYLLINE is an alkaloid structurally similar to caffeine, and found in small amounts in tea. Its main use is for the relief of bronchospasm, where beta-2 adrenoceptor stimulants have failed. It is given intravenously in combination with the stabilizing agent ethylenediamine (as aminophylline) for the treatment of severe asthma (q.v.) or paroxysmal nocturnal dyspnoea. Formerly used in the treatment of left ventricular failure, it has been largely superseded by more effective diuretics (q.v.). When indicated, aminophylline should be given by very slow intravenous injection; acute overdose may cause convulsions and cardiac arrhythmias (q.v.).

THERAPEUTICS is the general name applied to different methods of treatment and healing.

THERAPY means the treatment of disease.

THERIAC means an antidote or substance given to neutralize poison. The name was specially given to Venice treacle, a celebrated mixture of 64 drugs prescribed in olden times as an antidote for poisons and a preventive of disease.

THERMO- is a prefix implying some relation to heat.

THERMOGRAPHY is a method of detecting the amount of heat produced by different parts of the body. This is done with an infra-red sensitive photographic film. High blood flow in an area shows up as a heat zone and thus tumours such as breast cancer can be identified.

The process records such changes in temperature in a record known as a thermogram. Unfortunately, such hot areas of skin are caused by a number of other conditions. It is therefore a diagnostic method that can be used only as a rough screening procedure.

THERMOMETER SCALES (see TEMPERATURE).

THIABENDAZOLE is a drug that was the routine treatment for various parasitic infections, including those due to guinea-worm and certain nematodes, as well as strongyloidiasis (q.v.). Albendazole is now the preferred treatment with thiabendazole used only in certain circumstances. (See STRONGYLOIDIASIS).

THIAMINE is the *British Pharmacopoeia* name for vitamin B_1. Also known as ANEURINE, it is found in the husks of cereal grains. Its deficiency may be produced by too careful milling of rice in the East, or by a diet of white bread to the exclusion of brown bread and other cereal sources of this vitamin. The resulting disease is a form of neuritis with muscular weakness and heart failure, common in Japan and other parts of the East and known as beriberi (q.v.). Vitamin B_1 has been isolated in crystalline form, and a minute dose of this rapidly cures the symptoms of beriberi. The best sources of this vitamin are wholemeal flour, bacon, liver, egg-yolk, yeast and the pulses. The daily requirement is dependent, among other things, upon the total food intake, and has been estimated to be in the region of 0·5 mg of thiamine per 1000 Calories, increased during pregnancy to 2 mg daily as a minimum. (See APPENDIX 5: VITAMINS.)

THIAZIDES (see BENZOTHIADIAZINES).

THIERSCH'S GRAFT is the term given to a method of skin-grafting in which strips of skin are shaved from a normal area and placed on the abnormal area to be grafted. (See SKIN-GRAFTING.)

THIGH is the portion of the lower limb above the knee. The thigh is supported by the femur or thigh-bone, the longest and strongest bone in the body. This fits by a rounded head at its upper end into the acetabulum, a hollow at the side of the pelvis, and at the lower end two large rounded condyles or knuckles rest upon the head of the tibia, and, along with the patella, or knee-cap, form the knee-joint. A large four-headed muscle, the quadriceps, forms most of the fleshy mass on the front and sides of the thigh and serves to straighten the leg in walking and to maintain the erect posture of the body in standing. At the back of the thigh, lie the hamstring muscles; and on the inner side the adductor muscles, attached above to the pelvis and below to the femur, pull the lower limb inwards. The large femoral vessels emerge from the abdomen in the middle of the groin, the vein lying to the inner side of the artery. These pass downwards with an inclination inwards deeply placed between the muscles, and at the knee they lie behind the joint. The great saphenous vein lies near the surface and can be seen towards the inner side of the thigh passing up to the groin, where it joins the femoral vein. The femoral nerve accompanies the large vessels and controls the muscles on the front and inner side of the thigh; while the sciatic nerve, about the thickness of a lead pencil, lies close to the back of the femur and supplies the muscles at the back of the thigh and muscles below the knee.

Deep wounds on the inner side of the thigh are dangerous by reason of the risk of damage to the large vessels. Pain in the back of the thigh is often due to inflammation of the sciatic nerve. (See SCIATICA.) The veins on the inner side of the thigh are specially liable to become dilated. (See VEINS, DISEASES OF.)

THIOPENTONE SODIUM is the *British Pharmacopoeia* name for a commonly used intravenous anaesthetic. Its main use is for inducing anaesthesia, which it does rapidly and painlessly.

THIORIDAZINE is a tranquillizer that is a useful anti-psychotic drug. (See NEUROLEPTICS.)

THIOTEPA is one of the alkylating agents that is proving of value in the treatment of certain forms of malignant disease, including cancer of the breast and ovary. (See CYTOTOXIC.)

THIOUREA COMPOUNDS have the property of interfering with the synthesis of thyroxine in the thyroid gland and have been used with success, for the treatment of thyrotoxicosis, either as the propyl salt or as carbimazole (q.v.). The drugs are used in one of two ways: (*a*) to control thyrotoxicosis, and for this purpose it usually needs to be taken for long periods; (*b*) as a preoperative measure in patients undergoing thyroid surgery.

THIRST, like appetite, is an instinctive craving for something necessary to the continuance of bodily activity. The sensation of thirst is generally referred to the back of the throat, because, when there is a deficiency of water in the system, the throat and mouth especially become parched by evaporation of moisture from their surface. The mere swallowing of water, however, is not sufficient to abolish thirst, as appears in cases where a fistulous opening into the gullet exists, through which the water escapes. Thirst is increased by heat, and is a constant symptom of fever; it is also present in diseases which remove a considerable amount of fluid from the system, such as diarrhoea, diabetes mellitus, and after great loss of blood

by haemorrhage. A desire for water is also a feature of many conditions associated with great exhaustion.

THORACIC DUCT is the large lymph-vessel which collects the contents of the lymphatics proceeding from the lower limbs, the abdomen, the left arm, and left side of the chest, neck, and head. It is about the size of a goose quill, is provided with numerous valves, and opens into the veins at the left side of the neck. (See GLANDS; LYMPHATICS.)

THORACOCENTESIS means the withdrawal of fluid from the pleural cavity. (See ASPIRATION.)

THORACOPLASTY is the operation of removing a varying number of ribs so that the underlying lung collapses.

THORAX is another name for the chest.

THREADWORM (see ENTEROBIASIS).

THREONINE is one of the essential amino-acids (q.v.).

THRESHOLD: The degree of stimulation, or electrical depolarization, necessary to produce an action potential in a nerve fibre (see NERVES). Stimulation below this level elicits no conducted impulse and supramaximal stimulation will elicit the same response as a threshold stimulus (see NERVES).

THRILL is a tremor or vibration felt on applying the hand to the surface of the body. It is felt particularly over the region of the heart in conditions in which the valve openings are narrowed or an aneurysm is present.

THROAT is, in popular language, a vague term applied indifferently to the region in front of the neck, to the larynx or organ of voice, and to the cavity at the back of the mouth. The last-mentioned use of the word, to denote the pharynx or cavity into which the nose, mouth, gullet, and larynx all open, is the correct one. (See PHARYNX. Information will also be found under LARYNX; NECK; TONSILS; NOSE.)

THROMBIN (see COAGULATION).

THROMBOANGIITIS OBLITERANS, also known as BUERGER'S DISEASE after the American surgeon who gave the first co-ordinated description of it in 1908, is an inflammatory disease involving the blood-vessels of the limbs, particularly the lower limbs. The cause is not known, but the use of tobacco is an important factor. It is almost entirely confined to men, and is more common in Jews than in Gentiles. Pain is the outstanding symptom, accompanied by pallor of the affected part. Sooner or later ulceration and gangrene tend to develop in the feet or hands. There is no specific treatment, but, if seen in the early stages, considerable relief may be given to the patient.

THROMBOCYTE (see PLATELETS).

THROMBOCYTOPENIA A disorder in which the number of platelets (q.v.) in the blood is reduced. This predisposes to bruising and bleeding. It may be idiopathic (q.v.) but is also caused by malignant diseases (q.v.) (particularly haematilogical) and drugs. (See PLATELETS.)

THROMBOEMBOLISM The formation of a thrombus (blood clot) in one part of the circulatory system from which a portion becomes detached and lodges in another blood vessel partially or completely obstructing the blood flow (an embolism). Most commonly a thrombus is formed in the veins of the leg and the embolism lodges in the pulmonary (lung) circulation. A pulmonary embolus is a potentially fatal condition and requires urgent anticoagulant treatment and sometimes surgery. Venous thromboses in the legs may occur after surgery and preventive anticoagulant treatment with heparin (q.v.) and warfarin is often used. Similar treatment is needed if a thrombus develops. Streptokinase (q.v.) is also used to treat thromboembolism.

THROMBOLYSIS The breakdown of a blood clot by enzymic activity. Naturally occurring enzymes (q.v.) limit the enlargement of clots, and drugs – e.g. streptokinase (q.v.) – may be given to 'dissolve' clots – e.g., following a coronary thrombosis (q.v.).

THROMBOPHLEBITIS is the condition characterized by inflammation of the veins combined with clot formation. (See VEINS, DISEASES OF.)

THROMBOSIS means the formation of a blood-clot within the vessels or heart during life. The process of clotting within the body depends upon the same factors as in clotting of blood outside the body, involving the fibrinogen and calcium salts circulating in the blood, as well as blood platelets. The indirect cause of thrombosis is usually some damage to the smooth lining of the blood-vessels brought about by inflammation, or the result of atheroma, a chronic disease of the vessel walls. The blood is also specially prone to clot in certain general conditions such as anaemia, the ill health of wasting diseases like cancer, and in consequence of the feeble circulation of old age.

Thrombosis may occur in the vessels of the brain and thus causes stroke in people whose arteries are much diseased.

Thrombosis of a coronary artery of the heart is a very serious condition which affects, as a rule, middle-aged or elderly people. (See also ARTERIES, DISEASES OF; CLOT; COAGULATION; CORONARY THROMBOSIS; PULMONARY THROMBOSIS; STROKE; VEINS, DISEASES OF.)

THROMBOXANE is a substance produced in the blood platelets (see PLATELETS) which induces aggregation of platelets and thereby thrombosis (q.v.). It is also a vasoconstrictor (q.v.).

THROMBUS A clot of blood. Usually describing the formation of a clot within a vessel obstructing the flow of blood, but it can also describe blood which has escaped from a damaged vessel and clotted in the surrounding tissue.

THRUSH, or CANDIDIASIS, is a commonly occurring fungal infection caused by *Candida albicans*. It exists as a commensal in the gastrointestinal tract, but may become pathogenic in the very young, the elderly, and in disturbances of the natural microbiological flora due to other disease, antibiotic treatment, immunocompromised states, and diabetes (q.v.).

Symptoms In infants it may occur as oral thrush, presenting as a white deposit on the tongue or cheek, or as a napkin dermatitis, and may be rapidly controlled by a one-week course of oral nystatin (q.v.) or clotrimazole (q.v.). Elderly, obese patients often develop lesions in warm, moist areas such as under the breasts, the armpits, and the groins. Vaginal thrush is particularly common during pregnancy, and among diabetics. It generally causes an irritable erythema with copious discharge, and is treated with a combined course of topical (pessaries and creams) and oral fungicides. Patients should always be tested for glycosuria (q.v.) and lesions should be swabbed.

THUMB-SUCKING, or FINGER-SUCKING, is a universal and harmless habit in infancy. It is usually gradually given up during the pre-school period, but quite often persists after school age especially if the child is tired, lonely or unhappy. In these cases the remedy is to deal with the cause. Threats should not be used to try to stop the habit.

THYMUS GLAND The thymus gland was given its name by Galen in the second century AD because of its resemblance to a bunch of thyme flowers. It has two lobes and lies in the upper part of the chest. Each lobe is made up of a number of lobules divided into an outer portion, or cortex, and a central portion, or medulla. The cortex resembles lymphoid tissue and is made up of masses of small round cells called thymocytes. It is an area of intense lymphopoiesis and the rate of production of new cells is five times greater than that in lymph nodes and other lymphoid tissues. The medulla is more loosely cellular and consists of a stroma which contains far fewer lymphocytes than in the cortex but also contains epithelial cells and Hassall's corpuscles.

The thymus gland is now established as a vital part of the immunological system. Until 1960 the function of the thymus was completely unknown. Stem cells from the bone marrow come to the thymus where they develop into immunologically competent cells. They are then seeded out to the rest of the lymphoid tissue. There are two distinct populations of lymphocytes. One is dependent on the presence of the thymus (T lymphocytes) and the other is independent of the thymus (B lymphocytes). Both are concerned with immune responses. They differ in their distribution and in their life span. The thymus-dependent lymphocyte is a cell which in the absence of antigenic stimulation circulates through the blood, lymph nodes and back into the circulation again over a period of more than 10 years. It performs a policing role, awaiting recognition of foreign material which it is able to identify as such. It reacts by multiplication and transformation and these are the ingredients of the immune response. B lymphocytes are produced in the bone marrow and are concerned with the production of the circulating humoral antibodies.

The most common clinical disorder associated with abnormality of the thymus is myasthenia gravis (q.v.). Ten per cent of patients with myasthenia gravis will have a tumour of the thymus whilst the remainder will have inflammatory changes in the thymus called thymitis.

THYROID CARTILAGE is the largest cartilage in the larynx and forms the prominence of the Adam's apple in front of the neck. (See LARYNX.)

THYROID GLAND is a highly vascular organ situated in front of the neck. It consists of a narrow isthmus crossing the windpipe close to its upper end, and joining together two lateral lobes which run upwards, one on each side of the larynx. The gland is therefore shaped somewhat like a horseshoe, each lateral lobe being about 5 cm (2 inches) long and the isthmus about 12 mm (½ inch) wide, and it is firmly bound to the larynx. The weight of the thyroid gland is about 28·5 grams (1 ounce), but it is larger in females than in males, undergoes in many women a periodic increase at each time of menstruation, and often reaches an enormous size in the condition known as goitre (q.v.).

Minute structure The gland is enveloped in a layer of fibrous tissue and possesses a rich blood supply. It is composed of multitudes of closed vesicles, each formed by a layer of cubical cells and containing a thick yellow fluid (colloid). Round the vesicles there is a dense network of capillary blood-vessels, whilst the finest lymphatic vessels communicate with the interior of these vesicles.

Function The chief function of the thyroid gland is to produce a hormone rich in iodine. The main active ingredient of this hormone is thyroxine. This hormone, or secretion, which passes directly from the thyroid into the bloodstream, is de-iodinated in the body cells to triiodo-thyronine which exerts the physiological action of the thyroid hormone. The hormone is one of the most important in the body and controls the rate of metabolism. Thus, if it is deficient in children they fail to grow, a condition known as CRETINISM (q.v.). If the deficiency develops in adult life, the individual becomes obese, lethargic, and develops a coarse skin, a condition known as MYXOEDEMA (q.v.). Overaction of the thyroid, or HYPER-THYROIDISM, results in loss of weight, rapid heart action, anxiety, overactivity and increased appetite. (See THYROTOXICOSIS.)

The production of the thyroid hormone is controlled by a hormone of the pituitary gland – the thyrotrophic hormone.

THYROID GLAND, DISEASES OF (see CRETINISM; GOITRE; GRAVES' DISEASE; MYXOEDEMA).

THYROTOXIC ADENOMA is a variety of thyrotoxicosis in which one of the nodules of a multinodular goitre becomes autonomous and secretes excess thyroid hormone. The symptoms that result are similar to those of Graves' disease (q.v.), but there are minor differences. The first difference is that these autonomous adenomas tend to occur in long-standing nodular goitres so that the patients are older than those with Graves' disease. The symptoms of hyperthyroidism therefore tend to be more cardio-vascular, such as atrial fibrillation and heart failure. Exophthalmos and pre-tibial myxoedema do not occur as these are autoimmune manifestations of Graves' disease and toxic adenomas do not have an auto-immune basis.

Treatment The first line of treatment is to render the patient euthyroid by treatment with antithyroid drugs. Then the nodule should be removed surgically or annihilated by radioactive iodine treatment.

THYROTOXICOSIS is a disorder of the thyroid gland in which excessive amounts of thyroid hormones are secreted into the bloodstream. Resultant symptoms are tachycardia (q.v.), tremor, anxiety, sweating, increased appetite, weight loss and dislike of heat. The commonest cause is Graves' disease; others include toxic adenoma (q.v.) and multinodular goitre. For treatment see GRAVES' DISEASE.

THYROTROPHIN-RELEASING HOR-MONE A hormone produced and released by the hypothalamus (q.v.) which stimulates the release of thyrotrophin-stimulating hormone (q.v.) by the pituitary gland (q.v.).

THYROTROPHIN-STIMULATING HOR-MONE (TSH) A hormone manufactured and released by the anterior part of the pituitary gland (q.v.) which stimulates the thyroid gland (q.v.) to manufacture and release thyroid hormones (thyroxine and tri-iodothyronine, qq.v.).

THYROXINE is a crystalline substance, containing iodine, isolated from the thyroid gland and possessing the properties of thyroid extract. It has also been synthesized. It is used in cases of defective function of the thyroid, such as cretinism, and myxoedema.

TIA (see TRANSIENT ISCHAEMIC ATTACKS/EPISODES).

TIAPROFENIC ACID (see NON-STEROIDAL ANTI-INFLAMMATORY DRUGS).

TIBIA is the larger of the two bones in the leg. One surface of the tibia lies immediately beneath the skin in front and towards the inner side of the leg, forming the shin. Fractures of this bone are accordingly very liable to wound the skin and become compound. The thigh-bone rests upon the larger upper end of the tibia at the knee-joint, whilst below, the tibia and fibula together enter into the ankle-joint, the two bosses or malleoli at the ankle belonging, the inner to the tibia, the outer to the fibula.

TIC is the term applied to the habit spasm which forms a personal peculiarity in neurotic subjects. (See CRAMP.)

TICARCILLIN (see ANTIBIOTIC).

TIC DOULOUREUX is another name for facial, or trigeminal, neuralgia due to some affection of the fifth cranial nerve, and characterized by pain, situated somewhere about the temple, forehead, face, or jaw, and sometimes by spasm in the muscles of the affected region. (See TRIGEMINAL NEURALGIA.)

TICK is the general name given to a group of arachnid insects, some of which act as transmitters of diseases.

Ticks are blood-sucking arthropods which are responsible for transmitting a wide range of diseases to man, including Rocky Mountain spotted fever. African tick typhus and fièvre boutonneuse (see TYPHUS FEVER). Apart from being transmitters of disease, they cause intense itching and may cause quite severe lesions of the skin. The best repellents are dimethyl phthalate and diethyltoluamide. Once bitten,

relief from the itching is obtained from the application of calamine lotion. Tick-bites are an occupational hazard of shepherds and game-keepers. (See BITES AND STINGS.)

TIE (see TRANSIENT ISCHAEMIC ATTACKS/EPISODES).

TIMOLOL MALEATE is a beta-adreno-ceptor-blocking drug which of value in the treatment of angina pectoris, myocardial infarction, and hypertension. It is also used in the treatment of glaucoma. (See ADRENERGIC RECEPTORS.)

TINCTURE is an alcoholic solution, generally of some vegetable substance.

TINEA is the technical name for ringworm. (See RINGWORM.)

TINNITUS means a noise heard in the ear without any external cause. It is a frequent accompaniment of deafness.

Tinnitus is common, affecting about one in six adults at some time in their life. Only one-third of these consult a doctor and in less than one per cent does the tinnitus interfere with leading a normal life. The cause is damage to the auditory pathway and the most common part of the pathway to be damaged is the cochlea. Tinnitus may be a symptom of general diseases such as anaemia, high blood pressure and arterial disease. It may be the result of drugs, particularly aspirin, chloroquine, quinine and certain antibiotics. Investigation is necessary to exclude any underlying cause but in most cases no cause can be found, and the management depends on relieving the effects of tinnitus on the patient because it is not usually possible to abolish the tinnitus altogether. Drugs such as carbamazepine, tocainide amide and mexiletine may help. The use of tinnitus maskers and hearing aids can suppress tinnitus by masking it with other sounds which the patient learns to listen to. Hearing aids suppress tinnitus by amplifying background noise.

Under the auspices of the Royal National Institute for Deaf People, the RNID Tinnitus Helpline has been established (see APPENDIX 2: ADDRESSES). Calls are charged at local rates. (See DEAFNESS; MENIÈRE'S DISEASE.)

TISSUES OF THE BODY are the simple elements from which the various parts and organs are found to be built. All the body originates from the union of a pair of cells but as growth proceeds the new cells produced from these form tissues of varying character and complexity. (See CELL.) It is customary to divide the tissues into five groups:
(1) Epithelial tissues, including the cells covering the skin, those lining the alimentary canal, those forming the secretions of internal organs. (See EPITHELIUM.)

(2) Connective tissues, including fibrous tissue, fat, bone, cartilage. (See these headings.)

(3) Muscular tissues (see MUSCLE).

(4) Nervous tissues (see NERVES).

(5) Wandering corpuscles of the blood and lymph (see BLOOD: LYMPH).

Many of the organs are formed of a single one of these tissues or of one with a very slight admixture of another, such as cartilage, or white fibrous tissue. Other parts of the body that are widely distributed are very simple in structure and consist of two or more simple tissues in varying proportion. Such are blood-vessels (see ARTERIES; VEINS), lymphatic vessels (see LYMPHATICS), lymphatic glands (see GLANDS), serous membranes (see SEROUS MEMBRANES), synovial membranes (see JOINTS), mucous membranes (see MUCOUS MEMBRANE), secreting glands (see GLANDS; SALIVARY GLANDS; THYROID GLAND) and skin (see SKIN).

The structure of the more complex organs of the body is dealt with under the heading of each organ.

TISSUE PLASMINOGEN ACTIVATOR (TPA, tPA) is a natural protein that occurs in the body. It has the property of breaking down a thrombus (q.v.) in a blood vessel (see THROMBOLYSIS). It is effective only in the presence of fibrin (q.v.) and activates plasminogen, which occurs normally on the surface of the fibrin.

TITRATION is a form of chemical analysis by means of standard solutions of known strength.

TITRE The strength of a solution as determined by titration (q.v.). In medicine it is used to describe the amount of antibody (q.v.) present in a known volume of serum (q.v.).

TITUBATION means a staggering or reeling condition, especially due to disease of the spinal cord or cerebellum.

TNM CLASSIFICATION A method of classifying cancers to determine how far they have spread. This helps doctors to determine the best course of treatment and the prognosis; it is useful in research. Originally defined by the American Joint Committee on Cancer, the T applies to the primary tumour, the N to any lymph node involvement and the M to any metastatic spread.

TOBACCO is the leaf of several species of Nicotiana, especially of the American plant *Nicotiana tabacum.*

The smoking of tobacco is the major public health hazard in Britain today. It causes a hundred thousand premature deaths per year in the United Kingdom alone. In addition to the deaths caused by cigarette smoking, it is also a major cause of disability and illness in the form of myocardial infarction, peripheral vascular disease, chronic obstructive airways disease and emphysema. Action on Smoking and Health (ASH) is a small charity founded by the Royal College of Physicians in 1971 that attempts to alert and inform the public to the dangers of smoking and to try to prevent the disability and death which it causes (see ASH).

Cigarette smoking is the major cause of chronic obstructive lung disease morbidity and 80 to 90 per cent of chronic obstructive lung disease in the United States is attributable to it. In 1982 the United States' Surgeon General stated that cigarette smoking was the major single cause of cancer mortality in the United States. Tobacco's contribution to all cancer deaths is estimated to be 30 per cent. Cigarette smoking is also the most important of the known modifiable risk factors for coronary heart disease.

Composition In addition to vegetable fibre, tobacco leaves contain a large quantity of ash, the nature of this depending predominantly upon the minerals present in the ground where the tobacco plant has been grown. Of the organic constituents the brown fluid alkaloid known as nicotine is the most important. The nicotine content of different tobaccos varies, and the amount absorbed depends upon whether or not the smoker inhales.

Tobacco smoke also contains some sixteen substances capable of inducing cancer in experimental animals. One of the most important of these is benzpyrene, a strongly carcinogenic hydrocarbon. As this is present in coal-tar pitch, it is commonly referred to in this context as tar. Other constituents of tobacco smoke include pyridine, ammonia and carbon monoxide.

A very small amount of nicotine, such as that derived from a single cigarette, has a stimulating effect upon the mental and bodily powers.

In larger amount, the action is a depressant and narcotic one, which in habitual smokers is modified to a sedative.

The greatest hazard of smoking, however, is the fact that it is the major cause of lung cancer, coronary artery disease, peripheral vascular disease, chronic bronchitis and emphysema. It also has an adverse effect on the fetus when the pregnant mother smokes.

Another set of symptoms frequently arising in those who smoke is irritable cough and soreness of the throat. These symptoms pass off when smoking is discontinued. There is increasing evidence that passive smoking (inhaling smoke from someone else's cigarette) is also harmful. Children whose parents smoke are at increased risk of pneumonia and glue ear. There is growing pressure under health-and-safety-at-work legislation for employers to provide smoke-free working conditions for their staff.

The giving up of the smoking habit is largely a psychological problem, but there is some evidence that the use of nicotine chewing gum facilitates the process.

TOBRAMYCIN is an antibiotic related to gentamicin (q.v.) and with a similar range of activity. It is given by injection.

TOES (see CORNS AND BUNIONS; FOOT; NAILS).

TOLAZOMIDE (see SULPHONYLUREAS).

TOLBUTAMIDE is a sulphonamide derivative, or sulphonylurea, which lowers the level of the blood sugar in diabetes mellitus. As it is rapidly excreted from the body, it has to be taken twice daily. Like chlorpropamide (q.v.), it may induce undue sensitivity to alcohol. (See also DIABETES MELLITUS, SULPHONYLUREAS.)

TOLERANCE   This occurs when the response to a particular amount of a drug or physiological messenger decreases (i.e. a larger dose must be given to produce the same response as before).

TOLMETIN (see NON-STEROIDAL ANTI-INFLAMMATORY DRUGS).

TOLNAFTATE is a preparation which in the form of a 1-per-cent solution, is proving useful as a local application in the treatment of certain forms of ringworm, particularly ringworm of the foot. It may also be applied as a powder or cream. It is used, too, in the treatment of tinea versicolor (see RINGWORM) and erythrasma (q.v.).

TOLUENE, or METHYLBENZENE, is a product of the distillation of coal tar widely used as a solvent in the manufacture of paint and rubber and plastic cements.

TOMOGRAPHY   A technique using X-rays or ultrasound to build up a focused image of a 'slice' through the body at a given level. By producing a series of such slices at different depths a three-dimensional image of the body structures can be built up (see X-RAYS).

-TOMY is a suffix indicating an operation by cutting.

TONGUE   The tongue is made up of several muscles, is richly supplied with blood-vessels and nerves, and is covered by highly specialized mucous membrane. It consists of a free part known as the tip, a body, and a hinder fixed part or root. The under surface lies upon the floor of the mouth, whilst the upper surface is curved from side to side, and still more from before backwards so as to adapt it to the roof of the mouth. At its root, the tongue is in contact with, and firmly united to, the upper

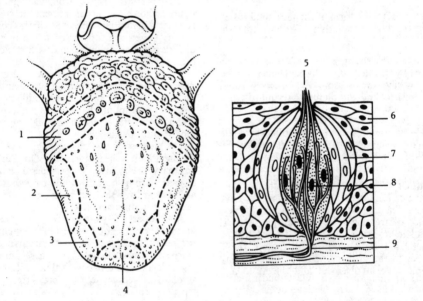

1 bitter	6 stratified epithelium
2 sour	7 sustentacular cell
3 salt	8 gustatory cell with hairlet
4 sweet	9 nerve
5 gustatory pore	

(Left) Tongue from above showing different areas of taste discrimination.
(Right) vertical section through surface of tongue showing taste bud (×400).

edge of the larynx; so that in some persons who can depress the tongue readily the tip of the epiglottis may be seen projecting upwards at its hinder part.

Structure The *substance* of the tongue consists almost entirely of muscles running in various directions. One runs along the upper surface and another along the lower surface from root to tip. Other fibres run vertically from the upper to the lower surface, whilst the chief bulk of the tongue is made up of muscle-fibres running from side to side. These various fibres are chiefly concerned in making changes in the shape of the tongue and moving it within the mouth. In addition to these, the tongue has numerous outside attachments; one muscle on each side unites it to the lower jaw-bone just behind the chin, and this muscle serves to protrude the tongue from the mouth; other muscles, which retract the tongue, attach it to the hyoid bone, the larynx, the palate, and the styloid process on the base of the skull.

The *mucous membrane* on the under surface of the tongue is very thin, so that the large blood-vessels on each side can easily be seen through it. In the middle line a fold of mucous membrane, the frenum, passes from the under surface to the floor of the mouth, and, when this frenum is attached too far forwards towards the tip of the tongue, the movements of the organ are impeded, and the condition is known as tongue-tie. On the upper surface or dorsum of the tongue the mucous membrane is thicker, and in its front two-thirds is studded with little projections of three kinds. The majority of these projections or *papillae* are of *conical* shape, and when the tongue becomes furred the apppearance is due to an unhealthy collection of epithelium upon them. Some of them end in long filaments, and are then known as *filiform* papillae. The roughness of the tongue in cats and other carnivorous animals is due to large backwardly directed conical papillae, which assist in cleaning the flesh off bones. On the tip, and towards the edges of the tongue, small red rounded *fungiform* papillae are seen, which act in all probability as end-organs for the sense of taste. On a line dividing the front two-thirds from the hinder one-third, and set in the shape of a V, is a row of seven to twelve large flat-topped *circumvallate* papillae, each placed in a corresponding depression and just visible, in most mouths, when the tongue is pressed firmly down with some flat instrument. These also act as end-organs for the nerves of taste. Each circumvallate papilla is surrounded by a trench, and upon both sides of the trench open numerous *taste-buds*. A taste-bud is shaped somewhat like a barrel, with an outer covering of flattened stave-like cells, enclosing a bundle of spindle-shaped cells which end in hairlike processes at the mouth of the bud, and are connected at their deeply placed end with some filaments from the nerves of taste. These taste-buds are also found in the fungiform papillae, though in smaller numbers, and they are scattered over the throat, fauces, and palate; so that the popular expression 'a fine palate', as applied to the sense of taste, is quite correct.

No fewer than five *nerves* supply branches to each side of the tongue. These are the *lingual* branch of the 5th nerve, which is the nerve of ordinary sensation, to the front two-thirds of the tongue; the *chorda tympani* branch from the 7th nerve, which is supposed to be the nerve of taste, for a similar extent; the *glossopharyngeal* or 9th nerve, which conveys sensations both of touch and taste from the hinder third: the *superior laryngeal* branch of the 10th nerve, also sensory; and the *hypoglossal* or 12th nerve, which supplies the muscles of the tongue.

Functions The chief uses of the tongue are of three kinds: (*a*) to push the food between the teeth for mastication, and then mould it into a bolus preparatory to swallowing; (*b*) as the organ of the sense of taste, and as an organ provided with a delicate sense of touch; and (*c*) to play a part in the production of speech. (See VOICE AND SPEECH.)

It is usual to classify any taste as:

1. Sweet   3. Bitter
2. Salt   4. Acid

since finer distinctions are largely dependent upon the sense of smell. The loss of keenness in taste brought about by a cold in the head, or even by holding the nose while swallowing, is well known. Sweet tastes seem to be best appreciated by the tip of the tongue, acids on its edges, and bitters at the back. It is possible, too, by chewing the leaves of an Indian plant, *Gymnaema sylvesive*, to do away with the power of tasting bitter and sweet substances, while the sensation for acids and salts remains, so that in all probability there are different nerve-fibres and end-organs for the different varieties of taste. Many tastes depend upon the ordinary sensations of the tongue, such as the constringent taste of tannin and the metallic taste of a weak galvanic current passed through the tongue. The sense of taste may be affected by certain drugs. Thus, penicillamine (q.v.) may reduce the sense of taste for sweet and salt, levodopa (q.v.) may induce a metallic or garlic-like taste, lithium (q.v.) may be accompanied by a rather vague unpleasant taste, captopril (q.v.) by a loss of the sense of taste, whilst metformin (q.v.) may cause a metallic taste.

Like other sensations, taste can be very highly educated for a time, as in tea-tasters and wine-tasters, but this special adaptation is lost after some years.

TONGUE, DISEASES OF (see MOUTH, DISEASES OF).

TONGUE, FURRING OF (see MOUTH, DISEASES OF).

TONICS, in effect, are placebos (q.v.). They may be used in conditions for which there is no known remedy, to strengthen and support the patient. While few doctors believe there is a genuine pharmacological basis for tonics – benefits are attributable to placebo effects – sufficient doctors and patients believe that tonics may be beneficial to justify their inclusion in the *British National Formulary* and prescription. Available tonics range from rhubarb compound mixture to various mineral and vitamin supplements.

TONSILLITIS is the inflammation of the tonsils.

ACUTE TONSILLITIS It must never be forgotten that the infection is never entirely confined to the tonsils; there is always some involvement of the surrounding throat or pharynx. The converse is true that in many cases of 'sore throat' the tonsils are involved in the generalized inflammation of the throat.

Causes Most commonly caused by the β-haemolytic streptococcus (q.v.), its incidence is highest in the winter months. Formerly an important precursor of rheumatic fever (q.v.), early diagnosis and treatment have made this disease rare in developed countries. Occasionally it is the presenting feature of diphtheria (q.v.), a disease now rare since the introduction of immunization (q.v.). Acute tonsillitis may also be associated with glandular fever, or infectious mononucleosis (q.v.). Caused by the Epstein Barr virus, this disease is mildly infectious and is often spread by direct oral contact ('the kissing disease').

Symptoms The onset is usually fairly sudden with pain on swallowing, fever and malaise. On examination, the tonsils are engorged and covered with a whitish exudate, consisting of a purulent discharge. This may occur at scattered areas over the tonsillar crypts (follicular tonsillitis), or it may be more extensive. The glands under the jaw are enlarged and tender, and there may be pain in the ear on the affected side. Although usually referred pain, it may indicate spread of the infection up the Eustachian tube to the ear, particularly in children. Occasionally an abscess, or quinsy, develops around the affected tonsil. Due to a collection of pus, it usually comes on four to five days after the onset of the disease, and requires specialist surgical treatment.

Treatment Penicillin or erythromycin is the drug of choice, together with paracetamol or aspirin, and plenty of fluids.

Removal of tonsils is indicated: (*a*) when the tonsils and adenoids are permanently so enlarged as to interfere with breathing; in such cases the adenoids are removed as well as the tonsils; (*b*) when the individual is subject to recurrent attacks of acute tonsillitis which are causing significant debility, absence from school or work on a regular basis; (*c*) when there is evidence of a tumour of the tonsil.

TONSILS are two almond-shaped glands situated one on each side of the narrow fauces where the mouth joins the throat. Each has a structure resembling that of a lymphatic gland,

and consists of an elevation of the mucous membrane presenting twelve to fifteen openings, which lead into pits or lacunae. The mucous covering is formed by the ordinary mucous membrane of the mouth, which also lines the pits; and the main substance of the gland is composed of loose connective tissue containing lymph corpuscles in its meshes, and packed here and there into denser nodules or follicles. The tonsils play an important rôle in the protective mechanism of the body against infection.

TOOTH, SUPERNUMERARY Malformed extra teeth are frequently found, particularly in the upper incisor region. They often do not erupt but prevent the eruption of the permanent teeth.

TOOTHACHE (see TEETH, DISEASES OF).

TOPHUS is the name given to the concretions which form in connection with joints or tendon sheaths as the result of attacks of gout. At first the tophus is a soft mass, but later becomes quite hard. It is composed of biurate of soda. (See GOUT.)

TOPICAL Pertaining to drugs or other treatment applied locally to the area being treated – e.g. the skin, eye, etc.

TORPOR is a condition of bodily and mental inactivity, not amounting to sleep, but interfering greatly with the ordinary habits and pursuits. It is often found in people suffering from fever, and is a common symptom in aged people whose arteries are diseased. It may annoy young people after meals when they are the subjects of constipation or of dyspepsia, due to eating too much indigestible food.

TORSION means twisting. The term is applied to the process in which organs, or tumours, which are attached to the rest of the body by a narrow neck or pedicle, become twisted so as to narrow the blood-vessels or other structures in the pedicle. (See TESTICLES, DISEASES OF.)

Torsion is also the term applied to the twisting of the small arteries severed at an operation, by which bleeding from them is stopped.

TORTICOLLIS This is shortness of the sternomastoid muscle on one side resulting in asymetry and limitation of movement of the neck. (See CRAMP; SPASMODIC TORTICOLLIS; WRY-NECK.)

TOUCH, according to the popular idea, is the fifth sense diffused all over the body, by which we become conscious of our surroundings otherwise than by the four special senses of hearing, seeing, tasting and smelling. But when this diffused sensitiveness is examined it is found to consist of a group of senses, several of which have special end-organs situated in the skin, muscles and elsewhere and special nerve-paths to convey their impressions to the brain. It is convenient, however, to adopt the popular view, and to consider all these under one heading. The cutaneous sense, then, is made up of the following:

Touch sense proper, by which we perceive a touch or stroke and estimate the size and shape of bodies with which we come in contact, but which we do not see.
Pressure sense, by which we judge the heaviness of weights laid upon the skin, or appreciate the hardness of objects by pressing against them.
Heat sense, by which we perceive that a body is warmer than the skin.
Cold sense, by which we perceive that a body touching the skin is cold.
Pain sense, by which we appreciate pricks, pinches and other painful impressions.

To these we may for convenience add:

Muscular sensitiveness, by which the painfulness of a squeeze is perceived. It is produced probably by direct pressure upon the nerve-fibres in the muscles.
Muscular sense, by which we test the weight of an object held in the hand, or gauge the amount of energy expended on an effort.
Sense of locality, by which we can, without looking, tell the position and attitude of any part of the body.
Common sensation, which is a vague term used to mean composite sensations produced by several of the foregoing, like tickling, or creeping, and the vague sense of well-being or the reverse that the mind receives from internal organs. (See the article on PAIN.)

The structure of the end-organs situated in the skin, which receive impressions from the outer world, and of the nerve-fibres which conduct these impressions to the central nervous system, have been described under NERVES.

Touch affects the Meissner's or touch corpuscles placed beneath the epidermis; as these differ in closeness in different parts of the skin, the delicacy of the sense of touch varies greatly. Thus the points of a pair of compasses can be felt as two on the tip of the tongue when separated by only 1 mm; on the tips of the fingers they must be separated to twice that distance, whilst on the arm or leg they cannot be felt as two points unless separated by over 25 mm, and on the back they must be separated by over 50 mm. On the parts covered by hair, the nerves ending round the roots of the hairs also take up impressions of touch.

Pressure is estimated probably through the same nerve-endings and nerves that have to do with touch, but it depends upon a difference in the sensations of parts pressed on and those of surrounding parts. Heat-sense, cold-sense and pain-sense all depend upon different nerve-endings in the skin; and thus, with care and delicate instruments like needles, bristles in holders and metal pencils through which hot or cold water can be made to circulate, the skin may be mapped out into a mosaic of little areas where the different kinds of impressions are registered. Whilst the tongue and finger-tips are the parts most sensitive to touch, they are comparatively insensitive to heat, and can easily bear temperatures which the cheek or elbow could not tolerate. The muscular sense, in all probability, depends on the sensory organs known as muscle-spindles, which are scattered through the substance of the muscles, and the sense of locality is dependent partly upon these and partly upon the nerves which end in tendons, ligaments and joints.

Disorders of the sense of touch occur in various diseases.

HYPERAESTHESIA is a condition in which there is excessive sensitiveness to any stimulus, such as touch. When this reaches the stage when a mere touch or gentle handling causes acute pain it is known as HYPERALGESIA. It is found in various diseases of the spinal cord immediately above the level of the disease, combined often with loss of sensation below the diseased part. It is also present in neuralgia, the skin of the neuralgic area becoming excessively tender to touch, heat or cold. Heightened sensibility to pain is seen sometimes in drunkards, who wince at a mere touch when not under the influence of alcohol. Heightened sensibility to temperature is a common symptom of neuritis. (See PAIN.)

ANAESTHESIA, or diminution of the sense of touch, causing often a feeling of numbness, is present in many diseases affecting the nerves of sensation or their continuations up the posterior part of the spinal cord. The condition of *dissociated analgesia*, in which a touch is quite well felt, though there is complete insensibility to pain, is present in the disease of the spinal cord known as syringomyelia, and affords a proof that the nerve-fibres for pain and those for touch are quite separate. In tabes dorsalis there is sometimes loss of the sense of touch on feet or arms; but in other cases of this disease there is no loss of the sense of touch, although there is a complete loss of the sense of locality in the lower limbs, thus proving that these two senses are quite distinct.

PARAESTHESIAE are peculiar forms of perverted sensation such as creeping, tingling, pricking or hot flushes.

TOURNIQUET is an instrument used for the temporary stoppage of blood supply to a limb, in order to control severe bleeding. Although serving its purpose, unless the tourniquet is untied after about 15 minutes gangrene may result, necessitating amputation. Tourniquets are rarely used nowadays because of this major hazard, and direct pressure on the bleeding points provides a simpler, safer, and equally effective means of controlling bleeding in emergencies.

TOW is a form of jute which is very hygroscopic, absorbing up to 25 per cent of moisture.

TOXAEMIA is a term applied to forms of blood-poisoning due to the absorption of bacterial products (toxins) formed at some local site of infection, such as abscesses. In other cases the toxaemia is due to defective action of some excretory organ, such as the kidney. As regards treatment, the most important consideration is to remove the source of infection.

Toxaemia of pregnancy is a term sometimes used to describe the two complications of pregnancy known as pre-eclampsia and eclampsia (q.v.).

TOXIC SHOCK SYNDROME is a syndrome, first described in 1978, characterized by high fever, diarrhoea, shock and an erythematous rash. It is frequently associated with the use of tampons, but has occasionally been reported in men. The disease is due to a staphylococcal toxin. The treatment consists of supportive measures to combat shock and eradication of the staphylococcus by antibiotics. A mortality rate of 10 per cent has been reported. The syndrome may recur.

TOXICOLOGY is the science dealing with poisons. (See POISONS.)

TOXINS are poisons produced by bacteria. (See IMMUNITY; IMMUNOLOGY; MICROBIOLOGY.) Toxins are usually soluble, easily destroyed by heat, sometimes of the nature of crystalline substances, and sometimes albumins. When injected into animals in carefully graduated doses, they bring about the formation of substances called antitoxins which neutralize the action of the toxin. These antitoxins are generally produced in excessive amount, and the serum of the animal when withdrawn can be used for conferring antitoxic powers upon other animals or human beings to neutralize the disease in question. The best known of these antitoxins are those of diphtheria and tetanus. Toxins are also found in many plants and in snake venom.

Some toxins are not set free by bacteria, but remain in the substance of the latter. They are known as endotoxins and are not capable of producing antitoxins.

TOXOCARIASIS is a disease acquired by swallowing the ova of a roundworm which lives in the intestine of cats (*Toxocara cati*) or dogs (*Toxocara canis*). In man, the small larval worms produced by these ova migrate to various parts of the body, including the retina of the eye, where they then die, and produce a small granuloma (q.v.) which in turn may produce allergic reactions. In the eye it may cause choroidretinitis. It is said that 2 per cent of apparently healthy people in Britain have been infected in this way. A course of treatment with diethylcarbamazine is said to kill the worm.

TOXOID is toxin (q.v.) which has been rendered non-toxic by certain chemicals, or by heat, or by being partly neutralized by antitoxin. The best-known example is diphtheria toxoid. (See IMMUNITY.)

TOXOPLASMOSIS is a disease which is due to infection with protozoa of the genus *Toxoplasma*. The infection may be acquired from eating raw or undercooked meat, from cats, or from gardening or playing in contaminated soil. It occurs in two forms: an acquired form and a congenital form. The acquired form may run such a benign course that it is not recognized, the patient scarcely feeling ill. In the congenital form the unborn child is infected by the mother. The congenital form, the incidence of which in the United Kingdom is 1 in 5000 pregnancies (1 in 2000 pregnancies in Scotland), may develop in one of two ways. The infant may either appear generally ill, or the brunt of the infection may fall on the nervous system causing hydrocephalus (q.v.), mental retardation, or loss of sight. In some cases the infection may be so severe that it kills the fetus, resulting in a miscarriage or stillbirth. In other cases the infection is so mild that it is missed until in later life the child begins to show signs of eye trouble. As the congenital form of the disease, which is most serious, seems to develop only if the mother acquires the infection during pregnancy, it would appear to be a wise precaution that pregnant women should avoid contact with cats and eating raw or undercooked meat foods.

TOY LIBRARIES The National Toy Libraries Association, founded to help handicapped children get suitable toys, now has links with several hundred toy libraries throughout the country. These libraries keep a wide range of toys that can either be played with at the Library or taken home. The range includes trucks for children to ride on, toys for babies, and others with an educational element. They also provide a convenient place for parents and child minders to meet, share common problems and seek advice if they want to. Further details can be obtained from: Play Matters National Toy Libraries Associations (see APPENDIX 2: ADDRESSES).

TRACE ELEMENTS are chemical elements that are distributed throughout the tissues of the body in very small amounts and are essential for the nutrition of the body. Nine such elements are now recognized: cobalt, copper, fluorine, iodine, iron, manganese, molybdenum, selenium and zinc.

TRACHEA is another name for the windpipe (q.v.). (See also AIR PASSAGES.)

TRACHEITIS means inflammation of the trachea. It may occur along with bronchitis, or independently, due to similar causes.

TRACHEOSTOMY, or TRACHEOTOMY, is the operation in which the windpipe is opened from the front of the neck, so that air may obtain direct entrance into the lower air passages. The opening is made through the second and third rings of the trachea (windpipe) (q.v.).

Reasons for operation Conditions in which the opening of the larynx is narrowed are treated by the appropriate means but, should these fail, some form of airway intervention is necessary. In the majority of cases this would involve the insertion of an endotracheal tube, i.e. a tube is inserted either through the nose or mouth and down the pharynx through the larynx to bypass the obstruction, or by a tracheostomy. The majority of tracheostomies performed nowadays are for patients in intensive-therapy-unit situations. These patients require airway intervention for prolonged periods to facilitate artificial ventilation which is performed by means of a mechanical ventilator. The presence of a tube passing through the larynx for a prolonged period of time is associated with long-term damage to the larynx, and therefore any patients requiring prolonged intubation usually undergo a tracheostomy to prevent further damage to the larynx. Endotracheal intubation is also the preferred method of airway intervention for acute inflammatory disorders of the upper airway as opposed to tracheostomy. Tracheostomy in these cases is performed only in the emergency situation if facilities for endotracheal intubation are not available or if they are unsuccessful. Tracheostomy may also be performed for large tumours which obstruct the larynx until some form of treatment is instituted. Similarly it may be needed in conditions whereby the nerve supply to the larynx has been jeopardized impairing its protective function of the upper airway and its respiratory function.

Tracheostomy tubes When the trachea has been opened it is necessary to introduce a tube in order to keep the opening from closing. The tubes are made either of hard rubber or more often of metal; and there is always an *outer tube* which is fixed in position by tapes passing round the neck, and an *inner tube* which slides freely out of and into the other, so that it may be removed at any time for cleansing, and is readily coughed out should it happen to become blocked by mucus.

A dressing is generally applied between the edges of the outer tube and the wound to prevent trauma to the skin of the neck.

The inner tube must be removed and washed several times daily, and if at any time it gets blocked by coughed-up mucus, it must be instantly removed and wiped. The outer tube is not removed till one or two days have elapsed after the operation, and then it is replaced by a fresh tube carefully introduced.

After-treatment When the operation has been performed for some permanent obstruction, the tube must be worn permanently; and the double metal tube is in such cases replaced after a short time by a soft rubber single one. When the operation has relieved some passing condition like diphtheria, the tube is left out now and then for a few hours, and finally, at the end of

a week or so, is removed altogether, after which the wound quickly heals up.

(See APPENDIX 2: ADDRESSES.)

TRACHOMA is a severe type of conjunctivitis (see EYE DISEASES). This chronic contagious condition is caused by *Chlamydia trachomatis*, a bacterium with virus-like characteristics. Trachoma is common in the Third World, where it is the leading cause of preventable blindness worldwide. The disease may be seen in immigrant populations in developed countries, though it is usually inactive. The bacterium is transmitted by flies and causes inflammation of the conjunctiva and cornea with consequent scarring. The active disease is treated with tetracycline tablets and eye drops and cure is usually satisfactory.

TRACTION The application of a pulling force to the distal part of a fracture in order to allow the fracture to heal with the bone in correct alignment. There are many different methods for applying traction, usually involving weights and pulleys.

TRAINING (see DIET; EXERCISE).

TRANCE is a profound sleep from which a person cannot for a time be aroused, but which is not due to organic disease. The power of voluntary movement is lost, though sensibility and even consciousness may remain. It is usually due to hysteria, and may be induced by hypnotism. (See CATALEPSY; ECSTASY; and SLEEP.)

TRANEXAMIC ACID is a drug used in the control of bleeding. Its mode of action is similar to that of aminocaproic acid (q.v.).

TRANQUILLIZERS A tranquillizer is a drug which induces a mental state free from agitation and anxiety, and renders the patient calm, serene and peaceful. Strictly speaking, tobacco, alcohol and the barbiturates might be included in this category, but the term 'tranquillizer' is usually restricted to certain new groups of drugs whose main action is the control of anxiety and psychomotor agitation without producing sleepiness, or clouding of consciousness. Among the more widely used drugs in this group are chlorpromazine, diazepam and chlordiazepoxide.

TRANSCUTANEOUS ELECTRICAL NERVE STIMULATION is a method of electrical stimulation that is being used for the relief of pain, including that of migraine, neuralgia and phantom limbs. Known as TENS, its mode of action appears to have some resemblance to that of acupuncture. Several controlled trials suggest that it provides at least a modicum of relief of pain after operations, thereby reducing the amount of analgesics that may be called for.

TRANSFUSION OF BLOOD has been practised since the 17th century, although with a high mortality rate. The main problems encountered have been the tendency of the transfused blood to clot and the liability of the red blood cells to break up, leading to haematuria and jaundice. Recipients often showed an allergic response, in severe cases leading to anaphylactic shock. It was only when incompatibility of blood groups (q.v.) was considered as a potential cause of this allergy that routine blood testing became standard practice. Since the National Blood Transfusion Service was started, in 1946, in the United Kingdom, blood for transfusion has been collected from voluntary, unpaid donors, screened for infections such as syphilis, HIV and hepatitis, sorted by group, and stored in blood-banks throughout the country. A standard transfusion bottle has been developed, and whole blood may be stored at 2–6 °C for three weeks before use. Transfusions may then be given of whole blood, plasma, blood cells, or platelets, as appropriate. Stored in the dried form at 4–21 °C, away from direct sunlight, human plasma is stable for five years, and is easily reconstituted by adding uninfected distilled water.

AUTOLOGOUS TRANSFUSION is the use of an individual's own blood, provided in advance, for transfusion during or after a surgical operation. This is a valuable procedure for operations that may require large transfusions or where a person has a rare blood group. Its use has increased because of the fear of AIDS.

EXCHANGE TRANSFUSION is the method of treatment in severe cases of haemolytic disease of the newborn (q.v.). It consists of replacing the whole of the baby's blood with Rh-negative blood of the correct blood group for the baby.

TRANSIENT ISCHAEMIC ATTACKS OR EPISODES (TIA, TIE) are episodes of transient ischaemia of some part of the cerebral hemispheres or the brain stem lasting anything from a few minutes to several hours and followed by complete recovery. By definition the ischaemic episode must be less than 24 hours. These episodes may be isolated or they may occur several times in a day. The cause is atheroma of the carotid or vertebral arteries and the embolization of platelets or cholesterol. These attacks present with strokes (q.v.) that rapidly recover.

TRANSLOCATION is the term used to describe an exchange of genetic material between chromosomes (q.v.). It is an important factor in the etiology, or causation, of certain congenital abnormalities such as, for example mongolism. It is one of the main abnormalities sought for in amnioscopy (q.v.).

TRANSPLANTATION of organs of the body has become a practical possibility within recent years. The major outstanding problem is how to prevent the recipient's body from rejecting and destroying the transplanted organ. Such rejection of a foreign body is part of the normal protective mechanism of the body and is essential for the maintenance of the integrity of the body.

If the transplant comes from another person it is known as an *allotransplant*. If it comes from the patient himself – for example, a skin graft – it is known as an *autotransplant*. If it comes from an animal it is known as a *xenotransplant*.

The pioneering success was achieved with transplantation of the kidney, and this has been most successful when the transplanted kidney has come from an identical twin. Less successful have been live transplants from other blood relatives, while least successful have been transplants from other live donors and cadaver donors. The results, however, are steadily improving. Thus the one-year functional survival of kidneys transplanted from unrelated cadaver donors has risen from around 50 per cent to over 80 per cent, and survival rates of 80 per cent after three years are not uncommon. For a well-matched transplant from a live related donor the survival rate after five years is around 90 per cent. And, of course, if a transplanted kidney fails to function, the patient can always be switched on to some form of dialysis (q.v.). In the United Kingdom the supply of cadaveric kidneys for transplantation is only about half that necessary to meet the demand.

Other organs that have been transplanted with increasing success are the heart, the lungs, the liver, bone marrow, and the cornea of the eye. Heart, lung, liver and pancreas transplantations are now carried out in specialist centres. It is estimated that in the United Kingdom approximately 200 patients a year between the ages of 15 and 55 would benefit from a liver transplant if an adequate number of donors were available. Over 100 liver transplants are carried out annually in the United Kingdom and one-year-survival rates of up to 80 per cent have been achieved.

Good progress has been made in techniques of tissue typing and immunosuppression to overcome the problems of organ transplantation. Drugs are now available that can depress the immune reactions of the recipient, which are responsible for the rejection of the transplanted organ. Notable among these is cyclosporin A. By these and other means, such as careful typing of the donor kidney, results are steadily improving. One of the more promising developments is the development of an anti-lymphocytic serum (ALS) which reduces the activity of the lymphocytes (q.v.), cells which play an important part in maintaining the integrity of the body against foreign bodies.

Donor cards are now available in all general practitioners' surgeries and pharmacies but, of the millions of cards distributed since 1972, too few have been used. The reasons are complex but include the reluctance of the public and doctors to consider organ donation, poor organization for recovery of donor kidneys and worries about the diagnosis of death. A code of practice for procedures relating to the removal of organs for transplantation was produced in 1978 and this code has been revised in the light of further views expressed by the Conference of Medical Royal Colleges and Faculties of the United Kingdom on the Diagnosis of Brain Death. Under the Human Tissue Act 1961 only the person lawfully in possession of the body or his designate can authorize the removal of organs from a body. This authorization may be given orally. Patients who may become suitable donors after death are those who have suffered severe and irreversible brain damage. Such patients will be dependent on artificial ventilation. Patients with malignant disease or systemic infection and patients with renal disease, including chronic hypertension, are unsuitable. If a patient carries a signed donor card or has otherwise recorded his wishes there is no legal requirement to establish lack of objection on the part of relatives, although it is good practice to take account of the views of close relatives. If a relative objects, despite the known request by the patient, staff will need to judge, according to the circumstances of the case, whether it is wise to proceed with organ removal. If a patient who has died is not known to have requested that his organs be removed for transplantation after his death the designated person may only authorize the removal if, having made such reasonable enquiry as may be practical, he has no reason to believe (*a*) that the deceased had expressed an objection to his body being so dealt with after his death, or (*b*) that the surviving spouse or any surviving relative of the deceased objects to the body being so dealt with. Staff will need to decide who is best qualified to approach the relatives. This should be someone with appropriate experience who is aware how much the relative already knows about the patient's condition. Relatives should not normally be approached before death has occurred but sometimes a relative approaches the hospital staff and suggests sometime in advance that the patient's organs might be used for transplantation after his death. The staff of hospitals and organ exchange organizations must respect the wishes of the donor, the recipient and their families with respect to anonymity.

Relatives who enquire should be told that some post-mortem treatment of the donor's body will be necessary if the organs are to be removed in good condition. It is ethical to maintain artificial ventilation and heart beat until removal of organs has been completed. This is essential in the case of heart and liver transplants and many doctors think it is desirable when removing kidneys. Official criteria have been issued in Britain to recognize when brain-stem death (q.v.) has occurred. This is an important protection for patients and relatives when someone with a terminal condition – usually as a result of an accident – is considered as a possible organ donor.

TRANS-SEXUALISM is the psycho-sexual abnormality characterized by feelings of be-

longing to the gender opposite to that of the genitalia and the secondary sex characteristics. Trans-sexuals or their families wanting help and guidance should contact the Gender Dysphoria Trust International or the Partner's Group for Partners and Families of Trans-sexuals (see APPENDIX 2: ADDRESSES).

TRANSURETHRAL RESECTION The use of a special cystoscope (q.v.) (a resectoscope) inserted through the urethra (q.v.) to resect the prostate gland (q.v.) or bladder tumours (see resection).

TRANSVERSE An anatomical description of a line, plane or structure at right angles to the long axis of an organ or the body.

TRANSVESTITISM, or TRANSVESTISM, is the term given to a psycho-sexual abnormality in which there is a repetitive compulsion to dress in the clothes of the opposite sex to achieve orgasm.

TRANYLCYPROMINE (see ANTIDEPRESSANTS).

TRAUMA is the term used to indicate disorders due to wounds or injuries.

TRAVEL MEDICINE Many countries have reciprocal health arrangements with Britain under which British visitors may receive emergency treatment free or at reduced cost. Information about these arrangements is available in leaflet SA40, available from any local DSS office. General and specific advice for travellers on such matters as immunizations needed can be obtained from their doctor, through travel agents or one of the high street travel 'health shops'. (See APPENDIX 3: TRAVEL AND HEALTH.)

TRAVEL SICKNESS is the sickness that is induced by any form of transport, whether by sea, air, motor-car or train. (See MOTION-SICKNESS.)

TRAVELLER'S DIARRHOEA is an all too common affliction of the traveller, which basks in a multiplicity of names: e.g. Aden gut, Aztec two step, Basra belly, Delhi belly, Gippy tummy, Hong Kong dog, Montezuma's revenge, Tokyo trots, turista. It is caused by a variety of micro-organisms, usually *E. coli*. Some people seem to be more prone to it than others, though for no good cause. Obvious preventive measures include the avoidance of salads, unpeeled fruit and ice cream, and never drinking unboiled or unbottled water. Two widely recommended preventive drugs are Streptotriad (one tablet twice daily for a week, and then one daily) and doxycycline (100 mg daily). Both are said to provide a satisfactory degree of protection, provided a fulminating infection is avoided, as long as taken.

TRAZODONE (see ANTIDEPRESSANTS).

TREMOR means a very fine kind of involuntary movement. Tremors may be seen in projecting parts like the hands, head and tongue, or they may involve muscles or even the individual fibres of a muscle here and there. They are of various grades of fineness. Very coarse tremors, which prevent a person from drinking a glass of water without spilling it, are found in multiple sclerosis and in chorea (see under these headings); somewhat finer tremors, which produce trembling of the hands or tongue when they are stretched out, are caused by alcoholism (see ALCOHOL), by poisoning with other substances like lead, by Parkinsonism (q.v.), and by the weakness which follows some acute disease or characterizes old age; a fine tremor of the outstretched fingers is a characteristic of thyrotoxicosis (q.v.); very fine tremors, visible in the muscles of face or limbs, and known as fibrillary tremors, are present in general paralysis of the insane, and in progressive muscular atrophy or wasting palsy. Tremors may occur at rest and disappear on movement as in Parkinsonism, or they may occur only on movement (intention tremors) as in cerebellar disease.

TRENCH FEVER is an infectious disease caused by *Rickettsia quintana* which is transmitted by the body louse. Large epidemics occurred among troops on active service during the 1914–18 War. It recurred on a smaller scale in the 1939–45 War, and is endemic in Mexico.

TRENCH, or IMMERSION, **FOOT** is due to prolonged exposure of the feet to water, particularly cold water. Trench warfare is a common precipitating factor, and it was rampant during the 1914–18 War. Cases also occurred during the 1939–45 War, particularly during the slow winter advance up through Italy after the Anzio landings. Cases occurred, too, during the Falklands campaign. The less common form due to warm water immersion occurred with some frequency in the Vietnam war. It is characterized by painful swelling of the feet accompanied in due course by blistering and ulceration which, in severe, untreated cases, may go on to gangrene. In mild cases recovery may be complete in a month, but severe cases may drag on for a year.
Treatment Drying of the feet overnight, where practicable, is the best method of prevention, accompanied by avoidance of constrictive clothing and tight boots, and of prolonged immobility. Frequent rest periods and daily changing of socks also help. The application of silicone grease once a day is another useful preventive measure. In the early stages treatment consists of rest in bed and warmth. In more severe cases treatment is as for infected tissues and ulceration. Analgesics (q.v.) are usually necessary to ease the pain. Technically, smoking should be forbidden, but the psychological effects in troops on active service may outweigh its advantages.

TRENDELENBERG POSITION First described by Frederick Trendelenberg in 1881, this is a steep head-down tilt so that the patient's pelvis and legs lie above the heart. It is used to improve access and limit blood loss during surgery to the pelvis. It has been used to treat shocked patients, but, as the position increases pressure on the diaphragm and embarrasses breathing, raising the legs by themselves is better.

TREPHINING, or TREPANNING, is an operation in which a portion of the cranium is removed. Originally the operation was performed with an instrument resembling a carpenter's brace and known as the trephine or trepan, which removes a small circle of bone; but now this instrument is only used, as a rule, for making small openings, whilst, for wider operations, gouge forceps, circular saws driven by electric motor, or wire saws are employed in order to give greater ease and speed.

The operation is one requiring nicety of manipulation, but is neither difficult nor serious, and was one of the commonest major operations of antiquity. It is said, from the appearances presented by skulls found in old French burial mounds, to have been practised by prehistoric peoples; at all events Hippocrates describes fully the operation and the conditions that call for it, whilst Galen mentions two varieties of the instrument in common use. Both among the Greeks and Romans, and in the Middle Ages, resort seems to have been made to trephining on very slight provocation for conditions traceable to the head.

At the present time, the conditions under which it may be thought advisable to trephine the skull are chiefly as follows. In cases of fracture, with splintering of the skull, the operation is performed to remove the fragments of bone and any foreign bodies, like a bullet, which may have entered, in order that the wound may be thoroughly cleansed. In compression of the brain with unconsciousness following an injury, the skull is trephined and any blood-clots removed, or torn vessels ligatured. When an abscess is present within the skull, the operation is called for in order to evacuate the pus. In certain forms of epilepsy, or in continued headache, when the symptoms point to a definite part of the brain being involved, the skull may be trephined over this area, so that any clot, scar, thickening of the bone or cyst, which is setting up the irritation, may be discovered and removed. For a cerebral tumour, trephining is often performed either with the view of removing the tumour, if possible, or at all events of relieving the great pressure within the skull caused by the growing mass.

TREPONEMA is the name of a genus of spirochaetal micro-organisms which consist of slender spirals and which progress by means of bending movements. *Treponema pallidum* (formerly called *Spirochaeta pallida*) is the causative organism of syphilis.

TRIAGE Derived from French word for 'sorting', a universal term applied to methods of allocating treatment prioritizations for casualties from disasters or in warfare. Triage helps a medical team to treat urgently casualties who, though badly injured, can be saved, to defer those whose treatment is less urgent and to provide care and comfort for those with fatal injuries.

TRIAMCINOLONE is a corticosteroid (q.v.), which has a potency equivalent to that of prednisone, but is less likely to cause retention of sodium.

TRIAZOLAM (see BENZOTHIAZEPINES).

TRICHIASIS A condition in which the eyelashes become ingrown. (See EYE DISEASES.)

TRICEPS A muscle of the posterior upper arm which acts to extend the forearm. So named because it originates from three heads.

TRICHINOSIS, or TRICHINIASIS, is the name of a disease set up by eating meat infected with the parasitic nematode worm, *Trichinella spiralis*. Although it infects over 100 animal species, this nematode usually infects humans via pig meat in which the immature *spiralis* is encysted. The full-grown female worm, which inhabits the intestine, is 3 mm in length, and the larvae, to whose movements the disease is due, are much smaller. The disease is acquired by eating raw or underdone pork from pigs that have been infected with the worm. When such a piece of meat is eaten, the embryos contained in it are set free, develop into full-grown trichinellae, and from each pair of these 1000 or more new embryos may arise in a few weeks. These burrow through the walls of the gut, spread throughout the body and settle in voluntary muscle.
Prevention is based on thorough inspection of meat in slaughter-houses, for even cooking, unless the meat is in slices, is not an efficient protection. Pigs should not be fed on unboiled garbage. Rats may be a source of sporadic outbreaks, as infected rats have been found near piggeries. The disease is widely distributed throughout the Americas, Asia, Africa and the Arctic. Sporadic cases and epidemics occur and outbreaks also appear in Europe, though rarely in Britain.
Treatment Thiabendazole or mebendazole are usually effective, while steroids help patients with systemic illness and muscle tenderness.

TRICHO- is a prefix denoting relation to hair.

TRICHOMONAS VAGINALIS is a protozoon normally present in the vagina of about 30 to 40 per cent of women. It sometimes becomes pathogenic and causes inflammation of the genital passages, with vaginal discharge. A man may become infected as a result of sexual intercourse with an infected woman and have a urethral discharge as a result; it may also cause prostatitis. Excellent results are being obtained from the use of metronidazole in its treatment. To obtain a satisfactory result it may be necessary to treat both partners.

TRICHOMONIASIS is the disease caused by infection with *Trichomonas vaginalis* (q.v.).

TRICHOPHYTON is the parasite that causes ringworm. (See RINGWORM.)

TRICHORRHOEA is the term applied to the falling-out of hair. It is usually due to some general disease such as scarlet fever or typhoid fever. When there is no obvious cause, such as this, treatment consists of attention to the general hygiene of the scalp. Vigorous massage is to be avoided.

TRICHOTILLOMANIA is the condition in which a person has an obsessional impulse to pull out his own hair.

TRICHURIASIS is a worldwide infection, particularly common in the tropics. It is caused by *Trichuris trichiura*, or whipworm, so called because of its shape, the rear end being stout and the front end hairlike, resembling the lash of a whip. The male measures 5 cm and the female 4 cm in length. Infection results from eating vegetables, or drinking water, polluted with the ova (eggs). These hatch out in the large intestine. The diagnosis is made by finding the eggs in the stools. The worms seldom cause any trouble unless they are present in large numbers when, especially in malnourished children, they may cause bleeding from the bowels, anaemia and prolapse of the rectum. The most effective drug at the moment is mebendazole: 100 mg twice daily for three days.

TRICUSPID VALVE is the valve, with three cusps or flaps, that guards the opening from the right atrium into the right ventricle of the heart. (See HEART.)

TRIFLUOPERAZINE (see NEUROLEPTICS).

TRIGEMINAL NERVE is the fifth cranial nerve. It consists of three divisions: (1) the ophthalmic nerve, which is purely sensory in function, being distributed mainly over the forehead and front part of the scalp; (2) the maxillary nerve, which is also sensory and distributed to the skin of the cheek, the mucous membrane of the mouth and throat, and the upper teeth; and (3) the mandibular nerve, which is the nerve of sensation to the lower part of the face, the tongue and the lower teeth, as well as being the motor nerve to the muscles concerned in chewing. The trigeminal nerve is of special interest, owing to its liability to neuralgia (q.v.), trigeminal neuralgia (q.v.), or tic douloureux as it is also known, being the most painful form known of neuralgia.

TRIGEMINAL NEURALGIA, or TIC DOULOUREUX, is one of the most severe forms of neuralgia. It affects the great nerve of sensation in the face (trigeminal nerve), and may occur in one or more of the three divisions in which the nerve is distributed. It is usually confined to one side. Women suffer, on the whole, more often than men, and they are usually over the age of 50. The attack is often precipitated by movements of the jaw, as in talking or eating, or by tactile stimuli such as a cold wind or washing the face. When the *first or upper division of the nerve* is involved, the pain is mostly felt in the forehead and side of the head. It is usually of an intensely sharp, cutting, or burning character, either constant or with exacerbations each day while the attack continues. There is also pain in the eyelid, redness of the eye and increased flow of tears. When the *second division of the nerve* is affected, the pain is chiefly in the cheek and upper jaw. When *the third division of the nerve* suffers, the pain affects the lower jaw, and the chief painful points are in front of the ear and above the chin. Attacks of tic douloureux, extremely distressing as they are, may recur for years; and, although interfering with sleeping and eating, they rarely appear to lead to any serious results. Nevertheless, the pain may be so intolerable as to make life a burden.
Treatment The outlook in trigeminal neuralgia was radically altered by the introduction of the drug carbamazepine, which usually relieves the pain. In view of its potential side-effects, it must only be taken under medical supervision. If the side-effects are intolerable or pain not relieved, phenytoin (q.v.) may help. Otherwise, surgery is needed in the shape of controlled, radiofrequency heat damage to the appropriate part of the trigeminal nerve.

TRIGGER FINGER, or SNAPPING FINGER, is the condition in which when the fingers are straightened on unclenching the fist one finger, usually the ring or middle finger, remains bent. The cause is obscure. In severe cases treatment consists of opening up the sheath surrounding the tendon of the affected finger. When confined to the thumb it is known as TRIGGER THUMB.

TRIGGER THUMB (see TRIGGER FINGER).

TRIGLYCERIDE One of the basic chemical 'building blocks' from which fats are formed. A triglyceride molecules consists of three fatty-acid molecules which have chemically reacted with glycerol.

TRIGONE is the base of the bladder between the openings of the two ureters and of the urethra.

TRI-IODOTHYRONINE is the substance which exerts the physiological action of thyroid hormone. It is formed in the body cells by the de-iodination of thyroxine (tetra-iodothyronine) which is the active principle secreted by the thyroid gland. It has also been synthesized, and is now available for the treatment of myxoedema (q.v.). It is three times as potent as thyroxine. (See also THYROID GLAND.)

TRIMESTER A period of three months. Normal human gestation is divided into three trimesters.

TRIMETHORIM is an anti-bacterial agent used in the treatment of infections of the urinary tract. It is also a constituent of co-trimoxazole (q.v.).

TRIMIPRAMINE is a relatively weak antidepressant drug which also acts as a sedative. (See ANTIDEPRESSANTS.)

TRIMUSTINE is a nitrogen mustard derivative (q.v.) used in the treatment of certain forms of malignant disease. It is administered intravenously.

TRINITRIN (see GLYCERYL TRINITRATE).

TRIPLETS (see MULTIPLE BIRTHS).

TRISMUS is another name for lockjaw. (See TETANUS.)

TROCAR is an instrument provided with a sharp three-sided point fitted inside a tube or cannula, and used for puncturing cavities of the body in which fluid has collected.

TROCHANTER is the name given to two bony prominences at the upper end of the thigh-bone. The *greater trochanter* can be felt on the outer side of the thigh. The *lesser trochanter* is a small prominence on the inner side of this bone.

TROCHES is another name for lozenges. (See LOZENGES.)

TROCHLEAR NERVE is the fourth cranial nerve, which acts upon the superior oblique muscle of the eye.

TROPHIC is a term applied to the influence that nerves exert with regard to the healthiness and nourishment of the parts to which they run. When the nerves become diseased or injured, this influence is lost and the muscles waste, while the skin loses its healthy appearance and is liable to break down into ulcers. (See NERVOUS DISEASES; BED SORES.)

TROPHOBLAST is the outer layer of the fertilized ovum which attaches the ovum to the wall of the uterus (or womb) and supplies nutrition to the embryo.

TROPICAL DISEASES Technically, those diseases occurring in the area of the globe situated between the Tropic of Cancer and the Tropic of Capricorn: pertaining to the sun. They include many 'exotic' infections – many of them parasitic in origin – which fall under the umbrella of 'Tropical Medicine'. However, disease in the tropics is far broader than this and includes numerous other infections, many of them with a viral or bacterial basis, e.g. the viral hepatidises, streptococcal and pneumococcal infections, and tuberculosis. The prevalence of other diseases, such as rheumatic cardiac disease, cirrhosis, heptocellular carcinoma ('hepatoma'), and various nutrition-related problems, is also much increased in most areas of the tropics. (See ANCYLOSTOMIASIS; BERIBERI; BLACKWATER FEVER; CHOLERA; DENGUE; DRACONTIASIS; DYSENTERY; ELEPHANTIASIS; FILARIASIS; HEAT STROKE; LEISHMANIASIS; LEPROSY; LIVER DISEASES; MALARIA; ORIENTAL SORE; PLAGUE; PRICKLY HEAT; SCHISTOSOMIASIS; SLEEPING SICKNESS; STRONGYLOIDIASIS; SUNBURN; YAWS; YELLOW FEVER)

TRUNK A major vessel or nerve from which lesser ones arise, or the main part of the body excluding the head, neck and limbs.

TRUSS is an device used to support a hernia; or to retain the protruding organ within the cavity from which it tends to pass. Every truss possesses a pad of some sort to cover the opening and a belt or spring to keep it in position.
  Before applying a truss the wearer must make certain that the hernia has been reduced. This may mean lying down before applying the truss. A truss will rarely control a hernia satisfactorily, and it should be considered as a temporary measure only until surgical correction is possible. In the past trusses have been supplied to patients considered too frail for surgery, but modern anaesthetic techniques means that most people can have their hernias surgically repaired.

TRYPANOSOMA is a genus of microscopic parasites, several of which are responsible for causing sleeping sickness and some allied diseases. (See SLEEPING SICKNESS.)

TRYPANOSOMIASIS (see SLEEPING SICKNESS.)

TRYPSIN is the chief protein enzyme of the pancreatic secretion. Secreted by the pancreas as trypsinogen (an inactive form), it is converted in the duodenum by another enzyme, enteropeptidase. It changes proteins into peptones and forms the main constituent of pancreatic extracts used for digestion of food. (See PANCREAS; PEPTONIZED FOOD.)

TRYPTOPHAN is an antidepressive drug that has helped some patients with resistant depression. Used as a supporting drug with other treatment, tryptophan was withdrawn because of side-effects. It may, however, soon be made available to patients for whom no alternative treatment is suitable.

TSETSE FLY is an African fly of the genus *Glossina*. One or more of these is responsible for carrying the trypanosome which causes sleeping sickness and thus spreads the disease among cattle and from cattle to men.

TSUTSUGAMUSHI, or JAPANESE RIVER FEVER, is a disease of the typhus group. (See TYPHUS FEVER.)

TUBAL PREGNANCY Implantation of the embryo in the fallopian tube (q.v.) rather than in the lining of the uterus (q.v.). The patient usually complains of pain between six and ten weeks' gestation and, if the Fallopian tube is not removed, there may be rupture with potentially life-threatening haemorrhage (also known as ectopic pregnancy).

TUBERCLE is a term used in two distinct senses. As a descriptive term in anatomy, a *tubercle* means a small elevation or roughness upon a bone, such as the tubercles of the ribs. In the pathological sense, a *tubercle* is a small mass, barely visible to the naked eye, formed in some organ as the starting-point of tuberculosis. The name of *tubercle bacillus* was originally given to the micro-organism that causes this disease but this has now been changed to *Mycobacterium tuberculosis*. The term tubercular should strictly be applied to anything connected with or resembling tubercles or nodules, and the term *tuberculous* to anything pertaining to the disease tuberculosis.
  When *Mycobacteria tuberculosis* have gained entrance to an organ, no matter whether inhaled, or whether absorbed from food and circulated through the lymphatics or bloodvessels, the following results ensue. The individual bacilli multiply, and around each group forms a minute tubercle, or granule, which is of a size almost invisible to the naked eye, and greyish in colour. These tubercles fuse together, and, at the same time, soften to a cheesy substance, so as to form yellow bodies about the size of pin-heads. Each grey tubercle, under

the microscope, shows the appearance of a group of cells of medium size (epithelioid cells), surrounded by many smaller cells (connective tissue cells and white blood corpuscles), attracted to the spot as a result of the inflammation set up. Scattered between these cells lie the mycobacteria. Near the centre of the older tubercles there are often seen one or more large cells with many nuclei (giant cells). The larger yellow tubercles form a more or less structureless mass in the centre, but show numbers of the small grey tubercles round their edge. Thus the process spreads, the healthy tissue being broken down and giving place to the soft, cheesy mass, which, in the case of the lungs, finally bursts into a bronchial tube, is coughed up, and leaves a ragged cavity in its place. Another change, however, takes place at the same time, for, in consequence of the irritation set up by the tubercle, strands of fibrous tissue are built up round its edge, and, when the process is a very chronic one, these come to form a dense capsule for the tuberculous area, cutting it off from further advance on healthy tissue, and forming a natural cure.

TUBERCULIDE is the term given to any skin lesion which is the result of infection with the tubercle bacillus, or *Mycobacterium tuberculosis* as it is now known.

TUBERCULIN is the name originally given by Koch in 1890 to a preparation derived from the tubercle bacillus, or *Mycobacterium tuberculosis* as it is now known, and intended for the diagnosis or treatment of tuberculosis.
Varieties *Old Tuberculin* (OT) is the heat-concentrated filtrate from a fluid medium on which the human or bovine type of *Mycobacterium tuberculosis* has been grown for six weeks or more. *Tuberculin Purified Protein Derivative* (Tuberculin PPD) is the active principle of Old Tuberculin, and is prepared from the fluid medium on which the *Mycobacterium tuberculosis* has been grown. It is supplied as a liquid, a powder, or as sterile tablets. The liquid contains 100,000 Units per millilitre, and the dry powder contains 30,000 Units per milligram. It is distributed in sterile containers sealed so as to exclude micro-organisms. It is more constant in composition and potency than Old Tuberculin.
Uses The basis of the tuberculin reaction is that any person who has been infected with the *Mycobacterium tuberculosis* gives a reaction when a small amount of tuberculin is injected into the skin. A negative reaction means that either the individual has never been infected with the tubercle bacillus, or that the infection has been too recent to have allowed of sensitivity developing.

There are various methods of carrying out the test, of which the following are the most commonly used. The *Mantoux Test* is the most satisfactory of all and has the advantage that the size of the reaction is a guide to the severity of the tuberculous infection. It is performed by injecting the tuberculin into the skin on the forearm. The *Heaf Multiple Puncture Test* is reliable. It is carried out with the multiple puncture apparatus, or Heaf Gun. The *Vollmer Patch Test* using an impregnated filter paper, is useful in children because of the ease with which it can be carried out.

TUBERCULOSIS is the general name for the whole group of diseases associated with the presence of the *Mycobacterium tuberculosis*, of which pulmonary tuberculosis is the most important. (See MICROBIOLOGY.)

Tuberculosis not only affects the lungs, but may invade almost any organ, being seldom found, however, in the muscles or in tissues with few blood-vessels, like cartilage and sinews. The disease spreads usually by way of the lymphatic vessels. The severity of the disease varies considerably, according to the organ attacked and its manifestations range from abscesses to meningitis. The enlargement of glands, most common in the neck, to which the name of scrofula was formerly given, seems to have been much more widespread in former times, and was known also as 'king's evil', from the superstition that a touch of the royal hand conveyed a cure to the affected person. The disfiguring skin disease known as lupus vulgaris is another of the manifestations of the disease.

Consumption was the popular name for tuberculosis because it was characterized by a rapid or gradual wasting away of the body.

The essential part of the disease, from which it receives its name of tuberculosis, is the formation in the substance of an organ of tubercles, fine granules of a size barely visible to the naked eye, these tubercles multiplying and changing in such a way as to lead finally to the destruction of the organ in which they are found.
Nature of the disease Tuberculosis has been recognized as a disease from the earliest times. Hippocrates (460–375 BC) bestowed the name of phthisis upon the disease as it affects the lungs, but not until 1882, when Koch announced the discovery of the tubercle bacillus, or *Mycobacterium tuberculosis* as it is now called, was the pathology of the disease understood.

The manner in which these bacilli gain access to the body is important. There are three possible channels: by innoculation through a knife contaminated with, say, tuberculous sputum; by inhalation of the aerosol discharges of infected persons; and by ingestion via products such as infected milk.

Tuberculosis is present throughout the world but it is especially prevalent in Asian countries where 60–80 per cent of children under 14 are infected. In 1994 the World Health Organization (WHO) declared the disease a global emergency. WHO estimates that each year 8 million new infections occur and 3 million people die, mostly in developing countries. Trends are upwards, however, in Europe and North America after decades in which the disease was declining. In England and Wales 5,920 cases were notified in 1993, a rise of 120 on the previous year. In Britain mortality is now about 5 per 100,000 cases. The main concerns in Europe and the USA focus on several factors, which include HIV infection (q.v.), migration of people, poverty, deprivation, homelessness, the likely emergence of drug resistance, failure of patients to comply with treatment and the protection of healthcare workers.

Causes The direct cause of the disease is the *Mycobacterium tuberculosis.* (See MICROBIOLOGY.) But, in view of the fact that many people suffer from the disease in a mild degree and afterwards recover, and that many limited cases of tuberculosis in bones, skin and glands are successfully treated, it appears that there are other factors such as age and heredity that determine the course of an infection.

Varieties The forms of tuberculosis other than pulmonary tuberculosis, such as tuberculous disease of joints, bones and spine, meningitis, intestine, lupus, are considered under these headings. The lung disease may present in different ways.

Treatment This falls very naturally into two classes: (*a*) preventive, and (*b*) remedial.

(*a*) PREVENTIVE TREATMENT The problem of prevention is partly social and partly medical. Abolition of overcrowding, provision of good homes, an adequate supply of protective foods and enough money to buy them went a long way towards diminishing the incidence of tuberculosis, but unemployment, increasing poverty and housing shortages have since the late 1980s provided an environment in which the disease may well increase in incidence in the Western world. To a considerable extent, tuberculosis is a social disease. On the medical side, the problem is essentially to prevent uninfected susceptible people – especially children – from coming into contact with the infecting agent – the *Mycobacterium tuberculosis.* The great risk to the child is coming into contact with an adult who has the causative organism in his or her sputum. Every attempt must therefore be made to detect and treat all sufferers from tuberculosis.

Two of the most important preventive measures have been BCG vaccination (q.v.) and mass miniature radiography (q.v.), although the latter is no longer provided in the United Kingdom.

(*b*) REMEDIAL TREATMENT For all practical purposes this now consists of chemotherapy.

Chemotherapy The outlook in tuberculosis was revolutionized by the introduction of effective antituberculous drugs. Since the isolation, in 1944, of streptomycin, the first chemotherapeutic substance to be of any value, several other drugs have been introduced. There are two important general aspects of chemotherapy. The first is that the *Mycobacterium tuberculosis* may become resistant to a drug given by itself. This can be prevented by using varying combinations of ethambutol, rifampicin and isoniazid, with streptomycin reserved for patients who fail to respond to these drugs. Most patients recover and suffer no recurrences; those who fail to respond – around 5 per cent – are usually the homeless and people who abuse alcohol and thus do not comply with treatment arrangements. The authorities are concerned, however, about appearance of tubercle bacilli resistant to known drugs.

TUBEROSE SCLEROSIS, or EPILOIA, also sometimes known as TUBEROUS SCLEROSIS, is a hereditary disease due to a developmental abnormality of the brain. The prevalence is 1 in 50,000 of the population. It is characterized by mental retardation (usually from birth), epilepsy which usually starts before 2 years of age and multiple small nodules or tumours in the face which usually appear around puberty. Relatives of those with this condition can obtain help and guidance from the Tuberous Sclerosis Association of Great Britain (see APPENDIX 2: ADDRESSES).

TUBOCURARINE is the active constituent of curare (q.v.). It is a muscle relaxant (q.v.) which is widely used in anaesthesia.

TULARAEMIA is a disease of rodents such as rabbits and rats, caused by the bacillus, *Francisella tularense*, and spread either by flies or by direct inoculation, for example, into the hands of a person engaged in skinning rabbits. In man the disease takes the form of a slow fever lasting several weeks, with much malaise and depression, followed by considerable emaciation. It was first described in the district of Tulare in California, and is found widely spread in North America and in Europe, but not in Great Britain. Streptomycin, the tetracyclines and chloramphenicol, have proved effective in treatment.

TULLE GRAS A dressing of gauze impregnated with soft paraffin to prevent it sticking to the wound.

TUMOUR means literally any swelling, but, by common consent, the term is held not to include passing swellings caused by acute inflammation, whilst the collections of diseased material arising in the course of chronic inflammation, like tuberculosis, syphilis, leprosy and glanders, sometimes are and sometimes are not classed as tumours, according to their size and appearance.

Varieties Some are of an infective nature, as already stated; some arise undoubtedly as the result of injury; several contributing factors are mentioned under the heading of CANCER, but for the rest, the causes of tumours are really still undiscovered.

Traditionally tumours have been divided into benign (simple) and malignant. Even benign tumours can be harmful because their size or position may distort or damage nerves, blood vessels or organs. Usually, however, they are easily removed by surgery. Malignant tumours or cancers are harmful and potentially lethal, not just because they erode tissues locally but because many of them spread, either by direct growth or by 'seeding' to other parts. Malignant tumours arise because of an uncontrolled growth of previously normal cells. Heredity, environmental factors and life-style all play a part in malignancy (see also ONCOGENES). Symptoms are caused by local spread and as a result of metastases – the distant secondary growths caused by the seeding. These metastases cause serious local damage, for example, in the brain or lungs, as well as disturbing the body's metabolism. Unless treated with chemotherapy or radiotherapy or surgery or a combination of these, malignant tumours are ultimately fatal. Many, however, can now be cured. The original site and type of a malignant tumour usually determine the rate and extent of spread. The type of cell and organ site determine the characteristics of a malignant tumour. The prognosis (outlook) for a patient with a malignant tumour depends largely on how soon it is diagnosed. Staging criteria have been developed to assess the local and metastatic spread of a tumour, its size and also likely sensitivity to the types of available treatment. The ability to locate a tumour and its metastases accurately has vastly improved with the introduction of radionucleide and ultrasound scanning (q.v.), CT scanning (q.v.) and magnetic resonance imaging (MRI) (q.v.).

Tumours are now classed according to the tissues of which they are built, somewhat as follows:

(1) Simple tumours of normal tissue
(2) Hollow tumours or cysts, generally of simple nature
(3) Malignant tumours: (*a*) of imperfect cellular structure, resembling the cells of skin, mucous membrane, or secreting glands; (*b*) of imperfect connective tissue.

TURGOR   Being or becoming swollen or engorged.

TURNER SYNDROME occurs in one in 2,500 live female births. It is caused by either the absence of or an abnormality in one of the two X chromosomes. Classical Turner Syndrome is a complete deletion of one X so that the karyotype is 45XO. Half of the people with Turner Syndrome have mosaicism with a mixture of Turner cells and normal cells or other abnormalities of the X chromosome such as partial deletions or a ring X. They are females, both phenotypically and sexually; clinical features are variable and include short stature, with final height between 1·295 m and 1·575 m and ovarian failure. However, a few women (fewer than 1 per cent) with Turner Syndrome do develop ovulatory menstrual cycles. Other clinical features may include a short neck, webbing of the neck, increased carrying angle at the elbow (cubitus valgus), widely spaced nipples, cardiovascular abnormalities of which the commonest is coarctation of the aorta (about 10 per cent), morphological abnormalities of the kidneys, including horseshoe kidney and abnormalities of the pelviureteric tracts, recurrent otitis media, squints, increased incidence of pigmented naevi, hypothyroidism and diabetes mellitus. Intelligence is across the normal range, although there are specific learning defects which are related to hand–eye co-ordination and spatial awareness.

Patients with Turner Syndrome may require therapeutic help throughout their life. In early childhood this may revolve around surgical correction of cardiovascular disease and treatment to improve growth. Usually puberty will need to be induced with oestrogen therapy. In adult life, problems of oestrogen therapy, prevention of osteoporosis, assessment and treatment of hypertension and assisted fertility predominate. For the address of the Turner Syndrome Society see APPENDIX 2: ADDRESSES.

TWINS (see MULTIPLE BIRTHS).

TYMPANIC MEMBRANE is the ear-drum, which separatees the external and middle ears. (See EAR.)

TYMPANITES means distension of the abdomen due to the presence of gas or air in the intestine or in the peritoneal cavity. The abdomen when struck with the fingers, gives under these conditions a drum-like (tympanitic) note.

TYMPANUM is another name for the middle ear. (See EAR.)

TYPHOID FEVER (see ENTERIC FEVERS).

TYPHUS FEVER is an infective disease of world-wide distribution, the manifestations of which vary in different localities. The causative organisms of all forms of typhus fever belong to the genus Rickettsia. These are organisms which are intermediate between bacteria and viruses in their properties and measure 0·5 micrometre or less in diameter.

LOUSE TYPHUS, in which the infecting Rickettsia is transmitted by the louse, is of world-wide distribution. More human deaths have been attributed to the louse via typhus, louse-borne relapsing fever and trench fever, than to any other insect with the exception of the malaria mosquito. Louse typhus includes Epidemic Typhus, Brill's Disease which is a recrudescent form of Epidemic Typhus, and Trench Fever (q.v.).

EPIDEMIC TYPHUS FEVER, also known as exanthematic typhus, classical typhus, and louse-borne typhus, is an acute infection of abrupt onset which, in the absence of treatment, persists for fourteen days. It is of world-wide distribution, but is largely confined today to parts of Africa. The causative organism is the

Rickettsia prowazeki, so-called after Ricketts and Prowazek, two brilliant investigators of typhus, both of whom died of the disease. It is transmitted by the human louse, *Pediculus humanus*. The rickettsiae can survive in the dried faeces of lice for 60 days, and these infected faeces are probably the main source of infection of man.

Symptoms The incubation period is usually 10 to 14 days. The onset is preceded by headache, pain in the back and limbs and rigors. On the third day the temperature rises suddenly, and the face and eyes become congested. At the same time the headache becomes more intense, and the patient is drowsy or delirious. Subsequently a characteristic rash appears on the abdomen and inner aspect of the arms, to spread over the chest, back and trunk. In cases which are not going to recover, death usually occurs from heart failure about the fourteenth day. In those who recover, the temperature falls by crisis about this time. In diagnosis the Weil-Felix reaction is helpful. The death-rate is variable, varying from nearly 100 per cent in epidemics among debilitated refugees to about 10 per cent.

FLEA TYPHUS, in which the infecting Rickettsia is transmitted by the flea, is represented by Murine Typhus.

MURINE TYPHUS FEVER, also known as flea typhus, is world-wide in its distribution and is found wherever individuals are crowded together in insanitary, rat-infested areas. Hence the old names of jail-fever and ship typhus. The causative organism, *Rickettsia mooseri*, which is closely related to *R. prowazeki*, is transmitted to man by the rat-flea, *Xenopsyalla cheopis*. The rat is the main reservoir of infection. Once man is infected, the human louse may act as a transmitter of the Rickettsia from man to man. This explains how the disease may become epidemic under insanitary, crowded conditions. As a rule, however, the disease is only acquired when man comes into close contact with infected rats.

Symptoms These are similar to those of louse-borne typhus, but the disease is usually milder, and the mortality rate is very low (about 1·5 per cent).

TICK TYPHUS, in which the infecting Rickettsia is transmitted by ticks, occurs in various parts of the world. The three best-known conditions in this group are Rocky Mountain Spotted Fever, Fièvre Boutonneuse and Tick-bite Fever.

MITE TYPHUS, in which the infecting Rickettsia is transmitted by mites, includes scrub typhus, or tsutsugamushi disease, and rickettsialpox.

RICKETTSIALPOX is a mild disease caused by *Rickettsia akari*, which is transmitted to man from infected mice by the common mouse mite, *Allodermanyssus sanguineus*. It occurs in USA, West and South Africa and the former Soviet Union.

Treatment The general principles of treatment are the same in all forms of typhus, and can be divided into prophylactic and curative. *Prophylaxis* consists of either avoidance of, or destruction of, the vector. In the case of louse typhus and flea typhus, the outlook has been revolutionized by the introduction of efficient insecticides such as DDT and Gammexane. The value of the former was well shown by its use after the Second World War. This resulted in almost complete freedom from the epidemics of typhus which ravaged Eastern Europe after the 1914–18 War being responsible for 30 million cases with a mortality of 10 per cent. Now only 10,000 to 20,000 cases occur a year, with around a few hundred deaths. Efficient rat control is another measure which reduces the risk of typhus very considerably. In areas such as Malaysia, where the mites are infected from a wide variety of rodents scattered over large areas, the wearing of protective clothing is the most practical method of prophylaxis.

Curative treatment was revolutionized by the introduction of chloramphenicol and the tetracyclines. These antibiotics altered the prognosis in typhus fever very considerably. Currently the most widely used is the long-acting tetracycline, doxycycline, one single oral dose of which is said to cure the disease.

TYROSINE An amino acid (q.v.) important in the production of catecholamines, melanin and thyroxine (qq.v.).

Louse-borne	Flea-borne	Tick-borne	Mite borne
Epidemic typhus	Murine (endemic) typhus	Rocky Mountain spotted fever	Tsutsugamushi fever
Brill's disease		African tick typhus (Tick-bite fever)	(Scrub typhus)
Trench fever		Fièvre boutonneuse	Rickettsialpox

Classification of the typhus fevers.

U

ULCER means a breach on the surface of the skin or on the surface of the membrane lining any cavity within the body, which does not tend to heal quickly.

An ulcer consists of a floor or surface, which, in consequence of the loss of tissue, is usually depressed below the surrounding healthy surface, and an edge where the healthy tissues end. The floor of a healing ulcer is composed of granulations, which are small masses of cells engaged in forming connective tissue and richly supplied with capillary blood-vessels that give the ulcer a bright-red appearance; whilst the edge shows a blue line of growing epithelial cells, which are constantly spreading inwards. In the process of healing, the fibrous tissue formed by the granulations contracts and thus draws the edges of the ulcer together and gives a puckered appearance to the scar. If anything interferes with these natural processes, the ulcer is prevented from healing.

Varieties VARICOSE ULCER generally comes on as the result of scratching the skin of a leg which has been rendered eczematous by the bad circulation. It will not heal so long as the patient walks about, and has a great tendency to develop into a callous ulcer.

INTERNAL ULCERS develop sometimes in the mouth (see MOUTH, DISEASES OF); in the stomach (see STOMACH, DISEASES OF); in the duodenum (see DUODENAL ULCER); in the bowels (see INTESTINE, DISEASES OF); and in other parts. SYPHLITIC ULCERS have the characters of possessing a very abrupt edge, as if punched out, and of leaving behind after healing a brownish discoloured scar. TUBERCULOUS ULCERS may arise from the bursting of a tuberculous abscess under the skin; whilst the skin disease known as lupus vulgaris is a variety of tuberculous disease.

MALIGNANT ULCERS are developed when a cancer spreads so as to involve the skin. Such an ulcer has often a very offensive smell, requiring the use of deodorant substances.

TROPHIC ULCERS are apt to appear as the result of weakened nerve influence: e.g. the deep perforating ulcer on the sole of the foot in locomotor ataxia, or bed sores in people sick of some lingering disease. (See BED SORES.)

Causes An ulcer may be set up by any cause which damages the surface of the body and prevents immediate healing. Naturally, any constitutional condition which diminishes the vitality or the healing power of the body acts in this way, and among these causes may be mentioned old age, general ill-health, scurvy, diabetes mellitus, gout, syphilis and tuberculosis, so that wounds produced in those suffering from any of these conditions are apt to form ulcers. Defective circulation in the direction either of a poor blood supply or of the stagnation which takes place in varicose veins is another important cause. Constant movement of any part on which there is a wound is quite sufficient to delay its healing and produce an ulcer.

Treatment In treating an ulcer, three objects must be kept in view: (1) to remove the cause of ulceration; (2) to render the floor and edge of the ulcer healthy so that healing may begin; (3) to assist the healing process and ward off any continuing source of irritation.

ULCERATIVE COLITIS (see COLITIS).

ULNA is the inner of the two bones in the forearem. It is wide at its upper end, and its olecranon process forms the point of the elbow. In its lower part it is more fragile and is liable to be broken by a fall upon the forearm while something is grasped in the hand. Chipping off of the olecranon process is a not uncommon result of falls upon the elbow. (See FRACTURES.)

ULOGLOSSITIS means inflammation of the gums and of the tongue.

ULTRAFILTRATION: Filtration carried out under pressure. Blood undergoes ultrafiltration in the kidneys to remove the waste products, urea and surplus water that constitute urine.

ULTRASOUND or ULTRASONIC WAVES comprise very high-frequency sound waves above 20,000 Hz that the human ear cannot hear. Ultrasound is widely used for diagnosis and also for some treatments. In obstetrics ultrasound can assess the stage of pregnancy and detect abnormalities in the fetus. It is a valuable adjunct in the investigation of diseases in the bladder, kidneys, liver, ovaries, pancreas and brain. Ultrasound also detects thromboses in blood vessels and enables their extent to be assessed. A non-invasive technique that does not need ionizing radiation, ultrasound is quick, versatile and relatively inexpensive, with scans being done in any plane of the body. There is little danger to the patient or operator and unlike, for example, X-rays, ultrasound investigations can be repeated as needed. A contrast medium is not required. Its reliability is dependent on the skill of the operator. It is replacing isotope scanning in many situations, and also radiography. Ultrasound of the liver can separate medical from surgical jaundice in approximately 97 per cent of patients. It is very accurate in detecting and defining cystic lesions of the liver but is less accurate with solid lesions and yet will detect 85 per cent of secondary deposits. This is less than CT scanning. It is very accurate in detecting gall-stones and more accurate than the oral cholecystogram. It is useful as a screening test for pancreatic disease and can differentiate carcinoma of the pancreas from chronic pancreatitis with 85 per cent accuracy.

It is the first investigation indicated in patients presenting with renal failure as it can quickly determine the size and shape of the kidney and whether there is any obstruction to the ureter. It is very sensitive to the presence of dilatation of the renal tract and it will detect space-occupying lesions, differentiating cysts and tumours. It can detect obstruction of the ureter due to renal stones by showing dilatations of the collecting system and the presence of the calculus. Adrenal tumours can be demonstrated by ultrasound though it is less accurate than CT scanning (q.v.). Ultrasound is now the first test for suspected aortic aneurysm and it can also show the presence of clot and delineate the true and false lumen. It is good at demonstrating sub-phrenic and sub-hepatic abscesses and will show most intra-abdominal abscesses. CT scanning is however better for the retro-peritoneal region. It has a major application in thyroid nodules as it can differentiate cystic from solid lesions and show the multiple lesions characteristic of the nodular goitre. It cannot differentiate between a follicular adenoma and a carcinoma as both these tumours are solid. Ultrasound cannot demonstrate normal parathyroid glands but it can identify adenomas provided they are more than 6 mm in diameter. Ultrasound can differentiate masses in the scrotum into testicular and appendicular and it can demonstrate impalpable testicular tumours. This is important as 15 per cent of testicular tumours metastasize whilst they are still impalpable.

Doppler ultrasound is a new technique which shows the presence of vascular disease in the carotid and peripheral vessels as it can detect the reduced blood flow through narrowed vessels.

Ultrasound has particular applications in obstetrics. A fetus can be seen with ultrasound from the seventh week of pregnancy, and the fetal heart can be demonstrated at this stage. Multiple pregnancy can also be diagnosed at this time by the demonstration of more than one gestation sac containing a viable fetus. A routine obstetric scan is usually performed between the sixteenth and eighteenth week of pregnancy when the fetus is easily demonstrated and most photogenic. The fetus can be measured to assess the gestational age and the anatomy can also be checked. Intra-uterine growth retardation is much more reliably diagnosed by ultrasound than by clinical assessment. The site of the placenta can also be recorded and multiple pregnancies will be diagnosed at this stage. Foetal movements and even the heart beat can be seen. A second scan is often done between the thirty-second and thirty-fourth weeks to assess the position, size and growth rate of the baby. The resolution of equipment now available enables pre-natal diagnosis of a wide range of structural abnormalities to be diagnosed. Spina bifida, hydrocephalus and anencephaly are probably the most important but other anomalies such as multicystic kidney, achondroplasia and certain congenital cardiac anomalies can also be identified. Foetal gender can be determined from twenty weeks of gestation. Ultrasound is also useful as guidance for amniocentesis.

In gynaecology polycystic ovaries can readily be detected as well as fibroids and ovarian cysts. Ultrasound can monitor follicular growth when patients are being treated with infertility drugs. It is also useful in detecting ectopic pregnancies.

Ultrasonic waves are one of the constituents in the shock treatment of certain types of gallstones (q.v.) and calculi (q.v.) in the urinary tract (see LITHOTRIPSY). They are also being used in the treatment of Menière's disease (q.v.) and of bruises and strains. In this field of physiotherapy, ultrasonic therapy is proving of particular value in the treatment of acute injuries of soft tissue. If in such cases it is used immediately after the injury, or as soon as possible thereafter, it is claimed, there is no question of delayed, chronic recovery. For this reason it is being widely used in the treatment of sports injuries. The sound waves stimulate the healing process in dameged tissue.

ULTRAVIOLET RAYS (UVR) are invisible light rays of very short wavelength. They are beyond the violet end of the spectrum and are the part of sunlight that causes the skin to tan or, in cases of overexposure, to burn (see SUNBURN). UVR helps the skin to produce vitamin D (see VITAMIN and APPENDIX 5: VITAMINS). The earth's atmosphere absorbs much of the ultraviolet radiation (see OZONE) and thus prevents sunlight killing off life. Reduction in the earth's ozone layer is allowing more UVR to reach the surface and one result is an increase in the incidence in skin cancer (see SKIN DISEASE; MELANOMA), particularly among fair-skinned people overexposed to the sun. Ultraviolet lamps produce UVR and are used to tan skin: as with sunlight, people should not overexpose themselves.

UMBILICAL CORD the fleshy tube containing two arteries and a vein through which the mother supplies the fetus with oxygen and nutrients. The cord, which is up to 60cm long, ceases to function after birth and is clamped and cut about 2·5cm from the infant's abdominal wall. The stump shrivels and falls off within two weeks, leaving a scar which forms the umbilicus.

UMBILICUS is the technical name for the navel.

UNCINATE FIT is a state in which a patient has a hallucination of smell or of taste; it may be a manifestation of epilepsy, or the result of a tumour pressing on that part of the brain concerned with the appreciation of smell and taste.

UNCONSCIOUS A state of unconsciousness (q.v.) or a description of mental activities of which an individual is unaware. Unconscious is also used in psychoanalysis to characterize that section of a person's mind in which memories and motives reside. They are normally inaccessible, protected by inbuilt mental resistance. This contrasts with the subconscious where a person's memories and motives, while temporarily suppressed, can usually be recalled.

UNCONSCIOUSNESS The brain is the organ of the mind. Normal conscious alertness depends on its continuous adequate supply with oxygen and glucose, both of which are essential for the brain cells to function normally. If either or both of these are interrupted, altered consciousness results. Interruption may be caused by three broad types of process affecting the brain stem (see BRAIN): the reticular formation (a network of nerve pathways and nuclei-connecting sensory and motor nerves to and from the cerebrum, cerebellum (see BRAIN), spinal cord (q.v.) and cranial nerves) and the cerebral cortex. The three types are diffuse brain dysfunction – for example, generalized metabolic disorders such as uraemia (q.v.) or toxic disorders such as septicaemia (q.v.) – direct effects on the brain stem as a result of infective, cancerous or traumatic lesions, and indirect effects on the brain stem such as a tumour or oedema in the cerebrum creating pressure within the skull. Within these three divisions are a large number of specific causes of unconsciousness.

Unconsciousness may be temporary, prolonged or indefinite (see PERSISTENT VEGETATIVE STATE), depending on the severity of the initiating incident. The patient's recovery depends on the cause and success of treatment where given. Memory may be affected, as may motor and sensory functions, but short periods of unconsciousness as a result, say, of trauma have little obvious effect on brain function. Repeated bouts of unconsciousness, which can happen in boxing, may, however, have a cumulatively damaging effect, as can be seen on CT scans of the brain.

Poisons such as carbon monoxide, drug overdose, a fall in the oxygen content of blood (HYPOXIA) in lung or heart disease, or liver or kidney failure harm the normal chemical working or *metabolism* of nerve cells. Severe blood loss will cause anoxia of the brain. Any of these can result in altered brain function in which impairment of consciousness is a vital sign.

Sudden altered consciousness will also result from FAINTING ATTACKS (SYNCOPE) in which the blood pressure falls and the circulation of oxygen is thereby reduced. Similarly an epileptic fit causes partial or complete loss of consciousness by causing an abrupt but temporary disruption of the electrical activity in the nerve cells in the brain.

As the brain's function progressively fails, in these events, drowsiness, stupor and finally coma (q.v.) ensue. If the cause is removed or, when the patient spontaneously recovers from a fit or faint, normal consciousness is usually quickly regained. Strokes (q.v.) are sometimes accompanied by a loss of consciousness. This may be immediate or come on slowly, depending on the cause or site of the strokes.

Loss of consciousness may be temporary – for instance, after a sharp blow on the head – but if a large area of brain tissue is damaged by anoxia, disease or trauma, it may be prolonged or even permanent (see PERSISTENT VEGETATIVE STATE). Comatose patients are graded according to the Glasgow Coma Scale in which the patient's response to a series of tests indicate numerically the level of coma.

Treatment of unconscious patients depends on the cause and range from first-aid care for someone who has fainted to hospital intensive-care treatment for a victim of a severe head injury or massive stroke.

UNDECYLENIC ACID is a long chain fatty acid which is of value in the treatment of tinea pedis. (See RINGWORM.)

UNDULANT FEVER is another name for brucellosis (q.v.).

UNGUAL An adjective relating to the finger nails or toe nails.

UNGUENTUM is the Latin name for ointment.

UNIT is the term applied to a quantity assumed as a standard for measurement. Thus, the *unit of insulin* is the specific activity contained in such an amount of the standard preparation as the Medical Research Council may from time to time indicate as the quantity exactly equivalent to the unit accepted for international use. The standard preparation consists of pure, dry, crystalline insulin. (See APPENDIX 6: MEASUREMENTS IN MEDICINE.)

URACHUS is a corded structure which extends from the bladder up to the navel, and represents the remains of the canal which in the fetus joins bladder with allantois.

URAEMIA describes the clinical state which arises from renal failure. It may be due to disease of the kidneys or it may be the result of pre-renal causes where a lack of circulating blood volume inadequately perfuses the kidneys. It may result from acute tubular necrosis and it may result from obstruction to the outflow of urine.

The word uraemia means excess urea in the blood, but the symptoms of renal failure are not due to the abnormal amounts of urea circulating but to the electrolyte disturbances and acidosis which are associated with impaired renal function. The acidosis results from a decrease in the ability to filter hydrogen ions from blood into the glomerular fluid and the reduced production of ammonia and phosphate means fewer ions capable of combining with the hydrogen ions so that the total acid elimination is diminished. The fall in glomerular filtration also leads to retention of sodium and water with resulting oedema, and to retention of potassium resulting in hyperkalaemia. The most important causes of uraemia are the primary renal diseases of chronic glomerular nephritis and chronic pyelonephritis. It may also result from malignant hypertension damaging the kidneys and amyloid disease destroying the kidneys. Analgesic abuse can cause tubular necrosis. Diabetes may cause a nephropathy and lead to uraemia as may myelomatosis and systemic lupus erythematosis. Polycystic kidneys and renal tuberculosis account for a small proportion of cases. (See KIDNEYS, DISEASES OF.)

Symptoms Uraemia is sometimes classed as *acute*, i.e. those cases in which the symptoms develop in a few hours or days, and *chronic*, including cases in which the symptoms are less marked and last over weeks, months, or years. There is, however, no dividing line between the two, for in the chronic variety, which may be said to consist of the symptoms of chronic glomerulonephritis, an acute attack is liable to come on at any time.

Headache in the front or back of the head, accompanied often by insomnia at night and drowsiness during the day, is one of the commonest symptoms, although it is apt to be attributed to some other cause. Unconsciousness of a profound type, which may be accompanied by convulsions resembling those of epilepsy, is the most outstanding feature of an acute attack and is a very dangerous condition.

Still another symptom, which often precedes an acute attack, is severe vomiting without apparent cause. The appetite is always poor, and the onset of diarrhoea is a serious sign.

Treatment The treatment of the chronic type of uraemia includes all the measures which should be taken by a person suffering from chronic glomerulonephritis. An increasing number of these patients, especially the younger ones, are treated with dialysis and/or renal transplantation. (See KIDNEY, ARTIFICIAL; TRANSPLANTATION.)

URATES (see URIC ACID).

UREA, or CARBAMIDE, is a crystalline substance of the chemical formula $CO(NH_2)_2$, which is very soluble in water or alcohol. It is the chief waste product discharged from the body in the urine, being formed in the liver and carried to the kidneys in the blood. The amount varies considerably with the quantity and nature of the food taken, rising greatly upon an animal (protein) dietary. It also rises during the continuance of a fever. The average amount excreted daily, during health, on a mixed diet is about 33 to 35 grams.

Urea is administered for its diuretic action, and also as a test of kidney action, in doses of 5 to 15 grams. It is used, too, as a cream in the treatment of certain skin diseases, characterized by a dry skin, such as ichythosis (q.v.).

Urea is rapidly changed, by a yeast-like micro-organism, into carbonate of ammonia; and to this chemical change the ammoniacal smell of badly kept latrines is due.

UREAPLASMA is a group of micro-organisms which plays a larger part in the causation of disease than was at one time suspected. One of them, *Ureaplasma urealyticum*, is now recognized as a cause of chronic prostatitis, nonspecific urethritis (see URETHRA, DISEASES OF.) and infertility.

URETER is the tube, about the thickness of a goose-quill, which on each side leads from the corresponding kidney down to the bladder. Each ureter begins above at the pelvis of its kidney and after a course of 25 to 30 cm (10 to 12 inches) through the loins and pelvis it opens by a narrow slit into the base of the bladder. The lower end pierces the wall of the bladder so obliquely (lying embedded in the wall for about 21 mm) that, though urine runs freely into the bladder, it is prevented from returning up the ureter as the bladder becomes distended.

URETHRA is the tube which leads from the bladder to the exterior, and by which the urine is voided. It is about 20 cm (8 inches) long in the male and 3·5 cm (1½ inches) long in the female.

URETHRA, DISEASES OF AND INJURY TO The urethra is the tube that runs from the bladder through which the urine is voided. Disease of or damage to the urethra interferes with the passage of urine.

TRAUMA Injury to the urethra is often the result of severe trauma to the pelvis – for example, in a car accident or as the result of a fall. Trauma can also result from catheter insertion or the insertion of foreign bodies into the urethra. The signs are the inability to pass urine, and blood at the end of the penis. The major complication of trauma is the development of a urethral stricture.

URETHRITIS is inflammation of the urethra from infection.

Causes The sexually transmitted disease gonorrhoea (q.v.) affects the urethra, mainly in men, and causes severe inflammation and urethritis. Non-specific urethritis (NSU), resulting from a chlamydial infection (q.v.), is a more common cause of urethritis.

Symptoms The classic signs and symptoms are a urethral discharge associated with urethral pain, particularly on micturition, and dysuria.

Treatment This involves taking urethral swabs, culturing the causative organism and treating it with the appropriate antibiotic. The complications of urethritis include stricture formation.

STRICTURE This is an abrupt narrowing of the urethra at one or more places. Strictures can be a result of trauma or infection or a congenital abnormality from birth. Rarely tumours can cause strictures.

Symptoms The usual presenting complaint is one of a slow urinary stream. Other symptoms include hesitancy of micturition, variable stream and terminal dribbling. Measurement of the urine flow rate may help in the diagnosis, but often strictures are detected during cystoscopy.

Treatment The traditional treatment was the periodic dilation of the strictures with 'sounds' – solid metal rods passed into the urethra. However, a more permanent solution is achieved by cutting the stricture with an endoscopic knife (optical urethrotomy). For more complicated long or multiple strictures an open operation (urethroplasty) is required.

URETHRITIS means inflammation of the urethra (see URETHRA, DISEASES OF).

URIC ACID is a crystalline substance, very slightly soluble in water, of chemical formula, $C_5N_4H_4O_3$. It is white in the pure state, but when found as a urinary deposit it is reddish-brown, presenting a supposed resemblance to cayenne pepper. The bi-urate of sodium and urate of ammonium occur in considerable amount in the urine during a feverish state or after great exertion, and produce, as the urine cools, a dense pink or yellow sediment. The average daily quantity of uric acid passed by human beings is 0·5 to 1 gram. In the urine of birds and reptiles uric acid is the chief nitrog-enous constituent, taking the place of the urea excreted by human beings. Uric acid is formed in the liver and removed by the kidneys from the blood. The amount is increased in the following conditions: (*a*) Excessive consumption of meat, combined with sedentary habits. (*b*) Gout (see GOUT). (*c*) Diseases in which the white corpuscles of the blood are increased: e.g. leukaemia.

Owing to their insolubility, uric acid and the various urates often produce deposits in the urinary passages, which are known as urinary sand, gravel, or stones according to their size.

URINALYSIS Analysis of the physical and chemical composition of urine (q.v.) to detect variations in the substances normally present and to identify abnormal constituents such as sugar, drugs, blood, or alcohol.

URINARY BLADDER The urinary bladder is a highly distensible organ for storing urine. It consists of smooth muscle known as the detrusor muscle and is lined with urine-proof cells known as transitional cell epithelium.

The bladder lies in the anterior half of the pelvis, bordered in front by the pubis bone and laterally by the side wall of the pelvis. Superiorly the bladder is covered by the peritoneal lining of the abdomen. The bottom or base of the bladder lies against the prostate gland in the male and the uterus and vagina in the female.

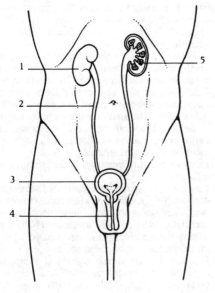 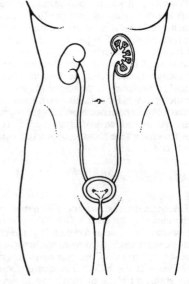

1 right kidney
2 ureter
3 bladder
4 urethra
5 left kidney (section)

Diagram of urinary system: (left) male; (right) female.

URINARY BLADDER, DISEASES OF

Diseases of the bladder are diagnosed by the patient's symptoms and signs, examination of the urine, and using investigations such as X-rays and ultrasound scans. The interior of the bladder can be examined using a cystoscope, which is a fibreoptic telescope (q.v.) that is passed into the bladder via the urethra.

CYSTITIS, or INFLAMMATION OF THE BLADDER Most cases of cystitis are caused by bacteria which have spread from the bowel, especially *Eschericia coli*, and entered the bladder via the urethra. Females are more prone to cystitis than males owing to their shorter urethra which allows easier entry for bacteria.

Symptoms Typically there is frequency and urgency of micturition, with stinging and burning on passing urine (dysuria) which is often smelly or bloodstained. In severe infection patients develop fever and rigors, or loin pain. Before starting treatment a urine sample should be obtained for laboratory testing, including identification of the invading bacteria.

Treatment This includes an increased fluid intake, analgesics, doses of potassium citrate to make the urine alkaline to discourage bacterial growth, and an appropriate course of antibiotics.

STONE OR CALCULUS The usual reason for the formation of a bladder stone is an obstruction to the bladder outflow – which results in stagnant residual urine, ideal conditions for the crystallization of the chemicals that form stones – or from long-term indwelling catheters which weaken the natural mechanical protection against bacterial entry and, by bruising the lining tissues, encourage infection.

Symptoms The classic symptom is a stoppage in the flow of urine during urination, associated with severe pain and the passage of blood.

Treatment This involves surgical removal of the stone either endoscopically (litholapaxy), by passing a cystoscope (q.v.) into the bladder via the urethra and breaking the stone, or by lithotripsy (q.v.) in which the stone (or stones) is destroyed by applying ultrasonic shock waves. If the stone cannot be destroyed by these methods, the bladder is opened and the stone removed (cystolithotomy).

CANCER Cancer of the bladder accounts for 7 per cent of all cancers in men and 2·5 per cent in women. The incidence increases with age, with smoking and with exposure to the industrial chemicals, beta-napththylamine, and benzidine.

Symptoms The classical presenting symptom of a bladder cancer is the painless passing of blood in the urine, haematuria. All patients with haematuria must be investigated with an X-ray of their kidneys, an intravenous urogram (IVU) (q.v.) and a cystoscopy (q.v.).

Treatment Superficial bladder tumours on the lining of the bladder can be treated by local removal via the cystoscope using diathermy (cystodiathermy). Invasive cancers into the bladder muscle are usually treated with radiotherapy or surgical removal of the bladder (cystectomy). Local chemotherapy may be useful in some patients with multiple small tumours.

URINE consists of the waste substances resulting from the body's metabolic processes, selected by the kidneys from the blood, dissolved in water, and excreted. Urine is around 96-percent water, the chief waste substances being urea (approximately 25 g/l), common salt (approximately 9 g/l), and phosphates and sulphates of potassium, sodium, calcium, and magnesium. There are also small amounts of uric acid, ammonia, creatinine, and various pigments. Poisons, such as morphine, may be excreted in the urine, and in many infections, such as typhoid fever, the causative organism may be excreted.

The daily urine output varies, but averages around 1500 ml in adults, less in children. The fluid intake and fluid output (urine and perspiration) are interdependent, so as to maintain a relatively constant fluid balance. Urine output is increased in certain diseases, notably diabetes mellitus (q.v.); it is diminished (or even temporarily stopped) in acute glomerulonephritis (see KIDNEY, DISEASES OF), heart failure, and fevers generally. Failure of the kidneys to secrete any urine is known as anuria, while stoppage due to obstruction of the ureters by stones, or of the urethra by a stricture, despite normal urinary secretion, is known as urinary retention.

Normal urine is described as straw to amber coloured, but may be changed by various diseases or drugs. Chronic glomerulonephritis or poorly controlled diabetes may lead to a watery appearance, as may drinking large amounts of water. Consumption of senna, beetroot, or rhubarb may lead to an orange or red colour, while passage of blood in the urine (haematuria) results in a pink or bright red appearance, or a smoky tint if just small amounts are passed. A greenish urine is usually due to bile (q.v.), or may be produced by taking quinine (q.v.).

Healthy urine has a faint aroma, but gives off an unpleasant ammoniacal smell when it begins to decompose, as may occur in urinary infections. Many foods and additives give urine a distinctive odour; garlic is particularly characteristic. The density or specific gravity of urine varies normally from 1015 to 1025. A low value suggests chronic glomerulonephritis, while a high value may occur in uncontrolled diabetes mellitus (q.v.) or a feverish state. Urine is normally acidic, which has an important antiseptic action; it may at times become alkaline, however, and in vegetarians, owing to the large dietary consumption of alkaline salts, it is permanently alkaline.

Chemical or microscopical examination of the urine is necessary to reveal abnormal drugs, poisons, or micro-organisms. There are six substances which must be easily detectable for diagnostic purposes. These are albumin, blood, glucose, bile, acetone, and pus and tube-casts. Easily used strip tests are available for all of these, except the last.

EXCESS OF URINE   It is important to distinguish urinary frequency from increase in the total amount of urine passed. Frequency may be due to reduced bladder capacity, such as may be caused by an enlarged prostate, or due to any irritation of the kidneys or bladder, such as cystitis (q.v.) or the formation of a stone. Increased total urinary output, on the other hand, is often a diagnostic feature of diabetes mellitus (q.v.). Passage of urine at night may result, leading to bed wetting, or nocturnal enuresis (q.v.) in children. Diagnosis of either condition, therefore, means the urine should be tested for glucose, albumin, gravel, and pus, with appropriate treatment.

URINE RETENTION occurs when urine is produced by the kidneys but is not voided by the bladder. It is generally less serious than anuria (q.v.), in which urine is not produced. **Causes**   Neurological injury, such as trauma to the spinal cord, may cause bladder weakness, leading to retention, although this is rare. Obstruction to outflow is more common: this may be acute and temporary, for example after childbirth or following surgery for piles, or chronic, for example, with prostatic enlargement (see PROSTATE). Commonly seen in elderly men, this leads to reduced bladder capacity, with partial emptying every few hours. Total retention is rare, but may result from a stricture, or narrowing, of the urethra – usually the result of infection or injury – or to pressure from a large neighbouring tumour.

Retention is generally treated by regular use of a catheter (q.v.), various types of which are available. Tapping of the bladder with a needle passed above the pubis is rarely necessary, but may occasionally be required in cases of severe stricture.

URINOMETER or DENSIMETER, is a simple instrument designed for estimating the specific gravity of urine.

UROBILINOGEN   Urobilinogen is a chemical compound formed when bacteria in the intestine act on bilirubin (q.v.). Some is reabsorbed and returns to the liver and some is eliminated in the faeces.

URODYNAMICS   The measurement of the pressures within the urinary bladder (q.v.) as well as the pressures of the urethral sphincter. The technique is useful in the investigation of patients with urinary incontinence. Special equipment is needed to carry out the procedure.

UROKINASE is an enzyme (q.v.) obtained from urine which dissolves blood clots. It is sometimes used in the treatment of pulmonary embolism (q.v.).

UROLOGY is that branch of medicine which treats of disorders and diseases of the kidneys, ureters, bladder, prostate, and urethra.

URSODEOXYCHOLIC ACID is a preparation used in the treatment of cholesterol gallstones (see GALL-BLADDER, DISEASES OF).

URTICARIA or NETTLE-RASH is a disorder of the skin characterized by an eruption resembling the effect produced by the sting of a nettle, namely, raised red or red-and-white patches, occurring in parts or over the whole of the surface of the body, and attended with great itching and irritation. It may be acute or chronic.
Causes   In some cases the attack appears to be connected with digestive upsets or eating certain protein foods like meat, fish, or shell-fish, also occasionally from the use of certain drugs, such as penicillin. In some it is due to the injection of sera, insect bites or exposure to cold – so-called cold urticaria – and occasionally may be the result of effort. The cause cannot always be identified but usually urticaria is an allergic reaction on the part of the affected individual to some substance to which he or she is hypersensitive. It comes into the same category as asthma and hay fever. In all three conditions the individual is allergic to some factor or factors, but the allergic response varies: in asthma it is the bronchioles of the lungs that are involved; in hay fever it is the mucous membrane of the nasopharynx, sinuses and eyes; whilst in urticaria it is the skin that gives the allergic response.
Symptoms   In severe cases there is fever and constitutional disturbance, together with sickness and faintness, which either precede or accompany the appearance of the rash. The eruption may appear on any part of the body, but is most common on the face and trunk. The attack may pass off in a few hours, or may last for several days, the eruption continuing to come out insuccessive patches. The lesions are accompanied by severe itching. Occasionally a similar process takes place in the throat, and there is then considerable danger from blockage of the larynx. (See also ALLERGY.)
Treatment   The treatment of urticaria has been revolutionized by the introduction of the antihistamine drugs. There is now a large number of these, and it is necessary to find which particular preparation suits a particular individual. In addition, it is necessary to discover, if possible, the causative factor and to remove it. For instance, if an attack always follows eating a particular food, this should be avoided in future. In severe cases attempts may be made to desensitize the individual to the allergen. Patients who become severely ill may need hospital admission and treatment with steroids (q.v.).

UTERUS or WOMB, is a hollow organ suspended in the cavity of the pelvis. In shape, it is triangular from side to side, and flattened from before backwards. The lower angle is prolonged into a rounded neck (*cervix*), about 2·5 cm (1 inch) long, which communicates through a narrow opening or mouth (*os uteri*) with the vagina, the passage leading to the exterior of the body. In size, the normal uterus is only about 7·5 cm (3 inches) long, 5 cm (2 inches) in its greatest width, and 2·5 cm (1 inch) in thickness from front to back, while the walls are so thick that the cavity consists of a mere slit. It weighs 30 to 40 grams. During pregnancy, however, it enlarges to an enormous extent, and the walls increase still further in thickness. (See MUSCLE.) The cavity is lined by a thick, soft, mucous membrane, and the wall is chiefly composed of muscle fibres arranged in three layers. The outer surface, like that of other abdominal organs, is covered by a layer of peritoneum. The uterus has a copious supply of blood derived from the uterine and ovarian arteries. It has also many lymphatic vessels, and its nerves establish wide connections with other organs. (See PAIN.) The position of the uterus is in the centre of the pelvis, where it is suspended by several ligaments between the bladder in front and the rectum behind. On each side of the uterus are the broad ligaments passing outwards to the side of the pelvis, the utero-sacral ligament passing back to the sacral bone, the utero-vesical ligament passing forwards to the bladder, and the round ligament uniting the uterus to the front of the abdomen.

UTERUS, DISEASES OF These may arise either in the body of the uterus or the cervix, usually as a result of abnormal development, infection or tumours. In rare instances the uterus may be completely absent as a result of abnormal development. In such patients secondary sexual development is normal but menstruation is conspicuously absent (primary amennorhoea). The chromosomal make-up of the patient must be checked. In a few cases the genotype is male (testicular feminization syndrome). No treatment is necessary, although the patient must be carefully counselled as she will be unable to conceive. The uterus develops as two halves which fuse together. If the fusion is incomplete, a uterine septum results. Such patients may have fertility problems which can be corrected by surgical removal of the uterine septum. Very rarely there may be two uteri with a double vagina.

Most women have uteri which are pointing forwards (anteversion) and bent forwards (anteflexion). About 25 per cent of women have uteri which are pointed backwards (retroversion) and bent backwards (retroflexion). This is a normal variant and very rarely gives rise to any problems. In the rare instance of a problem caused by a retroverted uterus, the attitude of the uterus can be corrected by an operation called a ventrosuspension.

The lining of the uterine cavity is called the endometrium. It is this layer that is partially shed cyclically in women of reproductive age giving rise to menstruation. Infection of the endometrium is called endometritis and usually occurs after a pregnancy or in association with the use of an intrauterine contraceptive device (IUCD). The symptoms are usually of pain, bleeding and a fever. Treatment is with antibiotics. Unless the Fallopian tubes are involved and damaged, subsequent fertility is unaffected. Very rarely, the infection is caused by tuberculosis. Tuberculous endometritis may destroy the endometrium causing permanent amenorrhoea and sterility.

Menstrual disorders are amongst the most common causes for a woman to consult her doctor. Heavy periods (menorrhagia) are often caused by fibroids (see below) or adenomyosis (see below) or anovulatory cycles. Anovulatory cycles result in the endometrium being subjected to unopposed oestrogen stimulation and occasionally undergoing hyperplasia. Treatment is with cyclical progestogens (q.v.) initially. If this form of treatment fails, endoscopic surgery to remove the endometrium may be successful. The endometrium may be removed using the laser (q.v.) (endometrial laser ablation) or electrocautery (q.v.) (transcervical resection of endometrium). Hysterectomy will cure the problem if endoscopic surgery fails. Adenomyosis is a condition in which endometrial tissue is found in the muscle layer (myometrium) of the uterus. It usually presents as heavy and painful periods, and occasionally pain during intercourse. Although medical treatment is often tried initially, hysterectomy is usually required.

Oligomennorhoea (scanty or infrequent periods) may be caused by a variety of conditions including thyroid disease (q.v.). It is most commonly associated with usage of the combined oral contraceptive pill. Once serious causes have been eliminated, the patient should be reassured. No treatment is necessary unless conception is desired in which case the patient may require induction of ovulation.

Primary amenorrhoea means that the patient has never had a period. It should be investigated, although usually it is only due to an inexplicable delay in the onset of periods (delayed menarche) and not to any serious condition. Secondary amenorrhoea is the cessation of periods after menstruation has started. The most common cause is pregnancy. It may be also caused by endocrinological or hormonal problems, tuberculous endometritis, emotional problems and severe weight loss. The treatment of amenorrhoea depends on the cause.

Fibroids (leiomyomata) are innocent tumours arising from the smooth muscle layer (myometrium) of the uterus. They are found in 80 per cent of women but only a small percentage give rise to any problems and may then require treatment. They may cause heavy periods and occasionally pain. Sometimes they present as a mass arising from the pelvis with pressure symptoms from the bladder or rectum. Although they can be shrunk medically using gonadorelin analogues, which raise the plasma concentrations of luteinizing and follicle-stimulating hormones (q.v.), this is not a long-term solution. In any case fibroids only require treatment if they are very large or if they are enlarging or if they cause symptoms. Treatment is either myomectomy (surgical removal) if fertility is to be retained or a hysterectomy (q.v.).

Uterine cancers tend to present after the age of 40 with abnormal bleeding (intermenstrual or postmenopausal bleeding). They are usually endometrial carcinomas. Eighty per cent present with early (Stage 1) disease. Patients with operable cancers should be treated with total abdominal hysterectomy and bilateral excision of the ovaries (q.v.) and Fallopian tubes (q.v.). Post-operative radiotherapy is usually given to those patients with adverse prognostic factors. Pre-operative radiotherapy is still given by some centres, although this practice is now regarded as out-dated. Progestogens (q.v.) may be extremely effective treatment in cases of recurrence but their value remains unproven when used as adjuvant treatment.

The cervix (neck of the womb) may produce an excessive discharge due to the presence of a cervical ectopy or ectropion. In both instances columnar epithelium – the layer of secreting cells – which usually lines the cervical canal is exposed on its surface. Asymptomatic patients do not require treatment. If treatment is required, cryocautery – local freezing of tissue – is the method of choice.

Cervical smears are taken and examined in the laboratory to detect abnormal cells shed from the cervix. Its main purpose is to detect cervical intraepithelial neoplasia (CIN) – the presence of malignant cells in the surface tissue lining the cervix – since up to 40 per cent of women with this condition will develop cervical cancer if the CIN is left untreated. Women with abnormal smears should undergo colposcopy, a painless investigation using a low-powered microscope to inspect the cervix. If CIN is found, treatment consists of simply removing the area of abnormal skin, either using a diathermy loop or laser instrument.

Unfortunately cervical cancer remains the most common of gynaecological cancers. Early cases may be treated by a radical or Wertheim's hysterectomy. This is a major operation in which the uterus, cervix, upper third of vagina and the tissue surrounding the cervix are removed together with the lymph nodes draining the area. The ovaries may be retained if desired. Most patients with cervical cancer are treated by radiotherapy, either because they present too late for surgery or because the surgical skill to perform a radical hysterectomy is not available. These operations are best performed by gynaecological oncologists who are gynaecological surgeons specializing in the treatment of gynaecological tumours.

In 1989 in England and Wales 4,147 cases of cancer of the cervix were registered and 4,073 cases of cancer of the uterus. In 1985 3,969 cases of cervical cancer were registered and 3,393 cases of uterine cancer.

UVEA is a term applied to the middle coat of the eye, including the iris, ciliary body and choroid.

UVEITIS An inflammation of the uveal tract. *Iritis* is inflammation of the iris, *cyclitis* inflammation of the ciliary body and *choroiditis* inflammation of the choroid. The symptoms and signs vary according to which part of the uveal tract is involved and tend to be recurrent. The patient may experience varying degrees of discomfort or pain, with or without blurring of vision. The eye may be red or appear white. In many cases a cause is never found. Some known associations include various types of arthritis, some bowel diseases, virus illnesses, tuberculosis, syphilis, parasites and fungi. Treatment is with anti-inflammatory drops and occasionally tablets (e.g. steroid eye drops and tablets), plus drops to dilate the pupil.

UVULA is the small mass of muscle covered by mucous membrane that hangs down from the middle of the soft palate on its posterior aspect. Very rarely the structure is excessively long and may require trimming. Generally though its function is not certain and it seldom causes problems.

V

VACCINATION, from *vacca*, Latin for cow, means inoculation with the material of cowpox, performed to afford protection to the inoculated person against an attack of smallpox, or at all events with the view of diminishing the seriousness of, and averting a fatal result from, any such attack. This is the strict sense of the term, but it is used nowadays to describe the process of inoculating with any vaccine to obtain immunity, or protection, against the corresponding disease.

VACCINE is the name applied generally to a substance of the nature of dead or attenuated living infectious material introduced into the body with the object of increasing its power to resist or to get rid of a disease. (See also IMMUNITY.)

In cases where healthy people are inoculated with vaccine as a protection against a particular disease, this is done to produce antibodies which will confer immunity against a subsequent attack of the disease. (See IMMUNIZATION for programme of immunization during childhood.)

Vaccines may be divided into two classes: stock vaccines, prepared from micro-organisms known to cause a particular disease and kept in readiness for use against that disease; and autogenous vaccines, prepared from micro-organisms which are already in the patient's body and to which the disease is due. Vaccines intended to protect against the onset of disease are necessarily of the stock variety.

AUTOGENOUS VACCINES are prepared from the cultivation of bacteria found in the expectoration, the urine, the faeces, and in areas of inflammation such as boils. This type of vaccine was introduced by Wright about 1903.

ANTHRAX VACCINE was introduced by Pasteur about 1882 for the protection of sheep and cattle against this disease. A safe and effective vaccine for use in human beings has now been evolved.

BCG VACCINE is used to provide protection against tuberculosis. BCG vaccination is usually considered for five main groups of people:

(1) Schoolchildren: the routine programme in schools usually covers children aged between 10 and 14

(2) Students including those in teacher training colleges

(3) Children and new-born infants in families of Asian origin because of the high incidence of tuberculosis in this ethnic group

(4) Health service workers and others liable to infection at work

(5) Household contacts of people known to have active tuberculosis and new-born infants in households where there is a history of tuberculosis.

(See BCG VACCINE.)

CHOLERA VACCINE was introduced by Haffkine in India about 1894. Two injections are given at an interval of at least a week; this gives a varying degree of immunity for six months.

DIPHTHERIA VACCINE is available in several forms. (See DIPHTHERIA.) It is usually given along with tetanus and pertussis vaccine in what is known as Triple Vaccine. This is given in three doses: the first at the age of 3 or 6 months, the second six to eight weeks later, and the third six months later, with a booster dose at the age of 5 years.

HAY FEVER VACCINE is a vaccine prepared from the pollen of various grasses. It is used in gradually increasing doses for prevention of hay fever in those susceptible to this condition.

INFLUENZA VACCINE: a vaccine is now available for protection against influenza due to the influenza viruses A and B. Its use in Britain is customarily based on advice from the health departments according to the type of influenza expected in a particular year.

MEASLES, MUMPS AND RUBELLA VACCINES are given in combination early in the second year of life.

PERTUSSIS (WHOOPING-COUGH) VACCINE is prepared from *Bordetella pertussis*, and is usually given along with diphtheria and tetanus in what is known as Triple Vaccine.

PLAGUE VACCINE was introduced by Haffkine, and appears to give useful protection, but the duration of protection is relatively short: from two to twenty months. Two injections are given at an interval of 4 weeks. A reinforcing dose should be given annually to anyone exposed to the disease.

POLIOMYELITIS VACCINE gives a high degree of protection against the disease.

This is given in the form of attenuated Sabin vaccine which is taken by mouth – a few drops on a lump of sugar. Reinforcing doses of polio vaccine are recommended on school entry, on leaving school, and on travel abroad to countries where poliomyelitis is endemic.

RABIES VACCINE was introduced by Pasteur in 1885 for administration, during the long incubation period, to people bitten by a mad dog, in order to prevent the disease from developing.

RUBELLA VACCINE, usually given with mumps and measles vaccine in one dose, now provides protection against rubella (German measles). It also provides immunity for adolescent girls who have not had the disease in childhood and so ensures that they will not acquire the disease during any subsequent pregnancy, thus reducing the number of congenitally abnormal children whose abnormality is the result of their being infected with rubella via their mothers before they were born.

SMALLPOX VACCINE was the first introduced. As a result of the World Health Organization's (WHO) successful smallpox eradication campaign – it declared the disease eradicated in 1980 – there is now no medical justification for smallpox vaccination.

TETANUS VACCINE is given in two forms: (a) In the so-called Triple Vaccine, combined with diphtheria and pertussis (whooping-cough) vaccine. This is used for the routine immunization of children, the first dose being given at the age of 3 to 6 months, a second dose six to eight weeks later, and a third dose six months later. A booster dose of tetanus vaccine is recommended on leaving school, on entering higher education, or on starting employment. (b) By itself to adults who have not been immunized in childhood and who are particularly exposed to the risk of tetanus, such as soldiers and agricultural workers.

TYPHOID VACCINE was introduced by Wright and Semple for the protection of troops in the South African War and in India. TAB vaccine, containing *Salmonella typhi* (the causative organism of typhoid fever) and *Salmonella paratyphi* A and B (the organisms of paratyphoid fever) has now been replaced by Typhoid Monovalent Vaccine, containing only *S. typhi*. The change has been made because the monovalent vaccine is less likely to produce painful arms and general malaise and there is no evidence that the TAB vaccine gave any protection against paratyphoid fever. Two doses are given at an interval of four to six weeks, and give protection for one to three years.

YELLOW FEVER VACCINE is prepared from chick embryos injected with the living, attenuated strain (17D) of pantropic virus. Only one injection is required, and immunity persists for many years. Reinoculation, however, is desirable every ten years.

The hazards of vaccination, or immunization are minimal, compared with its benefits. Complications, however, do occur.

VACCINIA is another term for cowpox, a disease in which vesicles form on the udders and teats, due to the same virus as is responsible for smallpox in man. It is also the term used to describe the reaction to smallpox vaccination.

VACUOLE A space inside the cytoplasm of the cell. It is formed by a folding in of the cellular membrane when the cell ingests material from the outside – for example, when white blood cells attack bacteria.

VAGINA is the lower part of the female reproductive tract. It is a muscular passage leading from the labial entrance to the womb. It is lined with mucous membrane and receives the erect penis during sexual intercourse. The semen is ejaculated into the upper part of the vagina and from there the sperms must pass through the cervix and uterus to fertilize the ovum in the fallopian tube.

VAGINISMUS is spasmodic contraction of the opening of the vagina on attempted coitus. It is usually psychological in origin, due, for instance, to frigidity, but it may also be due to some local inflammatory condition.

VAGINITIS is inflammation of the vagina. (See LEUCORRHOEA.)

VAGOTOMY is the operation of cutting the fibres of the vagus nerve to the stomach. It is sometimes performed as part of the surgical treatment of duodenal ulcer, the aim being to reduce the flow or acidity of the gastric juice.

VAGUS, or PNEUMOGASTRIC, nerve is the tenth cranial nerve. Unlike the other cranial nerves, which are concerned with the special senses, or distributed to the skin and muscles of the head and neck, this nerve, as its names imply, strays downwards into the chest and abdomen, supplying branches to the throat, lungs, heart, stomach, and other abdominal organs. It contains motor, secretory, sensory, and vasodilator fibres.

VALGUS means literally knock-kneed, and is a bending inward at the knees (*genu valgum*), or at the ankle, as occurs in flat-foot (*pes valgus*).

VALINE is an essential amino-acid (q.v.).

VALVES are found in the heart, veins, and lymphatic vessels, for the purpose of maintaining the circulation of the blood and lymph always in one direction. (See HEART; LYMPH; VEINS.)

VALVULAR DISEASE (see HEART DISEASES).

VALVOTOMY An operation that opens a stenosed heart valve and allows it to function properly again. Various techniques are used

including a dilating instrument, a balloon or open-heart surgery.

VANCOMYCIN is an antibiotic derived from streptomyces, which is active against a wide range of Gram-positive organisms, including the staphylococcus (q.v.).

VAN DEN BERGH TEST is one performed on a specimen of serum of the blood in cases of jaundice, to decide whether this is due to ordinary bile (immediate or direct reaction) or incompletely formed bile pigment (delayed or indirect reaction).

VAPORIZER A device that turns water or a drug into a fine spray, thus enabling medicine to be taken by inhalation. It is used, for example, in the treatment of asthma.

VARICELLA is another name for chickenpox (q.v.).

VARICOCOELE means a condition in which the veins of the testicle are distended. (See TESTICLE, DISEASES OF.)

VARICOSE VEINS are veins that have become stretched and dilated. (See VEINS, DISEASES OF.)

VARIOLA is another name for smallpox (q.v.).

VARIX means an enlarged and tortuous vein.

VARUS, meaning bow-legged, is the term applied to a bulging condition at the hip (*coxa vara*), at the knee (*genu varum*), or at the ankle (*talipes varus*).

VAS is the Latin term for a vessel, especially a blood-vessel.

VASCULAR Relating to the blood vessels.

VASCULITIS Inflammation of the blood vessels. This may damage the lining of the vessels and cause narrowing or blockage, thus restricting blood flow. This, in turn, may harm or destroy the tissues supplied by the affected blood vessels. Vasculitis is probably caused by small particles called immune complexes, circulating in the blood, that adhere to the vessel walls and provoke inflammation. Normally these complexes are consumed by the white blood cells.

VASECTOMY is the surgical operation performed to render men sterile, or infertile. It consists of ligating, or tying, and then cutting the ductus, or vas, deferens (see TESTICLE). It is quite a simple operation carried out under local anaesthesia, through a small incision, or cut (or sometimes two) in the upper part of the scrotum. It has no effect on sexual drive or ejaculation, and does not cause impotency. It is not immediately effective, and several tests, spread over several months, must be carried out before it is safe to assume that sterility has been achieved. Although, in those who desire it, fertility can sometimes be restored by a further operation, to restore the continuity of the vas, this cannot be guaranteed, and only seems to occur in about one-fifth of those so operated on.

VASO-ACTIVE INTESTINAL PEPTIDE (VIP) was isolated in 1970. It stimulates the intestinal secretion of water and electrolytes, inhibits gastric secretion and promotes hyperglycaemia. It also has a secretin-like action on the pancreas, stimulating the production of pancreatic juice. It is secreted by the non-beta cells of the pancreas. Tumours of these cells, which are uncommon, provoke a watery diarrhoea syndrome or what is sometimes called pancreatic cholera.

VAS DEFERENS A narrow tube that leads from each testis through the prostate gland to join a tube from the seminal vesicles to form the ejaculatory duct. Sperm and seminal fluid pass through this duct during ejaculation (see TESTICLE).

VASOCONSTRICTION Narrowing of blood vessels which results in the blood flow to a particular part of the body's being reduced. Cold will cause vasoconstriction of the vessels under the skin thus reducing heat loss. Shock due to injury or loss of blood will also provoke vasoconstriction.

VASODILATORS are substances that cause dilatation of the blood-vessels. They may be drugs, such as amyl nitrite (q.v.), or natural substances in the body, such as kinins (q.v.).

VASOMOTOR NERVES are the small nerve fibres that lie upon the walls of blood-vessels and connect the muscle fibres of their middle coat with the nervous system. Through these nerves the blood-vessels are retained in a state of moderate contraction. There are vasodilator nerves, through which are transmitted impulses that dilate the vessels, and, in the case of the skin-vessels, produce the condition of blushing. There are also vasoconstrictor nerves which transmit impulses that constrict, or narrow, the blood-vessels, as occurs on exposure to cold. (See HYPOTHERMIA.) Various drugs produce dilatation or contraction of the blood-vessels and several of the substances produced by endocrine glands in the body have these effects: e.g. adrenaline (q.v.).

VASOPRESSIN is the fraction isolated from extract of the posterior pituitary lobe which stimulates intestinal activity, constricts blood-vessels, and inhibits the secretion of urine. It is also known as the antidiuretic hormone because of this last effect, and its only use in medicine is, on account of this effect, in the treatment of diabetes insipidus (q.v.). (See also PITUITARY BODY.)

VASOVAGAL ATTACK The temporary loss of consciousness caused by an abrupt slowing of the heartbeat. This may happen following shock, acute pain, fear, or stress. A common cause of fainting in normal people, a vasovagal attack may be a consequence of overstimulation of the vagus nerve (q.v.) which is involved in the control of breathing and the circulation.

VEGANISM is a strict form of vegetarianism. Vegans do not eat meat, dairy produce, eggs or fish.

VEGETARIANISM is the principle of restricting one's diet, for health or humanitarian reasons, to foods of fruit or vegetable origin. Most vegetarians, while excluding meat and fish from their diets, include foods of animal origin, such as milk, cheese, eggs, and butter. Such a diet should supply an adequate balance of nutrients, although people with special dietary requirements, such as pregnant or feeding mothers, and very strict vegetarians, may require dietary supplements (see VITAMIN).

VEGETATIONS are roughenings that appear upon the valves of the heart, usually as the result of acute rheumatism. They lead in time to narrowing of the openings from the cavities of the heart, or to imcompetence of the valves that close these openings. (See HEART DISEASES.)

VEGETATIVE SYSTEM is a term applied to that part of the nervous system which acts in an involuntary manner, to a large extent independently of the brain and spinal cord, and which regulates and connects movements and secretions of internal organs. It is also known as the autonomic nervous system. The term includes the sympathetic and parasympathetic nervous systems (q.v.).

VEINS are the vessels which carry blood to the heart after it has circulated through the tissues of the body. In general the veins lie alongside corresponding arteries that carry outwards to the tissues the blood which afterwards returns by the veins. The veins are, however, both more numerous and more capacious than the arteries, and, as a rule, there are two accompanying veins for each artery of moderate size. In addition to these deeply placed veins, there are superficial veins in the limbs, which can be readily seen in their distended state lying immediately beneath the skin.

Structure A vein is of similar structure to an artery, consisting of three coats: outer of fibrous tissue, middle of muscular and elastic fibres, and inner composed of elastic membrane and flattened cells. Any vein has, however, a much thinner wall than its corresponding artery, especially as regards the middle coat. Most veins are provided with valves similar in structure to the valves of the heart, and consisting each of two segments or pouches, which lie flat against the wall of the vein as the blood passes in the proper direction, or which meet and close the passage whenever the blood tends to run backwards. The valves are most numerous in the veins of the lower limb, those in the arm stand next in point of numbers, whilst there are few valves in the veins of internal organs.

Chief veins Four *pulmonary veins* open into the left atrium of the heart, two coming from each lung. Into the right atrium there open some small veins from the walls of the heart, and two great vessels, superior vena cava and inferior vena cava, that bring back blood from the body generally.

The *superior vena cava* brings the blood from the head, neck, and upper limbs. It is formed by the union of two *innominate veins*, each of which results from the junction, at the root of the neck, of the internal jugular vein, from the neck, and the subclavian vein, from the upper limb. The *internal jugular vein* receives the blood from within the skull and collects branches from the face and neck as it runs downwards alongside the carotid artery under cover of the thick sternocleidomastoid muscle. One of its most important branches is the *external jugular vein*, which runs beneath the skin from the angle of the jaw straight downwards to the middle of the collar-bone. This vessel can be readily seen when the veins of the neck are distended, and is liable to be opened in wounds of this region. The *subclavian vein* is the last section of the system of veins that accompany the arteries in the arm, each vein being named after its corresponding artery. The superficial veins of the arm are of special interest, because the large *basilic vein* that runs up the inner side of the upper arm is the vein usually opened in blood-letting. Its tributary, the median cubital vein, is used for punctures to get blood for various tests or in order to give intravenous injections. (See VENESECTION.)

The *inferior vena cava*, which lies to the right side and in front of the spinal column, starting at the junction of the two common iliac veins about the level of the navel, collects the blood from the lower limbs and abdomen. In the lower limbs and in the pelvis, the deeply placed veins correspond in name and in position to the arteries, while the surface veins of the lower limb empty their contents into the *small saphenous vein* on the back of the leg, and the *great saphenous vein* that runs from the instep up the inner side of the leg, knee, and thigh. These veins, and especially the great saphenous vein, are of special interest because of their liability to become distended or varicose. Within the abdomen, the inferior vena cava receives branches corresponding to several branches of the aorta, its largest branches being the *hepatic veins*, which return not only the blood that has reached the liver in the hepatic arteries, but also blood which comes from the digestive organs in the *portal vein* to undergo a second capillary circulation in the liver. (See PORTAL VEIN.)

There are several connections between the superior and inferior cava, the most important being three *azygos veins* that lie upon the sides of the spinal column, the veins on the front of the abdomen, and some veins that emerge from the abdomen at the navel and connect the portal system with those of the inferior and superior vena cava. By these means the circulation is maintained even when one of these large vessels has been blocked by some disease within the chest or the abdomen.

VEINS, DISEASES OF Veins are the blood vessels that convey blood back from the tissues towards the heart. Two common conditions that affect them are thrombosis and varicosities. THROMBOSIS occurs when blood, which is normally a liquid, clots within the vein to form a semisolid thrombus (clot). This occurs through a combination of reduced blood flow and hypercoagulability (a reduced threshold for clotting). The commonest site for this to occur is in the deep veins of the leg where it is known as a deep-vein thrombosis (DVT).

Predisposing factors include immobility (leading to reduced blood flow) such as during long journeys (e.g. plane flights) where there is little opportunity to stretch one's legs, surgery (leading to immobility and hypercoagulability of blood), oestrogen administration (low-dose oestrogen oral contraceptives carry a very low relative risk) and many medical illnesses such as heart failure, stroke and malignancy.

Deep-vein thrombosis presents as a tender, warm, red swelling of the calf. Diagnosis may be confirmed by venogram (an X-ray taken following injection of contrast medium into the foot veins) or by ultrasound scanning looking for flow within the veins.

Diagnosis and treatment are important because there is a risk that the clotted blood within the vein becomes dislodged and travels up the venous system to become lodged in the pulmonary arteries. This is known as pulmonary embolism (q.v.).

Treatment is directed at thinning the blood with anticoagulants, initially with heparin and subsequently with warfarin for a period of time while the clot resolves.

Blocked superficial veins are described as superficial thrombophlebitis, which produces inflammation over the vein. It responds to anti-inflammatory analgesics. Occasionally heparin and antibiotics are required to treat associated thrombosis and infection.

VARICOSE VEINS are dilated tortuous veins. They most commonly occur in the legs but may also occur in the anal canal (haemorrhoids) and in the oesophagus (due to liver disease).

Normally blood flows from the subcutaneous

tissues to the superficial veins which drain via perforating veins into the deep veins of the leg. This flow, back towards the heart, is aided by valves within the veins. When these valves fail increased pressure is exerted on the blood vessels leading to dilatations known as varicose veins.

Treatment is needed to prevent complications such as ulceration and bleeding, or for cosmetic purposes. Treatment alternatives include injection with sclerosing agents to obliterate the lumen of the veins; surgery; and in the elderly or unfit an elastic stocking may suffice. One operation is the Trendelenburg operation in which the saphenous vein is disconnected from the femoral vein and individual varicose veins are avulsed.

VENA CAVA is the name applied to either of the two large vessels that open into the right atrium of the heart. (See VEINS.)

VENEPUNCTURE is the name applied to inserting a needle into a vein, usually for the purpose of injecting a drug or withdrawing blood for haematological or biochemical analysis.

VENEREAL DISEASES (See SEXUALLY TRANSMITTED DISEASES.)

VENESECTION, or BLOOD-LETTING, may be employed for two purposes. Most commonly, small quantities of blood may be required for analysis, as an aid to dagnosis or control of various diseases. For example, knowledge of the plasma glucose concentration is important in the diagnosis and management of diabetes mellitus (q.v.), or blood may be required in order to test for infections such as HIV or hepatitis. Blood may be obtained by pricking a finger tip, or inserting a needle into a vein, depending on the amount required. Controlled bleeding of larger amounts may also be used in certain cases of acute heart failure, as a rapid and temporary method of relieving the strain on the heart. It is also used in the treatment of polycythemia (q.v.).

Venesection was popular in the 19th century, and was commonly used to avoid the consequences of excessive eating or drinking. Techniques used, such as leeches and cupping (q.v.), were generally unhygienic. Many people died from the bleeding, rather than from the original disease, and such techniques are rarely used today.

VENOGRAPHY is the study of the veins, particularly by means of X-rays after the veins have been injected with a radio-opaque substance.

VENTILATION is the process by which air is purified and circulated in domestic, occupational, industrial, and other settings. Ideally, the air we breathe should be of the right temperature and humidity, and free of dust, smoke, pollen, and other contaminants. Ventilation aims to produce such an atmosphere.

Air-conditioning is frequently used in hospitals, offices, and other public places. Special filters may be used to reduce the risk of airborne infections and allergies (q.v.), but poorly maintained and contaminated systems may result in outbreaks of serious disorders, such as legionnaire's disease (q.v.). Sterilization of air is rarely required, but ultraviolet light is sometimes used to kill pathogenic organisms. (See ASTHMA, BRONCHITIS, HUMIDIFICATION.)

VENTILATION, ARTIFICIAL The procedure, usually carried out in an operating theatre or intensive-care unit, in which a device called a ventilator takes over a person's breathing. This is done for someone who is unable to breathe normally. Damage to the respiratory centre of the brain as a result of head injury, disease of the brain, or an overdose of sedative or narcotic drugs may affect the respiratory centre. Chest injuries, disease of the lungs, nerve or muscle disorders or surgery of the chest or abdomen can also affect breathing and require the use of a ventilator to maintain normal breathing. Artificial ventilation can also be carried out as an emergency by mouth-to-mouth resuscitation (see APPENDIX 1: BASIC FIRST AID and ARTIFICIAL VENTILATION OF LUNGS.)

VENTILATOR Machinery used to provide artificial ventilation. Also called respirator or life-support machine, it is an electric pump linked to a supply of air which it pumps into the patient through an endotracheal tube passed through the nose or mouth into the trachea. Sometimes the air is pumped straight into the trachea through an artificial hole called a tracheostomy (q.v.). During ventilation the patient's blood gases are closely monitored and other bodily activities such as pulse and heart pressure are regularly measured. Some patients need to be kept on a ventilator for several days or even weeks if their medical condition is serious. (See ARTIFICIAL VENTILATION OF LUNGS.)

VENTOUSE, or VACUUM EXTRACTOR, is used in obstetrics. It is based upon a suction-cup technique, whereby the baby is sucked out of the uterus instead of being drawn out by forceps.

VENTRAL means belonging to the belly.

VENTRICLE is the term applied to the two lower cavities of the heart (see HEART), and also to the cavities within the brain.

VENTRICULAR FIBRILLATION a dangerous and rapid arrhythmia of the ventricle.

VENTRICULOGRAPHY is the process of taking an X-ray photograph of the brain after the fluid in the lateral ventricles of the brain has been replaced by air; in this way any alteration in the outline of the ventricles (e.g. from pressure by a tumour) can be detected.

VERAPAMIL is a drug used in the treatment of disordered rhythms of the heart and angina pectoris (q.v.), and is also proving of value in the treatment of high blood-pressure. (See CALCIUM-CHANNEL BLOCKERS.)

VERATRUM, also known as green hellebore, Indian poke, and poke root, is the root of *Veratrum viride*, a plant of the United States. It acts as a sedative and depressant of the heart and nervous system by virtue of veratrine and other alkaloids that it contains. Alkaloids obtained from it are used in the treatment of high blood-pressure. (See HYPERTENSION.)

VERBIGERATION means the insane repetition of meaningless words and sentences.

VERMICIDES, or VERMIFUGES, are substances that kill, or expel, parasitic worms from the intestines.

VERRUCA is the Latin term for a wart.

VERRUCOSE means covered with warts.

VERSION, or TURNING, is the name given to an operation in obstetrics which consists in turning the child in cases in which the lie of the child is abnormal.

VERTEBRA is one of the irregularly shaped bones that together form the vertebral column. (See SPINAL COLUMN.)

VERTIGO, or giddiness, is a condition in which the affected person loses the power of balancing himself, and has a false sensation as to his own movements or as to those of surrounding objects. The power of balancing depends upon sensations derived partly through the sense of touch, partly from the eyes, but mainly from the semicircular canals of the internal ear. In general, vertigo is due to some interference with this mechanism or with the centres in the cerebellum and cerebrum with which it is connected. Giddiness is apt to be associated with headache, nausea, and vomiting.
Causes The simplest cause of vertigo is some mechanical disturbance of the body affecting the fluid in the internal ear; such as that produced by moving in a swing with the eyes shut, the motion of a boat causing sea-sickness, or a sudden fall. (See MOTION-SICKNESS.) The

cause which produces a severe and sudden giddiness is Menière's disease (q.v.), a condition in which there is loss of function of the labyrinth of the inner ear. An acute labyrinthitis may result from viral infection and produce a severe vertigo lasting 2 to 5 days. Because it often occurs in epidemics it is often called epidemic vertigo. Vertigo is sometimes produced by the removal of wax from the ear, or even by syringing out the ear. (See EAR, DISEASES OF.) A severe upset in the gastrointestinal tract may cause vertigo. Refractive errors in the eyes, an attack of migraine, a mild attack of epilepsy, and gross diseases of the brain, such as tumours, are other causes acting more directly upon the central nervous system. Finally, giddiness may be due to some disorder of the circulation, e.g. bloodlessness of the brain produced by fainting, or by disease of the heart. **Treatment,** while the attack lasts, requires the victim to lie down in a darkened, quiet room. Sedatives have most influence in diminishing giddiness when it is distressing. After the attack is over, the individual should be examined to establish the cause and, if necessary, to be given appropriate treatment.

VESICAL is the term applied to structures connected with, or diseases of, the bladder. (See URINARY BLADDER.)

VESICANTS are blistering agents. (See BLISTERS AND COUNTER-IRRITANTS.)

VESICLE means a small collection of fluid in the epidermis. The fluid in some cases consists of a drop of sweat collected at the mouth of a sweat-gland, but in general it is serum from the blood. The skin disease specially associated with the formation of vesicles is herpes; in this disease the vesicles usually burst and then scab over. Some infectious diseases show an eruption composed of vesicles: e.g. smallpox and chickenpox. When a large number of white corpuscles from the blood find their way into a vesicle, it becomes a pustule.
   The term vesicle is also applied to minute sacs of normal structure, such as the air-vesicles in which the finest bronchial tubes end in the lungs.

VESICULAR BREATHING Normal breath sounds heard in the lung by means of a stethoscope. These are soft regular sounds which become altered by disease and the changed characteristics may help the physician to diagnose a disease in the lung.

VESTIBULOCOCHLEAR NERVE is the eighth cranial nerve. It consists of two sets of fibres, which constitute two separate nerves. One is known as the vestibular nerve, which is the nerve of equilibration or balance. The other is known as the cochlear nerve, which is the nerve of hearing. Disturbance of the former causes giddiness, whilst disturbance of the latter causes deafness.

VESTIGIAL An adjective referring to an organ which exists in a rudimentary form and whose function and structure have declined during the course of evolution. An example is the appendix.

VIABLE The ability of an organism to survive on its own. In the UK the legal age of the viability of a fetus is 24 weeks.

VIBRATOR is an instrument used for vibratory massage in the mechanical treatment of disease. For its use see MASSAGE.

VIBRIO is a bacterium of curved shape, such as the vibrio of cholera.

VILLUS is the name given to one of the minute processes which are thickly planted upon the inner surface of the small intestine, giving it, to the naked eye, a velvety appearance, and greatly assisting absorption. (See DIGESTION, ABSORPTION AND ASSIMILATION; INTESTINE.)

VINBLASTINE is an alkaloid (q.v.) derived from the periwinkle plant (*Vinca rosea*) which is of value in the treatment of certain forms of malignant disease, particularly choriocarcinoma and Hodgkin's disease. (See CYTOTOXIC.)

VINCENT'S ANGINA is an ulcerative inflammation of the throat, often foul smelling, and caused by large, spindle-shaped bacilli and spirilla.

VINCRISTINE is an alkaloid derived from the common periwinkle which is proving of value in the palliative treatment of certain forms of malignant disease. (See CYTOTOXIC.)

VINEGAR (see ACETIC ACID.)

VINYL ETHER is an inhalational anaesthetic used in minor surgical procedures of short duration, and for the induction of anaesthesia (q.v.).

VIOMYCIN is an antibiotic which is active against the *Mycobacterium tuberculosis*, but less active than streptomycin or isoniazid.

VIRAEMIA A condition occurring at various times in some viral infections in which the infecting virus is present in large amounts in the blood. In other virus infections the organisms are merely transported in the blood on their way to target tissues or organs.

VIRAL HAEMORRHAGIC FEVER or EBOLA VIRUS FEVER, is a highly fatal disease due to a virus related to that of Marburg disease (q.v.). Two large outbreaks of it were recorded in 1976 (one in the Sudan and one in Zaïre), with a mortality, respectively, of 50 and 80 per cent, and the disease reappeared in the Sudan in 1979. After an incubation period of 7 to 14 days, the onset is with headache of increasing severity and fever. This is followed by diarrhoea, extensive internal bleeding and vomiting. Death usually occurs on the eighth to ninth day. Infection is by person-to-person contact. Serum from patients convalescent from the disease is a useful source of antibodies to the virus.

VIRILISM is the term applied to the condition in which masculine characteristics develop in the female, and is commonly the result of an overactive suprarenal gland, or of a tumour of its cortex. It may also result from an androgen-secreting ovarian tumour and also from the polycystic ovary syndrome.

VIRULENCE The power of a bacteria or virus to cause disease. Virulence can be measured by how many people the micro-organism infects, how quickly it spreads through the body, and how many people die from it.

VIRUS is the term applied to a group of infective agents which are so small that they are able to pass through the pores of collodion filters. They are responsible for some of the most important diseases affecting man: e.g. influenza, poliomyelitis, smallpox, and yellow fever. Some idea of their size may be obtained from the fact that the virus of influenza measures 80 nanometres, whereas the staphylococcus measures 1000 nanometres. (1 nanometre = one thousand-millionth of a metre.)

VISCERA is the general name given to the larger organs lying within the cavities of the chest and abdomen. The term 'viscus' is also applied individually to these organs.

VISION Broadly speaking, vision is the ability to see.
PATHWAY OF LIGHT FROM THE EYE TO THE BRAIN Light enters the eye by passing through the transparent cornea, then through the aqueous humour filling the anterior chamber. It then passes through the pupil, through the lens and the vitreous to reach the retina. In the retina the rod and cone photoreceptors detect light and relay messages in the form of electrochemical impulses through the various layers of the retina to the nerve fibres. The nerve fibres carry messages via the optic nerve, optic chiasm, optic tract, lateral geniculate body and finally the optic radiations to the visual cortex. Here in the visual cortex these messages are

interpreted. It is therefore the visual cortex of the brain that 'sees'.

VISUAL ACUITY Two points will not be seen as two unless they are separated by a minimum distance. This distance is such that the objects are so far apart that the lines joining them to the eye enclose between them (subtend) an angle of at least one minute of a degree. This amount of separation allows the images of the two points to fall on two separate cones (if the light from two points falls on one cone, the two points would be seen as a single point). There are many tests of visual acuity. One of the more common is the Snellen Test Type. This is made up of many letters of different size. Each letter is constructed in a specific manner so that the various components of the letter subtend an angle of one minute of one degree at the eye. Each letter when placed at specified distance from the patient subtends an angle of five minutes of a degree. Thus the top letter subtends an angle of 5 minutes when placed 60 metres from the eye, the lowest letter subtends the same angle when placed 4 metres away. By conventions the chart is placed 6 metres away from the patient. Someone able to see the lowest line at this distance has a visual acuity of 6/4. If they are only able to see the top letter they have 6/60 vision. 'Normal' vision is 6/6.

COLOUR VISION: 'White light' is made up of component colours. These can be separated by a prism, thereby producing a spectrum. The three cardinal colours are red, green, and blue. All other colours can be produced by a varying mixture of these three. Colour vision is a complex subject. The trichromat theory of colour vision suggests that there are three types of cones, each type sensitive to one of the cardinal colours. Colour perception is based on differential stimulation of these cone types. The opponent colour theory suggests that each cone type can generate signals of the opposite kind. Output from some cones can collaborate with the output from others or can inhibit the action of other cones. Colour perception results from these various complex interactions.

Defective colour vision may be hereditary or acquired and can occur in the presence of normal visual acuity. *Hereditary defective colour vision* is more common in men (7 per cent of males) than women (0·5 per cent of females). Men are affected, but women convey the abnormal gene to their children. It occurs because one or more of the photopigments of the retina are abnormal, or the cones are damaged. Red–green colour defect is the commonest. *Acquired defective colour vision* is the result of disease of the cones or their connections in the retina, optic nerve or brain, e.g. macular disease, optic neuritis. Colour vision can be impaired but not lost as a result of corneal opacification or cataract formation. *Tests of colour vision*: these include matching of coloured yarn, using specially designed numbers made of coloured dots surrounded by dots of confusing colour (e.g. Ishihara plates) and by means of coloured buttons which must be arranged in order of changing hue.

VISION, DISORDERS OF The list of disorders resulting in poor or dim vision is huge. Disturbance of vision can result from an uncorrected refractive error, disease or injury of the cornea, iris, lens, vitreous, retina, choroid or sclera. It may also result from disease or injury to the structures comprising the visual pathway from the retina to the occipital cortex (see VISION, Pathway of light from the eye to the brain) and from lesions of the structures around the eye, e.g. swollen lids, drooping eyelids.

VISION, FIELD OF When the eye looks at a specific point or object, that point is seen clearly. Other objects within a large area away from this fixation point can also be seen but less clearly. The area that can be seen around the fixation point, without moving the eye, is known as the field of vision. The extent of the field is limited inwards by the nose, above by the brow and below by the cheek. The visual field thus has its greatest extent outwards from the side of the head. The field of vision of each eye overlaps to a large extent so that objects in the centre and towards the inner part of each field are viewed by both eyes together. Because the eyes are set slightly apart, each eye sees objects in this overlapping part of the field slightly differently. It is because of this slight difference that objects can be perceived as three dimensional. Defects in the visual field (scotomas) can be produced by a variety of disorders. Certain of these produce specific field defects. For example, glaucoma, some types of brain damage and some toxins can produce specific defects in the visual field. This type of field defect may be very useful in diagnosing a particular disorder. The *blind spot* is that part of the visual field corresponding to the optic disc. There are no rods nor cones on the optic disc and therefore no light perception from this area. The blind spot can be found temporal (i.e. on the outer side) of the fixation point.

VISUAL ACUITY (see VISION).

VISUAL EVOKED RESPONSE Stimulation of the retina with light causes changes in the electrical activity of the cerebral cortex. These changes can be measured from outside the skull and can give valuable information about the state of the visual pathway from the retinal ganglion cells to the occipital cortex. Not only can it determine that function is normal, it can also help to diagnose some causes of poor vision.

VITAL CAPACITY The amount of air that can be forcibly exhaled from the lungs after a deep inspiration.

VITAMIN is a term applied to a group of substances which exist in minute quantities in natural foods, and which are necessary to normal nutrition, especially in connection with growth and development. Some, A, D, E and K, are fat soluble and can be stored in the body. The remainder, C, B_{12} and other members of the B complex, are water soluble and are quickly excreted. Most vitamins have now been synthesized. When they are absent from the food, defective growth takes place in young animals and children, and in adults various diseases arise; whilst short of the production of actual disease, persistent deprivation of one or other vitamin is apt to lead to a state of lowered general health. Certain deficiencies in diet have long been known to be the cause of scurvy, beriberi, and rickets. A diet containing foods such as milk, eggs, butter, cheese, fat, fish, wholemeal bread, fresh vegetables and fruit should contain sufficient vitamins. Details of the various vitamins are given in APPENDIX 5: VITAMINS.

VITILIGO are patchy areas of depigmentation of the skin surrounded by areas of increased pigmentation. It is seen in many auto-immune diseases such as Graves' disease, chronic thyroiditis and Addison's disease and it is due to the auto- immune destruction of the melanin-secreting cells in the skin.

VITREOUS BODY is a semi-fluid, transparent substance which fills most of the globe of the eye behind the lens.

VIVISECTION   For over a century the medical profession has aimed at maintaining as high a standard as possible for vivisection. It was the medical profession led by Dr James Paget that was responsible for the passing of the Cruelty to Animals Act 1876, which aimed to eliminate cruelty. The infliction of pain was reduced to a minimum by the use of anaesthetics, and the licensing and surveillance of animal experiments was ensured.

Most experiments are carried out on specially bred mice and rats. Fewer than 1 per cent are done on cats, dogs, non-human primates, farm animals, frogs, fish and birds. Control on experiments have recently been strengthened. The great majority of animal experiments is done without anaesthesia because feeding experiments, taking blood, or giving injection, do not require anaesthetics in animals any more than in man. Universities in Britain are responsible for less than one-fifth of animal experiments; commercial concerns and government institutions are responsible for most of the rest. Tests on cosmetics account for under 1 per cent of all animal work, but are necessary because such materials are often applied with great frequency – and for a long time – to the skin of adults and infants.

A common argument is that animal research should be replaced by work on tissue culture. This is a method of research and investigation that is being increasingly used, but there is a limit to the extent to which infection, cancer, or drugs can be investigated on cultures of tissue cells. Other methods involving computerized or mathematical modelling of experiments are also being developed.

VOCAL CORDS (see LARYNGOSCOPE; LARYNX; VOICE AND SPEECH).

VOCAL RESONANCE   The air carrying the voice produced in the larynx passes through the throat, mouth and nose. The shape and size of these structures will influence the timbre of the voice, or vocal resonance. This will vary from person to person and even within an individual; i.e. with a cold.

VOICE AND SPEECH are two terms applied to the system of sounds which are produced in the upper air passages and in the mouth, and which form one of the means of communication between human beings.

Voice means the set of fundamental notes and tones produced by the larynx which are modified in various ways during their passage through the mouth so as to form speech or song. Speech differs from song in being less sustained and of smaller compass with regard to pitch, and in presenting sounds which have not a musical character.

VOICE is produced in the larynx of most animals. Voice production may be studied with the laryngoscope (q.v.), an instrument which enables the changes that take place in the larynx, when different notes are sounded, to be clearly seen.

Musical notes vary in three characters: loudness, pitch, and quality or timbre. The *loudness* of the voice depends upon the volume of air which is available for agitating the vocal cords, and therefore upon the size of the chest and the vigour with which its muscles can be made to act.

The *pitch* of the voice is determined by several things, the chief points being the size of the larynx; the degree of tenseness at which the vocal cords are, for the time being, maintained by the laryngeal muscles; the fact as to whether the cords vibrate as a whole or merely at their edges; and the shape which is given to the cavity of the larynx by movements of the arytenoid and epiglottic cartilages. In any given voice, the range of pitch seldom exceeds two and a half octaves, although the particular part of the musical scale that can be produced varies according as the voice is bass, tenor, contralto or soprano. Generally speaking, a large larynx with long vocal cords produces low notes, and hence men have a deeper voice than women. For the same reason the small larynx of childhood produces a shrill voice, whilst the rapid growth of the larynx at the time of puberty, and consequent uncertainty of muscular control over the vocal cords, produces the breaking of the voice that occurs in boys at this time. This is occurring at an earlier age. Thus fifty years ago, treble lines in cathedral choirs were made up of boys aged 11 to 16. Today choir schools are rarely catering for boys over 13, and voices are breaking as young as 12. Changes in the voice also occur at other ages as a result of the secondary action of the sex hormones. Thus, during menstruation there may be a slight decrease in the quality of the singing voice, affecting especially notes in the highest register, and there may be a lowering of pitch during pregnancy. At the menopause the entire vocal range for speaking and singing may be lowered, and with the onset of old age there tends to be increasing virilism of the voice.

The manner in which the muscles of the larynx act upon the cords allows the pitch to change at will. Thus if the thick part of each cord be held rigid and only the sharp free edge be allowed to vibrate, a high note is the result, and a still higher note is reached in men when only the front part of this free edge is allowed to move, as in the falsetto voice. On the other hand, by allowing a greater thickness of the cord to vibrate, the person loads the vibrating edge, and so produces a much deeper note.

The *timbre* of the voice is partly due to these differences in the larynx, but chiefly to peculiarities and to voluntary changes in shape of the mouth and other cavities associated with the air passages. These changes in shape are chiefly concerned with the alterations of the fundamental notes which produce speech.

It should be remembered, however, that, while the muscular arrangements of the larynx are chiefly concerned with the pitch of the voice, and the shape of the mouth with its modulation, the *loudness* is varied by the movements of the chest. The neglect of this fact is often responsible for the bad voice-production which leads to great straining of the throat, and is largely responsible for the throat affections of many of those who use the voice much.

There are certain peculiar forms of voice production. The *falsetto voice* has been already mentioned. *Whispering* is a form of speech in which voice is completely absent, the larynx being wide open and the sound produced entirely in the mouth. *Ventriloquism* is a form of speech in which the voice is produced by the indrawing of air, instead of in the usual way of expiration. Since it is always difficult to localize the source of sound, the ventriloquist can easily suggest to his audience a false place of origin for the unusual voice.

SPEECH consists of a series of rapid modifications of the voice, produced by changes in position of the palate, tongue, and lips.

DEFECTS OF SPEECH: The act of speech has a very elaborate controlling mechanism in the nervous system. Further, the power of speech is gained in early life by children hearing the sounds made by others and mimicking them, so that the centres for speech in the brain are intimately connected with those concerned in the sense of hearing.

MUTISM, or the entire absence of the power to speak, may be due to various causes, the most effectual being some mental deficiency which denies to the child sufficient intelligence to mimic the actions of those around him. In other cases the child seems to be quite intelligent, but, owing apparently to some defect in the nervous control of the voice and speech organs, or in these organs themselves, he is unable to make any sounds. A common cause of mutism is complete deafness present at birth, or caused by some ear diseases in early childhood. The child in this case cannot learn to speak, simply because he cannot hear, but, if properly educated, he can be taught to speak fluently and to understand what is said by watching the lips and throat of others. (See SPEECH DISORDERS.)

STAMMERING is a bad habit of speech due to want of co-ordination between the different parts of the speech mechanism. (See STAMMERING.)

Such minor peculiarities in speech as burrs and lisps are due to peculiarities in the action of the tongue or palate, whilst the deformities of tongue-tie and cleft-palate are accompanied by still greater defects of speech. When the nose is blocked by any condition, such as a cold in the head or polypus, the pronunciation of the resonants *m, n,* and *ng* is interfered with, these being heard as *b, d,* and *g,* respectively.

DYSPHASIA is a condition in which various forms of inability to speak, or to understand speech, come on, usually late in life, as the result of brain disease. (See DYSPHASIA.)

APHONIA, or loss of voice, causes speaking to be carried on in a whisper. It is usually either due to some disorder of the vocal cords, as in the laryngitis which may form part of a cold, or is a symptom of hysteria. It is generally of short duration. (See also DYSARTHRIA.)

VOLAR means something pertaining to the palm or sole.

VOLKMANN'S CONTRACTURE is the condition in which, as a result of too great a pressure from splint or bandage in the treatment of a broken arm, the flexor muscles of the forearm contract and thus obstruct free flow of blood in the veins; the muscles then swell and ultimately become fibrosed.

VOLUNTARY MUSCLE Also known as skeletal muscle, this forms the muscles which are under a person's conscious control. Muscles that control walking, talking and swallowing are examples of those under such control (see INVOLUNTARY MUSCLE and MUSCLE).

VOLVULUS means an obstruction of the bowels produced by the twisting of a loop of bowel round itself. (See INTESTINE, DISEASES OF.)

VOMITING means the expulsion of the stomach contents through the mouth. When the effort of vomiting is made, but nothing is brought up, the process is known as retching. When vomiting occurs, the chief effort is made by the muscles of the abdominal wall and by the diaphragm contracting together and squeezing the stomach. The contraction of the stomach wall is no doubt also a factor, and an important step in the act consists in the opening at the right moment of the cardiac or upper orifice of the stomach. This concerted action of various muscles is brought about by a vomiting centre situated on the floor of the fourth ventricle in the brain.

Causes Vomiting is brought about by some irritation of this nervous centre, but in the great majority of cases this is effected through sensations derived from the stomach itself. Thus, of the drugs which cause vomiting some act only after being absorbed into the blood and carried to the brain, although most are irritants to the mucous membrane of the stomach (see EMETICS); various diseases of the stomach, such as cancer, and ulcer, and food poisoning, act in a similar way. Irritation, not only of the nerves of the stomach, but also of those proceeding from other abdominal organs, produces vomiting; thus in obstruction of the bowels, peritonitis, gall-stone colic, renal colic, and even during pregnancy, vomiting is a prominent symptom.

Severe emotional shock may cause vomiting, as may unpleasant experiences such as seeing an accident, suffering severe pain or travel sickness.

Direct disturbance of the brain itself is a cause: for example, a blow on the head, a cerebral tumour, a cerebral abscess, meningitis. Many cases of hysteria also show attacks of vomiting as one of their prominent symptoms.

Nausea and vomiting are common symptoms that may arise from local disease of the gastro-intestinal tract, but they are also associated with systemic illness and also with disturbances of labyrinthine function, such as motion sickness and acute labyrinthitis.

There are two centres in the brain concerned with vomiting. One is the chemo-receptor trigger zone. This centre is in contact with the blood and lies outside the blood-brain barrier. It is the site at which drugs such as apomorphine and toxins act. It is rich in dopamine receptors and hence dopamine antagonists are effective treatment for vomiting. The vomiting centre itself co-ordinates impulses received from the chemo-receptor trigger zone from the vestibular apparatus and the gastro-intestinal tract and also from higher centres in the cerebral cortex. The vomiting centre contains many cholinergic and histamine receptors and this is why anti-cholinergic drugs and anti-histamines are effective drugs in the control of vomiting.

Treatment The cause of the vomiting must be sought and treatment directed towards this. If the vomiting is due to local disease in the gastro-intestinal tract the old-fashioned remedies of sodium bicarbonate and bismuth may be helpful, along with rest. If the vomiting is vestibular in origin and due, for example, to motion sickness, hyoscine or antihistamines are the drugs of choice, though the side effects of sedation, dry mouth and constipation may be troublesome.

Nausea and vomiting are a common feature of migraine. Metoclopramide is the drug of choice. This drug acts by encouraging gastric emptying and gastro-intestinal motility is altered by nausea and vomiting. Domperidone is also effective.

Vomiting may occur after surgical operations and this is due to the combined effects of analgesics, anaesthetic agents and the psychological stress of operation. Various drugs can be used to prevent or stop postoperative vomiting.

Nausea and vomiting are common symptoms in pregnancy. Drugs are best avoided in this situation as they may damage the developing fetus. Simple measures, such as the taking of food before getting up in the morning and reassurance, are often all that is necessary.

VON RECKLINGHAUSEN'S DISEASE This description covers the inherited disease, multiple neurofibromatosis. About one new case occurs every 3,000 live births. The disease is characterized by tumours along the course of nerves which can be felt beneath the skin. Soft tumours may also develop beneath the skin. The condition may have other associated abnormalities such as scoliosis, decalcification of the bones due to overactivity of the parathyroid glands and fibrosis in the lungs. Surgery may be needed for cosmetic reasons or to relieve pressure on the nervous system.

VOYEURISM The regular viewing of people who are naked or part naked or who are taking part in sexual intercourse. The voyeur's subjects are unaware that they are being watched. The voyeur, nearly always a man, usually becomes sexually excited and may induce orgasm by masturbation.

VULVA is the general term applied to the external female genitals.

VULVO-VAGINITIS is inflammation of the vulva and the vagina. It is more common in young girls than in adult women. It may be a manifestation of infection elsewhere in the body, or may indicate the presence of some infection in the vagina.

W

WALK (see GAIT).

WARFARIN is an anticoagulant which is active whether given by mouth, intramuscularly, intravenously or rectally. It is usually given by mouth, when its maximum effect occurs within about 36 hours. Its action passes off within 48 hours of cessation of treatment. The dose is adjusted in the light of regular checks on the patient's coagulation time (see COAGULATION).

WARTS, or VERRUCAE, are small, solid growths, arising from the surface of the skin. They are due to a papovavirus infection of the skin. They are highly infectious, and it is estimated that 10 per cent of the population suffer from them. The infection is most likely to be spread in schools by hand-holding games, and among adolescents by walking barefoot on gymnasium floors and in swimming baths.
COMMON WARTS develop on the skin of children and young people on the knuckles, on the backs of the hands and on the knees. Occasionally such warts come out in a crop. In structure, they consist of a bundle of fibres produced by overgrowth of the papillae in the true skin, each bundle enveloped by a cap of the horny cells that cover the surface of the epidermis, and the whole mass being surrounded by a ring of thickened epidermis. PLANE WARTS, which are flat-topped, are commonest on the face and the back of the hands. PLANTAR WARTS occur on the soles of the feet, most commonly in older children and adolescents. Epidemics are not uncommon in schools. SENILE WARTS are usually hard, wrinkled, and slightly raised areas of skin found in old people. SOFT WARTS, consisting of little tags of skin, are found especially upon the neck, chest, ears, or eyelids of people whose skin has been subjected for long to some irritation. HORNS are formed sometimes upon the face or hands, as the result of the drying up of the sebaceous material exuding from the skin that covers a wart, and, as the secretion goes on, these horns occasionally reach a length of some inches. TUBERCULOUS WARTS are developed sometimes as the result of a wound in the skin of the hands, especially of those who have come in contact with persons or animals suffering from some form of tuberculosis: e.g. pathologists and butchers.
Treatment   There is much to be said for the old advice that the best way to manage warts is to let them manage themselves. Quite often they disappear spontaneously, which explains the large range of vaunted 'cures'. Warts can be treated with cryosurgery, electrocautery, curettage, laser treatment or by applying a preparation of salicylic acid or podophyllin.

WASHING (see DISINFECTION).

WASHING OUT OF THE STOMACH or GASTRIC LAVAGE is performed for various reasons, particularly in order to remove poison that has been recently swallowed, before it shall have had time to act. Expert opinion today differs as to the value and safety of washing out the stomach in cases of poisoning. If it is done for this purpose, it should only be done by a doctor, nurse or experienced first-aider. The elementary rules are as follows:
(1) Place the head of the patient over the side of the bed so that the mouth and throat are at a lower level than the larynx and trachea.
(2) Use a wide-bore stomach tube (Jaques gauge 30) and lubricate it well with glycerin or some similar lubricant. In the adult 50 cm (20 inches) will reach the stomach. Make sure the tube is in the gullet (oesophagus) and not the trachea.
(3) For the first wash use 300 ml water, or olive oil if a tar oil derivative has been taken. Repeat this process, using 300-600 ml at a time, at least three or four times, saving all washings for analysis.
(4) If the patient is conscious, leave in the stomach 600 ml water containing 20 ml sodium or magnesium sulphate. If the patients is comatose, leave the stomach empty, and leave a nasogastric tube in place to keep the stomach empty. In the unconscious patient it is necessary to protect the airway with a cupped endotracheal tube. (See STOMACH TUBE.)

WASSERMANN REACTION was a test introduced for the diagnosis of syphilis by examination of the blood. It has now been largely supplanted by other more specific tests.

WASTING (see ATROPHY).

WATERBRASH, or PYROSIS, is a symptom of dyspepsia; during the course of digestion, the mouth fills with tasteless or sour fluid, which is generally saliva, but sometimes seems to be brought up from the stomach. At the same time, a burning pain is often felt at the pit of the stomach or in the chest. The condition is a symptom of excessive acidity of the stomach contents, due sometimes to an irritating diet, and often characteristic of a duodenal ulcer. (See DYSPEPSIA.)

WATER-HAMMER PULSE is a name given to the peculiarly sudden pulse that is associated with incompetence of the aortic valve of the heart, and suggests the philosophical toy after which it is named. (See PULSE.)

WATER ON THE BRAIN was a traditional name for hydrocephalus and for meningitis. (See HYDROCEPHALUS; MENINGITIS.)

WAX is used in medicine as an ingredient of ointments, plasters, and suppositories. It is used either as yellow wax derived directly from honeycomb, or as white wax, which is the same substance bleached. It is also used in the form of paraffin wax to apply heat in the relief of rheumatic pains.

For wax in the ear, see EAR, DISEASES OF.

WEAKNESS (see ATROPHY; CACHEXIA; PARALYSIS; TONICS).

WEALS, or WHEALS, are raised white areas on the skin with reddened margins, which may result from sharp blows, or may be a symptom of nettle-rash.

WEANING The process by which a baby is introduced to solid foods after having only had breast milk or artificial milk to drink. The transfer usually starts at around 4 months of age. (See INFANT FEEDING.)

WEBBED FINGERS or TOES, or SYNDACTYLY, constitute a deformity sometimes present at birth, and liable to run in families. The web may be quite a thin structure, or the fingers may be closely united by solid tissue. In any case, separation is a matter of considerable difficulty, because, if the web is simply divided, it heals up as before. A special operation is necessary, consisting in turning back a flap of the web upon each of the united fingers, or some other device to produce healing in the new position.

WEBER'S TEST A test with a tuning fork that is used to assess a person's deafness.

WEIGHT AND HEIGHT Charts relating height to age have been devised and give an indication of the normal rate of growth. (See APPENDIX 6: MEASUREMENTS IN MEDICINE for more details.) The wide variation in normal children is immediately apparent on studying such charts. Deviations from the mean of this wide range are called percentiles. Centile or percentile charts describe the distribution of a characteristic in a population. They are obtained by measuring a specific characteristic in a large population of at least 1,000 of each sex at each age. For each age there will be a height, above and below which 50 per cent of the population lie and this is called the fiftieth centile. The fiftieth centile thus indicates the mean height at a particular age. Such tables are less reliable around the age of puberty because of variation in age of onset.

Minor variations from the mean do not warrant investigation but if the height of an individual falls below the third centile (3 per cent of normal children have a height that falls below the third centile) or above the ninety-seventh centile, investigation is required. Changes in the rate of growth are also important and skeletal proportions may provide useful information. There are many children who are normal but who are small in relation to their parents. The problem is merely growth delay. These children take longer to reach maturity and there is also a proportional delay in their skeletal maturation. The actual height must always be assessed in relation to maturity. The change in skeletal proportions is one manifestation of maturity but other features include the maturing of facial features with the growth of nose and jaw and dental development. Maturity of bone can readily be measured by the radiological bone age.

Failure to gain weight is of more significance. Whilst this may be due to some underlying disease, the commonest cause is a diet containing inadequate calories. Over the last six decades or so there has been quite a striking increase in the heights and weights of European children. Manufacturers of children's clothing, shoes and furniture have had to increase the size of their products. Growth is now completed at 20–21 years, compared with 25 at the turn of the century. This increase, and earlier maturation, it has been suggested, have been due to a combination of genetic mixing as a result of population movements, combined with the whole range of improvement in environmental hygiene, and not merely to better nutrition.

In the case of adults views have changed of recent years concerning 'ideal' weight. Life insurance statistics have shown that maximal life expectancy is obtained if the average weight at ages 25 to 30 years is maintained throughout the rest of life. These insurance statistics also suggest that it is of advantage to be slightly over average weight before the age of 30 years, to be of average weight after the age of 40, and to be under-weight from ages 30 to 40. In the past it has been usual, in assessing the significance of an adult's weight, to allow a 10 per cent range on either side of normal for variations in body build. A closer correlation has been found between thoracic and abdominal measurements and weight.

WEIGHTS AND MEASURES It is over a hundred years since the metric system was legalized in Britain, but it was not until 1969 that it became illegal to use any system of weights and measures other than the metric system for dispensing prescriptions.

A rationalization of the metric system is now in operation, known as the International System of Units (SI) (see APPENDIX 6: MEASUREMENTS IN MEDICINE).

WEIL'S DISEASE (see LEPTOSPIROSIS).

WERNICKE'S ENCEPHALOPATHY Also called the Wernicke-Korsakoff syndrome, this uncommon disorder is characterized by mental confusion or delirium that occurs in combination with an unsteady gait (q.v.), nystagmus (see EYE DISEASES), and paralysis of the eye muscles and eventually psychosis (q.v.). It is caused by a deficiency of vitamin B_1 (thiamine) which affects the brain and nervous system. It occurs in alcoholic individuals and in patients with persistent vomiting. As soon as the condition is diagnosed, it must be treated with large doses of thiamine. Unless the patient has developed symptoms of psychosis, the condition is usually reversible with treatment.

WERTHHEIM'S HYSTERECTOMY A major operation done to remove cancer of the uterus or ovary. The ovaries, fallopian tubes, the uterus and its ligaments, the upper vagina, and the regional lymph nodes are all excised.

WET PACK is a method of treatment popular in some countries for the purpose of applying a moderate degree of cold or of heat, for some time, to a patient's skin.

WHEEZING is a popular name applied to the various sounds produced in the chest when the bronchial tubes are narrowed. It is applied particularly to the long-drawn breathing of asthma, and to the whistling or purring noises that accompany breathing in cases of bronchitis. (See ASTHMA; BRONCHITIS.)

WHIPWORM is a popular name for *Trichuris trichiura*. (See TRICHURIASIS.)

WHITE BLOOD CELL (see LEUCOCYTE).

WHITE HAIR The greying or whitening of hair which takes place with age is due to a loss of its pigment, melanin (q.v.), and the collection of air bubbles in the shaft of the hair. There is no evidence that hair ever goes white overnight, whether in response to shock, strain or any other cause. Rapid whitening may occur patchily in a matter of days, but it is more often a matter of weeks or months. In the more rapid cases the cause is thought to be a form of alopecia areata (see BALDNESS), in which the dark hairs which fall out are replaced by white hairs. An alternative cause is vitiligo (q.v.). Certain drugs, including mephenesin and chloroquine (q.v.), may also cause whitening of the hair.

WHITE LEG is a fairly common and well-known condition in which a limb, usually one of the lower limbs, becomes enlarged, white, and painful as a result of thrombosis in a vein. (See VEINS, DISEASES OF.)

WHITES (see LEUCORRHOEA).

WHITLOW is a popular term applied to all acute inflammations of the deep-seated tissues in the fingers, whether the structure affected is the root of the nail, the pulp of the finger-tip, the sheaths of the tendons that run along the back and front of the fingers, or the bone.

WHOOPING-COUGH, or PERTUSSIS, is a respiratory-tract infection caused by *Bordetella pertussis* and spread by droplets. It may occur at all ages, but around 90 per cent of cases are children under 5 years, particularly girls. Most common during the winter months, it tends to occur in epidemics, with periods of increased prevalence occurring every three to four years. It is a notifiable disease.

Symptoms The first, or catarrhal, stage is characterized by mild, but non-specific, symptoms of sneezing, conjunctivitis (see EYE DISEASES), sore throat, mild fever and cough. Lasting 10 to 14 days, this stage is the most infectious; unfortunately it is almost impossible to make a definite clinical diagnosis, although analysis of a nasal swab may confirm a suspected diagnosis. This is followed by the second, or paroxysmal, stage with irregular bouts of coughing, often prolonged, and typically more severe at night. Each paroxysm consists of a succession of short sharp coughs, increasing in speed and duration, and ending in a deep, crowing inspiration, often with a characteristic 'whoop'. Vomiting is common after the last paroxysm of a series. Lasting two to four weeks, this stage is the most dangerous, with the greatest risk of complications. These may include pneumonia and partial collapse of the lungs, and fits may be induced by cerebral anoxia (q.v.). Less severe complications caused by the stress of coughing include minor bleeding around the eyes, ulceration under the tongue, hernia and prolapse of the rectum. Mortality is greatest in the first year of life, particularly among neonates, infants up to 4 weeks old. Nearly all patients with whooping-cough recover after a few weeks, with a lasting immunity. Very severe cases may leave structural changes in the lungs, such as emphysema (q.v.), with a permanent shortness of breath or liability to asthma (q.v.).

Treatment Antibiotics, such as erythromycin or tetracyclines, may be helpful if given during the catarrhal stage, but are of no use during the paroxysmal stage. Cough suppressants are helpful, and skilled nursing may be required to maintain nutrition, particularly if the disease is prolonged, with frequent vomiting. A vaccine (q.v.) is routinely given to infants as part of the triple vaccine, but should not be given to any child with a disorder of the central nervous system, or a history of convulsions (q.v.).

In an epidemic of whooping-cough, which extended from the last quarter of 1977 to mid-1979, 102,500 cases of whooping-cough were notified in the United Kingdom, with 36 deaths. This was the biggest outbreak since 1957 and its size was partly attributed to the fall in vaccination acceptance rates. In 1992 2,171 cases were notified in England.

WIDAL REACTION (see AGGLUTINATION).

WILMS' TUMOUR, or NEPHROBLASTOMA, is the commonest kidney tumour in infancy. It is a malignant tumour, which occurs in around 1 per 10,000 live births. The survival rate with modern treatment (removal of the kidney followed by radiotherapy and chemotherapy) is now around 80 per cent.

WILSON'S DISEASE or HEPATOLENTICULAR DEGENERATION, is a familial disease in which there is an increased accumulation of copper in the liver, brain, and other tissues including the kidneys. Its main manifestation is the development of tremor and rigidity, with difficulty in speech. In many cases there is improvement following the administration of dimercaprol, penicillamine, or trientine dihydrochloride; these substances cause an increased excretion of copper.

WINDPIPE is the popular name for the trachea, which extends from the larynx above to the point in the upper part of the chest where it divides into the two large bronchial tubes, one to each lung. It thus extends through the lower part of the neck and upper part of the chest, and is about 10 cm (4 inches) in length. It consists of a fibrous tube kept permanently open by about twenty strong horizontally placed hoops of cartilage, each of which forms about two-thirds of a circle, but is defective behind where the two ends are united by muscle-fibres. This fibro- cartilaginous tube is lined by a smooth mucous membrane, richly supplied with mucous glands and covered by a single layer of ciliated epithelium. (See also AIR PASSAGES.)

WINTER VOMITING DISEASE, or EPIDEMIC NAUSEA AND VOMITING, is a condition characterized by nausea, vomiting, diarrhoea and giddiness, which occurs during the winter. Outbreaks of it usually involve whole families or may affect communities like schools. It is due to parvoviruses (q.v.). The incubation period is 24 to 48 hours, and attacks seldom persist for more than 72 hours.

WISDOM TOOTH is a popular name for the last molar tooth on either side of each jaw. These teeth are the last to appear and should develop in early adult life, but often they do not cut the gum till the age of 20 or 25 or indeed they may sometimes remain permanently impacted in the jaw-bone. This occurs in up to 25 per cent of individuals. The lower third molar is often impacted against the second because of the direction in which it erupts. (See TEETH.)

WITCH-HAZEL is a preparation of the bark, twigs, and dried leaves from *Hamamelis virginiana*, a plant of the United States possessed of strong astringent properties. It is used to check haemorrhages and excessive mucous discharges, and also for piles.

WITHDRAWAL SYMPTOMS Unpleasant physical and mental symptoms that occur when a person stops using a drug or substance on which he or she are dependent. The symptoms include tremors, sweating, and vomiting which are reversed if further doses are given. Alcohol and hard drugs, such as morphine, heroin, and cocaine, are among the substances that induce dependence, and therefore withdrawal symptoms, when stopped. Amphetamines and nicotine are other examples.

WOLFFIAN DUCTS The Wolffian ducts and the Mullerian ducts are separate sets of primordia that transiently co-exist in embryos of both sexes. In the male the Wolffian ducts give rise to the vas deferens, the seminal vesicles and the epididymis, while the Mullerian ducts disappear. In female embryos the Mullerian ducts grow and fuse in the midline to produce the Fallopian tubes, the uterus and the upper third of the vagina, whereas the Wolffian ducts regress. The former phase of development requires a functioning testis from which an inducer substance diffuses locally over the primordia to bring about the suppression of the Mullerian duct and the development of the Wolffian duct. In the absence of this substance development proceeds along female lines regardless of the genetic sex.

WOMB (see UTERUS).

WOMB MUSIC is the name given to the playing to crying babies of sounds comparable to those by which the unborn babe is surrounded in the womb, such as the beating of the mother's heart, the bowel sounds of the babe and the like. The claim is that the replaying of these brings back the 'peaceful music of the womb', to which they have become conditioned, and thus 'sings' them to sleep.

WOOL-SORTERS' DISEASE is another name for anthrax. (See ANTHRAX.)

WORD BLINDNESS is a condition in which, as the result of disease in the brain, a person becomes unable to associate their proper meanings with words, although he may be quite able to spell the letters. WORD DEAFNESS is an associated condition in which, though hearing remains perfect, the patient has lost the power of referring the names he hears to the articles they denote. (See DYSPHASIA.)

WORMS (see ASCARIASIS, ENTEROBIASIS, TAENIASIS).

WOUNDS A wound is any breach suddenly produced in the tissues of the body by direct violence. An extensive injury of the deeper parts without corresponding injury of the surface is known as a bruise or contusion.

Varieties Classified according to the immediate effect produced, four varieties are usually described as *incised, punctured, lacerated*, and *contused*.

INCISED WOUNDS are usually inflicted with some sharp instrument, and are clean cuts, in which the tissues are simply divided without any damage to parts around. The bleeding from such a wound is apt to be very free, but it can be readily controlled.

PUNCTURED WOUNDS, or stabs, are inflicted with a pointed instrument. These wounds are the most dangerous, partly because their depth involves the danger of wounding vital organs, partly because bleeding from a stab is hard to control, and largely on account of the difficulty of sterilization. The wound produced by the nickel-nosed bullet is a puncture, much less severe than the ugly lacerated wound caused by an expanding bullet, or by a ricochet, and, if no clothing has been carried in by the bullet, the wound is clean and usually heals at once.

LACERATED WOUNDS are those in which tearing of tissues takes place, such as injuries caused by machinery. The blood-vessels being torn and twisted, little bleeding is apt to result, and a limb may be torn completely away without great loss of blood. Such wounds are, however, specially liable to infection.

CONTUSED WOUNDS are those accompanied by much bruising of surrounding parts, as in the case of a blow from a cudgel or poker. In these wounds also there is little bleeding, but healing is slow on account of damage to the edges of the wound. Any of these varieties may become infected.

First-aid treatment The first aim is to check any bleeding. This may be done by pressure upon the edges of the wound with a clean handkerchief, or, if the bleeding is serious, by putting the finger in the wound and pressing it upon the spot from which the blood is coming.

If medical attention is available within a few hours, it should not be interfered with further than is necessary to stop the bleeding and to cover the wound with a clean dry handkerchief or piece of lint. When expert assistance is not soon obtainable, the wound should be cleaned with an antiseptic such as chlorhexidine (q.v.) or boiled water and the injured part fixed so that movement is prevented or minimized. A wounded hand or arm is fixed with a sling (see SLING), a wounded leg with a splint (see SPLINTS). If the victim is in shock he or she must be treated for that (see SHOCK and APPENDIX 1: BASIC FIRST AID).

WRIST is the joint situated between the arm above and the hand below. The region of the wrist contains eight small carpal bones, arranged in two rows, each containing four bones. Those in the proximal row, that is the row nearest the forearm, are from the outside inwards when looking at the palm of the hand, the scaphoid, lunate, triquetrum, and pisiform. Those in the distal row, that is the row nearest the hand, are the trapezium, trapezoid, capitate and hamate. These intervene between the arm bones and the five metacarpal bones in the hand, and have the effect of diminishing jars communicated to the hand in virtue of a certain amount of sliding movement over one another, of which they are capable. These small bones are closely bound to one another by short, strong ligaments, and the wrist-joint is the union of the composite mass thus formed with the radius and ulna in the forearm. The wrist and the radius and ulna are united by strong outer and inner lateral ligaments, and by weaker ligaments before and behind, whilst the powerful tendons passing to the hand and fingers give it a great measure of strength.

The joint is capable of movement in all directions, and, on account of its shape and its numerous ligaments, is little liable to dislocation, although stretching or tearing of some of these ligaments is a common accident, constituting a sprain. (See JOINTS, DISEASES AND INJURIES OF.) Inflammation of the tendon-sheaths before and behind the wrist, causing the presence of fluid, also results occasionally from an injury, and produces a sense of weakness in the wrist. A fairly common condition is that known as a ganglion, in which an elastic swelling full of fluid develops on the back or front of the wrist in connection with the sheaths of the tendons. (See GANGLION.)

WRIST-DROP (see DROP WRIST).

WRITER'S CRAMP is a spasm which affects certain muscles when engaged in writing, and which may not occur when the same muscles are employed in other acts. Similar symptoms are observed in the case of musicians (guitar, clarinet and piano in particular), typists, word-processor and computer operators and artists.

WRY-NECK is a condition in which the head is twisted to one side. It may be caused by the contraction of a scar, such as that resulting from a burn or by paralysis of some of the muscles, but in the great majority of cases it is a spasmodic condition due to excessive tendency of certain muscles to contract. (See CRAMP; SPASMODIC TORTICOLLIS.)

X

XANTHELASMATA These are yellow plaques of lipid deposited in the skin. They tend to occur in the eyelids. They are often associated with hyperlipidaemia.

XANTHOMATA These are deposits of fatty tissue in tendon sheaths and over bony prominences such as knees, elbows and fingers. They are indicative of a state of hyperlipidaemia which may be a primary inherited disorder or secondary to such conditions as biliary cirrhosis, diabetes mellitus or nephrotic syndrome.

X CHROMOSOME One of two sex chromosomes. Every normal female body cell has a pair of X chromosomes. Men have only one X chromosome and this is paired with a Y chromosome. The sex cells in men and women each have one X and one Y chromosome. Certain diseases are linked to the presence of an X chromosome: these include haemophilia (q.v.) (see GENES).

XENOGRAFT is a transplant from one animal to another of a different species. It is also known as a heterograft.

XERODERMA is a rough, dry condition of the skin accompanied by the copious formation of scales.
XERODERMA PIGMENTOSUM is a rare hereditary affection of the skin appearing first in early childhood. It is characterized by a dry skin which is heavily freckled and hypersensitive to sunlight.

XEROPHTHALMIA (see EYE DISEASES).

XEROSIS means abnormal dryness, especially of the eye.

XEROSTOMIA is the condition of dryness of the mouth due to lack of saliva. Its most extreme form occurs following radiotherapy of the mouth, and in the condition known as Sjögren's syndrome. No satisfactory substitute for natural saliva has been found though some find a methyl-cellulose substitute gives partial relief, as may a glycerin mouth-wash.

XIPHISTERNUM (see XIPHOID PROCESS.)

XIPHOID PROCESS or XIPHOID CARTILAGE: Also known as the xiphisternum, this is the small oval-shaped projection forming the lowest of the three parts of the sternum or breast bone.

X-RAYS (RÖNTGEN RAYS) were discovered in 1895 by Wilhelm Conrad Röntgen. Their use for diagnostic *imaging (radiology)* and for cancer therapy (see RADIOTHERAPY) is now an integral part of medicine. Many other forms of diagnostic imaging have been developed in recent years, sometimes also loosely called 'radiology'. Similarly the use of chemotherapeutic agents in cancer has led to the term *oncology* which may be applied to the treatment of cancer by both drugs and X-rays.

The rays are part of the electro-magnetic spectrum; their wavelengths are between 10^{-9} and 10^{-13} metres; in behaviour and energy they are identical to the gamma rays emitted by radioactive isotopes. Diagnostic X-rays are generated in an evacuated tube contining an anode and cathode. Electrons striking the anode cause emission of X-rays of varying energy; the energy is largely dependent on the potential difference (kilovoltage) between anode and cathode. The altered tissue penetration at different kilovoltages is used in radiographing different regions, for example in breast radiography (25–40 kV) or chest radiography (120–150 kV). Most diagnostic examinations use kilovoltages between 60 and 120. The energy of X-rays enbles them to pass through body tissues unless they make contact with the constituent atoms. Tissue attenuation varies with atomic structure, so that air-containing organs such as the lung offer little attenuation, while material such as bone, with abundant calcium, will absorb the majority of incident X-rays. This results in an emerging X-ray pattern which corresponds to the structures in the region examined.

The recording of the resulting images – *radiography* – is achieved in several ways, mostly depending on the use of materials which fluoresce in response to X-rays. Initially the use of such materials, mounted on card and examined in darkness, allowed brief study of bodily structures or events. Permanent images were on photographic glass plates. However photographic amulsions are relatively insensitive to X-rays so X-ray film is now also excited by light emitted by substances which fluoresce in response to X-rays. The film, usually doubly coated with emulsion to increase its responsiveness, is placed in a light-tight cassette. It is firmly compressed between screens faced with materials responsive to X-rays. Originally barium platino-cyanide and calcium tungstate were used; now more responsive materials – rare-earth compounds – such as zinc-cadmium sulphide are employed. The result has been a marked reduction in the X-ray dose needed for a given examination.
CONTRAST X-RAYS Many body organs are not shown by simple X-ray studies. This has led to the development of *contrast* materials which can be used to make particular organs or structures wholly or partly opaque to X-rays. Thus barium-sulphate preparations are largely used for examining the gastro-intestinal tract, i.e. barium swallow, barium meal, barium follow-through (or enteroclysis) and barium

enema. Water-soluble iodine-containing contrast agents that ionize in solution have been developed for a range of other studies.

More recently a series of improved contrast molecules, chiefly non-ionizing, has been developed, with fewer side-effects. They can, for example, safely be introduced into the spinal theca for *myeloradiculography* – contrast X-rays of the spinal cord. Using these agents, it is possible to show many organs and structures mostly by direct introduction, e.g. via a catheter. In urography, however, contrast medium injected intravenously is excreted by the kidneys which are outlined, together with ureters and bladder. A number of other more specialized contrast agents exist, e.g. for cholecystography – radiological assessment of the gall bladder. The use of contrast and the attendant techniques has greatly widened the range of radiology.

IMAGE INTENSIFICATION The relative insensitivity of fluorescent materials when used for observation of moving organs – e.g. the oesophagus – has been overcome by the use of image intensification. A faint fluorographic image produced by X-rays leads to electron emission from a photo-cathode. By applying a high potential difference, the electrons are accelerated across an evacuated tube and are focused on to a small fluorescent screen, giving a bright image. This is viewed by a TV camera and the image shown on a monitor and sometimes recorded on videotape or cine.

TOMOGRAPHY X-rays images are two-dimensional representations of three-dimensional objects. Tomography (Greek *tomos* – a slice) began with X-ray imaging produced by the linked movement of the X-ray tube and the cassette pivoting about a selected plane in the body: over- and underlying structures are blurred out, giving a more detailed image of a particular plane.

In 1975 Godfrey Hounsfield introduced *computerized tomography* (*CT*). This involves (i) movement of an X-ray tube around the patient, with a narrow fan beam of X-rays; (ii) the corresponding use of sensitive detectors on the opposite side of the patient; (iii) computer analysis of the detector readings at each point on the rotation, with calculation of relative tissue attenuation at each point in the cross-sectional plant. This invention has enormously increased the ability to discriminate tissue composition, even without the use of contrast.

The tomographic effect – imaging of a particular plane – is achieved in many of the newer forms of imaging – *ultrasound* (q.v.), magnetic resonance imaging (see NUCLEAR MAGNETIC RESONANCE) and some forms of nuclear medicine, in particular *positron emission tomography* (*PET*) (q.v.). An alternative term for the production of images of a given plane is *cross-sectional imaging*.

While the production of X-ray and other images has been largely the responsibility of radiographers, the interpretation has been principally carried out by specialist doctors called radiologists. In addition they, and interested clinicians, have developed a number of procedures, such as *arteriography* (see ANGIOGRAPHY), which involve manipulative access for imaging, e.g. selective coronary or renal arteriography.

The use of X-rays, ultrasound or computerized tomography to control the direction and position of needles has made possible guided biopsies, e.g. of pancreatic, pulmonary or bony lesions, and therapeutic procedures such as drainage of obstructed kidneys (percutaneous nephrostomy), or of abscesses. From these has grown a whole series of therapeutic procedures such as angioplasty (q.v.), stent insertion (q.v.) and renal-stone track formation. This field of *interventional radiology* has close affinities with minimally invasive surgery.

Radiotherapy, or treatment by X-rays The two chief sources of the ionizing radiations used in radiotherapy are the gamma rays of radium (q.v.) and the penetrating X-rays generated by apparatus working at various voltages. For superficial lesions energies of around 40 kilovolts are used, but for deep-seated conditions, such as cancer of the internal organs, much higher voltages are required. X-ray machines are now in use which work at two million volts. Even higher voltages are now available through the development of the linear accelerator, which makes use of the frequency magnetron which is the basis of radar. The linear accelerator receives its name from the fact that it accelerates a beam of electrons down a straight tube, 3 metres in length, and in this process a voltage of eight million is attained. The use of these very high voltages has led to the development of a highly specialized technique which has been devised for the treatment of cancer and like diseases.

Like the photographic effect, the therapeutic effects were discovered almost accidentally. It was observed that prolonged exposures to the rays caused inflammation, and even ulceration of the skin, and further, that they caused loss of hair, and that they improved various diseased conditions. Repeated exposures, for example, of the hands of physicians using this method of treatment, have been observed to produce pigmentation of the skin, excessive growth of its horny layer, and even epithelioma. X-rays are particularly hurtful to the testes and ovaries of young people; and when these are exposed to the rays repeatedly, the genital glands must be covered by sheet-lead or some such protection, in case sterility should result. Too severe a reaction to the irritating effect of the rays upon the patient's skin at a single session must also be avoided. It is important to protect the surrounding areas, and this is done by the use of masks of sheet-lead, with a hole cut out over the affected area, and by enclosing the tube in a metal-lined box, with an opening opposite the affected spot. By these means, as well as by wearing lead-lined gloves, and by frequently anointing the skin with some simple ointment, people constantly applying the rays are effectually protected.

The greatest value of radiotherapy is in the treatment of malignant disease. In many cases it can be used for the treatment of malignant growths which are not accessible to surgery, whilst in others it is used in conjunction with surgery.

Leukaemia and other conditions, in which the spleen is enlarged, are often greatly benefited by exposure of the spleen or long bones to X-rays or radium. (See RADIOTHERAPY.)

In simple conditions, particularly superficial ones, X-rays have been used very successfully, but are being used less and less, in view of the increasing necessity to reduce to the absolute minimum the amount of irradiation to which people are exposed.

Y

YAWNING consists of an involuntary opening of the mouth, which is accompanied by marked dilatation of the pharynx, a characteristic distortion of the face and usually stretching of the limbs. The cause and function of yawning are quite obscure. It is classically regarded as a sign of drowsiness or boredom, but it not infrequently occurs following a severe haemorrhage, and it is also sometimes associated with indigestion.

YAWS, known also as FRAMBOESIA and PIAN. A non-venereal spirochaetal infection caused by *Treponema pertenue*; it was formerly widespread in most tropical and subtropical regions amongst the indigenous population, florid disease being more common in children than adults. The term is of Carib-Indian (native to north-eastern South America, the east coast of Central America, and the lesser Antilles) origin. It is directly contagious from person to person; infection is also transmitted by flies, clothing, and living in unclean huts. Clinically, the primary stage is characterized by a granulomatous lesion, or papule (framboesioma or 'mother yaw') at the site of infection – usually the lower leg or foot; this enlarges, crusts, and heals spontaneously. It appears some 2–8 weeks after infection, during which time fever, malaise, pains, and pruritus may be present. In the secondary stage, a granulomatous, papular, macular or squamous eruption occurs; periostitis may also be present. The late, or tertiary stage (which appears 5–10 years later), is characterized by skin plaques, nodules, ulcers, hyperkeratosis (thickening of the skin of the hands and feet) and gummatous lesions affecting bones. Recurrence of infection in individuals suffering from a concurrent infection (e.g., syphilis or tuberculosis) renders the infection more serious. Diagnosis is by demonstration of *T. pertenue* in exudate from a suspected lesion. Treatment is with penicillin,

to which *T. pertenue* is highly sensitive. Extensive eradication campaigns (initiated by the WHO in 1949) have been carried out in endemic areas; therefore, the early stages of the infection are rarely counted; only tertiary stages come to the attention of a physician. Failure of surveillance can lead to dramatic local recurrences.

Y CHROMOSOME One of two sex chromosomes that is present in every male body cell where it is paired with an X chromosome. The sex or germ cells in women as well as men contain one X and one Y chromosome (see GENES).

YEAST consists of the cells and spores of unicellular fungi belonging to the family of Saccharomycetaceae. The main species of yeast used in medicine is *Saccharomyces cerevisiae*, which is used in the fermentation industries, such as brewing. It is a rich source of the vitamin B complex (see VITAMIN), but its use has largely been given up since the various components of the vitamin B complex became available as separate entities.

YELLOW FEVER, also known as YELLOW JACK and VOMITO AMARILLI. An acute arbovirus infection caused by a flavivirus of the togavirus family, transmitted from animals to humans by various species of forest mosquito (jungle/sylvan yellow fever), and from human to human by *Aëdes aegypti* (urban yellow fever). Mosquito transmission was shown by Walter Reed and his colleagues in 1900. It is endemic in much of tropical Africa and Central and South America but does not occur in Asia. In the urban cycle, man constitutes the reservoir of infection, and in the jungle/sylvan variety, mammals – especially subhuman primates – are involved in transmission. Historically, yellow fever was enormously important, causing devastating epidemics; it also carried a high mortality rate in travellers and explorers. Differentiation from other infections associated with jaundice was often impossible.

Clinically, yellow fever is characterized by jaundice, fever, chills, headache, gastrointestinal haemorrhage(s), and albuminuria. The incubation period is 3–6 (up to 10) days. Differentiation from viral hepatitides, other viral haemorrhagic fevers, severe *Plasmodium falciparum* malaria, and several other infections is often impossible without sophisticated investigative techniques. Infection carries a high mortality rate. Liver histology (biopsy is contraindicated due to the haemorrhagic diathesis) shows characteristic changes; a fulminating hepatic infection is often present. Acute inflammation of the kidneys and an inflamed, congested gastric mucosa, often accompanied by haemorrhage, are also demonstrable; myocardial involvement often occurs. Diagnosis is primarily based on virological techniques; serological tests are also of value.

Yellow fever should be suspected in any travellers from an endemic area. Management consists of instituting techniques for acute hepatocellular (liver-cell) failure. The affected individual should be kept in an isolation unit, away from mosquitoes which could transmit the disease to a healthy individual. Formerly, laboratory infections were occasionally acquired from infected blood samples. Prophylactically, a satisfactory attenuated vaccine (17D) has been available for around 60 years; this is given subcutaneously and provides an individual with excellent protection for 10 years; international certificates are valid for this length of time. Every traveller to an endemic area should be immunized; this is mandatory for entry to countries where the infection is endemic.

YERSINIA is a genus of bacteria which includes the causative organism of plague, *Yersinia pestis*. (See PLAGUE.)

YOGHURT is sour milk curdled with one of the lactic-acid producing bacilli, such as *Lactobacillus acidophilus* or *Lactobacillus bulgaricus*. It contains all the protein, fat, calcium, and vitamins of the original milk, and is therefore a nutritious food, but there is no evidence that it has any unique beneficial properties of its own. In countries where standards of hygiene are low it has the advantage of having been sterilized by boiling and is therefore unlikely to be contaminated with dangerous micro-organisms.

YOHIMBINE is derived from the bark of *Pausinystalia yohimbie*, a West African tree. Once widely used as an aphrodisiac, an action for which there is no good evidence, it is now being used in the treatment of certain cases of postural hypotension and for the treatment of impotence. It is an alpha adrenoreceptor agonist.

YTTRIUM-90 An artificially produced isotope of the element Yttrium. The isotope is radioactive and emits beta rays which are utilized for the treatment of tumours.

Z

ZIDOVUDINE An antiviral drug, with the trade name of Retrovir, used to treat AIDS and its related conditions, such as pneumocystis pneumonia. The drug slows down the growth of human immunodeficiency virus (HIV) but does not cure the disease. It may be given intravenously or by mouth. The drug, also called AZT, has been in use since 1987, and it works by blocking the enzyme that simulates HIV to grow and multiply. It may cause anaemia so regular blood tests are necessary.

ZINC is a metal, several salts of which are used in medicine for external application. It is essential for growth and development in animals and plants. The average human body contains a total of 1 to 2 grams, and most human diets contain 10 to 15 mg. In human beings, deficiency of zinc results in lack of growth, slow sexual development and anaemia. Deficiency is also associated with a skin disorder known as acrodermatitis enteropathica.

Uses Zinc chloride is a powerful caustic and astringent which, combined with zinc sulphate, is used as an astringent mouth-wash. Zinc sulphate is also used in the form of eye-drops in the treatment of certain forms of conjunctivitis. (See EYE DISEASES.)

Zinc oxide, zinc stearate, and zinc carbonate are made up in dusting powders, in ointments, in paste bandages or suspended in water as lotions for the astringent action they exert upon abraded surfaces of the skin. Zinc and castor oil ointment of the *British Pharmacopoeia* is a well-tried treatment for napkin rash.

Zinc undecenoate is used as an ointment and as a dusting- powder in the treatment of ringworm (q.v.).

ZOLLINGER-ELLISON SYNDROME A rare disorder in which severe peptic ulcers recur in the stomach and duodenum (see DUODENAL ULCER; STOMACH, DISEASES OF). It is caused by a tumour in the pancreas that produces a hormone gastrin (q.v.) which stimulates the stomach and duodenum to produce excess acid and this causes ulceration. Treatment is by surgery.

ZONA and **ZOSTER** are two names for the eruption popularly known as shingles. (See HERPES ZOSTER.)

ZONULOLYSIS is the process whereby the zonule (see EYE) is dissolved by an enzyme (chymotrypsin) as part of intracapsular cataract surgery. Once the zonule has been dissolved the cataract can be lifted out of the eye (see CATARACT).

ZOONOSES are animal diseases which can be transmitted to man. There are over 150 infections of domestic and wild vertebrates which can be transmitted in this way, including bovine tuberculosis, brucellosis, hydatid cysts, ringworm, toxocariasis, toxoplasmosis, leptospirosis, listeriosis, and rabies. (See separate entries for details of these diseases.)

ZYGOMA, or ZYGOMATIC BONE, is the name given to a bridge of bone formed by the union of a process from the temporal bone with one from the malar bone. It lies in the region of the temple, gives attachment to the powerful masseter muscle which moves the lower jaw, and forms a protection to the side of the head.

ZYGOTE   This is the cell produced when an ovum is fertilized by a sperm. A zygote contains all the hereditary material for a new individual: half comes from the sperm and half from the ovum. After passing down the fallopian tube, when the zygote starts dividing, it becomes implanted in the uterus and develops into an embryo.

APPENDIX 1: BASIC FIRST AID

This appendix is designed to cover the basic principles involved in the immediate treatment of some common emergencies. It is not comprehensive, and anyone wishing to become proficient at first aid should attend a course run by a reputable organization such as the British Red Cross, St John Ambulance, and the St Andrew's Ambulance Association (see APPENDIX 2: ADDRESSES)

First-aid treatment in an emergency is intended:

- to preserve life and stop the victim's condition from deteriorating.
- to help recovery and save the victim from further harm.
- to make the casualty as comfortable as possible and reassure him/her and the family.
- to assess the events surrounding the illness or accident so that relevant facts can be given to a doctor, nurse or paramedical staff.

No ill or badly injured person should be moved without skilled assistance – especially if a neck or spinal injury is suspected – unless the individual's life is in immediate danger from the surroundings, for example, a fire. He or she should be kept warm; constricting clothing should be loosened; and a clear airway should be established, with any false teeth removed.

BLEEDING This may occur from arteries, veins or capillary beds. The former is easily recognized as the blood tends to spurt from the wound at the same rate as the pulse. With the latter two types the blood tends to flow from the wound. Minor bleeding is usually treated in the home by the application of bandages, etc. However, the basic principles of treatment for major haemorrhages may be applied. Pressure should be applied to the bleeding point, via gauze or a clean piece of cloth if available, firmly enough to stop the flow of blood. With the pressure applied, the wound should be raised above the level of the heart. The patient should then be transferred to a place where medical care is available. If the loss of blood is severe enough for the victim to have become shocked, he or she should be laid flat with the legs raised, if possible.

BURNS All but the most minor burns should be seen by a doctor as it is difficult to assess the severity of the burn immediately after it occurs. If the person or his or her clothing is actually on fire, then the first move must be to smother the flames by covering them with a blanket or coat, for example, and 'patting out' the flames without sustaining burns yourself. Many burns,

however, are caused by hot liquids, hot gases, flashes from explosions or contact with a very hot object so that the person is not actually on fire. The treatment for all these burns is the same – to remove any clothing over the affected area, if possible, and to put the affected area under cold running water until the pain has stopped or the ambulance has arrived (the cold water should be applied for several minutes as cooling of the tissues, particularly the deeper layers of the skin, will limit the extent of the burn). The burn should be left exposed or covered with a piece of clean wet linen, e.g. a pillowcase, for the transfer to hospital. No lotions or potions should be applied to the burn until it has been seen by a doctor or a nurse.

CHOKING Severe life-threatening choking occurs when a piece of food or a foreign object becomes lodged in the larynx or trachea (qq.v.) causing obstruction. The person may cough, gag, or wheeze and will become cyanosed (blue) as he or she fights to take a breath. Infants or small children should be held along the arm, head down, and several gentle blows with the flat of the hand should be delivered to the back between the shoulder blades. This will usually dislodge the foreign body. In older children or adults the Heimlich Manoeuvre should be employed. Stand behind the victim with your arms wrapped around the waist. Make a fist with one hand with the thumb placed at a point half way between the victim's navel and the bottom of the breastbone. Grasp the fist with your other hand and give a quick inward and upward thrust. This may be repeated several times if necessary. Alternatively, if the person is unconscious, he or she should be placed on the back, face up and the same thrust performed with the heel of the hand whilst kneeling astride the hips. If a choking person is alone, he or she can perform the manoeuvre by placing a fist in the correct position and delivering the thrust by pressing it against a firm surface.

CARDIAC/RESPIRATORY ARREST The measures described here are basic life-support procedures – they can be performed if necessary without any equipment. Before commencing cardiopulmonary resuscitation on a person who has collapsed, it is essential to establish that it is required. Performing artificial ventilation and cardiac massage on a person who is breathing and whose heart is still beating can be dangerous. The person's chest and abdomen should be observed for respiratory movement and the pulse should be checked either at the neck or groin or by feeling directly over the heart.

The technique for simple resuscitation may be remembered by means of the mnemonic 'ABC (Airway, Breathing and Circulation)'. The aim of basic resuscitation is to maintain the flow of oxygenated blood to vital organs until the person's heartbeat and breathing can be restarted, if that is possible.

AIRWAY: If the airway is obstructed, no air can enter the lungs; therefore the mouth should be checked for foreign bodies, which can be removed by hooking them out with an index finger. False teeth should be removed. To prevent the tongue from obstructing breathing, the jaw should be pulled forward (using a finger behind the angle or the chin) and the head extended on the neck so that the person looks as if he or she is 'sniffing the morning air'. *Care must be taken if there is any suspicion of neck injury.*

BREATHING If clearing the airway does not allow breathing to recommence, then artificial ventilation of the lungs must be started. Mouth-to-mouth ventilation, using the rescuer's expired air to inflate the victim's lungs, is probably the easiest and most satisfactory to use. The victim is positioned as described above. The rescuer uses one hand to obstruct the nose and steady the head and the other to pull the jaw forward and open the mouth. The rescuer then places his or her mouth completely over that of the victim and blows out so as to inflate the victim's lungs, starting with two slow breaths to reinflate the lungs. It is important to observe the victim's chest rise and fall normally before commencing the next breath. If the chest does not rise or there is marked resistance to the inflating breath, then the airway is probably obstructed and the head should be repositioned.

CIRCULATION Ventilating the lungs without any blood's circulating will not provide oxygenated blood to vital organs. Therefore, if there is no pulse or heartbeat, cardiac massage should be started to produce this circulation. The person performing cardiac massage, who should preferably have been trained in the technique, should kneel beside the victim with the heel of one hand over the lower two-thirds of the breastbone and the other hand placed on top. Downward pressure is applied, keeping the arms straight with the elbows locked, so as to depress the breastbone 4–5 cm. Pressure is released slowly so that it takes the same time as compression. The rate of compressions should be 80 per minute. If there are two rescuers, then the person performing cardiac massage should stop after every five compressions to allow the other to perform one cycle of artificial ventilation. A lone rescuer should perform two breaths after every 15 compressions.

Once spontaneous ventilation and cardiac output have returned, the patient should be placed in the recovery, or coma, position. This consists of rolling the person on to his or her side, with the lower arm and leg straight and in line with the body. The upper arm and leg are flexed and brought forward to prevent the patient from rolling on to his or her front.

DROWNING About 500 people die from drowning each year in Britain, and an unknown number survive a near drowning. About a fifth of drownings occur in salt water. Wet drowning (when water is aspirated into the lungs) occurs

in 85 per cent of cases. The remaining 15 per cent develop laryngo-spasm so that, although they also die of asphyxia, no water enters the lungs.

There has been some controversy about what type of water carries the worst prognosis, but it is now thought that salt and fresh water are equally bad. The effect of salt water is to draw fluid into the alveoli from the vascular compartment with concomitant damage to the lung. This results in pulmonary oedema and hypoxia. Fresh water washes out pulmonary surfactant (causing pulmonary atelectasis and leading to hypoxia) and is absorbed into the vascular compartment causing volume overload and electrolyte disturbances. Both types may result in acidosis and circulatory collapse and may be complicated by hypothermia and trauma (which may have precipitated the drowning).

Treatment Cardiopulmonary resuscitation (see CARDIAC/RESPIRATORY ARREST in this Appendix) should be started as soon as possible and the patient transferred to hospital. This should include people who recover consciousness fairly quickly as pulmonary oedema may develop over the next few hours. If the patient is hypothermic, resuscitation should continue until he or she has been warmed to normal body temperature. Patients may require admission to an intensive care unit for artificial ventilation, circulatory support, or correction of electrolyte imbalance or acidosis.

ELECTROCUTION People may be electrocuted when they touch an object which is live so that a current passes through them to earth. A lightning strike has a similar effect. The severity of the outcome depends on the frequency and amplitude of the current which flows through them. Below 2mA there is only a feeling of strong paraesthesia, 15–100mA will produce muscular contraction in the muscles near the point of contact, which makes letting go of the object impossible, and 50mA–2A is the threshold for producing ventricular fibrillation (q.v.). [These thresholds are for the mains electricity supply, which in Britain has a frequency of 50Hz, a frequency that is particularly liable to induce ventricular fibrillation]. Thus electrocution can cause burns to the tissues at the sites where the current enters and leaves the body and may also induce ventricular fibrillation. If a person is seen being electrocuted, no attempt should be made to touch the victim until the power supply is turned off, as the helper may also be electrocuted. If the switch or mains supply cannot be found, then the victim should be knocked away from the power source using a non-conducting object such as wood. Burns should be treated as described above and, if the patient has developed ventricular fibrillation, then cardiopulmonary resuscitation should be started (see CARDIAC/RESPIRATORY ARREST in this Appendix). Any person experiencing significant electrocution should be seen by a doctor.

FITS A major fit or seizure is known as a Grand Mal convulsion and consists of two phases: the tonic phase when the person may let out a cry, falls to the ground and is observed to be rigid, and the clonic phase when he or she shakes. At the end of the fit there is usually a period of unconsciousness. The most important task in looking after people undergoing a fit is to prevent them from doing any damage to themselves. Any objects which might cause harm, particularly hot food and liquids, should be moved out of their way, but there is no need to try to move them unless they are in danger. At the end of the fit, when they are unconscious, they should be placed in the coma position.

POISONING The number of substances with which people are poisoned, either deliberately or accidentally, is too great to list individually. This section will merely cover some basic principles to follow on discovering a person who has been poisoned.

If the person is unconscious, he or she should be nursed in the coma position [see CARDIAC/ RESPIRATORY ARREST in this Appendix]. Vomiting should never be induced at home except under medical supervision. If corrosive substances have been ingested, then water or milk should be drunk to dilute the effects on the oesophagus and stomach, and any remaining on the skin should be washed away with copious volumes of water. The container from which the tablets or other substance came should be taken to hospital with the patient to help medical staff correctly identify the poison. Likewise if it is a plant, a leaf or berry should be taken to hospital. (See POISONS.)

APPENDIX 2: ADDRESSES

ACCIDENT PREVENTION IN THE HOME Child Accident Prevention Trust, Clarkes Court, 18–20 Farringdon Lane, London EC1R 3AU (0171–608 3828).

Royal Society for the Prevention of Accidents, Cannon House, The Priory, Queensway, Birmingham B4 6BS (0121–200 2461).

ADOPTION See CHILD ADOPTION.

AGEING Age Concern England, Astral House, 1268 London Road, Norbury, London SW16 4ER (0181–679 8000, fax: 0181–679 6069).

AGORAPHOBIA See PHOBIAS.

AIDS National Aids Helpline: 0800–567123. Information leaflets: 0800–555777.

Communicable Diseases Surveillance Centre (PHLS), 61 Colindale Avenue, London NW9 5EQ.

ALCOHOL Alcoholics Anonymous, PO Box 1, Stonebow House, Stonebow, York YO1 2NJ (01904–644026/7/8/9).

Al-Anon Family Groups UK and Eire (including Alateen), 61 Great Dover Street, London SE1 4YF (0171–403 0888).

Alcohol Concern, Waterbridge House, Loman Street, London SE1 0EE (0171–928 7377).

Scottish Council on Alcohol, 137–145 Sauchiehall Street, Glasgow G2 3EW (0141–333 9677, fax: 0141–333 1606).

Accept (community services for problem drinkers and tranquillizer misusers), 724 Fulham Road, London SW6 5SE (0171–371 7477).

ALZHEIMER'S DISEASE Alzheimer's Disease Society, 2nd floor, Gordon House, 10 Greencoat Place, London SW1P 1PH (0171–306 0606).

ANOREXIA Anorexia Anonymous, 24 Westmoreland Road, Barnes, London SW13 (0181–748 3994).

ARTHRITIS Arthritis Care, 18 Stephenson Way, London NW1 2HD (0171–916 1500, helpline 0800–289170 weekdays 12.00–16.00).

ANKYLOSING SPONDYLITIS National Association for Ankylosing Spondylitis, 3 Grosvenor Crescent, London SW1X 7ER (0171–235 9585, fax: 0171–235 5827).

ASH (ACTION ON SMOKING AND HEALTH) ASH, 109 Gloucester Place, London W1H 4EJ (0171–935 3519, fax: 0171–935 3463).

ASTHMA National Asthma Campaign, Providence House, Providence Place, London N1 0NT (0171–226 2260, fax: 0171–704 0740).

AUTISM National Autistic Society, 276 Willesden Lane, London NW2 5RB (0181–451 1114, fax: 0181–451 5865).

BACKACHE National Back Pain Association, The Old Office Block, Elmtree Road, Teddington, Middlesex TW11 8TD (0181–977 5474, fax: 0181–943 5318).

BACUP See CANCER INFORMATION SERVICE.

BLINDNESS Royal National Institute for the Blind, 224 Great Portland Street, London W1N 6AA (0171–388 1266).

BRAIN INJURIES Headway National Head Injuries Association, 7 King Edward Court, King Edward Street, Nottingham NG1 1EW (0115–924 0800).

BREAST CANCER CARE Breast Cancer Care, 15–19 Britten Street, London SW3 3TZ (Freeline: 0500-245 345).

BRITTLE BONE DISEASE Brittle Bone Society, 112 City Road, Dundee DD2 3QT (01382–817771).

CALIBRE See TALKING BOOKS.

CANCER CARE Marie Curie Cancer Care, 28 Belgrave Square, London SW1X 8QG (0171–235 3325).

Cancer Relief Macmillan Fund, Anchor House, 15/19 Britten Street, London SW3 3TZ.

CANCER INFORMATION SERVICE British Association of Cancer United Patients, 3 Bath Place, Rivington Street, London EC2A 3JR (0171–696 9003, fax: 0171–696 9002; information service, from outside London: 0800-181199; London: 0171–613 2121, counselling service: 0171–696 9000).

CEREBRAL PALSY SCOPE, 12 Park Crescent, London W1N 4EQ (0171–636 5020).

Scottish Council for Spastics, 22 Corstorphine Road, Edinburgh EH12 6HP (0131–337 9876).

CHILD ADOPTION British Agencies for Adoption and Fostering (BAAF), Skyline House, 200 Union Street, London SE1 0LY (0171–593 2000).

Parent to Parent Information on Adoptive Services (PPIAS), Lower Boddington, Daventry, Northamptonshire NN11 6YB (telephone and fax: 01327–60295).

National Organisation for Counselling Adoptees and Parents, 3 New High Street, Headington, Oxford OX3 7AJ (01865–750554).

Office of Population Censuses and Surveys, Adoptions Section, Smedley Hydro, Trafalgar Road, Birkdale, Southport PR8 2HH (0151–471 4313, fax: 0151–471 4359).

CHIROPODY Society of Chiropodists, 53 Welbeck Street, London W1M 7HE (0171–486 3381, fax: 0171–935 6359).

CHIROPRACTIC Chiropractic Advancement Association, PO Box 1492, Trowbridge, Wilts. BA14 9YZ (01225–776052, fax: 01225–769842).

CLEFT LIP AND PALATE See PALATE MALFORMATIONS.

COELIAC DISEASE Coeliac Society of the United Kingdom, PO Box 220, High Wycombe, Bucks. HP11 2HY (01494–437278).

COLITIS AND CROHN'S DISEASE National Association for Colitis and Crohn's Disease, 98a London Road, St Albans, Herts. AL1 1NX (01727–44296).

COLOSTOMY British Colostomy Association, 15 Station Road, Reading, Berkshire RG1 1LG (01734–391537, fax: 01734–569095).

CYSTIC FIBROSIS Cystic Fibrosis Trust, Alexandra House, 5 Blyth Road, Bromley, Kent BR1 3RS (0181–464 7211, fax: 0181–313 0472).

DEAFNESS Royal National Institute for Deaf People, 105 Gower Street, London WC1E 6AH (0171–387 8033, fax: 0171–388 2346, Minicom: 0171–383 3154), tinnitus helpline: 0345–090210, weekdays 10.00–15.00.

Hearing Research Trust, 330–332 Gray's Inn Road, London WC1X 8EE (0171–833 1733, fax: 0171–278 0404).

Sense (National Deaf Blind and Rubella Association), 11–13 Clifton Terrace, Finsbury Park, London N4 3SR (0171–272 7774, fax: 0171–272 6012).

Sense in Scotland, 5/2 No. 8 Elliot Place, Clydeway Centre, Glasgow G3 8EP (0141–221 7577, fax: 0141–204 2797).

National Deaf Children's Society, 15 Dufferin Street, London EC1Y 8TD (0171–250 0123, fax: 0171–251 5020).

DERMATITIS National Eczema Society, 163 Eversholt Street, London NW1 1BU (0171–388 4097).

DIABETES British Diabetic Association, 10 Queen Anne Street, London W1M 0BD (0171–323 1531, fax: 0171–637 3644).

DISABLED LIVING Disabled Living Foundation, 380–384 Harrow Road, London W9 2HU (0171–289 6111).

British Red Cross, 9 Grosvenor Crescent, London SW1X 7EJ (0171–235 5454).

National Demonstration Centre, Department of Postgraduate Education Services, Pinderfields General Hospital, Aberford Road, Wakefield WF1 4DG (01924–814856, fax: 01924–814546).

Disability Scotland, Information Department, Princes House, 5 Shandwick Place, Edinburgh EH2 4RG (0131–229 8632, fax: 0131–229 5168).

Motability, Gate House, West Gate, Harlow, Essex CM20 1HR (01279–635666, fax: 01279–635677).

DONORS National Blood Transfusion Service: 0345–711711.

HM Inspector of Anatomy, Department of Health, Wellington House, 133–155 Waterloo Road, London SE1 8UG.

British Organ Donor Society, Balsham, Cambridge CB1 6DL (01223–893636).

DOWN'S SYNDROME Down's Syndrome Association, 155 Mitcham Road, London SW17 9PG (0181–682 4001, fax: 0181–682 4012).

DYSLEXIA British Dyslexia Association, 98 London Road, Reading, Berkshire RG1 5AU (01734–662677, helpline: 01734–668271, weekdays 10.00–12.00, 14.00–17.00).

DYSPHASIA Action for Dysphasic Adults, 1 Royal Street, London SE1 7LN (0171–261 9572).

Stroke Association, CHSA House, 123–127 Whitecross Street, London EC1Y 8JJ (0171–490 7999, fax: 0171–490 2686).

EATING DISORDERS Eating Disorders Association, Sackville Place, 44 Magdalen Street, Norwich NR3 1JE (01603–619090, helpline 01603–621414 Monday–Friday 9.00–18.30; under-18 helpline 01603–765050 Monday–Wednesday 16.00–18.00; fax: 01603–664915).

See ANOREXIA.

ECZEMA See DERMATITIS.

EPILEPSY British Epilepsy Association, Anstey House, 40 Hanover Square, Leeds LS3 1BE (0113–243 9393).

Epilepsy Association of Scotland, 48 Govan Road, Glasgow G51 1JL (0141–427 4911, fax: 0141–427 7414).

FIRST AID British Red Cross, 9 Grosvenor Crescent, London SW1X 7EF (0171–235 5454).

St John Ambulance, 1 Grosvenor Crescent, London SW1X 7EF (0171–235 5231, fax: 0171–235 0796).

St Andrew's Ambulance Association, Strachan House, 16 Torphichen Street, Edinburgh EH3 8JB (0131–229 5419).

HAEMOPHILIA Haemophilia Society, 123 Westminster Bridge Road, London SE1 7HR (0171–928 2020).

HEAD INJURIES See BRAIN INJURIES.

HEALTH AND SAFETY Health and Safety Executive, 2 Southwark Bridge Road, London SE1 9HS (0171–717 6104).

HEALTH EDUCATION Health Education Authority, Hamilton House, Mabledon Place, London WC1H 9TX (0171–383 3833).

HEALTH VISITORS Health Visitors' Association, 50 Southwark Street, London SE1 1UN (0171–378 7255).

HEARING AIDS See DEAFNESS.

HUNTINGTON'S CHOREA Huntington's Disease Association, 108 Battersea High Street, London SW11 3HP (0171–223 7000).

ILEITIS See COLITIS AND CROHN'S DISEASE.

ILEOSTOMY Ileostomy Association of Great Britain and Ireland, Amblehurst House, Black Scotch Lane, Mansfield, Notts. NG18 4PF (telephone and fax: 01623–28099).

LARYNGECTOMY Laryngectomee Clubs, Ground Floor, 6 Rickett Street, Fulham, London SW6 1RU (0171–381 9993).

LEARNING DISABILITY Mental Health Foundation, 37 Mortimer Street, London W1N 8JU (0171–580 0145, fax: 0171–631 3868).

British Institute of Learning Disabilities, Wolverhampton Road, Kidderminster, Worcs. DY10 3PP (01562–850421, fax: 01562–851970).

MENCAP (Royal Society for Mentally Handicapped Children and Adults), 123 Golden Lane, London EC1Y 0RT (0171–454 0454, fax: 0171–608 3254).

ENABLE (Scottish Society for the Mentally Handicapped), 9 Buchanan Street, Glasgow G1 3HL (0141–226 4541, fax: 0141–204 4398).

LUPUS Lupus U.K., 51 North Street, Romford, Essex RM1 1BA (01708–731251, fax: 01708–731252).

MARRIAGE GUIDANCE See RELATE.

MASSAGE Chartered Society of Physiotherapy, 14 Bedford Row, London WC1R 4ED (0171–242 1941, fax: 0171–831 4509).

MASTECTOMY See BREAST CANCER CARE.

MENTAL HEALTH MIND (National Association for Mental Health), Granta House, 15–19 Broadway, Stratford, London E15 4BQ (0181–519 2122).

Mental Health Act Commission, Maid Marian House, 56 Houndsgate, Nottingham NG1 6BG (0115–950 5998).

NSF (National Schizophrenia Fellowship), NSF Office and Life Skills Project, 197 King's Cross Road, London WC1X 9DB (0171–837 7003, fax: 0171–278 2262).

See ALZHEIMER'S DISEASE.

MIGRAINE British Migraine Association, 178a High Road, Byfleet, West Byfleet, Surrey KT14 7ED (01932–352468).

MOTOR NEURONE DISEASE See PARALYSIS.

MULTIPLE BIRTHS TAMBA (Twins and Multiple Births Association), PO Box 30, Little Sutton, South Wirral L66 1TH (telephone and fax: 0151–348 0020, TAMBA Twinline: 01732–868000).

MULTIPLE SCLEROSIS Multiple Sclerosis Society of Great Britain and Northern Ireland, 25 Effie Road, Fulham, London SW6 1EE (0171–736 6267, helpline: 0171–371 8000, fax: 0171–736 9861, counselling service, London: 0171–222 3123, 24 hours; Midlands: 0121–476 4229; Scotland: 0131–226 6573).

Multiple Sclerosis Resource Centre, 4a Chapel Hill, Stansted, Essex CM24 8AG (01279–817101).

SPOD (Association to Aid the Sexual and Personal Relationships of People with a Disability), 286 Camden Road, London N7 0BJ (0171–607 8851, Tuesdays and Thursdays 10.30 to 13.30, Wednesdays 13.30 to 16.30).

MUSCULAR DYSTROPHY Muscular Dystrophy Group of Great Britain, 7/11 Prescott Place, London SW4 6BS (0171–720 8055, fax: 0171–498 0670).

MYALGIC ENCEPHALITIS ME Association, Stanhope House, High Street, Stanford-le-Hope, Essex SS17 0HA (01375–642466, fax: 01375–360256).

MYASTHENIA GRAVIS Myasthenia Gravis Association, Keynes House, 77 Nottingham Road, Derby DE1 3QS (01332–290219).

MYOPATHY See MUSCULAR DYSTROPHY.

NARCOLEPSY Narcolepsy Association (UK), 1 Brook Street, Stoke-on-Trent ST4 1JN (telephone and fax: 01782–416417).

NATIONAL LISTENING LIBRARY See TALKING BOOKS.

NOTIFIABLE DISEASES See AIDS.

NURSING Royal College of Nursing, 20 Cavendish Square, London W1M 0AB (0171–409 3333, fax: 0171–355 1379).

OSTEOARTHRITIS See ARTHRITIS.

OSTEOGENESIS IMPERFECTA See BRITTLE BONE DISEASE.

OSTEOPATHY General Council and Register of Osteopaths, 56 London Street, Reading, Berkshire RG1 4SQ (01734–576585).

OSTEOPOROSIS National Osteoporosis Society, PO Box 10, Radstock, Bath BA3 3YB (01761–432472).

PAGET'S DISEASE National Association for the Relief of Paget's Disease, 207 Eccles Old Road, Salford M6 8HA (0161–707 9225).

PALATE MALFORMATIONS Cleft Lip and Palate Association, 1 Eastwood Gardens, Kenton, Newcastle-upon-Tyne NE3 3DQ (0191–285396).

Dental and Maxillofacial Department, Hospital for Sick Children, Great Ormond Street, London WC1N 3JH.

PARALYSIS Spinal Injuries Association, Newpoint House, 76 St James's Lane, Muswell Hill, London N10 3DF (0181–444 2121).

Spinal Injuries Scotland, Festival Business Centre, 150 Brand Street, Glasgow G51 1DH (0141–314 0056).

Motor Neurone Disease Association, PO Box 246, Northampton NN1 2PR (01604–25050/22269, fax: 01604–24726).

PARKINSONISM Parkinson's Disease Society of the UK, 22 Upper Woburn Place, London WC1H 0RA (0171–383 3513, fax: 0171–383 5754).

PHENYLKETONURIA National Society for Phenylketonuria (UK) Ltd, 7 Southfield Close, Willen, Milton Keynes MK15 9LL (01908–691653).

PHOBIAS Phobics Society, 4 Cheltenham Road, Chorlton-cum-Hardy, Manchester M21 9QN (0161–881 1937).

POISONS National Poisons Information Service:
Belfast 01232–24905
Birmingham 0121–554 3801
Cardiff 01222–709 901
Dublin 00–353 18 379966
Edinburgh 0131–536 2300
Leeds 0113–243 0715
London 0171–635 9191
Newcastle 0191–232 5131

PSORIASIS Psoriasis Association, Milton House, 7 Milton Street, Northampton NN2 7JG (01604–711129).

RELATE Relate Marriage Guidance, Herbert Gray College, Little Church Street, Rugby, Warwickshire CV21 3AP (01788–573241, fax: 01788–535007).

REMPLOY Remploy Ltd, 415 Edgware Road, Cricklewood, London NW2 6LR (0181–452 8020).

SICKLE-CELL ANAEMIA Sickle Cell Society, 54 Station Road, Harlesden, London NW10 4UA (0181–961 7795/4006, fax: 0181–961 8346).

SPEECH DISORDERS AFASIC (Overcoming Speech Impairment), 347 Central Markets, Smithfield, London EC1A 9NH (0171–236 3632/6487).

SPEECH THERAPY College of Speech and Language Therapists, 7 Bath Place, Rivington Street, London EC2A 3DR (0171–613 3855, fax: 0171–613 3854).

SPINA BIFIDA Association for Spina Bifida and Hydrocephalus, ASBAH House, 42 Park Road, Peterborough PE1 2UQ (01733–555988, fax: 01733–555985).

Scottish Spina Bifida Association, 190 Queensferry Road, Edinburgh EH4 2BW (0131–332 0743).

SPINE AND SPINAL CORD DISEASES See ANKYLOSING SPONDYLITIS.

STAMMERING AFS (Association for Stammerers), 15 Old Ford Road, London E2 9PJ (0181–983 3591, parents' helpline: 0181–981 8818).

Association for Research into Childhood Stammering, Michael Palin Centre for Stammering Children, Finsbury Health Centre, Pine Street, London EC1R 0JH (0171–837 0031).

STOMA See COLOSTOMY and ILEOSTOMY.

STROKE See DYSPHASIA.

SUDDEN INFANT DEATH SYNDROME Foundation for the Study of Infant Deaths, 35 Belgrave Square, London SW1X 8QB (0171–235 0965).

TALKING BOOKS Calibre, Aylesbury, Bucks. HP22 5XQ (01296–432339, 01296–81211).

National Listening Library, 12 Lant Street, London SE1 1QH (0171–407 9417, fax: 0171–403 1377).

TINNITUS See DEAFNESS.

TOY LIBRARIES Play Matters National Toy Libraries Associations, 68 Churchway, London NW1 1LT (0171–387 9592).

TRACHEOSTOMY Association for Children with Tracheostomies, 215a Perry Street, Billericay, Essex CM12 0NZ (telephone and fax: 01277–654425).

TRANS-SEXUALISM Gender Dysphoria Trust International, BM Box No. 7624, London WC1N 3XX (01323–641100).

Partners' Group for Partners and Families of Trans-sexuals, BM Box No. 6093, London WC1N 3XX (01323–641100).

TRAVEL See APPENDIX 3: TRAVEL AND HEALTH.

TUBEROSE SCLEROSIS Tuberous Sclerosis Association of Great Britain, Little Barnsley Farm, Catshill, Bromsgrove, Worcestershire B61 0NQ (01527–71898).

TURNER SYNDROME Turner Syndrome Society, 2 Mayfield Avenue, London W4 1PW (0181–995 0257/994 7625, fax: 0181–995 9075).

APPENDIX 3: TRAVEL AND HEALTH

INTRODUCTION
Whether a person is travelling abroad for business or pleasure or is going to live in another country, he or she should obtain information about the climate, environment and health risks at their destination (including any stopovers that involve personal contacts with local people). Certain risks to health in another country may always be present; sometimes hazards to health may be temporary because of a local epidemic or sudden adverse environmental circumstance, such as a drought, earthquake or volcanic eruption, any of which can cause problems in obtaining supplies of food, clean water and medicine.

Any intending travellers with an existing illness should find out from their doctors whether they are fit to travel, whether the country of destination will admit them and whether they will be able to obtain appropriate treatment and how it will be paid for.

Healthy travellers are also advised to inquire about health-care arrangements (including payments) in their destination country in case they fall ill while away. Some countries have reciprocal arrangements with the UK. Travellers should take sensible precautions about drinking water and food as hygiene standards vary widely throughout the world. Pharmacists are usually helpful with advice on over-the-counter remedies for travel sickness (q.v.) and traveller's tummy.

Travel agents have a responsibility to advise their clients about health risks, and the travel trade has access to directories giving up-to-date information on visa requirements, recommended immunizations, climate, current health hazards and currency allowances. They cannot, however, be expected to give detailed individual advice, especially if the traveller has an existing medical condition.

There are many publications of help to travellers and authoritative advice is available from organizations listed in this appendix.

Travellers returning home who fall ill – even several months later – should always tell their doctor where they have visited and when in case their illness originated in another country.

USEFUL ADDRESSES
Topical medical advice can be obtained by *those advising travellers* from PHLS Communicable Disease Surveillance Centre, 61 Colindale Avenue, London NW9 5EQ (0181–200 6868); Hospital for Tropical Diseases, 4 St Pancras Way, London NW1 0PE (0171–388 9600); Communicable Diseases (Scotland) Unit, and Department of Tropical Medicine, Ruchill Hospital, Glasgow G20 9NB (0141–946 7120); Department of Infectious and Tropical Diseases, Birmingham Heartlands Hospital, Bordesley Green East, Birmingham B9 5ST (0121–766 6611) (inquiries from doctors and pharmacists only); Department of Infectious Diseases and Tropical Medicine, North Manchester General Hospital, Delaunays Road, Manchester M8 6RB (0161–795 4567); Liverpool School of Tropical Medicine, Pembroke Place, Liverpool L3 5QA (0151–708 9393).

SOURCES OF 'OFFICIAL' ADVICE
The Department of health produces annually the T4 booklet *Health Advice for Travellers* and this is available free from post offices. It contains information on what compulsory and recommended immunizations apply to countries. Advice is given on reducing health risks and on entitlement to medical treatment at reduced cost. Certificate E111 entitles nationals of European Community countries to care in other member states and the leaflet explains how to get this.

The health departments in Scotland, Wales and Northern Ireland also produce information on immunization against infectious diseases; this is published by HMSO and referred to as the 'green book'.

The World Health Organization in Geneva issues annually *International Travel and Health Vaccination Requirements and Health Advice*, also available from HMSO. It is written primarily for a medical readership. Designated yellow-fever vaccination centres are distributed throughout the UK and details of these can be obtained from local departments of public health and in Scotland and Northern Ireland from health boards.

Most good bookshops contain a range of travel books and specific travel health guides that contain information relating to health. Books may, however, become quickly out of date because of changing circumstances and health regulations in different countries. *The Traveller's Handbook*, published by Wexas Ltd, is a good and comprehensive guide; *The Tropical Traveller*, published by Penguin in 1993, is also helpful.

Among several specialist organizations giving travel advice, for instance, to handicapped people, and publishing books and leaflets, are the following: International Association for Medical Assistance to Travellers, Gotthardstrasse 17, 6300 Zug, Switzerland (membership free but voluntary contributions welcome; publishes a directory of English-speaking doctors and leaflets on climate, acclimatization, immunization, etc.); Air Transport Users Council, 103 Kingsway, London WC2B 6QX (0171–242 3882) (*Care in the Air*, advice for handicapped travellers); Intermedic, 77 Third Avenue, New York, United States of America NY 10017 (members may obtain a list of recommended English-speaking doctors in many countries); British Airways Medical Service, Queens Building (N121), Heathrow Airport, Hounslow, Middlesex (0181–562 7070) (*Your Patient and Air Travel* is useful for medical practitioners); British Diabetic Association, 10 Queen Anne Street, London W1M 0BD (0171–323 1531) (leaflets including travel guide concerning the more popular destinations); Royal Association for Disability and Rehabilitation (RADAR), 12 City Forum, 250 City Road, London EC1V 8AF (0171–250 3222) (leaflets available to help the handicapped arrange their travels); National Association for Maternal and Child Welfare Ltd, 1st floor, 40–42 Osnaburgh Street, London NW1 3ND (0171–383 4117) (*The Care of Babies and Young Children in the Tropics* by D. Morley, *Travelling with Children*).

APPENDIX 4: COMMON MEDICAL TESTS AND PROCEDURES

ACETONE (URINE)
Aim Detection of diabetic ketoacidosis.
Method Using Acetest tablets, Chemstrip or Multistix.
Normal Negative.

ADRENOCORTICOTROPHIC HORMONE (ACTH) (PLASMA)
Aim Diagnosis of Addison's disease, Cushing's syndrome, etc.
Normal Sleep–wake cycle of ACTH production, with highest levels at 6.00–8.00 (soon after getting up) and lowest levels at 21.00–22.00 (after going to bed). Secretion is increased by pregnancy and stress.

AMNIOCENTESIS
Aim Assessment of fetal maturity and diagnosis of fetal abnormalities.
Method/hazards With ultrasound guidance, a needle is inserted through the mother's abdominal wall and uterus, and a specimen of amniotic fluid withdrawn. There is a small risk to the fetus and the test should only be performed when essential.

AMYLASE (SERUM)
Aim Investigation of pancreatic and hepatic disease.
Normal 25–125 U/1 (units per litre).

APGAR SCORE
Aim Assessment of neonate's physical health.
Method Evaluation at 1 minute and 5 minutes after delivery of skin colour, muscle tone, respiratory effort, heart rate, and response to stimulus. Points are awarded and appropriate action (such as resuscitation) started.

BICARBONATE (WHOLE ARTERIAL BLOOD)
Aim Investigation of acidosis and alkalosis.
Normal 18–23 mmol/l.

BIOPSY OF TUMOURS
Aim Histological diagnosis of type of tumour and malignancy.
Methods Fine-needle and large-needle aspiration biopsy – excision biopsy.

CALCIUM (SERUM)
Aim Diagnosis of hyperparathyroidism, hypoparathyroidism, etc.
Normal See table B1 (page 580). Range may be affected by other drugs.

CARDIAC STRESS TEST
Aim Assessment of cardiac efficiency.
Method Heart rate, blood pressure, and electrocardiograph are recorded continuously while the patient performs an incremental work test. The test is stopped whenever requested, e.g. in the presence of excessive dyspnoea, chest pain, etc.

Contraindications include acute infection, recent myocardial infarction, unstable angina, congestive heart failure, uncontrolled dysrhythmia, etc.

CERVICAL CANCER SCREENING
Aim Early detection of changes in cervical cells, allowing earlier treatment.
Method Starting 6 months after first intercourse, then at 3-yearly intervals for rest of life. The test involves a cervical smear with a spatula, the cells then being examined histologically.

CHORIONIC GONADOTROPHIN (URINE, FIRST MORNING SPECIMEN)
Aim Diagnosis of pregnancy.
Methods Agglutination inhibition assay: positive in pregnancy 8–14 days after first missed period. Monoclonal antibody test: positive in pregnancy 14–18 days from conception.

CHORIONIC VILLUS SAMPLING
Aim Ascertainment of fetal chromosome pattern.
Method A small sample of trophoblastic tissue is obtained from the placenta, by ultrasound guidance either transvaginally or transabdominally, taken between the 9th and 11th weeks of pregnancy. There is a small risk of abortion.

CORDOCENTESIS
Aim Investigation of the chromosome pattern and haemoglobinopathies in mid-pregnancy.
Method Blood is withdrawn from the umbilical cord at about the 18th week of pregnancy and extensively analysed.

ENZYME-LINKED IMMUNOSORBENT ASSAY (ELISA) (URINE)
Aim Diagnosis of pregnancy.
Method Measurement of human chorionic gonadotrophin in urine may give a positive result 8–10 days after fertilization. False negative results may be due to testing too early in pregnancy, to excessively dilute urine, or to a urine infection.

ERYTHROCYTE COUNT (WHOLE BLOOD)
Aim Investigation of anaemia.
Normal See table B1 (page 580).

ERYTHROCYTE SEDIMENTATION RATE (ESR)
Aim Investigation and monitoring of fever, inflammatory, malignant, or autoimmune disease.
Method Anticoagulated whole blood is used. The result obtained may be influenced by numerous factors, notably various conditions and different drugs. *See over.*

Normal	male	<50	<15 mm/h
		>50	<20 mm/h
	female	<50	<20 mm/h
		>50	<30 mm/h

GLASGOW COMA SCALE (MODIFIED)
Aim To test the depth of coma.
Method Opening of the eyes, best verbal response, and best motor response are scored separately, giving a total quantitative index of the level of cerebral dysfunction.

GLOMERULAR FILTRATION RATE (GFR)
Aim Investigation of renal function.
Method Plasma and urinary creatinine levels are measured and the creatinine clearance rate calculated. This corresponds closely to the GFR, normally 120 ml/min.

GLUCOSE (BLOOD, URINE)
Aim Diagnosis and monitoring of diabetes mellitus.
Method Stick tests available for urine and blood samples.
Normal See tables **B1** and **B4** (pages 580 and 581).

GLUCOSE TOLERANCE TEST (ORAL)
Aim Diagnosis of diabetes mellitus/impaired glucose tolerance.
Method Pretest patient, ensure no recent illness, accident, or surgery. Discontinue non-essential drugs. Patient fasts for 10–16 hours, then takes 75 g glucose over 5 minutes. Serum glucose level is measured at 0, 30, 60, 90 and 120 minutes. The test should be performed in the morning.

Normal	fasting	3.9–5.8 mmol/l
	30 minutes	6.1–9.4 mmol/l
	60 minutes	6.7–9.4 mmol/l
	90 minutes	5.6–7.8 mmol/l
	120 minutes	3.9–6.7 mmol/l

GLYCATED HAEMOGLOBIN (WHOLE BLOOD)
Aim Monitoring of diabetes mellitus.
Method The test reflects the mean blood-glucose concentration over the previous 4–8 weeks. It is a measure of long-term control and should be repeated at around 3-monthly intervals.
Normal (In insulin-dependent diabetic) 7–9 per cent.

HAEMATOCRIT (PACKED RED CELL VOLUME) (WHOLE BLOOD)
Aim Investigation of anaemia and polycythaemia.
Normal See table **B1** (page 580).

HEPATITIS A ANTIGEN (SERUM)
Aim Diagnosis of hepatitis A infection.
Normal Negative.
Anti-HAV IgG appears about four weeks after infection and persists indefinitely.

HEPATITIS B SURFACE ANTIGEN (SERUM)
Aim Diagnosis of active or chronic hepatitis B virus infection.
Normal Negative.

HUMAN IMMUNODEFICIENCY VIRUS (HIV) ANTIBODY (SERUM)
Aim Diagnosis of HIV infection.
Method HIV antibodies are usually detectable from 4 weeks to 4 months after infection, and persist indefinitely. The test is by enzyme-linked immunosorbent assay (ELISA).
Normal Negative.

IRON (SERUM)
Aim Investigation of anaemia.
Normal See table **B1** (page 580).

LUMBAR PUNCTURE
Aim To obtain samples of cerebrospinal fluid (CSF) for investigation of central nervous system diseases.
Method With the patient lying on his side, and under local anaesthesia, a long needle is inserted between the third and fourth lumbar vertebrae. When performed correctly, a small volume of fluid should flow out spontaneously; this is collected and analysed (see table **B2** (page 581) for normal values).
The test should never be carried out in the presence of a raised CSF pressure, since it may precipitate transtentorial or tonsillar herniation.

MYOGLOBIN (SERUM)
Aim Diagnosis of myocardial infarction.

Normal	men	19–92 µg/l
	women	12–76 µg/l

The increase in value begins 30–60 minutes after onset of myocardial infarction and continues for 2–3 days.

SKIN BIOPSY
Aim Histological or immunofluorescent examination of skin lesions, especially if there is any suspicion of malignancy.
Method Various techniques are used, depending on the amount of skin required and the degree of doubt of the diagnosis.

THYROXINE, FREE (FT4) (SERUM)
Aim Measurement of thyroid function.
Method Various methods are used. The normal value is 10–31 pmol/l, but varies with the technique used.

TUBERCULIN SKIN TESTS
Aim Diagnosis of tuberculosis.
Method Antigens of *Mycobacterium tuberculosis* are injected intradermally. In the Heaf test, six skin punctures are then made through the antigen. The test is read at 3–7 days and a positive result is the appearance of four or more papules.

APPENDIX 5: VITAMINS

INTRODUCTION

A general description of vitamins is in the main text. Vitamins are divided into those that are fat soluble and those that are water soluble. Fat-soluble vitamins are A, D, E and K, the water-soluble ones B group and C.

The water-soluble vitamin B group is complex. Although often found together in similar types of food – cereals, milk, liver, etc. – they are not related chemically. These vitamins are all coenzymes, organic (non-protein) compounds which, when the appropriate enzyme (q.v.) is present, have an essential function in the chemical reaction catalysed by the enzyme. The vitamin B group comprises B_1 (thiamine, aneurine), B_2 (riboflavin), B_3 (niacin, nicotinic acid), B_6 (pyridoxine), B_{12} (cobalamin, cyanocobalamin), biotin, folacin (folic acid) and pantothenic acid.

Unlike fat-soluble vitamins, the water-soluble ones are not stored in large amounts in the body so deficiency of these is more likely.

FAT-SOLUBLE VITAMINS

VITAMIN A (PREFORMED SPECIFIC COMPOUNDS: RETINOL, RETINAL, RETINOIC ACID. PRECURSOR: CAROTENE)

Functions Maintenance of epithelial cells and mucous membranes. Constituent of visual purple (for night vision). Necessary for normal growth, development and reproduction. Maintenance of immune system.

Symptoms of deficiency Keratinized skin, dry mucous membranes, xerophthalmia. Night blindness. Susceptibility to disease.

Symptoms of toxicity Dry skin. Loss of appetite and hair, enlarged spleen and liver, abnormal pigmentation of skin. Fetal malformations.

Food sources *Preformed vitamin A* Liver, especially cod and halibut liver oil; egg yolk; milk and butter. *Carotene* Dark-green, leafy vegetables, especially spinach, broccoli, kale. Deep orange vegetables and fruits, especially carrots, tomatoes, apricots.

Recommended daily amounts (IUs*)

Babies and children	1875–3500
Boys (>11 years) and men	5000
Girls (>11 years) and women	4000
Lactating women	6000–6500

*International Units

VITAMIN D (ERGOCALCIFEROL OR CALCIFEROL (VITAMIN D_2); CHOLECALCIFEROL (VITAMIN D_3); 25-HYDROXYCHOLECALCIFEROL (MAIN CIRCULATING FORM OF VITAMIN D); 1,25-DIHYDROXY-CHOLECALCIFEROL (MAIN ACTIVE FORM OF VITAMIN D). PRECURSOR OF VITAMIN D_2: ERGOSTEROL (PLANTS); OF VITAMIN D_3: 7-DEHYDROCHOLESTEROL (IN SKIN).

Functions Helps in absorption of calcium and phosphorus. Regulates blood concentrations of calcium. Promotes mineralization of teeth and bones.

Symptoms of deficiency Rickets in children. Osteomalacia in adults.

Symptoms of toxicity Calcification of soft tissues, hypercalcaemia, renal stones, loss of weight and appetite, nausea and fatigue, failure of growth.

Sources Cod and halibut liver oils, bony fish, egg yolk, fortified milk, butter and polyunsaturated margarine. Sunlight acts on ergosterol in plants to produce vitamin D_2 and on the skin to produce vitamin D_3.

Recommended daily amounts (IUs)

Babies and children	300–400
Subjects aged 11–25	400
Subjects over 25	200
Pregnant and lactating women	400

VITAMIN E (α-TOCOPHEROL)

Functions Prevents oxidation of vitamin A in gut. Protects red blood cells from haemolysis. Maintains cell membranes by reducing the oxidation of polyunsaturated fats.

Symptoms of deficiency Breakdown of red blood cells.

Symptoms of toxicity Headache, nausea, longer blood-clotting times.

Food sources Wheat germ, vegetable oils, legumes, nuts, whole grains, fish, green, leafy vegetables.

Recommended daily allowances (mg)

Babies and children	3–7
Boys (>11 years) and men	10
Girls (>11 years) and non-pregnant women	8
Pregnant and lactating women	10–12

VITAMIN K (PHYTOMENADIONE, PHYLLOQUINONE)

Functions Necessary for the formation of prothrombin and other factors necessary for blood clotting.

Symptoms of deficiency Haemorrhage.

Symptoms of toxicity Haemolytic anaemia, liver damage.

Sources Dark-green leafy vegetables, especially alfalfa, spinach, cabbage. Cauliflower. Egg yolk. Soybean oil. From synthesis by intestinal bacteria.

Recommended daily amounts (μg)

Babies and children	5–20
Boys (>11 years) and men (increasing with age)	45–80
Girls (>11 years) and women (increasing with age)	45–65
Pregnant and lactating women	65

CHOLINE

The basic compound participates in the synthesis of lecithin (q.v.) and other phospholipids as well as of acetylcholine. Choline, which helps to transport fat in the body, and is essential to life, is sometimes classed as a vitamin, but the body is able to produce the compound.

WATER-SOLUBLE VITAMINS

VITAMIN B₁ (THIAMINE, ANEURINE)
Functions Has role in carbohydrate metabolism. Helps nervous system, heart and muscles to function properly. Promotes appetite and functioning of digestive tract.
Symptoms of deficiency Polyneuritis, beriberi, fatigue, depression, poor appetite and functioning of digestive tract.
Symptoms of toxicity Anaphylactic shock, lethargy, ataxia, nausea, hypotension.
Sources Whole grains, wheat germ, enriched white-flour products, legumes. Brewer's yeast. Heart, liver, kidney; pork.
Recommended daily amounts (mg)

Babies and children	0.3–1.0
Boys (>11 years) and men	1.2–1.5
Girls (>11 years) and women	1.0–1.1
Pregnant women	1.5
Lactating women	1.6

VITAMIN B₂ (RIBOFLAVIN (FORMERLY VITAMIN G))
Functions Essential for certain enzyme systems important in the metabolism of food (carbohydrate, protein and fat).
Symptoms of deficiency Inflamed tongue, scaling and burning skin, sensitive eyes, angular stomatitis and cheilosis, cataracts.
Symptoms of toxicity None recorded.
Sources Green, leafy vegetables, peanuts, whole grains. Milk and its products, eggs, liver, kidney, heart.
Recommended daily amounts (mg)

Babies and children	0.4–1.2
Boys (>11 years) and men	1.4–1.8
Girls (>11 years) and women	1.2–1.3
Pregnant women	1.6
Lactating women	1.7–1.8

VITAMIN B₃ (NIACIN, NICOTINIC ACID (A DERIVATIVE OF PYRIDINE))
Functions Part of two important enzymes regulating energy metabolism. Promotes good physical and mental health and helps maintain the health of the skin, tongue and digestive system.
Symptoms of deficiency Pellagra, gastrointestinal disturbances, photosensitive dermatitis, depression.
Symptoms of toxicity Flushing, loss of appetite, nausea and vomiting, abnormal energy metabolism, anaphylaxis, circulatory collapse.
Sources Whole grain flour, enriched white flour, legumes. Brewer's yeast. Meat; heart, liver, kidney.
Recommended daily amounts (mg)

Babies and children	5–13
Boys (>11 years) and men	15–20
Girls (>11 years) and women	13–15
Pregnant women	17
Lactating women	20

VITAMIN B₆ (PYRIDOXINE (PYRIDOXAL IS A COENZYME DERIVATIVE OF PYRIDOXINE))

Functions Important in metabolism of proteins, amino-acids, carbohydrate and fat. Essential for growth and health.
Symptoms of deficiency Not fully known but possibly convulsions, peripheral neuropathy, secondary pellagra, depression and oral symptoms.
Symptoms of toxicity Reduces prolactin secretion, which is important for milk production. Damage to sensory nerves. Liver damage.
Sources Whole grains, potatoes, green vegetables, maize. Liver; red meat.
Recommended daily amounts (mg)

Babies and children	0.3–1.4
Boys (>11 years) and men	1.7–2.0
Girls (>11 years) and women	1.4–1.6
Pregnant women	2.2
Lactating women	2.1

VITAMIN B₁₂ (COBALAMIN, CYANOCOBALAMIN)
Functions Important for haemoglobin synthesis. Essential for normal functioning of all cells, especially of the nervous system, bone marrow, and gastrointestinal tract.
Symptoms of deficiency Pernicious anaemia, subacute degeneration of the spinal cord, various psychological disorders, possibly loss of appetite (anorexia).
Symptoms of toxicity Not known.
Sources Not found in significant amounts in plant foods. Eggs, dry milk and milk products. Meat; liver, kidney, heart.
Recommended daily amounts (μg)

Babies and children	0.3–1.4
Subjects over 11 years	2.0
Pregnant women	2.2
Lactating women	2.6

VITAMIN B COMPLEX (FOLATE, FOLIC ACID)
Functions Formation of red blood cells. Normal function of gastrointestinal tract. Helps in metabolism of protein.
Symptoms of deficiency Possible neural tube defect in fetuses, anaemia.
Symptoms of toxicity Possible hypersensitivity reactions.
Sources Dark-green, leafy vegetables, legumes, whole grains. Yeast. Glandular meats.
Recommended daily amounts (μg)

Babies and children	25–100
Boys (>11 years) and men	150–200
Girls (>11 years) and women	150–180
Pregnant women	400
Lactating women	260–280

VITAMIN B COMPLEX (BIOTIN)
Functions Takes part in amino-acid and fatty-acid metabolism.
Symptoms of deficiency Rare: dermatitis, soreness of the tongue, dependency.
Symptoms of toxicity Not known.
Sources Egg yolk, cauliflower, kidney, legumes, liver, nuts, yeasts.
Recommended daily amounts 150–300 μg.

VITAMIN B COMPLEX (PANTOTHENIC ACID)

Functions An essential component of coenzyme A, which is a key factor in many of the body's metabolic activities.

Symptoms of deficiency Rare, but in a trial on volunteers malaise, abdominal discomfort and sensory disturbances occurred.

Symptoms of toxicity Not known.

Sources Widely distributed in foodstuffs.

Recommended daily amounts Adults probably need about 4 to 7 mg/day.

VITAMIN C (ASCORBIC ACID, DEHYDROASCORBIC ACID)

Functions Protects against infection and helps in wound healing. Important for tooth dentine, bones, cartilage, connective tissue and blood vessels.

Symptoms of deficiency Scurvy, anaemia, swollen and bleeding gums, loose teeth, bruising (from rupture of small blood vessels).

Symptoms of toxicity Kidney stones.

Sources Citrus fruits, tomatoes, strawberries, currants, green, leafy vegetables, broccoli, cabbage, potatoes.

Recommended daily amounts (mg)

Babies and children	30–45
Subjects over 11 years	50–60
Pregnant women	70
Lactating women	90–95

APPENDIX 6: MEASUREMENTS IN MEDICINE

10^3	kilo	k
10^{-1}	deci	d
10^{-2}	centi	c
10^{-3}	milli	m
10^{-6}	micro	μ
10^{-9}	nano	n
10^{-12}	pico	p

INTRODUCTION

This appendix gives a brief description of the System of International Units (SI units) and tables of 'normal' values for the composition of body fluids and body wastes. In addition there are tables of desirable body weights according to age (infants) and height and body build (adults).

Readers should bear in mind that 'normal' values may vary, sometimes quite widely, in healthy individuals. Furthermore, the relationships between height, build and weight are flexible and should not be treated as absolute targets.

A SI UNITS AND MULTIPLES

The International System of Units (*Système International*) usually referred to as SI units, was introduced in the 1970s and has been expanded and developed since. Now the SI units and symbols and certain units derived from the system are used for measurements in most scientific disciplines and are an integral part of scientific language. The units comprise three classes: base units, supplementary units and derived units. The seven base units are the metre (length), kilogram (weight), second (time), ampere (electric current), kelvin (temperature), mole (amount of substance: one mole of a compound has a mass equal to its molecular weight in grams) and candela (luminous intensity). The SI units used commonly in medicine are shown below. Some traditional measurements are still used, one example being millimetres of mercury (Hg) which is the unit for blood pressure.

SI UNITS COMMONLY USED IN MEDICINE

Quantity	SI unit (abbreviation)
Length	metre (m)
Area	square metre (m²)
Volume	cubic metre (m³) = 100 litre (l or L)
Mass	kilogram (kg)
Amount of substance	mole (mol)
Energy	joule (J)
Pressure	pascal (Pa)
Force	newton (N)
Time	second (s)
Frequency	hertz (Hz)
Power	watt (w)
Temperature	degree Celsius (°C)

MULTIPLES AND SUBMULTIPLES

Factor	Prefix	Abbreviation
10^6	mega	m

B 'NORMAL' BODY VALUES

1 BLOOD (PLASMA, SERUM)

Biochemical values

Substance	Approximate adult range
Ammonium	24–48 μmol/l
Ascorbate	45–80 μmol/l
Base excess	0±2 mmol/l
Bicarbonate (serum)	23–29 mmol/l
Bilirubin, total (plasma)	5–17 μmol/l
Caeruloplasmin (serum)	1.5–2.9 μmol/l
Calcium (serum)	2.1–2.6 mmol/l
Carbon dioxide tension (Pco2)	4.5–6.1 kPa
β-carotene	0.9–5.6 mmol/l
Chloride (serum)	95–105 mmol/l
Cholesterol (serum)	3.9–6.5 mmol/l
Copper (serum)	13–24 mmol/l
Cortisol (plasma)	280–700 nmol/l
Creatine (serum)	15–61 μmol/l
Creatinine (serum)	62–133 μmol/l
Fibrinogen (plasma)	5.9–11.7 μmol/l
Folate (serum)	11–48 nmol/l
Glucose, fasting (serum)	3.9–6.4 mmol/l
Iron (serum)	13–31 μmol/l
Iron binding capacity, total (serum)	45–73 μmol/l
Lactate	0.6–1.8 mmol/l
Lipids, total (plasma)	4.0–10.0 g/l
Osmolality (serum)	280–295 mmol/kg
Oxygen tension (Po2)	11–14 kPa
pH	7.35–7.45
Potassium (serum)	3.5–5.0 mmol/l
Protein (serum)	
total	62–82 g/l
albumin	35–55 g/l
globulin	25–35 g/l
Pyruvate	45–80 μmol/l
Sodium (serum)	135–145 mmol/l
Triglycerides (serum)	0.3–1.7 mmol/l
Urate (serum)	0.1–0.4 mmol/l
Urea (serum)	4.0–8.0 mmol/l

Haematological values

Measurement	Adult daily range
Bleeding time (Ivy)	5 minutes
Cell counts	
Erythrocytes, men	4.6–6.2 × 10 12/l
women	4.2–5.8 × 10 12/l
Leucocytes, total	4.5–11.0 × 10 9/l
Differential:	
Neutrophils	3.0–6.5 × 10 9/l
Lymphocytes	1.5–3.0 × 10 9/l
Monocytes	0.3–0.6 × 10 9/l
Eosinophils	50–300 × 10 6/l
Basophils	15–60 × 10 6/l
Platelets	150–350 × 10 9/l
Reticulocytes	25–75 × 10 9/l

Haemoglobin, men	2.2–2.8 mmol/l
women	1.9–2.5 mmol/l
Haematocrit, men	0.40–0.54
women	0.37–0.47
Mean corpuscular haemoglobin (MCH)	0.42–0.48 fmol
Mean corpuscular volume (MCV)	80–105 fl
Mean corpuscular haemoglobin concentration (MCHC)	0.32–0.36
Red cell life span (mean)	120 days

2 CEREBROSPINAL FLUID

Measurement	Approximate adult range
Cells	5/µl; all mononuclear
Chloride	120–130 mmol/l
Glucose	2.8–4.2 mmol/l
Pressure	70–180 mm water
Protein, total	0.2–0.5 g/l
IgG	0.14 of total protein

3 FAECES

Measurement	Approximate adult range
Bulk	100–200 g/24 hours
Dry matter	23–32 g/24 hours
Fat, total	6.0 g/24 hours
Nitrogen, total	2.0 g/24 hours
Urobilinogen	40–280 mg/24 hours
Water	0.65 g/24 hours

4 URINE

Measurement	Approximate adult range
Albumin	0.2–1.5 µmol/24 hours
Calcium	2.5–7.5 mmol/24 hours
Catecholamines (adrenalin)	55 nmol/24 hours
Chloride	110–250 mmol/24 hours
Copper	0.8 µmol/24 hours
Creatine, men	300 µmol/24 hours
women	700 µmol/24 hours
Creatinine	9–17 mmol/24 hours
Glucose	11 mmol/l
Magnesium	3.0–4.5 mmol/24 hours
Osmolality	38–1400 mmol/kg water
pH	4.6–8.0
Phosphorus (inorganic)	20–45 mmol/24 hours
Porphyrins:	
Coproporphyrin	77–380 nmol/24 hours
Uroporphyrin	12–36 nmol/24 hours
Potassium	25–100 mmol/24 hours
Protein	10–150 mg/24 hours
Sodium	130–260 mmol/24 hours
Urate	1.2–3.0 mmol/24 hours

5 TEMPERATURE

Normal, adults	36.6–37.2 °C
children	36.5–37.5 °C
infants	37.5–38.5 °C
Hyperpyrexia (q.v.)	41.6 °C
Hypothermia (q.v.)	35.0 °C

NB The temperature in the axilla or groin is about 0.5 °C lower, and in the rectum about 0.5 °C higher, than the oral temperature.

C DESIRABLE BODY WEIGHTS

1 CHILDREN, BIRTH TO 5 YEARS, SEXES COMBINED

Age	Standard weight (kg)
0 (birth)	3.4
1 month	4.3
2 months	5.0
3 months	5.7
4 months	6.3
5 months	6.9
6 months	7.4
8 months	8.4
10 months	9.3
12 months	9.9
18 months	11.3
2 years	12.4
3 years	14.5
4 years	16.5
5 years	18.4

2 ADULTS, ACCORDING TO HEIGHT AND BUILD

Men

Height (m)	Build (weight in kg)		
	Small	Medium	Large
1.550	50.8–54.4	53.5–58.5	57.2–64.0
1.575	52.2–55.8	54.9–60.3	58.5–65.3
1.600	53.5–57.2	56.2–61.7	59.9–67.1
1.625	54.9–58.5	57.6–63.0	61.2–68.9
1.650	56.2–60.3	59.0–64.9	62.6–70.8
1.675	58.1–62.1	60.8–66.7	64.4–73.0
1.700	59.9–64.0	62.6–68.9	66.7–75.3
1.725	61.7–65.8	64.4–70.8	68.5–77.1
1.750	63.5–68.0	66.2–72.6	70.3–78.9
1.775	65.3–69.9	68.0–74.8	72.1–81.2
1.800	67.1–71.7	69.9–77.1	74.4–83.5
1.825	68.9–73.5	71.7–79.4	76.2–85.7
1.850	70.8–75.7	73.5–81.6	78.5–88.0
1.875	72.6–77.6	75.7–83.9	80.7–90.3
1.900	74.4–79.4	78.0–86.2	82.6–92.5

Women

Height (m)	Build (weight in kg)		
	Small	Medium	Large
1.425	41.7–44.5	43.5–48.5	47.2–54.0
1.450	42.6–45.8	44.5–49.9	48.1–55.3
1.475	43.5–47.2	45.8–51.3	49.4–56.7
1.500	44.9–48.5	47.2–52.6	50.8–58.1
1.525	46.3–49.9	48.5–54.0	52.2–59.4
1.550	47.6–51.3	49.9–55.3	53.5–60.8
1.575	49.0–52.6	51.3–57.2	54.9–62.6
1.600	50.3–54.0	52.6–59.0	56.7–64.4
1.625	51.7–55.8	54.4–61.2	58.5–66.2
1.650	53.5–57.7	56.2–63.0	60.3–68.0
1.675	55.3–59.4	58.1–64.9	62.1–69.9
1.700	57.2–61.2	59.9–66.7	64.0–71.7
1.725	59.0–63.5	61.7–68.5	65.8–73.9
1.750	60.8–65.3	63.5–70.3	67.6–76.2
1.775	62.6–67.1	65.3–72.1	69.4–78.5

An individual assessment of a person's size can be made by using the Body Mass Index (BMI) (q.v.). (See also OBESITY.)

040–623–1